Farquharson's Textbook of Operative Surgery

To
Margaret
and
Katharine

Farquharson's
Textbook of Operative Surgery

Edited by

R. F. Rintoul FRCSE FRCS

Consultant Surgeon, Nevill Hall Hospital, Abergavenny;
Examiner for the Royal College of Surgeons of Edinburgh

EIGHTH EDITION

CHURCHILL LIVINGSTONE
EDINBURGH HONG KONG LONDON MADRID MELBOURNE NEW YORK AND
TOKYO 1995

CHURCHILL LIVINGSTONE
Medical Division of Longman Group Limited

Distributed in the United States of America by Churchill
Livingstone Inc., 650 Avenue of the Americas, New York,
N.Y. 10011, and by associated companies, branches and
representatives throughout the world.

First edition 1954   Fifth edition 1972
Second edition 1962   Sixth edition 1978
Third edition 1966   Seventh edition 1986
Fourth edition 1969   Eighth edition 1995

ISBN 0 443 04712 X

British Library Cataloguing in Publication Data
A catalogue record for this book is available from the British
Library.

Library of Congress Cataloging in Publication Data
A catalog record for this book is available from the Library of
Congress.

For Churchill Livingstone

Commissioning Editor: Miranda Bromage
Indexer: Nina Boyd
Design Direction: Sarah Cape
Production: Kay Hunston
Sales Promotion Executive: Douglas McNaughton

The
publisher's
policy is to use
**paper manufactured
from sustainable forests**

Printed in UK

Contents

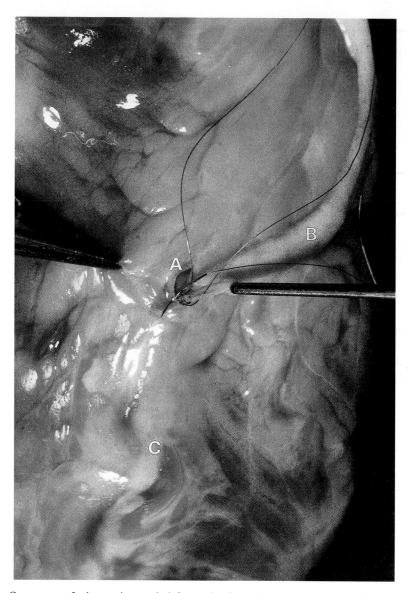

Coronary graft. A: arteriotomy in left anterior descending coronary artery; B: vein graft; C: native left anterior descending coronary artery. (Courtesy of Professor Wheatley)

Contributors

David C. C. Bartolo MS FRCS
Consultant Surgeon, The Royal Infirmary of
Edinburgh; Honorary Senior Lecturer, Edinburgh
University, Edinburgh, UK

David C. Carter Md FRCSE FRCS(Glasg) FRCP
Regius Professor of Clinical Surgery, Royal Infirmary,
Edinburgh, UK

J. Christie MB ChB FRCSE
Consultant Orthopaedic Surgeon, Royal Infirmary of
Edinburgh, Edinburgh, UK

O. James Garden MD FRCS(Glas) FRCSE
Senior Lecturer in Surgery, University Department of
Surgery, Royal Infirmary of Edinburgh, Edinburgh,
UK

Timothy B. Hargreave MS FRCS FEB(Urol)
Consultant Urological Surgeon, Western General
Hospital, Edinburgh; Part-time Senior Lecturer,
University of Edinburgh, Edinburgh, UK

Geoffrey Hooper FRCS
Consultant Orthopaedic Surgeon, Princess Margaret
Rose Hospital and the Royal Infirmary of Edinburgh,
Edinburgh; Honorary Senior Lecturer, Department of
Orthopaedic Surgery, University of Edinburgh,
Edinburgh, UK

J. M. S. Johnstone MB ChB FRCSE
Consultant Surgeon, Leicester Royal Infirmary NHS
Trust, Leicester, UK

Jeremy R. B. Livingstone MB ChB FRCSE FRCOG
Consultant Obstetrician and Gynaecologist and
Honorary Senior Lecturer, Simpson Memorial
Maternity Pavilion and Royal Infirmary of Edinburgh,
Edinburgh, UK

D. B. L. McClelland BSc(Hons) Mb ChB MRCP PhD
FRCP MRCPath
Regional Director, Edinburgh & South East Scotland
Blood Transfusion Service and Department of
Transfusion Medicine, Royal Infirmary, Edinburgh,
UK

I. M. C. Macintyre Md FRCSE
Consultant Surgeon, Western General Hospital,
Edinburgh, UK

Ian B. Macleod BSc FRCSE
Consultant Surgeon, Royal Infirmary of Edinburgh;
Honorary Senior Lecturer, Department of Clinical
Surgery, University of Edinburgh, UK; Editor, Journal
of the Royal College of Surgeons of Edinburgh

Carl H. A. Meyer FRACS
Consultant Neurosurgeon, The Midland Centre for
Neurosurgery and Neurology, Birmingham, UK

William G. Murphy MD MRCP MRCPath
Senior Lecturer in Medicine, University of Edinburgh,
UK

R. Forbes Rintoul FRCSE FRCS
Consultant Surgeon, Nevill Hall Hospital,
Abergavenny, UK; Honorary Clinical Teacher, Welsh
National School of Medicine

C. Vaughan Ruckley MB ChM FRCSE FRCPE
Professor of Vascular Surgery and Consultant
Surgeon, Royal Infirmary of Edinburgh, Edinburgh,
UK

J. H. Saunders MB ChB FRCS(Glas)
Consultant Surgeon, Western General Hospital,
Edinburgh, UK

David P. Taggart MD(Hons) FRCS(CTH)
Senior Registrar, Royal Brompton Hospital, London,
UK

A. C. H. Watson MB ChB FRCS(Ed)
Consultant Plastic Surgeon, Lothian Health Board;
Honorary Senior Lecturer, University of Edinburgh,
Edinburgh, UK

David J. Wheatley MD ChM FRCS
British Heart Foundation Professor of Cardiac
Surgery and Honorary Consultant Cardiothoracic
Surgeon, Royal Infirmary, Glasgow, UK

Janet A. Wilson BSc MB ChB FRCS FRCSE
Consultant ENT Surgeon, Royal Infirmary,
Edinburgh, UK

ARTISTS

Peter Cox
Medical Illustrator, Ledbury, Herefordshire

Gillian Lee
Medical Artist, Buckhurst Hill, Essex

Ian Lennox
Senior Medical Artist, University of Edinburgh
Medical School

Eddy Lowe
Medical Artist, The Midland Centre for
Neurosurgery, Smethwick

Stephen McAllister
Senior Medical Illustrator, Tenovus Institute for
Cancer Research, Cardiff

Jean MacDonald
Senior Medical Artist, Department of Medical
Illustration, Glasgow Royal Infirmary

Anne McNeill
Medical Artist, Department of Clinical Surgery, Royal
Infirmary of Edinburgh

Preface to the Eighth Edition

When the first edition of Mr Farquharson's textbook was published in 1954, many surgeons were capable of practising a wide spectrum of general surgical operations and it was possible for a single author to provide comprehensive advice within a single textbook. Since then, diagnostic methods have undergone constant change: standard radiology has largely been replaced by ultrasound scanning, computerized axial tomography (CAT scanning) and radioisotope scanning; nuclear magnetic resonance imaging is increasingly being used, as imaging quality improves. The scope for fibreoptics has been extended by the more effective imaging afforded by modern instruments, which has led to the increased safety of endoscopic and minimal access surgery. Some operations have now been replaced by percutaneous surgery, and the "interventional radiologist" may provide a preoperative percutaneous biopsy. The operating microscope with small instruments and appropriate atraumatic sutures has produced new surgical possibilities in moving or replacing tissues. In addition, many synthetic materials are available for prosthetic replacement of excised joints or other tissues so as to maintain normal body function or appearance.

However, the general surgeon of today must be aware of the basic techniques which are available and must have a sound understanding of the reasons for applying these methods; it remains the objective of this textbook to provide this information in a single volume.

The publication of this eighth edition has been made possible only with the willing assistance of many colleagues – some from previous editions and some new – in many hospitals throughout the UK. The text has been written particularly for the trainee surgeon to guide him through the operations which he will initially undertake. It includes many of the procedures with which he should be familiar on joining the staff of specialist units around the world, and may well

assist him in his choice of training. The book gives the trainee access to a basic knowledge of most specialties and allows him to benefit immediately on joining a new unit. It thus extends beyond the level of the basic FRCS examinations and introduces the trainee to higher specialist training.

The book is also aimed at surgeons practising in smaller hospitals at home and abroad, where more specialized advice would not otherwise be available. For the benefit of such readers, the simpler techniques have been described in sufficient detail to allow a surgeon of limited experience to operate with confidence and safety should the situation demand that he proceed. References have been selected as a stimulus to further reading by supplying, where possible, details of an original article or of a more recent publication which covers the subject more comprehensively. The overall objective has been to maintain the continuity of style which Mr Farquharson introduced into his earliest teaching so as to provide an easily comprehensible and practical text.

The list of contributors precedes this preface, together with the list of artists. Many of the drawings have been retained but a number have been added to accompany new text. The use of word-processing in preparation of this edition has had many benefits, including comprehensive resetting of the index. To all who have contributed to the new edition, I am profoundly grateful.

As with the previous edition, my wife has shared the enormous task of collecting, collating and checking the material from many sources. Without her help, this edition would never have appeared and she knows, I hope, how grateful I am.

Abergavenny, 1995   R. Forbes Rintoul

1
Incisions and sutures; plastic Surgery

R. F. RINTOUL & A. C. H. WATSON

INCISIONS

Very few operations can be carried out without cutting through the skin. Usually it is divided on the way to deeper structures but it is the first organ to be damaged by trauma and it may bear benign or malignant lesions that have to be removed. Every cut in the skin heals with a scar.

The integrity of the skin is essential as a barrier to bacteria and to control water and heat loss. Its mobility and elasticity are necessary for the proper functioning of the limbs, and its appearance has an important influence on the relationships between an individual and those around him. Wounds breach the skin's integrity and scars can restrict function and cause disfigurement. It is the duty of the surgeon who creates a wound to do so in such a way that when he closes it at the end of his operation the resulting scarring will cause the least possible disturbance to function and appearance.

All skin incisions should be carefully planned so as to give good access to the structures requiring surgical correction but, wherever possible, they should lie in or parallel to one of the 'lines of election' (see Fig. 1.1). They should not pass longitudinally across the flexor aspect of a joint. If they can be placed inconspicuously without compromising access, this should be done.

The surgeon has little choice in scar placement when dealing with a traumatic wound, but the eventual outcome depends very much on the way in which he treats it.

TISSUE HANDLING

All incisions through the skin must be made cleanly with a sharp knife held at right angles to the surface (Fig. 1.2). It is not necessary to use a fresh knife to incise the deeper layers since this has not been shown to affect contamination of deep structures with skin organisms. An incision of adequate length should always be made. Short incisions may be appreciated by the patient, but they cannot be justified if they add unnecessary difficulties to the operation. In certain abdominal and thoracic operations, however, the newer

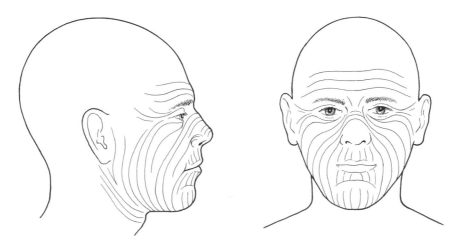

Fig. 1.1 Lines of election on the face

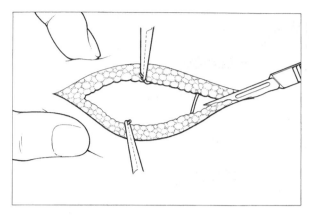

Fig. 1.2   Method of making skin incision and of arresting haemorrhage

techniques of minimally invasive surgery overcome the problem of adequate access by providing a television image of the operation through a single 'stab' incision while allowing the operative procedure to be carried out through one or more additional small incisions (p. 687). In all operations — but particularly in those involving manipulation of skin — tissues should be handled gently, the skin being held with hooks or delicate forceps.

Sometimes it is undesirable to close a wound immediately for reasons such as difficulty in achieving haemostasis, uncertainty about the viability of the deeper tissues or the adequacy of clearance of a malignant lesion. In these circumstances it may be wiser to pack the cavity, dress the wound and close the defect 48 hours later as a secondary procedure.

ARREST OF HAEMORRHAGE

All bleeding points should be secured with artery forceps or picked up with forceps which are connected to coagulating diathermy. In order to minimise haemorrhage, any larger vessels which cross the line of incision should be identified and clamped between two pairs of forceps, before they are divided. If diathermy is not available, small superficial vessels can be occluded by pressure alone, the forceps being retained for a minute or two. Larger vessels require to be ligatured or 'tied off' with fine thread or catgut. Every time this is done two foreign bodies are introduced — the ligature itself and strangulated tissue beyond it. Care should therefore be taken as far as possible to clamp the vessel alone, without taking up adjacent tissue; likewise the ligature should be of the finest material consistent with security, and the end should be cut as short as is practicable. When using diathermy, it is preferable to

coagulate the vessel alone *without a mass of surrounding tissue* so as to ensure correct haemostasis and to avoid unnecessary tissue damage.

For the 'tying off' of bleeding points close co-operation between surgeon and assistant is required. The surgeon passes the ligature material around the forceps; the assistant holds the forceps, depressing the handle and elevating the point as much as possible, so that the blood vessel which is clamped becomes encircled by the ligature (Fig. 1.3). Just as the surgeon is tightening the first hitch of the knot the assistant *slowly* releases the forceps. If the forceps are released suddenly the blood vessel is liable to slip out of the grasp of the ligature.

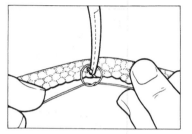

Fig. 1.3   Method of 'tying off' a bleeding point

KNOTS

Different types of knots
The simple and reliable *reef* knot is well known, and is universally advocated for surgical purposes. It is essential that it should be kept 'square' by being tightened in the correct directions, for an insecure slip-knot results if this precaution is not observed (Fig. 1.4). With slippery suture material such as catgut, nylon or other monofilaments, the ends should not be cut too short or the knot may slip. The *triple knot* is a modification of the reef knot giving additional security, and allows the ends to be cut very short. Multiple knots are, however, required to provide a safe knot with monofilament sutures. The *surgeon's knot* is best suited to the ligation of large vessels and pedicles, when ligature material of appropriate strength is employed.

Tying knots with the left hand
This easily-learned accomplishment saves much time, especially in the tying of sutures, since there is then no need to lay down the needle, which is held throughout in the right hand. It is useful, both for the initial knot of a continuous suture, and for interrupted sutures so that several of these can be obtained from the length of material.

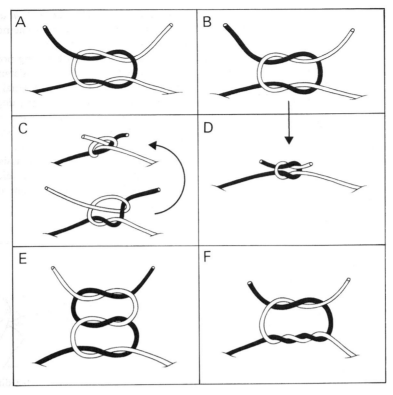

Fig. 1.4   Different varities of knots: (A) a *'granny knot*. An unsafe knot, which should never be used. (B) *A reef knot*. Must be kept 'square' by tightening in the correct directions. (C) *A reef knot* — spoiled by careless tightening, so that an insecure knot results. The white strand has been pulled to the left. (D) The white strand has been correctly pulled to the right, the black to the left — see (B). (E) *Triple knot*. (F) *'Surgeon's knot'* with an extra turn to the first loop

It is important to tie a reef knot, and to keep this 'square' by tightening it in the correct manner. A satisfactory technique is shown in Figures 1.5–1.10.

METHODS OF WOUND CLOSURE (see also RECONSTRUCTIVE PROCEDURES, p. 9)

After most operations the skin incision is closed by suture, in an attempt to obtain healing by first intention. Imperfect haemostasis leads to failure of healing since the formation of a haematoma prevents accurate coaptation of the cut surfaces and predisposes to infection. All bleeding vessels must therefore be dealt with before skin stitches are inserted. Should it be impossible to do this, or should further bleeding be expected, the wound should be drained by a fine tube to an evacuated bottle.

Sharp needles and fine suture materials should be used for all wound repairs, the sutures being evenly spaced and tied without strangulating the tissues (Figs 1.11 & 11.12). Carefully placed subcuticular sutures will give an excellent scar. Interrupted sutures should be removed early: 4 to 5 days on the face, 7 days else-

where, but longer in the lower limb below the knee and in vertical abdominal wounds.

Superficial stitches
Superficial stitches normally include only the skin and subcutaneous tissue. The needle should be made to pass perpendicularly through the skin in order that inversion of the edges may be avoided, and the stitches should be tied with only sufficient tightness to bring the skin edges together without constriction. Too tight stitches cause ischaemia of the tissue and result in delayed healing.

Suture material
Nonabsorbent material with a smooth surface should be employed for skin sutures. Silk and nylon are in general use. Silk allows accurate tension to be applied to each knot whereas nylon requires additional hitches for security. In many situations, subcuticular absorbable sutures (Fig. 1.13) may be used to approximate the dermal layer of the skin so that skin stitches do not require to be inserted *or* removed. Their insertion requires a careful technique to avoid an irregular scar and

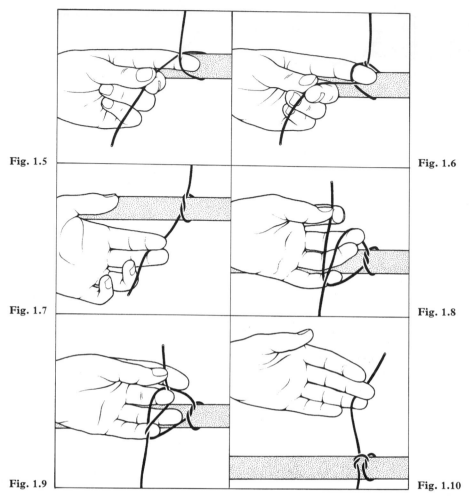

Fig. 1.5

Fig. 1.6

Fig. 1.7

Fig. 1.8

Fig. 1.9

Fig. 1.10

Figs 1.5–1.10 Method of tying a reef knot with the left hand. Note how the knot is kept 'square' by tightening in the correct directions. (The end of suture material passing off the edge of each drawing is held in the right hand.)

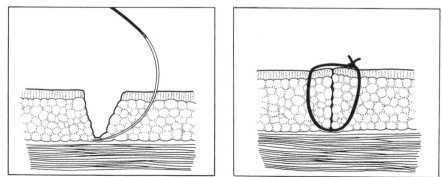

Fig. 1.11

Fig. 1.12

Figs 1.11 & 1.12 Correct method of suturing. The needle is introduced vertically through the skin, and traverses the entire thickness of subcutaneous tissue

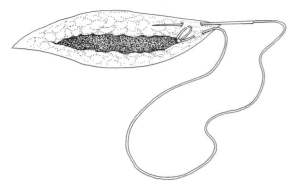

Fig. 1.13 Subcuticular absorbable suture

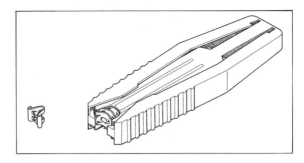

Fig. 1.16 Disposable skin clips and applicator

it is essential that the knots are placed well away from the wound edge. At some sites (e.g. in the head and neck), adhesive tapes (Figs 1.14 & 1.15) or Michel or alternative clips (Fig. 1.16) can be used to support the skin edges; they are removed after 3–4 days.

Needles (Fig. 1.17)

Except in certain situations, an ordinary round-bodied needle is not easily thrust through skin. Skin needles are usually triangular on cross-section, or have spear-shaped points. They may be straight or curved.

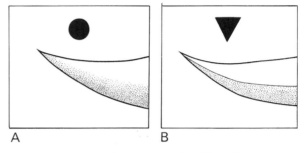

Fig. 1.17 Needle points: (A) Round bodied. (B) Reverse cutting

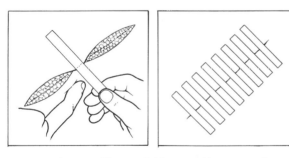

Figs 1.14 & 1.15 Closure of skin wound by means of *Steri-strips*

Types of suture

Various types of skin stitches in common use are shown in Figures 1.18 and 1.19. Superficial sutures may be either continuous or interrupted. All knots are placed to lie at one side of the wound, so that they do not become buried in the scar. Continuous suture saves much time in the closure of a long wound. However, should infection or haematoma formation occur, it is necessary to remove a part of the suture for drainage and secure the free ends with beads as in the subcuticular suture (Fig. 1.20).

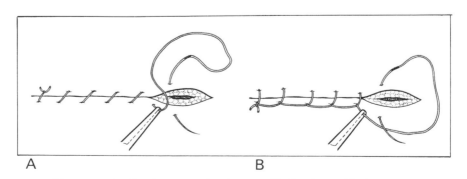

Fig. 1.18 (A) Continuous overhand suture. (B) Continuous blanket suture

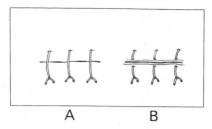

Fig. 1.19   (A) Ordinary interrupted sutures. (B) Eversion sutures

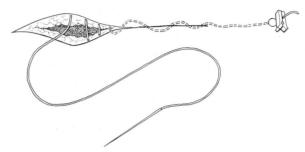

Fig. 1.20   Subcuticular suture of prolene held at each end

ANAESTHESIA FOR SIMPLE LESIONS

Local anaesthesia

For minor operations on the skin and superficial structures a local anaesthetic has many advantages. It is the least toxic of all anaesthetics and has no after-effects, so that the patient can resume full activity immediately afterwards.

The drug in most common use at present is *lignocaine* in its various proprietary forms — 0.5 to 1% solution is commonly employed. For infiltration (also used for post-operative pain control following incisions under general anaesthesia) the longer acting *bupivacaine* — 0.25 to 0.5% solution — is used. Its onset of action is slower than lignocaine but it is effective for up to 8 hours. A small quantity of adrenaline may with advantage be added to either solution. By its vasoconstrictor properties, this enhances the effect of the local anaesthetic and reduces bleeding. Proprietary solutions contain 1 part adrenaline in 200 000.

Infiltration anaesthesia aims at paralysing the nerve endings at the actual site of operation, the injection being made into the subcutaneous tissues immediately deep to the skin lesion and in the line of any incision that requires to be made. The infiltration of a small area can be carried out through one or two punctures with a fine hypodermic needle. Large needles, which are required for a wide infiltration, should not be introduced until the skin has been anaesthetized by injection through a fine needle. The best way of doing this is

to raise a cutaneous wheal by the injection of a small quantity of anaesthetic solution within the layers of the skin. The needle is introduced in a direction almost parallel with the surface. As soon as its bevel disappears a few drops of solution are injected under pressure, so as to raise a round white wheal with a pitted surface (Fig. 1.21). This area is immediately insensitive. Further wheals are raised according to the extent of the infiltration required. The needle for infiltration passes through the skin at the site of the wheal (Fig. 1.22).

Field block
By this method the anaesthetic solution is injected into the tissues at some distance from the actual site of operation, so that a zone of anaesthesia is created

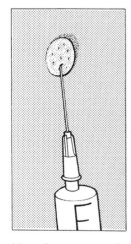

Fig. 1.21   The raising of a cutaneous wheal

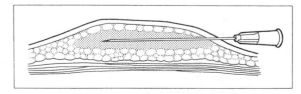

Fig. 1.22   Subcutaneous infiltration

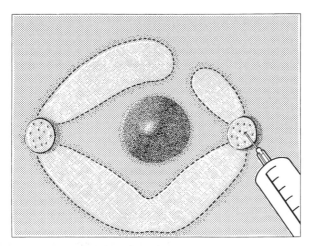

Fig. 1.23 Local anaesthesia by field block

surrounding the operation area (Fig. 1.23). A fairly long needle is required for the injection, and a suitable number of skin wheals are raised for its insertion. It usually suffices to make the injection into the subcutaneous tissue alone, but in certain cases it may be advisable to infiltrate the muscle or other tissue lying deep to the lesion. Before any injection is made into the deeper tissues an aspiration test should be made, in order to ensure that the needle has not entered a blood vessel. The injection is then made while the needle is slowly withdrawn. Field block has advantages over infiltration anaesthesia in that the lesion is not obscured by local swelling.

CONGENITAL DEFORMITIES OF THE SKIN

Haemangiomas

Characteristically these are not present (or are very small) at birth, but enlarge during the first two or three months of life, remain static for a year or more, and then gradually resolve. Those in the skin are known as 'strawberry naevi'. Most should be left alone and surgery be reserved for tidying up any redundant tissue after resolution. Injection of sclerosants, cryotherapy etc have been tried but are not of proven value and cause scarring which may impair the end result. Early surgery may occasionally be necessary for functional reasons, e.g. if vision is obscured.

Port wine stains
Excisional surgery is not advisable except for removing nodules and outgrowths in the adult. The treatment of choice is the laser: the *argon laser* has been widely used for adults but causes scarring in children. At present the pulsed tunable dye laser is showing the most promise for the treatment of children.

Vascular anomalies
These may be arterial, venous or capillary, and may be localised or diffuse. They enlarge only in response to changes in hydrostatic pressure. They may, however, be associated with enlargement of a limb. Embolisation can be effective for arterial lesions.

Congenital pigmented naevi
These may be large, hairy and very disfiguring. There is a small but well-documented risk of malignant change in giant congenital naevi. Therefore excision is advisable providing the size is not so large as to prevent reconstruction of the resulting defect using one of the techniques described later in this chapter. In the first few weeks of life the naevus cells are sometimes very superficial to the dermis, and later migrate more deeply. It is therefore sometimes possible to get rid of the pigmentation by very early tangential excision, dermabrasion or curetting of the outer layers of the skin. Unfortunately hairs persist and pigmentation often recurs.

BENIGN TUMOURS OF THE SKIN

Indications for operation may be cosmetic, functional, because of complications such as recurrent infection, or because of an uncertain diagnosis.

Sebaceous cysts

For the removal of small cysts under healthy skin a linear incision is employed. If the cyst is markedly protuberant, or if the skin is thin and unhealthy, an elliptical segment of skin should be removed along with the cyst. The skin overlying the cyst is raised by careful dissection (Fig. 1.24); thereafter the cyst can be shelled

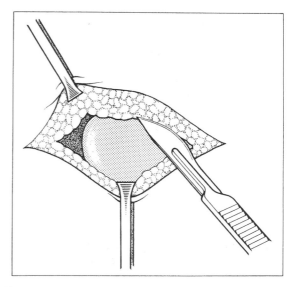

Fig. 1.24 Removal of a sebaceous cyst by dissection

out without difficulty using curved artery forceps to open the plane immediately adjacent to the cyst wall. An alternative method — that of *avulsion* — is particularly suited to the removal of sebaceous cysts on the scalp. A comparatively small incision is required, and the skin is raised for a short distance on one side only. The cyst is then deliberately opened and the contents squeezed out. A pair of non-toothed dissecting forceps, with one blade outside the cyst and one blade within, is insinuated round the side of the cyst wall until this can be grasped at its deepest part, which is much tougher than the superficial part and will not tear easily. By traction on the forceps (Fig. 1.25), the entire cyst wall can usually be avulsed with ease. The wound is sutured, and a pressure dressing is applied to prevent haematoma formation in the cavity.

Infected sebaceous cysts
If any inflammation is present, removal of the cyst should always be deferred until this has subsided. If an abscess forms it should be incised and the contents evacuated; a cyst so treated seldom recurs.

Dermoid cysts

Superficial dermoid cysts occur as a rule in the face or scalp, the superciliary region being a common site. They are often firmly attached to the periosteum or bone, and may even have fibrous connections through bone diploe with dura mater, so that their removal may present some difficulty, and should be attempted only with the strictest aseptic precautions (see p. 284).

Implantation (dermoid) cysts occur on the hands and fingers. Their removal is described on page 208.

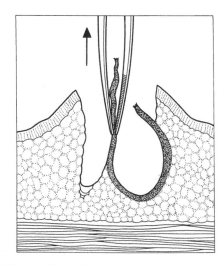

Fig. 1.25 Avulsion of a sebaceous cyst

Lipomata

Surgical removal offers no difficulty unless the growth lies in an intermuscular plane or lies close to a major nerve. Through an overlying skin incision, the tumour can usually be shelled out with ease from within its capsule, but care should be taken that all extensions are removed. If the tumour is pedunculated, an elliptical incision is made around its base.

Papillomata

'*Infective warts*' which occur usually in crops may be treated successfully by local application (salicylic acid paint or the cryoprobe), or they may be destroyed by the diathermy current. Occasionally they require to be excised.

True papillomata should be excised if they are subject to pressure or friction, or if their removal is desired for cosmetic reasons. All excised skin lesions should be submitted to histological scrutiny since clinical examination does not always give a reliable guide to the future potential of the growth. If the wart has suddenly enlarged or has become ulcerated, malignant change must be suspected. The site of the lesion may arouse the suspicion of the surgeon especially on the sole of the foot where the so-called amelanotic melanoma can occur. This highly malignant tumour is not pigmented as its name implies. An elliptical incision around a suspicious wart should include an adequate margin of surrounding skin of at least 5 mm.

Pigmented warts or naevi

The majority of these are benign, and remain so throughout life: occasionally they take on malignant characteristics as indicated by an abnormal growth pattern, variable pigmentation and an irregular edge. Depending on the site and the surgeon's suspicion of melanoma, excision should include a generous margin of surrounding skin (5–10 mm). Excision of a *simple* naevus requires a 2–3 mm margin so as to provide for adequate histological examination.

MALIGNANT TUMOURS OF THE SKIN

In all malignant tumours of the skin it is to be expected that permeation of the growth will have occurred, at least to some extent, into the tissue spaces at the periphery of the tumour, and in certain cases there will be evidence of spread to the regional lymph glands. Successful removal therefore requires the excision of a sufficiently wide margin of surrounding tissue along with the primary growth. The margin required varies with the nature of the tumour. If regional nodes are palpable, block resection is required.

Basal cell carcinoma (rodent ulcer)

This is the commonest malignant skin tumour. It is slow growing; it tends to infiltrate along tissue planes but, if untreated, may penetrate deeply and erode into the subcutaneous tissue, and even into bone. It does not disseminate to the regional lymph nodes except on vary rare occasions. Small basal cell carcinomas are sometimes treated by curettage or cryotherapy, but for most the choice of treatment lies between radiotherapy and excisional surgery, both of which have a cure rate of over 95%. Radiotherapists are reluctant to treat tumours in certain areas, e.g. the pinna, overlying the lacrimal gland or close to the lacrimal canaliculi. Good plastic reconstruction following excision carries no more scarring than radiotherapy and usually requires only a single outpatient procedure under local anaesthesia. If surgery is chosen, excision should include a margin of 5 mm on all aspects, including the deep surface.

Squamous cell carcinoma (epithelioma)

This tumour is usually sensitive to radiotherapy which may be used as an alternative to operation. Two different types of tumour can be recognized clinically : those arising in sun-damaged skin (often multiple, superficial and with an excellent prognosis), and those occurring in apparently normal skin, which are often more aggressive. Excision of the latter type of growth should include at least 10–15 mm of healthy skin on all sides. Squamous cell carcinoma of the lip is discussed more fully on p. 276.

Malignant melanoma

This is the most aggressive of the skin cancers and may spread early to lymph nodes. It may arise in previously normal skin or from a pre-existing naevus. A skin lesion with various degrees of pigmentation and nodularity should make the surgeon suspicious of malignant melanoma, especially if there are adjacent satellite nodules. All suspicious lesions should be subjected to excision biopsy with a margin of 10 mm except for a large lesion where major resection would result in unnecessary disfigurement in the event of the tumour being benign. Only in this situation is incision biopsy acceptable. Excision biopsy is necessary in order to establish a diagnosis of malignant melanoma and to plan any subsequent surgery. Since tumour thickness and degree of penetration are major determinants of survival (Breslow, 1970; Meyer, 1985) the pathologist must be able to report depth measurements of the melanoma and its level of invasion. This is not possible with an incision biopsy or frozen section.

A 10 mm excision is sufficient for a tumour up to 1 mm thick, and an excellent prognosis can be ex-

pected. If the pathologist's report shows the tumour to be thicker, a wider excision is necessary. As a guide, 10 mm width of excision for every 1 mm thickness is appropriate. Excision should be down to, but not through, deep fascia. Skin grafting or flap closure may be required.

Melanoma under or near the nail of a finger or toe (*subungual*) should be treated by amputation of the digit at a level to allow appropriate skin clearance, depending on the thickness of the tumour.

Melanomata of mucosa of mouth, vagina or anal canal are even more malignant than those in other situations. Those of the anal canal demand an abdominoperineal excision.

There is conflicting evidence regarding the value of *prophylactic* removal of regional lymph nodes (i.e. when they are not clinically involved by metastases). It is not generally done unless the primary lesion is thick and it lies close to the lymph nodes. In all other cases, the patient is closely followed up for examination of the regional lymph nodes so that block dissection can be advised when there is clinical evidence of their involvement.

Radiotherapy has no place in the primary treatment of melanoma, but can be valuable in palliation, particularly of spinal and intracranial metastases. There have been many clinical trials of chemotherapy and immunotherapy as adjuvants or for palliation. At the present time no systemic treatment has proved of value, but isolated limb perfusion, for disease limited to the limb, is showing promising results (Ghussen, 1984).

RECONSTRUCTIVE PROCEDURES

The reconstructive ladder

Not every wound can be closed directly, especially after trauma or tumour excision. Wounds should never be sutured under such tension that the skin edges go white. This indicates strangulation and ischaemia and the wound will not heal primarily. If direct closure without tension is impossible then a range of choices is available and each should be considered in turn, starting with the simplest and moving step by step to the more complex if the simpler procedure seems inappropriate (Fig. 1.26).

Simple undermining and advancement
Careful undermining of the adjacent tissues away from the edge of the wound may permit primary closure of quite a large defect without tension. The level at which this undermining should be carried out is important. In the face undercutting must be in the subcutaneous layer to avoid damage to the branches of the facial nerve (Fig. 1.28). In the limbs and over the trunk the

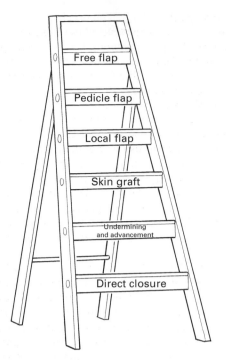

Fig. 1.26 The reconstructive ladder

most suitable plane lies on the deep fascia (Fig. 1.29); in the scalp, it is the layer between pericranium and the galea (Fig. 1.30). Carefully placed parallel incisions in the under surface of the galea may reduce tension on the suture line and give a little more advancement.

Skin grafts

If direct closure is not possible, even after undermining the skin edges, a skin graft should be considered. Grafts are completely detached from their origin and, to survive, must obtain adequate nourishment from the bed on which they are placed.

Split skin grafts

These are the general purpose skin grafts most frequently used. They can be taken from any part of the body but the commonest donor sites are the anterior surface of the thigh and the upper arm. The grafts may be cut at different depths. Thin grafts (*Thiersch grafts*) consist of little more than epidermis and are used mainly to cover granulating areas where the urgent need is wound healing. They 'take' well even in the presence of infection but their inability to stand up to wear and tear and their tendency to contract relegates them to the category of temporary grafts that will need replacement later by thicker grafts or flaps. Thicker grafts contain more dermis and are far more durable and pleasing in appearance. Indeed the thicker *split-skin grafts* are almost indistinguishable from a full thickness graft. However, the surgeon must be careful to select an unobtrusive donor site, since, the thicker the split-skin graft, the more unsatisfactory may be the healed donor surface.

Preparation of the recipient area

A clean 'tidy' freshly-made wound (created by accident or deliberately by the surgeon's knife) presents no

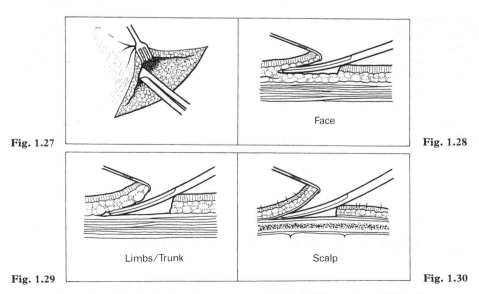

Fig. 1.27

Face   Fig. 1.28

Fig. 1.29   Limbs/Trunk   Scalp   Fig. 1.30

Figs 1.27–1.30 Techniques of undermining skin in different parts of the body

problems provided that complete haemostasis is secured by fine ligatures and careful use of the diathermy — preferably the bi-polar coagulator. The base of the wound should be as even as possible and any spaces between muscle bellies should be carefully obliterated by a few interrupted fine sutures. If these two criteria cannot be fulfilled it may be wiser to cut the skin graft, preserve it in the refrigerator, and apply it some 36–48 hours later or to dress the wound and perform a definitive grafting operation 7–10 days later.

By contrast, 'untidy' wounds and granulating areas may require careful preparation. Adherent sloughs must be excised and any crevices in the granulating area removed by scraping away the exuberant soft granulations. Frequent wet dressings with gauze soaked in saline, eusol or sodium hypochlorite (Milton) must be applied until a healthy, pink, flat granulating surface is produced. (In spite of statements to the contrary, hypochlorite dressings remain the best and cheapest way of eliminating slough.) The fitness of the wound for grafting is probably best judged by the clinical appearance; information obtained by bacterial investigation is not always helpful and may be misleading. Complete sterility is usually unobtainable and is not essential. The presence of B-haemolytic streptococci group A is a contraindication to grafting but can be dealt with by systemic antibiotic therapy. A heavy growth of any pathogenic organism can interfere with graft 'take' and frequent dressings, possibly containing an antibacterial agent such as povidone iodine, may first be required to reduce bacterial colonization. The indiscriminate local application of antibiotic powders, solutions and creams or various desloughing agents (enzymatic, chemical or hydrophillic) is an extremely expensive and largely worthless substitute for a good simple dressing technique.

In the operating theatre a healthy granulating area requires little extra preparation other than cleansing with povidone iodine or Hibitane followed by saline. If some of the granulations are still exuberant and unhealthy in appearance, they should be scraped away to leave a yellow firm base, or shaved down using a skin grafting knife. Bleeding is controlled by firm pressure with packs soaked in warm saline or hydrogen peroxide solution.

Cutting the graft

The donor site, which should have been shaved if the surface was hairy, is prepared like any other operation site with povidone iodine, chlorhexidine or cetrimide. The limb should be held firmly by the assistant whose hands give counter pressure from behind to present the surgeon with a flat surface from which the graft will be cut. The surgeon places a wooden board on the donor site just in front of the skin grafting knife (Fig. 1.31). After appropriate adjustment of the guard on the knife, the blade of the knife and the edge of the wooden board are coated with liquid paraffin to allow a smooth gliding motion on the skin. The skin grafting knife is held firmly in the hand, pressed firmly against the skin and, with a steady to and fro sawing motion, the knife and skin grafting board move steadily forwards (Fig. 1.32).

Although the blade in the knife may have been set at a predetermined depth, the thickness of the graft is also influenced by the pressure applied to the skin and the angle of the blade. The surgeon must check the thickness of the graft as he cuts it. This can be judged by the translucency of the graft and the pattern of bleeding and appearance of the donor site. A very thin graft is translucent so that the knife blade will appear bluish grey in colour. A thicker graft will appear whiter in colour, the bleeding points on the donor surface will be few, far apart rather than closely packed and confluent as with the thinner grafts (Fig. 1.33). If the skin graft has been cut at too deep a level and subcutaneous fat appears in the wound, the surgeon has two choices: (a) to resuture the graft in place and take a thinner graft elsewhere or (b) to use the thick graft as a full-thickness graft and place a thin split-skin graft on the unintentionally deep donor site. The donor site should be dressed as soon as the grafts have been cut, using a layer of tulle gras gauze, Gamgee tissue or cotton wool and a sterile crepe or elasticated cotton bandage carefully applied to exert even pressure, absorb any exudate and put the donor site at rest. The wound should be left undisturbed for 10–14 days and when the dressings are soaked off the donor site should be healed. Alternative donor site dressings such as alginate preparations may be used.

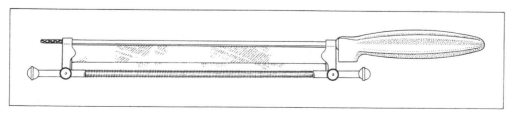

Fig. 1.31 A skin grafting knife (Bodenham's modification of the Humby knife)

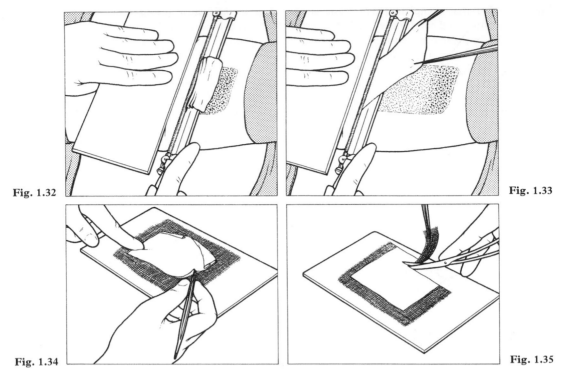

Figs 1.32–1.35 *Taking a skin graft*
Fig. 1.32 Cutting the graft. **Fig. 1.33** Various thicknesses demonstrated by change in pattern of bleeding.
Fig. 1.34 Spreading the graft on tulle gras. **Fig. 1.35** Trimming the graft

Preparation of the graft

The sheets of skin that have been cut are spread out evenly, with their deeper surface uppermost, on a large sheet of tulle gras laid neatly and taut on a wooden board. The skin is then trimmed as required (Figs 1.34 & 1.35). When used as a single sheet the graft is cut to a suitable size and tacked to the edges of the defect by a few well-placed sutures that can be left long, if required, to help fix a tie-over dressing (Fig. 1.36). When skin grafting a large area, the better sheets of skin should be reserved for the most important sites, namely across joints and flexion creases.

Storage of skin grafts

If some of the graft is left over after the defect has been covered, or if delayed grafting is planned, the skin can be preserved for up to two weeks in a refrigerator at about 4°C. After spreading the graft on tulle gras, the raw surfaces should be folded together, the graft rolled up and placed in a sterile universal container with a gauze swab wrung out in saline. It should then be placed on the top shelf of the refrigerator.

Mesh grafting

The most efficient technique of making a split-skin graft cover a large area is to pass the sheet of split skin through a meshing device that cuts the skin into a pre-determined lattice pattern which allows the skin to be expanded by a factor of 1.5, 3 or 6 (Fig. 1.37). The final result may show a fine mesh-work pattern but this ultra-economical use of skin when donor sites are limited is a major advance in the life-saving skin cover of extensive burns. The smaller degrees of expansion are valuable in the presence of exudate, which can pass through the gaps, or for giving the graft greater ability to conform to an irregular bed.

Where a mesher is not available, slits can be cut in the graft with a knife, or it can be cut into strips or squares. In large burns these can be applied alternately with allo- or xenografts. As the latter are rejected the patient's own epithelial cells grow out to replace them.

All these methods for expanding skin result in parts of the wound healing by secondary intention. Scarring and wound contraction are therefore greater than when the wound is completely covered by a sheet of skin.

Care of grafts: dressings or exposure

Failure of the split-skin graft to 'take' completely is due to:

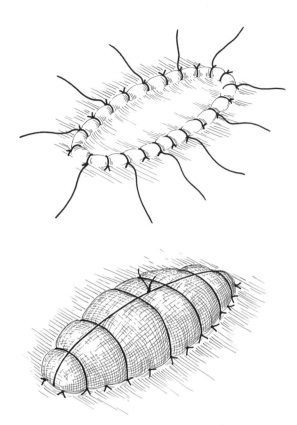

Fig. 1.36 Tie-over dressing

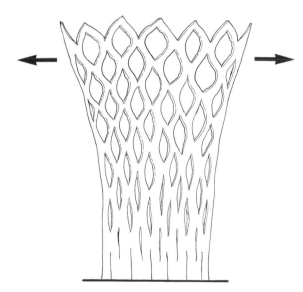

Fig. 1.37 Expansion of meshed skin

1. a collection of serum or blood beneath the graft
2. infection
3. accidental dislodgement of the graft, usually the result of a poor dressing technique or inadequate

attention to fixation when the grafts are treated by exposure.

Pressure is not essential for the take of a graft but a firm dressing will keep the parts at rest during the early healing stages and protect the graft from unnecessary outside interference, provided it does not slip and shear the graft from its bed. Sutures will help to keep it in place. On a flat or evenly convex surface, firm crepe bandaging suffices over a layer of dry gauze or Gamgee tissue. A layer of Elastoplast or light plaster cast may be added for better protection. On a concave or irregular surface, fluffed-out gauze or pieces of polyurethane foam or cotton wool wrung out in liquid paraffin or acriflavine emulsion may be used to fill the cavity before bandaging as before. Care must be taken to prevent movement of the dressing. A tie-over dressing (Fig. 1.36), which is held in place by tying the long ends of the sutures together over it, is often the best way to protect the graft. These dressings should be left undisturbed for at least 5–8 days and only removed earlier if there is pain, pyrexia or smell indicating infection.

Exposure of skin grafts allows exudate or haematoma to be expressed in the first few hours, prevents shearing by a dressing and reduces the risk of infection. It is particularly useful for large grafts on the trunk, perineum and face. However it requires expert nursing management and a co-operative patient to be effective.

Excision and grafting of full thickness burns
Split skin grafts are used to cover the raw areas produced by full thickness burns. Grafting may be delayed until the dead skin has separated spontaneously, with the help of dressing. However, in certain full thickness burns early excision of the burn followed by immediate or delayed skin grafting may save weeks of suffering and disability. In deep dermal burns tangential excision using a skin grafting knife down to the zone of punctate bleeding with immediate cover using thin split skin grafts was first advocated by Janzekovic (1970) in Yugoslavia, and this has revolutionised the treatment of this type of injury.

Full thickness skin grafts (Wolfe grafts)
These grafts, which are composed of the full thickness of the skin, are unsuitable for use on granulating areas but ideal for resurfacing clean surgical wounds produced by excision of scars or tumours. They are particularly useful where the texture and colour match or durability of the skin are important. For this reason they are widely used to correct facial deformities such as ectropion, scars and growths of the eyelids, nose and cheek and in the hand to correct deformities, burn contractures of the fingers, finger tip injuries and in the treatment of syndactyly.

The recipient site must be carefully prepared and absolute haemostasis achieved. An exact pattern is then made of the defect in metal foil or jaconet or paper. Any non-hairy part of the body can be chosen for the donor site, special preference being given to those sites where the donor site can be closed quickly and easily by primary suture. The postauricular sulcus (Figs 1.38 & 1.39), the supraclavicular and infraclavicular regions are good donor sites. So too, is the inframammary crease in the woman and the lateral groin in both sexes, provided care is taken not to transplant hairy skin. Flexion creases at the elbow or knee are best avoided as the resultant scars can be disfiguring. The pattern is laid on the donor site and the skin is cut at a superficial level, much as skin is raised in the dissecting room, taking care not to button-hole the skin or raise too much subcutaneous fat in the process. Any remaining fat must be trimmed away from the undersurface of the graft with sharp scissors. The donor defect is closed without tension. The graft is then sewn into the surgically-created defect with fine sutures to give exact apposition at the graft-to-skin junction. Depending on the recipient site the graft may be left exposed or protected by a tie-over dressing.

Composite grafts

There is a limit to the thickness of tissue which can survive by picking up a blood supply from a vascular bed, which is why fat is trimmed from a full thickness graft. However, in favourable circumstances, thicker free grafts can survive if they have a good vascular inset. This has particular application in reconstruction of the alar margin of the nose, using a composite graft from the pinna, consisting of two layers of skin sandwiching a strip of cartilage.

Flaps

In contrast to a free graft, which is completely detached from its donor site and is transposed to the recipient site, a flap at all times maintains an intact circulation. This allows skin, subcutaneous tissue and sometimes other tissues to be transferred to resurface areas that are unsuitable for free split-skin grafts, e.g. where the bed is avascular, where appearance is important, where there is a serious contour defect, or at sites where further reconstructive work may be necessary, such as tendon, nerve or bone graft repairs.

Local flaps

These are the first choice if a flap is necessary. When the defect is too large for simple undermining to allow closure, the local tissues can often be advanced, transposed or rotated to close it, using skin that is similar in texture and colour to the missing tissues.

V-Y advancement

This technique can be used to release some tight webs or contractions, and flaps with a subcutaneous pedicle can be advanced in this matter to close circular defects (Fig. 1.40) and in the closure of certain finger-tip injuries — the Kutler (Kutler, 1949; Fisher, 1967) or Kleinert (Atasoy, 1970) flaps.

Transposition flaps

Skin can often be transposed into a defect from an adjacent area of laxity at right angles to it (Fig. 1.41). Careful planning using a paper or jaconet pattern is essential to ensure that the flap is long enough.

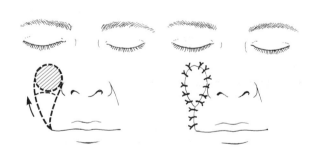

Fig. 1.40 V-Y advancement flap on subcutaneous pedicle

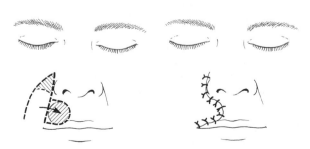

Fig. 1.41 Transposition flap from naso-labial fold to defect in upper lip

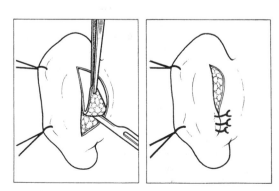

Fig. 1.38 Cutting a post-auricular full thickness skin graft
Fig. 1.39 Defect closed by suture

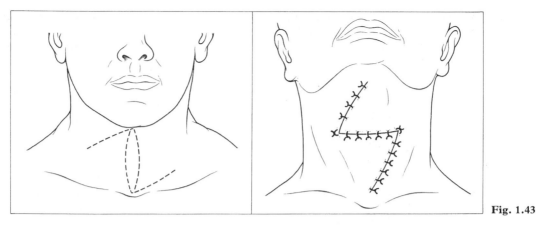

Fig. 1.42   **Fig. 1.43**

Fig. 1.42   Z-plasty to release contracture of neck
Fig. 1.43   Completed Z-plasty

Z-plasties

Contracted linear scars commonly occur in the neck, the axillary fold or in the neighbourhood of joints where they may restrict or prevent movement. Excision of the scar, combined with some plastic procedure to prevent recurrence of the contracture is required. Such a manoeuvre is the Z-plasty, in which two interdigitating triangular flaps are transposed. The scar is excised (or incised along its crest) and from each extremity an incision is made at an angle of 60° so that the markings resemble the letter 'Z' (Fig. 1.42). The triangular flaps are then raised, transposed and sutured in their new position (Fig. 1.43). The effect of this is to lengthen the original axis of the scar and place a new axis across the contracture. This procedure works best if the original scar is linear, with good quality skin on each side of the band. It is of no use in the release of broad thick contractures or in the closure of defects over convexities such as the skull. It is used widely as part of the treatment of Dupuytren's contracture in the hand, and plastic surgeons regularly use it in the closure of difficult wounds. The permutations and combinations of this and other types of flap are superbly described by McGregor (1989).

Rotation flaps are useful in some situations, depending on the anatomical site of the defect and the laxity of the surrounding tissues. Examples of appropriate sites are on the scalp, on the cheek (Figs 1.44 & 1.45) or for sacral pressure sores. A very large rotation flap is needed to close quite a small defect, as it depends on distribution of tension along the length of the incision.

Distant flaps

When a local flap is not available, a flap may be transferred from a distance, carrying its blood supply through a pedicle which bridges intact skin. When the

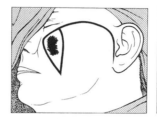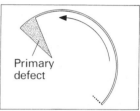

Primary defect

Fig. 1.44   Cheek rotation flap to cover facial defect
Fig. 1.45   Principle of rotation flap showing back cut (dotted line) that can be used to release tension

flap is soundly inset into the recipient defect and has picked up a new blood supply, the pedicle can be divided. This usually takes about three weeks. Details of distant flaps are beyond the scope of this book, but the cross finger flap is a commonly used example (Fig. 1.46).

Vascular anatomy of flaps

There are two types of flap distinguished by their vascular anatomy. Many traditional flaps belong to the category of '*random pattern*' flaps which are raised without consideration of the vascular distribution within them. For this reason the flap must conform to strict limitations in its length to breadth ratio, which should not be greater than 1:1. Most local flaps and the cross finger flap fall into this category.

By contrast, an '*axial pattern flap*' has an identifiable arteriovenous system in its long axis and long flaps can be raised with far fewer restrictions on their width. The axial vessels may lie in the subcutaneous tissue, e.g. the groin flap based on the superficial circumflex iliac artery (McGregor, 1972) and the hypogastric flap based on the superficial hypogastric vessels. The vascular pedicles of other flaps may lie more deeply.

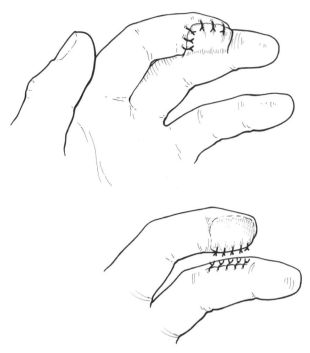

Fig. 1.46   Cross finger flap. Flap raised from dorsum of middle phalanx, middle finger and sutured to cover defect. (After three weeks, flap pedicle divided)

Interest in the vascular supply of other potential axial pattern flaps has encouraged a detailed re-examination and study of the blood supply not only to the skin and subcutaneous fat, but to the fascia, the underlying muscles, bones and nerves. Plastic surgeons now have at their disposal a very wide range of flaps, incorporating any number or all of these structures, that can be raised, transposed or rotated into local or distant defects. The deep fascia carries a rich blood supply and can nourish the overlying skin when included in a flap (*fascio-cutaneous flaps*). These can be invaluable in closing defects in the lower limb, where they have proved to be far safer than flaps of skin and fat alone. Vessels supplying the deep fascia run in the intermuscular septa or through the muscles, and these can be incorporated in the pedicles of flaps. For example, the pectoralis major muscle with or without the overlying skin, can be raised on its vascular pedicle and transposed into the neck or lower face (Bakamjian, 1965). The latissimus dorsi muscle can be transposed with or without some of its covering skin to reconstruct the breast following mastectomy, chest wall defects, defects in the neck or in the upper limb. These and other muscle flaps, such as the gastrocnemius, rectus abdominis, gracilis and gluteus maximus flaps, and fascial flaps,

can be used to close difficult chronic wounds and, when raised without overlying skin, can be covered with split skin grafts. The excellent blood supply of muscle gives it particular value in covering compound fractures.

Free tissue transfer

Many of these flaps, and others too, can be raised on their vascular pedicles as free flaps and transported to almost any site in the body provided there are suitable vessels at the recipient site to allow revascularization of the free flap by microvascular anastomoses (Fig. 1.47). Compound flaps can be designed to include segments of bone and nerve which can themselves be revascularized at the same time.

The tube pedicle flap, associated so intimately with the names of Gillies (in the U.K.) and Filatov (in the Soviet Union) was for many decades the standard way of reconstructing a complex of large defects. It has now been replaced by the newer techniques and is only rarely used.

Tissue expansion

This is a technique of gaining extra skin by the subcutaneous insertion of a silicone bag which can be gradually expanded by the injection of normal saline over a period of several weeks. This is done through a filling port attached by a tube to the expander, which may be buried under the skin or lie on the surface. The expanded skin may be used to provide a local flap (e.g. of hairy scalp to replace an area of alopecia) (Fig. 1.48) or to cover a silicone implant (e.g. in breast reconstruction).

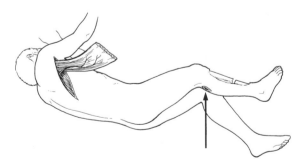

Fig. 1.47   Free latissimus dorsi muscle flap, based on the thoraco-dorsal vessels, transferred to cover compound tibial fracture with microvascular end-to-side anastomosis to popliteal vessels. The muscle is then covered with a split skin graft

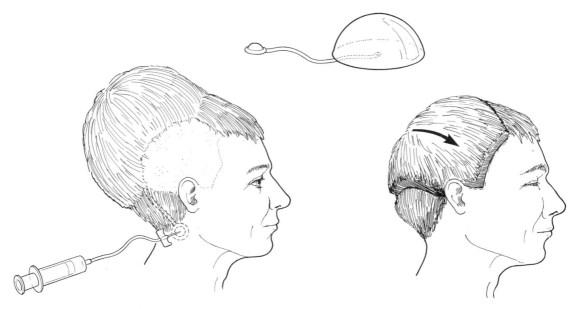

Fig. 1.48 Tissue expansion. (a) Silicone tissue expander with filling port and connecting tube. (b) Expander, inserted under hairy scalp, being filled to stretch scalp and produce enough to cover area of alopecia above right ear. (c) After removal of expander and excision of alopecia, expanded scalp advanced to fill defect

REFERENCES

Atasoy E, Ioakimidis E, Kasdan M, Kutz J, Kleinert H E 1970 Reconstruction of the amputated finger tip with a triangular volar flap. Journal of Bone and Joint Surgery 52A: 921–926

Bakamjian V Y 1965 A two-stage method for pharyngo-oesophageal reconstruction with a primary pectoral flap. Plastic and Reconstructive Surgery 36: 173–184

Breslow A 1970 Thickness, cross-sectional areas and depth of invasion in the prognosis of cutaneous melanoma. Annals of Surgery 172: 902–908

Fisher R H 1967 The Kutler method of repair of finger tip amputations. Journal of Bone and Joint Surgery 49A: 317–321

Ghussen F, Nagel K, Groth W, Muller J M, Stutzer H 1984 A prospective randomised study of regional extremity perfusion in patients with malignant melanoma. Annals of Surgery 200: 764–768

Janzekovic Z 1970 A new concept in the excision and immediate grafting of burns. Journal of Trauma 10: 1103–1108

Kutler W 1949 A new method for finger tip amputations. Journal of the American Medical Association 133: 29–31

McGregor I A 1989 Fundamental techniques of plastic surgery and their surgical applications, 8th edn. Churchill Livingstone, Edinburgh

McGregor I A, Jackson I T 1972 The groin flap. British Journal of Plastic Surgery 25: 3

Meyer K L, Childers S J 1985 The surgical approach to primary malignant melanoma. Surgery Gynaecology and Obstetrics 160: 379–386

FURTHER READING

Cason J A 1981 Treatment of burns. Chapman and Hall, London

Cormack G C, Lamberty B G H 1986 The arterial anatomy of skin flaps. Churchill Livingstone, Edinburgh

Grabb W C, Smith J W 1979 Plastic surgery, 3rd edn. Little, Brown, Boston

Mathes S J, Nahai F 1979 Clinical atlas of musculo- and musculo-cutaneous flaps. Mosby, St. Louis

Mathes S J, Nahai F 1982 Clinical applications for muscle and musculo-cutaneous flaps. Mosby, St. Louis

McCarthy J G 1990 Plastic surgery (8 vols). W B Saunders Co, Philadelphia

McCraw J B, Arnold P G 1986 A color atlas of muscle and musculo-cutaneous flaps. Hampton Press, Norfolk, Virginia

Muir I F K, Barclay T L, Settle J A D 1987 Burns and their treatment, 3rd edn. Butterworths, London

Mustarde J C, Jackson I T 1988 Plastic surgery in infancy and childhood, 3rd edn. Churchill Livingstone, Edinburgh

O'Brien B McC, Morrison W A 1987 Reconstructive microsurgery. Churchill Livingstone, Edinburgh

2

General preparations; intravenous fluids and blood products

D. B. L. McCLELLAND, W. G. MURPHY & R. F. RINTOUL

During the outpatient investigation of any patient who is to be admitted to hospital for an operation, the surgeon will have already offered advice regarding preparation of a general nature. In many cases, the patient need be admitted only on the morning of his operation, but this assumes that his fitness for anaesthesia has been considered and that little further preparation is required. A preadmission clinic will provide the opportunity for full and thorough assessment and minimise the patient's stay in hospital. Patients who require complex assessment or preparation for surgery will be admitted to hospital several days before operation and will then have the opportunity to become accustomed to their surroundings.

Respiratory complications are among the most common after abdominal surgery. It is a wise precaution to postpone a non-urgent operation in a patient with respiratory infection until the patient's lung function is at its optimum. X-ray of the chest is advisable in such cases and in all patients being prepared for major procedures, since underlying disease may be more clearly defined and postoperative changes may be compared with the initial X-ray.

Diet. A patient admitted to hospital on the day prior to operation follows an unrestricted diet except for a light supper. Fluids and food are withheld for the night if operation is arranged for the following morning. For operations later in the day, 4-6 hours of fasting is adequate. Those patients who require longer preparation may take the opportunity to improve their nutrition with a well balanced normal diet or with one of the many fluid substitutes now available. In cases where hepatic dysfunction may be present, e.g. in bilary disease (p. 425), a high carbohydrate diet should be prescribed in order to ensure adequate stores of liver glycogen. Glucose may be given orally — 100 to 200 g daily for 2–3 days before operation.

Gastric aspiration. In cases of vomiting, a nasogastric tube should be passed in order that all stomach contents can be withdrawn before the patient is taken to the theatre. The tube is left in situ during the operation, so that further aspiration can be carried out as

required. This is a valuable precaution in preventing vomitus being inhaled during induction of anaesthesia. Even in the absence of vomiting, there is a definite risk of acid regurgitation during induction and many anaesthetists prescribe an H2 blocking drug as an alternative to inserting a tube.

Renal function. Investigation of the blood chemistry is indicated in conditions of fluid and electrolyte imbalance, and in hypoproteinaemia. Preoperative measurement of blood urea should be routine since a high level requires investigation and correction if postoperative renal failure is to be avoided. Estimation of the specific gravity of the urine, and examination for albumin and sugar, should be carried out as routine before any operation. In conditions where the fluid or electrolyte balance may be disturbed (see below) it is important to keep a fluid balance chart to record input and output of body fluids. In many major procedures, this involves the insertion of a bladder catheter so that the urinary output can be measured accurately. The smallest possible size of catheter should be used so as to minimise damage and infection.

Bowel action. Provided that the bowel action has been regular, it is unnecessary to give an aperient. Where indicated, however, some mild laxative such as Lactulose may be prescribed not later than the morning of the day prior to operation. Alternatively, suppositories may be given on the evening before operation when a normal evacuation has not been obtained. For all operations on the colon or rectum where resection is likely to be carried out, special preparation (p. 479) is required.

Blood. Routine testing includes haemoglobin and white cell estimation. In many cases the underlying disease leads to anaemia, which it may be necessary to correct by transfusion, so that the patient is submitted to operation in the optimum condition to withstand blood loss. In all major abdominal cases a full blood examination should include determination of the blood group so that an individual compatibility test can be done against the blood of a prospective donor. Blood transfusion plays an integral part in saving life, and the blood may not be available when it is most urgently required unless the need is anticipated. In such cases it is an advantage to set up an intravenous infusion of dextrose or saline at the commencement of anaesthesia, so that blood transfusion may be substituted quickly and easily during operation should this prove necessary.

INTRAVENOUS INFUSION

Choice of vein

Cannulation of the venous system may be required for the administration of drugs, for the intravenous infusion of fluids, for transfusion of blood products or for parenteral feeding when alternative routes are unsuitable. Access is also required for measurement of the central venous pressure. The choice of vein thus depends on the individual requirements for each patient, and on the patency of the veins. In general, it is an advantage to use veins on the dorsum of the hand or on the forearm for isotonic fluids and central veins for irritant solutions. Whenever possible, the most peripheral vein should be used first in order to preserve more central veins for subsequent use. The cephalic vein on the radial side of the forearm (Fig. 2.1) can usually be identified even when the veins generally are collapsed and it is of convenient size. Since it lies between the wrist and elbow joints, the cannula is less likely to be disturbed by movement, and there is no need for splintage. In an emergency, veins of the cubital fossa are easily identified, but it is best to insert a long cannula which will not obstruct when the elbow is flexed. Splinting of the elbow should be avoided since the necessary bandaging may interfere with the smooth flow of the infusion. Three sites are available for rapid infusion or for the placement of a cannula within the right heart, namely the subclavian, jugular and basilic veins. Use of the cephalic vein in the upper arm or of the long saphenous vein anterior to the medial malleolus is not recommended because of the tendency of these veins to become thrombosed and because of the immobility imposed by an infusion in the leg. A careful aseptic technique is essential in all cases, especially for the insertion of a 'central venous line' where colonization of the catheter tip by bacteria can lead to septicaemia. This infection risk is higher for a triple-lumen catheter than for one with a single-lumen but 'tunnelled' central lines have reduced risk of infection. 'Tunnelling' is most appropriate with a subclavian catheter where the skin puncture and vein puncture are separated by several centimetres.

Percutaneous puncture of vein

Many types of intravenous needles and needle cannu-

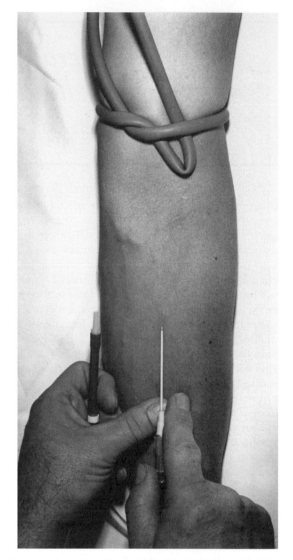

Fig. 2.1 Insertion of an infusion needle into the cephalic vein in the forearm. The tubing, emptied of air, is ready to be attached

lae are now available, most incorporating a needle within a plastic cannula. The combined needle and cannula may be introduced into a vein by percutaneous puncture. Examples are illustrated in Figure 2.2. No attempt will be made to describe the technique of entering a vein with a needle; this will usually be learned by demonstration and perfected by practice. Confirmation that the vein has been entered should be obtained by the backflow of blood into the cannula after withdrawal of its central needle and before connection of the infusion; otherwise infusion fluid may extravasate into the tissues around the vein. The needle or cannula should be secured by strapping, so that it

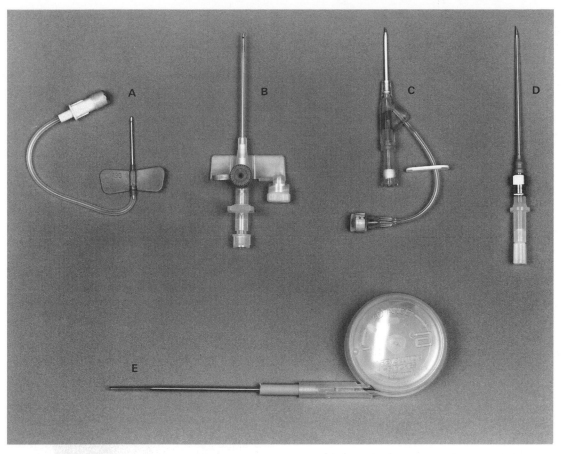

Fig. 2.2 Types of intravenous needle cannulae for percutaneous use: The Butterfly (A) and the Venflon (B) needles incorporate side plates to allow rigid fixation. Each can be used for intermittent drug administration (through a syringe) or for 'drip' infusion; the Venflon needle allows for both functions. The Y-can (C) is also dual purpose. Cannulae (B), (C) and (D) (Jelco) consist of a fine needle within a plastic cannulae. After it has been confirmed, by aspiration of blood, that the vein has been entered, the needle is withdrawn, and the infusion tubing is connected to the cannula. The 'drum cartridge catheter' (E) is advanced by rotation of the drum after the attached needle has been used to puncture the vein

will not be pulled out of the vein by minor strains or jerks on the tubing. Insertion of a cannula in a shocked patient, in whom the veins may be very collapsed is only achieved with the experience obtained from entering normal veins.

In the technique for central venous catheterization, the appropriate vein is punctured, an intravenous catheter is advanced towards the heart and both the needle and stylet are withdrawn. Some indication of the position of the catheter tip is obtained by comparing the length of the stylet with the length of catheter which is visible outside the vein. However, radiographic confirmation of the catheter position should be obtained whenever possible. The subclavian vein is more commonly entered below rather than above the clavicle and requires experience to avoid the risk of causing pneumothorax. With the patient's head rotated to the opposite side and tilted head downwards, the needle is introduced below the midpoint of the clavicle and advanced towards the back of the sternoclavicular joint keeping close to the clavicle. The internal jugular vein is punctured deep to the sternomastoid, aiming in the direction of the vein at the sternal end of the clavicle. Details of the technique are best learned from someone experienced in their use. Access through the basilic vein is obtained either by direct puncture at the medial border of the biceps muscle or through the median cubital vein and a 'drum cartridge' catheter is used so that its tip is advanced as far as the right atrium.

Cannulization by exposure of vein ('cut down')
With experience in percutaneous puncture, it is rarely necessary to require a 'cut down'. Its use is thus restricted to patients where superficial veins are thrombosed and the skill of placing a 'central line' is not available. It can also be used when a larger cannula is

required for rapid infusion of fluids. When the need for rapid blood transfusion can be anticipated, it is preferable to use a short wide diameter cannula or even the obliquely trimmed end of the transfusion set.

In a conscious patient a little local anaesthetic solution is infiltrated intradermally in a line transversely across the vein, and a small incision is made. The superficial fascia is cleared by inserting the points of sharp scissors, and opening them on each side of the line of the vein (Fig. 2.3). When the vein has been isolated in this way two ligatures are passed around it; the distal one is tied and held in forceps (Fig. 2.4), the proximal one is half tied in readiness to receive the cannula and its ends are left loose. With sharp pointed scissors a nick is made in the vein between the ligatures, the distal one being used as a retractor. The cannula, which should have been filled with the infusion solution in order to exclude air bubbles, is quickly inserted, and the proximal ligature is tied to enclose it. At this point, it is convenient to pass a stitch through the skin and to

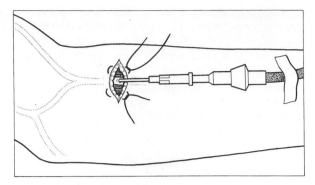

Fig. 2.5 The cannula is inserted and the wound sutured

tie it round the base of the cannula, in order to prevent it from being pulled out of the vein before the tubing can be fixed with strapping. The skin wound is closed with two mattress sutures (Fig. 2.5).

INTRAVENOUS FLUIDS

Fluid and electrolyte therapy is an essential part of surgical treatment, both pre- and postoperative.

The essentials of such therapy are (1) to make good any fluid deficit already incurred, (2) to ensure an adequate balance between the daily intake and output of fluid, replacing any continuing losses as they arise, and (3) to administer fluids which contain in solution the appropriate mineral constituents according to the patient's needs.

Dehydration. By far the commonest cause of dehydration is abnormal loss of fluid from the gastrointestinal tract. Such losses may occur before operation, and are then likely to be due to the primary condition which brings the patient for treatment, e.g. the profuse vomiting of pyloric obstruction, or the severe and prolonged diarrhoea of ulcerative colitis. Alternatively the fluid loss may occur as a complication of operation, e.g. prolonged aspiration of gastric contents or discharge from fistulae. In either case the deficit should be assessed, if possible, from the clinical state, from the haematocrit, or from the estimated amount of fluid lost. Serum analysis is not always helpful initially but is a guide to progress. (When fluid losses are large, laboratory analysis of each *fluid* is of value.) Early replacement of deficiencies should be the aim, firstly to ensure that the patient is in the best possible condition to withstand surgery, and secondly because the difficulties of replacement are greatly increased thereafter. As soon as the deficiency has been assessed, replacement should begin, the method and the quantity administered depending upon the circumstances. If adequate fluid can be administered orally (but this is rare in surgical

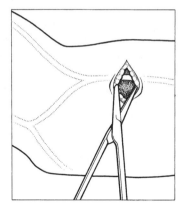

Fig. 2.3 Method of exposing a vein in the forearm

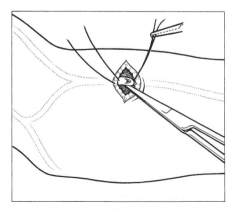

Fig. 2.4 The vein is controlled by ligatures and a nick is made with scissors

patients), few difficulties will arise. As a rule administration must be by the intravenous route, and the fluids to be infused must then be selected with care.

Solutions. The simplest solutions for intravenous infusion are isotonic (0.9%) saline and 5% dextrose solution. Some of each solution is necessary each day depending on losses likely to be sustained. In general, the *normal* requirement of the body for salt is in the region of 5 g per day, and this will be met very adequately by 600 ml of isotonic saline solution. For practical purposes this is given as either one or two 1/2 litres of saline. When the patient's main need is for water alone, any additional fluid should be given in the form of dextrose solution. Proportionately much larger quantities of saline will, however, be required when there is actual loss of gastrointestinal secretions, for in general such losses should be replaced with saline. Certain alternative solutions are mentioned in the following sections.

Quantity to be administered and rate of flow. When the fluid loss has been severe, it is obviously desirable to replace this as expeditiously as possible, and large quantities of intravenous fluid may then be required. Using central venous pressure measurements, over- and under-infusion can be avoided in such cases. Adequate replacement can also be judged by the patient's clinical state, a useful guide being a urine output of 1–2 ml per minute. Serum electrolytes should be measured frequently. Any marked degree of water and salt depletion leads to nitrogen retention, so that the blood urea level is a most useful and most sensitive index of the degree of depletion and the efficacy of replacement (le Quesne, 1967). The optimal basal intake of fluid in *average* conditions is in the region of 2–3 litres in the 24 hours, 0.75 to 1 litre for 'insensible' loss (via the expired air and by evaporation from the skin), and 1–2 litres to allow for an adequate urinary output, of which the acceptable minimum is 500 ml. A pyrexial patient will lose even more fluid, and sodium will be lost through sweating. If fluid cannot be taken orally, the whole amount should be given intravenously. Since the *normal* daily requirement of the body for salt is about 5 g, this will be adequately met by 600 ml of isotonic saline solution; thus two or three 1/2-litres of dextrose solution should be given for every one 1/2-litre of saline. Any abnormal losses by vomiting, etc., should be compensated for by a corresponding increase in the amount of saline infused, so that a daily balance is achieved (see below). For the first 24–48 hours after a major operation when sodium and water are retained by the body and urinary output is reduced, the amount of fluid infused should not normally exceed 2 litres per day unless it is necessary to compensate for abnormal losses. The rate of administration — in drops per minute — can be determined by multiplying the required number of litres per day by 11. Intravenous therapy should be discontinued when 2½ litres (i.e. 100 ml per hour) can be taken orally.

Daily fluid balance. The keeping of a daily fluid balance chart is an essential safeguard whenever a patient is being treated by continuous intravenous infusion — whether this be pre- or postoperatively. An exact record must by kept throughout the 24 hours of all fluid intake, orally or by intravenous infusion. The output — by urine, by vomiting or by gastric aspiration, by fistulous discharges or by diarrhoea — must be similarly recorded. (The fluid content of solid faeces can be disregarded.) To the total amount of the recorded output must be added 0.75 to 1 litre for 'insensible' loss, increasing the volume in a pyrexial patient. The intake and output should be compared after each 12 hours, and any fluid debt or *negative balance* should be replaced during the ensuing 12-hour period. A more frequent balance should be kept where losses are high, and in all cases a cumulative balance should be made daily, taking into account gains or losses during the preceding days of the infusion.

Acidosis (diminished alkali reserve) is commonly caused by loss of alkaline secretions of the alimentary tract below the stomach — as may result from the vomiting of high intestinal obstruction, intestinal fistulae, ileostomy or prolonged diarrhoea. The main deficiencies, besides that of fluid are of sodium and potassium. When, as is usually the case, the sodium loss predominates, there will be an associated fall in the plasma bicarbonate level, a fall in the CO_2 combining power, and a resulting acidosis. The administration of isotonic saline replaces losses in water and sodium, but not in potassium; Hartmann's solution containing potassium ions and bicarbonate (as lactate) — in addition to sodium and chloride — is thus ideal for the replacement of lower gastrointestinal losses. In severe acidosis, 500 ml of 1.26% sodium bicarbonate may be given by intravenous infusion over a period of 2 hours although a total of 2 litres of this solution may need to be given.

Alkalosis. Continued vomiting or aspiration of gastric secretions over a prolonged period leads to a state of alkalosis, since gastric juice normally contains excess of chlorides over sodium and potassium, and there is therefore a greater loss of acid radicles. When vomiting has continued for more than a few days, there is a considerable loss of sodium and potassium, due to loss in the urine, rather than in the vomit. The alkalosis leads to an increased bicarbonate concentration in the plasma, and therefore in the glomerular filtrate. In consequence there is an increased retention of hydrogen ions by the kidneys, hence secretion of bicarbonate in the urine along with potassium. The loss of water, chlorides and sodium is replaced very adequately by the infusion of isotonic saline solution. Potassium chloride should be added to the solution in divided doses.

Potassium deficiency. The management of potassium deficiency in the postoperative period is one of considerable importance. Immediately following an operation, and in direct proportion to its severity, there is an increased loss of potassium in the urine. This results from mobilisation of intracellular potassium as a result of sodium retention. Potassium loss also occurs from prolonged vomiting or loss of intestinal secretions. Possibly the most important loss follows the prolonged intravenous infusion of solutions containing no potassium, since this is secreted in larger quantities in the urine while sodium is conserved. There is probably little risk of potassium deficiency during the first 48 hours of infusion. When, however, the infusion is continued for a longer period, it is wise to give potassium, either orally or added to the infusion. Potassium deficiency, which presents clinically by intense drowsiness deepening to coma, muscular weakness and incoordination, should be suspected whenever there has been prolonged or severe loss of gastrointestinal secretions or if an intravenous infusion has been in use for over 48 hours without added potassium. Replacement should not await laboratory confirmation of the deficiency, which being mainly intracellular will not be accurately represented by the serum level. Potassium should be given orally if possible because of the risk of arrhythmias occurring from too rapid a rise in the plasma concentration. If oral administration is practicable the recommended dosage is 1 to 2 g of potassium chloride 8-hourly for the first 24 hours, followed by 2 g every 3 to 4 hours until the serum potassium reaches normal levels. If intravenous administration is necessary, 1.5 g (20 mmol) of potassium chloride should be added to 500 ml of dextrose solution, and infused over a period of four hours. Provided the urinary output is over 600 ml per day, further potassium infusion is safe, three or four such infusions being commonly given each day. Ready-prepared solutions containing 3 g of potassium chloride per litre are more convenient and supply an identical concentration. In circumstances where potassium loss is considerable, magnesium deficiency may also be present. This is recognized by serum measurement and is easily amenable to replacement therapy.

Protein deficiency

Many patients who require surgery, particularly as an emergency, are depleted of plasma proteins. Rapid depletion can result from severe haemorrhage or from serious burns or other injuries. Gradual depletion may be due to inadequate dietary intake of protein, resulting either from starvation or from defective absorption, as may occur in malignant disease, and in conditions such as Crohn's disease and ulcerative colitis. The deficient albumin content of the plasma gives rise to a decrease in the colloid osmotic pressure, so that, provided that severe dehydration is not present, extruded tissue fluid fails to return to the circulation, and some degree of oedema results. Such conditions give rise to increased susceptibility to infections and to diminished healing power. They, therefore, add considerably to the risk of operation and retard convalescence.

The normal level of plasma proteins is 65–85 g per litre, including 35 g per litre of albumin. Estimations made during protein deficiency may give a misleadingly high figure on account of the dehydration which may coexist, and this factor must be considered.

Acute protein deficiency cannot be corrected by blood transfusion although plasma, or plasma substitutes, are used in the treatment of burns to correct the colloid osmotic pressure and maintain the circulation. Chronic deficiency of protein can be treated by the administration of a high protein diet, comprising 200–250 g of protein daily. This should be combined with vitamin C in doses up to 1 g daily. If the patient cannot take food normally by mouth, protein hydrolysates may be given by 'drip' through a nasogastric tube. Proprietary solutions can be administered through a fine bore (1 mm) tube which has been passed into the stomach and which is well tolerated once it is in position (Fig. 2.6). For longer term enteral feeding, a fine needle catheter jejunostomy placed at operation (Humberstone, 1992) or a feeding gastrostomy (page 398) may be used.

It should be noted that all major operations lead to a considerable amount of protein catabolism, and, if hypoproteinaemia exists preoperatively, a serious deficiency may develop. It is obvious, therefore, that any protein replacement required should be effected if possible before operation.

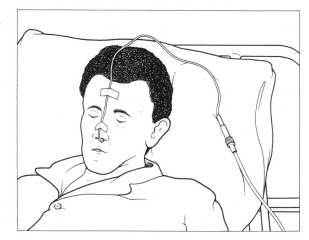

Fig. 2.6   Fine bore (1 mm) tube for nasogastric feeding

Total parenteral nutrition (TPN) may be considered to combat postoperative or post-traumatic negative nitrogen balance where normal feeding will be delayed for more than a few days but the advantages and risks should be carefully considered in each patient. It may also be given preoperatively to a malnourished patient but is less effective than enteral feeding. *Fat emulsions* and *glucose* provide essential calories and both are necessary for correct utilization of *amino-acid solutions* (Forrest, 1985). It is usual to mix together all the fluids for 24 hours in a single 3 litre bag and to administer the contents through a cannula placed in a central vein. This is helpful in minimising side effects but strict aseptic precautions must be maintained. A limited range of fluids can be given into a peripheral vein although problems with thrombosis of the drip vein may occur.

BLOOD TRANSFUSION AND BLOOD PRODUCTS

Transfusion of blood has been a well established part of clinical practice since the early nineteen hundreds. The crucial first development in safe transfusion was Landsteiner's discovery in 1901 of the major human blood group system (the ABO system). Since then transfusion has become an increasingly specialised therapy; safe transfusion requires access to specialist facilities for the collection, testing and processing of blood and for the necessary tests on the patient.

Transfusion of blood or blood components is indicated in surgical patients for:

1. acute blood loss leading to cardiorespiratory decompensation (red cell containing components)
2. critical haemostatic failure (platelets, plasma, whole blood).

Processed blood products, including albumin, specific clotting factor concentrates and immunoglobulin preparations may also be indicated for use in surgical patients. These are considered later in this section.

Acute blood loss leading to cardiorespiratory decompensation

The aim of replacement therapy should be to maintain the patient's circulatory volume and oxygen delivery capacity at an adequate or optimal level by the use of red cell preparations and other fluids. Replacing all blood loss with blood transfusion is neither necessary nor desirable and exposes the patient unnecessarily to the risks of blood transfusion.

The average healthy adult can lose 500 ml of blood rapidly and with no ill effects. Given adequate fluid replacement, a loss of one to two litres can be sustained without irreversible hypotension. Children, the elderly and patients with cardiac or pulmonary disease are less resistant to blood loss (and more susceptible to the risks of over-transfusion) and so require a more exacting approach to transfusion.

Having made a clinical assessment of blood loss the following points should be considered:

1. Does the patient need *blood* or can some *safer fluid* be used?
2. *Oxygenation* must be maintained; in the fit patient, a haematocrit of 30% with the associated reduction in blood viscosity provides optimal capillary flow and adequate tissue oxygenation. Low plasma viscosity will be better maintained by crystalloid or colloid solutions than by plasma.

A general replacement policy for the acutely bleeding patient should be based on a planned sequence of crystalloid solutions, colloid solutions and whole blood or red cell concentrates.

Transfusion of the anaemic surgical patient

There is no universal standard for a desirable haemoglobin level in surgical patients. Patients with a well-compensated chronic anaemia may tolerate lower haemoglobin levels than patients with normal preoperative haemoglobin. In general however, patients tolerate acute blood loss less well when the haemoglobin level is below 7 g/dl than when it is above that figure; the inability to replace blood losses with red cell transfusion to patients with a preoperative haemoglobin of 7 g or less (as has occurred in Jehovah's Witnesses undergoing surgery) is associated with a significant increase in mortality.

Critical haemostatic failure

Haemostatic failure leading to excessive bleeding in surgical patients may be present prior to the surgical or traumatic event, may arise during the course of surgery or resuscitation or may be anticipated because of the volume of blood loss or the presence of hypotension or of sepsis.

Pre-existing haemostatic defects in surgical patients should be sought by a detailed history with particular reference to previous major haemostatic challenges and administration of drugs such as aspirin or anticoagulants. A simple laboratory coagulation screen consisting of a prothrombin time and a platelet count should augment the clinical history where possible. The development of a coagulopathy during the course of an operation or resuscitation can be observed by the presence of unexpected bleeding from small vessels (microvascular bleeding) generally manifesting as a diffuse ooze in the wound or at intravascular cannulae insertion sites. A laboratory assessment including a prothrombin time and partial thromboplastin time, tests for the presence of disseminated intravascular coagulation such as d-dimers, a platelet count, and if reliably available, a bleeding time, may help clarify the underlying mechanism of such coagulopathy and help to direct the therapy.

Following massive blood loss and fluid replacement an acquired coagulopathy can arise due to dilutional thrombocytopenia and dilution of soluble clotting factors. Impairment of haemostatic function will arise after approximately one blood volume has been replaced with platelet-poor fluids (including whole blood and red cell concentrate). Critical dilution of soluble clotting factors will arise when approximately two blood volumes have been replaced. When the patient has had a period of hypotension the development of haemostatic failure will be accelerated by consumptive coagulopathy. Prophylactic use of platelets and plasma has not been shown to be of benefit in patients receiving large volume transfusion. However, where a coagulopathy does develop in these patients, platelet transfusions will be necessary. Plasma will be needed in addition (about 1 litre in an adult) to replace clotting factors if the clotting times are prolonged *and if the plasma fibrinogen is greater than 0.8 gm/l.* Fibrinogen replacement with cryoprecipitate (approximately 10 donor units in an adult) will be required if the plasma fibrinogen is less than 0.8 gm/l.

Aspirin causes irreversible platelet dysfunction. This can cause increased bleeding at surgery for several days after a single dose. Major surgery should be delayed for about a week after aspirin has been taken; if this is not possible *and* if a significant bleeding problem is encountered, platelet transfusion may be needed.

Patients with specific clotting factor deficiencies will require specific factor replacement and the expertise of a haematologist. Patients with multiple factor deficiencies secondary to liver disease may require factor replacement using fresh frozen plasma. For elective procedures in these patients the prothrombin ratio should be reduced to 1.7 or less. Since the *in vivo* half life of factor VII is only a few hours, close monitoring of such patients will be required. Patients on warfarin therapy can often be managed without the use of blood products unless urgent surgery is required or life-threatening bleeding develops. In these circumstances clotting factor concentrates (II, IX and X, and VII) should be used if available. Otherwise plasma infusion will be required, generally of the order of 1 litre for an adult. A combination of II, IX and X concentrate with smaller volumes of plasma (approximately 200 to 500 ml) can be used if factor VII only is unavailable.

Some surgical procedures, in particular cardio-pulmonary bypass surgery and liver transplantation, present peculiar haemostatic problems of their own and may require intensive blood product support with platelets and plasma.

BLOOD COMPONENTS AND BLOOD PRODUCTS (Table 2.1)

Collection and storage of blood

Blood for transfusion is collected into a citrate anti-coagulant solution, containing dextrose and adenine to prolong red cell viability: 400 to 500 ml of blood is

Table 2.1 Blood components

Product	Indications	Special precautions	Shelf-life
Whole blood	Massive haemorrhage	Must be ABO + Rh D compatible	35 days
Red blood cells (Red cell concentrate) (may be supplemented)	Most routine transfusions and for massive replacement as part of planned programme	Must be ABO + Rh D compatible	As above
Leucocyte-depleted red cells	Patients with transfusion reactions or risk of sensitisation to leucocyte antigens on long-term programmes	Must be ABO + Rh D compatible	Depends on method of preparation
Platelet concentrates	Bleeding due to thrombocytopenia	Should be ABO compatible	5 days
Fresh frozen plasma	Bleeding due to multiple coagulation factor deficiency or coumarin overdose (with II, IX, X)	Must be ABO compatible	1 year at −40°C
Cryoprecipitate	Bleeding with fibrinogen depletion (< 0.8 g/l)	Should be ABO compatible	1 year at −40°C
Albumin 5%	Acute volume expansion;		4 years
25%	impaired renal function associated with hypoproteinaemia		4 years
Factor VIII	Haemophilia A		2 years
Factor II, IX, X	Haemophilia B Coumarin anticoagulant reversal		2 years
Factor IX	Haemophilia B		
Immunoglobulins	Various indications (see text)		4 years

drawn from the donor into about 60 ml of anticoagulant mixture. The donation is either then used, stored as whole blood or processed in a number of different ways. The unit can be centrifuged to sediment the red cells; the plasma is then expressed into a second bag. The plasma-containing bag is then detached from the red cells for use as fresh frozen plasma, for the preparation of cryoprecipitate, or sent for bulk processing to yield blood products such as clotting factors or immunoglobulins. The residual red cell concentrate can be used as such, having a haematocrit of 60–80%. Commonly however, an *additive solution* is added to the red cell concentrate to improve storage characteristics and to reduce the haematocrit to 50–65%. The additive solution will vary depending on the supplier, but generally contains adenine and a high molecular weight sugar such as mannitol or sorbitol. Platelets for clinical use may be prepared at the plasma separation stage using a differential centrifugation technique.

Red cell preparations

Red cell concentrate, red cell concentrate supplemented with additive solution, and whole blood must be stored at 2–6°C in properly controlled refrigerators. During storage of red cell preparations there is progressive loss of in vitro function and loss of intracellular potassium into the extracellular medium. After 35 days of shelf life a unit of whole blood will contain approximately 10 mmol of extracellular potassium; this will be slightly less in stored red cell concentrate. Intracellular 2,3-diphosphoglycerate (2,3-DPG) is an essential cofactor for adequate haemoglobin function, in particular the release of bound oxygen at low oxygen tension. This cofactor decays with time during storage and will have fallen to negligible levels after two weeks of storage. Following transfusion of stored red cells, 2,3-DPG activity recovers within 24 hours.

Platelet preparations

These are provided either as pools of platelet concentrates from different whole blood donors, or from one or two donors by apheresis. Platelets are stored at 22°C. A platelet transfusion for an adult will be designed to contain approximately 3×10^{11} platelets suspended in up to 300 ml of plasma or synthetic platelet storage medium. Platelets can be transfused through a normal blood giving set, through most mechanical transfusion pumps, and through needles as fine as 23 gauge. Transfusion can be rapid, and unless the haemodynamic state of the patient precludes it, it should be complete within 30 minutes.

Plasma preparations

Preparations for transfusion are generally provided as fresh frozen plasma, stored plasma, or cryosupernatant. In surgical patients there is little to choose between these three products; stored plasma will have reduced amounts of factors VIII and V, and cryosupernatant plasma will also have reduced amounts of fibrinogen. Plasma is stored below –30°C in bags of 200–300 ml and may take 20–30 minutes to thaw. ABO compatibility is essential.

Essential transfusion immunology

Transfusion immunology is now a complex and specialised field. An understanding of certain aspects is essential to all clinicians involved in using transfusion therapy.

Red cell antigens and antibodies

The ABO system. By far the most important red cell antigens are those of the ABO blood group system. This is because most normal individuals have naturally occurring antibodies to red cell antigens of the ABO system in their plasma. These antibodies can cause rapid intravascular destruction of transfused red cells that are ABO-incompatible, frequently leading to a fatal haemolytic transfusion reaction. Group O patients, since they have antibodies to both A and B cells, are at the greatest risk.

The Rhesus (Rh) system. There are five principal antigens within the Rh system, designated C D E c e. The most important is the Rh D antigen, since this is the most immunogenic and most often associated with clinical problems. For this reason Rh typing is usually restricted to Rh D typing and individuals are designated as Rh D positive or negative.

The reasons for the importance of the Rh system are as follows:

1. Individuals who are Rh D negative can easily be stimulated to produce antibodies to Rh D by transfusion of Rh D positive red cells. These antibodies can produce severe transfusion reactions, which may be fatal.

2. Anti Rh D antibodies in pregnant women cause haemolytic disease in an Rh D positive fetus. It is therefore *essential* to avoid transfusion of Rh D positive blood to Rh D negative women of childbearing age.

3. Patients with anti Rh D antibodies must be transfused with Rh D negative blood. Because of the low incidence of Rh D negative individuals, this can cause serious problems for a blood bank.

Other red cell antigens. There are numerous other red cell antigen systems that can cause transfusion problems. Although these are quantitatively less important than the ABO and Rh systems, they can be involved in serious transfusion reactions. Safe transfusion therefore requires that all patients should be tested for the presence of unexpected antibodies against red cells that may lead to serious transfusion reactions. If a patient is known to have a red cell antibody that may cause a serious transfusion reaction, antigen-negative red cell donations must be found for that individual.

Leucocyte and platelet antigens and antibodies. Leucocytes and platelets also have complex antigen systems and patients can develop antibodies against them. Leucocyte antibodies are a common cause of transfusion reactions, although these are not normally severe. The development of platelet antibodies may make patients clinically resistant to platelet transfusion, which will necessitate the use of serologically compatible platelets.

The investigation and management of these problems require specialized advice and facilities.

THE PROVISION OF COMPATIBLE BLOOD

It cannot be overemphasised that the testing required to supply compatible blood is a specialized task which should be done by trained staff using appropriate techniques, reagents and equipment. The details of the compatibility testing method will depend on local practices and also on the urgency with which blood is required in emergency transfusion. It should very rarely be necessary to transfuse blood without some form of compatibility test. It is justifiable to transfuse uncrossmatched Group O blood, if delaying transfusion until a compatibility test is done will expose the patient to serious risk of exsanguination. Transfusion of uncrossmatched O blood is not without risk. The patient may have clinically significant anti red cell antibodies to other (for example Rhesus) blood group antigens from previous pregnancy or transfusion. However, an alternative to using uncrossmatched Group O blood in an emergency is to determine the patient's ABO and Rh D type and to transfuse blood of the same ABO and Rh D type. This carries the major hazard that any error in typing or in the subsequent identification of the patient can lead to a fatal ABO incompatible transfusion.

Elective transfusions

Compatibility testing
Clinical staff with access to a blood bank do not require detailed knowledge of laboratory procedures but should be aware of certain organisational aspects of the crossmatching laboratory. This will enable them to obtain the safest and most effective service from the blood bank.

Identification procedures
The aim of compatibility testing is to ensure that blood

of the correct type is transfused to the patient. The main cause of serious transfusion accidents is CLERICAL MISTAKES LEADING TO WRONG IDENTIFICATION OF THE PATIENT, BLOOD SAMPLE OR BLOOD TO BE TRANSFUSED. The person who takes a blood sample for compatibility testing must make sure that the sample tube is fully labelled with the patient's full identification, that the request form is fully completed and that the correct blood sample and request form are sent together to the blood bank.

The ward staff who set up a blood transfusion are responsible for checking that the blood which is supplied for a named patient is transfused to the correctly identified patient. The patient's name and blood group must be recorded on a label of each blood unit supplied, and this must be checked with the appropriate information on the patient's identity band.

'Group and antibody screen'
When surgery is planned and blood transfusion is unlikely but possible (probability of transfusion 2.5:1 or less), the patient's ABO and Rh D group can be determined in advance, and the serum screened for anti-red blood cell antibodies. If the patient does need transfusion, blood can be issued from the blood bank within 30 minutes or less with a very high degree of safety. This policy increases the efficiency of blood stock usage without compromising patient safety.

Response time of the blood bank
It is important to know how quickly the blood bank can respond to urgent requests for blood. It is also very important that surgical staff communicate clearly to the blood bank staff when blood is needed urgently. This will allow the blood bank to select the safest form of compatibility testing which can be carried out in the time available. Local arrangements will differ widely and transport delays may be a major factor in compromising the urgent supply of blood.

Information required by the blood bank
The blood bank should be told about any clinical features of the patient that indicate an increased possibility of problems with the transfusion. In particular, knowing that patients have had pregnancies, or have given birth to infants with haemolytic disease, or have had previous transfusions or transfusion reactions will alert the blood bank to look for anti red blood cell antibodies, and may help clarify the meaning of laboratory tests.

Samples required by the blood bank
The blood bank will require a sufficient volume of the patient's blood to carry out compatibility testing. Five

to ten ml of clotted or EDTA blood will be required in an adult. Where pre-existing antibodies are found in the patient's serum, the blood bank will usually require further specimens for complete identification.

AUTOLOGOUS TRANSFUSION

Many patients undergoing surgery can have their transfusion requirements met by the use of the patient's own blood.

Preoperative donation

For procedures where (a) there is a likelihood that blood transfusion will be required and (b) surgery can be reliably scheduled about 5–6 weeks ahead, patients can electively donate units of blood into the hospital blood bank for their own use at surgery. Donations of 2–4 units in the weeks before surgery will reduce the need for subsequent homologous blood transfusions. Careful medical assessment of patients is required to avoid risks of repeat venesections such as hypotensive or thrombotic episodes in the patient/donor population.

Ante normovolaemic haemodilution

Patients undergoing surgery can have a large volume of blood (0.5–1.0 l) drawn into blood bags containing citrate anticoagulant in the anaesthetic room, while circulating volume is maintained by crystalloid infusion (ratio 3 volumes crystalloid to 1 volume blood). This technique can provide 1–2 units of fresh autologous blood (including functional platelets and clotting factors) for transfusion should the need arise without compromising the oxygen delivery to the tissues, provided the post dilution haematocrit is kept in the region of 0.30.

Intraoperative blood salvage

Several techniques exist by which blood shed during surgery can be retrieved and re-infused into the patient. All of these techniques are contraindicated if the operating field is not sterile (for example contaminated by bowel flora), or if the field may be contaminated by malignant cells. In decreasing order of sophistication the available techniques are:

1. Cell washers. These machines require trained personnel. Blood sucked from the operation field or postoperative drain is anticoagulated, washed, filtered and directed into a bag for subsequent or immediate re-infusion into the patient. The machine is in the operating theatre during use.

2. In a modification of the above technique, blood is drawn into special containers from the operation field or drain, and then taken to a central site for washing,

filtering and re-suspension. The processed blood is then returned to the patient.

3. In the simplest method, blood is drawn into an evacuated container, containing citrate anticoagulant. Without any further processing the blood is returned to the patient through a blood filter. For all its apparent lack of sophistication, this appears to be quite an effective and cheap method.

Autologous transfusion techniques used either singly or in combination can greatly reduce the need for stored blood. Where the blood supply is erratic and where adequate biological screening is absent these techniques can be life saving.

Use of autologous blood does not preclude the risk of severe haemolytic transfusion reactions due to failure properly to label the blood at donation or identify the patient at transfusion. In addition bacterial contamination of stored autologous blood may occur, with disastrous consequences.

HAZARDS OF BLOOD TRANSFUSION

The relative risks and benefits of transfusion therapy must be assessed by the clinician in each case before taking the decision to transfuse. The main risks are as follows:

Haemolytic transfusion reactions (Table 2.2)

These reactions occur when there is an incompatibility between donor red cells and preformed antibodies in the recipient plasma. They are usually due to an ABO mismatch, and are almost always due to avoidable human error. Errors in the clinical unit are due either

- to putting the patient's blood sample drawn for compatibility testing into a sample tube on which some other patient's name is written, or more commonly
- to erroneous transfusion of blood that has been issued for one patient, to another patient.

The mortality associated with an ABO incompatible transfusion is approximately 10%. In a severe case the reaction will begin after a very small volume of blood has been transfused and will be characterised by shock, chills, fever, dyspnoea, back pain, pain at the infusion site and headache. This may be followed by disseminated intravascular coagulation with haemoglobinuria, oliguria, renal failure and jaundice. The essential steps in the management of an acute haemolytic transfusion reaction are shown in Table 2.1.

Delayed haemolytic febrile transfusion reactions

IgG antibodies to minor blood groups such as Rhesus, Kell, or Kidd can result in haemolysis of the transfused

Table 2.2 Management of acute haemolytic transfusion reaction

Investigation	Treatment
1. Check all documentation for errors. Return blood to blood bank and request urgent investigation 2. Take blood for Blood bank (10 ml) Blood urea and electrolytes Coagulation tests (10 ml) 3. Do an ECG — look for evidence of hyperkalaemia 4. Repeat biochemical and coagulation screens 2–4 hourly until patient is stable.	1. Stop transfusion immediately 2. Hydrocortisone 100 mg i.v. 3. Insert bladder catheter, drain bladder and monitor urine output 4. Start infusion of physiological saline 5. Frusemide 150 mg i.v. 6. If urine output is still below 100 ml/hour after 3–4 hours start treatment for acute renal failure 7. If evidence of hyperkalaemia start insulin–glucose, or resonium therapy 8. If evidence of disseminated intravascular coagulation seek advice on blood product replacement

unit. This may occur very shortly after transfusion, but more commonly there is an interval of several days after the transfusion. Usually, but not invariably, the patient has been exposed to the blood group antigen in the past by transfusion at pregnancy. Although these reactions are often mild, presenting with a low grade fever, jaundice, and anaemia, they can be associated with serious morbidity and even death.

Febrile reactions

These occur in about 1% of transfusions, and are generally due to sensitisation to leucocyte or platelet antigens by pregnancy or previous transfusion. Since they are clinically indistinguishable from an ABO incompatibility at an early stage, the transfusion must be stopped. An antipyretic, generally paracetamol, should be given. If possible the transfusion should not be restarted until a red cell mismatch has been excluded. Patients with a history of repeated reactions of this type should receive leucocyte-poor red cell or platelet transfusions.

Allergic reactions

Allergic reactions and anaphylactic reactions varying from urticaria to anaphylactic shock may arise. Severe anaphylactic reactions are rare, and sometimes associated with the presence of anti IgA antibodies in IgA deficient individuals. Such severe reactions must be managed by stopping the transfusion and administering adrenalin, hydrocortisone and oxygen. Continued blood transfusion in such patients is extremely hazardous until washed red cells can be provided, and must not be attempted. For milder reactions administration of an antihistamine usually allows resumption of the transfusion, and premedication with antihistamine should prevent recurrence.

Bacterial contamination of blood

This is a rare hazard, but the risk is always present, especially if blood is not stored constantly at 4°C and if blood bags are carelessly handled. A heavily conta-

minated blood donation may appear almost black in colour, although this may be missed; if the red cells and plasma have been allowed to separate there may be a layer of haemolytic staining above the red cell layer. Transfusion will cause a rapid, severe and often fatal collapse due to endotoxic shock. The transfusion must be stopped immediately and intensive therapy for septicaemic shock initiated, with inclusion of high doses of antibiotics active against Gram-positive and Gram-negative organisms.

Fluid overload

In the anaemic, the elderly, the very young, or in patients with cardiopulmonary disease, careful observation is required to avoid this complication. Red cell concentrates should be used in preference to whole blood, and administration of diuretics will often be required.

Transmission of disease

Transfusion of blood and blood components, or infusion of blood products may carry a risk of transmission of viral, bacterial, or protozoal disease. Viruses that can be transmitted include HIV I and II, HTLV I and II, hepatitis A, B and C, cytomegalovirus, Epstein-Barr virus, human parvovirus B19, and very rarely other viruses, including yellow fever.

HIV transmission. Current screening tests, if properly applied, will identify almost all donors who are infectious for HIV. Occasionally individuals will donate blood during the window period, the time between becoming infected with the virus and developing a detectable antibody response. This period is typically about 28 days but may be prolonged. Careful exclusion of donors who have been exposed to known risk behaviour will minimise the risk of this event, but it cannot be totally eliminated. Where there is a high rate of transmission of disease in the population, and where such transmission is occurring within groups considered to be at low risk (for example the unsuspecting partners of individuals who are unaware that they are infected) the risk of viral transmission will be greater. More importantly, where blood donations are drawn from donors who are not wholly motivated by altruism the risk of transfusing a seronegative infected unit is increased.

HTLV I and II. Human T-lymphocytotrophic viruses are transmissible by blood transfusion. These viruses have a latent period of many years. HTLV I can cause adult T-cell leukaemia or spastic parapheresis; the clinical consequences of infection with HTLV II are presently uncertain.

Blood donations are routinely screened for *hepatitis B* and *hepatitis C* infectivity markers. Occasional transmission of these viruses can still occur from marker-negative donations.

Transmission of *cytomegalovirus or Epstein-Barr virus* from transfusions to non-immune individuals can cause an acute transient mononucleosis syndrome. In immunocompromised patients, particularly those undergoing bone marrow transplantation, cytomegalovirus can cause a severe and sometimes fatal infection.

Parvovirus B19 infection causes a mild acute febrile illness, particularly in children. It occurs in outbreaks in the community, spread as a respiratory tract infection. It can also be transmitted by blood transfusion. It is invariably associated with a transient red cell aplasia which usually goes undetected in those with otherwise normal marrow function. In patients with a severe haemoglobinopathy it can precipitate critical exacerbations of anaemia. In patients with symptomatic HIV infections, B19 superinfection can cause a persistent life-threatening marrow suppression. This virus causes particular transfusion-related problems, since it is highly resistant to inactivation by current methods of neutralisation of viruses in blood products prepared from pooled human plasma.

Transmission of virus infection by processed blood products
With the exception of early reports of transmission of hepatitis C from some preparations of IVIgG, immunoglobulin preparations and human albumin preparations have a remarkable record of viral safety. Since the introduction of solvent detergent treatment or terminal heat treatment of the other blood products, transmission of disease-causing viruses, with the exception of B19, is a rare event.

Hepatitis A may rarely be transmitted by blood transfusion when donations are drawn from asymptomatic donors during the viraemic phase. Occasional outbreaks of hepatitis A from coagulation factor concentrates have occurred.

A number of protozoal infections can be transmitted by blood transfusion, including malaria, babesiosis, leishmaniasis, toxoplasmosis, and South American trypanosomiasis.

BLOOD PRODUCTS

Albumin solutions
Stable Purified Protein Solution (SPPS) or Plasma Protein Fraction (PPF) contains 4–5% albumin, 85–90% of the total protein being albumin, with a sodium concentration of 140 mmol/l. These preparations are sterilised and do not transmit virus infections. They have the major disadvantage of high cost. The indications for use of albumin solution are listed below.

Volume replacement in shock or hypovolaemia. Large volumes of crystalloid solutions (Ringer's lactate) have been used successfully to replace massive extra and intravascular fluid losses, but excessive volumes may lead to pulmonary oedema. Initial volume replacement should therefore employ crystalloid solutions (1–2 litres, depending on the size, age and fitness of the patient). Thereafter, a colloid may be used before transfusion of blood. Albumin solutions are satisfactory but costly for this phase of resuscitation and for most patients synthetic volume expanders such as gelatin or hydroxyethyl starch may be used. Initial resuscitation with albumin solutions should be avoided since this may increase pulmonary complications in some groups of patients.

Burns. Albumin solutions may be used to replace the protein loss in burned patients.

Ascites. Albumin solutions may be useful in maintaining the intravascular volume following drainage of ascites.

Hypoproteinaemia. Concentrated (25%) albumin solutions can be used to promote renal function when this is compromised by a decreased intravascular volume and an expanded extravascular space in the presence of hypoalbuminaemia. Albumin solutions should not be used to correct chronic hypoproteinaemic conditions such as liver failure, and are not effective in correcting nutritional hypoproteinaemia, since the amino acids of albumin are poorly metabolized, and the infused albumin increases the catabolism of endogenous albumin.

Fibrin sealant
In some countries preparations of fibrin sealant are available. These consist of a two phase preparation, a fibrinogen concentrate, and a thrombin preparation that clots the fibrinogen when mixed with it. The two solutions are made up separately immediately before use, and are brought into contact with each other using a dual syringe with a single nozzle or an aerosol spray, during direct application to the bleeding site. Fibrin sealant has found a widespread use in almost all surgical specialties. In addition it can induce local haemostasis in patients with acquired or congenital

coagulopathies undergoing surgery or after trauma. There have been no identified adverse effects in man, although animal studies have suggested that fibrin sealant may impair nerve repair.

Clotting factor concentrates
Currently available clotting factor concentrates do not carry a significant risk of transmission of viral disease. They are generally used under the supervision of haematologists, for patients with established isolated clotting factor defects. Patients with coagulopathies associated with liver disease or warfarin therapy can be treated with concentrates of factors II, IX and X, and factor VII, as discussed above.

Immunoglobulin preparations made from pooled normal human plasma
Immunoglobulin preparation made from pools of normal donor plasma are available for intravenous (IVIgG) or intramuscular (Human Normal Immunoglobulin) use.

IVIgG is used in physiological doses to treat hypogammoglobulinaemia or in pharmacological doses (high dose IVIgG) for autoimmune (idiopathic) thrombocytopenic purpura. The indications for the use of high dose IVIgG are being extended to other autoimmune and immune conditions. Among these are Guillain-Barré syndrome, myasthenia gravis, autoimmune haemolytic anaemia, and other forms of immune thrombocytopenia.

Normal human immunoglobulin can be used in conjunction with hepatitis A vaccine following exposure to hepatitis A in non-immune individuals.

Specific immunoglobulin preparations, prepared from donors with high titres of the relevant antibody in their serum, are available for a number of conditions.

Human anti-D immunoglobulin for prophylaxis of rhesus haemolytic disease of the newborn.

Human tetanus immunoglobulin for tetanus prophylaxis in conjunction with adequate wound toilet and tetanus vaccine in patients with a significant degree of devitalized tissue, a puncture type wound, or contact with soil or manure likely to harbour tetanus organisms in a wound.

Human varicella zoster immunoglobulin for the prophylaxis of non-immune individuals exposed to varicella zoster in whom there is an increased risk of serious complications of a varicella zoster infection. These patients include: patients receiving corticosteroid or immunosuppressive treatment, patients suffering from malignant conditions such as lymphoma or leukaemia or with congenital or primary immune deficiency, premature infants whose mother lacks a prior history of varicella, premature infants born before 28 weeks gestation or with birth weight of less than 1000 g, regardless of maternal history of varicella, newborn babies of mothers who develop varicella within five days before birth or up to 48 hours after delivery, pregnant contacts of varicella.

THROMBOSIS PREVENTION

Thrombosis in the deep veins of the calf (DVT) occurs in over 20% of general surgical patients unless prophylaxis is used on a regular basis. The risks increase with age and duration of the operation but patients most at risk are those over 40 years of age, obese patients and those with malignant disease. For prophylaxis, anti-embolism (graduated compression) stockings can be used on all patients and are free from side effects; subcutaneous low dose heparin is more effective but must be given selectively and can lead to troublesome haemorrhage. A combination of heparin and stockings should be used for high risk patients — especially those who have had a previous DVT. *Intermittent pneumatic compression* of the legs during operation gives protection for patients less at risk and may be used along with anti-embolism stockings. Alternatively, the heels may be raised on a sponge rubber pad during surgery (Fig. 20.7) to avoid pressure on the calf muscles. After all operations, early mobilization encourages the return of normal leg circulation and helps in the full recovery of the patient.

REFERENCES

Forrest A P M, Carter D C, Macleod I B 1985 Principles and practice of surgery. Churchill Livingstone, Edinburgh, Ch 10

Humberstone D A, Hill G L 1992 Fluids, nutrition and transfusion. In: Kyle J, Smith J A R, Johnston D H (eds),

Pye's Surgical Handicraft, 22nd edn Butterworth-Heinemann Ltd, Oxford

le Quesne L P 1967 Fluid and electrolyte balance. British Journal of Surgery 54: 449–452

FURTHER READING

American association of blood banks technical manual 1990, 13th edn. American Association of Blood Banks, Washington DC, USA (This manual describes the full range of technical procedures)

Fleck A, Ledington I McA 1988 Fluid and electrolyte balance. In: Ledingham I McA, MacKay C (eds) Jamieson and Kay's Textbook of surgical physiology, 4th edn. Churchill Livingstone, Edinburgh, Ch 3

Mollison P L 1992 Blood transfusion in clinical medicine, 9th edn. Blackwell, London (A comprehensive text dealing with the theoretical basis of transfusion)

Handbook of Transfusion Medicine 1990 HMSO, London

World Health Organization (1989) Essential blood components, plasma derivatives and substitutes. Global Blood Safety Initiative Consultation on Developing and Strengthening Blood Transfusion Services, World Health Organization, Geneva

World Health Organization (1989) Use of plasma substitutes and plasma in developing countries. Global Blood Safety Initiative Consultation on Developing and Strengthening Blood Transfusion Services, World Health Organization, Geneva

World Health Organization (1989) Essential consumables and equipment for a blood transfusion service. Global Blood Safety Initiative Consultation on Developing and Strengthening Blood Transfusion Services, World Health Organization, Geneva

3

Vascular surgery

C. V. RUCKLEY

Anatomy

An artery consists of three coats. The outer coat or *tunica adventitia* is composed of fibrous and elastic tissue, and contains the periarterial sympathetic nerves; it is attached only loosely to the middle coat, and can be stripped from it without difficulty. The middle coat or *tunica media* constitutes the main thickness of the arterial wall; it is composed of smooth muscle with a proportion of elastic tissue, this proportion being greater in the large vessels. The inner coat or *tunica intima* lines the lumen of the vessel. It consists of a layer of endothelial cells, supported on a basement membrane of elastic tissue.

When an artery is completely divided, its cut ends contract and retract, as the result of spasm of the muscular coat. In this way spontaneous arrest of haemorrhage may be brought about. The tunica adventitia, which has less power of contraction, and which may also be loosely attached to surrounding tissues, remains projecting beyond the other coats at the cut ends, and requires to be trimmed away before end-to-end repair of the vessel can be effected.

A vein has a structure very similar to that of an artery, except that all coats, especially the tunica media, are much thinner. The bicuspid valves, although little more than a single cell layer in thickness, are able to withstand gravitational pressures in excess of 100 mmHg but may be rendered incompetent if the vein becomes dilated or involved in thrombus. Valves are absent from the inferior vena cava, the pulmonary veins and the portal system.

The concept of *collateral circulation*, important in all areas of surgery, is particularly relevant to vascular operations. The surgeon should be constantly aware of the alternative channels by which blood can bypass vessels obliterated by disease, by trauma or by the surgeon. Branches which can provide collateral circulation should, if possible, be preserved during dissection.

BASIC TECHNIQUES IN ARTERIAL SURGERY

The exposure of specific arteries is dealt with in later sections; there are however certain principles common to all vascular operations, attention to which should enable the inexperienced surgeon to avoid serious trouble.

The dissection and control of arteries

When exposing an artery it is important to mobilize enough of the vessel and its branches to ensure complete proximal and distal control. The inexperienced surgeon is advised to place slings of plastic, umbilical tape or stout ligature material around a vessel to aid dissection and give control of a vessel which has been opened. However vascular surgeons often dispense with slings in order to simplify and expedite the operation. Once an artery has been exposed the best plane of dissection for mobilization and control is deep to the adventitia. This does not apply to veins. Vessels should always be handled gently, since trauma to the wall commonly leads to thrombosis, and in particular they should never be grasped or clamped with an instrument likely to cause damage. Remember that the soft elastic intima can easily be split without visible damage to the adventitia. Any clamp should be applied with the minimal compression required to control flow.

Modern vascular clamps have relatively atraumatic jaws. Particularly good in this respect is the Fogarty hydragrip clamp with its compressible disposable plastic inserts which clip into the jaws of the instrument (Fig. 3.1A). There is no clamp that will avoid causing damage if it is applied to a heavily calcified vessel, in which case a soft area of wall should be sought before a clamp is applied or a sling drawn tight. If vascular clamps are not available in the emergency situation, a serviceable substitute can be made by sheathing a non crushing gastro-intestinal clamp with cloth or rubber tube. Better still a sling of tape or fine silastic tube can be passed through a length of stiff plastic tube to act as a 'snub' as shown in Figure 3.1E. A small branch is readily controlled by a ligature passed twice round it.

As a general rule, and particularly in the case of aneurysms, the distal clamps should be applied before the proximal ones and before the vessels are mobilized in order to minimize distal embolism.

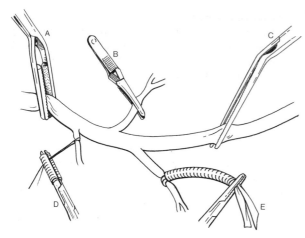

Fig. 3.1 Methods of controlling blood vessels. (A) Fogarty soft jaw clamp. (B) Bulldog clamp. (C) Atraumatic metal jawed vascular clamp. (D) Double ligature sling. (E) Sling with snub

Haemorrhage

Bleeding can usually be controlled by direct compression at the bleeding point while the vessel is exposed and controlled above and below. Where this is not practicable, as in the case for example of ruptured aortic aneurysm, the aorta can be compressed by the assistant above the neck of the aneurysm while the neck is identified and clamped. If there is difficulty finding the neck or if there is serious bleeding a quick method is for the aneurysm to be opened and the surgeon's index finger inserted into the neck of the sac to give immediate control of bleeding and provide a guide to the positioning of a clamp. An alternative method of controlling aortic bleeding from within is by means of a Foley catheter, while Fogarty catheters (p. 55) can be used for the same purpose in smaller arteries.

Arteriotomy (incision into an artery)

This should, as a general rule, be made longitudinally, allowing one to see a greater area of the inside of the vessel; it can readily be extended and it gives access to the orifices of branches, advantages which outweigh the only benefit of a transverse incision which is that it can be closed with less tendency to narrow the lumen. However, in vessels of 4 mm or less, especially if made simply for the purpose of embolectomy, a transverse incision may be preferable and unlike an arteriotomy in a large vessel it should be closed with interrupted sutures. A longitudinal incision in an artery smaller in diameter than the common femoral generally requires to be closed with a small patch of vein, taken usually from the long saphenous.

Suturing and suture materials

Nonabsorbable sutures must be used for arteries, although absorbable monofilament sutures are being tried in vein reconstruction. Teflon coated braided dacron is a satisfactory material but the best, especially for small vessels is soft, pliant, monofilament polypropylene. A useful standard size of suture for femoral and popliteal arteries and others of equivalent size is 5/0. Finer sutures are used for smaller vessels while as large as 2/0 may be used on the aorta.

Needles should be round bodied or, in the case of dense graft material or heavily diseased arterial wall, tapercut. During closure special care must be taken to include the intima every stitch (unless of course an endarterectomy has been performed) since the dissection of an intimal flap is probably the commonest cause of early thrombosis after reconstruction. When closing an arteriotomy a continuous suture is used, seeking to obtain slight eversion of the cut edges. As one approaches the end of the closure it may be difficult to see the end of the arteriotomy and to ensure that all layers are included in the stitch. It is therefore advised that a separate end stitch should be placed at the opposite end of the incision, as shown in Figure 3.2. Accurate suturing is more important in vascular surgery than in most other areas. When dealing with medium to small vessels (as distinct from microvascular surgery) the use of magnification ($\times$ 2–4) by means of a loop, or spectacles fitted with binocular lenses, is often advisable.

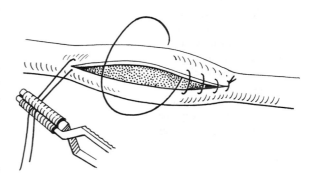

Fig. 3.2 Closure of arteriotomy

Vascular anastomoses

There are many different techniques for joining blood vessels to each other or to synthetic grafts. In constructing an end-to-end anastomosis care must be taken to avoid narrowing the lumen and it is always preferable, especially when dealing with small vessels, to bevel the ends as shown in Figure 3.11. It is usually more convenient to use continuous sutures but interrupted sutures may be preferred when dealing with an unusually difficult part of an anastomosis especially if the artery is friable or when joining vessels of very small diameter.

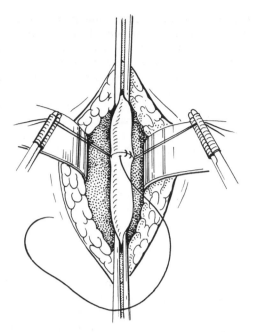

Fig. 3.3 Standard end to end anastomosis. Note the stay sutures and the continuous suture which slightly everts the edges

Broadly, there are two techniques for either end-to-end or end-to-side anastomosis. The first is to place anchoring sutures at the beginning as shown in Figure 3.3. This has the advantage of stabilizing the vessels and grafts, but may limit access. The second is to take advantage of the remarkable frictionless qualities of the newer polypropylene monofilament suture materials to use a 'parachute' or 'purse-string' method. With the cut ends some distance apart a posterior row of continuous sutures is placed and then drawn tight, purse-string fashion, to approximate the vessels (Fig. 3.11). The anterior layer is then easily completed. A similar principle can be applied to end-to-side anastomosis (Fig. 3.13).

EXPOSURE OF THE MAIN VESSELS OF THE NECK AND LIMBS

The commonest indication for exposure of a main artery is elective reconstruction for chronic obliterative disease.

Emergency exploration may be undertaken in acute occlusion or when arterial injury is suspected. Reconstruction is less frequently attempted in veins owing to the liability to thrombosis but may be needed in a case of severe trauma to ensure limb survival or avoid severe swelling. Venous thrombectomy is rarely performed. Venous interruption by means of filter has moved into the province of the radiologist.

The carotid arteries

Endarterectomy for the prevention of stroke is perhaps the most frequent vascular operation in the neck. Others include excision of carotid body tumour and exploration in cases of trauma.

Anatomy

The common carotid artery begins its course in the neck behind the sternoclavicular joint. Thence it passes upwards in a line towards the lobe of the ear, but ends opposite the upper border of the thyroid cartilage by dividing into external and internal carotid arteries. It is enclosed along with the internal jugular vein and the vagus nerve in the carotid sheath of deep cervical fascia; the vein is lateral to it, and the nerve lies in the groove behind the two vessels.

Superficial relations. These are sternomastoid, sternohyoid, sternothyroid and omohyoid — this last muscle crossing it obliquely at the level of the cricoid cartilage; at this level also, the ansa hypoglossi and the superior and middle thyroid veins lie in front of the artery. It is overlapped to a variable extent by the lobe of the thyroid gland.

The external carotid artery

This begins at the bifurcation of the common carotid artery, at the upper border of the thyroid cartilage, and runs upwards to end behind the neck of the mandible, by dividing into maxillary and superficial temporal arteries. It leaves the carotid triangle by passing under cover of the posterior belly of the digastric, and its upper part occupies a groove on the deep surface of the parotid gland.

The internal carotid artery

This begins at the bifurcation of the common carotid artery, and ascends to enter the skull through the carotid canal, which lies opposite the lower border of the external auditory meatus. It is at first posterolateral to the external carotid artery, and then deep to it. It is enclosed in the carotid sheath, with the internal jugular vein posterolaterally, and with the vagus nerve deep to the interval between them. Sternomastoid overlaps it laterally. *It has no branches in the neck.*

Superficial relations. These, in the carotid triangle, are the cervical branch of the facial nerve, the hypoglossal nerve, and the common facial and lingual veins, as these pass backwards to join the jugular.

Exposure

For exposure of the carotid arteries the head is turned to the opposite side and slightly extended. A sand bag is placed between the shoulder blades. The ideal incision from the cosmetic point of view is placed in the skin crease, and there are few neck operations for which

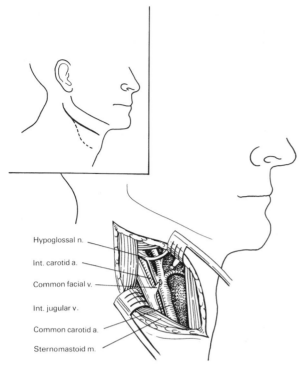

Hypoglossal n.
Int. carotid a.
Common facial v.
Int. jugular v.
Common carotid a.
Sternomastoid m.

Fig. 3.4 Exposure of the great vessels on the right side of the neck

adequate exposure cannot be thus obtained, but if greater longitudinal exposure is required the middle part of the incision may run parallel to the anterior border of sterno-mastoid (Fig. 3.4). In order to avoid damage to the cervical branch of the facial nerve the upper end of the incision should not approach nearer than 1.5 cm to the angle of the mandible. Platysma and deep fascia are divided in the line of the incision and the flaps are dissected a little way upwards and downwards. The anterior border of sternomastoid is freed and the muscle retracted posteriorly. The common facial vein crosses the field and if it is large is transfixed before it is divided between ligatures. The internal jugular vein is displaced backwards to expose the carotid arteries. The descendens hypoglossi nerve on the anterior surface of the carotid sheath can be divided without detriment. Fluctuations in blood pressure due to disturbance of baroreceptors can be avoided by infiltration of the tissues in the carotid bifurcation with 0.5 mls of 1% Xylocaine. In the case of carotid endarterectomy there is a danger that mobilization of the arteries will release thrombus into the cerebral circulation. Extreme gentleness should therefore be used in dissection.

Care must be taken to avoid damaging the hypoglossal nerve, which can be mobilized by division and ligation of the small vessels which tether it posteriorly

before it crosses the carotid arteries. To extend the access superiorly the posterior belly of the digastric can be divided. Further measures to give access to the carotid artery at the base of the skull include pernasal endotracheal intubation, fracture of the styloid process and anterior subluxation of the temporo-mandibular joint. Care must also be taken to avoid damage to the vagus nerve and the internal jugular vein which can be retracted gently on slings.

The exposure of the common carotid artery and internal jugular vein in the lower part of the neck is essentially similar. A skin crease incision is made at the level of the cricoid cartilage. The carotid sheath is exposed above the omohyoid which can be retracted downwards. The internal jugular vein, the descendens hypoglossi and the vagus nerves should be identified and separated before any attempt is made to pass a sling round the artery.

Subclavian and axillary arteries

Exposure may be necessary for the arrest of haemorrhage, the treatment of aneurysms (generally associated with a cervical rib) or for atheromatous occlusion.

Anatomy

The subclavian artery crosses the front of the cervical pleura at the root of the neck. It arches from the sterno-clavicular joint to the outer border of the first rib, where it becomes the axillary artery. It rises to a level 1–2 cm above the clavicle, when the shoulder is depressed. Scalenus anterior crosses the artery, dividing it into three parts. The subclavian vein lies in front of scalenus anterior, at a lower level than the artery, and behind the clavicle.

Superficial relations of third part. Skin; superficial fascia; platysma; supraclavicular nerves; deep fascia; external jugular vein and its tributaries (transverse cervical, suprascapular and anterior jugular veins); suprascapular artery; nerve to subclavius.

The axillary artery runs downwards and laterally behind the clavicle to become the brachial artery. Its second part lies deep to the pectoralis minor with the axillary vein just below and medial to it throughout its course.

Superficial relations of axillary artery. These, encountered after fascial layers, are pectoral muscles and nerves; acromiothoracic vessels; termination of cephalic vein.

Exposure (Fig. 3.5)

The third part of the subclavian artery is the most accessible and may be exposed in the first instance. The arm is placed at the side and is drawn downwards in order to depress the shoulder; the head is turned to the opposite side. An incision is made 1–2 cm above the clavicle

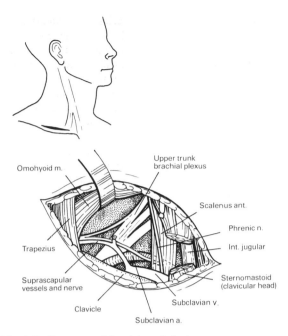

Fig. 3.5 Exposure of the right subclavian artery

exposed, with the scalenus anterior muscle medially, and with the upper and middle trunks of the brachial plexus to its lateral side. The transverse cervical artery, lying under cover of omohyoid, and the suprascapular artery, crossing the subclavian, are preserved.

Exposure of the *second and third parts* of the subclavian artery and the *axillary artery* is normally required for aneurysms and atheromatous occlusion. The upper limb is abducted and is supported on an arm board or on a small table (Fig. 3.6). A long incision is made, beginning at the anterior edge of the sternomastoid and continuing in the line of the vessels to the anterior axillary fold. The first stage of the dissection has already been described. Division of the sternomastoid and scalenus muscles, with care to avoid damage to the phrenic nerve, brings the second part of the subclavian artery into view. If necessary the middle third of the clavicle may be resected and pectoral muscles divided in the line of the incision to complete the exposure of the arteries.

The root of the neck is a hazardous area for the inexperienced surgeon. The subclavian artery is relatively thin walled and bleeding from it or one of the great veins is very difficult to control. In emergency situations to gain rapid control of the third part of the subclavian and the first part of the axillary artery there should be no hesitation in resecting the middle third of the clavicle. To gain control of the proximal subclavian or the brachiocephalic trunk a sternal split is necessary.

from sternal head of sternomastoid to anterior border of trapezius. Superficial fascia and platysma are incised in the same line and the deep fascia is divided. The external jugular vein may cross the field and have to be divided between ligatures. Omohyoid is retracted upwards, and the third part of the subclavian artery is now

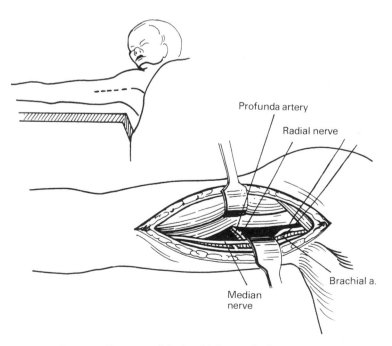

Fig. 3.6 Exposure of the brachial artery in the upper arm

Brachial artery

The brachial artery may be exposed easily anywhere in its course. Exploration is most likely to be required for embolism or iatrogenic trauma inflicted in the course of cardiological investigations. Exposure may also be necessary to investigate possible damage associated with fractures of the humerus.

Anatomy

The brachial artery begins as a continuation of the axillary artery at the level of the lower border of teres major. It runs downwards and slightly laterally, at first medial to the humerus and then in front of it. It ends in the cubital fossa, at the level of the neck of the radius, by dividing into radial and ulnar arteries. The artery is accompanied by venae comites in its lower part and by the basilic vein in the upper part.

Relations in the upper arm. The artery lies successively on the long and medial heads of triceps, the insertion of coracobrachialis, and brachialis. The biceps overlaps it on the lateral side. The median nerve, at first lateral, crosses in front of the artery in its middle third, and then runs along its medial side. The ulnar nerve is on the medial side of the artery in its upper half but diverges from its lower half. The medial cutaneous nerve of the forearm also lies to its medial side in the upper half of the arm.

Relations at the bend of the elbow. The brachial artery enters the cubital fossa, with the tendon of biceps on its lateral side, and the median nerve on its medial side. These structures lie on the brachialis muscle, which forms the upper part of the floor of the fossa. They are roofed over by deep fascia containing the bicipital aponeurosis, which stretches from the tendon of biceps to blend with the fascia over the medial side of the forearm. The superficial fascia overlying the fossa contains the median cubital and other veins.

Branches. The branches of the artery are the profunda, which arises near its commencement and accompanies the radial nerve spirally round the humerus; the ulnar collateral artery, which arises in the middle of the arm, and accompanies the ulnar nerve to the back of the medial epicondyle; the supratrochlear artery, which arises just above the elbow and runs also to the medial epicondyle.

Exposure in the upper arm

The upper limb is abducted and rotated laterally and is supported with the forearm resting on a small table (Fig. 3.6). The upper arm should be entirely free; if it is supported in any way, displacement of the muscles will render the approach more difficult. An incision is made along the medial edge of the biceps, and the deep fascia is divided in the same line. Care is taken to avoid the basilic vein which pierces the deep fascia in this situa-

tion. The biceps is mobilized and drawn laterally to expose the artery with its venae comites and the median nerve in close relationship (see anatomical description above).

Exposure at the bend of the elbow

The arm is abducted and supported on a table in the position of lateral rotation. An incision is made in the antecubital region along the medial border of the biceps tendon. The deep fascia, including the bicipital aponeurosis, is incised vertically, and the biceps tendon is retracted to the lateral side to display the contents of the fossa. (This is accomplished more easily if the elbow is flexed slightly to allow relaxation of the muscle.) The brachial artery lies in the centre of the fossa, between the tendon of biceps and the median nerve (Fig. 3.7).

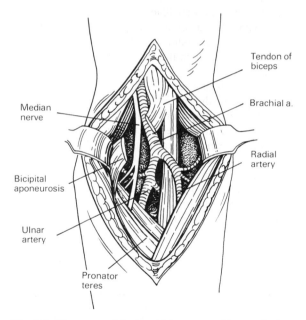

Fig. 3.7 Exposure of the brachial artery and its terminal branches in the cubital fossa (for the sake of clarity the veins have been omitted)

Iliac arteries

Exposure of the three iliac arteries is most often required for atheromatous occlusion. Temporary or permanent control of the external iliac may be required for high wounds of the femoral artery or septic wounds in the upper thigh, and ligature of the internal iliac artery may be indicated for secondary haemorrhage after hysterectomy.

Anatomy

The external iliac artery begins at the pelvic brim as a terminal branch of the common iliac artery, and runs downwards to pass deep to the midinguinal point, where it becomes the femoral artery.

Relations in the inguinal region. The artery lies on psoas, with its vein to the medial side. The femoral nerve is 1–2 cm lateral, with the small genitofemoral nerve in between. Anteriorly, it is in contact with the peritoneum; below the peritoneal reflection it is related to the muscles of the abdominal wall immediately above the inguinal ligament–transversus, internal oblique, and external oblique from within outwards.

Branches. These branches are the inferior epigastric which runs upwards into the rectus sheath, and the deep circumflex iliac which courses laterally along the back of the inguinal ligament.

Exposure

Exposure by the extraperitoneal route is the method of choice where the lesion is unilateral. The common, external and internal iliac arteries can be exposed in their whole length by an oblique muscle cutting incision in the lower abdomen, displacing the peritoneum and its contents forwards and medially out of the iliac fossa.

For extraperitoneal exposure of the external iliac artery alone, the patient is placed in a moderate Trendelenburg position and an incision is made 1–2 cm above and parallel to the middle of the inguinal ligament. The inguinal canal is opened and the muscular fibres of internal oblique are divided just above the inguinal ligament. Transversalis fascia is incised and the spermatic cord is retracted medially and upwards. The inferior epigastric artery should, if possible, be preserved as the peritoneum is gently raised to display the external iliac artery and vein (Fig. 3.8).

Intraperitoneal exposure

This is required where the lesion is bilateral or involves the bifurcation of the aorta. The small intestine is packed off within the peritoneal cavity or, if that is not possible, it is wrapped in moist towels or exenterated into a polythene bag over the right side of the wound. The aorta and right iliac vessels are exposed by division of the overlying peritoneum followed by blunt dissection. The right ureter must be seen and mobilized out of the way. The left iliac arteries are exposed by dividing the peritoneum lateral to the pelvic mesocolon.

Femoral artery

The common femoral artery is most frequently exposed during embolectomy or reconstruction. Wounds of the femoral artery are among the most common vascular lesions encountered. Exposure of the artery, in order that its condition may be investigated, is an integral part of the exploration of most penetrating wounds of the thigh.

Anatomy

The femoral artery, beginning as a continuation of the external iliac at the midinguinal point, runs obliquely downwards through the femoral triangle and subsartorial canal. Surgeons refer to the proximal portion, above the origin of the profunda, as the common femoral and the distal as the superficial femoral artery. It ends at the junction of the middle and lower thirds of the thigh by passing through the opening in adductor magnus, to become the popliteal artery. Its position is indicated by the upper two-thirds of a line drawn from the midinguinal point to the adductor tubercle, the thigh being slightly flexed and rotated laterally.

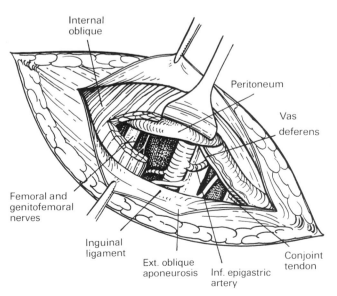

Fig. 3.8 Extraperitoneal exposure of the external iliac vessels at the groin

Relations in the femoral triangle. The femoral vein is on its medial side; the femoral nerve is 1–2 cm lateral. Four small branches arise near its origin — the superficial epigastric, the superficial circumflex iliac, and the superficial and deep external pudendal. The profunda femoris artery arises from the lateral side of the femoral artery 3–4 cm below the inguinal ligament; it runs medially behind the femoral artery to disappear between the adductor muscles.

Relations in subsartorial canal. The canal is formed by adductor longus and magnus posteriorly, vastus medialis anterolaterally, and the fibrous roof and sartorius anteromedially. Within the canal the femoral vein is posterolateral, the saphenous nerve is anteromedial, and the nerve to vastus medialis is lateral.

Exposure in the upper two-thirds of the thigh

An incision is made in the line of the artery. The long saphenous vein, lying in the superficial fascia, is preserved, in case it may be required for reconstruction. The deep fascia is incised, and the sartorius muscle is mobilized. To expose the upper part of the femoral vessels, and the profunda vessels, sartorius is retracted laterally. To expose the femoral vessels in their lower part, sartorius is retracted medially and the underlying bridge of fibrous tissue which roofs over the subsartorial canal is divided. In this way the femoral vessels may be exposed in their entire length.

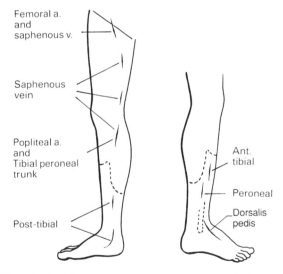

Fig. 3.9 Incisions for arterial reconstructions in the leg. Note that the incisions avoid potential flaps for amputation

Exposure at the femoropopliteal junction

The limb is flexed slightly at hip and knee joints, and is rotated laterally. The operator may find it more convenient to stand at the opposite side of the table, so that he faces the field of operation. An incision is made extending upwards from the adductor tubercle for 20 cm in the line of the artery and downwards along the posterior border of the tibia for 10 cm. The long saphenous vein is identified and held aside. The sartorius is mobilized and retracted backwards. The underlying fascia is divided in the line of the incision, to open up the subsartorial canal. The femoral vessels are now exposed, the vein lying posterolateral to the artery. The saphenous nerve and a branch of the artery, the descending genicular, are seen and preserved. The proximal part of the popliteal artery may be exposed by retracting or dividing the tendon of adductor magnus. The popliteal fascia is then incised and dissection is carried out through the popliteal fat, keeping close to the popliteal surface of the femur so as to avoid disturbing the popliteal vein. To expose the artery distally, the origin of the medial head of gastrocnemius is divided and retracted backwards.

Popliteal artery

Exposure of this artery may be indicated as part of an arterial reconstruction, an exploratory operation in wounds of the popliteal fossa, or for the treatment of aneurysms.

Anatomy

The popliteal artery begins as the continuation of the femoral at the opening in adductor magnus. It runs downwards in the popliteal fossa to end at the lower border of popliteus by dividing into anterior tibial and the tibial-peroneal trunk which in turn divides into posterior tibial and peroneal branches. It gives off small branches to the knee joint and to the surrounding muscles.

Relations. The popliteal vein is medial to the artery in its lower part, but crosses it posteriorly to lie posterolateral to it in its upper part. The medial popliteal nerve crosses the vessels posteriorly from lateral side above to medial side below.

Exposure

The popliteal artery can be approached through a longitudinal posterior incision directly over the line of the vessel, with the patient lying prone. An alternative approach to the distal popliteal and the tibial peroneal trunk is a lateral one with excision of the upper end of the fibula. The best approach however in the majority of cases is through a medial incision which, as well as giving access to the popliteal artery and tibial peroneal trunk, also facilitates removal of the saphenous vein which is commonly required for reconstruction or repair.

With the patient supine, the thigh is externally rotated and the knee is flexed 30 to 60°. A longitudinal

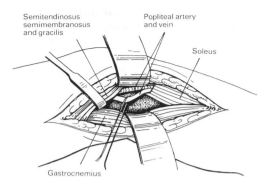

Fig. 3.10 Medial approach to the lower popliteal artery

incision is made beginning 1 cm posterior to the medial condyle and carried down parallel to and 1 cm behind the posteromedial border of the tibia (Fig. 3.10). Care must be taken to avoid damage to the saphenous vein which is close to the skin at this level. The crural fascia is divided to expose the tendons of semitendinosus, gracilis and semimembranosus. These may be retracted anteriorly, or divided to give access to the popliteal space. The medial head of gastrocnemius is retracted and the fat gently separated to expose the neurovascular bundle covered with a thick layer of fascia which is incised longitudinally. The popliteal vein is retracted posteriorly and must be separated with great care since venous bleeding in the popliteal fossa can be difficult to control and damage to the vein is likely to lead to thrombosis. The artery is then separated from the tibial nerve and encircled with a sling. For exposure of the origins of the tibial arteries the anterior tibial vein which crosses the artery must be divided and the soleus muscle incised at its origin from the posterior surface of the tibia.

Distal reconstruction
If the popliteal artery is obstructed it may be feasible to take a vein or synthetic graft down to a tibial or peroneal artery in mid or lower calf or at the ankle. If this is to be successful there should be an intact arterial arch in the foot and micro-surgical techniques should be employed. Although they are deeply placed and difficult to expose in mid calf, the tibial and peroneal vessels at the ankle are easily accessible. Appropriate incisions are illustrated in Figure 3.9.

WOUNDS OF BLOOD VESSELS

Control of bleeding
As a first aid measure profuse bleeding from a limb should be controlled by elevation, pressure pad and bandage rather than by tourniquet, a potentially

dangerous implement. No attempt should be made to apply artery forceps within a wound that is bleeding profusely since it is impossible to identify the damaged vessel with any accuracy, and there is a serious risk of injuring neighbouring structures.

The patient should be prepared for a definitive operation, carried out with adequate lighting and with all necessary facilities. If the bleeding has been temporarily arrested by packing or by local pressure, it may be possible, after gently removing the dressings, to explore the wound in a relatively bloodless field. If, however, there is still profuse bleeding it should be controlled by local pressure while the main artery is exposed at a proximal level, where it can be clamped or temporarily ligated.

Permanent ligature
In the case of the larger vessels of the limb — axillary, brachial, common femoral and popliteal, permanent ligature should be avoided if possible, because of the risks of subsequent ischaemia, if not of actual gangrene. (The subclavian and superficial femoral arteries constitute exceptions to this general rule. Because of abundant collateral circulations, they can usually be ligated with safety when necessary).

Reconstruction is usually possible and reversed saphenous vein is preferred to synthetic materials, especially if there is wound contamination. Where there is associated bone damage fractures should, if possible, be stabilized prior to reconstruction of the vessels (the two being done at the same operation); but if this means delay, temporary cannulae can be used to connect the vessels and maintain viability of the limb until definitive reconstruction is performed. The smaller arteries — i.e. those below the elbow and knee — normally have an adequate collateral circulation, so that reconstructive measures, which are very difficult because of the small size of the vessel, do not usually require to be considered. If both vessels of the forearm or lower leg are injured, an attempt should be made to reconstruct the larger.

Arterial haematoma
This may occur in cases of arterial injury where the extravasated blood cannot escape to the surface — either because there is no external wound, or because the external wound is too small. The resulting haematoma may be either circumscribed or diffuse, depending upon the resistance offered by the tissues. If the vessel wound is small it may become sealed off and the haematoma gradually absorbed. A large haematoma, by exerting pressure on the smaller vessels, may cause obstruction to the collateral circulation. When the haematoma is not absorbed its outer layers become organized, and the central part forms a cavity constantly

distended by the circulating blood; it shows expansile pulsation, and may now be described as a *traumatic arterial aneurysm* or false aneurysm.

Ultrasonography can be used to verify the patent connection with the artery. Furthermore local pressure with the ultrasound probe for 15 to 30 minutes over the leaking point can often induce thrombosis in the aneurysm and therefore avoid the necessity for operation. If ultrasound is not available or fails to close the leak, surgery will have to be considered especially if the haematoma is increasing in size, or if the circulation of the limb is embarrassed. If the surgeon is inexperienced in vascular surgery it may be necessary to expose and clamp the main vessel at a proximal level. The haematoma is then explored. Clots are removed, so that the bleeding point can be identified. If necessary, the proximal clamp can be cautiously released after the vessel has been exposed.

In the case of arteries at or above the elbow or knee, an attempt should usually be made to reconstruct the damaged vessel. If the operator lacks the necessary experience or facilities, he may have to be content with simple ligation, as close to the injury as possible. Although this entails some risk of ischaemia of the limb, such risks will have been lessened if the operation has been successful in arresting the bleeding, and in evacuating the haematoma which may have been embarrassing the collateral circulation. Vessels below the elbow or knee can usually be ligated with impunity although many surgeons believe that these too should be repaired wherever possible.

When there is no obvious increase in the size of the haematoma, and when the circulation of the limb remains satisfactory, it is best to postpone operation to permit the transfer of the patient to a centre where vascular surgery is undertaken.

A contracted and empty artery

This may result from the pressure of bone fragments after fracture, from crushing injuries without fracture, or from the disruptive force of a high velocity missile traversing the tissues in close proximity.

It was formerly believed that the condition of the vessel was due to a state of spasm, which involved also the distal ramifications of the artery, and, by reflex action, vessels forming the collateral circulation. It is now thought that simple contusion of the artery is the most important factor; this leads to rupture of the intima, localized contusion of the media, thrombosis and occlusion. Spasm may play a part in producing ischaemia, especially in the smaller vessels, but it should never be assumed to be solely responsible if signs of circulatory deficiency persist in the distal part of the limb for more than 2 to 3 hours after the injury. Failure to explore the artery and relieve underlying damage within 6 hours of

the onset may result in permanent ischaemic muscle damage.

Operation
This is the only effective treatment, and, in the absence of spontaneous recovery, should not be delayed. Arteriography is not required unless there is difficulty in deducing, from the site of the injury or fracture site on X-ray, where the artery has been damaged. The vessel is exposed and the incision enlarged until a normally pulsating length of vessel is seen above the pulseless segment. If there is doubt as to what part spasm may be playing this segment may then be covered with a warm 2% solution of papaverine sulphate (a smooth muscle relaxant) and left for a few minutes. Alternatively, an attempt may be made to inject the solution directly into the lumen of the artery, this method being used also to test the patency of the vessel. The damaged segment is the proximal end of the contracted part of the artery. It should be excised and a reconstruction performed.

TECHNIQUES IN ARTERIAL REPAIR

Damaged major arteries should be repaired wherever it is anatomically possible. When direct repair is impracticable, reconstruction by means of autogenous vein graft or a plastic prosthesis is advised. Even if the artery becomes occluded later, it may remain open long enough to ensure wound healing and a viable limb.

The successful repair of vascular injuries demands a meticulous technique, which includes gentleness in handling, absolute asepsis and scrupulous care in the placing of sutures.

Before any attempt is made to repair a damaged artery, attention must be paid to the toilet of the wound in the soft parts, and all bruised and devitalized tissue should be excised. The damaged vessel is exposed and is mobilized sufficiently to allow temporary ligatures or arterial clamps to be applied above and below the site of injury. Any unstable fracture is dealt with by some form of internal fixation prior to arterial reconstruction. If there is delay and the viability of the limb is at risk, a temporary cannula or shunt can be inserted. Treatment of the arterial wound depends essentially on the degree of damage to the vessel wall. Clean cut wounds without bruising are uncommon; if they are placed longitudinally or have caused only partial division of the vessel, they may be closed by direct suture; a cleanly severed vessel may be repaired by immediate end to end anastomosis. Usually, however, there is bruising or destruction of a segment of the vessel wall, with or without complete severance of continuity. If there is the slightest doubt about arterial damage, for example if there is any diminution of pulse volume distal to a contused area, an arteriotomy must be made in order that the intima can be examined. A contused segment should be excised, so that clean cut ends can be approximated for suture. The resultant gap does not necessarily preclude end-to-end anastomosis, since it can sometimes be bridged by mobilization of the vessel above and below. Excessive tension however will cause a repair to fail and if in doubt it is better to bridge the gap with a graft. Monofilament or fine teflon coated braided dacron are suitable suture materials. Carrel's method of everting sutures, which bring intima into contact with intima, is generally advocated, although a simple over and over suture may be equally effective. Small calibre vessels should be repaired with interrupted sutures. A combination of the two may also be used.

End-to-end anastomosis

The two segments are milked free of blood clot, and a few ml of heparin solution (10 units per ml of saline) are irrigated into each: some of the same solution may also be injected into the vessel on the far side of each clamp. The cut ends are then approximated by two stay sutures inserted at equidistant points. These sutures, held on forceps, are used to steady the vessel and to rotate it as required, while the anastomosis is completed around the entire circumference (Fig. 3.3). Stitches, which may be horizontal mattress to evert the edges or over and over, are placed about 2 mm apart and 2 mm from the cut edge. Heparin solution is used to irrigate the vessel which is flushed out by temporary release of clamps before the arteriotomy is closed. After the suture has been completed, the distal clamp is released first. The resulting retrograde flow is at a relatively low pressure: any obvious leaks are at once recognized, and are closed by additional sutures. The proximal clamp is then released, light gauze pressure being maintained on the outside of the anastomosis throughout. Oozing generally ceases spontaneously within a few minutes, but one or two further sutures may be required (Figs 3.11–3.13).

ARTERIAL RECONSTRUCTION

Most restorative operations on arteries take one of two forms — disobliteration or graft. The remarkable expansion of vascular surgery in recent years can largely be attributed to the development of a variety of synthetic grafts which provide admirable substitutes for arteries.

Indications for arterial reconstruction

The strongest indications arise in the case of congenital abnormalities, such as coarctation of the aorta

(although this is often dealt with by direct anastomosis) and in arterial injuries which include aneurysms and arteriovenous fistulae of traumatic origin. In obliterative vascular disease the indications are less clearcut since this is usually a widespread and progressive condition. Atherosclerosis being a generalised disease these patients are by definition high risk, carrying particular risk of complications due to obliterative disease in vessels supplying vital organs — particularly brain, kidneys

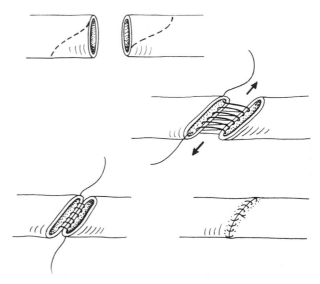

Fig. 3.11 An alterative technique for end-to-end anastomosis. The ends are bevelled to reduce the risk of constriction. A running posterior monofilament suture draws the ends together and is continued around the front of the vessel

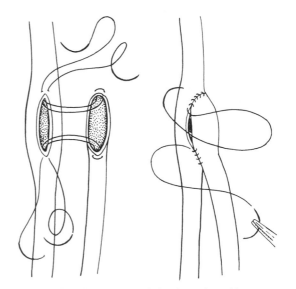

Fig. 3.12 Vascular anastomosis by the end-to-side technique

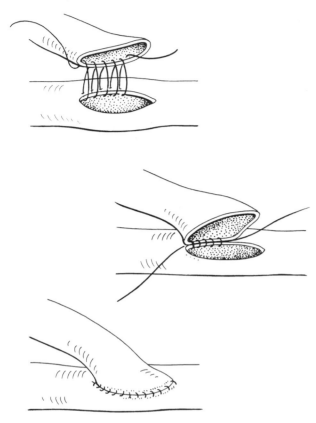

Fig. 3.13   An alternative technique for end-to-side anastomosis using a monofilament pursestring to approximate the posterior layer

and heart; myocardial infarction being the commonest cause of death in patients who undergo surgery for atherosclerosis. As a general rule the more localised the occlusion and the larger the vessel affected the better the outlook for reconstruction.

Autogenous vein

This is the material of choice for the reconstruction of small and medium sized arteries. As a rule a suitable vein is readily available, and will often survive in the presence of mild infection. A successful vein graft eventually becomes thickened to take on many of the characteristics of an artery. The long saphenous vein (when normal) is the ideal substitute for an artery of comparable size. It may be used either to bridge a gap resulting from the excision of an injured segment or to bypass a diseased segment. For bypass operations in the lower limb the saphenous vein may be reversed to avoid the effects of its valves, or it may be used 'in situ' or orthotopically in which case the valves have to be cut individually with a valvulotome.

For reversed vein graft the vein is exposed throughout its length by single or multiple incisions. Its branches are tied with fine silk 2–3 mm from the main vessel to avoid 'crimping' the adventia. It is removed, its distal end cannulated and gently distended with heparinized blood to check for haemostasis. It is reversed (because of the valves) and sutured end-to-end in the case of trauma or end-to-side in the case of bypass for obliterative disease by the methods of suture already described. The vein should be sutured under a moderate degree of tension, otherwise it stretches when arterial blood is admitted and may become tortuous and liable to thrombose.

In the in situ technique the saphenous vein is detached from the femoral vein, including a small cuff to increase the size of the orifice, great care being taken not to narrow the femoral vein. The upper end of the saphenous vein is then anastomosed end-to-side on to the common femoral artery. All tributaries are ligated in continuity. Release of the proximal clamp distends the graft with blood and shows the locations of the valves which are then cut with a valvulotome inserted from below. In some centres valvulotomy is done under direct vision using angioscopy. Finally the distal end-to-side anastomosis is constructed.

Synthetic prostheses

Tubes of woven or knitted dacron (Terylene) are now accepted as the ideal grafting material for arteries the size of the external iliac or larger. For smaller arteries vein should be preferred since this carries higher patency rates and lower risk of infection. Alternatives, if vein is not available, include expanded polytetrafluoroethylene (PTFE), human or animal biografts and other as yet unevaluated synthetic products. A graft will thrombose unless there are also patent distal vessels to ensure good run-off flow, and this is especially true of the reconstruction of small calibre arteries.

Fate of plastic prostheses

It has been shown that dacron is an effective arterial substitute, and that the grafts can remain patent and function well for many years. Grafts removed many years after implantation have shown a smooth glistening luminal surface, consisting mainly of collagen bundles and compressed fibrin and a surface layer of flattened epithelial cells. The plastic fibres of the prosthesis remain unchanged as an intermediate layer, but are permeated by cells growing from the adventitia to form a densely adherent covering or sheath of fibrous tissue. Muscle and elastic fibres appear to be absent, or are present only in very small quantities.

Thrombo-endarterectomy

This is an alterative method of restoring flow through a thrombosed artery, provided that the affected segment is short, and the cases are carefully selected. The artery is opened longitudinally, and the thrombus, together with the diseased intima and its atheromatous plaques,

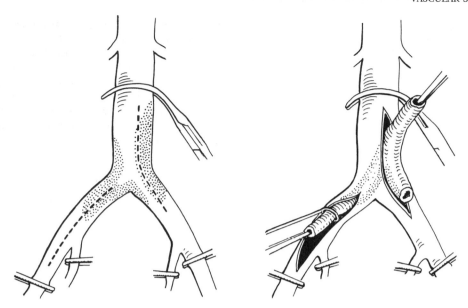

Fig. 3.14 Thrombo-endarterectomy of the aorta and iliac arteries. The thrombus and atheromatous material are removed through a plane of cleavage in the media, the adventitia and the outer layer of the media being left in situ

is removed through a plane of cleavage in the media, the adventitia and the outer layer of the media being left behind. The incision in the artery may be closed by a patch graft of vein or synthetic material if direct suture appears to narrow the lumen (Fig. 3.14).

Bypass grafting

This term denotes the insertion of a graft or synthetic prosthesis, by end to side anastomosis, to short-circuit an obstructed segment of artery — usually the femoral (Fig. 3.15). Certain advantages are claimed for the method. Exact matching of the calibre is unnecessary. There is less narrowing of the vessel than occurs at the points of end-to-end anastomosis of a replacement graft, since, owing to the oblique cutting of the bypass graft, the suture line represents the widest part of the union. There is less interference with the collateral circulation and the operation imposes less strain on the patient, since the vessel requires to be exposed only through a small incision above and below the obstructed segment. The graft can be tunnelled deeply, or sometimes a subcutaneous route serves better. As noted earlier autogenous vein is the graft material of choice in limb vessels. When vein is not available synthetic alternatives, as described above, may be considered. These materials, like vein, can if necessary be used to bypass diseased arteries right down to the level of the ankle provided that there is adequate run off in the form of a patent arterial arcade in the foot. The patency rates, especially for small calibre vessels are inferior to vein, although the interposition of a vein cuff or patch between synthetic graft and host artery may improve the patency.

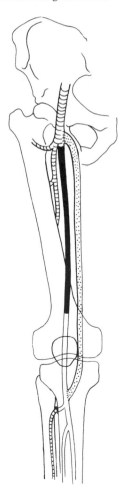

Fig. 3.15 Bypass graft for blocked femoral artery

Profundaplasty

This operation, first described in 1972, may help to preserve an ischaemic limb if the popliteal vessel is unsuitable to receive a bypass graft from the femoral artery. It can be combined with a graft from a higher level. Biplane arteriography is usually required to demonstrate profunda origin stenosis. The arteriotomy in the common femoral artery is extended into the profunda femoris, and closed with a vein patch or with the distal toe of a dacron graft.

Arterial dilatation

A recent innovation in the management of obliterative arterial disease is the development of percutaneous transluminal angioplasty (PTA), the dilatation of a stenosed or occluded segment, under local anaesthesia and radiological control, by means of a balloon (Gruntzig) catheter. The results appear to be superior in large arteries, e.g. the iliacs, but the technique is increasingly being employed to treat stenoses or short length occlusions at many sites throughout the body. Where follow up studies have shown a tendency to early re-occlusion, such as in calcified common femoral lesions, patency can be improved by the insertion of a metal stent at the time of the angioplasty.

Microvascular surgery

Advances in operating microscopes, miniature instruments, suture materials and surgical techniques have led to the development of the new speciality of microvascular surgery. Opportunities to apply these techniques may arise in several different fields including bypasses to the small arteries of ankle or foot, nerve and vessel repair, digit or limb reimplantation, hand surgery, free grafts in plastic surgery and organ transplantation. The practical details of microvascular surgery are beyond the scope of this text. Training courses are now available in a number of centres.

ANTICOAGULANT THERAPY

Anticoagulant therapy is indicated in all conditions where it is considered desirable to reduce the normal clotting power of the blood — i.e. in most thromboembolic states. These include coronary thrombosis, pulmonary embolism, mesenteric embolism and thrombosis, peripheral arterial embolism and peripheral phlebothrombosis. In treatment of these conditions, anticoagulant therapy is employed in order to prevent extension of the thrombosis and to encourage retraction and shrinkage of the clot; prophylactically, it serves to prevent further thrombotic episodes.

Contraindications

Contraindications to anticoagulant therapy are the presence of an actual or potential bleeding surface (as may occur for the first 2 or 3 days after operation) and blood dyscrasias involving impairment of the normal mechanism for the prevention of bleeding. Old and frail patients, and those with severe liver or kidney damage, should be given the drugs in much reduced dosage. It is frequently necessary, however, to weigh the risks in these conditions against those of pulmonary embolism; as a rule the latter consideration will override the former. If operation is intended on a patient who is being maintained on an oral anticoagulant the latter should be replaced by heparin several days before the operation. Heparin can be quickly reversed by protamine sulphate if perioperative bleeding is a problem.

Heparin

Heparin has at least two modes of action on the coagulation system. In combination with heparin cofactor it inhibits Factor Xa. This is thought to be the main mechanism of action of low dose subcutaneous heparin, a proven prophylactic against postoperative pulmonary embolism. In a dose of 5000 units twice or thrice daily it is given by deep subcutaneous injection into the fat of the abdominal wall. The first dose is given approximately 1 hour before operation and it is continued postoperatively until the patient is mobile. Such doses do not alter the clotting time.

Low molecular weight heparin appears to have better prophylactic effects in high risk patients such those undergoing major orthopaedic operations, but there is no proven advantage over unfractionated heparin in general surgical cases.

In large dosage heparin also blocks the thrombin-fibrinogen reaction. Doses of around 5000 units intravenously, are used to prevent thrombosis during arterial operations and generally do not require reversal. Larger doses, 10–15 000 units, are used for the initial treatment of acute thrombotic or thromboembolic episodes. Heparin is excreted rapidly by the kidneys, and when used in 'therapeutic' doses is controlled by estimation of the activated partial thromboplastin time, which should be maintained at between one and a half and two and a half times control value. Continuous intravenous infusion is the usual method of administration, 1–3000 units can be administered each hour by means of a low volume infusion pump. Deep subcutaneous injection into the fat of the abdominal wall may be used to replace intravenous administration after the first day, an injection of 15–25 000 units being given twice daily. In severe forms of thrombosis, such as extensive venous thrombosis, heparin should be continued for a week to 10 days before converting to oral anticoagulant. During conversion the two should be overlapped by 3 to 4 days.

Antidote

The half life of heparin in the circulation is 1.5 hours so that withdrawal is followed by restoration within a few hours of the normal clotting time. If, however, severe haemorrhage should occur, or should operation become urgently necessary, reversal with protamine sulphate will be required. In 0.1% of individuals protamine can cause quite severe sensitivity reactions, it must therefore be given by slow injection. The dose depends on how recently the heparin was administered. If protamine is required within a few minutes of heparin the appropriate neutralising dose is 1.0 mg per 100 IU of heparin. An hour after heparin administration only 50% of the neutralising dose will be required.

Oral anticoagulants

These drugs owe their anticoagulant action, partly to their ability to reduce the blood prothrombin by inhibiting its formation in the liver, and partly by lowering the concentration of Factors VII, IX and X. They differ from heparin in three important respects. Firstly, they can be given by mouth; secondly, their action is not fully developed for 48 hours or more; thirdly, since they are metabolized slowly and have a cumulative action, there is some danger of haemorrhage. Because of this, the dosage must be carefully controlled by regular estimation of the prothrombin time, which should be maintained at one and a half to two and a half times that of normal plasma. In the UK, warfarin sodium is at present the preparation of choice.

Dosage

Warfarin is usually started with an initial dose of 10 mg. Thereafter, doses must be carefully controlled by estimation of prothrombin time, carried out at first daily and then at increasing intervals of time until the desired prolongation of prothrombin is established. The usual maintenance dose of warfarin is 5–7.5 mg daily to achieve a prothrombin ratio of 2.0–4.5. Different ratios are chosen depending on the clinical indication and therefore the advice of the haematologist should be sought. It is clear that these drugs should not be used unless laboratory facilities of a high order are available — disadvantage which offsets to some extent their low cost as compared with heparin — but blood samples for the estimation of prothrombin time can now be sent by post to most laboratories.

Antidote

Since 48 hours may elapse after withdrawal of the drug before the prothrombin time returns to normal, a specific antidote is more necessary than in the case of heparin, should severe haemorrhage occur or an emergency operation be required. Such an antidote is found in *Vitamin K1 (phytomenadione)*, 15 to 25 mg of which can be administered either by mouth or by intravenous injection.

Thrombolytic therapy

Streptokinase and urokinase achieve their effect by activating circulating plasminogen as does the newer agent TPA (tissue plasminogen activator). Urokinase is derived from human urine. TPA is derived from a melanoma cell line or more recently from gene cloning techniques. Streptokinase is derived from streptococcal cultures. These agents are relatively expensive, particularly TPA.

They are however increasingly being used in acute arterial occlusion where they are administered in low dosage directly into the thrombus by means of a selectively positioned catheter. In deep vein thrombosis (DVT) thrombolysis may be considered in major iliofemoral thrombosis if it is of recent onset, i.e. within 4 to 5 days, and there is no potential source of bleeding such as a peptic ulcer, recent operation or fracture. Most DVTs however have been established for longer than that when they present clinically. DVT of the axillary or subclavian veins or the superior cava respond particularly well to thrombolysis which can be delivered locally by catheter or systemically.

Lytic therapy is indicated in massive pulmonary embolism. The cooperative study of the National Heart and Lung Institute in the U.S.A. (1970) showed that urokinase in comparison with heparin significantly accelerated the resolution of pulmonary thrombo-emboli at 24 hours as demonstrated by pulmonary arteriogram, lung scans and right heart pressures. However, no significant difference in 2 week mortality was noted (a larger trial would have been required), moreover bleeding occurred in 45% of patients receiving urokinase in contrast to 27% of those receiving heparin alone. In subsequent trials no difference in therapeutic effect was observed between urokinase and streptokinase. These agents should not be used without expert haematological advice.

ARTERIOGRAPHY

Outlining of an entire arterial system can be obtained by radiography after the injection of an opaque medium into the parent trunk. This method of investigation may give valuable information in cases of arterial injury or disease. It may demonstrate the site of any narrowing or constriction, or aneurysm or of arterio-venous fistula. It may indicate the extent of occlusive vascular disease, and the state of any collateral circulation. The opaque media commonly used at the present time are organic iodine compounds in which the pharmacological action of iodine is suppressed. They are radioinactive and are not retained in the body; they have some irritant action although this has been greatly reduced since the introduction of nonionic contrast media.

New arteriographic techniques include Digital Subtraction Imaging (DSI) and Nuclear Magnetic Resonance Imaging (NMRI). DSI uses computer enhancement of the radiographic image so that small volumes of contrast by small calibre intra-arterial injection are sufficient to provide high quality images. Intravenous injection can also be used to obtain arterial images but large volumes of contrast are required and the image quality is seldom of diagnostic standard for most clinical situations. There are substantial economies in film when using DSA, and the technique is becoming widely available.

Nuclear Magnetic Resonance (NMR) imaging, which does not require the injection of contrast material, is being developed but is very expensive and not as yet generally available.

Conventionally, after arteriography, the patient has been observed in hospital overnight in case of bleeding or local damage to the artery. With the advent of small calibre catheters and Digital Subtraction techniques arteriography, in many centres, is becoming a day care technique.

Aortography

This is used to investigate the circulation, not only in the aorta and its main branches, but also in the arteries of both lower limbs. It is of special value in demonstrating occlusive lesions at the aortic bifurcation or in the iliac arteries, and in outlining the renal blood vessels and parenchyma in cases of suspected tumour or essential hypertension. It is also being used extensively in the diagnosis of many other abdominal conditions. Direct injection of contrast material into the aorta by translumbar aortography has virtually disappeared. The great majority of arteriograms are performed by the perfemoral route and where this is impractical the transbrachial route is employed.

Transfemoral arteriography

By percutaneous puncture of one or other femoral artery, and by the introduction of a fine polythene catheter in a cardiac direction, an aortogram can be taken at any desired level without difficulty. The use of appropriately shaped catheters allows the selective catheterization of aortic branches — including mesenteric and renal vessels and the branches from the aortic arch to the head and upper limbs.

Transbrachial or transaxillary aortography

This method, whereby a catheter is introduced proximally into the brachial or axillary artery, percutaneously or by open operation, is used to outline the aortic arch and its branches and the descending thoracic aorta when the transfemoral route is not available.

Peripheral arteriography

For investigation of the distal circulation in the lower limb, 10 to 15 ml of contrast medium may be injected into the femoral artery, by percutaneous puncture just below the inguinal ligament, either general or local anaesthesia being employed. If there is any difficulty in entering the artery by percutaneous puncture or the operator lacks the necessary experience, the artery can be exposed through a small incision.

Renal arteriography is described on page 550.

ARTERIAL ANEURYSMS

Traumatic aneurysms may follow penetrating wounds of arteries, or they may occur as a late result of simple contusion when the injured segment of vessel subsequently gives way. Non-traumatic aneurysms are usually associated with generalized arterial degeneration.

In the early stages of development of a traumatic aneurysm — when the condition is better described as an *arterial haematoma* (p. 43) — conservative treatment should be employed, unless there is a progressive increase in the swelling or acute circulatory failure due to compression of the collateral vessels. Should these conditions be present, immediate operation is indicated. After evacuation of the haematoma, continuity of the artery is restored if at all possible, either by simple repair, or by one of the reconstructive methods which have been described — except in the case of vessels below the elbow or knee, where simple ligation is the procedure of choice.

In most cases, however, it is desirable to postpone operation until the primary wound has healed, and the inflammatory reaction to the haematoma settled. The optimum time for intervention will vary with each case. If the condition is progressive, operation may be demanded within a few days; if it is relatively quiescent, operation may be delayed for several months. The aneurysm may be induced to thrombose spontaneously by sustained occlusive pressure over the leaking point for 15 to 30 minutes with a duplex ultrasound scanning probe. This can be tried before deciding on the need for surgery.

For larger arteries, if ischaemia is to be avoided, reconstruction is generally required.

Ligature with obliteration of the sac

This is an appropriate procedure, in the case of vessels below the elbow or knee. It is best carried out from within the aneurysmal sac, and the term 'obliterative endo-aneurysmorrhaphy' is applicable. The method is as a rule effective in preventing recurrence; in addition it combines simplicity and safety, since surrounding structures are not disturbed and possible interference with the collateral circulation is reduced to a minimum. The steps in the operation are shown in Figure 3.17.

Ligature with excision of the sac

This is a more certain method of preventing recurrence, but, owing to the extent of the dissection required, damage may be inflicted upon the collateral circulation on which the nutrition of the part depends. It may be simpler and safer to ligate above and below the aneurysm, leave it in situ and construct a bypass graft.

Reconstructive procedures

Advances in the reconstructive surgery of arteries (pp. 45 & 46) have revolutionized the treatment of aneurysms. This applies particularly to aneurysms of the aorta. Most aortic aneurysms prove fatal within a limited time, either by rupture, by embolism or by pressure on surrounding structures, and there is no medical treatment which will influence the natural course of the disease.

Aneurysms of the aorta and large arteries

The surgical treatment of these aneurysms has advanced rapidly in recent years so that it is impossible to do more than lay down certain general principles for guidance.

Arch of aorta

Aneurysms of the arch (especially of the central part) carry the problem of maintaining an adequate cerebral circulation during the reconstructive procedure. A temporary bypass may be constructed — usually to the innominate artery. In the case of dissecting aneurysms treatment using hypotensive agents may be the first choice in the hope of effecting intramural thrombosis failing which the condition is dealt with either by division and suture of the aorta (thus effecting closure of the dissection) or by replacement of the affected segment with a prosthesis. These procedures may have to be combined with reconstruction of the aortic valve.

Descending thoracic aorta

The risks of temporarily clamping this vessel concern,

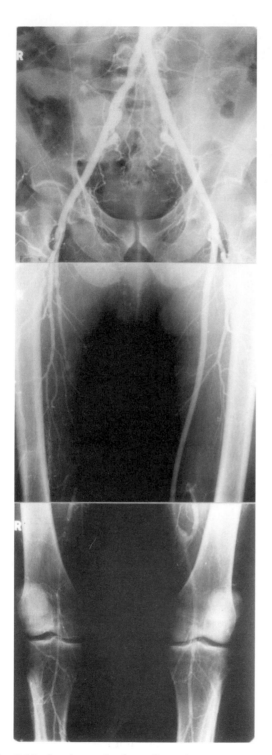

Fig. 3.16 Arteriogram by the perfemoral route

Choice of operation

For aneurysms in arteries of small calibre e.g. beyond the knee or elbow simple ligation will normally suffice.

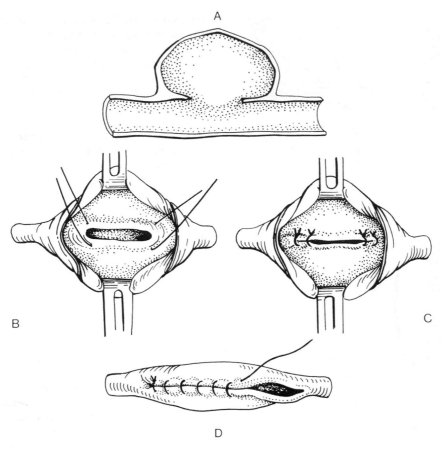

Fig. 3.17 Obliterative endo-aneurysmorrhaphy
(A) Cross-section of artery with false sac.
(B) Sutures placed to close the arterial openings within the sac.
(C) Sutures tied.
(D) Closure of the sac

not the brain, but the spinal cord and kidneys. This may be avoided by the construction of a temporary bypass. When there is associated coarctation, much less risk arises, for a collateral circulation has already been established.

Abdominal aorta

Fortunately it is uncommon for aneurysms of the abdominal aorta to develop above the level of the renal arteries, so that these vessels, together with the coeliac and superior mesenteric, are usually unaffected. The repair of thoraco-abdominal aneurysms is a formidable procedure which can only be undertaken in major vascular centres. Infra-renal aneurysm on the other hand is common and its repair constitutes one of the commonest vascular operations, both elective and emergency. The standard treatment is replacement with a plastic prosthesis, either a simple tube or less commonly a bifurcation graft. No attempt should be made to excise the posterior part of the aneurysmal sac. After

exposure through a long midline or transverse abdominal incision, by the intraperitoneal route described on page 41, the aorta above the sac and the iliac arteries distally are controlled with suitable clamps. Most surgeons give 5000 units of heparin intravenously in elective cases prior to cross clamping. There is usually no need to reverse the heparin. Pre-clotting of grafts is no longer required as either woven or sealed knitted grafts are used. The sac is opened in the midline and the contents evacuated. The mouths of any bleeding lumbar arteries are closed with stitch ligatures. The inferior mesenteric artery is usually found to be occluded at its origin and reimplantation is only rarely indicated.

The prosthesis is laid in the sac and sutured as an inlay. The great majority of abdominal aortic aneurysms can be treated with a simple tube graft, occasionally iliac anastomosis is required and rarely femoral (Fig. 3.18). The passage of Fogarty embolectomy catheters down both limbs prior to completion of the distal anastomoses is a recommended precaution against

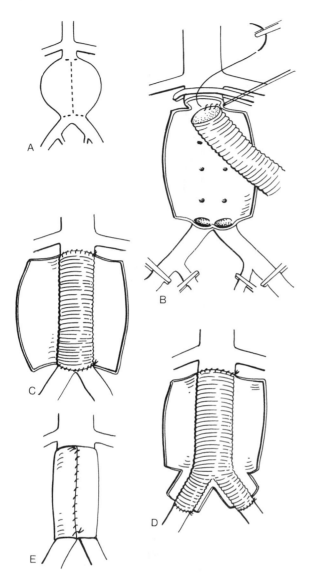

Fig. 3.18 Graft replacement for aneurysm of the abdominal aorta. The graft, which may be simple tube or bifurcation, is laid within the aneurysmal sac. The sac and peritoneum are closed over the graft

postoperative ischaemia, especially if systemic heparin has not been used. The sac is sutured around the graft in order to separate it from overlying bowel, if necessary by interposing a pedicle of omentum, because of the danger of later aorto-enteric fistula.

The natural history of aneurysm is still not well documented, size being the most important risk factor. The probability of rupture of a 6 cm aneurysm is generally regarded as around 50% within 2 years, however there are no reliable recent epidemiological data. However the probability of rupture of a 4 cm aneurysm is probably less than 5% in 5 years. Aneurysms expand at an average of 0.4 cms per year. The operative mortality of elective aneurysm surgery is around 5% and of surgery for ruptured aneurysm around 50%. The life expectancy and quality of life of survivors of both elective and emergency operations is excellent, being similar to those of an age and sex matched population.

Iliac, femoral and popliteal aneurysms
A restorative operation, with either replacement or by-pass, is the ideal treatment. The indications for replacement are increasing size, distal embolism or acute occlusion. If gangrene has developed by the time the patient seeks treatment, amputation will of course be required.

Innominate, subclavian and axillary aneurysms
The subclavian artery can usually be ligated with safety, provided that this is done beyond the first part, the branches of which provide an adequate collateral circulation. For aneurysms of the innominate and axillary arteries, a reconstructive operation should if possible be attempted.

Arteriovenous aneurysms (fistulae)
Fistulous communication between an artery and a vein is a common sequel to a penetrating injury, such as a knife wound. Depending on the presence or absence of an aneurysmal sac between the communicating vessels, the terms *varicose aneurysm* or *aneurysmal varix* may be employed, but the distinction is a somewhat arbitrary one.

Natural cure is most unlikely — indeed the condition is usually progressive. When the fistula involves the main vessels of a limb, signs of defective circulation develop in the distal part of the limb. In carotido-jugular fistulae, cerebral and ocular effects may predominate. The effects on the general circulation may be even more serious. The diversion of blood from the normal arterial bed results in a marked fall in the diastolic pressure, with a corresponding rise in pulse pressure. Increased venous return to the heart gives rise to progressive left ventricular enlargement. The larger the fistula, and the nearer it is to the heart, the more serious will be its effects. Operation is indicated before cardiac decompensation has become established.

Quadruple ligature
This is a suitable method for the smaller vessels. The artery and vein are exposed above and below the fistula, and each vessel is ligatured in both situations. Ligatures are applied also to any other vessels communicating with the sac. Thereafter the sac may be obliterated with further ligatures (Fig. 3.19). Every effort is made to avoid damage to important collateral vessels, on which the circulation of the limb depends.

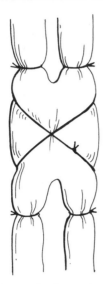

Fig. 3.19 Arteriovenous fistula; quadruple ligation and obliteration

Reconstructive operations

These are indicated in the case of the larger vessels. Direct repair may be possible especially in the early stages using a vein or dacron patch on the artery if necessary (Fig. 3.20). Later, it is advisable to excise the affected segment of the artery or to ligate above and below and to bypass it with an autogenous vein or synthetic graft.

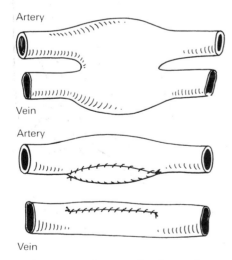

Fig. 3.20 A reconstructive operation for arteriovenous fistula

Simple ligation of the artery alone, proximal to the fistula, is contraindicated in the case of the main vessel of a limb, for it will almost invariably be followed by gangrene. The reason for this is that the pressure differential favours the short circuiting of the capillary bed via the fistula (Fig. 3.21).

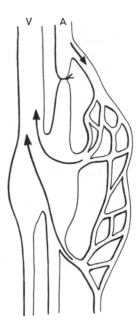

Fig. 3.21 Ligature of the artery alone, in arteriovenous fistula, is likely to cause gangrene

---

ACUTE ARTERIAL OCCLUSION

The advent of thrombolytic therapy has seen a marked change in the management of acute arterial occlusion in recent years, so that urgent operation is no longer the automatic first choice to revascularize a threatened limb.

Thrombosis can usually be distinguished by an antecedent history of claudication and is sometimes precipitated by a hypotensive episode. Arterial embolism is usually secondary to heart disease, especially auricular fibrillation or recent myocardial infarction, the embolus lodging at major arterial bifurcations — the aortic, the common iliac, the femoral or the popliteal. It occurs often in elderly and unfit patients, so that the mortality is high, and major surgical procedures are contraindicated. Following lodgement of the embolus, there is propagation of thrombosis both proximal and distal to the site of embolism, hence the view that intravenous heparin should be given early in management.

Management depends on available resources and vascular expertise. If an acutely ischaemic limb displays severe pain, pallor, coldness, loss of sensation and loss of power then immediate surgical exploration with a view to embolectomy/thrombectomy is essential, since these symptoms indicate inevitable limb loss within 4 to 6 hours of onset and there may not be time to try thrombolysis. In the majority of cases however the extremity is less critically affected and there is time to obtain an arteriogram with selective catheterization of the affected artery so that local low dose thrombolytic therapy (e.g. streptokinase 5000 units per hour) can be delivered into the thrombus. The response to lytic therapy can be monitored with serial angiograms and the patient converted to heparin when sufficient clearance has been achieved. This treatment is usually effective for both embolism and thrombosis. In the case of the latter, successful lysis generally has to be followed by balloon angioplasty of the stenosis which has given rise to the acute occlusion.

When expert radiology and thrombolytic therapy are not available, and the limb is severely ischaemic, removal of thrombus by means of the Fogarty embolectomy catheter should be attempted, especially when there are strong grounds for suspecting embolism rather than thrombosis. In the case of the latter the surgeon should be prepared to go on to an arterial reconstruction, if attempts to clear the thrombus are unsuccessful.

Once infarction has occurred in the calf muscles, evidenced by tenderness and fixed planter flexion, salvage is unlikely and should not be attempted on account of the dangers of the reperfusion syndrome with renal failure (Gregg, 1983).

Embolectomy catheters

The slender balloon catheter, devised by Fogarty (1963, 1971) has been a most significant advance in vascular surgery, and is now an indispensable instrument for embolectomy. This catheter is 80 cm long and is available in sizes 3 to 7F. It has a delicate inflatable balloon close to its tip, the balloon being of varying sizes. The catheter is threaded into the artery to a level beyond which no clots are thought to be present. The balloon is then inflated with sterile saline until slight resistance is felt, and the catheter is withdrawn with the balloon inflated, bringing with it any clots present within the lumen. The inflation should be gradually increased to match the widening calibre if the catheter is being withdrawn proximally and vice versa. After removal of thrombus a completion, on-table angiogram should be obtained. An X-Ray plate is positioned under the limb and a bolus of 20–40 mls of contrast fluid is injected by hand through an umbilical catheter inserted through the arteriotomy, the proximal inflow being clamped off. Often this will reveal residual thrombus requiring re-passage of the embolectomy catheter. If this is unsuccessful further clearance can often be obtained by the instillation of streptokinase (100 000 U), while the inflow remains clamped off. A repeat on-table angiogram after half an hour will frequently show substantial improvement. Alternatively the arterial tree can be explored more distally to effect removal of thrombus.

Over-vigorous use of the embolectomy catheter can result in arterial damage, which is another reason why completion angiography should be routine.

Aortic and iliac embolectomy

Aortic bifurcation and iliac emboli, together with any distal thrombi, can now be removed via the femoral arteries, which are approached below the inguinal ligament, and the procedure can be carried out very expeditiously under local anaesthesia. The entire neck, thorax and abdomen should, however, be prepared and draped and an anaesthetist should be present since, if extraction of the clot by the embolectomy catheter is unsuccessful, it may be necessary to construct an aorto-femoral, axillo-femoral or femoro-femoral bypass.

Through incisions below the inguinal ligaments, the femoral arteries are exposed; they are elevated with tapes passed above and below the origin of the profundae, and these branches are controlled in the same way. An incision 1–1.5 cm in length is made into the femoral artery just above the origin of the profunda. Attention should first be paid to removal of thrombi in the distal arterial tree i.e. both from the distal part of the femoral artery and from the profunda. After the catheter has been passed as far distally as possible, the balloon is inflated until mild resistance is felt, and is then withdrawn, additional fluid or air being injected gradually as the calibre of the vessel increases. Ideally the clearance of the distal arterial tree should be checked by peroperative arteriography. It can be misleading to rely on good backflow alone. Arteriography can be done simply by positioning a cassette, draped in a sterile towel, under the limb and the hand injection of 20 ml of contrast fluid through a cannula into the distal lumen. After all thrombi have been removed, a solution of heparin (10 units per ml of saline) is injected into the distal vessels, which are then occluded by atraumatic arterial clamps. A larger size balloon catheter is now introduced into the main trunk, and is passed upwards into the aorta to a level well above the embolus. The balloon is then inflated with the appropriate amount of fluid, and is extracted as previously described, bringing the clot, or a considerable part of it, with it. The catheter should be passed repeatedly until no further clots can be delivered, and until a forceful blood flow is obtained. After one side has been cleared (Fig. 3.22), the procedure should be repeated from the opposite femoral artery. If the embolus has been a saddle-shaped one at the bifurcation of the aorta, about half of it can be expected to be removed through each femoral artery. Finally the arteriotomy incision is sutured. Anticoagulant therapy is continued after operation, not only to prevent further embolization, but also to prevent venous thrombosis, which is a frequent sequel to arterial embolization.

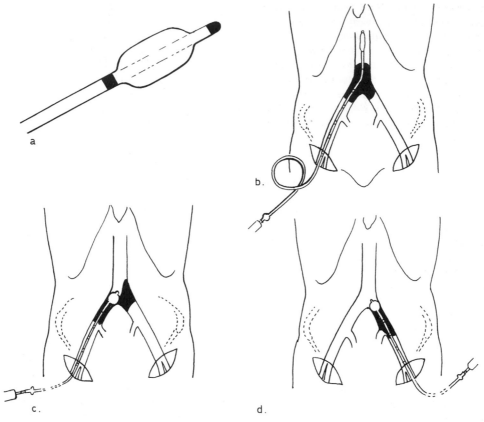

Fig. 3.22   Balloon catheter embolectomy.
(a) Tip of Fogarty catheter showing inflatable balloon. (b) Catheter tip above embolus after introduction through right femoral artery. (c) Clot being dislodged by withdrawal of inflated balloon. (d) Residual clot being removed through left femoral artery

Peripheral arterial embolism
The common femoral artery is the most frequent site for peripheral embolism (40% of all cases), the clot lodging at the point where the profunda artery branches off. Localized bulging, with pulsation above the embolus and a state of immobile constriction below, may be seen but this sign is by no means always present. The circulation is controlled by means of slings applied to the artery above and below; a longitudinal incision is made in the arterial wall, when, if the diagnosis is correct, clot will be present in the lumen. From the groin the Fogarty catheter can be passed down the profunda to the lower thigh and down the superficial femoral artery as far as the ankle. Thrombus is removed as described above. Completion angiography, as described above, is important at this level.

Mesenteric embolectomy
Acute mesenteric ischaemia is usually fatal. Occasionally however it is diagnosed sufficiently promptly to permit revascularization of the bowel by extraction of

thrombus from the superior mesenteric artery. This vessel is exposed in the root of the mesentery below the third part of the duodenum. Branches are controlled with slings or small bulldog clips. A transverse incision is made in the artery and embolus extracted as described above. The procedure may have to be combined with bowel resection. Regardless of apparent success there should always be a second look operation to check bowel viability after 24 to 48 hours.

Pulmonary embolectomy and venous thrombectomy
These are discussed in the section on venous thrombosis (p. 63).

VARICOSE VEINS

Anatomy
The venous outflow from the lower limb follows three main pathways; the superficial veins, the deep veins

and the interosseous veins. The deep veins, usually paired in the lower leg accompany the arteries. The superficial veins of the lower limb are collected into two main trunks — the long saphenous vein, which extends the whole length of the limb and the short saphenous vein, which extends upwards only as far as the knee. They connect with the deep system via connecting or perforating veins. The interosseous pathway is of little clinical significance, although it was formerly often used as a route for phlebography.

The long saphenous vein

This is formed by the union of veins on the medial side of the foot. It passes in front of the medial malleolus, and ascends to the medial side of the knee, lying just behind the femoral condyle. In the thigh it inclines laterally and forwards towards the saphenous opening, which lies 3–4 cm below and lateral to the pubic tubercle. It pierces the cribriform fascia, and passes deeply through the saphenous opening to join the femoral vein.

Tributaries. The more important of these, together with their usual anatomical arrangement, are shown in Figure 3.23. Considerable variations however exist; a high medial or lateral superficial femoral vein may be mistaken for the main trunk, and very occasionally this latter is double. Special note should be made of the tributary (J in Fig. 3.23) which ascends along the medial side of the calf, behind and parallel to the main trunk, and joining this just below knee level. This vessel has important communications with the deep veins, through 'perforators' (usually three in number) which traverse the deep fascia at fairly constant levels. It is in relation to this tributary, rather than to the main trunk of the long saphenous vein, that varicosities and ulcers in the lower leg commonly develop.

The short saphenous vein

This is formed by the union of veins on the lateral side of the foot. It crosses behind the lateral malleolus, and then ascends obliquely backwards towards the middle of the popliteal fossa, where, after receiving several small tributaries, it pierces deep fascia to enter the popliteal vein. It frequently communicates with the deep veins through a 'perforator' a handsbreadth above the lateral malleolus (Fig. 3.23).

Variations from the normal arrangement frequently occur. The vein may pierce the deep fascia in the upper part of the calf, or occasionally it may remain superficial throughout, joining the long saphenous vein as one of its medial tributaries near the knee. Before any treatment of varicose veins can be planned, it is essential to determine by careful examination whether the varices involve the long or short saphenous system, and to what extent they have developed in relation to com-

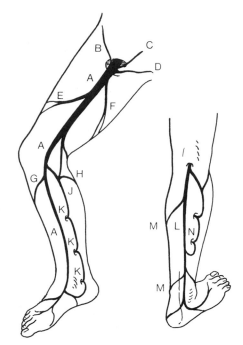

Fig. 3.23 Anatomy of long and short saphenous veins A = Long saphenous vein, main trunk; B = Superficial external iliac vein; C = Superficial epigastric vein; D = Superficial external pudendal vein; E = Lateral superficial femoral vein; F = Medial superficial femoral vein; G = Anterior vein winding round tibia below knee; H = Posterior vein, joining (or occasionally replacing) short saphenous vein; J = Posteromedial vein, which lies parallel to and behind main trunk of long saphenous vein, and anastomoses with arches arising from; K = perforating veins — usually three in number and constant in position; L = Short saphenous vein, with M = medial tributaries which may communicate with medial perforators; N = connection with lateral perforating vein, a handsbreadth above malleolus

municating or *perforating* veins which pass through fascia and muscle to connect with the deep veins of the limb.

Special tests have been designed in order to determine the choice of treatment. They fall into three main groups: (1) tests for valvular incompetence at the saphenofemoral and saphenopopliteal junctions; (2) tests for incompetent perforating veins; (3) tests for patency of the deep veins.

Assessment

The first and most important thing is for the surgeon to learn to recognize the patterns of varices which are characteristic of particular sites of incompetence. For example, if there are primary varices on the medial side of the thigh it can usually be assumed, even if it is not immediately obvious, that there is saphenofemoral incompetence. Indeed one of the commonest mistakes in varicose vein surgery is failure properly to deal with incompetence at the sapheno-femoral junction. Prominent varices in the lower half of the medial side of the calf are usually associated with incompetent perforators, especially if there are associated skin changes of pigmentation, eczema or ulceration. The presence of a retromalleolar venous flare extending down on to the foot is a clear sign of the existence of an incompetent perforator at its apex. Varices on and skin changes on the lateral side of the calf may stem from short saphenopopliteal incompetence or from connections with an incompetent long saphenous vein. Careful examination will distinguish the two, provided that the surgeon bears in mind the variations which may occur in the termination of the short saphenous vein.

Before the operation, with the patient standing, the main venous channels are palpated, percussed and marked with an indelible marker. The simplest and most widely used test (*Trendelenburg*) depends on observation of the filling of varices before and after systematic removal of rubber tourniquets (the most distal first) which have been applied with the leg elevated. *Doppler ultrasound* is a valuable noninvasive tool, simple in application, which can be used to demonstrate saphenofemoral or saphenopopliteal reflux, perforator incompetence and patency of deep veins.

When there is a history of deep vein thrombosis phlebography is the most reliable method of confirming patency of deep veins. If however there is no oedema, venous claudication or severe skin changes it can be assumed that there is not a deep vein occlusion sufficient to preclude varicose vein surgery. Ascending phlebography is performed by injection of contrast medium into a foot vein. The medium is directed into the deep veins by tourniquet above the ankle. *Phlebography* can be used to locate perforating veins but in primary varicose veins is seldom justified for this indication, physical examination being preferred.

An important recent advance in the investigation of venous disease is colour coded Duplex scanning. This makes possible the non-invasive mapping of the superficial and deep venous systems. Blood flow velocity can be measured, the direction of venous flow observed and by this means the sites of valvular incompetence identified.

Sclerotherapy

Injection therapy is not necessarily an alternative to operation. It has a useful place for the abolition of minor varices unrelated to saphenous incompetence and is particularly effective in dealing with residual or recurrent varices postoperatively. If saphenofemoral or saphenopopliteal incompetence is present the sclerosis of distal varicosities offers no prospect of long term benefit.

Many different solutions have been employed during the past 50 years. The common objective is to induce endothelial damage and so initiate a chemical phlebitis. The injected vein eventually shrinks and becomes organized into fibrous tissue so that complete obliteration of the vein results. The most frequently used solution in the UK is sodium tetradecyl sulphate (STD). In the technique of compression sclerotherapy the sites of incompetent perforators are located as accurately as possible.

Up to eight 2 ml syringes are each loaded with 0.5 ml of sclerosing solution. The patient sits on a waist high couch with the legs horizontal. In this position the vein usually contains sufficient blood for venepuncture. The lowest injection site is selected first. The needle is inserted, the leg is elevated to empty the vein and the sclerosant injected while the vein is compressed with the fingers above and below the needle. Compression is then applied by means of a cohesive elastic bandage over Sorbo rubber pads or cotton wool balls. The procedure is repeated at several sites, working proximally.

Great care must be taken not to inject in the region of major arteries such as the tibial or peroneal vessels at the ankle. Severe pain at the time of injection, passing down into the foot, should alert to the possibility. The injection should be immediately stopped, intravenous heparin administered, the patient admitted to hospital and the advice of a vascular specialist obtained.

After sclerotherapy the importance of walking immediately and extra walking each day is emphasized. Provided that the patient remains relatively comfortable and the bandages firm they are not disturbed for 3 weeks.

Choice of operation

The various components of varicose vein surgery are (i) saphenofemoral ligation and/or saphenopopliteal ligation, (ii) saphenous stripping, (iii) multiple phlebectomy, (iv) ligation of perforators.

Crucial to the correct choice of operation is careful physical examination, as described above, with the aim of detecting the points at which there is reflux from the deep to the superficial system. When varices stem from saphenofemoral incompetence, as is the case in the great majority of both primary and secondary varicose veins, sapheno-femoral ligation is indicated. Since saphenofemoral reflux and perforator incompetence frequently coexist it is usually necessary to add multiple small incisions through which the major tributaries of the saphenous systems are interrupted, perforators ligated and varices ligated or avulsed.

Stripping of the long saphenous vein is less popular than hitherto owing to the importance of that vein as arterial replacement. However failure to remove the saphenous stem predisposes to varicose recurrence. The author's policy is not to strip the saphenous veins if the patient is diabetic, has a family history of arterial disease or is a smoker.

If stripping is performed without incompetent perforators being ligated the varicose condition will, in the long run be worse rather than better. Stripping should only be performed from knee to groin. Removal of the long saphenous vein in the calf serves no proven additional benefit (since perforators do not connect directly with it, see Fig. 3.23) but simply adds to the morbidity and carries a high probability of damage to the saphenous nerve.

Sapheno-femoral ligation

This operation, sometimes referred to as the Trendelenburg procedure or 'high ligation', is considered to be an essential part of any surgical treatment for varices involving the long saphenous system. It must be done in such a way that varicose recurrence is unlikely. This implies full and careful dissection of the area, removal of a segment of the proximal end of the long saphenous vein, together with the ligation of all tributaries entering this segment. For many years it was employed as the sole method of operative treatment for such varices, but at the present time it is usually combined with other procedures, such as stripping and multiple phlebectomies. The operation may be performed on an outpatient, but it is not one which an inexperienced surgeon should undertake. The entire varicose system including the position of the upper end of the long saphenous vein is mapped out with indelible marker before the operation is commenced.

An incision 5 to 8 cm in length is made below and parallel to the medial half of the inguinal ligament, at the level of the saphenous opening which is 3 cm below and lateral to the pubic tubercle — just medial to the femoral pulsation. As soon as a small cut has been made in the deep fascia, the fat can be separated by blunt dissection in the line of the saphenous vein. The vein is then cleared to a level of 7 to 8 cm below the opening.

The saphenous trunk must not be divided until it has been unequivocally identified. Once the surgeon is certain he has clarified the anatomy the saphenous vein is divided between clamps. Using the clamp as a convenient tractor, the upper segment of vein is raised from its bed; its three named upper tributaries — the superficial external iliac, the superficial epigastric and the superficial external pudendal — and any others discovered, are clamped and divided. The tributaries should not simply be divided flush with the saphenous vein but should be followed out at least to their first divisions. This makes varicose recurrence less likely by interrupting potential connecting channels between veins of lower abdominal wall, perineum and pelvis and those of the thigh. The superior margin of the saphenous opening is retracted upwards, so that the vein can be cleared right up to its junction with the femoral. The latter is carefully inspected for tributaries. The deep external pudendal vein is carefully ligated in continuity.

Although traction with a haemostat on the proximal stump of the long saphenous vein is very helpful for dissection, care must be taken when it comes to ligation not to tent up and thus constrict the common femoral vein. A nonabsorbable transfixion suture, e.g. 3/0 Vicryl, is used for the proximal ligation (Fig. 3.24). Attention is then turned to the distal stump. An important step is ligation of the medial superficial femoral tributary (F in Fig. 3.23). This can usually be reached

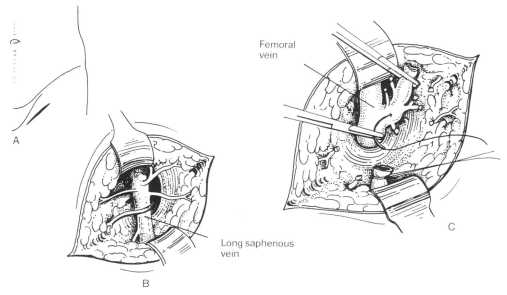

Fig. 3.24 Saphenofemoral ligation (Trendelenberg). (A) The incision is centred on a point 3–4 cm below and lateral to the pubic tubercle. (B) All the tributaries of the upper end of the long saphenous vein are exposed, ligated and divided. (C) The proximal stump of the long saphenous vein is transfixed and ligated

by retraction on the lower margin of the wound with the knee flexed. Sometimes a separate incision is required. A 1–2 cm incision is made just below the knee to locate the long saphenous vein and a stripper passed to the groin.

The groin wound is closed with absorbable subcutaneous and subcuticular sutures. The stripper is led out of the lateral end of the wound and the adjacent skin suture left untied until the leg has been bandaged (vide infra).

Difficulties and complications
Difficulty in finding the saphenous vein is overcome by enlarging the incision. A high medial or lateral superficial femoral tributary may be mistaken for the main trunk. If the main trunk of the saphenous vein is double, both divisions should be ligated. Mistaken identification of the main vein, or any anatomical variations from the normal will at once become apparent as the vein is traced upwards towards the saphenous opening.

Tearing of the femoral vein or slipping of the ligature on the saphenous stump causes alarming haemorrhage. The greatest danger is that the surgeon, in his anxiety to arrest haemorrhage, may apply forceps blindly in the depths of the wound, and by so doing may cause damage to the femoral artery or vein. All that is required is to pack gauze firmly into the wound, and to lower the head of the table. *The gauze is left in situ for at least 5 minutes*: when it is removed the haemorrhage will

be reduced to a mere trickle. If the ligature has slipped, the stump of the saphenous vein can then be picked up without difficulty.

A tear in the femoral vein should be sutured with fine nonabsorbable material on a round bodied needle. This is best achieved by using a fine nozzle suction close to the tear to clear blood from the field unless bleeding can be controlled by finger compression of the vein above and below the wound.

Tourniquet
On completion of the sapheno-femoral ligation the author's preference is to conduct the remainder of the operation under tourniquet. If it is intended to strip the long saphenous vein the stripper is passed first. The leg is exsanguinated by elevation and by the application of an Esmarch bandage or a pneumatic exsanguinator and a pneumatic or bandage tourniquet applied around the upper calf. This provides a bloodless field for the remainder of the operation. The majority of surgeons however do not employ tourniquet, relying on local pressure and elevation of the limb to control bleeding.

Vein stripping
The stripper consists of wire or plastic 85–90 cm in length with an olivary tip on one end and acorn-shaped head on the other. Modern disposable strippers have detachable acorns of various sizes which allows the stripping to be done in either direction (Fig. 3.25).

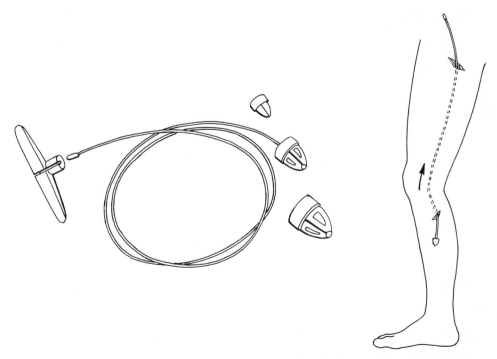

Fig. 3.25   The plastic disposable stripper has a range of sizes of olive heads. It is passed from knee to groin

Technique

For stripping of the upper half of the long saphenous vein, it is advised that sapheno-femoral ligation should first be carried out at the groin, i.e. the vein is exposed and all tributaries entering its upper segment are divided as described above. The vein is then transfixed and ligated at its junction with the femoral and is divided below the ligature. The distal end is temporarily controlled with a loosely tied ligature held in a haemostat (Fig. 3.26). The long saphenous vein is now exposed through a small skin crease incision three finger breadths below the knee joint; the stripper is introduced (Fig. 3.26B) and is passed upwards until it emerges through the upper end of the vein in the groin incision (Fig. 3.26A). A small acorn is attached and the vein tied on to the stripper (Fig. 3.26C). The stripper is drawn a short distance upwards so that the acorn-head is draw in through the incision. The vein is then divided below the ligature and the lower cut end is tied off. The vein is not stripped out at this stage. It will usually be necessary for further incisions to be made in the leg for avulsions or ligations. The groin

and knee wounds are closed with absorbable subcuticular sutures. In the groin incision the suture alongside the stripper is left untied, the loose ends being controlled by haemostats.

The remaining part of the operation — multiple phlebectomy is now performed — after which wounds are closed with skin strips, dressed and the leg elevated and bandaged with cohesive bandage as the stripper is withdrawn through the top incision and the last suture is tied, sterility being maintained by using the haemostats to tie the knot. If a tourniquet has been used the sequence is:

1. elevate the leg
2. bandage up to the lower border of the tourniquet
3. release the tourniquet
4. strip out the long saphenous vein
5. tie the final suture in the groin wound
6. complete the bandaging
7. return the leg to the horizontal position.

If this procedure is followed, and if during the sapheno-femoral ligation the medial superficial femoral vein has been dealt with as described above, there should be no haematoma formation — a common cause of postoperative discomfort after stripping.

Ligation of the short saphenous vein

This is indicated when varices involve this vein or its tributaries. A transverse incision is made across the lower part of the popliteal fossa at the level of the head of the fibula. (A vertical incision is liable to heal with keloid formation.) The short saphenous vein is identified, and is ligated and divided at the level where it pierces deep fascia to join the popliteal vein. The surgeon must be aware of the anatomical variations which commonly occur. Other superficial veins of the region, entering either the short saphenous or the popliteal vein, are dealt with in the same way.

Multiple phlebectomies

In most operations for varicose veins it is not sufficient simply to carry out saphenous ligations with or without stripping. It is necessary also to remove varices, ligate varicose tributaries at their junctions with the saphenous veins and to ligate perforating veins at the point at which they traverse the deep fascia. If it is intended to follow high ligation with a course of sclerotherapy then the need for multiple phlebectomies may be less.

Incisions near to joints should be made transversely; other incisions, being very small (around 0.5–1.0 cm), may be either transverse or longitudinal. Where perforators are suspected, for example at the medial border of soleus, an incision is made big enough to admit the tip of the little finger which is advanced down to the

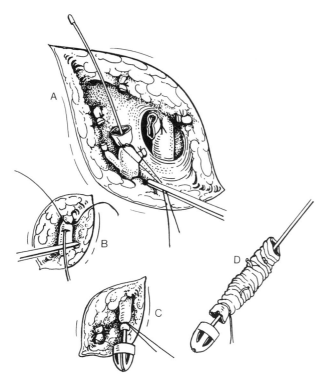

Fig. 3.26 Stripping operation for varicose veins
(A) Trendelenberg operation. Long saphenous vein ligatured and divided at junction with femoral. Tributaries divided between ligatures. (B) Long saphenous vein exposed just below knee. A ligature is placed around the vein and the stripper inserted. (C) Ligature tied to anchor vein against acorn head of stripper and vein divided. (D) The complete vein after avulsion telescoped against the head of the stripper

level of the deep fascia and swept around to identify any perforators in the area. These are then ligated.

Subfascial ligation

A variety of methods of obliterating perforating veins have been described including subfascial endoscopy. However, described here is a simple surgical method. This operation is reserved for patients whose legs are so scarred or inflamed that it is not possible to dissect the perforators outside the deep fascia. It is done under tourniquet as described above. The patient is usually positioned prone. A posterior calf stocking seam incision is made, veering off the tendo Achilles inferiorly to one or other side, depending where the main perforators are. The incision is carried straight down through the deep fascia. The circulation to the skin should not be jeopardized by any superficial dissection.

The deep fascia is easily separated from the underlying muscle and the perforators can be seen passing through holes in the deep fascia. They are ligated and divided. The deep fascia is not closed — in fact some surgeons believe that part of the benefit of this operation is derived from the fasciotomy. The skin is closed with a fine absorbable continuous subcuticular suture. These wounds are slow to heal and prone to complications, so the patient must be confined to bed rest for several days until it is clear that sound healing is taking place. Thrombo-embolism prophylaxis with subcutaneous heparin commenced pre-operatively is advised. Graduated elastic compression stockings are prescribed as soon as the patient begins to mobilize.

Post-operative management

Patients who have undergone minor operations, such as a few ligatures, can usually remain completely ambulant, since exercise obviates stasis in the deep veins, and reduces the risk of thrombosis. For the same reasons, however, they should avoid standing for any length of time for the first few days after operations, and, when seated, should keep the limb elevated. When more extensive procedures, involving multiple ligations of varices, stripping, skin grafting etc. have been employed, a more restful convalescence is advised, and a firm supporting bandage should be worn until healing is complete. In this group prophylactic subcutaneous heparin is advised, begun before operation and continued until the patient is mobile. It is the author's policy to prescribe graduated compression hose to be worn for at least 3 months after operation.

VENOUS ULCERS

Hypertension in the superficial veins is an important factor in the majority of ulcers in the lower third of the calf — the so-called 'ulcer-bearing area'. However, most patients with ulcers in the lower leg have other causative or aggravating disorders of which the more important are arterial insufficiency, obesity, arthropathy at the knee or ankle, rheumatoid vasculitis, hypertension, neurological deficit, chronic skin disorders and diabetes.

Venous ulcers are most commonly located on the medial side in relation to the main perforating veins. When the valves of these perforating veins become incompetent the rise in deep venous pressure caused by each calf contraction is transmitted outwards to the overlying superficial veins. Occlusion of the deep veins by thrombus aggravates the problem. Incompetence of valves in deep veins, an alternative sequel to deep vein thrombosis, results in excessive pressure being transmitted to the superficial veins not only at rest while standing or sitting but also during exercise.

Chronic hypertension in the venous side of the capillary circulation results in the skin changes characteristic of venous insufficiency: pigmentation, eczema, induration and ulceration. Contact dermatitis commonly supervenes as a result of sensitivity to antibiotics or other locally applied medicaments. These changes are the consequence of increased capillary permeability with escape of blood constituents into subcutaneous tissue. Lysis of red cells and haemosiderin deposition leads to pigmentation. Protein leaches into the extravascular space disturbing the osmotic equilibrium and giving rise to oedema. There has been much interest of late in the observation that venous insufficiency is associated with white cell sequestration in the tissues of the lower legs and the possibility that white cell activation may be responsible for the some of the observed pathological changes.

The basis of all *conservative treatment* is to counteract venous hypertension by elevation of the part if the patient can be kept at rest, or by means of firm compression by bandages or elastic stockings if he or she is ambulant. The importance of correctly applied high quality elastic bandage or properly fitting hosiery cannot be overemphasized. The patient will rapidly discard items which are uncomfortable or ill fitting.

Elastic bandages seldom provide sustained compression unless they are cohesive and applied by an expert bandager. Such bandages must always include the forefoot and extend to the knee. Compression should graduated, that is maximal in the lower calf and diminishing as the bandage ascends. The same is true of stockings of which the most generally useful types are of knee length.

A full account of the management of leg ulcers is beyond the scope of this book. However, it may be said that provided that the associated conditions are treated and the venous hypertension counteracted by physical measures the nature of the ulcer dressings are of secondary importance. Paste-impregnated bandages are the most generally useful dressing but a proportion of patients are sensitive to the constituents of the pastes. All agents which tend to cause allergy, especially local antibiotics, should be avoided. *Operation* is usually advocated without undue delay for the younger patient, but a preliminary period of conservative treatment is advisable, in order to reduce oedema and to obtain complete or partial healing of the ulcer before surgical intervention. In the case of older patients, operation may be reserved for those in whom conservative treatment is unsuccessful. It should not, however, be postponed for too long, for the results are less favourable when the ulcer is of long standing; in such cases, where irreversible changes may have occurred, skin grafting is likely to be an essential part of the treatment.

If varices are present in the superficial venous system, and if the deep veins have been shown to be patent, the superficial varices should be treated by one of the methods already described. It is usually advised that such treatment should include ligation or injection of perforating veins in the vicinity of the ulcer. Where there are advanced skin changes the subfascial method of perforator ligation is preferred.

Should venous ulceration persist despite well performed surgery to the superficial veins then it is likely that there is incompetence in the deep system. The surgical restoration of competence to deep valves is still in the realms of experimental surgery.

VENOUS THROMBOSIS AND EMBOLISM

The effective management of this condition depends very much on accurate diagnosis; the unreliability of clinical diagnosis is well known. For the detection of venous thrombosis Doppler ultrasound, the radio-iodine uptake tests and various types of plethysmography all have their place but if active treatment, especially thrombolytic therapy or surgery is planned, phlebography is still the most important investigation. Similarly, lung scanning or pulmonary angiography are of prime importance if pulmonary embolism is suspected. The opportunities for successful pulmonary embolectomy are, however, rare.

The majority of patients with venous thrombosis and/or pulmonary embolism can be satisfactorily treated with a week to 10 days of intravenous heparin overlapped with and followed by oral anticoagulants. Life threatening pulmonary embolism or major deep vein thrombosis of recent onset (within 4 days) which carries the risk of lethal embolism or post-thrombotic problems should be treated with thrombolysis, provided that there is no major bleeding risk such as an active peptic ulcer, fracture or major operation within the last 10 days. The choice of thrombolytic agent is largely determined by cost and availability. Tissue Plasminogen Activator (TPA) has the quickest action and avoids allergic reaction but is the most expensive. Urokinase is also expensive. Streptokinase is the least expensive but is slower to act and frequently causes considerable systemic upset. All carry a bleeding risk.

There are two possible surgical approaches to venous thrombosis: venous thrombectomy and venous interruption.

Venous thrombectomy

This operation is seldom performed today although some authors still recommend it for phlegmasia caerulea dolens. While it is not technically difficult to remove thrombus from an occluded vein, especially since the advent of the Fogarty catheter, there is a high frequency of rethrombosis, despite anticoagulation and the construction of an arteriovenous fistula, and follow-up studies have shown the majority of results to be disappointing. Furthermore, the patients in whom thrombectomy carries the best chance of success, those with newly formed iliofemoral deep vein thrombosis (DVT), are those who are most likely to respond to thrombolytic therapy with streptokinase.

Venous filter insertion

The prime indication for filter insertion is pulmonary embolism which has occurred despite properly controlled anticoagulation. It should also be considered where there is phlebographically demonstrated recent thrombus in a patient in whom thrombolytic therapy or anticoagulation is contraindicated. Any patient who requires abdominal surgery and who has a well documented history of thrombo-embolism should be considered for caval plication at the same operation. Venous interruption carries the theoretical risk of precipitating a post-thrombotic syndrome but in fact, in the majority of cases, modern filters remain widely patent. The filter is inserted percutaneously as a radiological procedure.

LYMPHOEDEMA

It is rare for lymphoedema to be treated surgically since the results are seldom cosmetically attractive or of long term benefit.

Primary lymphoedema is common, especially in its milder forms and may develop in childhood (lymphoedema praecox) or in early or middle adult life (lymphoedema tarda). It is still unclear in fact whether primary lymphoedema is the result of vascular dysplasia in utero or an acquired vascular disorder.

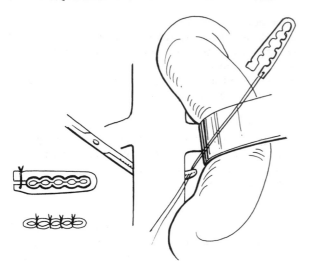

Fig. 3.27 Caval plication. Clip and suture plication are shown in cross-section. The Miles serrated clip is placed around the inferior vena cava below the renal vein, with the help of a silk ligature

Lymphangiography generally shows the lymphatics to be deficient or obliterated but occasionally an obstructed pattern may be seen. Secondary lymphoedema is the result of recurrent infections, malignant invasion, radiation, surgery or trauma.

Skin complications are those of hyperkeratosis and fissuring. Patients with lymphoedema are prone to recurrent episodes of spreading cellulitis, commonly precipitated by fungal infection, each of which causes further damage to the lymphatic drainage.

The diagnosis is made clinically. Lymphangiography is seldom indicated since management is almost invariably conservative with postural drainage, pneumatic compression and elastic graduated compression therapy. Skin care is important including the regular use of antifungal preparations and the control of bacterial infections with antibiotics.

Various operations to enhance lymphatic drainage have been describe with little evidence of success. When the bulk of the limb is so severe, despite vigorously applied conservative measures, as to constitute a serious disability then excisional surgery, such as the Charles or the Thompson operation, is indicated. The reader is referred to specialist texts.

OPERATIONS ON THE SYMPATHETIC NERVOUS SYSTEM

General considerations
Sympathectomy is less popular than formerly but is occasionally carried out (1) to improve the circulation in the limbs by the abolition of vasoconstrictor tone; (2) for the relief of visceral and causalgic pains; and (3) as a cure for hyperhidrosis.

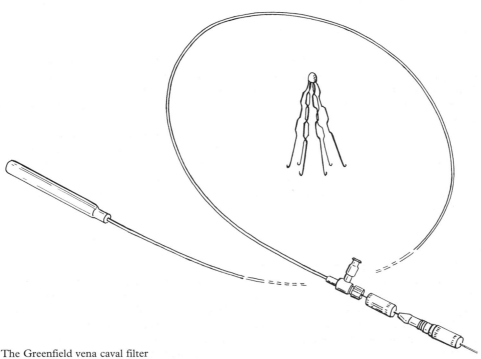

Fig. 3.28 The Greenfield vena caval filter

Anatomy

Sympathetic fibres to the lower limb, emerging from the cord between T.9 and L.2, pass through the lumbar ganglia. Removal of the lumbar 2 and 3 ganglia will thus cut off the entire sympathetic supply to the limb concerned. All sympathetic fibres to the upper limb emerge from the spinal cord between the 2nd and 8th thoracic segments, and thereafter pass through the upper three thoracic ganglia, removal of which abolishes the sympathetic supply to the upper limb. However, removal of the whole 'stellate' ganglion (the fused inferior cervical and 1st thoracic ganglia) interferes with the sympathetic supply to the head and neck and causes Horner's syndrome.

The sympathetic nerves control the tone of all arteries which have a considerable amount of smooth muscle in their walls. For practical purposes this means the medium sized and small arteries and arterioles of the limbs and the arteriovenous anastomoses. Sympathectomy may be indicated to obtain vasodilatation where the peripheral vessels show an excessive response to cold or emotion or where there is already obstruction of the main artery and dilatation of the resultant collateral circulation is desirable.

Raynaud's syndrome, acrocyanosis and erythrocyanosis

These are conditions where the vasoconstrictor response is excessive. Sympathectomy is rarely indicated in true primary Raynaud's in young women, but may provide symptomatic relief should the attacks continue and become more frequent or prolonged. Improvement may also follow cervicodorsal sympathectomy in secondary Raynaud's syndrome, but is liable to be temporary and be followed by relapse. Removal of the second and third lumbar ganglia improves the circulation in the cold, blue leg syndromes of young women and in neurological disorders where muscular paralysis may be associated with vasoconstriction and low blood flow to the distal part of the limb.

Thrombo-angeitis obliterans (Buerger's disease)

This involves the arteries distal to the knee and the elbow, but sympathectomy may help to delay the progress of the disease in the early stages and to lead to more limited amputations when these become necessary.

Critical ischaemia

In atherosclerosis, there is slow and often widespread occlusion of the main vessels to the limb. In cases where direct reconstructive surgery is not possible, sympathectomy may be done with the intention of dilating the collateral circulation. This often makes the foot warmer, brings temporary relief of pain, or improves ulceration.

Causalgia

This is the term is used to designate the persistent and intense pain which may follow minor amputations, or partial injury to a mixed nerve. The aetiology of the pain is obscure, but complete relief can often be obtained by sympathectomy.

Hyperhidrosis

Excessive sweating of the limbs can be completely abolished by sympathectomy. When sweating is sufficiently profuse to cause significant social or occupational inconvenience the operation should be advised.

Tests for vasomotor release

The potential response to sympathectomy can be tested by inducing reflex vasodilatation, by spinal anaesthesia or by paravertebral block. However, these tests are not always reliable and are seldom thought to be a necessary preliminary to sympathectomy today.

Paravertebral block

Surgical lumbar sympathectomy has been largely superseded by paravertebral injection. Similarly surgical cervicodorsal sympathectomy has been replaced by transthoracic endoscopic sympathectomy. A single injection of local anaesthetic can be used as a diagnostic or therapeutic test and may give immediate (albeit temporary) relief of causalgic pain or it may abolish vasospasm in a limb for a sufficiently long time to tide the patient over some circulatory crisis. The injection of phenol under radiological control may confer lasting benefit.

Cervicothoracic block

Long slender needles of the type used for lumbar puncture are employed. The patient should be placed in the lateral position with his spine fully flexed. The head is supported on a pillow to prevent lateral bending of the cervical spine. Three wheals are raised 4 cm lateral to the spinous processes of C.7, T.1 and T.2. A long needle is introduced through each wheal perpendicular to the skin surface until it makes contact with the neck of the rib (usually the one below). It is then manipulated so that it passes below the rib, and is inclined medially at an angle of 25° towards the sagittal plane, so that it impinges on the side of the vertebral body. This contact should be obtained at a depth of not more than 3 cm beyond the rib; in the absence of contact within this limit of penetration, the needle should be directed more medially. A rubber marker transfixed by the needle is a useful way of ensuring that the safe depth of penetration is not exceeded. After an aspiration rest to ensure that the needle has not entered a blood vessel, 5 ml of 1% procaine is injected slowly. It is an advantage to insert all three needles before any injection is made, since the direction of the first needle, if correctly placed, serves as a useful guide to the insertion of the remaining two needles. After a successful injection the upper limb and the face and neck on the affected side should become hot and dry; in addition there should be enophthalmos and constriction of the pupil (*Horner's syndrome*).

Lumbar block

This procedure is best carried out in a department of Radiology so that the position of the needle can be checked by screening. The injection of a small volume of radiological contrast material helps to confirm the appropriate site for injection.

The patient lies in the lateral position with the spine fully flexed and the waist supported by a pillow; wheals of local anaesthetic are raised 7–10 cm lateral to the upper extremities of the spinous processes of L.2 and 3. A 19 gauge needle 12–18 cm in length is introduced perpendicularly through each wheal until it makes contact with the transverse process. It is then partially withdrawn and re-inserted in a more upward direction so that it passes above the transverse process. At a depth of 2 to 3 cm beyond the process its point should be felt to scrape against the side of the vertebral body; if such contact is not obtained the needle is directed more medially. Local anaesthetic is infiltrated at each stage. A rubber marker should be used for the correct measurement of penetration. Any sharp pain indicates that the needle has struck a lumbar nerve, and its direction should at once be changed. After the needles have been placed and aspiration tests carried out 5 ml of 1% procaine (temporary block), or 4 ml of 8% phenol in Urografin (permanent block) is injected through each. If the injection has been correctly placed, there should be immediate cessation of sweating in the lower limb on the affected side; the degree of improvement in the circulation will depend upon the capacity of the vessels to dilate.

Cervicothoracic sympathectomy

This implies the removal at least of the 2nd and 3rd thoracic ganglia, which contain the cells of most of the postganglionic fibres supplying the upper limb. Preganglionic fibres are believed to reach these ganglia by one or two routes. They may travel by white rami communicantes from the 2nd and 3rd thoracic nerves (the sympathetic outflow from T.1 being distributed mainly to the head and neck). If they are derived from spinal roots lower than T.3, and enter corresponding ganglia of the sympathetic chain, they must thereafter ascend in the chain in order to synapse with post-ganglionic fibres supplying the upper limb. For complete denervation of the upper limb, it may be thought advisable

to remove the small lower part of the stellate ganglion (the part representing the 1st thoracic ganglion), the division being made below the level where the rami communicantes from the 1st thoracic nerve join the ganglion, so that a Horner's syndrome is avoided. For hyperhidrosis affecting the head and neck, it is necessary to remove the whole stellate ganglion (or at least to divide the rami from T.1) and thus to accept a Horner's syndrome. For axillary hyperhidrosis or for anginal pain, the upper four or five thoracic ganglia should be removed.

The procedure of choice for cervicodorsal sympathectomy today is transthoracic endoscopic sympathectomy.

Transthoracic endoscopic thoracic sympathectomy

Pre-operative investigations include a chest radiograph. Previous apical lung disease will preclude this procedure. Equipment includes a Veres needle, trochar and cannula and a catheterizing laparoscope with insulated electrode. General anaesthesia with a double lumen endotracheal tube is employed and the patient positioned supine with the arm abducted to 90°. The Veres needle is introduced into the 3rd or 4th intercostal space in the mid axillary line, the ipsilateral lung allowed to collapse and a total of 2 litres of carbon dioxide insufflated in four batches of 500 ccs. The Veres needle is then withdrawn and the trochar and cannula introduced, the trochar withdrawn and the laparoscope introduced through the cannula. The telescope itself may be used to push the lung out of the way or a separate retracting rod introduced through an anterior intercostal space. The sympathetic cord is identified as a pale pink structure traversing the heads of the ribs. It is coagulated from the neck of the third rib up to the pleural vault. The laparoscope is withdrawn and the pleural cavity vented while the anaesthetist re-expands the lung. The entry hole is closed with a mattress suture and a chest radiograph on the operating table taken to verify lung expansion. The procedure may now be repeated on the other side.

Anterior surgical approach

This method involves a somewhat difficult dissection but produces less post-operative pain than the alternative approaches. Both sides can be done at the one sitting, and convalescence is rapid. The ganglia are approached above the arch of the subclavian artery. The first part of the operation is similar to that described for exposure of the third part of the subclavian artery (p. 38) except that the clavicular head of sternomastoid is divided to expose scalenus anterior and the phrenic nerve. Thereafter (the phrenic nerve being safeguarded) scalenus anterior is divided at its insertion

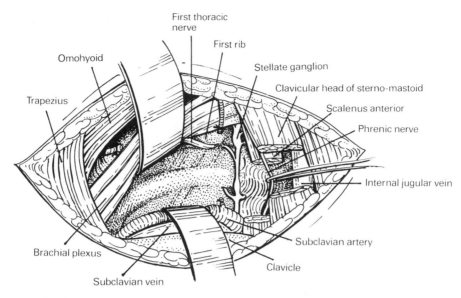

Fig. 3.29 Cervicothoracic sympathectomy by the anterior route above the arch of the subclavian artery

into the 1st rib. The subclavian artery, which is now exposed in the greater part of its length, is gently mobilized (Fig. 3.29) and retracted downwards. The thyrocervical artery is seen and ligated with silk. The vertebral artery does not appear at all in the field, and the internal mammary artery remains medially. The suprapleural membrane is detached from the inner border of the 1st rib, and the pleura is displaced downwards and laterally to expose the bodies of the upper three thoracic vertebrae and the posterior ends of the corresponding ribs. The sympathetic trunk is identified crossing the necks of the ribs (the 'stellate' ganglion lying on the 1st rib) and is divided just below the 3rd thoracic ganglion. The upper segment is drawn upwards and laterally, and the rami passing to and from the 2nd and 3rd ganglia are divided, after which these ganglia are removed. The lower third of the stellate ganglion is also removed.

Axillary approach

This method gives easy and direct access to the upper thoracic ganglia, but is a less convenient approach to the stellate ganglion. It should only be considered if endoscopic equipment is not available or if apical lung pathology would make endoscopy difficult. An incision 10–12 cm in length is made in the medial wall of the axilla along the line of the 2nd intercostal space, and is deepened through the fibres of serratus anterior until the space is reached. The only structure of importance to be avoided here is the nerve to serratus anterior, but this is usually behind the posterior end of the wound,

and is therefore not seen. The pleural cavity is entered after division of the intercostal muscles. A rib spreader is introduced, and the intercostal space is forcibly enlarged to an extent of 5–6 cm. This must be done very slowly to obviate postoperative pain. By means of a gauze roll and a suitable retractor, the lung is drawn downwards. The sympathetic chain should now be seen through the parietal pleura (Fig. 3.30), and the various ganglia are identified — the stellate, from its position on the neck of the first rib. The overlying pleura is then incised, and the sympathetic chain is divided below the 3rd thoracic ganglion (or, when indicated, below the 4th or 5th). The ganglia above the level of section are now mobilised and turned upwards, care being taken to avoid damage to the delicate intercostal veins, and the rami communicantes attached to these ganglia are divided. The chain is finally divided above the 2nd ganglion, or through the lower part of the stellate ganglion if desired. Any bleeding from intercostal vessels is carefully arrested. An intercostal drain is inserted. After inflation of the lung, the wound is closed.

Lumbar sympathectomy

Preganglionic fibres for the lower limb leave the spinal cord in the lower four or five thoracic and upper two lumbar nerves. They enter corresponding ganglia of the sympathetic chain, and descend in the chain to synapse around postganglionic cells in the lower lumbar ganglia and in the sacral ganglia. Removal of the 2nd and 3rd ganglia denervates the limb from the middle of the

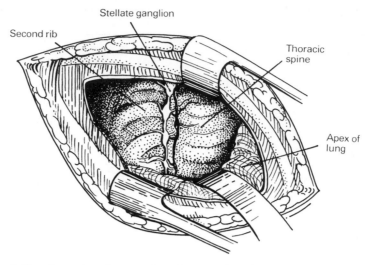

Fig. 3.30 Axillary (transpleural) approach to the upper thoracic ganglia of the sympathetic chain

thigh distally: removal of the 1st ganglion denervates the groin and the upper half of the thigh. It should be noted that, in regard to the sympathetic innervation of vessels below the knee (i.e. in the sciatic distribution) this is a preganglionic operation, for the fibres supplying these vessels have their cell stations in the sacral ganglia, which are not disturbed. In a bilateral operation, the 1st lumbar ganglion on at least one side should be left, since removal of both ganglia may cause sterility, due to paralysis of the ejaculatory mechanism.

The extraperitoneal approach is now accepted as the standard method, since it entails no intra-peritoneal disturbance. Both sides can be done at the one sitting without adding materially to the operative risk. The patient lies partly on his side and a transverse or oblique incision is made in the loin extending from the anterior axillary line to the lateral border of the rectus. The muscles are divided in the same line, and the peritoneum is displaced medially and forwards off the posterior abdominal wall, the genital vessels and the ureter being raised with it. The sympathetic chain is found lying in the groove between the vertebral bodies and the psoas muscle. On the right side it is behind the inferior vena cava (Fig. 3.31); on the left side it is overlapped by the aorta. The first lumbar ganglion must be sought for high up under cover of the crus of the diaphragm; the 4th ganglion may be obscured by the common iliac vessels. The intraperitoneal approach may be employed when the abdomen has to be opened on account of some earlier condition. With the patient in the Trendelenburg position the peritoneal cavity is opened by a lower midline or paramedian incision, and

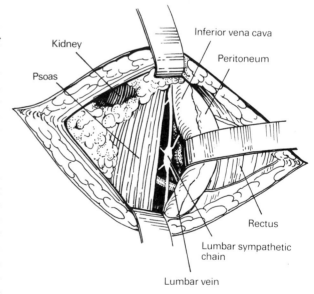

Fig. 3.31 Right-sided lumbar ganglionectomy by the extraperitoneal route

the intestines are packed off into the upper abdomen. For exposure of the left sympathetic chain, the peritoneum is incised along the lateral side of the descending colon, which is then raised from the posterior wall and retracted medially. For exposure of the right sympathetic chain the caecum and ascending colon may be mobilized in a similar manner, or a more direct approach may be made by incising the overlying peritoneum lateral to the inferior vena cava.

REFERENCES

Fogarty T J, Cranley J J, Krause R J, Strasser E S, Hafner C D 1963 A method for extraction of arterial emboli and thrombi. Surgery Gynaecology and Obstetrics 116: 241

Fogarty T J, Daily P O, Shumway N E et al 1971 Experience with balloon catheter technic for arterial embolectomy. American Journal of Surgery 122: 231

Gregg R O, Chamberlain B E, Myers J K, Tyler D B 1983 Embolectomy or Heparin therapy for arterial emboli? Surgery 93: 377

National Heart and Lung Institute, Bethesda, USA 1970 Urokinase pulmonary embolism trial. Phase I Results. Journal of the American Medical Association 214: 2163

FURTHER READING

Rutherford R B (ed) 1989 Vascular surgery. W B Saunders, Philadelphia

Bell P R F, Jamieson C W, Ruckley C V (eds) 1992 Surgical Management of Vascular Disease. W B Saunders, London

Browse N L, Burnand K G, Lea Thomas M 1988 Diseases of the veins. Arnold, London

4

Cardiac surgery

D. P. TAGGART & D. J. WHEATLEY

Open heart surgery using cardiopulmonary bypass is now one of the most frequently performed major operations in the Western world, the majority (approximately 70%) being coronary artery bypass grafting for ischaemic heart disease. Valve replacement accounts for a further 20% of operations while 5%–10% of operations are for congenital heart disease, disease of the great vessels (aneurysm of the ascending and/or transverse aortic arch) and transplantation. With the exception of atrial myxomas cardiac tumours are very uncommon and operations for cardiac trauma account for less than 1% of all operations.

In the developing world closed procedures without cardiopulmonary bypass, particularly commissurotomy for mitral stenosis, still account for the bulk of surgery. The number of open heart operations is however increasing largely due to an increase in valve replacements.

CARDIOPULMONARY RESUSCITATION

Cardiac arrest, the cessation of coordinated electromechanical activity, is the consequence of ventricular asystole or ventricular fibrillation which can only be distinguished by electrocardiography. The clinical picture is of sudden loss of consciousness, absence of peripheral pulses, dilatation of the pupils and cessation of respiration. The persistence of cardiac arrest for more than a few minutes leads to respiratory arrest and vice versa.

Management
Ideally, management of cardiac arrest requires one experienced practitioner and an assistant. In order of sequence, attention is paid to ventilation, restoration of cardiac output and correction of biochemical abnormalities. Electro-cardiographic leads are attached to the patient in order to monitor cardiac rhythm, a central or peripheral venous cannula is inserted for drug administration and a peripheral artery cannulated to monitor blood gases and blood pressure.

Airway. Establishment of an airway to ensure adequate oxygenation is crucial as irreversible hypoxic cerebral damage occurs within three to four minutes of cardiac arrest. Intubation with an endotracheal tube optimizes ventilation and prevents aspiration of vomitus but requires someone experienced in the technique. Blind attempts at tracheal intubation by an inexperienced practitioner are futile and frequently result in oesophageal intubation. Administration of 100% oxygen through an oral airway usually permits adequate ventilation until the arrival of an anaesthetist but an efficient suction disposal unit must be available to prevent aspiration.

Circulation. External cardiac massage consists of mechanical compression of the precordium towards the vertebral column and its adequacy is confirmed by the presence of a peripheral pulse (radial, femoral or carotid). It is conventional practice to alternate each respiratory effort with five mechanical compressions. When properly conducted it achieves an effective

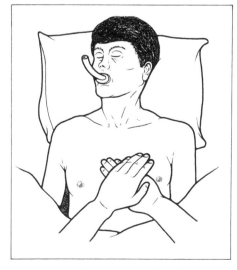

Fig. 4.1 External cardiac massage. With the patient lying on a firm surface, the sternum is pressed rhythmically towards the vertebral column 60 times per minute

cardiac output and internal cardiac massage is rarely indicated.

Ventricular asystole and fibrillation are indistinguishable in the absence of electrocardiography. In asystole a cautious blow to the precordium with a clenched hand may restore electrical rhythm. If electrical activity returns but is bradycardic (less than 50 beats per minute) atropine is administered (3 mg to 6 mg i.v. bolus). If there is no electrical response adrenaline is administered every few minutes (1 mg–2 mg i.v. bolus), between massage, until the restoration of electrical activity. Adrenaline frequently converts asystole to ventricular fibrillation suitable for cardioversion. Primary ventricular fibrillation or that occurring as a consequence of adrenaline administration requires defibrillation to restore a coordinated electrical rhythm. Direct current discharges from 200 joules up to 360 joules are administered until a satisfactory rhythm is restored. Electromechanical dissociation refers to the electrocardiographic restoration of an electrical rhythm but without accompanying mechanical cardiac activity. During resuscitation and after restoration of an apparently satisfactory electrocardiograhic rhythm it is essential, therefore, to check for the presence of a peripheral pulse confirming an adequate blood pressure.

Biochemistry. Persistence of (or recurrence of) fibrillation is treated with lignocaine (100 mg i.v. bolus followed by an infusion if necessary). Blood biochemistry is checked to ensure satisfactory serum potassium and arterial blood gases. Hyperkalaemia is an invariable consequence of prolonged cardiac arrest and if serum potassium is greater than 6.5 mmol/L calcium chloride is administered (10 ml of 10% solution as i.v. bolus). The presence of a profound acidosis requires administration of sodium bicarbonate (50–100 ml of 8.4% solution intravenously).

Consolidation. After successful resuscitation the patient is transferred to an intensive care or coronary care unit. Minimum requirements for monitoring are a triple-lumen central venous cannula (for blood sampling and fluid and drug administration) and radial artery cannula (for continuous blood pressure monitoring and arterial gas sampling). Other requirements, depending on particular circumstances, may include a Swan-Ganz catheter (for serial measurements of cardiac output), temporary pacing lines, inotropic support and intra-aortic balloon counter-pulsation.

Failure of cardiopulmonary resuscitation. Prompt application of the above measures usually achieves successful resuscitation. Failure to restore adequate cardiac output, in the presence of normal biochemistry, raises the possibility of one of the following conditions.

TENSION PNEUMOTHORAX is suspected with unilateral or bilateral absence of breath sounds, tracheal shift and the persistence of severe hypoxia. There is no time for radiological confirmation and treatment consists of placing a venous cannula in the mid-clavicular line in the second intercostal space of the suspected side. If the diagnosis is correct there is an immediate audible escape of air accompanied by an improvement in cardio-respiratory status. An underwater-seal chest drain is placed as soon as practical.

PULMONARY EMBOLISM is suggested by the absence of cardiac output despite effective external cardiac massage, the persistence of severe hypoxia despite adequate ventilation and a very high central venous pressure. The patient is ventilated with 100% oxygen while theatre is prepared for pulmonary embolectomy.

HYPOVOLAEMIA is suggested by the inability to achieve an effective cardiac output despite effective external cardiac compression and an abnormally low central venous pressure. It may result from unsuspected rupture of a major vessel as with aneurysms of the thoracic or abdominal aorta or from a bleeding duodenal ulcer. Treatment consists of correction of hypovolaemia with plasma expanders until blood is available (ABO O Rhesus negative blood may be used in dire circumstances) and the source of bleeding is identified.

SURGICAL APPROACH TO THE HEART

In the vast majority of operations on the heart and great vessels the approach is through a median sternotomy incision which provides easy, rapid and excellent exposure of the pericardial sac immediately behind the sternum. Left anterolateral thoracotomy is used for certain closed procedures (e.g. closed mitral valvotomy, systemic to pulmonary shunts, approach to patent ductus arteriosus and aortic coarctation) and for urgent access to the pericardium (e.g. tamponade following myocardial injury). Right thoracotomy is used to perform certain systemic to pulmonary shunts. The technique of thoracotomy is described in Chapter 5.

Median sternotomy (Fig. 4.2)
The skin *incision* runs from the suprasternal notch vertically in the midline to the xiphisternum. The incision is deepened in the midline, avoiding the origins of the pectoral muscles, to the sternal periosteum. The suprasternal ligament is divided with diathermy avoiding the brachio-cephalic vein deep to the sternal notch. Inferiorly the xiphisternum is divided with scissors and finger dissection is used to sweep clear any diaphragmatic or pleural attachments.

Mechanical ventilation is temporarily interrupted during sternal division to avoid inadvertent opening of the pleural sac(s). The sternum is divided in the mid-

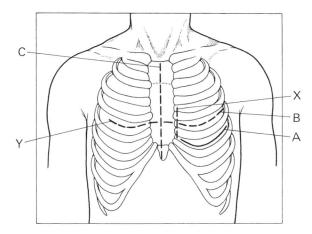

Fig. 4.2 Incisions for exposure of the heart. Median sternotomy (C) is most commonly used. A & B – lateral thoracotomy – extended to X or Y if necessary

line using either a vertical sternotome or an oscillating saw (particularly important in repeat surgery where the heart may be stuck to the back of the sternum). In the absence of a mechanical saw, the sternum can be split with a Gigli saw, passing the wire behind the length of the sternum with a long pair of forceps. Bleeding from the sternal marrow is reduced by sparing application of bone wax and bleeding from the periosteal edges by diathermy.

A self-retaining retractor is used to separate the sternal edges and the pleural sacs are swept off the pericardium. The thymus lying on the pericardium in the superior mediastinum is divided avoiding the innominate vein superiorly.

The pericardium is divided vertically in the midline from the aorta superiorly to the diaphragm inferiorly where the incision is extended bilaterally to give an inverted 'T' incision. The pericardial margins are sutured to the sternal edges elevating the heart from the pericardial cavity.

The sternum is *closed* with 6 or 8 interrupted steel wires being careful not to puncture the internal mammary arteries. The soft tissues are approximated in the midline ensuring there is no 'dead space' over the sternal periosteum.

PRINCIPLES AND TECHNIQUES OF CARDIOPULMONARY BYPASS

Cardiopulmonary bypass (CPB) using an extracorporeal circuit is essential for all open cardiac operations. The aim is to provide a systemic circulation so that precise surgery can be performed while the heart is arrested and emptied of blood.

There are various methods of achieving CPB but the general principle involves gravitational drainage of venous blood from the right heart to an extracorporeal perfusion circuit where, after gas and temperature exchange, it is returned to the arterial circulation.

The heart is prepared for CPB by cannulation of the ascending aorta and the right atrium after administration of heparin (3 mg/kg of body weight) to produce an Activated Clotting Time in excess of 400 seconds. A purse string suture is placed in the adventitia of the ascending aorta and passed through a tourniquet. An arterial cannula is then passed into the aorta through the purse string suture and secured to the tourniquet by a heavy suture. A large bore cannula for venous drainage is then passed through a purse-string suture in the right atrial wall and tied to a tourniquet. For most operations a single venous cannula provides satisfactory drainage but when considerable retraction is necessary (mitral valve replacement) or if there is a risk of air entrapment (when opening a cardiac chamber) then the inferior and superior vena cavae are cannulated separately and snared with cotton tapes.

The key components of the perfusion circuit (the 'pump') include (Fig. 4.3):

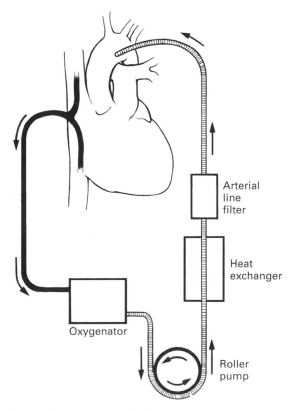

Fig. 4.3 Extracorporeal circuit

1. An *oxygenator* where oxygen is added to and carbon dioxide removed from blood (as both heart and lungs are excluded from the circulation during CPB).

2. A *heat exchanger* to cool blood initially and subsequently rewarm it.

3. *Cardiotomy suction* — the use of sump suckers placed in the pericardial cavity to return spilled heparinised blood to the pump.

4. A *roller pump* to return blood to the patient via the aorta. The pump can return blood at a steady rate (non-pulsatile perfusion) or in a pulsed mode (pulsatile perfusion) which may more accurately mimic the physiological situation.

5. An *arterial line filter* to remove debris and particulate matter from the arterial line of the pump returning blood to the patient.

On commencement of CPB the surgeon ensures that the heart empties and that the arterial line pressure is not excessively high (suggesting misplacement or poor positioning of the aortic cannula). The heart is therefore perfused but performing little mechanical work. Systemic blood temperature is usually reduced to between 28 and 32°C (moderate hypothermia) reducing metabolic rates and providing a safety margin, particularly for the brain, in case of pump failure.

The aorta is clamped proximal to the aortic cannula (Fig. 4.4) but distal to the coronary arteries so that, with the exception of some mediastinal collateral blood flow, little blood enters the heart or lungs if venous drainage is adequate. A cardioplegia solution

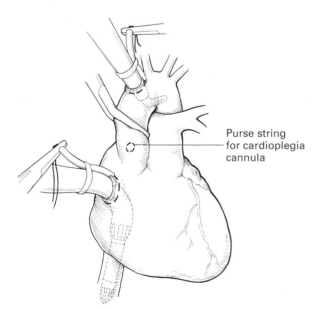

Fig. 4.4 Cannulation of right atrium and aortic arch for extracorporeal circuit

Purse string for cardioplegia cannula

(Hartmann's solution with a high potassium concentration) at a temperature of 4°C is then infused into the aortic root proximal to the cross clamp to produce asystolic arrest. At this stage the heart is ischaemic, as it is not receiving oxygenated blood, but because it is flaccid and cold its metabolic requirements are reduced to less than 5% of normal. Further myocardial cooling is achieved with topical slushed ice or a cooling jacket. Repeated administration of cardioplegic solution at 20 to 30 minute intervals permits ischaemic times of up to one hour before there is significant irreversible myocardial injury. The surgeon can therefore operate on the coronary arteries or valves of the heart in a quiet bloodless field.

There are many variations on the technique of CPB and detailed discussion is beyond the scope of this book. One common variation is to use the femoral artery for arterial return when access to the mediastinum is difficult due to previous surgery or in the presence of an ascending aortic aneurysm. Some surgeons prefer potassium-enriched blood rather than crystalloid cardioplegia and some administer the cardioplegic solution retrogradely through the coronary sinus rather than antegradely through the aortic root. The need for routine systemic and topical hypothermia has been challenged but for certain complex congenital operations and for surgery of the aorta involving the head and neck vessels profound hypothermia to a systemic temperature of 15–20°C permits total arrest of the circulation for thirty to sixty minutes.

Complications of CPB
CPB is a safe procedure and the mortality directly attributable to its effects are considerably less than 1%. CPB does, however, result in a 'whole body inflammatory' response due to systemic activation of a myriad of inflammatory mediators including complement and white blood cells in the extracorporeal circuit. The syndrome is characterised by temporary and usually reversible deficiencies in coagulation as well as cardiac, cerebral, respiratory and renal function.

The most worrying complication of cardiac surgery is overt cerebral damage in 1%–2% of patients. This is more common in elderly patients, in those with proven cerebrovascular disease and in patients undergoing valve replacement (due to embolization of air or calcific debris from the valve). One-third of patients suffer subtle neuropsychological impairment which recovers in the majority within 3–6 months.

TRAUMA TO THE HEART AND GREAT VESSELS

Blunt cardiac trauma usually results from road traffic

accidents or crush injuries to the chest and its consequences may be minor or catastrophic. Minor cardiac contusion, suggested by myocardial irritability and electrocardiographic changes, usually runs a benign course. Severe blunt injury may result in thrombosis of a coronary artery due to intimal tears, valvular or ventricular septal disruption, or even myocardial rupture.

Exsanguination is the usual consequence of myocardial gunshot wounds whereas penetrating stab wounds often result in cardiac tamponade and circulatory shock. In such circumstances emergency thoracotomy through the left fifth intercostal space to open the pericardium relieves the tamponade and produces an immediate improvement in cardiac output.

Penetrating injuries of cardiac muscle can usually be sutured with 3/0 prolene. Damage to a distal coronary artery is unlikely to produce major myocardial instability but laceration of a proximal coronary artery requires bypass grafting.

Thoracic aorta

Blunt injury to the thoracic aorta is frequently fatal. Injuries of the ascending aorta are almost invariably fatal and the majority (85%) of patients with descending thoracic aortic disruption die outside hospital. The usual site of aortic injury following blunt trauma is immediately distal to the left subclavian artery (the aortic isthmus) between the relatively fixed distal aortic arch and mobile descending aorta. Sudden deceleration, as in road traffic accidents, produces shearing at the isthmus resulting in a transverse linear tear. Complete aortic rupture results in exsanguination but occasionally aortic adventitia and mediastinal pleura maintain continuity between the transected aortic ends resulting in a false aneurysm which is at imminent risk of further rupture.

A history of deceleration injury and/or signs of significant chest injury such as sternal fracture, fracture of the first two ribs or multiple fractures raise the possibility of aortic injury. There may be few clinical features to suggest aortic disruption but hypertension in the upper limbs and weak femoral pulses accompanied by a widened mediastinum on chest radiography are highly suggestive. Aortography or CT scanning is necessary to confirm aortic dissection as a widened mediastinum may result from haematoma due to bleeding from small vessels of the sternum, ribs or thymus.

ISCHAEMIC HEART DISEASE

Ischaemic heart disease is the most common cause of death in the Western world and coronary revascularization is now one of the most frequently performed major operations. In 1990 almost one quarter of a million coronary artery operations and an equal number of coronary angioplasties were performed in the USA.

Pathologically, ischaemic heart disease results from atherosclerosis which predominantly affects the proximal segments of coronary arteries leaving the distal segments relatively disease free. The symptoms of ischaemic heart disease can be treated with drugs, angioplasty or surgery depending on the angiographically documented nature and extent of disease.

Percutaneous transluminal coronary angioplasty or balloon dilatation of localized coronary artery stenoses was initially described in 1976 by the cardiologist Gruntzig. A guide wire is inserted into the femoral artery and passed retrogradely up the aorta, under radiological control, to the stenosis in the coronary artery. A balloon catheter is advanced over the guide wire to the stenosis and inflated for a few minutes. Symptomatic improvement is initially achieved in 90% of patients but not all lesions are suitable for angioplasty and the technique is complicated by a re-stenosis rate of 30%–50% within 6 months. Angioplasty has also been used in the treatment of multi-vessel coronary disease but with less successful results. Complications of angioplasty include arterial dissection, occlusion of the dilated artery with a 1%–2% mortality and the need for urgent surgery in 2%–4% of patients.

The indications for surgical treatment of ischaemic heart disease are:

- symptomatic (severe symptoms of angina unresponsive to optimal medical therapy)
- prognostic (angiographic demonstration of stenoses known to adversely affect prognosis and with distal vessel(s) suitable for bypass grafting).

The rationale for coronary artery surgery is based on anatomical, pathological and clinical grounds. The left anterior descending, left circumflex and right coronary arteries lie on the epicardial surface of the heart in relatively constant anatomical positions. Atherosclerosis predominantly affects the proximal vessel leaving the distal vessel suitable for bypass grafting. Coronary revascularization has repeatedly been shown to be very effective in relieving angina and improving life expectancy for certain anatomical disease patterns (left main stem stenosis, three vessel disease, two vessel disease involving the proximal left anterior descending coronary artery particularly in the presence of impaired ventricular function).

The mortality of elective coronary surgery in the UK is currently 1%–2% but varies with age, symptomatic status and severity of left ventricular dysfunction. *Angiography* is essential for accurate identification of the number and severity of stenoses in the coronary arteries (Fig. 4.5). Most patients require three grafts

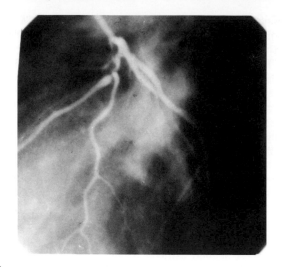

A

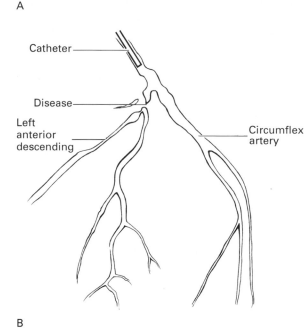

B

Fig. 4.5 Coronary angiogram showing severe disease at origin of left anterior descending coronary artery

Technique

The technique of vein grafting involves an oblique end-to-side anastomosis between the distal bevelled portion of a *reversed* segment of vein to an arteriotomy in the coronary artery distal to the stenosis (Fig. 4.6). Subsequently the proximal portion of the vein is anastomosed to the ascending aorta. The distal end of the internal mammary artery is usually anastomosed to the left anterior descending coronary artery while its proximal portion is left attached to the subclavian artery.

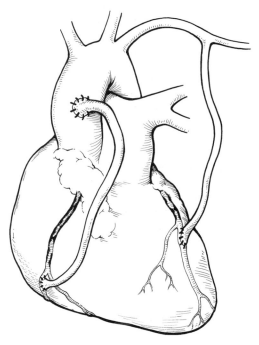

Fig. 4.6 Anastomosis of saphenous vein to right anterior descending coronary artery from aorta; anastomosis of internal mammary artery to left anterior descending coronary artery

Cardiac surgery after myocardial infarction

The vast majority of patients with acute myocardial infarction are managed medically. Immediate administration of streptokinase restores vessel patency and reduces early and late mortality. There is no evidence that emergency angioplasty or surgery is of benefit in patients with established myocardial infarction whereas both may be beneficial in unstable angina.

Acute complications of myocardial infarction which may require urgent surgery are ventricular septal defect or papillary muscle rupture causing mitral incompetence. The mortality of both these conditions is very high without surgery but operation also carries a significant mortality. Ventricular aneurysm is a chronic complication of myocardial infarction which may produce

and the most commonly used conduits are long saphenous vein (rarely short saphenous or cephalic vein) and internal mammary artery. Ten years after coronary surgery more than 90% of internal mammary artery grafts remain disease free while approximately 50% of vein grafts are occluded and a further 25% significantly diseased. In view of better long term patency rates with arterial conduits both internal mammary arteries and also the gastroepiploic artery can be used to perform total arterial revascularization.

profound ventricular dysfunction, with or without ventricular dysrhythmias. Repair of discrete ventricular aneurysms may produce considerable improvement in ventricular function.

VALVULAR HEART DISEASE

Replacement of the aortic or mitral valve (and rarely the tricuspid valve) accounts for approximately 20% of the workload of most cardiac surgical centres. With the decline in rheumatic fever in the Western world, aortic valve disease is increasingly due to calcification in a congenitally bicuspid valve or to calcific degeneration with advanced age. Mitral valve disease is still frequently a late sequela of rheumatic heart disease but increasingly due to mitral valve prolapse or to degenerative or ischaemic disease.

In the developing world aortic and mitral valve disease are still most frequently due to rheumatic heart disease. Mitral stenosis due to fused but otherwise pliable leaflets and uncomplicated by significant valve calcification, incompetence or fusion of the subvalvular apparatus can be treated by 'closed' valvulotomy with excellent results. The valve can be split either with a finger introduced through a purse-string in the left atrium or a dilator introduced through a purse-string in the apex of the left ventricle (Fig. 4.7).

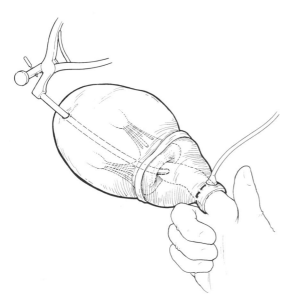

Fig. 4.7 Closed mitral valvotomy with transventricular dilator, guided by finger in left atrium

Valve replacement
The most important decisions about valve replacement are (i) timing of the operation and (ii) nature of the valvular prosthesis. Optimal timing of surgery is deter-

mined by a combination of clinical, echocardiographic and cardiac catheterization data. The natural history of aortic and mitral valve disease, for both stenotic and regurgitant lesions, was well established before valve replacement was a widely available option. Many patients remain well for a number of years with valvular heart disease because of cardiac compensatory mechanisms such as hypertrophy and dilatation. Thus, a modestly diseased valve may still be a better option than an artificial valve with its inherent disadvantages such as limited durability of tissue prosthesis and the need for anticoagulant therapy with mechanical prosthesis. On the other hand surgery should not be inappropriately delayed until there is severe irreversible myocardial damage.

Choice of valve
There is an increasing trend towards repair rather than replacement of the native mitral and aortic valve as this may result in better preservation of left ventricular function and reduce some complications associated with prosthetic valves. Not all valves are suitable for reconstruction and the spectrum of repair procedures varies from commissurotomy at its simplest to transfer of the chordae tendineae and valve leaflets.

The choice of mechanical or tissue valve depends largely on patient characteristics and often there is no absolute advantage of one over the other. Essentially there is a balance of risks between limited durability of tissue valves (but the possibility of avoiding anticoagulants) and the risks of long term anticoagulation with mechanical valves (but a lower incidence of structural failure reduces the chances of requiring further valve replacement). Mechanical valves may be of a tilting disc, bileaflet or ball and cage variety (Fig. 4.8).

Tissue valves do not require long-term anticoagulation if the patient remains in sinus rhythm. Tissue valves do, however, deteriorate with time and the failure rate is inversely proportional to age at implantation being at least 50% by 10 years in patients less than 40 years of age at implantation, 20% at 10 years in patients less than 60 years of age at implantation but negligible in patients aged over 70 years. Tissue valves are more prone to failure in the mitral than the aortic position (because of greater haemodynamic stress across the mitral valve). While failure of a tissue prosthesis is usually a slow procedure over months or years, allowing time for a further elective operation, failure of a mechanical valve, although rare, is sudden and catastrophic and patients frequently die before reaching hospital.

Tissue valves are used if there is a contraindication to warfarin (e.g. bleeding duodenal ulcer) and may be preferable in younger women who have not yet completed their family because of concerns over the poten-

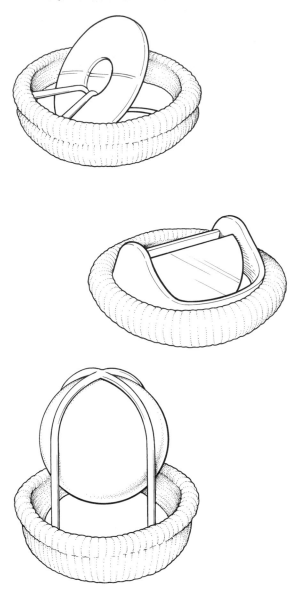

Fig. 4.8 Mechanical valves

tial teratogenicity of warfarin during pregnancy. Tissue valves may be the prosthesis of choice in patients aged over 70 years, particularly in the aortic position, as the failure rate is very low and the chances of avoiding anticoagulation high.

In general terms *mechanical valves* are indicated in younger patients because of their better durability as long as there is no strong contraindication to anti-coagulant therapy. Certain mechanical valves may have better haemodynamic function than tissue valves in smaller sizes and may therefore be preferable in patients with small aortic roots.

Technique

The surgical techniques for aortic or mitral valve re-placement are fairly standardized and variations in the technique are largely influenced by the underlying pathological process, the type of valve used and the surgeon's preference.

Most valve replacements involve the following steps:

1. The aortic valve is exposed by aortotomy in the anterior wall of the aorta. The mitral valve is exposed by an incision in the left atrium posterior and parallel to the inter-atrial groove.

2. The native valve is excised ensuring no debris falls into the ventricular cavity. In mitral valve replacement preservation of part of the posterior leaflet reduces the risk of ventricular disruption and minimises ventricular dysfunction.

3. The annulus of the prosthetic valve is sutured to the native annulus with interrupted or continuous su-tures. If the annulus is friable (e.g. in endocarditis) sutures are buttressed with teflon pledgets to reduce the chance of 'cutting out' which results in paravalve leak.

4. On completion of valve insertion, and before the aortotomy or atriotomy is closed, particular atten-tion is paid to removing all debris and air to prevent embolization.

Complications

Cerebrovascular accident. This major complication of valve replacement occurs in 2%–5% of patients and is usually due to debris from a heavily calcified valve or to air embolism.

Paravalve leaks. A paravalve leak is a regurgitant jet of blood between the valve sewing ring and the native annulus and is usually due to a stitch cutting out, particularly in the presence of severe calcification or infection.

Thromboembolic and bleeding complications. The fre-quency of these complications are inversely related, so that the greater the degree of anticoagulation the less the incidence of thromboembolic complications but the higher the incidence of spontaneous bleeding. Rigorous control of anticoagulation is necessary to minimise these complications.

Valve failure. Structural failure is much more likely with a tissue than a mechanical prosthesis particularly in younger patients and in valves inserted in the mitral position.

Endocarditis. Artificial valves, like diseased native valves, are prone to endocarditis. There is no evidence that mechanical or tissue valves are more prone to endocarditis but prophylactic antibiotics are mandatory prior to any invasive procedure.

CONGENITAL CARDIAC SURGERY

Detailed description of the pathophysiology and surgical treatment of all congenital cardiac defects is beyond the scope of this book but some of the more common conditions are described.

The incidence of congenital heart disease is approximately 8 cases per 1000 live births and advances in all aspects of management means that most defects are now amenable to surgical correction. The predominant clinical presentations of congenital heart disease are with cyanosis, cardiac failure or both. Cyanotic congenital heart disease is likely in a child without parenchymal lung disease with an arterial oxygen tension of less than 20 kPa while breathing 100% oxygen. Certain structural abnormalities which are initially acyanotic may become cyanotic with the development of pulmonary hypertension and reversal of left to right shunts (Eisenmenger syndrome). Cardiac failure is indicated by the presence of tachypnoea, tachycardia, poor perfusion, acidosis and hepatomegaly accompanied by increased vascular markings on chest radiology.

The age of presentation of a child with congenital heart disease is dependent on the underlying structural abnormality. All structural defects can occur in isolation or in association with other cardiac defects. Of every 8 children with congenital heart disease 1 or 2 will present with life-threatening symptoms immediately after birth (e.g. transposition of the great arteries) while others may not present until after the first year of life (e.g. Fallot's tetralogy). Presentation of congenital heart disease in the neonate is often related to closure of the ductus arteriosus soon after birth by a prostaglandin dependent mechanism in response to increasing circulating oxygen levels. Maintenance of duct patency is essential in certain forms of congenital heart disease. If pulmonary blood flow is duct dependent then closure results in cyanosis (e.g. pulmonary atresia, critical pulmonary stenosis, severe Fallot's tetralogy). If systemic blood flow is duct dependent then closure results in cardiac failure and acidosis due to poor tissue perfusion (e.g. critical aortic stenosis or aortic atresia). In such situations maintenance of duct patency with an infusion of prostoglandin E2 is vital until definitive treatment can be undertaken.

Palliative procedures

There is an increasing tendency to earlier definitive repair of cardiac structural abnormalities. Nevertheless, occasionally a child is too small or too ill to survive major corrective surgery and a palliative procedure 'buys time' for improvement in the child's health and growth when definitive surgery can be undertaken with less risk.

Systemic to pulmonary shunts for cyanotic congenital disease (Fig. 4.9)

Systemic to pulmonary shunts are performed to relieve cyanosis in right sided obstructive lesions or where pulmonary blood flow is duct dependent. The shunts are usually performed through a thoracotomy and do not require CPB. The success of a shunt can be judged by the presence of a shunt murmur, a decrease in cyanosis and polycythaemia, an improvement in exercise tolerance and an increase in the radiological size of the pulmonary artery.

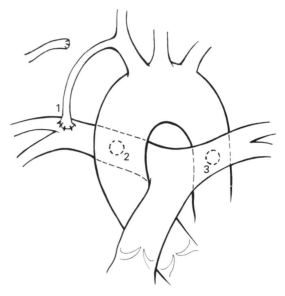

Fig. 4.9 Shunt operations for cyanotic congenital heart disease. 1 = Blalock–Taussig shunt (either subclavian artery to respective pulmonary artery. 2 = Waterston shunt (back of ascending aorta to pulmonary artery). 3 = Potts anastomosis (back of pulmonary artery to descending aorta)

Blalock–Taussig shunt. The original operation described anastomosis of the proximal end of the divided subclavian artery to the ipsilateral proximal pulmonary artery. Excessive pulmonary blood flow is limited by the diameter of the subclavian artery. The shunt is now commonly established using a prosthetic conduit between the subclavian and pulmonary arteries with the advantages of avoiding division of the subclavian artery and being easier to close at the time of definitive surgery.

Waterston shunt. This consists of a side-to-side anastomosis between the posterior wall of the ascending aorta and the anterior wall of the right pulmonary artery. It is rarely performed now because of its tendency to produce excessive ipsilateral pulmonary blood flow and because of difficulty in reconstruction of the pulmonary artery at definitive surgery. The Potts shunt, consisting of a side-to-side anastomosis between the thoracic aorta and the left pulmonary artery, has been abandoned for the same reasons.

Glenn shunt. This cavopulmonary anastomosis, between the superior vena cava and the right pulmonary artery, allows approximately 30% of systemic venous return to flow directly to the right lung bypassing the right side of the heart. If the confluence between the right and left pulmonary artery remains intact then blood flow to both lungs is increased (i.e. bi-directional). The Glenn shunt is used as part of the Fontan procedure (see below).

Banding of the pulmonary artery

Banding of the pulmonary artery limits excessive pulmonary blood flow (and therefore the risk of pulmonary hypertension) in large left to right shunts at ventricular level before definitive surgery is undertaken. The operation is performed through a left thoracotomy and the pulmonary artery is constricted with a heavy silk suture until the distal pulmonary artery pressure is 30%–50% of the systemic pressure (although this is partly dependent on systemic arterial oxygen saturation).

Atrial septectomy (Blalock–Hanlon)

Surgical atrial septectomy was previously performed to increase inter-atrial mixing in certain conditions such as complete transposition of the great arteries. It is now rarely performed as a similar effect can be achieved by balloon atrial septostomy (of Rashkind).

Common forms of congenital heart disease

Patent ductus arteriosus (PDA)

PDA is the persistence of the foetal communication between the arch of the aorta and the pulmonary artery (Fig. 4.10) and may be an isolated abnormality or occur in association with other structural defects. Failure of closure does not result in cyanosis (as the shunt is from the systemic to pulmonary circulation) but leads to volume overload of the left heart. PDA is commonly seen in premature infants and may close with indomethacin, a prostaglandin synthetase inhibitor. Closure of a PDA is necessary to avoid heart failure in early life or the risk of endocarditis or pulmonary vascular disease in later life.

It is now possible to close a PDA in some patients with an 'umbrella' introduced percutaneously through the large veins to the right side of the heart and advanced into the pulmonary artery under radiological control. *The surgical approach* is through the fourth or fifth left intercostal space, dividing or ligating the duct, after identification of the recurrent laryngeal nerve.

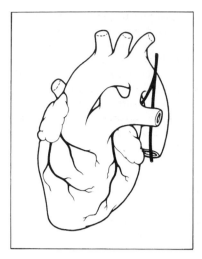

Fig. 4.10 Patent ductus arteriosus. Treated by division of the ductus, and closure of the cut ends

Coarctation of the aorta

This refers to a variable degree of constriction of the thoracic aorta, from a modest narrowing to virtually complete obliteration. It occurs immediately distal to the origin of the left subclavian artery (Fig. 4.11) and occasionally extends proximally into the arch. It may be an isolated abnormality or occur in association with other structural defects. Presentation may be in the neonatal period with severe heart failure or later in life with the classic features of hypertension in the upper limbs and weak, delayed femoral pulses provided through a collateral circulation. Repair delayed until after the first year of life may increase the risk of permanent hypertension.

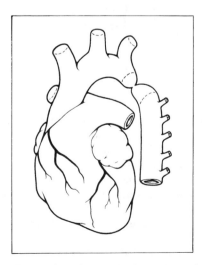

Fig. 4.11 Coarctation of the aorta. Treated by resection of the stenosed segment and end-to-end anastomosis

It is now possible to perform balloon dilatation of discrete coarctations under radiological control although there are concerns over recurrent stenosis and aneurysm formation in the long term.

The *surgical approach* is through a left thoracotomy with resection of the stenosed segment and end-to-end anastomosis. Some surgeons use the subclavian artery to fashion a patch enlargement of the coarctation to reduce the incidence of recurrent stenosis after an end-to-end resection.

Atrial septal defect (ASD)

An ASD (Fig. 4.12) results from maldevelopment of the interatrial septum and may be of three types (secundum, primum and sinus venosus) although some classifications include patent foramen ovale. An ASD leads to volume overload of the right heart because compliance differences favour increased flow across the defect from left to right. Chronic overload of the pulmonary circulation may produce vascular damage resulting in fixed pulmonary hypertension and shunt reversal (Eisenmenger syndrome).

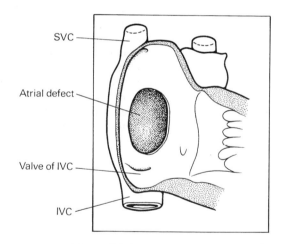

Fig. 4.12 Atrial septal defect — ostium secundum defect in inter-atrial septum can be closed by suture or patch

The most common and simplest defect is the secundum defect which is centrally placed in the septum. The primum ASD is a defect in the inferior septum often including a defect in the atrioventricular valves (being part of the spectrum of atrioventricular canal defects). The sinus venosus defect is a high ASD often associated with anomalous venous drainage of one of the pulmonary veins into the superior vena cava or high right atrium.

Closure of an ASD is indicated when the pulmonary to systemic flow ratio is greater than 2:1. It is now possible to close the small secundum ASD using a percutaneous umbrella technique. *Surgical repair* of an ASD is through a median sternotomy using CPB, cannulation and snaring of both vena cavae, and a right atrial incision. Small secundum defects can be closed by direct suture but larger defects require closure with a patch of pericardium. Sinus venosus defects require a patch to close the defect and to redirect anomalous pulmonary venous drainage to the left atrium. In primum ASD, in addition to closing the atrial defect, the mitral valve may require repair or occasionally replacement.

Ventricular septal defect (VSD)

VSD is the most common isolated structural abnormality which causes symptomatic heart disease in infancy and is an important cause of cardiac failure in the first year of life.

VSD is classified according to its relationship to the membranous portion of the ventricular septum (Fig. 4.13). The perimembranous VSD, in which the membranous portion of the septum is deficient, is the most common defect and may extend into the inlet, muscular or outlet septum. Infundibular VSD refers to a defect immediately below the pulmonary valve which may produce aortic incompetence because of prolapse of the right coronary cusp of the aortic valve. Muscular VSDs occur in the muscular portion of the septum, may be multiple and often close spontaneously.

A VSD produces volume overload of both ventricles. The magnitude of the shunt depends on the size of the defect (a small VSD may be restrictive) and the degree of pulmonary hypertension. Chronic volume overload of the pulmonary circulation may lead to fixed pulmonary hypertension with a reduction in the shunt and, finally, shunt reversal.

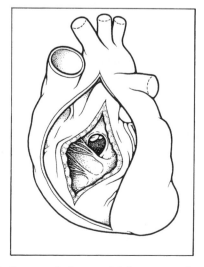

Fig. 4.13 Interventricular septal defect as seen through incision in wall of right ventricle. Requires patch closure

Surgical closure of a VSD is through a median sternotomy, cannulating and snaring both vena cavae. Depending on its precise location the VSD can be approached through the right atrium and tricuspid valve, through a right ventriculotomy or through the pulmonary artery. The VSD is closed with a patch of pericardium or prosthetic material. Sutures are placed to avoid the bundle of His on the posterior aspect of a perimembranous VSD or the superior aspect of an inlet VSD.

In very small infants in cardiac failure unlikely to survive more major surgery the pulmonary artery can be banded to restrict pulmonary artery and eventually left ventricle overload. This protects the pulmonary circulation from hypertension and corrects left ventricular failure. The band is tightened until the distal pulmonary artery pressure is less than 30 mmHg. The band is subsequently removed at the time of definitive corrective surgery.

Transposition of the great arteries (TGA)

TGA may occur in various forms but in the simplest type the right ventricle gives rise to the aorta and the left ventricle to the pulmonary artery. The two circuits are thus in parallel and mixing through a PDA, ASD or VSD is essential for survival. TGA is the commonest cause of cyanotic heart disease in the first week of life and an urgent atrial balloon septostomy (Rashkind) is necessary to increase intracardiac mixing unless a patent ductus arteriosus allows adequate mixing of the circulations.

Surgical repair is either by an arterial 'switch' or by inter-atrial repair. The arterial switch is an anatomical and physiological corrective operation in which the aorta and pulmonary artery are transected and re-anastomosed, the aorta to left ventricle and pulmonary artery to right ventricle. The technical difficulty in the operation lies in transferring the coronary arteries to the new aorta. The operation must be performed within the first few weeks of life before the left ventricle involutes.

In the atrial repair operation (Mustard, Senning), a baffle of pericardium or atrial wall is constructed within the atrium so that pulmonary venous blood is channelled anteriorly through the tricuspid valve to the right ventricle (and then to aorta). Systemic venous blood is channelled behind the baffle, through the mitral valve to the left ventricle and then to the pulmonary artery. The disadvantage of these operations is a high incidence of atrial arrhythmias in the long-term and concern over the ability of the right ventricle to support the systemic circulation for the rest of life.

Tetralogy of Fallot (TOF)

Fallot's tetralogy is the most common form of cyanotic heart disease in children surviving past infancy. The basic abnormality in Fallot's tetralogy is failure of the bulbis cordis to rotate adequately resulting in abnormal development of the infundibulum of the right ventricle so that the aorta is more anterior and to the right than normal and 'over-rides' the septum with a malalignment VSD beneath the aortic valve. Obstruction of the right ventricular outflow tract is usually due to a combination of infundibular stenosis (due to hypertrophy of the septal and parietal bands of infundibular muscle) and valve stenosis. In summary Fallot's tetralogy consists of a VSD, overriding aorta, pulmonary stenosis and right ventricular hypertrophy.

As the VSD is large and unrestrictive the ventricular pressures are equal. The degree of shunting is therefore dependent on the severity of infundibular stenosis and the level of the systemic vascular resistance. Right to left shunting increases with progressive infundibular obstruction and decreasing systemic vascular resistance (e.g. after exercise).

As the infundibular obstruction is mild at birth most children do not present within the first year of life. Parents of older children commonly report post-exercise cyanosis (increased right to left shunting) and squatting (compression of the femoral arteries reduces right to left shunting). Propranolol is used for prophylaxis and treatment of cyanotic attacks, which may be sudden and severe, and are a consequence of infundibular spasm.

The *surgical procedure* depends on age at presentation: children less than one year old are best treated initially with a systemic to pulmonary shunt (see above). Definitive surgery consists of patch closure of the VSD and relief of the right ventricular outflow obstruction.

Pulmonary atresia

The pathophysiology of pulmonary atresia is largely dependent on the absence or presence of an associated VSD. With a VSD the anatomy is similar to that of Fallot's Tetralogy but there is no continuity between the right ventricle and the pulmonary artery. Mixing of blood occurs at the ventricular level and blood reaches the pulmonary tree either through a PDA or through collaterals from the descending aorta.

With an intact septum, mixing of blood takes place at the atrial level and reaches the pulmonary tree by a PDA after traversing the left side of the heart. As the ductus begins to close within a few days of birth the child becomes profoundly cyanotic and immediate management consists of a prostaglandin infusion to maintain duct patency followed by a systemic to pulmonary shunt. The nature of definitive correction is dependent on the degree of abnormality of the tricuspid valve and right ventricle which can vary from mild hypoplasia to virtual absence.

Anomalous venous drainage

Anomalous venous drainage refers to the inappropriate drainage of the four pulmonary veins to the right atrium and may be total or partial. It is always accompanied by an ASD. The pulmonary veins form a confluence behind the heart and drain to the right atrium by a variety of routes which may be supracardiac (via a left superior vena cava, the innominate vein and right superior vena cava), cardiac (to the coronary sinus through a persistent left sided SVC) or infracardiac (via the portal vein and inferior vena cava).

The usual presentation is in infancy with cyanosis and breathlessness. There is a high volume flow through the right atrium and some desaturated blood crosses the ASD to the left atrium producing systemic desaturation.

Surgical correction involves closure of the ASD, division of the anomalous connections and diversion of blood to the left atrium.

Complex congenital heart disease

This term covers a large number of structural abnormalities and in particular hearts with only one functional ventricle. The long term aim of surgical treatment is to use the single ventricle to support the systemic circulation and to direct systemic venous blood to the pulmonary artery without the need for a right ventricle (Fontan operation).

TRANSPLANTATION

The first successful human heart transplant was performed in 1967 but the operation was only widely adopted after introduction of the immunosuppressive agent cyclosporine in 1981 led to a dramatic improvement in results. The improvement in results of heart transplantation has enticed many centres to institute heart-lung and lung transplantation programmes.

Most recipients are less than 60 years of age with advanced cardiac failure unresponsive to conventional medical or surgical therapy (and consequently have a very limited life expectancy). The aetiology of the cardiac failure is usually ischaemic heart disease or cardiomyopathy (idiopathic, postviral or postpartum).

The current one-year survival following heart transplantation is above 80% and five-year survival above 70%. There are a few absolute contraindications to transplantation — malignancy, severe renal, hepatic or respiratory disease or diabetes mellitus.

The donor heart is checked for ABO blood group and size compatibility and is ideally obtained from a donor less than 50 years of age, on minimum inotropic support and without sign of active infection.

Technique

Good communication between the retrieval and recipient surgical teams is crucial and cardiopulmonary bypass in the recipient should begin only when the donor heart arrives in theatre.

The donor heart is removed with a good length of superior vena cava (thereby avoiding damage to the sino-atrial node), inferior vena cava (thereby avoiding damage to the coronary sinus), pulmonary veins (ensuring left atrium is adequate size), pulmonary artery and aorta.

The recipient's heart is prepared for bypass by cannulating and snaring both vena cavae. The aorta is clamped and the native heart excised by dividing the aorta and pulmonary artery above the valves. The left and right atria are divided proximal to the atrioventricular groove leaving most of the recipient atria behind to which the respective donor atria are anastomosed. The operation is completed by pulmonary and aortic anastomoses.

Complications

Early complications are failure of the donor heart either because of poor protection during harvesting and transport or because of elevated pulmonary vascular resistance in the recipient causing failure of the donor right ventricle.

Intermediate term complications are rejection or infection which are respectively due to inadequate or excessive immunosuppression.

The most common long-term complication is accelerated coronary artery atherosclerosis in the donor heart which is believed to be a consequence of chronic rejection. This diffuse disease affects the distal coronary vessels and is therefore unsuitable for conventional bypass grafting and requires re-transplantation.

Long-term cyclosporine therapy is known to be associated with an increased risk of malignancy.

FURTHER READING

Anderson R H, McCartney F J, Shinebourne E A, Tynan M 1987 Terminology. In: Paediatric cardiology. Churchill Livingstone, Edinburgh

Califf R M, Harrell F E, Lee K I, et al 1989 The evolution of medical and surgical therapy for coronary disease. A 15 year perspective. Journal of the American Medical Association 261: 2077–2086

Christakis G T, Weisel R D, David T E et al 1988 Predictors of operative survival after valve replacement. Circulation 78 (suppl I): I.25 –I.34

Crawford S E, Svensson L G, Coselli J S, Safi H J, Hess K R 1989 Surgical treatment of aneurysm and/or dissection of the ascending aorta, transverse aortic arch, and ascending aorta and transverse aortic arch. Journal of Thoracic and Cardiovascular Surgery 98: 659–674

Edwards B S 1990 Recent advances in cardiac transplantation. Current Opinion in Cardiology 5: 295–299

Ellis L B, Harken D E 1964 Closed valvuplasty for mitral stenosis. A twelve year follow up study of 1571 patients. New England Journal of Medicine 270: 643–650

Gersh B J, Holmes D R 1993 Percutaneous transluminal coronary angioplasty or coronary bypass surgery in the management of chronic angina pectoris. Journal of Cardiology 40: 81–88

Grondin C M 1986 Graft disease in patients with coronary bypass grafting. Why does it start? Where do we stop? Journal of Thoracic and Cardiovascular Surgery 92: 323–329

Kirklin J K, Westaby S, Blackstone EH et al 1983 Complement and the damaging effects of cardiopulmonary bypass. Journal of Thoracic and Cardiovascular Surgery 86: 845–857

Loop F D, Lytle B W, Cosgrove D M et al 1986 Influence of the internal mammary artery graft on 10 year survival and other cardiac events. New England Journal of Medicine 314: 1–6

Murphy J G, Gersh B J, McGoon M D et al 1990 Long term outcome after surgical repair of isolated atrial septal defect. New England Journal of Medicine 323: 1645–1650

Rome J J, Keane J F, Perry S B, Spevak P J, Locke J E 1990 Double-umbrella closure of atrial septal defects: initial clinical applications. Circulation 82: 751–758

Rutherford J D, Braunwald E 1988 Selection of patients for the surgical treatment of coronary artery disease. Quarterly Journal of Medicine 67: 369–385

Standards and guidelines for cardiopulmonary resuscitation (CPR) and emergency cardiac care (ECC). Journal of the American Medical Association 1986 255: 2905–2932

Taggart D P, Wheatley D J 1990 Mitral valve surgery: to repair or replace? British Heart Journal 64: 234–235

Wheatley D J 1986 Surgery of coronary artery disease. Chapman and Hall, London

5

Thoracic surgery

D. P. TAGGART & D. J. WHEATLEY

Surgical anatomy and physiology (Fig. 5.1)

Trachea

The trachea is approximately 10 cm long and runs from the cricoid cartilage (opposite C6) to its intrathoracic division at the carina (opposite T5) into the right and left main bronchus. The anterior and lateral tracheal walls are composed of fibro-elastic tissue containing cartilaginous rings which prevent collapse while the posterior wall, composed of the trachealis muscle, is in contact with the oesophagus. The trachea is lined with columnar ciliated epithelium with mucous and serous glands.

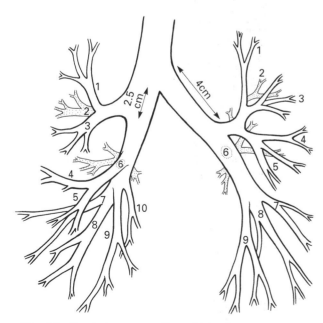

Fig. 5.1 Surgical anatomy of bronchial tree

Bronchi

The *right main bronchus* is shorter and wider than the left and is almost a direct continuation of the trachea. It is only 20° from the midline and tends to be the site where inhaled foreign material becomes lodged. The right upper lobe bronchus arises from the lateral wall of the right main bronchus one centimetre after its origin from the trachea. The middle lobe bronchus arises three centimetres distally, from the anterior wall of the intermediate bronchus (i.e. the part of bronchus between the origins of the right upper and middle lobes). Immediately below the middle lobe, the bronchus continues as the lower lobe bronchus.

The *left main bronchus lies* 40° from the midline. The left upper lobe bronchus arises from the lateral wall of the left main bronchus 4 cm below the carina. There is no separate middle lobe bronchus on the left and the equivalent of the right middle lobe is the lingula which is the first segmental branch of the left upper lobe bronchus.

Lungs

Both lungs are similar in structure. The right lung has three lobes: a major oblique fissure separates the lower lobe from the upper and middle lobes and the latter two lobes are separated by a minor horizontal fissure. The left lung has an upper and lower lobe separated by an oblique fissure (seen only on the lateral chest X-ray).

The basic anatomic unit of the lung is the bronchopulmonary segment. There are 19 bronchopulmonary segments (10 on the right and 9 on the left) linked together by connective tissue. Each segment behaves as an individual unit with its own bronchus and artery and, although they follow a general anatomic pattern, variations are common. The segmental pulmonary arteries run with the bronchial tree and do not cross the intersegmental plane while the segmental veins do.

The upper lobe of each lung consists of apical, anterior and posterior segments. On the right side the middle lobe has medial and lateral segments while the lingular equivalent on the left has superior and inferior segments. The lower lobe is composed of an apical segment (which on the right arises directly opposite the middle lobe) and anterior, lateral and posterior basal segments (and a further medial basal segment on the right). In addition to the pulmonary arteries lung parenchyma also receives a blood supply through the bronchial arteries. These arise from the aorta and intercostal arteries and form an arterial confluence in the hilum before following the branching bronchial tree. Bronchial arteries account for 1–2% of the cardiac output and drain mostly to the pulmonary veins (explaining the 'physiological shunt') or to bronchial veins which drain to the azygos and hemiazygos venous systems.

GENERAL PROCEDURES IN THORACIC SURGERY

Bronchoscopy

Indications
Bronchoscopy is performed for diagnostic or therapeutic reasons using a rigid or flexible instrument. The flexible instrument allows better visualization of the bronchopulmonary segments but the rigid instrument is better for therapeutic procedures such as removal of foreign bodies and tracheal toilet after aspiration.

Procedure
Flexible bronchoscopy can be performed at the bedside in fully conscious or sedated patients or through an endotracheal tube in ventilated patients. Rigid bronchoscopy (Fig. 5.2) requires general anaesthesia, except in critical circumstances, and while there are no absolute contra-indications particular care is exercised in patients with a rigid neck or in the presence of superior vena cava obstruction for fear of precipitating laryngeal oedema. The patient lies supine on the

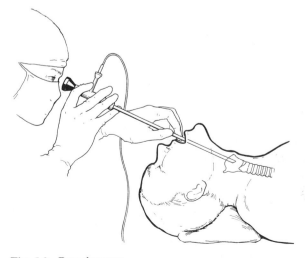

Fig. 5.2 Bronchoscopy

operating table with the head moderately extended and the neck flexed (with a single pillow under the head). A towel is wrapped around the head covering the eyes but leaving the nose exposed. A swab is used to protect the upper lip and the neck is extended by gentle traction on the upper jaw. The lightly lubricated bronchoscope is passed into the pharynx in the midline (but occasionally from the side in patients with very prominent teeth), past the uvula, until the epiglottis is visualized. The tip of the bronchoscope is passed behind the epiglottis and then used to lift the epiglottis forward thereby exposing the vocal cords. The bronchoscope is then rotated so that its tip can be easily passed through the vocal cords into the trachea. A Venturi jet ventilator is attached to the bronchoscope and the patient manually ventilated at frequent intervals. Many anaesthetists use a peripheral oxygen saturation meter clipped to a finger or the lobe of the ear to ensure satisfactory ventilation during the procedure.

A systematic examination of the trachea, carina (which forms a sharp angle unless splayed by subcarinal lymph nodes) and bronchial tree is carried out starting with the presumed normal side. Diagnostic bronchoscopy includes assessment of the mobility of the vocal cords (and mobility of the tracheobronchial tree with a rigid instrument), the quantity and nature of any secretions, the condition of the mucosal lining, whether the carina is splayed, and the presence of tumours or foreign bodies. Examination of the segmental bronchi requires a flexible bronchoscope or the use of angled telescopes with the rigid bronchoscope. A biopsy is taken of any suspicious lesion.

Complications
Rigid bronchoscopy is carried out uneventfully in most patients. Bleeding is common after biopsy procedures but rarely presents serious problems. If significant bleeding occurs the patient is turned on to the affected side and placed head down to prevent obstruction of the contralateral lung by blood. A pledget soaked in dilute adrenaline can be compressed against the bleeding site with biopsy forceps.

Pleural aspiration

Indications
Pleural aspiration is indicated for diagnostic and/or therapeutic reasons (a large effusion may compress the lung and cause respiratory embarrassment). Pleural effusion refers to the presence of fluid within the pleural cavity without specifying its nature. Depending on aetiology an effusion may be serous, purulent (empyema), bloody (haemothorax) or contain chyle (chylothorax). A transudate is an effusion with a low protein content (i.e. less than 30 g/L) as in cardiac failure and an exudate an effusion with a high protein

content (over 30 g/L) as in infection. The most common causes of pleural effusion are malignancy, congestive cardiac failure, pneumonia and/or empyema, and following operation or trauma. Rarely an effusion may consist of chyle due to injury to the thoracic duct during thoracic surgery. Any aspirate is sent for biochemical (protein content, pH, amylase if there is a suspicion of pancreatic pseudocyst, cholesterol if there is a suspicion of chyle) bacteriological and cytological analyses.

Pleural aspiration is often combined with *pleural biopsy and thoracoscopy* unless the aetiology of the effusion has already been established. Thoracoscopy is the introduction of a telescope into the pleural cavity, under general anaesthesia, allowing direct visual biopsy of visceral or parietal pleural lesions resulting in a very high diagnostic yield.

Procedure
The appropriate intercostal space for aspiration is determined from clinical and radiological examination (posteroanterior and lateral chest radiology is mandatory). The patient sits astride a chair and the proposed site of aspiration is chosen by counting intercostal spaces anteriorly, following the appropriate space posteriorly and confirming the presence of the effusion by dullness to percussion. The skin, subcutaneous tissues, muscle and parietal pleura over the effusion are anaesthetized with 10 ml of 1% lignocaine. A long spinal needle is introduced into the effusion, along the superior border of the inferior rib (avoiding the neurovascular bundle on the inferior border of the superior rib). Connecting the aspirating needle to a two-way tap permits aspiration into and emptying of the syringe without disconnection from the needle. Drainage of loculated effusions may require more than one puncture.

Large effusions are gradually evacuated through a basal chest drain which is clamped intermittently to avoid producing respiratory distress.

Complications
Failure of aspiration is usually due to inappropriate localisation of the effusion which can be avoided by careful clinical and radiological examination. If the aspirating needle is introduced too low it may penetrate the diaphragm, liver or spleen. Inadequate drainage of the effusion occurs if the needle is introduced too high or if the collection is solidified or loculated.

Mediastinoscopy
Mediastinoscopy is used in the investigation of superior mediastinal masses or lymphadenopathy especially where other diagnostic techniques have failed to establish a histological diagnosis (see also lung cancer).

Anterior mediastinotomy
This procedure is indicated in the assessment of masses lying in the anterior mediastinum, which are therefore anterior to the great vessels and inaccessible by mediastinoscopy. Its limitation is that it can only be used to explore one side of the mediastinum because of the presence of the sternum. A limited horizontal incision is made in the second intercostal space, through which excision of the second costal cartilage and ligation of the internal mammary artery can be performed. By blunt dissection behind the sternum the pleura and phrenic nerve are pushed laterally exposing the anterior mediastinal space. The pleura may be opened to inspect the hilum of the lung and to biopsy pulmonary tissue thereby converting the procedure to a limited thoracotomy.

Complications are uncommon but are those of any open thoracic procedure.

Intercostal drainage

Indications
The usual indication for intercostal drainage is collapse of the underlying lung secondary to pleural collections of air or fluid.

The ability to insert a chest drain safely and efficiently should be in the repertoire of all doctors as it may be a life saving manoeuvre. While a small pneumothorax can usually be managed conservatively tension pneumothorax requires immediate drainage. In the emergency situation insertion of a peripheral venous cannula into the second intercostal space 5 cm from the midline is sufficient until formal drainage can be performed.

Procedure
Prior to insertion of the drain both posteroanterior and lateral chest X-rays (CXR) are carefully examined. In most situations insertion of the drain into the fourth to sixth intercostal space in the mid-axillary line successfully evacuates air or fluid as well as being of maximum comfort to the patient. This site proves easy for drain insertion in adults as it lies posterior to the muscle bulk of pectoralis major and anterior to that of latissimus dorsi. Ideally the drain is angled apically to remove air or basally to remove fluid but, in the absence of pleural adhesions or a loculated collection, pleural air or fluid will find the drain.

The patient sits upright in bed or astride a chair leaning forward, with the arm on the proposed site of insertion held across to the opposite shoulder.

After cleaning the proposed area of insertion with antiseptic 10 ml of 1% lignocaine is used to infiltrate skin (producing a subcutaneous bleb), subcutaneous tissues, intercostal muscles and pleura. Parietal pleura

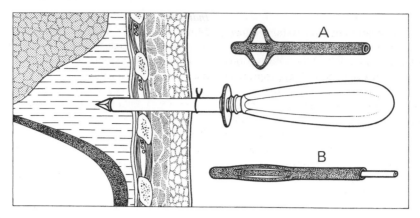

Fig. 5.3 Chest drainage by Malecot self-retaining catheter, introduced by trocar and cannula through an intercostal space. Note the suture placed around the cannula to mark the proposed depth of penetration

is very sensitive and must be anaesthetized. As the pleura is entered air or fluid should be freely aspirated and if not an alternative site is used.

A 1 cm oblique skin incision in the direction of the ribs is continued through subcutaneous tissue. The intercostal muscles are separated with blunt edged scissors until pleura is breached on the superior border of the underlying rib (to avoid the intercostal bundle on the inferior aspect of the superior rib). The drain, mounted on a trocar, is inserted through this track and angled apically to drain air and basally to drain fluid (Fig. 5.3). The drain, anchored with a securing stitch, is connected to an underwater seal and air will be seen to bubble on expiration or fluid will drain.

The simple underwater-seal bottle (Fig. 5.4) is still the most commonly used drainage system. This system effectively allows one-way escape of air and fluid from the pleural cavity. Occasionally the drainage system consists of three interconnected sealed bottles: the first bottle acts as a trap for collecting fluid, the second bottle acts as the underwater seal and the third bottle is used to regulate suction. This system is increasingly being replaced with commercially available disposable drainage units which have the same functions as the three sealed bottles but are more compact and less susceptible to introduction of infection.

A chest X-ray confirms satisfactory position of the drain. Usually connection to an underwater seal permits adequate passive drainage of air or fluid. Occasionally suction up to 35 cm of water can be applied to encourage expansion of a collapsed lung. The drainage system is kept at floor level and changed daily and the quantity and quality of any effluent is recorded. Daily radiology confirms successful removal of pleural air and/or fluid accompanied by expansion of the underlying lung. The presence of bubbling in the underwater

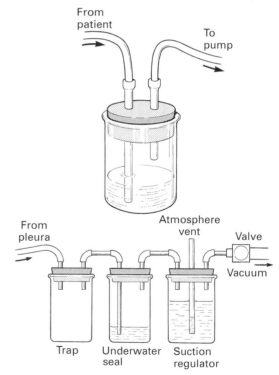

Fig. 5.4 Underwater seal drainage — single and three bottle methods

seal when the patient coughs suggests a continuing air leak even if the lung appears expanded on CXR.

It may be possible to increase patient mobility by replacing the underwater seal system with a Heimlich one-way valve (connected to a drainage bag if there is an effusion).

Complications

The most frequent complication of intercostal drainage is failure to drain a pleural collection either because the drain is wrongly sited or too small. The most serious complication of intercostal drainage is inappropriately low siting of the drain resulting in injury to the liver or spleen. Excessive blood loss suggests damage to the underlying lung or intercostal neurovascular bundle. Appearance of surgical emphysema implies blockage of the drain with exudate and is relieved by 'milking' the drain with rollers. If a chest tube is required for more than 7 days there is a significant risk of infection of the track and subsequently the pleural space.

Minitracheotomy

Minitracheotomy is the insertion of a narrow (4 mm) cannula into the trachea through the cricothyroid membrane for tracheal toilet. It can be inserted under local anaesthesia in spontaneously breathing or mechanically ventilated patients (Fig. 5.5). The cannula is well tolerated without sedation and allows effective removal of tracheal secretions with a 10 Fr suction catheter. Because of the narrow bore of the cannula there is minimal air leak during respiration and the patient can cough, speak and swallow comfortably. Supplemental oxygen can also be delivered through the cannula as necessary.

Indication

Minitracheotomy is indicated for tracheal toilet in patients with excessive tracheal secretions whose expectoration is ineffective (e.g. vocal cord palsy, bulbar palsy etc). In surgical patients with a high risk of pulmonary complications a minitracheotomy may be inserted prophylactically (Matthews, 1984).

Procedure

The patient is positioned supine with a sandbag under the shoulders to extend the head and the relevant landmarks are identified. The cricothyroid membrane is the small palpable depression immediately inferior to the thyroid cartilage. Local anaesthesia is achieved with 2 ml of 1% lignocaine. The skin is tensed over the membrane and a one centimetre stab through the membrane with a guarded scalpel is followed by passage of the cannula over its introducer. There is no resistance to passage of the cannula if it enters the trachea. The cannula is secured through its flanges with tapes tied behind the neck (Fig. 5.6). When the minitracheotomy is removed the skin hole closes within a few days.

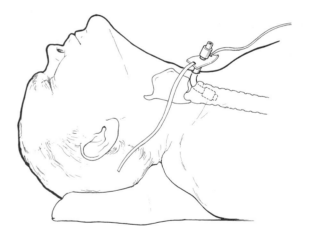

Fig. 5.6 Minitracheotomy — tube held by tapes which are tied behind the neck

Complications

Complications are uncommon. Occasionally there is excessive bleeding from engorged neck veins but this is minimal if the incision is in the midline and there is no loss of alignment between the skin incision and the hole in the cricothyroid membrane. Difficulty with insertion may be encountered in individuals with a short fat neck or in elderly patients with a calcified cricothyroid membrane. In such situations the minitracheotomy can be placed under direct vision after making a 2 cm incision in skin overlying the membrane.

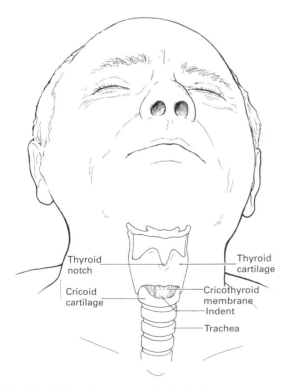

Fig. 5.5 Minitracheotomy — site for incision

Tracheostomy (see also Chapter 12)

Tracheostomy is performed less commonly than in the days prior to the availability of modern, high-volume, low pressure, cuffed endotracheal tubes and minitracheotomy. Endotracheal intubation safely provides an airway in the vast majority of emergency situations.

Indication

The usual indication for tracheostomy is the patient who requires prolonged mechanical ventilation because it optimises tracheal toilet and patient comfort, and assists in subsequent weaning from ventilation (by eliminating the dead space).

Procedure

Tracheostomy is ideally performed under sterile conditions in an operating theatre. As most patients who require tracheostomy are critically ill coagulation abnormalities are very common and should be corrected prior to surgery. The surgeon ensures that an appropriate range of cuffed tracheostomy tubes (uncuffed for small children) is available. Good lighting, assistance and diathermy are very useful for tracheostomy.

The patient is placed supine on the operating table and the neck extended by a sandbag under the shoulders. A 3 cm horizontal incision mid-way between the sternal notch and the cricoid cartilage is continued through subcutaneous tissue to the strap muscles which are separated vertically in the midline to reveal the cricoid cartilage and the first 4 tracheal rings. If the thyroid isthmus obstructs visualization it can usually be retracted but occasionally requires division.

The trachea can be incised in various ways but the first tracheal ring must be avoided. A heavy suture is placed transversely between the second and third cartilages and a Bjork flap ('n') fashioned around the second to fourth tracheal rings care being taken not to puncture the underlying cuffed endotracheal tube. The flap is retracted by securing the suture to the lower skin edge with tape and allows speedy replacement of an inadvertently displaced tracheostomy tube. A vertical midline incision in the second to fourth tracheal rings is used in infants and young children and some surgeons prefer this technique in adults. The tracheostomy tube is secured by tapes passed through its flanges and tied behind the neck.

Complications

Life-threatening complications of tracheostomy include blockage of the tube (by secretions, over-inflation of the cuff or tube displacement) and haemorrhage as a consequence of infection causing pressure necrosis or erosion into the brachiocephalic artery. Tracheal stenosis is now uncommon with high volume, low pressure cuffs but over-inflation of the endotracheal cuff, infection and excessive drying of the tracheal mucosa may lead to scarring and subsequent stenosis.

THORACIC TRAUMA

Chest wall and intra-thoracic visceral trauma can result from blunt or penetrating chest injuries. Blunt injuries are usually a consequence of crush injuries or road traffic accidents while penetrating wounds usually result from assault with knives or firearms. While penetrating or blunt chest wall trauma usually produces an obvious external injury simultaneous visceral injury may be less apparent particularly if the patient is unconscious.

Damage to specific structures

Chest wall

Isolated fractures of the clavicle or rib(s) are common and do not require specific treatment except for pain control to allow effective expectoration. In contrast, fracture of the sternum or scapula requires such force that there is frequently associated damage to the thoracic viscera. Multiple rib fractures and/or fracture of the sternum may result in 'flail chest' with paradoxical movement of the flail segment in inspiration and expiration. Flail chest may result in severe respiratory embarrassment both as a consequence of paradoxical chest movement as well as contusion of the underlying lung. In such circumstances mechanical ventilation may be required while, occasionally, operative fixation is indicated for large flail segments.

Pneumothorax/haemothorax

The clinical diagnosis of pneumothorax (ipsilateral decreased breath sounds and hyper-resonance to percussion) and tension pneumothorax (as above, accompanied by deviation of the trachea and apex beat to the contralateral side implying mediastinal shift) can be difficult without radiological confirmation. Tension pneumothorax arises when a tear in visceral pleura acts like a valve, allowing air into the pleural cavity in inspiration but preventing escape of air in expiration. This results in progressive collapse of the ipsilateral lung, mediastinal shift, collapse of the contralateral lung and cardiac/respiratory arrest. Ideally, radiology is performed to confirm the diagnosis but immediate uni- or bilateral intercostal drainage may be indicated in the moribund patient.

Haemothorax is usually due to laceration of one of the vessels of the chest wall (intercostal or internal mammary artery) and can often be managed by intercostal drainage alone. Thoracotomy becomes increasingly likely if there is an initial blood loss in excess of

1 litre followed by continued bleeding greater than 200 ml/hour over the next 4 consecutive hours.

Diaphragmatic injury

Diaphragmatic rupture due to blunt abdominal or chest trauma requires such force that many patients die of associated injuries before reaching hospital. In approximately 80% of patients reaching hospital alive the central or posterior portion of the left hemi-diaphragm is the site of injury. Both the peritoneal and pleural covers of the diaphragm are involved in the disruption so that abdominal viscera herniate into the pleural cavity. Stomach, omentum, spleen or colon can herniate on the left while on the right the liver minimises herniation of abdominal contents. Surgical repair of diaphragmatic rupture is always indicated to prevent long-term complications but its timing is dictated by associated injuries. Suspected injury of abdominal or thoracic viscera or cardiac or respiratory distress due to massive visceral herniation are indications for early repair.

Tracheobronchial tree

Disruption of the tracheobronchial tree is suggested by haemoptysis, surgical emphysema, mediastinal air on chest radiology and massive air leak on intercostal drainage. Most disruptions occur within a few centimetres of the carina and are confirmed at bronchoscopy. Lung contusion is difficult to diagnose except at thoracotomy but is suggested by unexpectedly severe respiratory insufficiency.

Trauma to the heart and great vessels

This is discussed in Chapter 4.

Management

The initial management of trauma patients concentrates on assessment of neurological, haemodynamic and ventilatory status. Patients who are unconscious, unable to maintain adequate ventilation or who are haemodynamically unstable are intubated and ventilated. Simultaneously, basic resuscitative measures are established while a complete assessment of associated injuries is made.

Initial management consists of:

1. Rapid general assessment to determine the need for mechanical ventilation (neurological, haemodynamic or respiratory insufficiency).

2. Basic resuscitative measures including central venous access (for fluid and drug administration) and radial artery cannulation (for haemodynamic and arterial blood gas monitoring).

3. Examination of the chest wall and assessment of visceral injury (knowledge of the nature of the injury provides valuable clues to the likely organ damage e.g.

aortic rupture following deceleration injury in road traffic accidents or the weapon responsible for penetrating chest injury).

4. Examination of abdomen (especially after blunt injuries) and limbs.

5. Urgent radiological examination of thorax (intercostal drainage may be necessary before radiology is available, e.g. tension pneumothorax).

6. Consider need for bronchoscopy (suspected disruption of upper airway) or aortography (widened mediastinum).

7. Consider need for emergency thoracotomy (massive bleeding from chest drains, cardiac tamponade causing circulatory shock etc.).

SPONTANEOUS PNEUMOTHORAX

Pneumothorax may occur in patients with known lung disease (e.g. bronchiectases or cystic fibrosis) or in otherwise healthy individuals due to rupture of a subpleural cyst. One third of patients with a spontaneous pneumothorax develop a further pneumothorax often on the opposite side. Some degree of tension (see above), which is potentially lethal, occurs in up to 40% of spontaneous pneumothoraces.

The management of a spontaneous pneumothorax depends on its size and whether it has occured more than once. In patients presenting for the first time a small pneumothorax which produces no respiratory distress can be managed conservatively as air will be gradually reabsorbed from the pleural cavity or can be aspirated with a needle and syringe. A larger pneumothorax requires intercostal drainage (see page 87) particularly if there is some degree of tension.

In patients with underlying lung disease or with recurrent pneumothorax other measures may be required to ensure lung re-expansion and to prevent recurrence. These measures, designed to produce inflammation in the visceral and parietal pleura so that the lung becomes adherent to the chest wall, include:

Chemical pleurodesis

An irritant chemical such as tetracycline is introduced into the thoracic cavity to promote generalised pleural inflammation. Adequate analgesia is vital as chemical pleurodesis produces intense pain. The chemical can be insufflated as a powder in the pleural cavity or dissolved in 50 ml of saline and allowed to track around the pleural cavity for a few hours by clamping the chest drain and instructing the patient to rotate 90°C every 15 minutes with the foot and the head of the bed alternatively elevated. The drain is then unclamped and suction applied for 48 hours to ensure apposition of the visceral and parietal pleura.

Pleurectomy

Pleurectomy is the stripping of parietal pleura from the thorax to produce a large raw area to which visceral pleura will stick thereby obliterating the pleural space. It is indicated for recurrent pneumothorax especially if chemical pleurodesis has failed. Parietal pleura is easily stripped from the apex and posterolateral aspects of the thoracic cavity but with greater difficulty elsewhere and particularly over the diaphragm. Inflammation can be promoted in areas where pleura is difficult to strip by abrasion with a gauze swab. Bilateral pleurectomies can be performed through separate thoracotomies or through a median sternotomy incision. Adequate analgesia is essential to permit postoperative chest expansion and expectoration.

There is currently great interest in performing pleurectomy through video assisted procedures avoiding the need for thoracotomy.

Bullae

Bullae are air-filled blebs which may occur as an isolated congenital abnormality or in association with other pulmonary disease such as emphysema, bronchiectases or tuberculosis (Potgieter, 1981). Rupture of a small apical sub-pleural bleb is the usual reason for 'spontaneous' pneumothorax. When associated with other pulmonary disease bullae are frequently multiple and bilateral and may be clearly demonstrated by CT scanning. A solitary large bulla may, however, be very difficult to distinguish from a pneumothorax on chest radiology although the treatment is very different.

Surgery may be indicated for isolated sub-pleural cysts which are responsible for recurrent pneumothorax which has not responded to chemical pleurodesis. In such cases access may be limited to a small axillary incision through the second or third intercostal space. Any apical cysts can be oversewn, excised or stapled. If the visceral pleura is markedly thickened with fibrinous exudate or following a failed attempt at chemical pleurodesis, a limited decortication may be necessary. An apical pleurectomy is advisable to encourage obliteration of the pleural space and to reduce the chance of recurrent pneumothorax.

Surgery may also be indicated for a giant bulla even when part of generalised pulmonary disease if it is thought to be responsible for compression of otherwise functional lung tissue. The principle of surgery is decompression of the bulla with preservation and recruitment of as much functional lung tissue as possible in these patients who are frequently respiratory cripples. The mortality may be as high as 30% but successful treatment can result in a significant improvement in respiratory function as demonstrated by an improvement in pulmonary function tests. General anaesthesia must be induced carefully to prevent development of

tension within the large bulla. After incision of the wall of the bulla all bronchial openings are identified and sutured before performing a parietal pleurectomy. Apical and basal chest drains are mandatory as there is often a substantial air leak which requires high volume, low-pressure suction to encourage the lung to remain expanded and to adhere to the pleurectomised thorax.

Monaldi decompression

Decompression of large solitary bulla under local anaesthesia can be performed in patients too ill to withstand general anaesthesia. A short segment of rib overlying the bulla is excised (Fig. 5.7). A purse-string

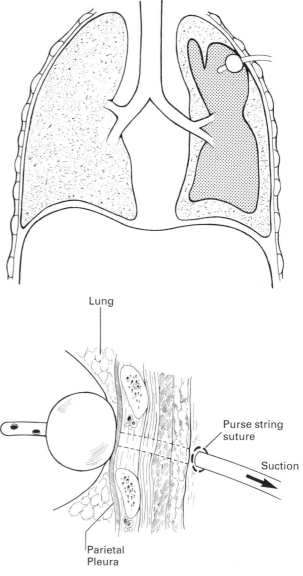

Fig. 5.7 Mondali procedure for drainage of large bulla with a Foley catheter

suture is placed through both the parietal and the visceral pleura of the underlying bulla through which a Foley catheter is passed. The catheter balloon is inflated and then retracted against the chest wall to prevent pneumothorax and the catheter connected to an underwater seal. The bulla decompresses over the following four to six weeks.

INFECTION IN THE PLEURAL SPACE

In Western countries lung resection for infection is now uncommon due to earlier presentation and treatment of such infections. In the developing world late presentation of infective lung disease resulting in destroyed pulmonary tissue and empyema occurs with tuberculosis, bronchiectases and widespread necrotizing pneumonia.

Empyema

Empyema is now less common in affluent societies because of earlier treatment of pulmonary infection and the widespread availability of potent antibiotics. Nevertheless empyema still occurs following acute lung infection, in association with chronic lung infections (e.g. tuberculosis, aspergillosis, actinomycosis) and in the presence of debilitating conditions such as malignancy. Empyema also occurs as a consequence of bronchopleural fistula following lung resection and subphrenic abscess complicating intra-abdominal sepsis (Le Roux, 1965).

The initial treatment of empyema is *intercostal drainage* with a large bore chest drain (32 Fr gauge) sited in the most dependent part of the infected collection (Fig. 5.8). The drain is best placed under general anaesthesia after a finger has been used to break down any loculi in the pleural space. Daily irrigation with dilute antiseptics or antibiotics is continued until the underlying lung is completely expanded and there is a minimal sterile effluent.

Intercostal drainage is successful in most patients. It is likely to fail if drainage is inadequate because the pus is particularly thick or if the intercostal drain is too small, sited wrongly or removed too soon. Conservative management may also fail when empyema is associated with malignant disease, infections such as tuberculosis or actinomycosis, or an underlying bronchopleural or oesophageal fistula.

Decortication

Decortication is the removal of thickened visceral and/or parietal pleura and any intervening empyema which restricts expansion of the underlying lung, diaphragm or chest wall. It is a major procedure and should not be performed in the presence of active sepsis.

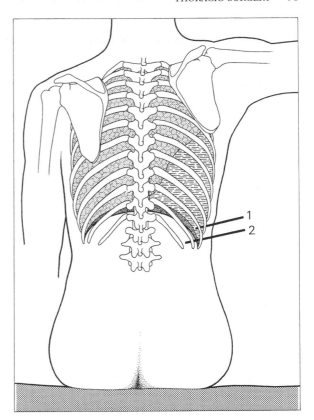

Fig. 5.8 Drawing to show the customary site for drainage of an acute pleural empyema. A needle introduced into the 10th or 11th intercostal space is liable to penetrate the diaphragm and to enter the abdominal cavity. Correct (1) and incorrect (2) positions of the needle are shown

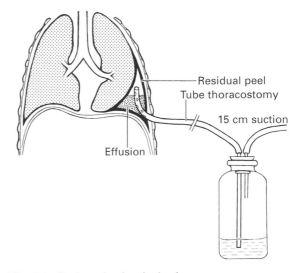

Fig. 5.9 Drainage by closed tube thoracostomy

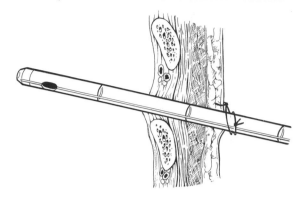

Fig. 5.10 Details of tube

Procedure

The patient is positioned as for standard thoracotomy (see below) and intubated with a double lumen endotracheal tube. Thoracotomy through the fifth or sixth intercostal space provides access to the whole pleural cavity which is important as adhesions may be most dense at the apex and the costophrenic angle. Parietal pleura is usually most easily stripped from the apex and posterolateral chest wall but less easily over the diaphragm. Pleural stripping and dissection in the correct plane is crucial or damage to extrapleural structures may occur. After mobilization of parietal pleura thickened visceral pleura is dissected from the lung surface. This is often difficult but is essential for re-expansion of the lung. Haemostasis and closure of lung air leaks must be meticulous and apical and basal chest drains are mandatory.

Complications

Extrapleural dissection may inadvertently injure blood vessels (internal mammary, intercostals, azygos, superior vena cava, aorta, brachiocephalic vein), nerves (phrenic, vagus, recurrent laryngeal), the thoracic duct or oesophagus. Bleeding in excess of 200 ml/hour

for 3 consecutive hours requires re-exploration. Atelectasis and bronchopneumonia result from excessive lung handling and air leakage may continue for a considerable period after surgery.

Rib resection

Rib resection is indicated in the treatment of empyema only if more conservative measures have failed. The rib to be resected is determined from posteroanterior and lateral CXRs after injection of contrast medium to show the most dependent part of the empyema cavity.

Procedure

Rib resection is usually carried out under general anaesthesia (and with a double lumen endotracheal tube if a bronchopleural fistula is present) but can be performed under local anaesthesia in sick patients. Aspiration through the proposed site of resection confirms location of the empyema cavity. A 5–10 cm incision is made over the rib to periosteum which is elevated with a rugine, taking care to avoid damage to the neurovascular bundle inferiorly. The rib is divided and 5–8 cm removed. The periosteum and pleura deep to the rib are incised and a specimen of pleura sent for histological examination. All loculi are broken down to ensure complete drainage of the cavity. A wide bore tube, of at least 2 cm external diameter with large terminal and side holes, is placed in the most dependent part of the cavity and the pleura and deep periosteal layers sutured around it. The superficial layers are approximated and the drain is secured to the skin by suture. The tube is gradually shortened as radiography, with or without contrast medium, shows gradual obliteration of the empyema cavity.

Complications

Failure of an empyema to resolve is usually because an inappropriately high rib is chosen for resection or because of the nature of the underlying infection.

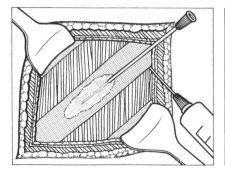
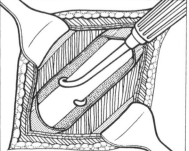

Fig. 5.11 Rib resection under local anaesthetic. Injection of solution below the periosteum, which, after being stripped upwards and downwards, is cleared from the deep surface of the rib by means of a curved elevator

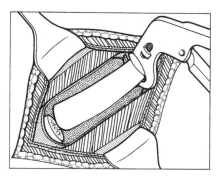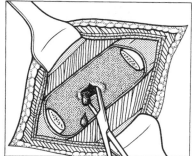

Fig. 5.12 Drainage of empyema after rib resection. Division of rib with special guillotine. Exploration of pleural cavity by sinus forceps introduced through incision in deep periosteum of rib and parietal pleura

Thoracostomy

Thoracostomy is the formation of a skin-lined track through the chest wall after rib resection to allow permanent pleural drainage. The track is sited in the mid axillary line at the most dependent part of the pleural cavity for maximum patient comfort and ease of access.

There are few indications for thoracostomy in modern surgical practice as most pleural space infections can be successfully managed by more conservative means. Thoracostomy is occasionally indicated for antibiotic resistant infection (e.g. actinomyces or aspergillosis) or for a malignant bronchopleural fistula in a patient with a limited life expectancy.

Procedure

The principle of thoracostomy is to provide an opening in the chest wall which will remain of sufficient size even after fibrotic contraction. An 'H' shaped incision is made in the mid axillary line with the transverse limb over the intercostal space between the two ribs to be resected. Both the transverse and the vertical limbs are approximately 8 cm long thereby producing rectangular skin flaps and a pleural opening of approximately 8 cm × 8 cm after resection of two adjacent ribs, their periosteum and the intervening neurovascular bundle. The skin flaps are sutured to the pleural margins with non-absorbable sutures and the cavity eventually becomes epithelialized.

Complications

Inadequate rib resection results in stenosis of the stoma, fibrotic contraction and an empyema cavity which does not drain properly.

Thoracoplasty

Thoracoplasty is the subperiosteal resection of a number of adjacent ribs allowing the mobilized chest wall to collapse on to underlying lung thereby obliterating the pleural space.

Thoracoplasty was commonly performed as part of the surgical treatment of tuberculosis in the pre-antibiotic era. Although now rarely performed it may be indicated in patients with chronic pleural space infection when the lung cannot be expanded because of previous resection or pulmonary disease.

Procedure

The aim is to perform subperiosteal resection of a number of adjacent ribs, from the costochondral junction anteriorly to the costotransverse ligament posteriorly to allow collapse of the chest wall, e.g. the 2nd to 5th ribs for apical collapse.

Complications

These include inadvertent opening of the pleural sac, bleeding and infection. Paradoxical movement of the mobilized chest wall may require firm strapping for a few days.

Chest wall reconstruction

Intrathoracic transfer of muscle flaps or omentum is increasingly being used in the management of chronic pleural infection rather than thoracostomy or thoracoplasty. Pectoralis major and serratus anterior are particularly suitable for apical and anterior defects while latissimus dorsi is more suitable for lateral, posterior and basal sites. Omentum may be used to fill pleural defects even in the presence of a bronchopleural fistula which has remained resistant to closure by other techniques.

LUNG CANCER

Bronchial carcinoma is the most common pathological condition requiring pulmonary surgery in Western society where it accounts for more than 90% of all lung resections. Bronchial carcinoma is currently 3 times more common in men than women but this ratio is changing because of reduced cigarette smoking in men and increased cigarette smoking in women.

The histologic types of bronchial carcinoma recognised in the WHO classification are squamous cell (45%), small cell (25%), large cell or undifferentiated (15%), adenocarcinoma (10%) and others (10%). In some series of lung carcinoma from the USA and Japan adenocarcinoma is the most common. There is, however, a large degree of intraobserver variation in the histologic typing of lung tumours even amongst expert pathologists.

From a practical point of view the management of bronchial carcinoma can be divided into small cell and non-small cell carcinoma. The small cell group grow and spread rapidly and often produce endocrine effects although such paraneoplastic syndromes can also occur with non-small cell carcinoma. In view of their tendency to metastasise early, less than 5% of small cell carcinomas are suitable for surgery although they are often sensitive, at least temporarily, to chemotherapy. The non-small cell group comprises all other histologic types and surgery, where feasible, is the treatment of choice. Non-small cell tumours are rarely sensitive to chemotherapy but may show some response to radiotherapy.

The overall five-year survival from diagnosis for all patients with bronchial carcinoma is less than 10%. Less than one third of patients with bronchial carcinoma are suitable for surgical resection because of evidence of metastatic disease at presentation. The overall five-year survival in patients undergoing resection is approximately 30% but much better in select subgroups (e.g. in patients with a solitary peripheral squamous lesion and no evidence of nodal involvement, five-year survival approaches 80%).

Thorough evaluation of tumour spread within and outwith the thoracic cavity is essential to minimise unnecessary thoracotomy in patients whose malignancy is inoperable. Staging (i.e. quantitative assessment) of tumour extent according to the TNM (tumour, node, metastases) classification indicates which patients are likely to benefit from surgery and permits an informed estimate of prognosis. Metastatic disease precluding surgical cure is frequently apparent on clinical examination or after simple investigation and includes:

1. evidence of extra-thoracic spread, e.g. cerebral or hepatic metastases
2. tracheal involvement or the presence of a malignant pleural effusion
3. involvement of cervical and mediastinal lymph nodes
4. superior vena cava obstruction
5. recurrent laryngeal nerve palsy (hoarse voice) and phrenic nerve palsy (raised hemidiaphragm) may indicate incurable disease.

Investigations

Appropriate investigations for bronchial carcinoma include radiology, sputum cytology, bronchoscopy, mediastinoscopy, anterior mediastinotomy and scalene node biopsy. The presence of a pulmonary mass greater than 3 cm diameter on chest radiology, especially if it has irregular or spiculated borders and an absence of calcification, is highly suggestive of bronchial carcinoma.

Sputum cytology is positive for malignant cells in 80% of central tumours and 50% of peripheral tumours but frequently cannot distinguish the histological type.

Bronchoscopy (see page 86) is essential to obtain adequate specimens for histology, to assess suitability for resection and to exclude synchronous tumours. The majority of bronchial carcinomas arise in the major airways and approximately two-thirds are visible at bronchoscopy. In general terms tumours more peripheral than the lobar bronchus are removed by lobectomy (unless growing across the fissure or involving the pulmonary artery). If the tumour involves the lobar orifice or the main bronchus then pneumonectomy but occasionally 'sleeve resection' (lobectomy plus partial resection of the main bronchus) is performed.

Mediastinoscopy

Mediastinoscopy is the percutaneous telescopic examination and biopsy of superior mediastinal contents.

Indications

The technique is particularly useful in assessing the operability of bronchial carcinoma when computerized axial tomography has identified enlarged superior mediastinal lymph nodes (conventionally greater than 1 cm in diameter) which may either be reactive (implying potentially curable disease) or contain metastatic tumour (implying incurable disease). N2 disease describes the presence of involved ipsilateral mediastinal lymph nodes and fewer than 20% of such patients are suitable candidates for surgical resection. N3 disease, the presence of ipsilateral scalene or mediastinal nodes implies incurable disease.

Procedure

Mediastinoscopy is usually performed after rigid bronchoscopy. With the patient lying supine the neck is extended by a sandbag under the shoulders. A 3 cm incision is made immediately above the suprasternal notch and the subcutaneous fat divided to the pretracheal muscles which are separated vertically in the midline and retracted laterally to expose pretracheal fascia. The fascia is divided transversely and the index finger used to 'burrow a tunnel' below the fascia towards the mediastinum. The finger sticks to the anterior surface of the trachea to the origin of the main bronchi where the pretracheal fascia ends. Anterior to the finger, pulsation of the brachiocephalic artery on the right and the aortic arch on the left can be appreciated.

The mediastinoscope is introduced into the tunnel and further blunt dissection is performed to expose pretracheal, superior tracheobronchial and inferior tracheobronchial (subcarinal) lymph nodes. It may be difficult to distinguish lymph nodes from vessels and it is sensible to aspirate with a fine gauge needle before biopsy.

Complications of mediastinoscopy are uncommon. In the event of bleeding, which may be venous (from the superior vena cava, azygos or brachiocephalic veins) or arterial (from the great vessels), the mediastinum should be tightly packed with a swab introduced through the mediastinoscope. Rarely, pneumothorax or recurrent laryngeal nerve injury may occur.

Anterior mediastinotomy (see page 87)

Scalene node biopsy

Scalene node biopsy has largely been superseded by computerized axial tomography and mediastinoscopy but aspiration or biopsy of palpable nodes remains useful. The nodes lie deep, medial and inferior to supraclavicular nodes and, although usually impalpable, are often involved in mediastinal and pulmonary disease and may prove diagnostic when other investigations are negative. The nodes lie in a fat pad in the scalene triangle whose floor is formed by the scalenus anterior muscle bounded medially by the internal jugular vein, inferiorly by the subclavian vein and superiorly by the omohyoid muscle.

Procedure. The patient lies supine with the head turned to the opposite side (and head down in case of inadvertent injury to the great veins resulting in air embolism) and a sandbag under the shoulders. A 5 cm incision, 2 cm above and parallel to the clavicle, begins at the clavicular head of sternomastoid. The incision is deepened through platysma to the fat pad between the sternomastoid and external jugular vein avoiding the supraclavicular nerves. The boundaries of the triangle are followed and the thoracic duct node between the internal jugular and subclavian veins removed (ensuring no leak of chyle) along with 4 or 5 other nodes in the fat pad.

Complications include damage to nerves or the thoracic duct and air embolization following venous damage.

Mediastinal tumours

Mediastinal tumour refers to the presence of any mediastinal mass which may or may not be neoplastic. While the anatomic position of a mass is a strong clue to its likely aetiology tumours of lymphatic origin and aortic aneurysms may occur in any position. Masses which occur in the:

- superior mediastinum may be thyroid, parathyroid and thymus
- anterior mediastinum may be dermoid, teratoma, seminoma, pericardial cyst
- central mediastinum may be foregut duplications (bronchial or intestinal) or lymph nodes (tuberculosis, lymphoma, sarcoidosis, bronchial carcinoma)
- posterior mediastinum may be neurogenic tumours.

A mediastinal mass may present as an asymptomatic finding on chest radiology. Less commonly the mass presents because of pressure symptoms (especially after haemorrhage into the mass) or as a consequence of malignant change.

Before resection of a mediastinal mass the surgeon must ensure that it is not a vascular swelling or a manifestation of generalised lymphadenopathy. Superior mediastinal masses are approached through a median sternotomy incision, anterior mediastinal masses by median sternotomy or lateral thoracotomy and central and posterior mediastinal masses by lateral thoracotomy.

PREOPERATIVE ASSESSMENT FOR THORACOTOMY

In addition to clinical examination preoperative assessment includes:

1. review of all investigations, especially radiology
2. estimation of respiratory function and reserve
3. evidence of lung sepsis and need for preoperative physiotherapy
4. adequacy of nutritional status.

Investigations

Good quality chest radiology is essential in the investigation of thoracic surgical patients and comparison with previous films is particularly useful. Chest films should be obtained in the posteroanterior and lateral views.

In addition to identifying the exact site of pathological lesions, examination of the position of the trachea, right horizontal fissure and diaphragm will give clues as to loss of lung volume (as in lobar collapse or consolidation) or excess volume (as in emphysema). As previously stated the presence of solitary masses greater than 3 cm in diameter with irregular or spiculated borders and the absence of calcification are highly suggestive of carcinoma.

Computerized axial tomography is gradually replacing conventional linear tomography in providing cross-sectional anatomical information on pathological lesions as well as identifying enlarged mediastinal nodes (which may be reactive, inflammatory or neoplastic).

Bronchography may be useful in quantifying the extent of destroyed pulmonary tissue in bronchiectases prior to surgical resection. Bronchography uses a contrast medium, injected into the trachea through cricothyroid puncture (or via an endotracheal tube) or directed to a specific lung segment at bronchoscopy, to delineate the bronchial tree and the extent and severity of diseased segments.

Pulmonary function tests
Respiratory function measurements provide some estimate of the likelihood that the patient will survive the proposed lung resection without becoming a respiratory cripple. In most patients the ability to climb a flight of stairs comfortably suggests adequate respiratory reserve but this assessment may be supplemented by preoperative pulmonary function tests. Unfortunately, no single test assesses all components of respiratory function or accurately predicts the probability of respiratory complications in a particular individual.

Pulmonary function is dependent on age, sex and body size but the following abnormalities imply respiratory impairment and an increased likelihood of postoperative complications:

1. a forced expiratory volume in one second (FEV1) of less than 2 L (for pneumonectomy), less than 1 L (for lobectomy) and less than 600 ml (for wedge resection)
2. a forced vital capacity (FVC) less than 1 L per minute
3. FEV1/FVC ratio less than 50% of predicted (should exceed 85%)
4. forced expiratory flow between 25% and 75% of expiration (FEF 25–75), is less effort dependent than FEV1, and impairment reflects small airways obstruction. It should normally be 3–4 L/sec.
5. maximum mandatory ventilation, equivalent approximately to 30 times FEV1, normally exceeds 150 L/min.
6. arterial oxygen tension less than 60 mmHg or carbon dioxide tension exceeding 45 mmHg breathing room air.

Depending on clinical assessment and the results of basic pulmonary function tests, more sophisticated investigations may be necessary, e.g. divided lung function tests (using spirometry and radioisotope perfusion scanning) estimate the likely respiratory capacity after the proposed lung resection.

Physiotherapy
All patients undergoing lung resection require physio-therapy. This is of particular importance in the presence of preoperative lung sepsis (e.g. bronchiectases) where intensive physiotherapy prior to surgery reduces postoperative mortality, morbidity and length of hospital stay.

Nutritional status
Many patients requiring lung resection are nutritionally deplete through the debilitating nature of chronic infection or malignancy and some patients will have lost significant amounts of body mass (more than 10% of pre-illness weight). Although operative mortality is directly related to the loss of body weight there is little evidence that preoperative nutritional support favourably alters this situation.

THORACIC INCISIONS AND LUNG RESECTION

Although a number of thoracic incisions are described, in practice only the lateral thoracotomy (extended posteriorly or anteriorly) and the median sternotomy (described in Chapter 4) incisions are commonly used.

Lateral thoracotomy
On the right this provides access to the lung and to the right side of the anterior and posterior mediastinum. Division of the azygos vein gives access to the whole length of the intrathoracic oesophagus and trachea. Lateral thoracotomy on the left provides access to the lung, to the left side of the anterior and posterior mediastinum, to the descending thoracic aorta and to the lower third of the thoracic oesophagus.

Procedure
Correct *positioning* is vital (Fig. 5.13). The patient is supported in the lateral decubitus position with sandbags or adhesive tape. Pressure areas such as the elbows and knees are protected with padding or pillows.

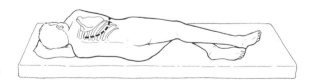

Fig. 5.13   Position for lateral thoracotomy

The skin *incision* starts midway between the spine of the scapula and the thoracic vertebral spines and runs vertically down, midway between the posterior border of the scapula and the spines of the vertebral column (Fig. 5.14). About 2 cm below the inferior angle of

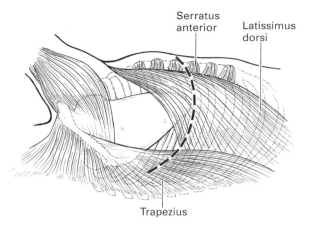

Serratus
anterior   Latissimus
dorsi

Trapezius

Fig. 5.14 Landmarks for lateral thoracotomy

the scapula the incision curves anteriorly to run to the sternal end of the fifth or sixth intercostal space.

The incision is deepened through the subcutaneous tissues to the muscle layer. The more superficial muscle layer comprises (from posteriorly to anteriorly) trapezius, latissimus dorsi and serratus anterior. The latissimus dorsi is divided as low as possible to minimize denervation while the fibres of serratus anterior need only be separated over the fifth and sixth ribs anteriorly. Posteriorly the rhomboids, which lie deep to trapezius, are divided to expose the subscapular fascia which is separated from the inferior aspect of the scapula anteriorly to serratus anterior.

The fifth or sixth intercostal space provides adequate access for most pulmonary procedures (but higher and lower intercostal spaces may be more appropriate for particular procedures). The periosteum of the rib is divided with diathermy and elevated and stripped with a rugine to expose the pleura. Alternatively some surgeons divide the intercostal muscle directly along the upper border of the rib. Rib resection is unnecessary but division of the costo-transverse ligament posteriorly allows greater mobility of the superior rib reducing the risk of fracture when a self-retaining retractor is introduced.

The use of muscle sparing incisions, by mobilization and retraction of latissimus dorsi laterally and retraction of serratus anterior medially, also provides adequate exposure but without consistent benefit over judiciously performed muscle splitting incisions.

Conventionally an apical and basal drain are sited following partial lung resections and one basal drain following pneumonectomy. Stab incisions are placed below the wound to site an *A*pical chest tube *A*nteriorly to drain *A*ir (AAA) and a *B*asal tube *B*ehind to drain *B*lood (BBB). Intercostal drains size 28 Fr to 32 Fr are adequate.

An intercostal nerve block to 3 intercostal spaces above and below the incision with 0.5% bupivicaine helps control post-thoracotomy pain. Cryoanalgesia of the neurovascular bundle causes long-term thoracotomy wound pain and is no longer recommended. The ribs above and below the incision are approximated with 4 perichondral sutures before closing the muscle layer with a continuous 1 or 0 suture.

Median sternotomy

This is the most frequently used incision for open heart surgery and is described in detail in the Cardiac Surgery chapter. In thoracic surgery median sternotomy may be the incision of choice for procedures requiring access to both hemi-thoraces such as bilateral pleurectomy, simultaneous resection of metastatic lesions in both lungs and for excision of thymic or anterior mediastinal tumours.

Lung resection

The extent of lung resection depends on the nature and magnitude of the underlying pathological process. Lung resection may be of the whole lung (*pneumonectomy*), a single lobe (*lobectomy*) or part of a lobe (*segmentectomy or wedge resection*). In selected cases, resection of a lobe including its bronchial origin with re-anastomosis of the proximal and distal bronchus ('sleeve' resection) can be performed.

In the Western hemisphere more than 90% of lung resections are performed for primary bronchial carcinoma. Less commonly resection may be undertaken for bronchiectasis, chronic infection (including tuberculosis), benign tumours (carcinoid or hamartoma) or metastatic carcinoma (for limited secondary deposits and no other evidence of systemic spread).

In the developing world, resection is still most commonly performed for pulmonary infection due to tuberculosis, bronchiectasis and necrotizing pneumonia.

General principles of lung resection

1. Effective postoperative analgesia is essential to permit coughing and chest expansion thereby reducing the risks of pulmonary infection.

2. Prophylactic antibiotics reduce wound infection rates but do not influence other complications such as bronchopleural fistula.

3. One lung anaesthesia with a double lumen endotracheal tube has two benefits. It improves exposure by allowing collapse of the operated lung and by blocking the bronchus it minimises the risk of spill-over contamination to the contralateral lung.

4. A posterolateral thoracotomy through the bed of the fifth, sixth or seventh rib provides excellent exposure for most pulmonary resections.

5. The surgeon is aware that variations in anatomy, especially in the pulmonary vasculature, are common.

6. The minimum procedure which achieves the goals is the best option. Lobectomy, or possibly segmentectomy, for peripheral carcinomas is as effective as pneumonectomy but with reduced mortality and morbidity.

7. For carcinoma it is theoretically preferable to divide the vein draining the malignancy as the initial stage so as to minimise the risk of tumour embolization.

8. Inability to separate tumour from aorta, superior vena cava, vertebral bodies or trachea or intracardiac spread along the pulmonary veins or artery implies irresectability.

9. In resection for malignancy sampling of lymph nodes in various anatomical sites is important to allow accurate staging of the tumour.

10. The lung should be handled gently, particularly those segments which are not to be resected, to minimise postoperative atelectasis.

11. All hilar structures should be oversewn or doubly ligated before division.

Pneumonectomy

Differences in the right and left hilum (see Fig. 5.15) must be appreciated. Standard pneumonectomy is performed without entering the pericardium but if tumour extends along the major pulmonary vessels an intrapericardial resection (radical pneumonectomy) allows more complete tumour clearance.

Any pleural adhesions and the inferior pulmonary ligament are initially divided to allow mobilization of the lung and the pleura is then divided around the hilum posterior to the phrenic nerve. If tumour location permits, the pulmonary veins are divided first (the superior vein most easily from in front and the inferior vein most easily from behind) to minimize the risk of tumour embolization. The pulmonary artery is then divided between double ligatures and oversewn proximally. As the adventitia around the main bronchus contains bronchial arteries which are responsible for its blood supply, excessive clearance of adventitia prior to division of the bronchus is avoided so as to minimize the likelihood of a subsequent bronchopleural fistula. On the left, particular caution is necessary to avoid the recurrent laryngeal nerve as it hooks around the obliterated ductus arteriosus. The bronchus is divided by an open technique with subsequent suture closure of the bronchial stump or by using a stapling gun. The closed bronchial stump lies flush with the trachea, avoiding a blind stump which predisposes to bronchopleural fistula. The thoracic cavity is filled with saline and the anaesthetist generates an airway pressure of 40 mmHg to ensure there is no air leak from the bronchial stump which is then buried in adventitial tissue.

Lymph nodes are sampled from specific anatomical

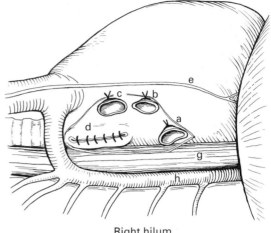

Right hilum

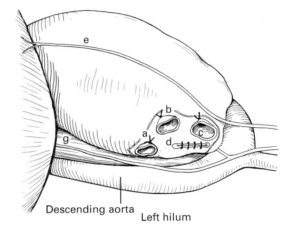

Descending aorta　Left hilum

Fig. 5.15 Anatomy of each hilum. (a = lower vein; b = upper vein; c = artery; d = bronchus; e = phrenic nerve; g = oesophagus; h = azygos vein)

sites for tumour staging and labelled in separate containers for pathological examination.

Following pneumonectomy it is conventional practice to place one basal drain connected to an underwater seal without suction (otherwise there is excessive mediastinal shift) for 24 hours.

Lobectomy

The general and operative principles for lobectomy are similar to those for pneumonectomy. Lobectomy is usually possible for resection of peripheral carcinomas which do not cross fissures, benign tumours, bronchiectases and chronic suppurative pulmonary disease, large emphysematous bullae and bronchopulmonary sequestration.

It is beyond the scope of this text to describe all types of lobectomy but the key to safe lobectomy is knowledge of the anatomy of the bronchopulmonary segments and their common variations. The hilar contents must be clearly exposed so that vessels to and from each lung segment are clearly delineated before any structure is divided. Fissures are frequently incomplete but dissection within the fissure still allows identification and division of the pulmonary arterial branches to a specific lobe.

Segmentectomy

Segmentectomy is indicated for peripheral lesions confined to a single bronchopulmonary segment particularly in patients with significantly impaired respiratory reserve. Segmentectomy is feasible because of the relatively avascular plane between the various bronchopulmonary segments which are supplied with their own bronchus and artery (although venous drainage may be shared).

Complications of lung resection

The mortality of pneumonectomy is around 6% being three times greater for right than for left pneumonectomy. The mortality from lobectomy is approximately 2%. The major causes of mortality are pneumonia, respiratory failure, myocardial infarction, bronchopleural fistula, empyema and pulmonary embolism.

The incidence of bronchopleural fistula following lung resection is approximately 5% after pneumonectomy but much less common after lobectomy. It usually presents between the first and third postoperative weeks and its clinical consequences are dependent on its size. A very small fistula, due to a pinhole leak around the suture line, may be demonstrated by radiological change in the volume of air in the pneumonectomy space without clinical manifestation. In contrast, large fistulae which allow fluid from the pneumonectomy space to re-enter the airway produce severe respiratory embarrassment and require urgent drainage of the pleural space and closure of the fistula.

The overall incidence of empyema following lung resection is approximately 5% and in half of such cases there will be a bronchopleural fistula.

Early complications following lung resection
1. Haemorrhage (minimised by oversewing all hilar ends of vessels).
2. Sputum retention leading to collapse-consolidation and bronchopneumonia (minimized by adequate analgesia and vigorous physiotherapy) may require rigid bronchoscopy and minitracheotomy.
3. Atrial fibrillation. Occurs in up to one-third of patients within ten days of a lung resection particularly if the pericardium is opened. Depending on clinical status treatment is by digitalization and/or cardioversion.
4. Persistent air leak. Air leaks from the raw surface of

the lung are common for up to two weeks after partial lung resection. Treatment is expectant and consists of intercostal drainage.

OESOPHAGEAL SURGERY

Surgical anatomy of the oesophagus

In the adult the oesophagus is a 25 cm muscular tube running from the lower border of the sixth cervical vertebra (opposite the cricoid cartilage) to the eleventh thoracic vertebra. The oesophagus passes through the diaphragm in a hiatal sling formed mainly by fibres of the right crus. At its upper end is the anatomically defined cricopharyngeal sphincter which relaxes on swallowing. At the gastric end is the lower oesophageal sphincter which is not a separate anatomical entity but a short length of oesophagus with a higher resting tone than the remainder of the oesophagus.

The oesophagus consists of 3 layers:

1. an outer longitudinal and an inner circular muscle layer without a serosal coat; the upper few centimetres of oesophagus contains striated voluntary muscle which gradually merges with smooth involuntary muscle
2. a submucosal layer of areolar tissue with numerous mucous glands
3. a mucous membrane of stratified squamous epithelium which becomes junctional columnar epithelium in the distal 2 cm of oesophagus before merging with gastric mucosa.

The *arterial blood supply* to the upper oesophagus comes from the inferior thyroid artery. The middle portion of oesophagus receives its blood supply from bronchial arteries and directly from small branches of the aorta. The lower oesophagus derives its blood supply from the left gastric and inferior phrenic arteries. These arterial branches form a longitudinal anastomosis in the muscular and submucosal layers so that devitalization of the oesophagus is rare even after extensive mobilization. *A submucosal venous* network connects with that of the stomach and becomes varicose in portal hypertension allowing portal venous blood to pass via the azygos vein to the superior vena cava.

The oesophagus receives *sympathetic and parasympathetic* innervation which form the myenteric plexus of Auerbach (between the muscle layers) as well as the plexus of Meissner. The vagus nerves form a plexus on either side of the oesophagus; towards the hiatus the left vagus lies anteriorly and the right vagus posteriorly.

Specific oesophageal investigations

Barium swallow and oesophagoscopy are the most frequently performed oesophageal investigations. Computerised axial tomography can assess extra-oesophageal spread of tumour and lymph node involvement. Manometry (see below) is often diagnostic in oesophageal motility disorders.

Oesophagoscopy

Oesophagoscopy, like bronchoscopy, has diagnostic and therapeutic indications and can be performed with a rigid or flexible instrument. Oesophagoscopy is used for biopsy of tumours, dilatation of strictures, intubation of carcinomas, sclerosing of varices, balloon dilatation of achalasia and intracavitary irradiation of cancer.

Prior to oesophagoscopy a barium swallow can assess the degree of obstruction (and therefore the likelihood of successfully passing the oesophagoscope). In chronic severe obstruction of the distal oesophagus producing mega-oesophagus (e.g. achalasia) repeated washouts may be necessary to remove debris prior to endoscopic examination.

Three indentations of the oesophagus, measured by distance from the incisor teeth at oesophagoscopy, are identifiable; the upper oesophageal sphincter (15 cm), a middle indentation caused by the aortic arch and left main bronchus (25 cm) and the lower oesophageal sphincter (40 cm). At oesophagoscopy the distance of any lesion (tumour, oesophagitis, hernia, stricture, perforation, diverticulum etc) from the incisor teeth is recorded.

Rigid oesophagoscopy requires general anaesthesia and the instrument is passed through the cricopharyngeus under direct vision. The rigid endoscope is better for removal of foreign bodies, obtaining large biopsies and passing bougies for stricture dilatation. Flexible endoscopy can be performed with intravenous sedation or general anaesthesia. It permits better examination of the distal oesophagus, stomach and duodenum and can be used to pass guide wires through strictures.

With experience, *complications* of oesophagoscopy are uncommon but include bleeding and perforation. The latter is suspected if the patient complains of excessive chest pain or if surgical emphysema is present. The diagnosis is confirmed radiologically; management is discussed below.

Oesophageal function tests

Manometry involves simultaneous measurement of intra-luminal pressure in three distinct oesophageal segments so that resting tone and generation and propagation of peristaltic waves can be monitored. Oesophageal manometry is used to establish a precise diagnosis in oesophageal motility disorders such as diffuse spasm, achalasia and scleroderma.

Measurement of pH in the distal oesophagus quantifies the frequency and severity of oesophageal reflux and is useful in complex diagnostic problems.

HIATUS HERNIA AND GASTRO-OESOPHAGEAL REFLUX

Although hiatus hernia and gastro-oesophageal reflux are frequently associated they are distinct entities. While a sliding hiatus hernia can be demonstrated radiologically in up to 90% of patients by head down tilt and abdominal compression, in only few is any associated reflux pathological. On the other hand the majority of patients with pathological reflux will be shown to have a hiatus hernia. Reflux is normally prevented by a number of anatomical and physiological features although there is controversy as to which are most important. Anti-reflux mechanisms include the physiological lower oesophageal sphincter, the intra-abdominal portion of the oesophagus, the oblique angle of the gastro-oesophageal junction (and its mucosal rosette) and the pinchcock effect of the diaphragm.

Hiatus hernia can be classified into three types:

- Type I or sliding hiatus hernia is the most common type and consists of a dilatation of the oesophageal hiatus and the phrenoesophageal membrane so that a portion of the gastric cardia slides upwards into the hiatus. There is however no true peritoneal sac and oesophageal length is initially normal. A sliding hiatus hernia is of little significance unless accompanied by pathological reflux. Severe oesophagitis complicating reflux leads to scarring and shortening of the intra-abdominal oesophagus promoting further reflux.

- Type II or rolling hiatus hernia is much less common and is characterised by a defect in most of the phrenoesophageal membrane so that part of the stomach and the peritoneal sac herniate into the chest. Initially the cardia remains fixed by a portion of the phrenoesophageal membrane and oesophageal length is maintained. As intrathoracic pressure is less than intra-abdominal pressure there is a progressive enlargement in the size of a rolling hiatus hernia and eventually most of the stomach may migrate to the chest. As the stomach is then susceptible to dilatation, torsion, volvulus and bleeding a rolling hiatus hernia is repaired even in asymptomatic patients.

- Type III hiatus hernia consists of a combination of Type II and Type I.

Disturbances of oesophageal peristalsis and lower oesophageal sphincter function which allow pathological reflux can be demonstrated in manometry studies while continuous oesophageal pH monitoring over 24 hour periods can delineate the frequency and severity of reflux. Endoscopy provides objective assessment of the severity of oesophagitis from Grade 0 (normal), 1 (erythema), 2 (patchy ulceration), 3 (confluent ulceration and patchy scarring) to 4 (stricture).

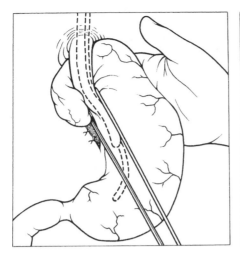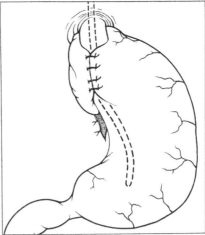

Fig. 5.16 Nissen fundoplication

Management

Conservative. Medical measures are used to treat the majority of patients with hiatus hernia and reflux. Simple measures include losing weight, stopping smoking, avoiding meals late at night and raising the head end of the bed. Antacids, H2 receptor antagonists (cimetidine, ranitidine) and proton pump blockers (omeprazole) alleviate symptoms and promote healing.

Surgical. Surgery is only considered in the severely symptomatic patient where medical therapy has failed and where there is objective evidence of oesophagitis or its complications such as bleeding and stricture. Because of the potential for complications in the rolling hiatus hernia, surgery is indicated even in the asymptomatic patient (Skinner, 1967).

Principles of surgery

Of the variety of surgical procedures described for hiatus hernia, most operations include an anti-reflux mechanism. The principles of surgery are:

- to restore an intra-abdominal portion of oesophagus and to maintain it as a narrow tube
- to perform a partial wrap of fundus around the gastro-oesophageal junction to minimise the tendency to reflux
- to narrow the oesophageal hiatus to prevent herniation of the gastro-oesophageal junction.

While some repairs can be performed from an abdominal approach, thoracotomy provides better access for mobilization of the oesophagus. Adequate mobilization is essential if the oesophagus has been shortened by fibrosis due to severe oesophagitis or if there has been a previous attempt at repair.

The long-term results of surgery are satisfactory in approximately 90% of patients. The side effects of the various operations are similar and consist of dysphagia, inability to belch and gaseous distension from too tight a repair.

Nissen fundoplication (Fig. 5.16)

This can be performed through the chest or abdomen. After complete mobilization of the oesophagus and cardia from the diaphragm, the gastric fundus is mobilized by dividing the short gastric arteries between the stomach and the spleen on the greater curvature and branches of the left gastric artery in the gastrohepatic ligament on the lesser curvature. A 40 Fr size bougie is passed into the oesophagus and the fundus of the stomach is passed behind the oesophagus and then sutured anteriorly forming a 360°C wrap over the lower 4 cm of oesophagus. It should be possible to pass a finger between the wrap and the anterior oesophagus (ensuring the wrap is not too tight). Sutures are placed posteriorly in the crura to narrow the hiatus.

Belsey mark IV (Fig. 5.17)

This name refers to Belsey's fourth modification of an operation initially described by Allison. This operation can only be performed by a thoracic approach (usually through the sixth intercostal space). The oesophagus is mobilized to the level of the aortic arch and the cardia completely freed from its diaphragmatic attachments. The gastric fundus is mobilized — as in the Nissen operation — and then plicated on to the lower 4 cm of oesophagus for 270° anteriorly and laterally, leaving the vagus nerves posteriorly. The repair is done in two layers, the first suturing the gastric fundus to the lower 2 cm of oesophagus and the second taking bites of oesophagus, fundus of stomach and the tendinous portion of the diaphragm. The posterior segment of oesophagus not included in the wrap is buttressed against the hiatus. Sutures are placed posteriorly in the crura to narrow the hiatus.

Hill's posterior gastropexy (Fig. 5.18)
This operation is performed through an abdominal approach. The oesophagus is mobilized from its hiatal attachments and the gastro-oesophageal junction anchored to the arcuate ligament followed by a partial plication of stomach around the junction.

Leigh–Collis gastroplasty (Fig. 5.19)
This refers to lengthening of a shortened intra-abdominal oesophagus by dividing the fundus of the stomach as a continuation of the oesophageal tube before performing an anti-reflux procedure.

Neuromuscular disorders of the oesophagus
The major function of the oesophagus is coordinated peristaltic activity to ensure delivery of food to the stomach. Disorders of this function result in oesophageal emptying problems and include:

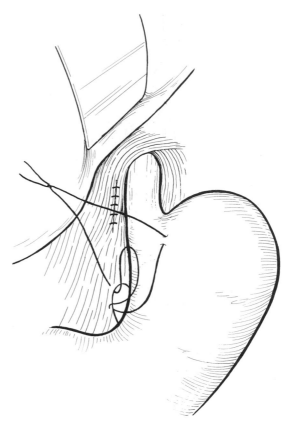

Fig. 5.18   Hill's gastropexy

Hiatus hernia — discussed separately

Achalasia
Achalasia is a disease of uncertain neurogenic aetiology characterised histologically by absence of Auerbach's plexus resulting in loss of peristaltic activity and failure of relaxation of the lower oesophageal sphincter. In 10% of patients it eventually gives rise to malignancy.

In the early stages achalasia typically presents with dysphagia for liquids (compared to carcinomas and organic strictures where there is initially dysphagia for solids) before progressing to total dysphagia. In later stages it gives the characteristic radiological appearance of a mega-oesophagus and typical manometry findings of absent peristalsis and failure of relaxation of the lower oesophageal sphincter.

Initial management is repeated passage of oesophageal bougies which can provide prolonged symptomatic relief. Dilatation with a hydrostatic bag under general anaesthesia provides good symptomatic relief for up to ten years in two-thirds of patients.

Heller's procedure is a longitudinal myotomy through the muscle fibres of the lower oesophagus down to the mucosal layer. The myotomy extends across the gastro-

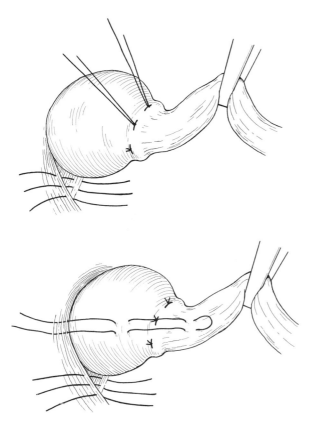

Fig. 5.17   Belsey mark IV

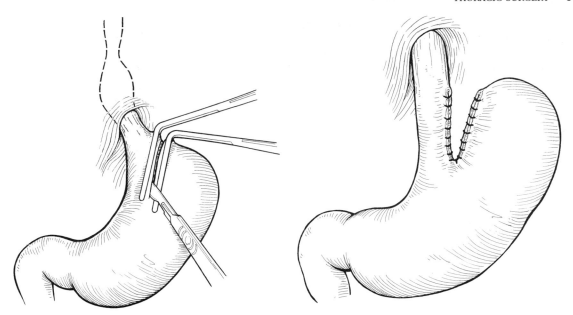

Fig. 5.19 Leigh–Collis gastroplasty

oesophageal junction for 5–7 cm to ensure division of all constricting muscle fibres. This procedure gives excellent long-term relief but is complicated by reflux oesophagitis in 5% of patients.

Pharyngeal diverticulum (see also Chapter 12)
In this condition, also known as Zenker's pulsion diverticulum, there is posterior herniation of the mucosal layer of the oesophagus between the inferior constrictor above and the cricopharyngeus below (Fig. 5.20). It most frequently occurs in elderly patients due to incoordination of relaxation of the cricopharyngeus muscle.

The diverticulum arises in the midline and usually enlarges to the left to produce dysphagia by compressing the oesophagus against the vertebral column. Clinical presentation may be with chronic pulmonary aspiration as the neck of the diverticulum lies above the cricopharyngeus and allows spillage of its contents into the respiratory tree when the patient is supine. There is also a risk of malignant transformation in the epithelial lining presumably due to stasis of potential carcinogens.

The *surgical approach* is by a left cervical incision retracting the thyroid gland and the larynx medially and the carotid sheath laterally. For the small diverticulum a cricopharyngeal myotomy may suffice. For the large diverticulum the sac is excised and a cricopharyngeal myotomy performed to prevent recurrence.

Diffuse spasm of the oesophagus
This condition may produce chronic chest pain and is often mistaken for angina. The aetiology of this condi-

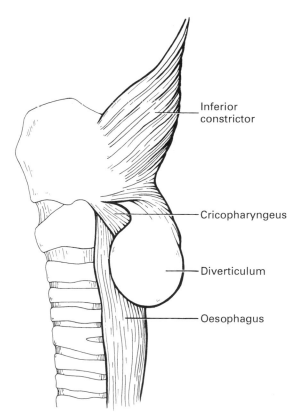

Inferior constrictor

Cricopharyngeus

Diverticulum

Oesophagus

Fig. 5.20 Pharangeal diverticulum

tion is uncertain but manometry demonstrates repeated high pressure peristaltic waves with normal relaxation of the lower oesophageal sphincter (cf. achalasia). Radiologically the oesophagus may have a 'corkscrew' appearance. Surgical treatment consists of an extended myotomy as in Heller's procedure but the results are less successful.

OESOPHAGEAL TUMOURS

Benign tumours

Benign tumours account for less than 10% of oesophageal tumours and most are leiomyomas or pedunculated intraluminal tumours. Leiomyomas are intramural tumours with an intact overlying mucosa most frequently occurring in the lower third of the oesophagus and giving a characteristic radiologic appearance of a sharply demarcated ovoid mass.

Malignant tumours

Oesophageal carcinoma usually occurs in men after the age of 50 years and is particularly common in China, Japan and in some native populations of South Africa. Aetiological factors in the development of oesophageal carcinoma are cigarette smoking, excessive alcohol intake, columnar-lined lower oesophagus (Barrett oesophagus) and conditions predisposing to oesophageal stasis such as achalasia.

Histologically most malignancies (80%–90%) are squamous cell. Adenocarcinoma accounts for approximately 10% of malignancies and occurs particularly in the columnar-lined Barrett oesophagus. Oat cell carcinomas, melanomas and malignant change in leiomyomas are very rare. Malignant tumours of the oesophagogastric junction are invariably gastric adenocarcinomas and account for half of all oesophageal malignancies. Approximately 10% of malignancies occur in the upper third of the oesophagus, 25% in the mid third and 65% in the lower third (Fig. 5.21). Oesophageal cancers invade locally and can produce systemic metastases but the predominant method of spread is through lymphatics.

Oesophageal carcinoma is a potentially curable disease as it does not metastasize in its early stages. Unfortunately it is usually advanced at the time of presentation so that prognosis is poor. The overall one-year survival is less than 15% and the five-year survival less than 4% although the prognosis is better in selected subgroups (Matthews, 1990).

In deciding treatment the following points should be considered:

1. Patients are often elderly and debilitated with marked weight loss and are therefore poor candidates for major surgical resection (which has a 10% mortality

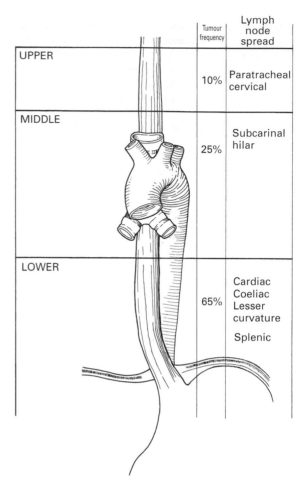

Fig. 5.21 Carcinoma of oesophagus — frequency and lymph node spread

even in the best patients and in the best surgical hands).

2. The position and local spread of tumour influence suitability for resection. Growths in the lower or middle third of oesophagus are more suitable for resection than growths in the upper third.

3. The majority of tumours are squamous cell and are usually radiosensitive while adenocarcinomas and small cell carcinomas are not.

Treatment options

Radiotherapy. Squamous tumours are variably sensitive to radiotherapy and good symptomatic relief and a 5%–10% five year survival can be expected with radical radiotherapy. Radiotherapy is especially indicated in elderly patients, in those unfit for surgery and for growths in the upper third of oesophagus where surgical results are poorer.

Chemotherapy. Few patients with oesophageal carcinoma show any significant response to chemotherapy.

Oesophageal intubation. This technique involves transoral passage of a plastic tube (e.g. Celestin (1981), Mousseau et al (1956)) which is then retrieved and secured through a gastrostomy (Fig. 5.22). More recently, endoscopic techniques for placing such tubes (pulsion intubation) without the need for laparotomy and gastrostomy have become popular. Oesophageal intubation does not provide as effective palliation as resection and still has a significant mortality and morbidity. Nevertheless, it is less traumatic than resection, especially in frail elderly patients, who can leave hospital within a few days.

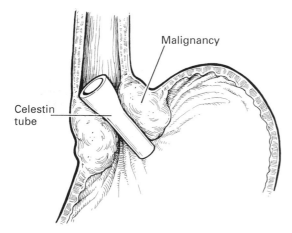

Malignancy

Celestin tube

Fig. 5.22   Oesophageal intubation for carcinoma

Surgery

Surgery offers the best prospect of cure in patients who present at an early stage of the disease and the best palliation for dysphagia even if complete cure is not possible. There is, however, little benefit from oesophagectomy in patients with liver and peritoneal metastases who have a very limited life expectancy. Operative mortality for oesophagectomy varies from 10%–40% depending on the surgeon's experience and should therefore only be undertaken by surgeons who perform the operation regularly.

Preoperative assessment includes oesophagoscopy to define the site and extent of tumour spread, simultaneous bronchoscopy to exclude invasion of the bronchial tree and computerised axial tomography to exclude hepatic and abdominal lymph node masses. Preoperative physiotherapy is useful in patients with 'spillover' respiratory infection but there is little evidence that preoperative nutritional support is beneficial. Prophylactic antibiotics are given during surgery to cover both aerobic and anaerobic organisms which proliferate in the obstructed oesophagus.

Numerous *techniques* of oesophageal resection are described but tumour location and local spread dictate

the optimal surgical approach. McKeown (1985) emphasised the tendency for submucosal and longitudinal lymphatic spread so that a ten centimetre resection margin is desirable. For tumours in the lower third, left thoraco-laparotomy allows oesophagogastrectomy removing the lower oesophagus and upper part of the stomach, with oesophagogastric anastomosis below the aortic arch. The classic resection for growths in the middle or upper third is the two-stage approach of Ivor Lewis (Lewis, 1946) which allows complete oesophageal resection and anastomosis higher in the thorax. This entails a laparotomy to mobilize stomach (as this cannot be done from the right thorax because of the presence of the liver) and to palpate for intrahepatic or peritoneal metastases. This is followed by a right thoracotomy which allows access to the whole intrathoracic oesophagus after division of the azygos vein. Some surgeons prefer the three-stage approach of McKeown (1985) where there is an additional cervical incision to permit anastomosis in the neck thereby avoiding the disastrous consequences of a leaking anastomosis in the thorax.

Thoracolaparotomy

Indication. Oesophageal tumours below the aortic arch or high gastric tumours extending to the lower oesophagus. This approach permits resection of spleen and pancreas as well as radical resection of lymphatic nodes along the left gastric artery in the lesser curvature.

Procedure. A double lumen endotracheal tube allows collapse of the lung and facilitates the intrathoracic oesophageal dissection. The patient is positioned as for a left thoracotomy with a slight dorsal tilt.

The skin incision starts midway between the umbilicus and xiphisternum and is continued obliquely up over the left costal margin and along the eighth intercostal space to end 2 cm below the angle of the scapula (Fig. 5.23). It is sensible to complete the abdominal portion of the incision first as the presence of palpable liver or peritoneal metastases implies that further resection will be unhelpful. The cartilaginous costal margin is divided and the pleural cavity entered through the eighth intercostal space. The diaphragm is separated 2 cm from the chest wall by a circumferential incision (thereby preserving its innervation and leaving a cuff for subsequent re-attachment). The inferior pulmonary ligament is divided to allow mobilization of the left lower lobe and to confirm that tumour invasion into mediastinal structures does not preclude resection. After opening the mediastinal pleura (without opening the right pleural cavity) the oesophagus and its surrounding fat and lymph nodes are mobilized from the pericardium anteriorly and the aorta posteriorly up to the level of the aortic arch.

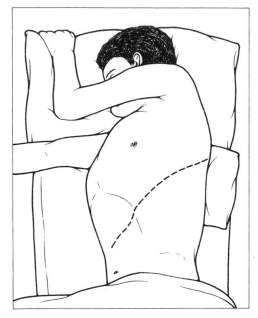

Fig. 5.23 Position of the patient for a combined abdomino-thoracic approach to the lower oesophagus. The line of incision is shown

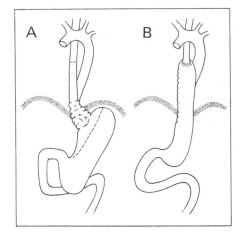

Fig. 5.24 Operation for carcinoma of the distal oesophagus. (A) Extent of resection. (B) Tube constructed from gastric remnant amd joined to oesophagus

Division of the left triangular ligament of liver provides access to the hiatus and the stomach is mobilized, through the gastrocolic omentum, to the pylorus. The duodenum is mobilized if necessary (Kocher manoeuvre) to permit the pylorus to reach the hiatus. To ensure continuity of vasculature around the mobilized stomach it is important to preserve the right gastro-epiploic arch along the greater curvature of the stomach and to divide the left gastric vessels close to their origin from the coeliac axis. The short gastric vessels between stomach and spleen are divided carefully to avoid injury to both the stomach and the spleen.

After tumour resection with a clear margin of oesophagus and stomach the proximal end of the gastric remnant is closed with sutures or staples to form a tube. The pylorus is stretched or a pyloromyotomy is carried out since vagotomy will, of course, have resulted from the resection. The oesophagus is anastomosed in an end-to-side fashion to a 2 cm incision in the anterior wall of the gastric remnant (Fig. 5.24B) and a naso-gastric tube passed to ensure decompression in the postoperative period. The oesophagus and stomach are sutured to mediastinal structures to prevent torsion and the hiatus reconstructed. The diaphragm is re-attached and the chest wall is closed in layers, leaving an intercostal drain at the lung base.

It is conventional practice to avoid solids by mouth for the first 5 postoperative days when a barium swallow is performed to ensure integrity of the anastomosis.

OESOPHAGEAL PERFORATION

The most common cause of oesophageal perforation is oesophagoscopy, particularly when attempting to dilate a stricture. Oesophageal perforation may also occur after trauma, impaction of foreign bodies, violent vomiting (Boerhaave syndrome) and spontaneously in association with malignancies. The mortality of oesophageal perforation may be as high as 30% even in specialised units and is largely related to delay in diagnosis (Skinner, 1980).

Perforation may occur at any site in the oesophagus but usually where it is narrowest i.e. at its upper (cricopharyngeus sphincter) and lowest portions (where it is most frequently diseased). The upper two-thirds of the oesophagus lie in close proximity to the right pleural cavity while the lower third lies closer to the left pleural cavity. The presence of a right or left sided pleural effusion is therefore a clue to the likely site of perforation.

Perforation at the time of oesophagoscopy is suspected if the patient complains of undue pain on swallowing (when the sedation or anaesthetic has worn off) even in the absence of surgical emphysema or radiological signs such as fluid levels or mediastinal gas. The diagnosis is confirmed by a barium swallow using dilute barium (water soluble contrast media may be excessively diluted in mediastinal or pleural fluid and fail to demonstrate a perforation as well as being intensely irritant to the trachea if aspirated).

Management of oesophageal perforation is dependent on:

- whether the tear is full or partial thickness
- the site of the tear

- duration since perforation (exploration is better within 12 hours)
- the presence or absence of a distal obstructing lesion.

Partial thickness tears are always managed conservatively. Management consists of nasoenteric feeding (parenteral nutrition is rarely indicated) and broad spectrum antibiotics to cover aerobic and anaerobic flora.

Transmural perforation of the cervical oesophagus is usually treated conservatively unless extensive. If a cervical abscess forms it can be drained along the anterior border of sternomastoid. Transmural perforation of the thoracic oesophagus requires surgery to control the local leak and therefore the risk of mediastinal infection. The principles of surgery are to repair the oesophageal tear and to establish free drainage for the false passage. The presence of a distal obstruction may require a more extensive resection.

Oesophageal resection has been described in detail previously but the following points should be considered in patients with perforations:

- the posterior mediastinal pleura between the right and left pleural sacs is left intact to minimise the risk of infection in both pleural cavities
- the oesophageal muscle coat is dissected to allow complete identification of the edges of the mucosal tear
- any repair is reinforced with a flap of pleura
- the pleural cavity is adequately drained with well sited drains
- the stomach is kept empty in the early postoperative period by intraoperative placement of a nasoenteric tube.

Patients who present late after perforation (i.e. more than 24 hours after occurrence) or who develop a fistula after an initial attempt at repair may be too ill — as a consequence of gross sepsis — to withstand major resection. In such circumstances an exclusion procedure may be life-saving: the thoracic oesophagus is closed proximal and distal to the perforation and a large pleural drain is directed to the site of perforation. A cervical oesophagostomy is fashioned proximally and a gastrostomy distally to permit enteral feeding. Oesophageal resection or reconstruction can await subsequent improvement in the patient's general condition.

OTHER OESOPHAGEAL CONDITIONS

Oesophageal atresia

Oesophageal atresia is one of the more common congenital abnormalities, the incidence being 1 for 3250 live births. Although the problem continues to challenge the surgeon, few conditions can be more rewarding to treat.

Embryogenesis

The respiratory system develops from a diverticulum which first appears in the embryo at 4 weeks as a longitudinal groove on the ventral surface of the foregut. Lateral ridges in the wall of the foregut on either side of the groove fuse in the midline so as to separate the two structures. The process of separation starts at the caudal end of the groove and extends incompletely to the cranial end. Oesophageal atresia and tracheo-oesophageal fistula are probably established at this early date and this would explain the high incidence of associated anomalies.

The structural form of the anomaly is variable (Figs 5.25–5.28). In 70% of babies, oesophageal atresia is associated with a fistula between the trachea and the distal limb of the oesophagus. In 10% oesophageal atresia is present without fistula; these babies have a characteristically scaphoid abdomen as the bowel is empty of gas. In a few there may be fistulae between the trachea and both proximal and distal segments of the oesophagus and, in others, a tracheo-oesophageal fistula may be present in the absence of an atresia.

Clinical presentation

The condition is apparent soon after birth. Maternal hydramnios and low birth weight are common. The baby collects excessive frothy saliva in the mouth and inadvertent feeding causes choking and respiratory distress. An unsuccessful attempt to pass a firm 12 French gauge nasogastric catheter will confirm the diagnosis. The major risk to the baby is that of atelectasis and pneumonia from overspill of saliva and, in the presence of a fistula, reflux of gastric secretion. The risks can be reduced by continuous suction of the nasopharynx, by physiotherapy and by nursing the baby horizontal in either a prone or lateral position. A plain X-ray should be taken of both chest and abdomen. A radio-opaque catheter in the oesophagus will indicate the length of the upper pouch and gas in the bowel will confirm the presence of a fistula and may demonstrate an associated intestinal abnormality.

Operation

In a fit baby an attempt should be made to close the fistula and repair the oesophagus during the first 36 hours of life. It may, however, be necessary to delay the procedure, either to treat respiratory problems or to investigate further an associated anomaly. At operation the mediastinum is reached by an extrapleural approach using a right thoracotomy incision through the fourth or fifth intercostal space. The proximal and distal segments of the oesophagus are mobilized with

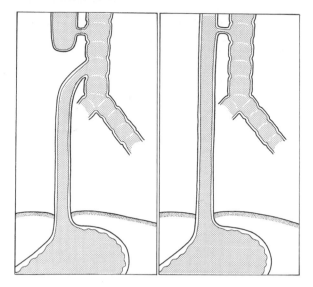

Fig. 5.25   Fig. 5.26

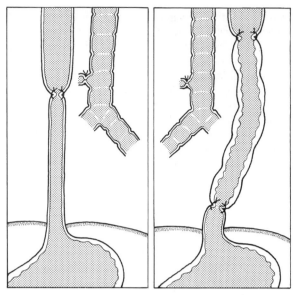

Fig. 5.29   Fig. 5.30

Fig. 5.29 Ligation and division of fistula and primary anastomosis of oesophagus
Fig. 5.30 Colonic interposition between proximal and distal oesophagus

In some babies, the gap between the proximal and distal oesophagus may be marginally too great to allow a primary anastomosis and in this situation some surgeons advocate a delayed procedure. It is hoped, during an interval of some weeks, that further growth of the oesophagus and daily stretching of the proximal segment with a bougie will result in the gap becoming relatively smaller, so that a primary anastomosis can again be attempted.

In other babies, particularly those without a tracheo-oesophageal fistula, the distal oesophagus is short and a primary anastomosis is impractical. In this situation a cervical oesophagostomy is fashioned together with a feeding gastrostomy. The oesophagostomy allows the baby to clear secretions and to be sham fed. After an interval of 12 months the gap between the proximal oesophagus and stomach can be bridged by one of three methods: a segment of colon can be interposed (Fig. 5.30) (Waterston, 1964), a gastric tube can be fashioned from the greater curvature of the stomach (Cohen, 1974) or the stomach can be mobilized and brought up to the neck through the mediastinum.

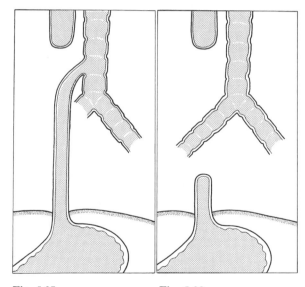

Fig. 5.27   Fig. 5.28

Figs 5.25–5.28 Anatomical variations of oesophageal atresia and tracheo-oesophageal fistula

care so as to preserve both the blood supply and the right vagus which runs along the lateral wall of the distal segment. The fistula, which normally lies between the distal segment and the lateral wall of the trachea just above the carina, is transfixed and divided. Continuity of the oesophagus is achieved by an end-to-end anastomosis of the two segments with fine interrupted sutures (Fig. 5.29). A fine nasogastric tube placed down the lumen of the oesophagus allows early feeding. Finally, the wound is closed with a drain in place.

DIAPHRAGMATIC HERNIA

Congenital malformations

The diaphragm is formed in the fetus between eight and ten weeks from the middle part of the septum transversum, the pleuroperitoneal folds and the dorsal mesentery of the foregut. A hernia is most commonly associated with failure of fusion of these components and the persistence of the pleuroperitoneal canal though, on occasions, the hernia may he within the foramen of Morgagni or the posterolateral foramen of Bochdalek (Sutton, 1982). The left dome of the diaphragm is more commonly affected than the right, presumably because the latter is protected by the liver. The underlying lung is hypoplastic and bowel fixation is abnormal. In eventration of the diaphragm, abdominal viscera lying within the thorax are covered with a hypoplastic structure and this condition mimics a true diaphragmatic hernia.

Presentation

The incidence of diaphragmatic hernia is approximately one per 5000 births. The condition presents with respiratory distress in the newborn. There is limited movement of the affected side of the thorax, the mediastinum is displaced to the opposite side and the abdomen appears scaphoid. A chest X-ray shows bowel within the thorax and an abdominal film may show reduced bowel content. The accumulation of gas in bowel lying in the thorax reduces the ventilatory capacity and aggravates the mediastinal displacement.

Management

For the immediate management a nasogastric tube is passed to empty the stomach and the baby nursed on the affected side in an incubator. Positive pressure ventilation through an endotracheal tube may be necessary. A face mask should not be used since it results in more gas being introduced into the stomach. Previously, emergency surgery was regarded as critical. More recently it has become accepted that, where necessary, the condition of the baby should be stabilised over 24–48 hours. In some babies, adequate oxygenation is difficult to achieve because of the patho-physiological problems associated with pulmonary hypoplasia, pulmonary hypertension and persistence of fetal circulation with right to left shunting. In this situation Tolazoline may be helpful. In other babies it is possible that adequate oxygenation can only be maintained by extracorporeal membrane oxygenation (ECMO) and the efficacy of this technique is at present being studied. Mortality in babies with a diaphragmatic hernia remains high (Simson, 1985).

Operation

The diaphragmatic hernia is repaired through a transverse upper abdominal incision. The bowel is gently withdrawn from the thorax. Incomplete rotation is inevitable and the duodenum may be partially obstructed by Ladd's bands (see p. 468). The hernia sac, if present, should be either excised or plicated, the underlying hypoplastic lung inspected and a thoracotomy drain placed in position. The anterior and posterior rims of the diaphragm can then usually be defined and brought together without difficulty, using interrupted nonabsorbable sutures. However, occasionally the deficit is such that the diaphragm needs to be replaced with a sheet of synthetic material. Sometimes reduction of gut from the thorax increases the visceral abdominal volume so that primary skin closure is impractical and can only be achieved with a synthetic pouch as in the repair of gastroschisis (p. 540).

Postoperative care

After operation, the nasogastric tube is left in position to ensure that the stomach remains empty and an intravenous infusion continues. Respiratory function is monitored by serial blood gas and bicarbonate analysis and assisted ventilation may be necessary. Sudden collapse in the postoperative period may be due to a pneumothorax on the normal side of the chest and is an indication for an immediate chest X-ray.

REFERENCES

Celestin L R, Campbell W B 1981 A new and safe system for oesophageal dilatation. Lancet 1: 74–75

Cohen D A, Middleton A W, Fletcher J 1974 Gastric tube oesophagoplasty. Journal of Paediatric Surgery 9: 451

Le Roux B T 1965 Empyema thoracis. British Journal of Surgery 52: 89–99

Lewis I 1946 The surgical treatment of carcinoma of the oesophagus, with special reference to the new operation for growths of the middle third. British Journal of Surgery 34: 18

McKeown K C 1985 The surgical treatment of carcinoma of the oesophagus: a review of the results of 478 cases. Journal of the Royal College of Surgeons of Edinburgh 30: 1–14

Matthews H R, Hopkinson R B 1984 Treatment of sputum retention by minitracheotomy. British Journal of Surgery 71: 147–150

Matthews H R, Walker S J 1990 Oesophageal carcinoma: the view from East Birmingham. Journal of the Royal College of Surgeons of Edinburgh 35: 279–283

Mousseau M M, Le Forestier J, Barbin J, Hardy M 1956 Place de l'intubation a demeure dans le traitment palliatif du cancer de l'oesophage. Archives Francaises des Maladies de l'Appareil Digestif et des Maladies de la Nutrition 45: 208

Potgieter P D, Benatar S R, Hewitson R P, Ferguson A D 1981 Surgical treatment of bullous lung disease. Thorax 36: 885–890

Simson J N L, Eckstein H B 1985 Congenital diaphragmatic hernia: a 20 year experience. British Journal of Surgery 72: 733–736

Skinner D B, Belsey R H 1967 Surgical management of oesophageal reflux and hiatus hernia: long term results

with 13 000 patients. Journal of Thoracic and
Cardiovascular Surgery 53: 33–54

Skinner D B, Little A G, DeMeester T R 1980 Management
of oesophageal perforation. American Journal of Surgery
139: 760–764

Sutton P P, Longrigg N 1982 Strangulated Bochdalek hernia
in an adult. Journal of the Royal College of Surgeons of
Edinburgh 27: 58–59

Waterston D 1964 Colonic replacement of the oesophagus
(intrathoracic). Surgical Clinics of North America 44: 6

FURTHER READING

Bains M S 1991 Surgical treatment of lung cancer. Chest
100: 826-837

Ellis F H 1986 Hiatus hernia. Clinical Symposia
38: 2–31

Jackson J W, Cooper D K (eds) 1986 Thoracic surgery. In

Rob and Smith's Operative Surgery, 4th edn.
Butterworths, London

Paneth M, Goldstraw P, Hyams B 1987 Fundamental
techniques in pulmonary and oesophageal surgery.
Springer-Verlag, London

6

Orthopaedic surgery

J. CHRISTIE

The introduction of infection at a bone or joint opera-tion leads to consequences which may well be disas-trous. Meticulous attention must, therefore, be paid to the aseptic ritual. Elective operations should not be performed in the presence of any systemic infection or of septic skin conditions, even although these are well removed from the site of operation. Preparation of the skin should be especially thorough, but the ritual of shaving and enclosing the limb in sterile drapes for 24 hours prior to surgery is no longer practised. There is now much evidence to show that shaving the skin at an interval before surgery is undertaken increases the risk of infection by creating small nicks or abrasions, which may harbour organisms. Shaving, if required, should be carried out immediately before operation and be limited to the operation site. The only preopera-tive skin preparation which is necessary is thorough cleansing with soap and water.

'No-touch' technique

This technique was at one time used by many orthopaedic surgeons. It requires that the gloved hand should be regarded as potentially contaminated, since sweating of the hands within the gloves carries to the surface organisms from the deeper layers of the skin, and gloves frequently become perforated at operation. The theatre sister should not touch any instruments or swabs by hand, but only with sterile forceps. Needles are threaded with forceps, and are passed to the surgeon in a needle holder. The skin incision is made through surgical adhesive film and the knife is dis-carded. The surgeon must not introduce his fingers into the wound, and should avoid touching the busi-ness end of the instruments. Needles are held in hold-ers, and forceps are used throughout for swabbing and for the tying of ligatures and sutures; blood on the glove is evidence of failure of the technique. Few surgeons now adhere to the full discipline since the fingers, used carefully and judiciously, provide the most delicate and sensitive surgical instruments. The use of double gloves in high risk situations overcomes most of the potential hazards of perforated gloves.

Nevertheless, tradition dies hard and most orthopaedic surgeons still practise a modified technique, which might be described as 'not much touch'.

Identifying the operation site

In orthopaedic surgery there is frequently no external evidence of disease of a joint once the patient is anaesthetised and accidents have occurred in which the wrong limb has been operated upon. To avoid such disasters the surgeon should personally confirm the site of surgery prior to anaesthesia and mark the operation site with a skin pencil.

Tourniquets

Tourniquets are used where possible in limb surgery except in cases of peripheral vascular disease. Properly used they limit blood loss and provide a dry operative field. Improperly used, they can cause damage to nerve or vessel. If applied too tightly, or too loosely, they may increase bleeding by impeding venous return without occluding the arterial circulation. Only pneumatic tourniquets with a pressure gauge should be used. The cuff should be applied to the upper arm, the proximal thigh or mid calf where muscle bulk will protect the nerves. Before inflating the tourniquet the limb should be ex-sanguinated by elevation for a few minutes or by applying an Esmarch bandage from the periphery proximally. Elevation is sufficient in most circum-stances and has the advantage of leaving a small amount of blood in the limb which helps to identify the vessels and allow their control during the operation. The tourniquet should be inflated to 50 mmHg above the arterial pressure. The safe duration of tourniquet time varies with the age of the patient and the health of his blood vessels. In experimental animals tourniquets have been retained for three hours without lasting ill effect but in practice an hour and a half is probably a wise limit. Tourniquets are not a substitute for haemos-tasis and it is important that all cut vessels should be ligated or coagulated. In major wounds particularly around vascular areas, such as the elbow or knee, it is wise to release the tourniquet before wound closure to confirm that satisfactory haemostasis has been secured, for a wound haematoma creates an environment favourable to infection and may cause wound breakdown.

In addition to careful haemostasis, wound drainage for 1 or 2 days is indicated in most orthopaedic operations. Suction drainage is most effective and represents one of the major advances in operative technique in recent years.

Antibiotic cover

With the introduction of major joint replacement surgery there has been a new incentive to control operative infection which is a major hazard in this type of surgery. Among the various measures which have been tried are the use of ultra clean air enclosures which have proved of value but are expensive additions to operating rooms and are not generally available. The use of appropriate antibiotic cover during and after operation has proved almost as valuable and has reduced the incidence of sepsis to less than 1% in some series. For maximal effect the antibiotic should reach high circulating blood levels during surgery and is best given intravenously at the time of anaesthetic induction. Wide spectrum antibiotics such as Cefuroxime have been most widely used and a suggested routine is 750 mg intravenously at induction and repeated intramuscularly or intravenously at 6 and 12 hours after surgery. None of these measures however is a substitute for gentle, careful surgical technique with good haemostasis and excision of any traumatised or devitalised tissues at the completion of the operation.

Aspiration of joints

Joint aspiration is frequently required for diagnostic or therapeutic purposes. As the synovial cavity is a continuous one, aspiration may be carried out on any aspect of a joint. The site should be selected therefore so as to avoid important anatomical structures and cause least discomfort to the patient. The tissues at the chosen site are infiltrated with local anaesthetic such as 1% lignocaine using a fine bore needle; the skin and joint capsule are the most sensitive structures. The infiltrating needle is left in situ for 2 minutes to mark the track while the anaesthetic is taking effect. With thin serous effusions the fine infiltrating needle may be adequate to allow diagnostic aspiration, but for thicker effusions such as blood or pus a wider bore needle is selected and introduced along the anaesthetised track.

Osteotomy

Osteotomy is the surgical division of bone. It may be performed to correct deformity of a bone or joint and to relieve pain in osteoarthritis. Common indications are metatarsal osteotomy to correct hallux valgus or to relieve pressure on a prominent metatarsal head, upper tibial osteotomy for osteoarthritis of the knee, supracondylar osteotomy for deformities resulting from polio-myelitis, intertrochanteric osteotomy for osteoarthritis of the hip, spinal osteotomy for kyphotic deformity in ankylosing spondylitis and osteotomy of any bone to correct congenital deformities or malunited fractures. Many of these procedures will be considered in the subsequent sections, but a few general principles may be considered here.

Osteotomies are in general precise operations designed to produce a specific realignment of a bone. It is necessary therefore to study the patient and the X-rays before operation and plan the exact level of bone section or the amount of bone removal required before surgery. The bone section should be done with minimal trauma so as to avoid bone necrosis. Thus it is best to avoid power saws, which may generate heat, and use sharp osteotomes or hand operated drills or saws. When the osteotomy has been completed internal fixation is usually applied to hold the correction.

A useful technique which has application particularly in children is the two stage procedure of 'osteotomy-osteoclasis'. In this procedure which is most widely used for supracondylar osteotomies of the femur, an appropriate wedge is removed leaving a small part of the cortex intact. The wedge is then broken into chips which are reinserted into the defect and a plaster cast is applied. Two weeks later under anaesthesia the plaster is wedged to complete the osteotomy and to produce the desired correction. No internal fixation is required.

OPERATIONS ON THE UPPER ARM AND SHOULDER

Exposure of humerus

Anterior approach to upper half

The patient lies on his back with the shoulder slightly raised by a flat sandbag placed beneath the lower part of the scapula. An incision is made as shown in Figure 6.1. For a full exposure it begins *behind* the highest point of the shoulder over the spine of the scapula, crosses the shoulder anteriorly to the coracoid, and then descends in the line of the medial border of the deltoid as far as the insertion of this muscle. The cephalic vein is identified lying in the delto-pectoral sulcus. Injury to the vein is avoided by deepening the incision through the medial fibres of deltoid, thus leaving a narrow strand of muscle protecting the vein. To obtain full exposure of the upper end of the humerus, the anterior part of deltoid should be mobilized at its origin from the anterior border of the lateral third of the clavicle. Henry (1973) advises that a sliver of

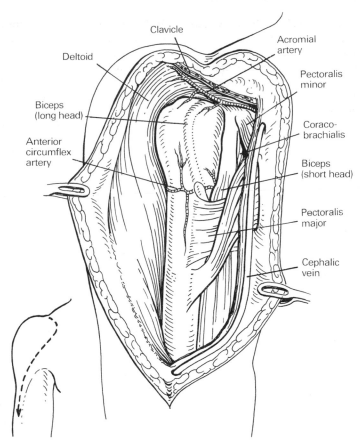

Fig. 6.1   Anterior exposure of shoulder and proximal humerus. The approach passes between deltoid and pectoralis major using the cephalic vein as a guide; the deltoid may be detached from the clavicle

bone comprising this border should be severed with a chisel, and swung laterally with the muscle fibres attached 'like a curtain on a rod'. This procedure allows very full exposure of the upper half of the humerus and of the shoulder joint (Fig. 6.1). At the close of the operation, the strip of bone bearing the deltoid origin is easily reattached with a single stitch.

Anterior approach to the lower half
The incision lies just lateral to the sulcus marking the lateral border of biceps, and so avoids the cephalic vein which lies in the sulcus (Fig. 6.2). The biceps is mobilized and retracted medially to expose the brachialis. The fibres of this muscle are then split by means of a blunt dissector, which is directed towards the front of the humerus in the midline. In this way the lateral strip of brachialis acts as a buffer protecting the radial nerve, while the medial strip protects the musculocutaneous nerve and, farther away, the main neurovascular bundle (Fig. 6.2). The split in brachialis may be carried down to within 2.5 cm of the epicondyles without opening the elbow joint. Flexion of the joint

relaxes the muscles, and allows them to be retracted to give wide exposure of the bone.

Exposure of the shoulder joint

Anterior approach
The anterior approach utilizes the upper part of the Henry exposure of the upper part of the humerus. It is not always necessary to detach the anterior fibres of the deltoid from the clavicle but, having retracted the deltoid laterally, the front of the shoulder is still obscured by the coracoid process and its attached muscles. These may be mobilized and retracted laterally; alternatively exposure may be obtained either by dividing the muscles (coracobrachialis, the short head of biceps and pectoralis minor) 1 cm below their origins, or by dividing the tip of the coracoid with an osteotome and displacing it medially with its muscles still attached. It simplifies reattachment at a later stage if the coracoid is first drilled and tapped with a screw, which is then removed before osteotomy and used to reattach the coracoid on completion of the operation. The front

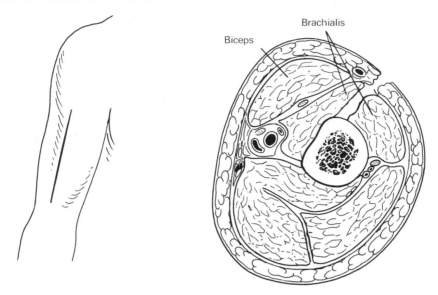

Fig. 6.2   Anterior exposure of distal humerus. The approach is made lateral to biceps and splits brachialis

of the shoulder joint now lies exposed, covered only by the subscapularis muscle.

Posterior approach to the shoulder joint

The patient lies on his side with the affected arm uppermost. The arm is freely draped to allow an assistant to change the position as required. The skin incision follows the spine of the scapula, extending laterally to the tip of the acromion. The deltoid muscle is mobilized from the spine of the scapula and from the ac-romion and is reflected distally and laterally (Fig. 6.3), care being taken to avoid damage to the axillary nerve, which emerges through the quadrilateral space distal to the teres minor. The shoulder joint is now hidden by the tendons of teres minor and infraspinatus and is exposed by separating these muscles or, if need be, by dividing the tendons 1 cm from their insertion and re-flecting them medially, care being taken to avoid injury to the suprascapular nerve, which enters infraspinatus at the base of the acromion.

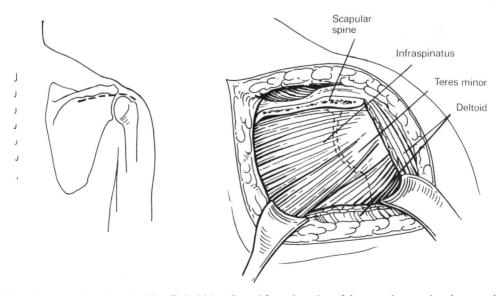

Fig. 6.3   Posterior approach to the shoulder. Deltoid is reflected from the spine of the scapula exposing the posterior muscles of the rotator cuff

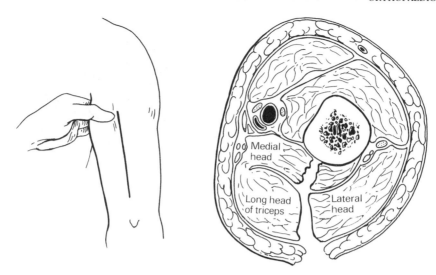

Fig. 6.4 Posterior approach to humerus

Posterior approach to the humerus

The posterior approach is more widely used than the anterior approach, being more appropriate for the reduction and internal fixation of fractures. In this approach, the radial nerve is at risk and its course must be constantly borne in mind. It crosses the middle third of the humerus obliquely from the medial to lateral side, lying deep to the long and lateral heads of triceps and lateral to the medial head of triceps. It enters the anterior compartment by passing through the lateral intermuscular septum to enter brachialis in the distal third of the upper arm. Both the nerve and its branches to the triceps must be carefully preserved.

The patient lies in the lateral position. The incision extends vertically down the middle of the posterior surface of the upper arm. The deep fascia is divided and the long head of triceps is identified in the proximal part of the wound by virtue of its mobility when compared with the lateral head and deltoid. The plane between the long and lateral heads is developed and the radial nerve and profunda artery are identified deep to these heads and carefully protected. As these muscle bodies become fused in the lower part of the wound, they have to be separated by sharp dissection. This then exposes the medial head of triceps, lying more deeply, and this muscle is split vertically in the mid-line to expose the posterior shaft of the humerus (Fig. 6.4).

Transacromial approach to the shoulder

This approach gives good access for surgery to the rotator cuff and fixation of fractures of the greater tuberosity. The skin incision is made in the coronal plane centred over the most prominent lateral point of the acromion and extending 5 cm both proximally and distally. The trapezius and deltoid muscles are split in the line of their fibres up to the acromion. Short flaps of conjoint aponeurosis, periosteum and bone are raised with an osteotome, as shown in Figure 6.5, and the acromion is then split with an oscillating saw and separated with a self-retaining retractor, exposing the subdeltoid bursa and the underlying rotator cuff. Rotation of the arm allows access to the whole of the rotator cuff. When closing the wound, the acromion is repaired by suture of the overlying aponeurotic and periosteal flaps.

Recurrent dislocation of the shoulder

In the great majority of cases, the dislocation is anterior and is due either to stretching of the anterior capsule,

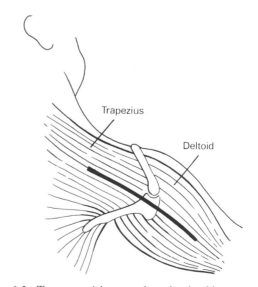

Fig. 6.5 Transacromial approach to the shoulder

or more commonly, to separation of the glenoid labrum from its bony attachment. Although recurrent posterior dislocation is very rare, accounting for only 2% of shoulder dislocations, it is nevertheless important to recognize that it can occur, for the operative treatment of the two types is, of course, entirely different.

In *recurrent anterior dislocation* a wedge-shaped defect may arise in the posterior part of the head of the humerus as a result of its repeated contact with the anterior margin of the glenoid and this notch, when present, facilitates redislocation. The surgical correction of recurrent anterior dislocation involves the repair or reinforcement of the anterior capsular structures and also limits external rotation and so prevents the humeral notch from engaging with the anterior margin of the glenoid.

The standard anterior approach to the shoulder is used (p. 115). The subscapularis tendon is divided 2 cm medial to its insertion. Before the division is completed, a holding suture is placed in the proximal part of the muscle, for otherwise it will retract and be difficult to recover. Ideally the tendon should be divided separately from the underlying capsule, but this can be difficult for the two structures are frequently fused at this level. The anterior capsule is then incised and the nature and extent of the capsular damage inspected by external rotation of the arm. The periosteum overlying the front of the neck of the scapula is elevated and the underlying bone is roughened with an osteotome so as to allow subsequent adhesion of the soft tissues. The distal stump of the subscapularis tendon and the underlying capsule are then sutured to the periosteum or labrum at the front of the neck of the scapula by means of 3 strong, but absorbable, mattress sutures which are all placed in position with the arm externally rotated and tied with the arm internally rotated. The medial capsular flap is brought to overlap the subscapularis tendon and sutured under moderate tension; the medial cut end of the subscapularis is brought as a separate layer to overlap the capsule and is in turn sutured to the soft tissues in the region of the lesser tuberosity. There are thus 4 overlapping layers reinforcing the front of the shoulder joint and limiting external rotation (Fig. 6.6). The coracoid process is then reattached and the wound closed. The arm is thereafter bandaged in internal rotation for 3 weeks, following which gentle, progressive mobilization of the shoulder is begun.

The above operation is known as the *Putti-Platt procedure* after the two eminent surgeons, who independently described it. It remains the most widely used operation for it combines simplicity with a high success rate.

Alternative procedures include the *Bankhart operation* in which the detached labrum is reattached to the

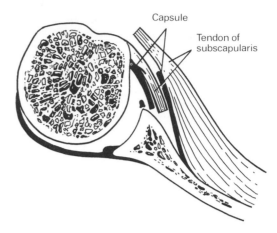

Fig. 6.6   The Putti–Platt repair of recurrent dislocation of the shoulder. The anterior capsule and subscapularis tendon are overlapped

glenoid margin by sutures passed through drill holes in the margin of the glenoid made with a right-angled dental drill. This is usually combined with a double breasting of the subscapularis as in the Putti-Platt procedure. Anterior bone blocks may also be used, utilizing the tip of the detached coracoid process, which is screwed to the anterior surface of the neck of the scapula or a free bone graft is taken from the iliac crest and placed intracapsularly. The latter is secured by tucking it into the pocket which lies in front of the neck of the scapula, or it may be placed anterior to the capsule and fixed to the neck of the scapula by means of a screw.

There are many other operative procedures described for correcting recurrent anterior dislocation of the shoulder. *Arthroscopic surgery* is being increasingly used not only to inspect the joint but also to allow stapling of the anterior capsule of the joint to the anterior aspect of the glenoid.

Recurrent posterior dislocation of the shoulder
The standard posterior approach is used. The infraspinatus tendon is divided 2 cm from its insertion and the posterior capsule incised. The pathology is usually a detachment of the posterior labrum from the glenoid and repair is effected by means of a bone block, which can be tucked into the space beneath the detached labrum and left projecting 1 cm. Alternatively it may be placed outside the capsule and secured in position by screwing it to the neck of the scapula, as in the anterior bone block procedure.

Operations on the rotator cuff
These may be required for ruptures or avulsion of the rotator cuff, for calcium deposits in the cuff or for supraspinatus tendonitis. Acute ruptures or avulsions

are recognized by inability to initiate abduction of the shoulder, although passive abduction is free and active abduction can be sustained above 90°. The transacromial approach to the shoulder is used and the tear in the rotator cuff is then identified by rotating the arm to bring it into view. The retracted proximal ends of the torn tendons are mobilized, brought laterally and sutured under an osteoperiosteal flap, the sutures passing through drill holes in bone at the point of attachment or alternatively using special sutures that anchor in the bone. The arm may be supported by the side in a sling following this operation and passive movements commenced within a few days. Active movements are delayed for 3 weeks.

Supraspinatus calcification occasionally requires surgery, either because of intense local pain, which has failed to respond to injections of local anaesthetic and hydrocortisone (which should always be attempted in the first place), or because the size of the calcified mass may be so great as to produce an actual block to abduction by engaging against the undersurface of the acromion. These lesions may be approached through a short coronal incision placed over the lesion distal to the acromion process. The deltoid fibres are split in the line of the incision and the chalky, inflamed area of the rotator cuff is then immediately identified. The calcified mass is incised and the chalk-like material curetted. No postoperative immobilization is required.

Acromioclavicular joint lesions
Subluxation of the acromioclavicular joint is a minor displacement limited by the integrity of the conoid and trapezoid ligaments. It causes few symptoms and requires no surgical repair. If these ligaments are completely disrupted, the outer end of the clavicle displaces upwards and backwards producing an ugly shoulder contour, but little disability. There is no conservative treatment. Many surgical procedures have been described, including insertion of a lag screw through the clavicle into the coracoid process, or transfixation of the reduced acromioclavicular joint by means of a Rush pin or stout Kirschner wire, the latter being bent over at its lateral extremity to prevent medial migration. The screw, or wire, should be removed after 8 weeks to allow restoration of the normal movement which takes place between the clavicle and the scapula. Some surgeons prefer synthetic or fascial loop repairs between the clavicle and the coracoid process combined with primary repair of the conoid and trapezoid ligaments.

Arthrodesis of the shoulder
This operation is rarely performed but may be indicated in chronic arthritis or to stabilize the shoulder in certain paralytic disorders such as poliomyelitis or brachial plexus injuries.

It is essential that the shoulder be fixed in the optimum position for the patient's needs. In general this is in 40° of abduction, 20° of flexion and 25° of internal rotation, i.e. a position in which the hand may readily be brought to the mouth. Many techniques of shoulder fusion are described. A simple and effective method consists simply of denuding the joint surfaces of articular cartilage and transfixing them in the desired position with a compression screw, with or without a bone graft fashioned from the fibula or the spine of the scapula. An anterior approach is used with a proximal extension to the incision to allow detachment of the deltoid from the acromion. The subscapularis and anterior capsule are then divided and the cartilage removed from the joint surfaces with gouges and osteotomes. A guide wire is then inserted through the lateral aspect of the upper end of the humerus to reach the centre of the glenoid and over this a cannulated trifin nail or cannulated screw is inserted, the length having been judged by X-ray. Following wound closure, the arm is immobilized in a shoulder spica. It greatly facilitates the application of the spica if the body part of the jacket is applied to the conscious patient prior to surgery. The spica is retained for at least 8 weeks, or until there is radiological evidence of union.

OPERATIONS ON THE ELBOW AND FOREARM

Exposure of the elbow joint
The *lateral approach* gives wide access to the elbow joint with minimum damage to the soft parts. It is performed with the patient's arm across his chest. The incision is centred on the lateral epicondyle and extends 5 cm proximally and distally. The lateral intermuscular septum is identified above the epicondyle, and, using it as a guide, the anterior muscles, brachioradialis and the common extensor origin are separated from the posterior muscles, triceps and anconeus (Fig. 6.7). The inci-

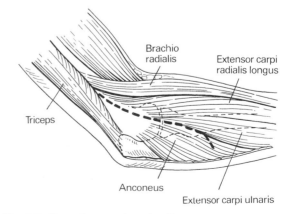

Brachio radialis

Extensor carpi radialis longus

Triceps

Anconeus

Extensor carpi ulnaris

Fig. 6.7 Lateral approach to the elbow

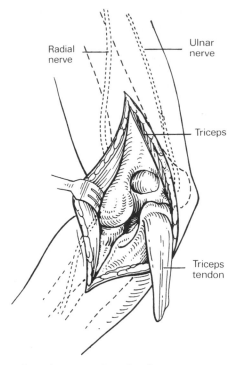

Fig. 6.8 Posterior approach to the elbow

sion is deepened to bone and to the capsule of the elbow between these muscles. If the operation is to be limited to the front of the elbow as for removal of a loose body, an incision is made in the anterior capsule. Conversely if access is required to the posterior part of the joint, the capsule is opened behind the epicondyle. Very wide exposure of the entire elbow may be obtained by dividing the lateral ligament and hinging the elbow open. Postoperatively a sling is worn for ten days.

The posterior approach

This approach is particularly useful if a very wide exposure of the elbow is required for reconstruction of comminuted fractures involving the elbow joint or for elbow arthroplasties. With the arm supported on a rest across the trunk, an incision is made, starting in the midline, 8 cm proximal to the olecranon and passing close to the lateral margin of the olecranon and distally for a further 5 cm along the posterior aspect of the ulna. The skin flap is retracted medially to allow exposure of the ulnar nerve behind the medial epicondyle and the position of the nerve is kept constantly in mind throughout the operative procedure. A tongue-like flap of triceps tendon is turned down to its insertion into the olecranon and the triceps incised in the midline down to bone. The capsule and muscular attachments to the epicondyles are then elevated as widely as may

be required by the operative procedure, great care being exercised to protect the ulnar nerve (Fig. 6.8).

Arthrodesis of the elbow

This operation is rarely performed and the indications and individual requirements of the patient are so varied that there is no standard technique. The optimal functional position must be established before operation by trial fixation in plaster casts.

Through the posterior approach, the joint surfaces are denuded of cartilage and transfixed in the predetermined position by means of a screw or strong Kirschner wires. Circumstances may require the head of the radius to be excised.

Arthroplasty of the elbow is still undergoing development. Many different models are being used at the present time and many difficulties have been encountered although some success is being achieved. Until time has established the worth of these various procedures they are best left in the hands of their innovators.

Exposure of the radius

The best approach to the shaft and lower end of the radius is through an incision overlying the medial border of the brachioradialis (Fig. 6.9). Distally, the incision should reach the radial styloid; proximally, it is carried up as far as is thought necessary. The cephalic vein, which crosses the line of incision in the middle

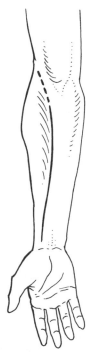

Fig. 6.9 Incision for exposure of the radius

third of the forearm, is divided between ligatures. The three long muscles which form the radial border of the forearm: brachioradialis, extensor carpi radialis longus and extensor carpi radialis brevis, and the radial nerve which lies on the deep aspect of brachioradialis, are mobilised and retracted laterally to expose the lateral surface of the shaft of the radius. The insertion of pronator teres to the middle of this surface, and the muscles arising from the anterior and posterior surfaces, are detached subperiosteally. The radial artery is displaced medially with the anterior muscles, and is carefully safeguarded. If the hand is now turned into full pronation, the lower two-thirds of the radius is widely exposed.

For *exposure of the upper third of the radius*, the incision, which still overlies the medial border of brachioradialis, is carried up into the upper arm to a point 8 cm above the elbow. The cleft between brachioradialis and the tendon of biceps is opened up, the radial recurrent vessels being divided between ligatures. The radius is exposed by a longitudinal incision made upon its anterior surface, through the most anterior fibres of supinator, the knife being kept immediately lateral to the biceps tendon. A rougine is now worked laterally around the bone to detach the fibres of supinator inserted into its anterior, lateral and posterior surfaces. In order to avoid the possibility of injury to the posterior interosseous nerve, which winds around the bone in the substance of supinator, it is essential that the instrument should be kept close to the bone throughout. If only the head and neck of the radius require to be exposed, and if wide access is not essential, a better approach is through an incision made directly over the posterior surface of the upper end of the bone.

Exposure of the ulna

The ulna is subcutaneous in its entire length, and can be exposed by an incision made along or adjacent to its posterior border.

OPERATIONS ON THE WRIST

The most commonly performed operations about the wrist are those on nerves and tendons described on pages 181 & 192. The wrist may be exposed from any aspect, according to the needs of the particular procedure. The *dorsal approach* gives widest access and is most suitable for arthrodesis. A longitudinal dorsal incision is made curving obliquely across the wrist. The extensor retinaculum is detached from its ulnar extremity and mobilized towards the radial side. The wrist is exposed by separating the digital extensors towards the ulnar side, and the extensor pollicis longus tendon

(which is freed from its groove on the dorsal aspect of the radius) and the radial wrist extensors towards the radial side. The capsule is then incised and reflected as required to expose the carpus.

Removal of ganglia

The term ganglion, apart from its use in reference to nerve tissue, is employed to denote a tense cystic swelling containing gelatinous material, which may develop in relation to joints and tendon sheaths. Although it may occur about any of the joints of the extremities, by far the commonest site is the dorsal surface of the wrist. It is therefore convenient to consider it here.

Ganglia frequently disappear spontaneously as a result of rupture and it is always worthwhile attempting this procedure therapeutically. The ganglion and its surroundings are injected with local anaesthesia and its contents dispersed either by manual pressure or by insertion of a wide bore needle. Many ganglia are painless and are best left alone, if they do not respond to this simple treatment. Where a ganglion continues to recur, and produces symptoms such as pressure on adjacent nerves or justified cosmetic concern, excision is indicated, but the patient should be warned that recurrence is fairly frequent.

The excision of a ganglion can sometimes be a difficult and time-consuming operation, which must always be carried out under a tourniquet and with full awareness of the anatomical relations in the vicinity. Bier's regional anaesthesia is ideal. A transverse incision is usually made so that the underlying cutaneous nerves can be easily identified and avoided. The investing fascia is incised longitudinally and the adjacent tendons are mobilized. Resection of the ganglion is then proceeded with, great care being taken to try and identify its communication with a synovial cavity. Not infrequently a ganglion can migrate some distance from its point of origin and if its connecting neck is not identified and excised, it may recur.

Arthrodesis of the wrist

This may be indicated to treat a painful wrist which has been disorganized by chronic arthritis or by trauma. The extent of the arthrodesis is determined by the extent of the disease. Thus in traumatic arthritis resulting from fractures of the distal radius, it may be necessary only to fuse the radius to the proximal bone of the carpus, which leaves a small amount of wrist movement from the remaining carpal joints. If the arthritis is more widespread, the arthrodesis may have to be extended to include the metacarpals and it may be necessary also to excise the lower end of the ulna. So long as forearm rotation is maintained, a stiff and painless wrist causes very little disability.

The dorsal approach, as described above, is used and

by flexing the wrist the residual articular cartilage is removed from the carpal joint surfaces, using gouges, osteotomes and sharp curette. Chips of cancellous bone obtained from the iliac crest are then packed into the residual gaps and crevices, with the wrist in flexion. The wrist is brought into the ideal position of 20° of extension, thus compacting the bone grafts. The joint capsule is repaired as far as possible and the extensor retinaculum, which has been carefully preserved, is placed deep to the extensor tendons and resutured at its ulnar attachment. The wrist is immobilized in plaster for 8 weeks.

Many prefer to elaborate the above procedure by the addition of an onlay bone graft. This is obtained from the outer aspect of the wing of the ilium at a site selected to give the correct curvature required by the operation site. A bed is prepared for the graft from the distal radius to the bases of the middle 3 metacarpals and the graft is cut and shaped to match (Fig. 6.10). If it fits well, no internal fixation is required. If it appears unstable, it may be temporarily transfixed by Kirschner wires, which are removed when the plaster is changed at 2 weeks.

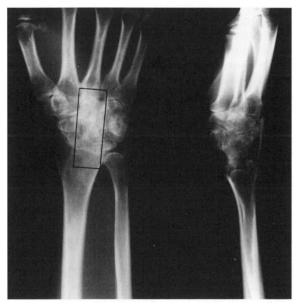

Fig. 6.10 X-ray showing the position of the posterior onlay graft for wrist fusion

OPERATIONS ON THE HIP AND THIGH

Aspiration of the hip joint
The needle may be inserted perpendicular to the skin at a point 2.5 cm below and lateral to the midinguinal point. The femoral artery, which lies deep to this point, should be safeguarded by palpation.

An alternative method is to introduce the needle just above the tip of the greater trochanter, and to pass it upwards and medially in the line of the femoral neck, following the bone until the joint is reached.

Exposures of the hip joint

The anterior approach
This gives excellent exposure with minimal muscle damage, and is widely used. The incision passes from just below the middle of the iliac crest to the anterior superior spine, and then extends vertically downwards for 10 to 12 cm (Fig. 6.11). Superficial and deep fascia are divided in the line of the incision. Gluteus medius and tensor fasciae latae are detached sub-periosteally from the iliac crest and are reflected downwards. The dissection is continued distally in the thigh in the interval between tensor fasciae latae laterally, and the sartorius and rectus femoris medially, care being taken to preserve the lateral cutaneous nerve of the thigh. The joint capsule is now exposed and is incised or excised according to the needs of the operation.

The anterolateral exposure of the hip
This approach gives more generous access to the hip joint than the anterior and is widely used for arthroplasty procedures. The operation can be done with the patient supine, a sandbag being placed under the buttock on the side of operation, or it may conveniently be done with the patient on the orthopaedic table, which allows greater freedom of manipulation of the leg by an unsterile assistant at the foot of the table, if required. The incision commences just below the iliac crest at a point 2.5 cm posterior to the anterior superior spine. It passes to the midpoint of the greater trochanter and then distally along the line of the femur for 5 cm. The fascia lata is then incised in the lower part of the wound just posterior to the insertion of tensor fasciae latae. Continuing the dissection upwards in the line of the skin incision, the plane between the muscle bellies of tensor fasciae latae anteriorly and gluteus medius and minimus posteriorly is then defined and the overlying fascia divided up to the iliac crest. The plane between these muscles is developed down to the side wall of the pelvis securing a number of vessels which cross the line of dissection. The nerve to tensor fascia femoris also crosses between the muscle groups and may be preserved if a limited operation is being carried out but usually has to be sacrificed if a major arthroplasty is being undertaken. No disability appears to result from denervation of this muscle. At the proximal end of the wound, the origins of the glutei and tensor are fused together and have to be separated by sharp dissection. If need be the exposure can be increased by stripping the glutei posteriorly off the iliac crest. The capsule of

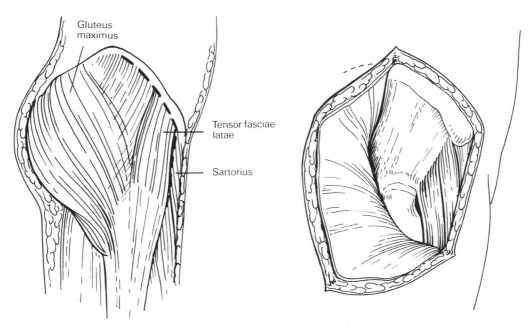

Fig. 6.11 Anterior approach to the hip

the hip joint is concealed at first by a very constant fat pad. When this is removed, the entire anterior and superior capsule of the hip joint is exposed and may be incised or excised as widely as the operation requires. The reflected head of rectus femoris may be removed but it is rarely necessary to detach the direct head.

The posterolateral approach

There are a number of variations of this approach but the most widely used is the 'Southern' approach of Austin Moore. The patient is supported in a true lateral position with the lower leg flexed to 90° at the hip and knee. The incision (Fig. 6.12a) starts in front

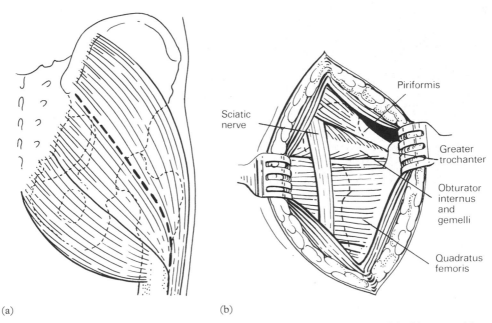

(a)   (b)

Fig. 6.12 (a) Incision for posterior approach to the hip. (b) Structures on posterior aspect of the hip exposed by splitting the fibres of the gluteus maximus

of the posterior superior iliac spine and extends to the midpoint of the greater trochanter and then distally in the line of the femur for a similar distance. The fascia lata and the gluteal insertion to it are divided in the line of the lower part of the incision and the split is extended proximally separating the fibres of gluteus maximus in the line of the proximal part of the skin incision. The split gluteus maximus is then held apart by a self-retaining retractor exposing the short external rotator muscles covering the posterior surface of the hip joint. These are from above downwards: piriformis, the obturator internus with the gemelli and quadratus femoris. The sciatic nerve which emerges below piriformis to lie on the posterior surface of the other rotators midway between the greater trochanter and the ischium should be identified and protected throughout the operation (Fig. 6.12b). By internally rotating the hip, the short rotator muscles become better defined and are divided close to their insertion, the proximal ends having first been secured by stay sutures. It is not always necessary to divide the piriformis or the quadratus femoris, nor is it necessary to detach gluteus medius and minimus from the greater trochanter. Having divided the external rotator muscles, the capsule of the hip joint is exposed and is incised as necessary for the procedure. If hip dislocation is required, it is achieved by internal rotation of the leg which must be carried out gently in osteoporotic elderly patients. If there is resistance to dislocation, it is best to divide the neck with the head in situ and remove it piecemeal thereafter.

Exposure of the shaft of the femur

The posterolateral approach causes minimal damage to the quadriceps and therefore is least likely to cause knee stiffness. It is now the standard approach to the femur and supersedes Henry's anterior approach. The patient lies on his side and a skin incision is made along the axis of the femur just behind the midlateral line of the thigh and is extended as far as may be required to give access to the objective of the operation (Fig. 6.13). The fascia lata is incised along the length of the skin incision just posterior to the iliotibial band. This exposes the vastus lateralis which is separated by blunt dissection from the lateral intermuscular septum as far as its origin from the linea aspera. The muscle is detached from its origin by an incision made about 0.5 cm lateral to the linea aspera since this allows the perforating vessels to be secured as they are encountered. If the muscle is detached from the linea itself the cut vessels may retract out of sight and be more difficult to find. The vastus lateralis and the remaining quadriceps muscles can then be mobilized from the lateral aspect and front of the femur by bone levers giving good access to the bone.

At wound closure only the fascia lata and skin require to be sutured. A conventional tourniquet can only be used for lesions of the distal femur, but it is possible to secure a tourniquet at a high level by passing a Steinmann pin into the lateral aspect of the femur in the upper thigh and placing the cuff of the tourniquet above it.

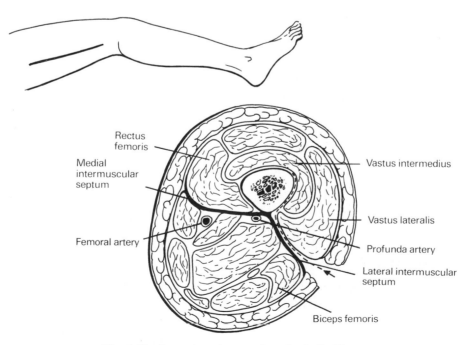

Fig. 6.13 Posterolateral approach to the shaft of femur

Total prosthetic replacement of the hip joint

One of the greatest advances in orthopaedic surgery in recent years has been the development of prosthetic joint replacements. The hip joint was the first to be developed and has remained the most successful of all joint replacements with a success rate exceeding 90% in many large series. The most widely used model is that developed by Charnley (1979) (Fig. 6.14). The two components of the prosthesis are secured to bone with methylmethacrylate cement. Although highly successful in properly selected cases, the prosthesis can fail mechanically either by breakage of the femoral component or, more commonly, loosening of the cement/bone bond. The other important cause of failure is infection, which, if it becomes established, requires a major revision operation with a much reduced success rate. The consequences of these complications are so serious that it follows that this operation should only be carried out where the clinical indications are unequivocal and where the surgeon is confident in the sterility of his theatre environment. The operation is indicated for severe pain or disability in the hip joint of an elderly patient despite conservative treatment. The common underlying pathological conditions are osteoarthritis, rheumatoid arthritis, avascular necrosis of the head of the femur or failure of primary treatment of a fractured neck of femur. The operation should not be carried out

for chronic arthritis due to an infectious cause unless the infection has been eradicated. Occasionally the operation may become necessary in a younger patient who suffers from bilateral hip joint disease, for example rheumatoid arthritis or ankylosing spondylitis, but in these circumstances the patient should always be advised that the procedure may not last indefinitely because of wear and loosening.

The operation is normally carried out under antibiotic cover (p. 114). The incision used depends on the surgeon's preference; both the anterolateral and posterior approaches are suitable. Charnley recommends the true lateral approach with division of the greater trochanter, which allows very generous exposure both of the acetabulum and of the shaft of the femur and is of particular value in a difficult case but has the disadvantage that the trochanter has to be firmly secured at the end of the operation which adds to the operative time and to the possible complications. This approach is not widely adopted for routine use. Nevertheless the inexperienced surgeon may well find this the easiest and safest approach and would do well to read Charnley's description. Having dislocated the hip, the head is removed with an osteotome or Gigli saw. The acetabulum is prepared by removal of all soft tissue, sclerotic bone and residual cartilage down to the level of the acetabular fossa, using cranked gouges. Two or three holes are made in the roof of the acetabulum and in the ischium to provide additional anchoring points for the cement. The blood and bony fragments are washed out of the acetabulum, using an antibiotic solution, and the acetabulum thoroughly dried. An acetabular cup of appropriate size is then selected. A mix of methylmethacrylate cement is firmly pressed into the exposed cancellous bone of the acetabulum and into the anchorage holes and the acetabular component is inserted using the appropriate guide to ensure correct placement, which should be at an angle of 45° from the longitudinal axis of the body. A common fault is to have the cup facing too laterally. Excess cement should be removed before it hardens. The femoral shaft is then reamed with the appropriate reamers and again thoroughly irrigated with antibiotic solution. A trial reduction of the femoral component is carried out without use of the cement to ensure correct fit. Stability is best achieved by a fairly tight reduction and a range of prostheses with different femoral neck lengths is available as required. Cement is inserted into the femoral canal either by a cement syringe or by digital pressure. During the insertion process the shaft is vented by a plastic catheter which is removed when the filling is complete. The femoral component is inserted with the neck pointing medially to the normal axis of the femur. Once the cement is hardened, the hip is reduced and the wound closed in layers over a suction

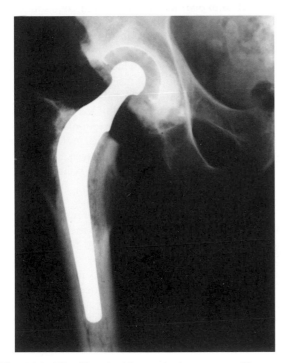

Fig. 6.14 The Charnley hip prosthesis as seen on X-ray. The acetabular component is made of high density polyethylene and the femoral of stainless steel

drain. The patient mobilizes quickly and is allowed to walk after 2 days and may leave hospital in 10 or 12 days when the wound has healed. Prolonged physiotherapy is not usually required.

There are many different designs of hip replacement and some of these are inserted without bone cement. There is no good evidence yet that they are superior to Charnley's original design.

Arthrodesis of the hip

Arthrodesis of the hip is now rarely performed as arthroplasty is in general a more acceptable solution to a chronic hip problem. Nevertheless, there remain some indications for this procedure, notably severe post-traumatic arthritis in a young and active person in whom an arthroplasty would be unlikely to last long. A satisfactory arthrodesis of the hip allows a comfortable, painless gait but an awkward sitting posture and, as with arthrodesis of any joint, it throws greater stress on neighbouring joints. Thus the spine and knee of the same leg tend to develop degenerative changes over a period of years. However, it is now possible to convert an arthrodesed or ankylosed hip to replacement arthroplasty when a patient reaches an appropriate age and the arthrodesis may then be regarded as an interim procedure, which will carry a patient through his most active working years.

Many techniques of arthrodesis are described, the one to be described here has the merit of simplicity and safety.

Ischiofemoral or V-arthrodesis

With the patient supine upon the orthopaedic table, the hip joint is carefully positioned to lie in 20° of flexion, 5° of external rotation and no abduction or adduction. If contraction of the hip joint prevents this position from being achieved, then an osteotomy must be carried out as described later. A midlateral incision is made extending from the greater trochanter distally for 10 cm. The lateral aspect of the upper femur is exposed subperiosteally and a guidewire is inserted under X-ray control as described in the internal fixation of fractures of the neck of femur (p. 153). The guidewire is aimed to cross the hip joint and enter the thick bone in the roof of the acetabulum just above the pelvic rim, and is advanced towards the sacro-iliac joint for about 6 cm. The length of nail is measured from the guidewire and a nail or hip screw is driven across the hip joint into the pelvis, thus stabilizing the hip in its optimal position. A lateral incision is then made over the fibula of the same leg and the bone is exposed between the lateral and posterior muscle groups. The midportion is stripped of soft tissues and an 8 cm length is removed for use as a graft. The

bone should be cut with a Gigli saw or oscillating power saw since it tends to splinter if divided with an osteotome or bone cutters. The fibular wound is closed and the patient turned to the prone position and retowelled. The hip wound is then extended as for the conventional posterior approach to the hip joint (p. 123). The gluteus maximus is split in the line of its fibres and the posterior aspect of the hip joint covered by the external rotators is exposed. The sciatic nerve is identified as it emerges from the lower border of piriformis and a tape is passed round it. A guidewire is inserted from the lateral aspect of the femur, 1 cm below the point of entry of the nail. The wire is advanced medially, proximally and posteriorly aimed towards the thick part of the ischium just below the hip joint, which is identified by finger palpation. Cannulated drills are advanced over the guidewire, across the femur and into the ischium, the largest drill being slightly less then the diameter of the fibular graft. The graft, which has been pointed by means of a file at one end, is then punched through the hole in the femur into the ischium for a distance of 3 cm. In order to prevent a fracture occurring at the site of the hole in the femur, it is prudent to attach a short plate to the triflange nail as in the fixation of an intertrochanteric fracture. The V formed by the graft and nail both traversing the femur and penetrating the pelvis give great stability to the arthrodesis and no additional immobilization is required. The patient may get up on crutches soon after the operation and protected weight-bearing is allowed with the help of crutches. Full weight-bearing should be possible in 6 weeks. Fusion takes place progressively through the fibular graft which hypertrophies and ultimately the hip joint itself fuses (Fig. 6.15).

The purpose of turning the patient from supine to prone position during the course of the operation is to enable the identification and protection of the sciatic nerve, which can be damaged if the graft is inserted blindly. The operator will be impressed by the close relationship between the graft and the sciatic nerve.

Arthrodesis combined with osteotomy

If the ideal position of the hip joint cannot be obtained (because of uncorrectable deformity) the above procedure should be carried out with the hip joint in its deformed position and a corrective subtrochanteric osteotomy is performed with the patient supine on the orthopaedic table, as a secondary procedure two weeks later — the osteotomy site being secured by a 7 hole plate. Some surgeons prefer to combine the arthrodesis and osteotomy as a one stage procedure but it can be difficult to get the ideal position by this means and the two stage procedure described above is safer and simpler.

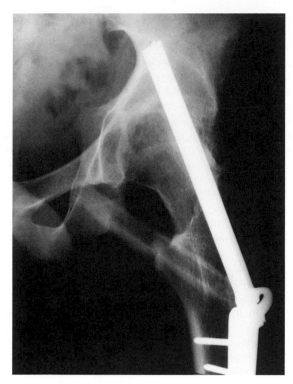

Fig. 6.15 X-ray showing V-arthrodesis of the hip. Note the hypertrophy of the fibular graft

Intertrochanteric osteotomy
Division of a bone in the vicinity of an osteoarthritic joint with correction of deformity may relieve pain in a high proportion of cases and in many instances produce an improved radiological appearance, at least for a number of years. This well tried procedure can be a useful interim procedure in patients too young for arthroplasty, but who have failed to respond to conservative measures. Intertrochanteric osteotomy for osteoarthritis of the hip and upper tibial osteotomy for osteoarthritis of the knee, (p. 135) are the most common procedures of this kind. The ideal indications for this procedure are severe pain with preservation of at least 50% of movement in the affected joint.

The patient is placed on the orthopaedic table and two-plane X-ray control is established as for pinning a fractured neck of femur (p. 153). A midlateral incision is made extending distally to the greater trochanter for about 10 cm and the shaft of the femur is exposed as for internal fixation of an intertrochanteric fracture (p. 155). It is useful to place the anterior bone lever just above the lesser trochanter, to serve as a guide for the osteotomy. A guidewire is inserted into the centre of the neck of the femur under X-ray control, and a second guidewire is passed across the femur to confirm the

level of the osteotomy, which should lie just above the level of the lesser trochanter. A flanged nail is driven into the neck of the femur, the length being measured to stop short of the articular surface by 2 cm to ensure that no penetration of the joint takes place. The osteotomy is carried out at the selected level either by using a Gigli saw or by perforating the bone with a series of drill holes, completing the osteotomy with an osteotome. The use of a power saw tends to produce some heat necrosis at the site of osteotomy which may delay healing.

In the past it has been the practice to displace the shaft of the femur medially at the osteotomy site by at least half the diameter of the bone; however there is no evidence which supports the need for this displacement and subsequent replacement arthroplasty, if required, is made more difficult if the osteotomy site has been displaced. It is therefore customary now simply to correct any pre-existing deformity at the osteotomy site, and achieve stabilization by the attachment of seven hole plate to the nail. Other techniques of fixation may be used, such as compression plate or fixed angle nail plate, according to the preference and experience of the surgeon.

Early mobilization is allowed, the patient taking part-weight for the first 6 weeks and full-weight thereafter.

Excision arthroplasty of the hip (Girdlestone pseudarthrosis)
Excision of the head and neck of the femur is an operation originally developed for the management of septic arthritis of the hip. It may appear of historic interest only in these days of artificial hip joints. Nevertheless, in many parts of the world where the facilities for hip joint replacement are lacking and where social customs, particularly the need to adopt the squatting posture, demand a very full range of hip movement, excision arthroplasty may still have a place in the management of a severely disorganized hip joint resulting from infection or chronic arthritis. The operation may be performed through the anterolateral or posterior approach. The head and neck of the femur are cleanly removed to leave a smooth intertrochanteric surface. The superior margin of the acetabulum is likewise resected to leave a smooth lateral surface to the pelvis (Fig. 6.16). The limb is then supported postoperatively in Hamilton Russell traction (Fig. 6.17). This form of traction maintains length and correct rotation of the limb and is applied for 4–6 weeks until a fibrous scar has formed at the operation site, so as to limit subsequent telescoping. The patient mobilizes, at first non-weight-bearing and gradually taking increased weight. Inevitably the limb will shorten and an appropriate shoe raise will subsequently be required. The patient will usually

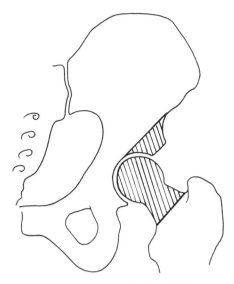

Fig. 6.16 Extent of bone resection in a Girdlestone pseudarthrosis

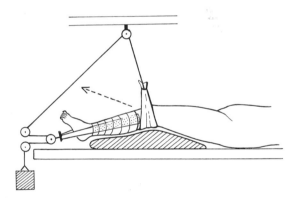

Fig. 6.17 Hamilton Russell traction. The resultant force shown by the arrow corresponds to the axis of the femur

need the support of a walking stick in his opposite hand.

Congenital dislocation of the hip

Congenital dislocation of the hip is theoretically a preventable condition and in an ideal world surgical procedures should rarely be required. Potentially unstable hips may be recognized at birth by Barlow's modification of Ortolani's test, and if the hips are splinted in a position of abduction, flexion and lateral rotation for 8–12 weeks, they will usually stabilize in the reduced position. If they escape detection at birth, subluxation or dislocation is then not usually recognized until the child begins to walk at a year. Even at this stage conservative treatment with gentle traction and progressive abduction may achieve reduction. Forceful attempts at manipulative reduction cause avascular

necrosis of the upper femoral epiphysis with disastrous results. The older the child at diagnosis the higher the incidence of imperfect reduction because of soft tissue obstruction within the acetabulum, usually an inturned fibrocartilaginous labrum or limbus. Operative reduction is then required. Excessive anteversion of the femoral neck may have developed which must also be corrected by lateral rotation osteotomy of the femur, otherwise recurrent subluxation is likely. If concentric reduction and correction of anteversion is achieved before the age of 3 by either conservative or surgical means, there is good prospect that the acetabulum will develop normally and give good containment of the femoral head. If perfect reduction has not been obtained by this age, the acetabular roof is unlikely to develop fully and an innominate osteotomy may be required to stabilize the joint.

Open reduction of congenital dislocation of the hip
This operation is normally performed between 1 and 3 years in infants in whom conservative reduction has failed. A preoperative arthrogram will confirm the displacement and indicate the nature of the obstruction. The anterior approach (p. 122) is used. A transverse skin incision below the anterior superior spine may be used to leave a less conspicuous scar. The anterior capsule is exposed and opened through an H incision. Careful probing or digital palpation will confirm the nature and extent of the soft tissue obstruction which is then excised. An inturned limbus may be identified and lifted up with a blunt hook. At operation it is possible to assess the degree of anteversion by flexing the knee and hip to 90° and measuring the angle between the neck and the axis of the tibia. When the head of the femur has been reduced the position of maximal stability is assessed, usually abduction with some flexion and internal rotation, and a plaster cast is applied to hold the legs symmetrically in this position for four weeks. At the end of this period, if excessive anteversion is present, a lateral rotation osteotomy is carried out through the upper femur. A lateral approach (p. 124) is made to the upper end of the femur which is exposed subperiosteally. Two guide wires are inserted, above and below the osteotomy site, at an angle to each other which corresponds to the desired amount of correction. An osteotomy is then carried out between the wires at a level about 2 cm below the lesser trochanter using a sharp osteotome and the bone is derotated until the two wires are parallel. A 4-hole plate is used to stabilize the osteotomy site, and a hip spica is applied for 4 weeks. Some surgeons add an element of varus at the osteotomy site by bending the plate a few degrees believing that this gives greater containment of the femoral head and in older children a small segment of the femur may be removed to

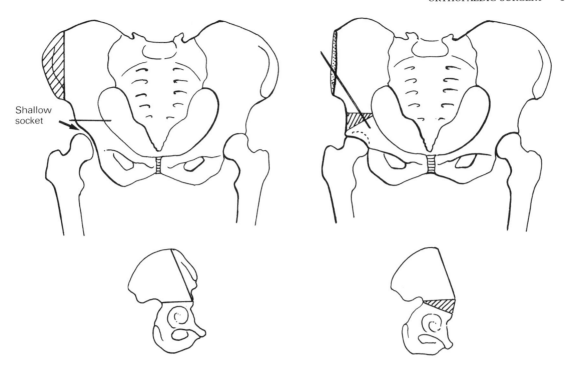

Fig. 6.18 Diagram of the salter innominate osteotomy

produce some femoral shortening and so reduce the tension of the soft tissues at the hip joint.

Iliac osteotomy

Many techniques of pelvic osteotomy have been described. The most widely adopted is that of Salter (1961) (Fig. 6.18) which may be combined with open reduction of the dislocation. The hip is exposed through the anterior incision which is extended backwards to the mid point of the iliac crest. The iliac apophysis is split along the line of the crest and the lateral half with the periosteum of the external surface of the ilium is stripped as far as the sciatic notch and the acetabulum and the medial half with the periosteum of the inner aspect is stripped for a similar extent. After open reduction of the hip joint and lengthening of the adductors and iliopsoas if required, an osteotomy is performed from the anterior superior spine to the sciatic notch using a Gigli saw or thin osteotomes, great care being taken to protect the sciatic nerve and superior gluteal vessels as they pass through the sciatic notch. The distal fragment is tilted outwards and forwards and wedged open in this position by means of a suitably shaped graft cut from the iliac crest. Stability is further ensured by placing a Kirschner wire across the osteotomy site through the graft. The split iliac apophysis is then sutured together and after wound closure a single hip spica is applied with the hip in slight abduction flexion and medial rotation. The plaster is removed after 6 weeks and mobilization commenced.

OPERATIONS ON THE KNEE

Aspiration of the knee

Effusion occurs more commonly in the knee than any other joint. Aspiration is required to relieve discomfort of a large effusion or for diagnostic purposes. The knee joint cavity extends at least 3 cm proximal to the upper pole of the patella and aspiration is most comfortably and easily carried out in this suprapatellar pouch by the technique described on page 114.

Arthroscopic surgery of the knee

In recent years, techniques of arthroscopic surgery have been developed for such procedures as the removal of torn cartilages, loose bodies and joint biopsies. These endoscopic procedures may be performed as day case surgery and the patient experiences less discomfort and speedier convalescence.

Arthroscopic surgery has now almost abolished the need for other than minimal arthrotomy during meniscectomy; removal of loose bodies, biopsy, joint débridement and surgery for osteochondritis is undertaken in those centres with adequate equipment.

Technique. An arthroscope portal (a transverse

incision of approximately 1 cm) is made 5 mm above the lateral joint line at the lateral border of the patellar tendon. The trochar and arthroscopic cannula are passed through this incision, the trochar is removed and a blunt probe is passed through the cannula into the joint; finally the blunt probe is removed and the arthroscope is passed through the cannula. The joint is thoroughly inspected before any arthroscopic surgery commences. First the suprapatellar pouch is inspected for synovial hypertrophy, loose bodies or synovial plicae, then the anterior compartment looking particularly for chondromalacia or plicae; the medial and lateral gutters are examined for loose bodies and then the medial and lateral compartments of the joint, the intercondylar notch and the posterior recesses are inspected. A very comprehensive examination of the knee may be accomplished and a wide range of surgical procedures carried out, including partial or total meniscectomy, removal of loose bodies, stabilisation of osteochondrial fragments, articular cartilage shaving and débridement, débridement of osteophytes, synovial biopsy, synovectomy, meniscal repair, cruciate substitution, and arthroscopic washout. A number of separate arthroscopic portals may be required to accomplish the surgery. Instruments available to the arthroscopic surgeon include straight and angles punches, straight and angled scissors or basket cutters, grabbers, powered instruments including shavers and cutters and laser cutting instruments. Clearly arthroscopic surgery is highly specialized and, although many surgeons practise diagnostic surgery, the surgery itself is becoming increasingly specialized.

Exposure of the knee joint

The knee joint is so superficial and accessible surgically that the possible surgical approaches are infinite. The one approach which may be regarded as standard is the anteromedial approach, which allows wide access and is appropriate for such procedures as synovectomy and replacement arthroplasty of the joint. The incision commences in the midline, 8 cm proximal to the patella and curves distally about 1 cm medial to its medial border, ending near the tibial tubercle. The vastus medialis and joint capsule are divided in the line of the skin incision and the synovial membrane is incised throughout its length. The patella may then be everted and dislocated laterally to expose the entire anterior aspect of the knee joint (Fig. 6.19). Flexing the knee increases exposure of the intercondyle area and the lateral recesses. Sometimes it is necessary to detach the medial third of the patellar tendon from the tibial tubercle in order to displace the patella fully.

Replacement arthroplasty of the knee joint
(Fig. 6.20)

This is now established as a standard and remarkably successful procedure, proving to be almost as durable as hip replacement. The antero-medial approach to the knee is used and the femur and tibia are prepared using standard cutting jigs to accept the femoral and tibial components of the knee replacement. The articulating surface of the patella may be replaced with a plastic 'button' though this is not usually felt to be necessary. As in hip replacement, the components of the prosthesis are held in place by polymethylmethacrylate cement

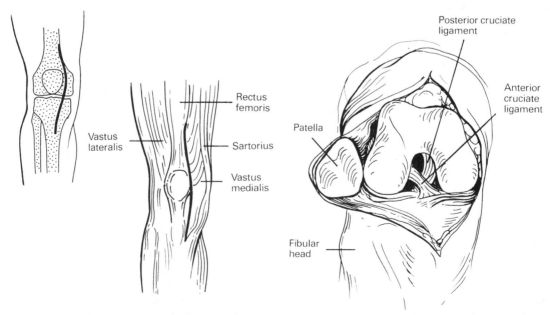

Fig. 6.19 Anteromedial exposure of the knee joint. The patella is rotated laterally

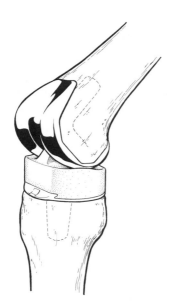

Fig. 6.20   Knee replacement

and stability is enhanced by short femoral and tibial stems in the medullary canal. The patient is allowed to mobilise the knee almost immediately after surgery and may weight bear after 2 or 3 days. Any surgeon contemplating knee replacement should have specialized training and should be familiar with specialist literature. As for all types of replacement arthroplasty, these operations are best restricted to the elderly and severely disabled. They are not procedures for the young and active.

Synovectomy of the knee

Synovectomy may be useful in patients suffering from rheumatoid arthritis who experience severe pain in association with marked synovial reaction, persistent effusion, in whom good joint movement is retained and in whom the X-rays show good preservation of the joint surface. It also has an established place in the management of haemophilic arthropathy (in patients who experience frequent bleeds) before advanced joint disorganization has occurred. The anteromedial approach (p. 130) is used. All accessible synovial membrane is stripped from the undersurface of the capsule and from the underlying bone, commencing with the suprapatellar pouch and extending to the lateral recesses and to the intercondylar area as far as can be reached. Through this approach about three-quarters of the synovial lining of the knee can be removed. Bone nibblers are useful for clearing the synovium in the more remote recesses of the joint. In rheumatoid arthritis a clear plane of separation is easily developed between the synovium and the underlying tissues. In haemophilic patients this plane tends to be obliterated.

Post-operative management is important. The knee must be splinted for the first few days until the quadriceps has regained control and thereafter knee mobilization is pursued with active physiotherapy. Manipulation under anaesthesia may be required in two weeks, if 90 degrees of flexion has not been achieved by then.

Removal of the medial meniscus

The menisci of the knee perform a valuable weight distributing function. Following their removal, the weight transmitted across the knee joint is concentrated at much smaller areas of contact of the incongruous articular surfaces and degenerative arthritis will usually develop after an interval of some years. For this reason menisci must be conserved if at all possible. Meniscectomy should only be undertaken when the meniscus is so damaged that it no longer performs its useful function. Clinical diagnosis of a torn meniscus can be difficult and in one large series was accurate in only 60% of cases. Arthrography or arthroscopy greatly increase the diagnostic accuracy and should be used whenever the diagnosis is in doubt. In recent years, it has also been recognized that degeneration of the meniscus is a common accompaniment of ageing and that in most cases it is not a source of lasting symptoms. The finding of degenerative changes therefore in a meniscus is not per se an indication for meniscectomy. Meniscectomy is indicated when the cartilage tear produces mechanical instability or locking of the knee or gives rise to persistent localized pain and tenderness. *Open* medial or lateral meniscectomy is mainly undertaken in departments that do not have access to appropriate arthroscopic equipment. This is the type of operation described below.

Preoperative treatment

The patient should be taught how to carry out quadriceps exercises before operation. These exercises, which are essential to prevent wasting of the muscles, are difficult to learn after operation when the knee is painful and heavily bandaged.

Operation

A pneumatic tourniquet should be used. The knee is flexed over the end of the operating table. The surgeon sits facing it with the foot resting in his lap. An anteromedial incision is made, which may be vertical or oblique (Fig. 6.21), the latter having the advantage of avoiding the infrapatellar branch of the saphenous nerve which if injured can cause postoperative discomfort. The capsule is divided in the line of the skin incision. The synovial membrane is picked up most easily at the proximal end of the incision over the femoral condyle and is incised in its turn. The margins of the wound are retracted and the meniscus inspected. A

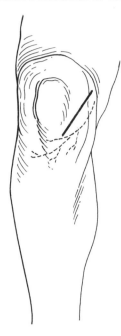

Fig. 6.21 Incision for removal of medial meniscus. The oblique incision avoids the infrapatellar branch of the saphenous nerve

bucket handle tear may be found displaced into the intercondylar area or a longitudinal split may be identified in the undisplaced cartilage. The anterior horn of the cartilage is hooked forward with a blunt hook and this may disclose marginal or parrot beak tears or a posterior peripheral tear. If no pathology is identified, the diagnosis is incorrect and the cartilage should be left in situ. The knee must then be carefully inspected for other abnormality which might have caused the patient's symptoms.

If the damage is a bucket handle tear, only the displaced portion need be removed and this is done by dividing its two points of attachment. This simple, atraumatic procedure leaves a rim of healthy meniscus which may still perform a useful function. If total meniscectomy is required, the anterior horn is hooked upwards with a blunt hook, a knife is passed beneath the meniscus sweeping laterally and upwards into the intercondylar area to detach the anterior horn. This is then grasped with a Kocher's or similar forceps and the meniscus firmly drawn forwards. The peripheral attachments are divided with a sharp knife. This is easily accomplished for the anterior half because it is under direct vision but the posterior half of the meniscus is largely out of sight and is much more difficult to mobilize. Powerful retraction and the use of Smillie knives with an end-cutting surface are useful here. The cartilage should be pulled onto the cutting edge of the knife by means of the Kocher's forceps and gradually mobilized and pulled into the intercondylar area. Once

this displacement has been achieved, the posterior attachment is easily divided. If a substantial part of the posterior horn breaks away and is left behind, a separate posteromedial incision may be required. The site for this incision is identified by passing a curved artery forceps through the anterior wound so that its point can be felt at the joint line on the postero-medial aspect. A short, vertical incision is then made centered on the point of the forceps. The fragment of posterior horn is seen and removed under vision. The synovium, capsule and skin are closed with absorbable sutures, a compression bandage is applied and the knee splinted in extension with a plaster slab or a canvas splint. The splint and bandage are retained for 10 days, during which time the patient practises quadriceps exercises. He may take weight on the limb or use crutches according to his inclination and can be discharged from hospital the day after operation. Following removal of the plaster, a short period of supervised physiotherapy will speed his recovery.

Removal of the lateral meniscus
Injuries of the lateral meniscus are less common but can occur and cystic change within the meniscus may also necessitate meniscectomy.

Operation
This is similar to that described for the removal of the medial meniscus. The central portion of the lateral meniscus is free of capsular attachment and therefore peripheral dissection may be slightly easier. The lateral geniculate artery should be looked for and cauterised as it can cause troublesome bleeding after the tourniquet is removed.

Removal of loose bodies from the knee
The knee is a large and complex joint and only a small part of it can be inspected through any one incision if arthroscopic surgery is not available. It is important that a loose body be located either by the patient or by X-ray prior to surgery. A blind exploration of the knee to find a loose body is likely to be unsuccessful. When the loose body has been located, a short incision is made directly over it and the loose body removed. In the case of non-radio opaque loose bodies, these should be located prior to surgery and securely transfixed with a needle before the joint is opened.

Operation for osteochondritis dissecans
Osteochondritis dissecans usually involves the intercondylar aspect of the medial femoral condyle. The fragment, if not separated in young children, may go on to spontaneous healing following a period of immobilization of the joint. Surgical treatment is not required. If, in the adolescent, the fragment is clearly mobile and

causing symptoms it should be removed, or if very large, repositioned and secured by Smillie pins or by Herbert screws. The incision is the same as that for medial meniscectomy. The softened and mobile area of cartilage, if not detached, can be easily identified by palpation with a blunt dissector. An incision is made through the margin of the loose fragment, which is then removed. If very large, the fibrotic, sclerotic bed is curetted and drilled at a number of points to improve vascularity. The fragment is then repositioned and pinned, using Smillie pins and the appropriate introducer (Fig. 6.22). If the fragment has been separated from its bed for some time, it will no longer fit the bed from which it came and no attempt should then be made to reposition it. Following removal of an osteochondritic fragment, the defect heals remarkably well with fibrocartilage in time. Fortunately the lesion usually occupies a non-weight bearing area. The postoperative management is as described for meniscectomy.

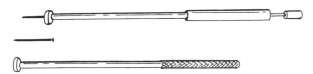

Fig. 6.22 Instruments used for the insertion of the Smillie pin (see also Fig. 6.43)

Patellectomy

Patellectomy is indicated for comminuted fractures and occasionally in severe cases of chondromalacia patellae and when osteoarthritic change is concentrated in the patellofemoral joint. A transverse incision is made over the patella and the vertical incision is made in the retinacular fibres which cover the bone. Using sharp dissection with a scalpel, the patella is carefully shelled out of its tendinous attachments, preserving them as far as possible. The aponeurotic flaps are overlapped with mattress sutures, a compression bandage is applied and the knee supported in a plaster splint until the quadriceps have recovered their activity. Mobilization can be commenced usually at the end of two or three weeks, except in traumatic cases in which the lateral expansions of the quadriceps mechanism have also been injured, in which case they must be splinted for 6 weeks to allow healing of the extensor mechanism.

Recurrent dislocation of the patella

This occurs most commonly in young girls in whom there is some minor congenital abnormality such as excessive genu valgum, poor development of the lateral femoral condyle, small and high patella or joint laxity. As many of these minor anomalies are inherited, it may be familial and is often bilateral. Recurrence may also follow traumatic dislocation of the patella which has not been protected sufficiently after the first incident to allow the capsule to heal.

Many operations are described for the treatment of this disorder and the selected procedure must take account of the underlying pathology: for example, in the presence of severe genu valgum, a supracondylar osteotomy would be appropriate. An operation widely practised in the past has been the distal and medial displacement of the insertion of the patellar tendon into the tibial tubercle, which may be appropriate where the patella is high and laterally displaced (*Hauser's operation*). However, it is becoming increasingly recognized that re-routing of the patella in this way leads to later degenerative arthritis in the patellofemoral joint and this procedure must now be rarely indicated. It must never be carried out in a growing child for it would damage the upper tibial growth plate causing tibial recurvatum.

A less traumatic procedure consists of the formation of a check ligament from the lateral third of the patellar tendon — the *Roux-Goldthwait procedure*. This was originally developed for the younger child but it works well at all ages.

Operation

A midline incision is made from the lower pole of the patella to the tibial tuberosity. A release incision is made in the lateral capsule, the patellar tendon is identified and a vertical split is made separating the lateral third from the medial two-thirds. The lateral portion is detached from the tibial tuberosity and passed underneath the tendon to be sutured to an osteoperiosteal flap on the anteromedial aspect of the upper tibia (Fig. 6.23). The knee is immobilized in a plaster cylinder for 6 weeks, quadriceps exercises being maintained throughout and continued during the post-plaster mobilization period.

Popliteal cyst (semimembranosus bursa)

This appears as a tense cystic swelling in the popliteal fossa to the medial side of the midline. It is the result of a one-way valvular mechanism which allows the escape of synovial fluid from the knee into the normal semimembranosus bursa. The condition is usually painless and tends to resolve with time and rarely requires treatment. Very large and painful cysts may be excised through a transverse incision. It is important to identify and close the communication with the knee joint.

Arthrodesis of the knee

This operation is occasionally indicated in a joint destroyed by infective arthritis or by degenerative arthritis in a young person who is unsuited for replacement arthroplasty.

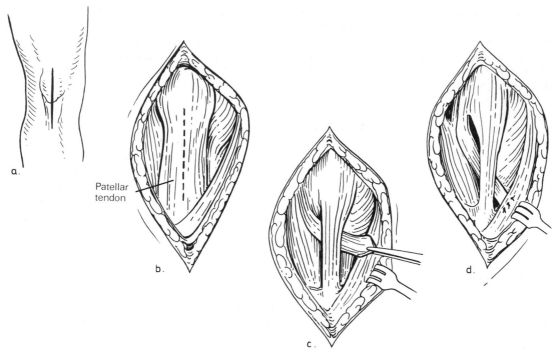

Fig. 6.23   Roux–Goldthwait procedure for recurrent dislocation of the patella

The most satisfactory and consistently effective technique is the compression arthrodesis as described by Charnley.

Operation

With the patient supine, a transverse or S-shaped incision is made at the level of the middle of the patella. The incision is deepened through the joint capsule at both sides and the infrapatellar tendon is divided. The knee is then flexed to expose the collateral and cruciate ligaments which are divided, allowing the tibia to be displaced forward in relation the femur. The joint surfaces are then resected with a tenon saw removing as little bone as possible. The cut surfaces should be flat and so shaped that, when coapted, the limb is in normal alignment with regard to abduction and adduction and in about 15° of flexion. Steinmann pins are inserted transversely through the distal femur and upper tibia at their mid points about 5 cm from the bone ends. The compression apparatus (Fig. 6.24) is applied to the ends of the pins and the wing nuts tightened to produce moderate bowing of the Steinmann pins; this will produce rigid stability at the site of the arthrodesis. The wound is closed and a plaster cylinder applied. At 4 weeks, the compression apparatus is removed and a new plaster reapplied for a further 4 weeks, by which time the arthrodesis should be consolidated.

Muscular imbalance of the knee

Isolated paralysis of the quadriceps does not give rise to great disability for the knee may be stabilized in extension through the action of gluteus maximus in extending the femur when the foot is securely balanced on the ground. Even slight flexion contracture at the knee may render this mechanism incompetent however and a supracondylar osteotomy to correct the flexion

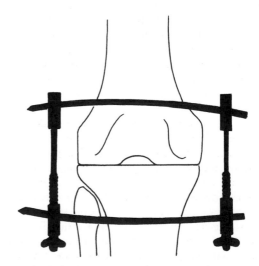

Fig. 6.24   Arthrodesis of the knee using the Charnley compression apparatus

deformity may then be required. When gluteus maximus is also paralysed and the foot muscles are incompetent, a caliper is necessary to stabilize the knee.

A persistent tendency to flexion deformity at the knee due to imbalance between overacting hamstrings and weak quadriceps — characteristic of spastic paralysis — can be corrected by *Egger's operation*, in which the hamstring muscles are detached from the tibia and reattached to the distal femur, where they reinforce hip extension rather than knee flexion.

Flexion deformities in the knee may also develop in chronically sick and elderly patients, who are bed- or chair-bound and neglected. If their deformities cannot be corrected by continuous traction, tenotomy of the hamstring tendons may be required, and if this proves inadequate, the origin of the two heads of gastrocnemius and the proximal attachment of the posterior capsule of the knee joint are erased from the bone and allowed to slide distally.

Supracondylar osteotomy

Severe genu valgum or varum and knee flexion deformity may be corrected by supracondylar osteotomy. The technique of osteotomy-osteoclasis described on page 114 may be used. Alternatively, in older children or adults, a complete osteotomy may be carried out with the removal of an appropriate wedge of bone to allow correction of the deformity and the osteotomy site is then stabilized by internal fixation, either with metal staples or a short plate. A plaster cast is applied and maintained for 5 or 6 weeks until there is radiological evidence of union.

Quadricepsplasty

Occasionally following fractures of the distal femur, adhesions may develop between the quadriceps mechanism and the underlying bone, which limit knee flexion. If this gives rise to significant disability, the operation of quadricepsplasty is indicated. This operation is a major undertaking and should only be carried out in patients who are well-motivated to cooperate with the extensive and often painful postoperative physiotherapy which is required.

Operation. A midline vertical incision is made in the front of the distal thigh continuing into the anteromedial incision of the knee (p. 130). The knee joint is first opened and any adhesions, which may be present within the knee joint itself, are divided. Sometimes these constitute the main source of contracture and no further dissection is required. However, usually it is necessary then to isolate the rectus femoris from the remaining components of the quadriceps and adhesions between the quadriceps and the bone are separated, as they are identified. After operation the knee is immobilized in a plaster splint in 90° of flexion. The

splint is removed at intervals throughout the day to allow the knee to be extended but the flexed position is retained throughout the night. Splintage is discarded when the patient has regained active control of the range of movement gained during the operation. Physiotherapy may have to be continued for several months.

High tibial osteotomy

High tibial osteotomy is carried out for osteoarthritis of the knee in patients with varus or valgus deformity. It is particularly successful in cases in which the arthritis is largely confined to one compartment of the knee. The osteotomy is carried out just above the patellar tendon insertion about 2 cm below the tibial articular surface. A wedge of bone is excised to restore the normal alignment of the limb. It is essential, before the operation is undertaken, to measure precisely the amount of correction required so that the correct thickness of wedge is removed. X-ray control is required during the operation.

The operation of lateral wedge osteotomy will be described as this is more commonly performed. The exposure for medial wedge osteotomy is easier because of the absence of the fibula, but otherwise is similar.

Lateral wedge osteotomy. A transverse incision is made over the upper tibia extending from the head of the fibula to the tibial tuberosity. It is prudent to identify the common peroneal nerve on the lateral aspect of the neck of the fibula and mobilize it so that it can be kept out of harm's way during the rest of the operation.

The lateral surface of the upper tibia is exposed subperiosteally as far as the patellar tendon and the lateral ligament and biceps tendon are detached carefully from the head of the fibula preserving the continuity of their attachment to the fascia on the lateral aspect of the upper fibula. The proximal 1.5 cm of the head of the fibula is then removed with an osteotome. This allows access to the posterior surface of the tibia. A guidewire is inserted at the level of the proposed osteotomy 2 cm below the articular surface and passed medially to emerge from the medial cortex at the same level. Its position is confirmed by X-ray. Bone spikes are then placed in front of the tibia deep to the patellar tendon and posteriorly passing it in contact with the bone while the knee is flexed. This ensures that the popliteal vessels and nerves are held out of the way. While an assistant holds the soft tissues away from the bone with these spikes, the surgeon, with broad osteotomes, carefully cuts a wedge of predetermined thickness, using the guidewire to mark the proximal surface of the wedge. This avoids the risk of drifting too close to the articular surface. When the wedge removal is completed the guidewire is withdrawn. The osteotomy is held closed by the assistant and is secured by

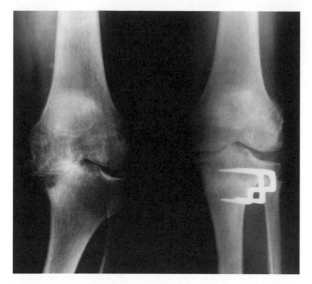

Fig. 6.25   X-ray showing upper tibial osteotomy for medial compartment osteoarthritis with genu varum

two offset staples (Fig. 6.25). The soft tissues are repaired and a compression bandage and plaster backslab applied.

Early weight-bearing is allowed and knee mobilization is commenced at 2 weeks, but a protective plaster slab is retained while weight-bearing for a further 2 weeks. Thereafter unprotected weight-bearing is allowed.

OPERATIONS ON THE ANKLE

Exposure of the ankle joint

The anterolateral approach gives excellent exposure of the ankle and tarsal joints, and causes minimal disturbance to the soft parts. The incision, shown in Figure 6.26, begins in front of the fibula 5 cm above the joint, and is carried downwards between the lateral malleolus and peroneus tertius, to end over the base of the fourth metatarsal. The superior and inferior extensor retinacula are divided as far as is necessary to expose the capsule of the ankle joint.

Arthroplasty of the ankle

At the present time, replacement arthroplasties of the ankle are being developed and undergoing trial. The value of these procedures is not yet established.

Arthrodesis of the ankle

This may be required for post-traumatic arthritis following intra-articular fractures involving the ankle joint and occasionally in chronic arthritis of inflammatory origin.

Many techniques for ankle arthrodesis are described. Charnley has developed a compression technique similar to that which is now standard for the knee. His approach to the ankle joint is through the transverse anterior incision, dividing all the extensor tendons and the anterior joint capsule and lateral ligaments, which

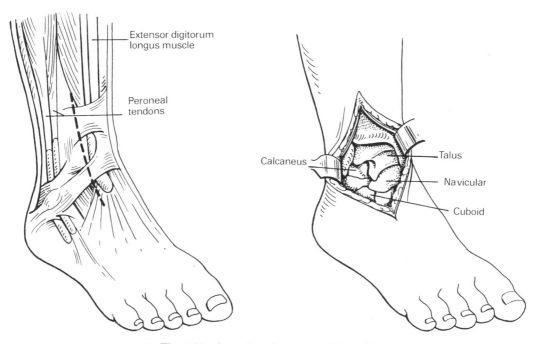

Fig. 6.26   Anterolateral exposure of the ankle

allows the ankle to be opened widely. The joint surfaces are then resected and Steinmann pins passed through the distal tibia and the talus and the compression apparatus attached as in the knee arthrodesis. The extensor tendons are repaired and the wound closed. Charnley states that this very radical approach does not give rise to any lasting disability. A compression arthrodesis, can, however be satisfactorily performed through 2 lateral incisions with preservation of all tendons, although the more limited access undoubtedly makes the resection of the bone ends more difficult. A simpler, noncompression method works well in most instances.

Technique

The ankle joint is exposed through the anterolateral approach. The ankle joint is opened and the articular surface is excised from the distal tibia and from the talus. The dissection is carried down on the medial side removing the articular cartilage from the medial malleolus and from the medial surface of the talus. The lateral surface of the talus is dealt with similarly but it is not usually possible nor necessary to excise so much on the lateral side as on the medial side. Cancellous chips are removed from the anterior iliac crest. With the foot in full planter flexion the cancellous chips are packed into the resultant gap and the foot is then brought up to neutral or a position of 5° of planter flexion if there is some shortening. The foot and ankle are immobilized in a below knee plaster for 8 weeks or until arthrodesis is sound. Weight-bearing is allowed after 2 weeks.

OPERATIONS ON THE HINDFOOT

Calcaneal osteotomy

Inversion of the calcaneus may exist as an isolated deformity or be part of a residual club foot deformity in which case it may be associated with a short tendo-Achilles. Correction of the deformity is obtained by eversion osteotomy of the calcaneum.

Operation

The patient lies prone. The incision extends obliquely across the medial aspect of the heel and proximally along the medial border of the tendo-Achilles for 3 cm. The tendo-Achilles is divided in a stepcut manner. The neurovascular bundle behind the medial malleolus is identified and preserved and the calcaneum is exposed subperiosteally on its superior and medial aspect. An osteotomy is carried out as shown in Figure 6.27. A wedge of cortical bone obtained either from the tibia or from the bone bank is driven into the osteotomy site from the medial aspect, holding it open in the desired position. The tendo-Achilles is repaired, if necessary

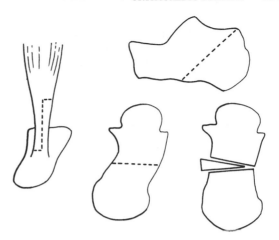

Fig. 6.27   Correction of heel inversion by an opening wedge osteotomy of the calcaneum

with lengthening, and a knee plaster is applied and weight-bearing allowed after 2 weeks. The plaster is retained for 8 weeks.

In pes cavus deformities associated with heel inversion, where the os calcis is of normal length, it is better to obtain correction by removing a wedge from the lateral aspect of the os calcis, producing slight shortening of the bone and relaxation of the plantar soft tissues.

Triple fusion

In this operation arthrodesis of the subtalar and midtarsal joints is carried out. The operation is designed to produce a well shaped and stable foot and is indicated in a wide range of deformities and paralytic disorders of the foot. The operation should not be carried out until skeletal growth has ceased. The incision is shown in Figure 6.28 and is deepened to expose the lateral and dorsal aspects of the tarsus, care being taken to preserve the extensor tendons. The soft tissues are mobilized as close to the bone as possible until the subtalar and midtarsal joints are fully exposed. Using thin osteotomes, the joint surfaces are resected in parallel to each other, exposure of the medial parts of the joints being obtained by an assistant forcibly inverting the foot. Appropriate wedges may be removed to correct any deformity. Sometimes a short medial incision over the talonavicular joint is necessary to allow complete clearance of the joint surfaces. If the joint excision has been accurately performed the bone surfaces should then be closely opposed with correction of deformity. The 3 joints are stabilized by transfixion with Kirschner wires or by use of small staples. Any residual gaps between the bone surfaces should be packed with cancellous bone graft. A below knee plaster is applied over a padded dressing and this is changed to a close fitting plaster at two weeks when the Kirschner wires can be withdrawn. Weight-bearing is allowed at four

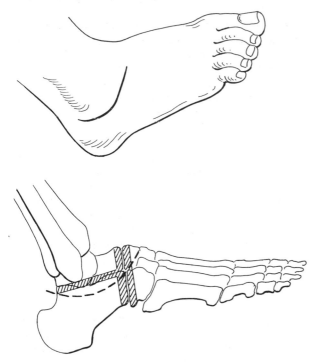

Fig. 6.28 Incision and extent of bone resection in the operation of triple fusion

weeks; the plaster cast is removed at 8–10 weeks, when there is radiological evidence of union.

Pes planus

Mobile flat foot does not require surgical correction. Spasmodic flat foot due to a congenital tarsal coalition may be cured before the age of 14 by excision of the anomalous bar. In older children, if the symptoms warrant it, a triple fusion may be required.

Pes cavus

Most cases of pes cavus cause little disability and do not require surgical treatment. There is no entirely satisfactory surgical correction for this deformity. *Steindler's operation,* which involves division of the shortened structures of the sole at their attachment to the calcaneum, produces temporary benefit only. Correction of heel inversion (p. 137), if present, may improve the posture of the foot as a whole and likewise correction of the associated toe clawing may also improve foot function. Occasionally a triple fusion or wedge resection of the midtarsal joint may be required, but the results of this procedure in pes cavus are disappointing.

Congenital talipes equinovarus

Club foot, which does not respond readily to conservative manipulation and corrective strapping, should be released surgically at an early stage, ideally between

2–4 months. If the deformity is allowed to exist for a longer period, adaptive changes occur in the bony skeleton, which makes full correction thereafter difficult and triple fusion may become necessary at a later stage. Early soft tissue release is therefore ideal.

The incision is made from the medial border of the tendo-Achilles to below the medial malleolus and forward to the medial border of the foot. The tibialis posterior, flexor digitorum longus, the neurovascular bundle and the flexor hallucis longus are identified behind the medial malleolus in that order from front to back. The neurovascular bundle is traced to its terminal branching in the sole of the foot and carefully preserved throughout the subsequent operation. The tendo-Achilles is then lengthened in a stepcut manner. The tibialis posterior, flexor digitorum longus and flexor hallucis longus tendons are lengthened in the same way. The capsule and ligaments on the medial and inferior aspects of the talonavicular joint are widely opened to allow correction of the talonavicular subluxation, which is a feature of the club foot deformity, and the ligaments on the medial aspect of the subtalar joint are similarly divided. Finally division of the capsular ligaments on the plantar aspect of the midtarsal joint are divided and it is now possible to manipulate the foot into full correction of its varus and inversion deformities. The stepcut tendons are now repaired with appropriate lengthening. The foot is immobilized in the correct position in a well padded plaster cast. The corrective plaster is maintained for at least 10 weeks.

Paralytic drop foot deformity

Paralytic drop foot may result from poliomyelitis of injury to the lateral popliteal nerve. The deformity can be controlled by one of the many varieties of drop splint but, if the patient finds this unacceptable, surgical correction is possible. If the tibialis posterior muscle is acting normally, triple arthrodesis may be carried out, the tendon tibialis posterior being then transferred through the interosseous membrane to be attached to the dorsum of the foot where it will act as a dorsiflexor. If this muscle is paralysed, a Lambrinudi variation of the triple arthrodesis is carried out in which a wedge of bone is removed from the plantar aspect of the talus, as shown in Figure 6.29 and the triple fusion is carried out with the talus in full equinus and the rest of the foot in dorsiflexion.

OPERATIONS ON THE FOREFOOT

Ingrowing toenail

Persistent ingrowing toenail is best treated by wedge resection as illustrated in Figure 6.30. In carrying out

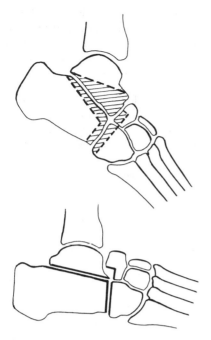

Fig. 6.29 Lambrinudi modification of the triple arthrodesis to correct paralytic drop foot deformity

this procedure, care must be taken to remove the entire nail fold and the germinal zone related to the piece of nail which is being removed. This fans out laterally at the base of the nail and meticulous dissection must be carried out to ensure that an irregular spike of nail does not recur.

Radical excision of the nail bed (Zadek's operation)
This is indicated for more general deformities of the nail such as onychogryphosis. The nail is first avulsed. The flap of skin overlying the base of the nail is elevated proximally and the sub-adjacent germinal layer

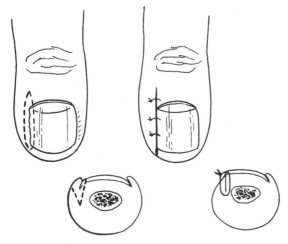

Fig. 6.30 Wedge resection for ingrowing toenail

of the nail bed is excised, paying particular attention to the lateral extensions, which are loosely attached to the bony expansion at the base of the terminal phalanx. The flap of skin is then sutured back to the base of the nail bed. If the skin underlying the nail is metaplastic and unhealthy, it is better to excise this entirely and to cover the residual defect with a skin graft.

Claw toes
Clawing of the toes is usually a feature of pes cavus but can occur independently. The common cause is a muscle imbalance resulting from weakness in the intrinsic muscles of the foot. If the clawing is severe and giving rise to symptoms, surgical correction is possible. If the toes can be corrected passively, the operation of choice is a flexor to extensor transfer whereas, if the deformity is fixed, interphalangeal fusion is preferred.

Flexor to extensor transfer in toes — Girdlestone's operation
Through separate dorsolateral incisions at the base of each toe, the fibrous flexor sheath is exposed and incised. The flexor tendons are divided as far distally as possible and the long flexor alone is brought to the dorsal aspect of the toe. It is passed through the extensor expansion and sutured to it with fine, non-absorbable suture. Thereafter the flexor tendon will act in the manner of the intrinsics, i.e. it will flex the metatarsophalangeal joint and extend the interphalangeal joint. Following the operation, the toes are held in the correct position by means of a plaster cast which extends forward to the tip of the toes. The plaster cast is retained for 4 weeks.

Interphalangeal fusion
Through mid-dorsal incisions in each toe, the extensor tendon is split longitudinally, the dorsal capsule of each joint is incised and the articular surface of the bone ends resected. Small, sharp chisels and gouges are useful here. When the 2 joints have been cleared in each toe, a Kirschner wire is used to transfix them. This is first inserted into the proximal surface of the middle phalanx and guided through the distal phalanx to emerge at the tip of the toe. It is then driven retrogradely across the proximal interphalangeal joint. The wire is removes after 4 weeks, during which time the patient may walk in an open-toed sandal.

Hammer toe
This term is applied to a flexion deformity at the proximal interphalangeal joint of the toe, usually the second. The condition is best treated by arthrodesis of the affected joint using a peg in socket procedure, which has the additional advantage of shortening the toe slightly, for a hammer toe is usually excessively long.

The first step in the operation consists in subcutaneous tenotomy of the extensor tendon in order to correct the dorsiflexion deformity of the first phalanx. The dorsal corn is excised by a longitudinal elliptical incision and the extensor tendon and dorsal capsule are incised. The head of the proximal phalanx is cleared and, with small bone shears and an osteotome, is shaped into a peg which should include the dorsal cortex to give increased strength. Then using a suitably sized drill or burr, a hole is bored into the base of the middle phalanx. This phalanx is now impacted on to the peg and no additional fixation should be required, although it is prudent to support the toe with a collodion splint for the first week or two. Weight-bearing in an open-toed sandal is allowed immediately.

Mallet toe

This is a flexion deformity of the terminal joint. The bones are too small at this level to allow a spike arthrodesis and it is sufficient simply to resect the joint surfaces and stabilize them with a short Kirschner wire, as in the Lambrinudi procedure.

Hallux valgus

Hallux valgus is exceedingly common, particularly among women in the Western world. Only a minority of cases produce significant symptoms and operative treatment should therefore be very selectively used. There is no point in carrying out any operative procedure for this condition, unless the patient agrees thereafter to wear shoes designed for function rather than fashion, for unsuitable footwear with high heels and narrow toes is undoubtedly a constant aggravating factor in the production of this deformity. Once the toe begins to deviate from its normal alignment, the condition tends to get progressively worse because the long tendons now bowstring to the lateral side and the mechanical advantage of the adductor is increased whereas that of the abductor is diminished. Any operative correction of hallux valgus must take these factors into account.

Many operations have been described to correct this deformity and the choice of procedure depends to some extent on the age and sex of the patient and on the degree of the deformity. Correction of the alignment by metatarsal osteotomy is indicated in young people in whom the joint remains relatively healthy. In older women, a Keller's arthroplasty is the operation of choice; while in men and when faced with a very gross deformity, arthrodesis is likely to produce the most satisfactory result.

Metatarsal osteotomy

There are many ways of carrying out this procedure; some exceedingly complex. The *Wilson osteotomy* has

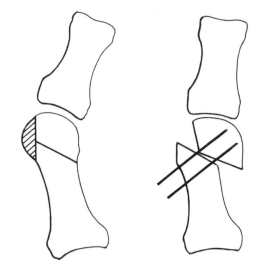

Fig. 6.31 Diagram of Wilson's osteotomy

the virtue of simplicity and in a recent review proved to be as satisfactory as any. A dorsomedial incision is made over the distal half of the first metatarsal, which is then exposed subperiosteally. An oblique osteotomy is then carried out through the neck of the metatarsal, as illustrated in Figure 6.31. The osteotomy can be performed with an oscillating saw or by multiple drilling completed with an osteotome. The hallux and the metatarsal head are then rotated into nominal alignment and the metatarsal head is displaced laterally in relation to the metatarsal shaft where it may be stabilized by 2 Kirschner wires. It is important that no dorsal angulation should take place at the osteotomy site. The medial bony projection from the stump of the metatarsal is removed and after wound closure a plaster is applied with the hallux held in slight overcorrection. A new weight-bearing plaster is applied in 2 weeks and retained for a further 2 weeks and thereafter the patient may walk in an orthopaedic sandal. At 8 weeks the osteotomy is united and the Kirschner wires are removed.

In older patients hallux valgus deformity is usually part of a more widespread disorganisation of the forefoot, characterized by collapse of the transverse arch with excessive pressure and pain under the metatarsal heads and frequently dorsal and lateral subluxation of the metatarsal phalangeal joints of one or more of the small toes with consequently poor toe function, which again puts excessive pressure on the metatarsal heads. The hallux valgus deformity may be so severe that the hallux comes to lie over or under the neighbouring toes. In such a foot, surgery confined to the hallux valgus deformity alone would relieve only one component of the patient's discomfort and additional procedures, such as metatarsal osteotomies and excision of the dislocated proximal phalanges may also be required. No operative procedures, however, are going to restore such a foot to its pristine condition, and the patient must be made fully aware of this before surgery is undertaken.

Keller's arthroplasty

A dorsomedial incision is made over the base of the proximal phalanx and the metatarsal head and neck. The soft tissues are stripped from the bones by sharp dissection. The structures which must be mobilized include the joint capsule and the 4 short muscles, which are attached to the base of the proximal phalanx. The medial prominence of the metatarsal head is trimmed as shown in Figure 6.32 and at least half of the proximal phalanx is removed. The skin only requires closure. The toe is then bandaged in slight overcorrection and the patient may walk in a wooden soled sandal within a few days. The patient should when possible maintain the foot in elevation until the postoperative swelling has subsided. Intrinsic exercises should be maintained postoperatively until maximal toe function is restored. It is sometimes useful to keep a small silicone rubber wedge between the first and second toes for some months after operation, if there is any tendency towards recurrence.

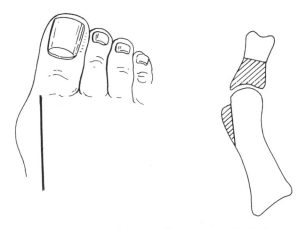

Fig. 6.32   Incision and extent of bone removal in Keller's arthroplasty

Hallux rigidus

Stiffness of the metatarsophalangeal joint may occur during adolescence when the common pathology is osteochondritis dissecans of the metatarsal head. At this age it is rarely painful and no treatment is usually required, although, if the patient finds the condition limiting, removal of a dorsal wedge at the base of the proximal phalanx may give a more useful arc of movement by allowing increased dorsiflexion.

In older people hallux rigidus is caused by osteoarthritis. It is extremely common and only a minority of people have symptoms sufficiently troublesome to warrant surgery. In some, discomfort is due simply to pressure on the marginal osteophytes which develop around the osteoarthritic joint, and simple removal of the osteophytes will bring sufficient relief. When the pain arises from the joint itself, Keller's arthroplasty or arthrodesis is carried out. Arthrodesis is probably the better procedure in the working man but should only be performed when some dorsiflexion is possible at the interphalangeal joint. Keller's arthroplasty is more suitable in women, who in general prefer to retain some movement in the metatarsophalangeal joint to allow them to wear varying heights of heel.

Arthrodesis of metatarsophalangeal joint

The joint is exposed as in the Keller's operation. Marginal osteophytes are removed and the articular surfaces are denuded of cartilage and then shaped to form close contact. The arthrodesis is stabilized by means of a transfixion screw with 5 or 10° of dorsiflexion in men and rather more in women. Slight valgus should also be allowed in women to facilitate subsequent shoe fitting. A below knee walking plaster extended forward to support the toe is worn for 6–8 weeks.

Clawing of the hallux

Flexion deformity of the interphalangeal joint of the big toe may develop following tibialis anterior paralysis, or more commonly as part of the generalized clawing associated with pes cavus resulting from weakness of the intrinsic muscles. The first metatarsal is abnormally flexed and painful callosities tend to develop under the metatarsal head and over the dorsum of the clawed toe. *Jones' operation* is designed to correct both aspects of the deformity by interphalangeal fusion and tendon transfer of extensor hallucis longus tendon to the neck of the first metatarsal. A transverse incision is made on the dorsal aspect of the interphalangeal joint and the joint surfaces are resected using sharp chisels. The joint is stabilized in a straight position by 2 crossing Kirschner wires. The extensor hallucis longus tendon is divided as distally as possible and a hole is drilled through the neck of the first metatarsal large enough to allow the tendon to be passed through and sutured back on itself in moderate tension. A below knee walking plaster is retained for 5 weeks. The Kirschner wires are removed at 8 weeks when the arthrodesis is solid.

Overlapping fifth toe

This is a common congenital deformity in which the fifth toe overlies the fourth and is subject to pressure from shoe wear. It is best corrected by the *Butler opera-*

tion. The skin incision starts in the dorsal aspect of the foot at the base of the fifth toe and passes distally to encircle the toe near its base. Care must be taken to ensure that the digital nerves and vessels are preserved. The incision then extends on to the plantar pad at the base of the toe, where a small circle of skin is removed to match the diameter of the toe. Through the dorsal incision, the extensor digitorum longus tendon and dorsal capsule of the metatarsophalangeal joint are divided. This allows the toe to be displaced into its correct position, where it is anchored by suturing the skin of the toe to the margin of the circular skin defect. This leaves a small deficiency of skin on the dorsal aspect of the toe but the skin in this region is loose and readily closed.

Metatarsal head resection or forefoot arthroplasty

Patients with rheumatoid arthritis frequently develop disabling metatarsalgia due to loss of toe function, dislocation of the metatarsophalangeal joints and excessive weight borne by the metatarsal heads. Excision of all the metatarsal heads may produce marked relief of pain. Such an operation does not, however, improve the function of the forefoot and it must be reserved for people with rheumatoid arthritis, who generally have multiple joint problems and restricted walking ability. The operation is not suitable for forefoot disorganization in non-rheumatic cases, nor is it suitable for patients when there is any doubt about the peripheral circulation as delay in wound healing is a feature of this procedure.

Technique

Three longitudinal incisions are made in the dorsal aspect of the foot at the level of the metatarsophalangeal joints. One is placed on the dorsomedial aspect of the big toe, as for Keller's arthroplasty, and the other two between the remaining toes. Through these incisions, the bases of the proximal phalanges of the toes, which are usually dislocated dorsally, are exposed and at least half of the proximal phalanx of each toe is excised. The metatarsal heads are exposed and excised with an oblique cut, as shown in Figure 6.33. The trimmed metatarsal necks should then present a smooth and uniform curve. If one projects beyond this alignment, it will certainly give rise to pain subsequently. Finally, an ellipse of skin, transversely orientated, is removed from the sole of the foot just behind the weight-bearing pad, which in this deformity has been drawn forwards to face anteriorly rather than plantarwards. When this elliptical plantar wound is closed, the weight-bearing pad is drawn back to its proper position and the now rather floppy toes fall into better alignment. A light compression bandage is applied to hold the toes in this

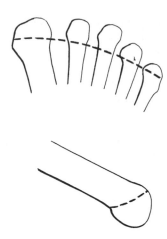

Fig. 6.33 Metatarsal head resection showing the amount of bone to be removed

position and when the wounds are healed a below knee walking plaster is applied for 3 weeks. Physiotherapy is directed towards strengthening the foot and toe muscles during the period of immobilization and subsequently to restore a moderate degree of toe function.

Not infrequently, some toes are more severely affected than others and the surgeon may in this event be tempted to carry out a metatarsal head resection only in the more troublesome toes. This, however, is invariably unwise for the remaining toes then become painful in turn.

In the non-rheumatic foot, in which only one or two metatarsal heads are displaced into the sole, a dorsal displacement osteotomy of the affected metatarsal may give relief. This operation is frequently indicated in conjunction with Keller's arthroplasty where one or more of the adjacent metatarsophalangeal joints may be affected in this way. Through a short incision the dorsal aspect of the neck of the affected metatarsal is divided obliquely. No fixation is required and immediate weight-bearing is allowed. The osteotomy will unite with dorsal displacement thus relieving pressure on the offending metatarsal head.

OPERATIONS FOR OSTEOMYELITIS

Improved social conditions and more effective treatment of primary foci of infection have greatly reduced the frequency and severity of osteomyelitis in developed countries. Elsewhere it continues to be a major problem. If infection is allowed to become established in bone it tends to cause extensive bone necrosis as a result of toxaemia and by interruption of the local blood supply. This is caused by pressure exerted by the inflammatory products together with periosteal stripping produced by the abscess when it escapes from bone under pressure. When large areas of bone death occur the organisms can linger there safe from the natural defences of the body and from antibiotics which cannot penetrate in the absence of a good blood supply. A state of chronic osteomyelitis is then established which may last for a lifetime. Other serious complications include damage to the adjacent growth plate and involvement of neighbouring joints.

Typically acute osteomyelitis is a disease of childhood and the common sites of involvement are the metaphyses frequently of the femur and upper tibia, but no bone is immune. In the adult the haemopoietic bones of the spine and pelvis are the most common locations. The infection usually reaches bone by the blood stream from a focus elsewhere such as a boil or infected wound or a urinary tract infection. The organism is the staphylococcus aureus in over 90% of cases but the rest are due to a wide range of organisms and the pattern may vary in different countries. Salmonella infections, for example, are common in countries with a high incidence of sickle cell disease.

Treatment is directed towards aborting the infection before it has a chance to become entrenched and involves both conservative and surgical measures. The first step is to try to identify the organism by blood culture, swabbing any obvious superficial source of infection or by local aspiration of the infected site. Antibiotic therapy is commenced immediately thereafter, before the bacterial confirmation is available. The antibiotic selected must be effective against staphylococcus aureus which may be assumed to be penicillin resistant, but should also cover the less common organisms including the coliforms which may occasionally be responsible. They must be administered intravenously and in high concentration initially. Developments in chemotherapy are so rapid that it is difficult to recommend in a textbook a drug regime that can be guaranteed to endure to the next edition, however at the time of writing, cloxacillin coupled with gentamycin or one of the injectable cephalosporins would be appropriate. Once the organism is identified and its sensitivity known the antibiotics can be varied accordingly. Chloramphenicol is of value if *Salmonella typhi* is suspected. Once the acute illness has subsided the drugs may be administered orally and must be continued for at least 3 weeks after the symptoms and signs have settled. Surgery is indicated if an abscess is detectable when the child is first seen or if the antibiotic therapy has not produced a dramatic improvement in the patient's condition within 24 hours. The operation consists of a surgical incision down to bone at the level of maximal swelling and tenderness. Any subperiosteal abscess is evacuated and several drill holes are made in the metaphysis to allow the release of an intraosseus abscess. The wound is irrigated with an antibiotic solution and then closed over a vacuum drain. The limb should be splinted in a plaster cast to relieve pain and prevent pathological fracture, but the site of infection must be windowed to allow observation.

Osteomyelitis may also arise from infection introduced through compound wounds or during the course of surgery. This should be preventable by good surgical technique and by meticulous wound excision (p. 165).

Chronic osteomyelitis

Once chronic osteomyelitis is established, chemotherapy will do no more than control the recurrent exacerbations of infection. The key to management is surgical removal of sequestra and the eradication of abscess cavities and dead space by saucerisation and filling the resulting defect with viable soft tissue such as a muscle flap. Sometimes the chronic infection takes the form of diffuse sclerosis with multiple sinus tracks but no large cavities or sequestra. In such cases surgical excision of the entire area of infected bone offers the only prospect of cure. This may be possible if the bone is expendable such as the clavicle or fibula but is obviously more difficult in the major weight-bearing bones, although the development of microsurgical techniques, which enable the transplant of a living fibula with attachment of it's blood supply, now offers the prospect of repairing large defects in any long bone following excision for chronic infection or tumour. Operations for chronic osteomyelitis have therefore to be varied according to circumstance. It is useful at the outset to inject the sinus track with a dye such as methylene blue. The incision should excise the sinus and the surrounding scar and follow the sinus to the bone which is exposed subperiosteally as widely as may be necessary. X-ray can help to identify the site of the sequestrum or cavity during the operation. Once this has been located, the cavity is saucerised — that is completely deroofed, using osteotomes and gouges and the margins bevelled as extensively as may be required to produce a crater whose opening is wider than its base. Sequestra, which are usually easily identified by their white and crenated appearance, are lifted out and the wall of the cavity closely examined for other loculi or communicating sinuses. A local flap of muscle is then mobilized with care to preserve its blood supply and this is used to fill the cavity. If no muscle is available the wound should be dressed and left open. A few days later, when clean and granulating, a split skin graft may be used to line the cavity. At a later date when all signs of infection have subsided, the cavity may be filled by cancellous bone.

It must be recognized that many cases of chronic osteomyelitis will recur, despite such radical surgery.

Table 6.1 Classification of primary bone tumours

Histological type	Benign	Frequency	Malignant	Frequency
Haemopoietic			Myeloma	XX
			Reticulum cell sarcoma	X
Chondrogenic	Osteochondroma	XXXX	Primary chondrosarcoma	X
	Chondroma	XXXX	Secondary chondrosarcoma	X
	Chondroblastoma	X		
	Chondromyxoid fibroma	X		
Osteogenic	Osteoid osteoma	X	Osteosarcoma	X
	Benign osteoblastoma	X	Parosteal osteosarcoma	X
Unknown	Giant cell tumour	X	Malignant giant cell tumour	X
			Ewing's tumour	X
			Adamantinoma	X
			Malignant fibrous histiocytoma	X
Fibrogenic	Fibroma	XX	Fibrosarcoma	X
	Fibrous cortical defect	XXXX		
Notochordal			Chordoma	X
Vascular	Haemangioma	X	Haemangioendothelioma	X
	Aneurysmal bone cyst	X		

The number of X's gives an approximate indication of frequency; X implying rarity and XXXX common occurrence.

OPERATIONS FOR BONE TUMOURS AND CYSTS

Bone tumours are exceedingly varied in their histogenesis and in their behaviour. Table 6.1 lists the more common of these tumours and gives some indication of their frequency. Malignant primary bone tumours are exceedingly rare, and with advances in endoprosthetic replacement and in chemotherapy, it is desirable that these should be managed in specialized units if available.

Benign tumours and cysts are much more common and easier to manage. Many show a tendency to spontaneous healing; these include most fibrous cortical defects, some chondroblastomas, aneurysmal bone cysts and simple cysts. Others are symptomless and therefore require no treatment except perhaps bone biopsy if their nature is uncertain.

Surgery is required for those which cause significant symptoms such as pain, pathological fracture or swelling sufficient to be disfiguring or to cause mechanical effects on other tissues. Surgery consists of simple excision or curettage with, if necessary, the repair of a residual defect with bone grafts. If a pathological fracture due to a benign tumour or cyst has occurred, it is often wiser to delay surgical treatment until the fracture has healed. Some illustrative examples are listed below.

Osteochondromas

These cartilaginous capped exostoses arising at the metaphyses may be solitary lesions or multiple in the

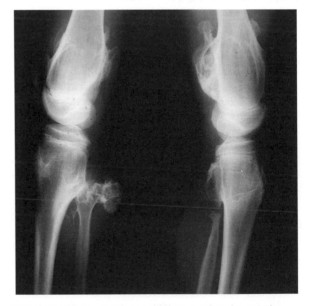

Fig. 6.34 X-ray showing multiple osteochondromata in diaphyseal aclasis. Note that some are sessile and others pedunculated

condition of diaphyseal aclasis. Only large and troublesome tumours (Fig. 6.34) require treatment and these are simply excised by dividing their origin from bone; as a rule they are devoid of soft tissue attachment. Growth of an osteochondroma in adult life suggests the possibility of malignant transformation to chondrosarcoma and a wider local resection is then indicated.

Chondromas

These cartilaginous tumours may be left if they are asymptomatic. Otherwise they are treated by curettage and bone graft replacement if large. The small chondromas which occur so commonly in the phalanges will heal following curettage without the need of bone graft.

Osteoid osteomas

These are small and intensely painful tumours of osteoblastic derivation. Frequently they may be overlooked on routine X-ray because of their minute size, but a bone scan will always reveal them as a 'hot spot'. Local excision is indicated and is invariably curative provided that the osteogenic nidus is removed.

Giant cell tumour

This often gives rise to problems of management because of its common subarticular location in major joints. Although it responds to radiotherapy, there have been so many reports of irradiation induced sarcoma following this treatment that it is no longer recommended. Although most giant cell tumours behave in a benign fashion, a minority assume malignant characteristics and this raises a further difficulty in treatment. If the tumour occurs in a bone which may be resected without loss of function, such as the distal ulna or proximal fibula, then local resection is the treatment of choice. When the tumour occurs in an epiphysis around the knee or hip and major fracture has not occurred, then curettage and packing with bone grafts should be tried in the first instance (Fig. 6.35). The success rate with this simple procedure can be high but it depends on the thoroughness with which the curettage is done. It is important to obtain the bone graft (if autogenous graft is used) with separate instruments and gloves to avoid the possibility of tumour transfer to the donor site. If the tumour presents with a major fracture or if it recurs following surgery, then wide local resection with major bone graft or endoprosthetic replacement is required (Fig. 6.36).

Malignant bone tumours

Malignant bone tumours tend to present with pain, swelling or pathological fractures — symptoms which are common to many other benign orthopaedic conditions such as osteomyelitis or stress fracture. It is of absolute importance therefore that a biopsy be obtained before radical treatment is undertaken. It is wise also to make a routine of sending biopsy specimens for both histological and bacteriological examination. Ewing's tumour and osteomyelitis, for example, may present in an identical fashion with pain, fever, raised ESR and similar X-ray appearance, and the diagnosis may be missed if biopsy is sent to the inappropriate laboratory.

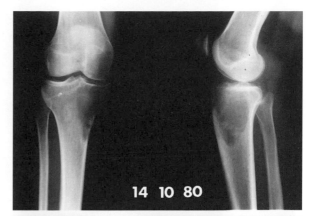

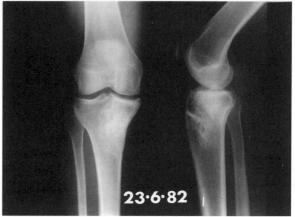

Fig. 6.35   X-rays showing giant cell tumour of upper tibia treated by curettage and bone graft

The biopsy wound should be small, and so situated that it may be excised during subsequent surgery. Ideally several specimens should be obtained from the tumour, for bone tumours frequently vary in their histological characteristics from place to place. Trephine needle biopsies are of value in situations such as the vertebral bodies where open biopsy would involve a major operation.

The management of these rare tumours has altered greatly in recent years. Amputation is no longer regarded as the only surgical procedure available and chemotherapy in conjunction with surgery or radiotherapy has significantly improved the prognosis of osteosarcoma and Ewing's tumour in particular. Historically patients suffering from these tumours had a survival rate of less than 20%, whereas recent series with survival rates at five years in excess of 50% are being reported.

Radical local surgery without amputation for malignant bone tumours should be undertaken only if it is possible to remove the tumour with a wide margin of normal tissue and yet leave enough useful function in the limb to make it better than a prosthesis. Limbs

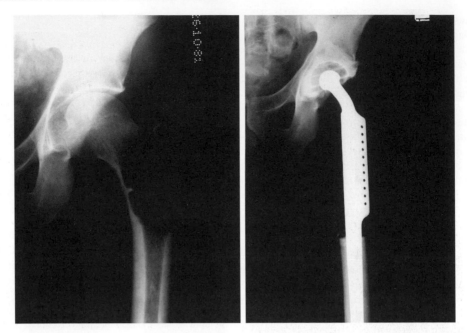

Fig. 6.36   X-rays showing giant cell tumour of proximal femur treated by endoprosthetic replacement

should not be preserved at a risk to the patient's life unless metastatic spread has already occurred.

To assess resectability of a tumour, it is desirable to have preoperative arteriography and CT scans of the limb in order to establish the tumour extent, and an endoprosthesis must be constructed to replace the resected bone or joint. Frozen sections at the time of surgery are useful to confirm that the limits of resection are tumour free. Chondrosarcomas, which in general are more slowly growing and less invasive than osteosarcomas, are most suitable for this type of surgery, but some osteosarcomas, fibrosarcomas and aggressive giant cell tumours may also be treated in this way. If the criteria for local resectability cannot be met then amputation well above the level of tumour must be performed. Chemotherapy, usually involving a combination of drugs including Adriamycin, Methotrexate, Vincristine and Cisplatin, is now given additionally in most cases of bone sarcoma. The optimal therapeutic regime has still not been established and many different courses of treatment are being evaluated. It is best that such treatment be supervised by an oncologist.

Metastatic bone tumours

These are much more frequent than primary malignant tumours. Breast, bronchus, prostate, thyroid and kidney are the common primary sites, although most malignant tumours will occasionally involve bone.

The treatment of these lesions is inevitably only palliative and depends on the nature of the primary tumour. Breast and prostatic secondaries, for example, may be controlled by hormonal therapy and by local radiotherapy. If pathological fractures occur or appear inevitable, it is often possible to stabilise the bone by curetting the local tumour and packing the resulting defect with methylmethacrylate cement incorporating an internal fixation device such as shown in Figure 6.37.

Bone cysts

Simple bone cysts and aneurysmal bone cysts both may undergo spontaneous healing with time and symptomless lesions do not necessarily require treatment. If large, painful and a source of repeated pathological fracture, they should be treated by curettage and bone grafting, although a high recurrence rate may be anticipated and the operation may have to be repeated.

Recent reports suggest that simple bone cysts may be cured by the injection into the cyst of Methylprednisolone in doses ranging from 40 to 200 mg. Two needles are introduced into the cyst, one to allow fluid to escape and the other for the introduction of the steroid. The healing response may not be apparent for several months and repeat injections may be necessary.

OPERATIONS ON FRACTURES

Surgeons tend to polarise into two groups with regard to fracture management — the conservative school take pride in the closed treatment of fractures, while others regard most fractures as a surgical challenge. To a very

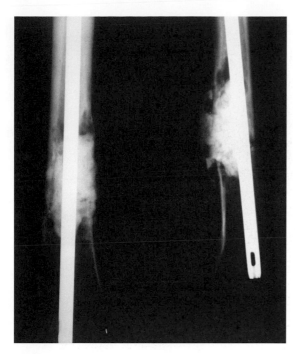

Fig. 6.37 X-ray of pathological fracture through a metastatic deposit stabilized by intramedullary nail and methylmethacrylate cement

great extent the surgeon's view will be coloured by his training and perhaps, more critically, by the equipment available to him. Techniques of internal fixation require expensive equipment but produce increasingly impressive results. Both approaches, conservative and operative, require skilled management. Both can lead to good functional results and each has its range of complications. Conservative management avoids the risk of introducing infection to the fracture site but it involves more prolonged immobilization of the limb or patient with complications of stiffness or osteoporosis, sometimes referred to as 'plaster disease' by the surgically disposed. Surgical treatment often permits earlier mobilization and more accurate reduction of a fracture but at the risk of introducing infection and devitalizing bone as a result of the soft tissue stripping required.

There are some broad areas of agreement, however, which may be used as guidelines. Most fractures in children heal readily and can be well managed conservatively. Minor malalignments will, in general, remodel with growth. Fractures which cannot be reduced or maintained in reduction because of soft tissue interposition or muscle forces are best openly reduced and internally fixed — examples are certain fractures of the olecranon, patella, radius and ulna and fractures involving weight-bearing joints where perfect reduction is desirable if subsequent degenerative arthritis is to be avoided. Fractures in the elderly which, if treated

conservatively, would involve prolonged immobilization in bed, are best treated by surgical means, if this will permit earlier mobilization. A hospital bed is a dangerous environment for the elderly and infirm. In patients with multiple injuries, particularly those with severe head or spinal injuries, internal fixation of limb fractures facilitates nursing care and reduces pulmonary complications and is considered mandatory if there is a high injury severity score. Pathological fractures due to malignant disease should, where possible, be treated by internal fixation for natural healing rarely occurs. Ideally the surgeon should be familiar with both methods and be prepared to select the technique most appropriate to the individual patient.

A bewildering wide range of internal fixation devices is now available, many incompatible with each other in the type of metal used and in the calibre and type of screws and bolts and each requires its own range of instrumentation. It is desirable therefore that each surgeon should decide on one compatible system and become thoroughly familiar with its use. It need hardly be said that an atraumatic and aseptic technique is essential. With composite implants, such as plates and screws, it is important that all components be of the same metal, otherwise electrolytic reaction may occur. Titanium, chromium cobalt alloys and certain standards of stainless steel are acceptable.

Open fractures

The principles governing the management of open fractures are the same as those which obtain for any wound. Surgical excision of dead or severely damaged tissue and the removal of foreign material is essential, if infection is to be avoided. Infection of bone is in general much more intractable than infection of soft tissue and fracture healing is likely to be delayed or to fail altogether in the presence of infection. If possible, a tourniquet is used in the initial stages of the operation. The injured part is thoroughly cleansed with a mild antiseptic solution, such as hibitane or cetavlon, and the wound irrigated with saline. The wound is extended, if necessary, to allow adequate inspection and excision of the deeper layers. Failure to enlarge the wound is the most common fault in the management of a compound fracture. Not infrequently a sharp spike of bone may have caught up fragments of clothing, earth or other highly contaminated materials which are then drawn back into the tissues when the limb is straightened. Small wounds associated with fractures are the tip of the iceberg and should alert the surgeon to the larger area of potential trouble beneath the surface.

Following wound extension, each layer is then carefully excised, removing the contaminated and damaged tissues, but respecting the major nerves and vessels.

The fractured bone ends must be delivered to view and any completely detached fragments of bone be removed. Soiled bone must be curetted or nibbled away and the wound again irrigated with saline. At this stage, the tourniquet should be released and the vitality of the tissues confirmed — healthy muscle should contract when lightly pinched with forceps.

Wound closure should rarely if ever be carried out and the wound should be simply dressed and left open for delayed primary closure or skin grafting after an interval of about 4 days, as discussed in the management of wounds in general on page 164.

Wide spectrum topical antibiotics applied by spray or in irrigation fluid are of value at the completion of the wound excision and systemic antibiotics are recommended but not essential in well excised wounds of limited extent. Specifically cephalosporins should be given and it is also prudent to give penicillin to counter tetanus or gas gangrene in extensive wounds where the adequacy of the excision is in doubt.

It is essential to stabilise the fracture after wound excision and external fixation, internal fixation or splintage may be used. Fractures involving joints almost invariably require accurate reconstruction despite the wound and similarly open fractures involving the patella or olecranon should be immediately fixed by some appropriate technique.

It is now well known that open diaphyseal fractures of long bones may also be treated by primary internal fixation with excellent results and increasing numbers of surgeons employ these techniques in combination with early plastic surgery to gain early full thickness skin cover of the wound. There is strong evidence that primary medullary nailing of open femoral shaft fractures is not only acceptable but is positively indicated, particularly in conjunction with major vessel injury. Open fractures of the tibia remain more controversial and external fixation, using skeletal pins mounted to a rigid external scaffold, as shown in Figure 6.38, may be of great value in the management of severe injuries with extensive soft tissue loss, requiring multiple dressings and skin grafting procedures. This technique maintains the fracture in good position while allowing free access to the wound.

Some surgeons in specialized units use intramedullary nailing or plating techniques with early plastic surgery for these open tibial fractures and report excellent results; external fixators are more widely favoured and are probably more generally applicable. Plaster management of open tibial fractures is very much less used now that better methods of stabilisation are available.

Skeletal traction

Skeletal traction may be used as an alternative to skin

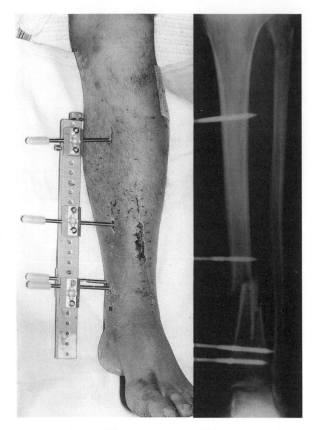

Fig. 6.38 External fixator used to stabilize a compound tibial fracture

traction as a means of maintaining length and alignment and rotation of a fracture. It is now less commonly used for fractures of the femoral shaft, but has occasional applications elsewhere.

The traction is applied by a metal pin passing through bone. The *Steinmann pin* — a sharpened pin, 3 mm in diameter — or the *Denham pin*, are used. The latter is similar to the Steinmann but has a central threaded segment which, when screwed into cortical bone, resists lateral movement and hence reduces the risk of infection.

The usual site for the application of skeletal traction is through the upper end of the tibia. Under general anaesthesia, the pin is inserted by hand using the T shaped introducer through the cortical bone just below the tibial tubercle. It is important that the pin is placed at right angles to the axis of the shaft of the tibia, otherwise asymmetric traction may result in undue stress on the ligaments on one side of the knee. The points of emergence of the pin through the skin should be left exposed but may be protected with a mild antiseptic, such as betadine cream. A metal stirrup or U-loop, to which the traction cord is attached, is fixed to the pin.

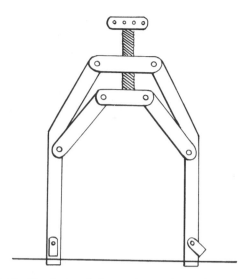

Fig. 6.39 Tensioning device used to apply traction to a Kirschner wire

Figure 6.39 illustrates one method of use. The traction should not exceed 10 kg except for short intervals and should never be so great as to cause distraction of the fracture — usually 5–8 kg is sufficient. It is important that the stirrup rotates freely about the pin so that the pin itself is not turned with every movement, otherwise pin tract infection will develop.

Other sites which are occasionally used for skeletal traction include the olecranon, the supracondylar region of the femur and the calcaneum. In these sites the finer Kirschner wire, which has its own telescopic introducer and stirrup attachment, may be preferred.

TECHNIQUES OF INTERNAL FIXATION

Having decided that internal fixation is required, the surgeon must then decide when the operation should be performed and which technique should be used. In general, surgery need not be delayed if the patient's general condition is satisfactory unless there is gross local swelling or local infection. Superficial skin abrasions and blisters are likely to become more infected with time and indicate early, rather then delayed, surgery.

Early stabilisation of long bone fractures is particularly important in patients with high injury severity scores in order to reduce pulmonary complications. There is evidence that intramedullary fixation does cause marrow substance to embolise to the lungs but the precise clinical significance of this finding is not yet clear. There appears to be no doubt that early stabilization of the skeleton is beneficial in patients with

multiple and severe injuries. Delaying surgery for up to 2 weeks has no adverse effect on subsequent fracture healing and it has even been suggested that healing may be enhanced by this period of delay in single fractures though the evidence for this is not definite.

Choice of technique
Ideally internal fixation should not only hold the fracture reduced, but it should be strong enough to support the fracture and allow early mobilization of the part and of the patient without need of additional splintage. The methods available include Kirschner wire transfixation (suitable for fractures of small bones or for small intra-articular fragments) screws and bolts (suitable for larger fragments as in comminuted fractures of the tibial plateau) metal plates and screws, with or without compression and intramedullary nails and rods which are useful for long bone fixation and for fractures of the neck of the femur. Most of these techniques are illustrated in the subsequent sections on individual fractures. Figure 6.40 illustrates some of these devices.

Note on screw fixation
Various types of screws are available for different purposes and it is important that the surgeon should understand the principles of their use. There are two basic types — self-tapping and those which require the hole to be pre-tapped. A self-tapping screw has a point designed to cut its own thread in bone. The bone is pre-drilled with a drill which is smaller than the diameter of the screw so that the thread of the screw will engage in the bone. Thus a standard screw of 4 mm diameter requires a 3 mm drill. A self-tapping screw should be long enough to allow the point to emerge from the distal bone surface, otherwise bone may grow into the cutting grooves of the point and make subsequent removal difficult. A non-self-tapping screw requires that the bone be pre-drilled and then pre-threaded with a tapping cutter. It is claimed that this latter method gives better fixation but in practice both types are satisfactory. Cortical bone screws have a shallow thread and cancellous bone screws a deeper thread and it is obviously essential that the correct tap be used for each.

When joining 2 pieces of bone together by means of screws, it is essential to overdrill the proximal fragment with a drill wider than the thread of the screw so that the 2 fragments can be impacted together (Fig. 6.41). If the screw thread engages in each fragment, tightening the screw cannot approximate them.

Compression fixation
Compression has been shown to promote bone healing in arthrodesis of the knee, (p. 134) and it is suggested

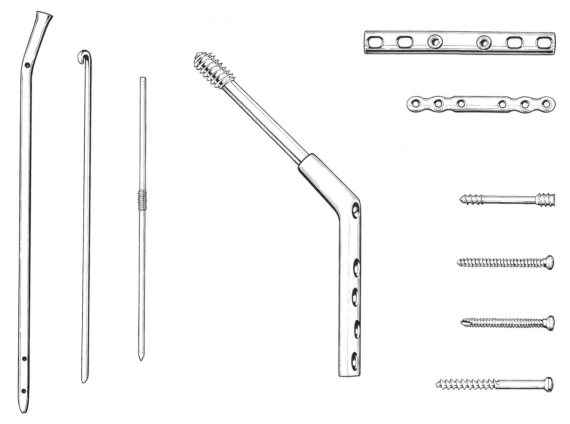

Fig. 6.40 Various internal fixation devices referred to in text. From *left* to *right*: locking intramedullary nail, Rush pin, Denham pin, compression hip screw. From *top* to *bottom*: compression plate (oval holes), standard plate, Herbert screw, cortical screw, cortical self tapping screw, cancellous screw

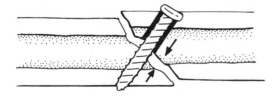

Fig. 6.41 Screw fixation of a cortical bone fracture (see text)

that it is of value in the management of fractures also. Whether this is due to any effect on the biology of fracture healing, or simply to secure fixation and close coaptation which results from compression, is a matter of debate. An accurately reduced, compressed fracture will heal with minimal external callus but it has the disadvantage that bone being so firmly splinted becomes locally osteoporotic from lack of stress so that refracture may occur following the removal of the fixation device. Nevertheless, compression techniques are acquiring increasing popularity. Two methods of compression plating are illustrated in Figure 6.42.

Illustrative examples of internal fixation of fractures

Intra-articular osteochondral fractures

These fractures may occur in the elbow, where they usually involve the capitellum or the radial head, and in the knee, where the lateral condyle of the femur or the undersurface of the patella are the common sites, usually complicating dislocation of the patella. They can be overlooked on X-ray, because the bone component may be a small inconspicuous flake while the larger cartilage component is, of course, invisible on X-ray. If neglected, they form loose bodies in the joint and the residual crater in the joint surface may lead to later osteoarthritis. Operative treatment is therefore necessary. The joint is opened at the site of injury, the loose fragment, if small, is removed and, if large, restored and fixed by Smillie's pins, Herbert screws or Kirschner wires, which are driven through the fragment into the subadjacent bone the head of the pin being buried below the cartilage surface (Fig. 6.43).

Fractures of the lateral condyle of the humerus, even in children, usually fail to unite and, unless internally

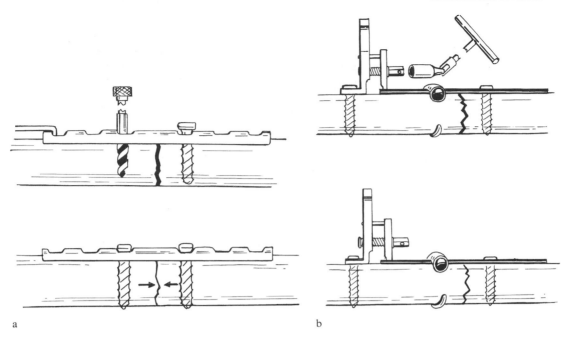

a   b

Fig. 6.42a & b Two techniques of compression plating. a. Uses a self-compression plate with oval slots for the screws. The first two screws are inserted in the end of the slot away from the fracture. As the sloping shoulder of the screw is tightened against the plate, the fracture is compressed. b. A conventional plate with round screw holes is attached to one side of the fracture with a single screw. The tensioning device is then fixed to the bone as shown and tightened to apply the desired pressure at the fracture site. The remaining screws are then inserted and the tensioning device is removed

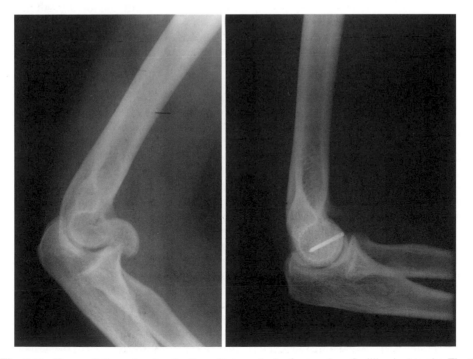

Fig. 6.43 X-way of elbow showing fixation of intra-articular fracture by a Smillie pin (see also Fig. 6.22)

fixed by means of a screw or Kirschner wire, cubitus valgus will develop and tardy ulnar palsy is likely to ensue. When using Kirschner wires to fix small fragments or small bones it helps to insert them with a power drill, rather than with the hand introducer, for the force required by the latter may displace the fragments.

Olecranon fractures

In fractures of the olecranon, the proximal fragment is pulled away by the action of triceps and healing by bone will not occur. Fibrous union may suffice for an elderly person but, if strong extension power is to be restored, internal fixation is necessary.

Through a curved lateral incision, the fracture site is exposed, the proximal fragment is drawn proximally with a bone hook and the fracture surfaces curetted of loose fragments or blood clot. The fracture is then accurately reduced and held by 2 towel clips. The bone fragments are stabilized by means of an oblique screw. The screw must be directed obliquely to engage the opposite cortex of the ulna (Fig. 6.44).

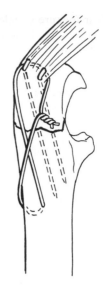

Fig. 6.45   Tension band wiring of olecranon fracture

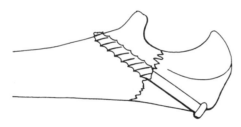

Fig. 6.44   Screw fixation of olecranon fracture

An alternative method, known as tension band wiring is illustrated in Figure 6.45. Having reduced the fracture, the surgeon inserts 2 Kirschner wires across the fracture site and bends the projecting ends over to prevent their migration down the shaft. A small hole is then drilled transversely through the posterior cortex of the ulna about 2 cm distal to the fracture site. A wire is passed through the hole and round the projecting Kirschner wires in a figure-of-eight fashion and tightened with tension. Early mobilization is encouraged for elbow movement increases the compression across the fracture.

Fractures of the radial head

Severely comminuted fractures of the radial head should be excised. The posterolateral approach minimizes risk of injury to the posterior interosseous nerve. An incision is made from the tip of the lateral epicondyle, in the direction of the subcutaneous border of the ulna, about 4 cm from the tip of the olecranon. The interval between the anconeus muscle and the common

extensor origin is identified and developed. Deep to this lies the capsule of the elbow joint. On opening the capsule, the radial head is readily visualised and can be removed. Displacement of the upper radial epiphyses occurs in children. If manipulative reduction fails the upper end of the radius is exposed and the displaced head of the bone is pressed into position. The radial head should never be removed during the growing period for this will result in relative overgrowth of the ulna with disorganization of the inferior radio-ulnar joint. Less severe fractures of the radial head can be treated conservatively, although loose displaced marginal fragments may be excised, or if large, internally fixed by small screws.

Fractures of the radius and ulna

These fractures are difficult to manage conservatively because of the opposing muscle forces, which act on the radius at different levels. In adults, internal fixation is usually required, for near perfect reduction must he achieved if forearm rotation is to be maintained. The bones are approached separately, otherwise cross union may occur. The fractures are then manipulated into reduction with bone forceps and stabilized by six-hole plates and screws. Compression plating may give sufficient stability to allow external fixation to be dispensed with. In other circumstances a full arm plaster should be used for at least 5 weeks.

Fracture of the ulna with dislocation of the radial head (Monteggia fracture)

This fracture has a bad reputation because of the common complication of persistent dislocation of the head of the radius. The key to management lies in perfect reduction of the ulnar fracture coupled with repair or reconstruction of the annular ligament of the radial head, if this remains unstable. Postoperative fixation in plaster is required for five weeks.

Plaster fixation for forearm fractures. It is sometimes stated that in order to obtain or maintain reduction of forearm fractures, it may be necessary to immobilize the forearm in full supination or pronation. These extreme positions are dangerous, for, if the arm should stiffen in either of these positions, severe functional disability will result. Forearm plasters should therefore always immobilize the arm in a mid-position of rotation where subsequent stiffening will be less of a handicap. If extreme positions of rotation are necessary in order to maintain reduction of any fracture, then internal fixation is undoubtedly a preferable method of treatment.

Fractures of the upper end of the femur

Fractures of the upper end of the femur occur most commonly in elderly women, usually as a result of a relatively minor injury, such as a simple stumble. Most are pathological fractures, the common underlying abnormality being osteoporosis but sometimes with a component of osteomalacia. A high proportion of the affected patients have associated illnesses which add to their infirmity and complicate the management of their fracture.

Less frequently these fractures occur in younger individuals, usually as a result of considerable violence.

These fractures may be classified as *transcervical* (intracapsular) or *trochanteric* (extracapsular). With intracapsular fractures many of the nutrient vessels which run proximally to the head from the base of the neck are disrupted leaving only a small variable contribution from the artery of the ligamentum teres. As a result, delayed healing of this fracture is common and avascular necrosis of the femoral head a frequent complication. Fractures of the trochanteric region, on the other hand, maintain a good blood supply on both sides of the fracture line and healing is rarely a problem.

Transcervical fractures may be further classified according to Garden's classification: (I) incomplete fracture, in this the inferior cortex remains intact while the superior cortex is impacted; (II) complete fracture without displacement; (III) complete fracture with partial displacement; (IV) complete fracture with full displacement. The prognosis worsens and the complication rate increases through stages I to IV and this classification therefore is a useful guide to management and treatment.

Transcervical fractures

There is no satisfactory conservative treatment for these injuries. Garden grade I fractures may sometimes heal spontaneously but a proportion of them come unstuck in the first 2 or 3 weeks and it is therefore prudent to internally fix them all. As transcervical fractures occur generally in the elderly and debilitated in whom the consequences of prolonged bed rest and immobilization are most damaging, surgical treatment, which will allow early mobilization, is almost routinely performed. The timing of operation is important. Many of these patients arrive in hospital dehydrated and hypothermic, having been lying helpless on the floor for some hours before being discovered. Others may have cardiac failure, respiratory infection, recent stroke, etc. and a day or two spent in assessing the patient thoroughly and in treating any remediable disorder, is time well spent. The mortality in this group of patients is high but can be reduced by careful preoperative preparation.

Choice of operation. Two types of procedure are available:

1. internal fixation with an intramedullary device, and
2. excision of the head of femur with prosthetic replacement.

The high failure rate of internal fixation in displaced subcapital fractures both in terms of union and in the complication of avascular necrosis, has popularised prosthetic replacement, but this also has its range of complications: the acetabulum may fail to stand up to the unyielding pressure of a metallic femoral head and infection and dislocation may occur in this elderly and unfit group of patients. In general, internal fixation is preferred for younger and fitter patients and for fractures in the Garden grades I and II. A replacement may be preferred for the elderly (over 80 years) and unfit and for grades III and IV, particularly in those patients with severe osteoporosis in whom the bone is too weak to support internal fixation devices.

Internal fixation. Many techniques of internal fixation are described, which is a sure indication that none is entirely satisfactory. A single Smith Peterson pin is usually inadequate and some form of multiple fixation is preferable (Fig. 6.46). No form of fixation will, however, succeed unless an accurate reduction of the fracture is obtained.

To achieve reduction of an intracapsular fracture the patient is anaesthetized and placed on an orthopaedic table. The affected limb is put on gentle traction and slight internal rotation. Anteroposterior and lateral X-rays are taken and the position assessed. If reduction has not been achieved, adjustment of the position of the leg can be simply made using the controls of the orthopaedic table. Forceful manipulative reduction of these fractures can be harmful by further jeopardising the blood supply.

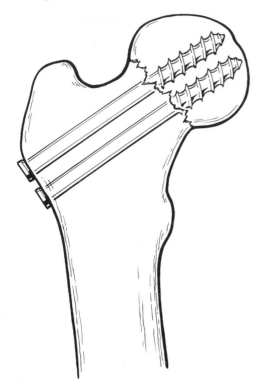

Fig. 6.46 Fixation of fractured neck of femur. Two flanged nails or one nail and a cannulated screw, as shown, give better fixation than a single device

In a small percentage of cases in which a satisfactory reduction is not achieved by such simple manoeuvres, open reduction may be required.

With the patient on the orthopaedic table and the fracture reduced, X-ray tubes or the image intensifier are positioned to allow AP and lateral projections of the hip. A straight lateral incision is made over the upper end of the femur from the tip of the greater trochanter distally some 6–10 cm depending on the obesity of the patient. The tensor fasciae latae and the fascia lata itself are split in the line of the skin incision, the vastus lateralis muscle is split longitudinally or reflected forwards from its origin and the lateral aspect of the shaft of the femur is thus exposed. Two or three guidewires are inserted into the femoral neck from the lateral aspect of the femur across the fracture site and into the head of the femur under X-ray control. The wires should be separated sufficiently to allow the internal fixation devices to be inserted and should diverge slightly. The placing of the guidewires becomes easier with increasing experience. When the cortical bone is hard, pre-drilling of the lateral cortex with a 4 mm drill simplifies the insertion of the guidewire and any subsequent adjustments that may be necessary. Two or three cannulated screws of a length carefully measured

from the guidewires to give maximal fixation in the head are then driven into position, checking at frequent intervals during their insertion that the guidewire is not advancing with the screw as may sometimes happen if the screw becomes slightly off line. When the screws (or alternative fixation devices) have been inserted, the guidewires are removed and the wound closed. Rapid mobilization is allowed and the patient encouraged to walk with assistance within 48 hours.

Femoral head replacement. If this procedure is selected, either the anterolateral or posterior approaches (pp. 122 & 123) may be used according to the preference of the surgeon. The posterior approach gives better access to the femoral shaft in stocky, obese patients. The joint capsule is opened, the femoral head removed and the neck of femur trimmed, if required, with bone cutters or reciprocating saw, to present a flat, smooth surface angled to match the flange of the prosthesis and allowing slight anteversion. It is of paramount importance that the prosthesis selected should match as closely as possible the size of the original head, otherwise high points of pressure will develop within the acetabulum, which will lead to early acetabular erosion. The correct size is measured by means of graded templates. The femoral shaft is then reamed using a notched broach corresponding to the stem of the prosthesis. No force should be used for it is easy to penetrate the shaft in these elderly patients with fragile bones. If difficulty in passing the broach is experienced the usual cause is inadequate removal of the superior cortex of the neck. With the Moore's prosthesis, particularly, it is necessary to excise the superior cortex of the stump of the neck as far as the face of the trochanter. The prosthesis is then inserted into the shaft of the femur and gently reduced into the acetabulum. Excessive force on the shaft of the femur during this manoeuvre may cause it to fracture. Tissue forceps are first placed on the cut margins of the capsule so that it can be held out of the way and, using the appropriate plastic punch, pressure is placed on the prosthetic head in the direction of the acetabulum, while gentle traction is maintained by the assistant on the femur. The femur is rotated to follow the head into the acetabulum rather than being used as a lever to rotate it in. The Moore's prosthesis (Fig. 6.47) is used without cement; the Thomson prosthesis — like a bipolar prosthesis (which articulates at a prosthetic interface as well as with the acetabulum) — may be used with or without cement. If it is to be cemented, a preliminary trial reduction should be carried out to ensure the correctness of the fit. With the posterior approach particularly, dislocation may occur in the early postoperative period if the hip is allowed to flex acutely as when sitting in a low chair or on a low toilet seat and this is therefore to be avoided for the first few days. Walking, however, is per-

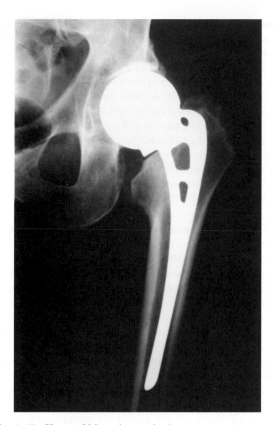

Fig. 6.47 X-ray of Moore's prosthesis

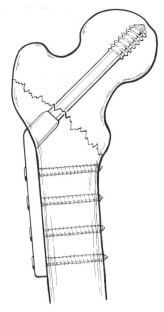

Fig. 6.48 Method of fixation of a trochanteric fracture

fectly safe and should be encouraged when the patient's condition allows.

Hip replacement. Hip replacement (see page 125) may be used in fitter elderly patients rather than hemi or bipolar arthroplasty.

Trochanteric fractures

Although these fractures have a good blood supply and healing is rarely a problem, stabilization can present technical difficulties, particularly if there is much comminution involving the medial cortex. Reduction is carried out on the orthopaedic table and usually presents no problems. If there is any difficulty, it is easy to expose the fracture site and obtain reduction under direct vision. The approach is similar to that for internal fixation of the removal neck fractures but requires to be extended distally down the shaft of the femur for 15 cm or more according to the length of plate selected. The most commonly used fixation device consists of a compression screw inserted into the femoral neck attached to a plate which is screwed to the shaft of the femur (Fig. 6.48). Protected weight bearing may be started early but full weight-bearing is avoided in the unstable fractures for at least six weeks.

Complications of fractures of the upper end of the femur

Avascular necrosis. Some degree of avascular necrosis develops in all displaced fractures of the femoral neck. In about 30% of those who survive long enough, the necrosis is sufficiently extensive to allow segmental collapse of the femoral head to take place. This complication does not always give rise to distressing symptoms or require treatment but, for those patients who have persistent and severe pain and progressive disability, total replacement arthroplasty of the hip joint is the appropriate solution.

Non-union. A certain percentage of displaced fractures of the femoral neck will not unite even with what appears to be adequate internal fixation. In this event the pins may cut out of the head and the fracture displaces once more. If the acetabulum remains healthy, a femoral head replacement is appropriate. If a penetrating nail has damaged the acetabulum, a total hip replacement arthroplasty is preferred. If non-union occurs in a young patient without gross displacement, a subtrochanteric osteotomy may allow healing to take place.

Penetration of the acetabulum by a fixation device. With both intracapsular and extracapsular fractures, settling at the fracture site may result in the fixation device penetrating through the femoral head into the acetabulum. This complication can be reduced if the nail is 0.5 to 1 cm short of the joint surface at the initial fixation or by using a sliding nail. If penetration occurs while the fracture remains ununited, the fixation device should be left in situ unless pain is severe. When the fracture has united, the fixation device can then be removed.

Subtrochanteric femoral fractures

Transverse fractures occurring just below the lesser trochanter are particularly characteristic of Paget's disease and osteomalacia but may occur in normal bone when subjected to sufficient trauma. The proximal fragment tends to flex, abduct and externally rotate due to the unopposed action of iliopsoas and the hip abductors. Conservative management is consequently difficult. Internal fixation with pin and plate or with a locking intramedullary nail is therefore usually indicated. The plate must be long enough to allow at least 6 screws to be attached to the distal fragment and if there is much comminution or if the bone is pathologically soft, it is wise to support the limb on Hamilton Russell traction (see Fig. 6.17) for the first few weeks.

Femoral shaft fractures

With fractures of the shaft of the femur 'closed' intramedullary nailing is normally used although the surgeon also has the option of conservative treatment for example using skeletal or skin traction with the limb supported on a Thomas splint. This option is only used when facilities for adequate intramedullary nailing are not available. Internal fixation may be achieved by intramedullary nailing or occasionally by plating, though this latter technique is in fact seldom used. Locked intramedullary fixation may be achieved with minimal or no exposure of the fracture site and will control rotational forces even if there is a lot of comminution of the fracture.

In femoral shaft fractures in adults intramedullary fixation with a locking nail is now the most widely adopted procedure.

Intramedullary nailing of femoral shaft fractures. Before embarking on intramedullary fixation of any bone the surgeon must ensure that he has available all the instruments necessary for insertion *and the removal* of a nail in the event of the nail becoming jammed. It is useful also to know the length of the nail required by taking an X-ray of the intact opposite limb bone with a measuring rod taped on the skin surface at the same level as the bone. Closed locked intramedullary nailing can be done successfully in practised hands, but requires an orthopaedic table which allows intraoperative skeletal traction with patient in the lateral position, image intensification and extensive instrumentation including flexible power drive cannulated reamers. Any surgeon embarking on this procedure should read a full description beforehand.

Open intramedullary nailing of the femur is still practised in centres that do not have facilities for 'closed' nailing. The patient is placed on his side with the fractured leg uppermost. The fracture site is then exposed through a posterolateral approach (p. 124) and the bone ends immobilized and cleared of loose fragments. The proximal fragment is then reamed retrogradely from the fractured surface using a hand or power driven reamer, starting with the smallest that will comfortably fit and increasing up to 14 or 15 mm for an adult. The reamers should be advanced to penetrate through the greater trochanter. The distal fragment is reamed to the same diameter, care being taken not to penetrate the knee joint. The nail is selected of the same diameter as the largest reamer used and of a length which will reach to the level of the upper pole of the patella and proximally to emerge 2 cm above the greater trochanter.

The nail is then inserted into the proximal fragment and driven proximally until it can be felt to reach the subcutaneous tissues of the buttock; this is facilitated by flexing and adducting the hip joint. The nail is exposed in the buttock through a small stab wound and is withdrawn until the end reaches the level of the fracture. The fracture is then reduced and stabilized by a bone clamp while the nail is driven distally until only 2 cm are left emerging above the greater trochanter (Fig. 6.49). If the nail is allowed to project further from the bone it causes discomfort and damage to the gluteal muscles, while burying the nail too deeply will make its removal difficult if this should subsequently become necessary.

Force should never be used when driving a nail, for a jammed nail can be very difficult to extract. If the nail is not passing easily it should be withdrawn and replaced with one 1 mm narrower. A check X-ray should be taken before wound closure to confirm the correct length and location of the nail. While the fracture site is still exposed the stability of the fracture should be tested, particularly with regard to rotation. If rotational stability is not secured, the limb should be supported on Hamilton Russell traction for a few weeks, otherwise early mobilization and weight-bearing is allowed.

Supracondylar fractures of the femur may be managed conservatively but can prove troublesome because of the tendency of the distal fragment to flex due to the pull of the gastrocnemius. Internal fixation is consequently often preferred and the condylar blade plate (illustrated in Figure 6.50) or a locking nail may be suitable.

Closed locked femoral intramedullary nailing. The patient lies supine on a traction table and a Steinmann pin is placed transversely through the femoral condyles. Traction is applied to the leg and reduction of the fracture is achieved using an image intensifier. A 10 cm incision is made proximal to the tip of the greater trochanter which is exposed and broached at its tip at the mid-anteroposterior point, and on the inner side of the trochanter. The proximal femoral canal is reamed with hand reamers and a guide wire is passed down the femoral canal and across the fracture site. The femoral canal is then reamed using power reamers and the

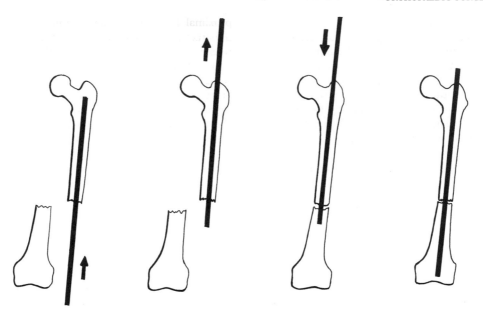

Fig. 6.49   Open method of insertion of intramedullary nail

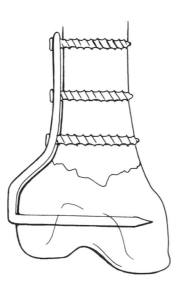

Fig. 6.50   Supracondylar fracture of femur stabilized by a condylar blade plate

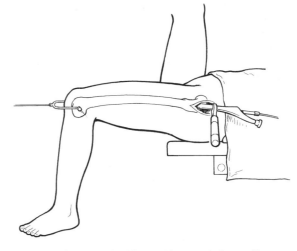

Fig. 6.51   Closed locked femoral intramedullary nailing

reamer's guide wire is changed for a nail guide wire. An approximately sized nail is inserted down the medullary canal over the nail guide wire thus stabilising the fracture. A jig attached to the proximal end of the nail (Fig. 6.51) allows a locking screw to be passed through the femur and the nail at the proximal end, and further locking screws are passed through the femur and nail at the distal end using an image intensifier based technique. The locked nail controls length as well as rotation at the fracture site.

Fractures of the patella
A similar principle may be used in transverse fractures of the patella (Fig. 6.52), but comminuted displaced fractures of the patella must be excised (p. 133).

Tibial fractures
Fractures of the tibial plateau. These are common injuries particularly among pedestrians struck by a car and in elderly patients who sustain a valgus strain to the knee. The fractures are often associated with ligamentous injury and both knees may be involved. Treatment depends on the severity of the injury and on the age and activity of the patient.

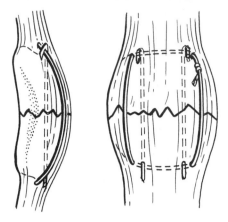

Fig. 6.52   Tension band wiring of patella

Ideally, as with all fractures involving the joint surface, perfect reduction should be the objective but severe comminution makes this difficult to achieve and in the old and inactive surprisingly good results can be obtained by a conservative routine of early mobilization. In younger patients in whom degenerative arthritis has more opportunity to develop, an attempt should be made to restore the joint surface and stabilize major fragments. Depressed segments of articular surface should be elevated to their normal situation and supported there by packing bone graft beneath. Major fragments are secured with cancellous screws or a reconstruction plate (Fig. 6.53). Major ligamentous injuries should be repaired at the same operation.

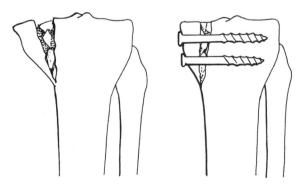

Fig. 6.53   Fixation of fracture of tibial plateau with cancellous screws

Tibial shaft fractures. More controversy surrounds the management of these fractures than any other and large series of successful results are reported by advocates of both the conservative and the surgical schools. Clearly both can work and the arguments outlined on page 147 should guide the decision. Improved plaster techniques allowing early knee movement (Sarmiento, 1981) have overcome many of the criticisms of plaster fixation although there is still some concern that midfoot stiffness is a problem after plaster or brace treatment.

If internal fixation is used there is a choice as with most long bones between plate and screws, and locked intramedullary nailing. The latter enjoys increasing popularity and can be done as a closed procedure with considerable facility, although it still requires modifications to the operating table and a range of specialized instruments. Closed intramedullary nailing has a smaller theoretical risk of infection than tibial plating because of the relatively small and distant surgical approach and is associated with relatively few complications in skilled hands.

The *technique of closed intramedullary nailing* of the tibia requires that the patient is placed on a traction table with the knee held at about 90° and traction is applied to the leg through a calcaneal pin. Reduction of the tibial fracture usually occurs with traction alone and it is only occasionally necessary to undertake reduction manoeuvres. A transverse incision is made over the patellar tendon which is then split vertically allowing access to the tibia immediately above the insertion of the patellar tendon. The tibia is breached at this point and guide wires are passed down the medullary canal. The cavity is then reamed to the appropriate size and an intramedullary nail is driven down the medullary canal thus stabilising the fracture. Transverse screws may be passed through special holes at the proximal and distal ends of the intramedullary nail thus controlling length and rotation.

Plate or screw fixation has the disadvantage of requiring an open operation on a superficial bone with the possibility of skin breakdown and infection. This risk, however, can be largely avoided if the skin incision is curved over the anterior muscle compartment where any difficulties in closure or subsequent breakdown will expose muscle rather than fracture and skin graft, if required, will have a receptive bed.

The deep fascia is incised in the line of the skin incision and is reflected medially to the periosteum which is incised along the lateral surface of the tibia and mobilised to expose the fracture site. A 6-hole heavy duty plate is then applied to the lateral surface, preferably with compression by the technique illustrated on page 151. The lateral surface is chosen when possible because it avoids a subcutaneous situation but all aspects of the tibia are accessible to fixation if the circumstances of the fracture dictate. Plate fixation, unlike intramedullary nailing, is not secure enough to allow unprotected weight bearing for several weeks.

Ankle fractures

Ankle fractures are exceedingly common, second only in frequency to the Colles fracture of the wrist. They may involve the medial or lateral malleoli alone or together, and in severe displacements, the posterior margin of the tibial articular surface. These fractures may be associated with ligamentous disruption. In general an ankle injury becomes unstable only if 2 or more of the stabilising components are broken, i.e. a malleolus plus a major ligament or two malleoli, and by the same token stability may be restored even if one of these structures is left unrepaired.

Unstable ankle injuries should be treated routinely by internal fixation for perfect reduction is required, as in all weight-bearing joints, and this is difficult to maintain by plaster alone. Isolated displaced medial malleolar fractures require fixation otherwise non union is common because of the pull of the powerful deltoid ligament which holds the bone fragments apart. Isolated fractures of the lateral malleolus on the other hand without demonstrable joint instability under anaesthesia may be managed conservatively by a below knee walking plaster.

Medial malleolar fractures are treated by screw fixation as in Figure 6.54, or, if the fragment is too small, 2 Kirschner wires inserted from different angles may be used.

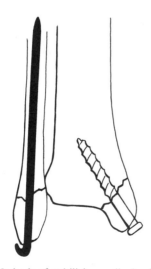

Fig. 6.54 Methods of stabilizing malleolar fractures

Lateral malleolar fractures may be fixed by screw or plate or intramedullary rod such as the Rush pin according to the fracture pattern.

Diastasis of the inferior tibiofibular joint should be stabilized by a transverse tibiofibular screw as shown in Figure 6.55 but it is important to remove this screw when the plaster is removed at 8 weeks for normal ankle motion requires a mobile inferior tibiofibular joint in order to accommodate to the variable width of the talar articular surface during flexion and extension.

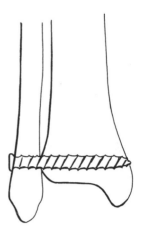

Fig. 6.55 Screw fixation of tibiofibular diastasis

Posterior marginal fragments of the tibial articular surface if small may be ignored but if large, i.e. representing more than a quarter of the tibial articular surface, they should be accurately reduced and internally fixed. The fragment is usually posterolateral and is therefore exposed through a vertical incision between the tendo-Achilles and the fibula. The flexor hallucis muscle obscures the fracture and is retracted proximally, the fracture surfaces are then cleared and accurate reduction is obtained under vision. Two cancellous screws are used to secure fixation.

Tibial plafond (complete distal end articular) fractures require complex reconstructive surgery using a plate and screws or external fixation and ligamentotaxis (traction across the joint).

Treatment of non-union
Non-union of a fracture is usually the result of infection, poor blood supply, inadequate fixation, soft tissue interposition or unrecognized bone pathology. Non-union is easy to recognize when the bone ends become sclerosed and a pseudo joint develops, but this may not occur for many months or even years and for practical purposes it is better to define non-union as failure of healing within a reasonable arbitrary period of 10 weeks for an upper limb fracture or 16 to 20 weeks for a lower limb fracture. It is recognized that some ununited fractures at this stage may be examples of delayed union which if immobilized for a further period might go on to spontaneous healing, but the distinction between delayed and non-union at this stage is impossible and in order to ensure healing with minimal further delay, all fractures at this stage which are unhealed should be considered for further treatment.

Non-unions of the femoral neck have been considered on page 155.

Other common sites of non-union are the tibial shaft, the humerus especially in obese elderly individuals, the forearm bones if the initial fixation was inadequate and the scaphoid, but no fracture is immune from this complication. Treatment consists of rectifying the causal factor and promoting union by the addition of cancellous bone graft or by adequate internal fixation such as intramedullary nailing which is known to stimulate a periosteal response and bone healing. Closed intramedullary fixation of the tibial or femoral non-union has the advantage that immediate weight bearing is allowed. It is not possible to describe the infinite variety of procedures which may be required but one treatment of tibial non-union will serve as an illustration.

The fracture site is exposed by the curved incision described on page 158. If infection is encountered, all dead and unhealthy tissue is excised, the wound irrigated with an antibiotic solution and methylmethacrylate beads containing Gentamicin are placed in the infected area and the wound closed. Once the organism has been identified systemic antibiotics are given and further surgery delayed for two weeks. By that stage the infection should be under control. The wound is opened, the antibiotic beads removed and cancellous strip grafts applied. Systemic antibiotics are continued until union occurs. If at the first operation no infection is encountered cancellous strip grafts (p. 160) are applied as a primary procedure without disturbing the fracture site if it is in good position and well stabilised by fibrous scar (Fig. 6.56). If the position requires ad-

justment or if the fracture is grossly unstable, internal fixation is used together with cancellous strip grafting. Unless the internal fixation is absolutely secure, external plaster fixation is also used until the fracture is healed, usually within 8 to 12 weeks. During this time weight-bearing is encouraged within the plaster.

Principles of bone grafting

Microscopic areas of bone death occur constantly throughout the skeleton as a result of minor trauma or focal vascular occlusion. These necrotic areas are continually repaired by a process of revascularisation, resorption of the dead bone and its replacement by new living bone which subsequently undergoes remodelling to restore the normal architecture of the part. In this way a constant process of skeletal renewal goes on throughout life. Larger areas of bone death resulting from more extensive vascular insult such as occurs in Perthes disease or as a result of fracture, is dealt with in the same way; although the larger the fragment the slower its eventual replacement. There is then a fundamental biological reaction to dead bone which attempts to replace it with living bone. This property is made use of in the operation of bone grafting. Bone taken from one situation and transplanted to another inevitably dies and is consequently replaced by living bone. By appropriately shaping and locating the graft it is possible for the surgeon to create new bone formation where he wishes. Thus cavities in bone may be induced to heal and defects in bone resulting from trauma or disease may be repaired. Bone may be used to bridge joints to create arthrodesis and in the case of ununited fracture, where the natural healing process has for some reason lost its impetus, bone may be conducted across the fracture site through the medium of the graft to restore bony union.

Although allografts of bone produce the same immunological reactions as the allografts of other tissues, this is of little consequence as all free grafts of bone, whether from the same individual or another, die and are treated in the same way. Thus allografts of bone, and bone which has been preserved by freezing or freeze drying, can be used surgically without regard to immunological reaction.

In bone grafting operations the following points are of importance: small grafts are more rapidly replaced than large and the least possible amount of bone should be used. Cancellous bone is more readily revascularised and offers less volume of bone to be resorbed than cortical and should be used unless there is some overriding mechanical requirement which demands cortical bone.

Bone grafts are at their weakest during the process of resorption and replacement by immature living bone and they must be supported by splintage until remodelling occurs.

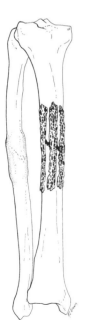
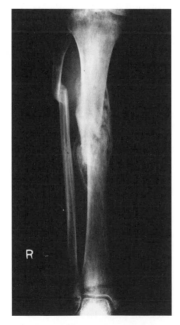

Fig. 6.56 Techniques of cancellous strip grafting for non-union

Cancellous strip grafting

This is a standard operation for an ununited fracture and may be used in conjunction with internal fixation. It is not used as frequently now that adequate intramedullary techniques have been introduced for treating tibial and femoral delayed unions. The iliac crest is used as the donor site. An incision is made parallel to and just below the crest extending from the anterior superior spine posteriorly as far as required. The lateral surface of the ilium is exposed subperiosteally, the crest with its attached muscles is detached with an osteotome and reflected medially, care being taken to leave the anterior superior spine undisturbed. The medial aspect of the ilium is exposed subperiosteally. Using a sharp chisel rather than an osteotome, thin slivers of cancellous bone are cut from the exposed margin of the ilium, 5 or 6 slivers, 6–10 cm in length being sufficient for most fractures. The detached crest is then carefully sutured back to the periosteum and muscles on the outer face of the ilium over a vacuum drain and the wound closed.

The fracture site is then exposed subperiosteally on all its aspects and the cancellous slivers are placed around it like barrel staves (see Fig. 6.56). Thin slivers long enough to reach healthy living bone on either side of the fracture site are ideal and will form a guide and stimulus to conduct the new bone across the fracture site. The scar tissue between the bone ends should be left undisturbed unless it is necessary to alter the position of the fracture for this confers some stability to the fracture site and does not act as a barrier to healing. If the position requires alteration, internal fixation should be used together with bone grafting.

It is important to obtain the graft before exposing the fracture site, otherwise unrecognized infection at the latter might contaminate the donor area.

REFERENCES

Charnley J 1979 Low friction arthroplasty of the hip, theory and practice. Springer Verlag, Berlin
Henry A K 1973 Extensile exposure, 2nd edn. Churchill Livingstone, Edinburgh
Salter R B 1961 Innominate osteotomy in the treatment of congenital dislocation and subluxation of the hip. Journal of Bone and joint Surgery 43B: 518
Sarmiento A, Latta C L 1981 Closed functional treatment of fractures. Springer Verlag, Berlin

FURTHER READING

Adams J C 1992 Standard orthopaedic operations, 4th edn. Churchill Livingstone, Edinburgh
Apley A G, Murphy W 1981 Where do we stand in the treatment of fractures? In: Hadfield J, Hobsley M (eds) Current surgical practice, vol 3. Arnold, London, ch 13
Barlow T G 1962 Early diagnosis and treatment of congenital dislocation of the hip. Journal of Bone and Joint Surgery 44B: 292
Burrows H J, Wilson J N, Scales J T 1975 Excision of tumours of humerus and femur with restoration by internal prostheses. Journal of Bone and Joint Surgery 57B: 148
Crenshaw A H (ed) Campbell's operative orthopaedics, 7th edn. C V Mosby Co, St Louis
Freeman M A R 1981 Reconstructive surgery in arthritis. In: Hadfield J, Hobsley M (eds) Current surgical practice, Vol 3. Arnold, London, ch. 14
Hooper G 1984 A colour atlas of common operations on the foot. Wolfe Medical Publications Ltd, London
Hooper G 1985 A colour atlas of minor operations of the hand. Wolfe Medical Publications Ltd, London
Hoppenfeld S, de Boer P 1984 Surgical exposures in orthopaedics — the anatomic approach. J B Lippincott Co, London
Hughes S P F 1983 Second generation joint replacements. British Journal of Hospital Medicine 30: 234
Muller M E, Allgower M, Schneider R, Willenegger H 1979 Manual of internal fixation, 2nd edn. Springer Verlag, Berlin
Rockwood C A, Green D P (eds) 1984 Fractures in adults, 2nd edn. J B Lippincott Co, London
Sweetnam R 1983 Limb preservation in the treatment of bone tumours. Annals of the Royal College of Surgeons of England 65: 3

7

Soft tissue injury

J. CHRISTIE

Tissue devitalization contamination and infection
Whenever a wound is inflicted, some devitalization of tissue (cellular damage) is inevitable. When the wound is made with a sharp knife the damage is comparatively slight and interferes little with healing. The majority of accidental wounds, however, are inflicted by contact with some blunt or ragged object, or by crushing, and in these wounds tissue devitalization may be extensive. All wounds which are not made under the aseptic conditions of an operating theatre are potentially infected and most accidental open injuries, whether civilian or military, cause contaminated foreign material to enter the tissues. Organisms lie on the surface of the wound for a period of time and multiply in that situation. During this period of 12 or 24 hours there will be no local evidence of infection and there is unlikely to be any constitutional disturbance that might suggest sepsis. A certain number of wounds however will develop evidence of infection after this period if left untreated. Organisms will flourish locally, enter the lymphatics and the characteristic signs of local inflammation will appear along with signs of a general systemic disturbance.

Many variables determine whether wound infection supervenes. It is well known for instance that organisms can be cultured from the surface of some 25% of apparently clean surgical wounds, but that this contamination is not inevitably followed by infection. Infection is more likely to supervene when there is devitalized or injured tissue present, when foreign material is left behind or when highly virulent organisms are involved. The resistance of the patient is also critical and it is known that in conditions of immunodeficiency, or when there is vascular disease or diabetes present, infection is more likely to occur. The wound should be treated as soon as practicable, as delay also leads to an increasing incidence of infection.

TYPES OF WOUNDS

Wounds caused by sharp instruments
Frequently sharp instruments, knives, cut glass, or ragged pieces of metal, will cause an incised wound with comparatively little tissue destruction. It must be remembered though that this kind of wound may penetrate deeply causing sharp injury to important structures, making careful and critical examination essential. By and large however there does not tend to be the kind of massive tissue destruction that is caused by blunt injury.

Wounds caused by blunt force
Many wounds are caused by bludgeoning force so that the skin and underlying tissues are opened, usually by shearing stress, and tearing injury may occur as a result of the considerable violence involved. As a general rule, the amount of tissue damage that occurs relates to the degree of violence involved. When this type of blunt wound has occurred, shearing and devitalization of the skin, as well as of underlying fat and muscle, should be suspected and treatment should take account of this. Table 7.1 shows energy levels in open fractures from different mechanisms (Chapman quoted by Gustilo, 1982) and gives an idea of the severity of violence that is to be expected.

Table 7.1

	Joules
Fall from a pavement	135
Skiing injury	400–700
High-velocity gunshot wound	3000
Bumper injury at 20 mph	135 000

Gunshot wounds

Shotgun injuries
Injuries caused by a shotgun vary very much in their severity. For the first few feet after discharge from the barrel of a shotgun the pellets will travel in a 'shot-cloud' and are closely followed by the wadding. A patient struck by the discharge at this close range will sustain severe penetrating injury at the point of impact and the pellets will spread rapidly through the soft tissue causing widespread damage. The wadding will also

enter the wound but usually remains fairly discrete within the soft tissues.

After shotgun injury it is usually fruitless to attempt to remove more than a small proportion of the retained pellets. It is however of great importance to remove the wadding if this has been injected into the wound, as the material from which it is made is usually irritating; also the central entrance wound should be laid widely open.

Low velocity gunshot wounds
Many pistols and rifles discharge bullets which have a relatively low velocity (< 360 m (1200 feet) per second). Unless these are soft nosed or hollow bullets which break up and cause widespread injury, relatively little damage may occur within the tissues, though of course major and vital structures can be injured. A low velocity bullet passing through the soft tissues will tend to leave a track which is not surrounded by much tissue necrosis. There may be small entrance and exit wounds though a larger exit wound may occur if the bullet breaks up. The bullet is sometimes retained within the tissues.

The form of surgical treatment required will depend upon whether major structures have been damaged. In general, though, a low velocity injury through soft tissue, with small entrance and exit wounds, does not need to be laid open unless some underlying vital structure is involved. The entrance and exit wounds should be adequately débrided and cleaned with iodine, and it is wise for the patient to be given an antibiotic. Removal of a retained bullet is not essential.

High velocity gunshot wounds
High velocity missiles, with a speed of greater than 900 m (3000 feet) per second, may cause considerable tissue destruction. The higher velocity bullet carries a great deal of kinetic energy which may be imparted into the tissues. Furthermore the faster bullet tends to wobble as it passes through soft tissue and resistance to its passage is increased; thus a greater proportion of its kinetic energy is transferred causing increased damage.

As the bullet passes through flesh, a phenomenon occurs (first reported by Woodruff in 1898) known as *cavitation*. The tissues are accelerated away from the bullet during its passage, and a momentary cavity forms filled with water vapour, immediately behind the travelling missile (Fig. 7.1). The tissues become stretched and sheared from their blood supply. The cavity, if deep, will close rapidly but not before air and debris have been sucked in through the bullet track. Tissues sheared from their blood supply become necrotic for up to several centimetres around the bullet track. These bullet tracks must be laid open and excision of necrotic tissue undertaken.

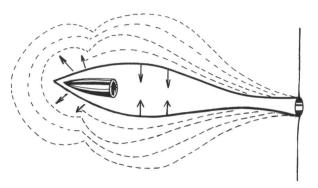

Fig. 7.1 Illustrating the passage of a high velocity missile through soft tissue

Usually a high velocity bullet causes a small entrance wound and when it passes through flesh over a large distance, it may cause a relatively small exit wound, but cavitation will have occurred within the tissues. When the bullet passes through a relatively short track, as through a limb, the site of exit may coincide with the site of maximum energy transfer, causing a large exit wound.

A large exit wound also occurs when the bullet shatters bone, and multiple fragments exit along with the metal.

Lawnmower injuries
Injuries caused by lawnmowers are becoming relatively common in most Western communities. The blades usually revolve in a circular fashion on a vertical axis and cause fairly extensive injury, commonly of the feet. There are a number of virulent bacteria particularly Gram negative organisms, which may be injected into the tissues, so that these wounds are probably best left open primarily.

Injuries caused by teeth
Injuries caused by biting (particularly human tooth wounds) are also rife with relatively aggressive organisms. Here again it is wise to leave the wound open in the first instance, secondary suture being carried out later.

TREATMENT OF WOUNDS

The primary and most important aspect of the treatment of all recent accidental civilian and war wounds is careful and expert surgery. Appreciation of the severity and extent of tissue damage is critical, and the surgical procedure must always take account of this.

Surgical wound excision is the treatment of choice for all significant wounds in both civilian and military practice, whenever practicable.

Surgical débridement is a procedure originally described during the Napoleonic wars, and is not so formal nor so extensive as excision of the wound.

It cannot be stressed enough that wound excision is the single most important step in preventing wound infection. The operation is exacting and consists of careful excision of the wound edges, fat, fascia and underlying muscle to the furthest depth and cavity of the wound.

Débridement on the other hand refers to the excision, in a looser way, of necrotic and unhealthy looking tissue. There are situations in which débridement is more appropriate than wound excision, particularly after a lengthy period of time has elapsed between wounding and surgery, for the treatment of wounds of the face, or in the management of wound infection.

The retention of dead tissue or inanimate foreign material within the wound poses the greatest single threat to uncomplicated healing. Wound excision will undoubtedly remove a relatively small number of healthy cells but its primary intent is to remove dead or inanimate matter, also abraded and potentially infected surfaces. Only viable and healthy tissue should be left behind except in exceptional circumstances.

Many high energy shearing, or bullet wounds, will leave dead tissue behind, and it is important to appreciate the potential consequences of injury; only a high index of suspicion will frequently allow the surgeon to make an adequate exploration and excision of all the injured areas.

Antibiotics are now established as having an important role to play (Gustilo, 1982) in the prevention of wound infection. By and large they should be given in high doses intravenously, as soon as possible after injury, and should be continued over the period of surgery. High doses of intravenous cephalosporins in particular have been shown to diminish the risk of infection following injury. These should be started almost as soon as the patient is admitted and should be continued for at least 3 days.

Wound excision

This is a carefully planned operation designed to remove all devitalized and contaminated tissues which might predispose to the development and spread of infection. It involves therefore, the excision, not only of the skin edges, but of all tissues lining the wound cavity. Primary excision is the treatment of choice in all significant recent wounds whether military or civilian. It is important to remember that shearing injuries may have caused devitalization of skin and underlying muscle which will require adequate exposure and excision. High velocity bomb or bullet wounds should also be laid open, and the dead and necrotic tissue underneath carefully excised.

The operation should be attempted only if it can be performed during the first 18 hours or so after injury. Beyond that time it is probably wiser to revert to the less extensive procedure of wound débridement. After 12 hours or so considerable judgement may be required in deciding which of the two operations is most appropriate.

Operation

Except after hand injury where a bloodless field is particularly desirable, the use of a tourniquet is not usually advised. The tourniquet tends to obscure potential bleeding points and makes the recognition of devitalised tissue somewhat difficult; theoretically also it may reduce the resistance of the part to infection.

Skin preparation is carried out over a wide area around the wound. Soap and water is the best agent for preliminary cleansing, and is usually effective in removing ingrained dirt and grease; subsequently an iodine preparation or Cetavlon wash may be used with advantage. Care should be taken to prevent washings from the surrounding skin entering into the wound by light gauze packing if necessary. After cleansing, the skin is dried with spirit and is prepared with one of the commonly used antiseptics.

The edges of the wound are now excised with a sharp knife (Fig. 7.2). Where the skin is only lightly injured it

Figs 7.2–7.5 *Stages in the operation of primary wound excision*

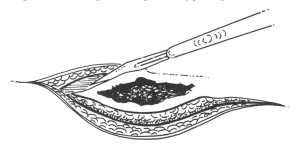

Fig. 7.2 Excision of the skin edges

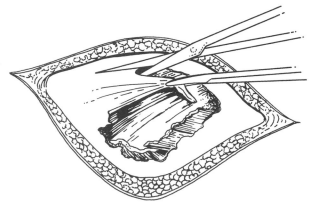

Fig. 7.3 Excision of wound in deep fascia

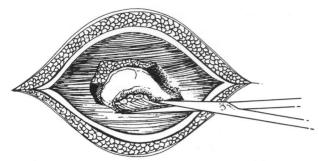

Fig. 7.4   Removal of the devitalized muscle

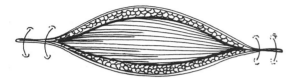

Fig. 7.5   Wound partially sutured

is adequate to excise a strip some 2 mm or 3 mm wide. Where there is more extensive abrasion and injury a wider margin of skin must be removed. Once the skin has been excised subcutaneous tissues are similarly carefully excised with the knife. The skin wound is enlarged, should this prove to be necessary, by further incisions which should usually be made in the long axis of a limb. Deep fascia is excised in a similar way, and muscle is trimmed back also using a knife or scissors. Devitalized muscle tissue carries the greatest danger of infection, and the colour, contractile response and the bleeding capacity of the muscle will determine how much should be excised. Bruised and ischaemic muscle fibres are usually darker than normal, do not contract when cut, and do not bleed. All devitalized fibres are excised with scissors. Successive snips are made in a direction away from the damaged area until healthy fibres are encountered; these are recognized by brisk response to the stimulus of cutting, and by oozing of blood from the cut ends. When wide retraction of severed muscles has occurred, it may be necessary to enlarge the wounds considerably through skin and deep fascia in order to obtain access to all damaged tissues. Foreign bodies are removed along with small detached fragments of bone. Bone fragments with a periosteal or muscular attachment should be left behind. Larger bone fragments that contribute to stability should only be retained if they have a blood supply. The treatment of arterial or nerve injuries has been discussed in Chapters 3 and 8. Careful arrest of haemorrhage is most important. Bleeding points are clipped as they appear, and are ligatured with fine sutures, or are coagulated with diathermy. On completion of the excision the wound should have only viable tissues left behind.

During the procedure, the tissues should be copiously washed with saline, and should be handled delicately.

Wound débridement (surgical toilet)

This operation consists of the removal of foreign bodies and debris from the wound, together with the excision of any devitalized skin tags and of obviously necrotic tissue. Many surgeons use the term débridement to describe the operation undertaken primarily after injury. It should be stressed that wound excision is nearly always to be preferred in the early period after injury and that the simpler removal of foreign material and debris from the wound, along with excision of devitalized tissue is a procedure that is appropriate when significant time has elapsed before the patient can be taken to surgery, or in special circumstances such as wounding of the face. The preparation of the skin around the wound is similar to that described for wound excision, and the operation is different only in that formal excision of the wound edges is not undertaken. The more obviously abraded or injured tissues are removed along with foreign material and dirt. Healthy tissues are not disturbed.

Wound closure

After wound excision or débridement has been carried out, the surgeon has to decide whether the wound should be completely sutured, partially sutured or left widely open and packed with gauze. The decision is one which requires considerable judgement. It is frequently tempting to suture the wound throughout its length in an attempt to obtain healing by first intention. Successful primary healing is pleasing to the patient and surgeon alike, but the risk of infection is always greater after primary wound closure. Infection may be disastrous particularly when there is an underlying fracture; therefore wounds overlying open fractures should be left open.

Extensive wounds of any kind after severe violence, particularly when there is impregnation of foreign material with extensive tissue necrosis, should also be left open after wound excision has been completed. Similarly wounds that are more than 18 hours old and that have been dealt with by débridement should also be left open, as should high velocity bullet injuries whose track has been laid wide open in order to excise necrotic tissue. Experience in the Second World war, in the Korean war and Vietnam conflicts, has again established that many wounds are best treated open after appropriate excision (Dudley, 1973).

After the first 4 or 5 days of being left open, wounds develop a remarkable resistance to infection and many may be closed relatively safely. It is also striking that wounds left open and allowed to discharge freely ab initio rarely become infected.

Primary suture

Many cleanly incised wounds may be closed by primary suture after excision. It is unwise however to close a wound that has been untreated for about 18 hours since injury. When a wound is closed by primary suture there should be no large underlying cavity and the tissues within the wound should be entirely healthy. When there is a large cavity which cannot be obliterated it is usually wiser to leave the wound open, or to use a system of closed irrigation for some days. Interrupted nonabsorbable sutures may be used to close a cleanly incised wound.

No wound should be closed under tension. Tension is liable to occur whenever there is significant swelling after injury, particularly after crushing injury of a limb or when there is an underlying fracture. When a medium suture breaks before drawing the wound edges together, skin tension is likely to be too great to allow safe closure. In these circumstances the wound is best left open. It is also wise to leave wounds caused by lawnmowers, or by human or animal bites, open for a period of days before formal secondary suture and it is worth repeating that wounds overlying open fractures should be left open.

Partial primary suture

The centre of the wound may, on occasion, be left open. This is safer than wholly closing the wound and allows many extensive injuries, also those that have had to be extended in order to gain adequate access, to be closed up to the point that skin tension develops. The central part of the wound or indeed one of its ends may be left open, and is usually covered by a light gauze dressing. Alternatively a small drain may be left in the depths of the wound. This is a wise precaution when a cavity remains in the wound, as it will prevent the retention of blood, serum or other exudate. It is rare that a wound which is allowed adequate drainage in this way becomes infected. Retention of infected exudate and bacterial toxins are the most potent factors allowing further spread of infection.

Gauze packing

Gauze packing of an open wound may be necessary when there has been heavy contamination or much devitalization of tissue. It is also necessary when, due to tissue loss, a large cavity is left behind. Usually only light packing is used so as to hold the wound open. Tullegras, or Sofratulle gauze is laid on the tissues and the packing is laid into the dressing. It is important that the cavity is only lightly packed and that free drainage is allowed from the wound. When a wound is packed open, secondary suture or some plastic procedure such as skin grafting, may be required at a later date.

Delayed primary suture

Delayed primary suture is the optimum treatment for a wound which has been left open and packed with gauze in the first instance. This is not always possible and some wounds, particularly those with skin loss, may require skin grafting procedures, rotation or free vascularised flaps.

Delayed primary suture is usually undertaken some 5 days after the original procedure. The wound should be free from infection on clinical inspection and culture, and the surfaces of the wound should be clean. When there is a copious discharge present or obvious dead tissue and slough, the procedure should be delayed.

The technique is similar to that described for primary suture. When there is a large cavity and dead space cannot be obliterated, it is wiser not to close the entire wound but to allow drainage from the area of the cavity. Alternatively the wound may be closed over the cavity but irrigation should be used. The wound should only be closed secondarily if tension can be avoided.

Immobilization

All severe soft tissue wounds should be immobilized after initial treatment. Rest encourages healing by preventing movement and muscle spasm. Immobilization is particularly useful when it is necessary to transport the patient after initial treatment, and will considerably diminish mortality. Immobilization is best achieved by a splint which includes the joints above and below the wound in a suitable position of function.

When an open fracture is present, other forms of immobilization such as an external or internal fixation, or formal traction within a splint may be more appropriate if other facilities are not available.

When a plaster cast is used, certain rules should be stringently observed:

1. When considerable swelling of the limb is anticipated the plaster cast should be split throughout its length. If the cast is not split initially, the surgeon should ensure that there will be regular observation of the limb during the period in which the swelling may be anticipated, and the cast should be split whenever there is the remotest suspicion of ischaemia.

2. Encircling dressings, bandages or wool are liable to become saturated with hardened and dried blood, and thus become rigid. When a plaster cast is split, the underlying dressings must also be divided so that skin is visible throughout the length of the split. The plaster must be split from end to end.

3. A window may be cut in the plaster so that regular inspection can be carried out. It is important that the plaster window is retained and that, after inspection of the wound is completed, the plaster window is replaced

and held in place with firm compression bandaging, otherwise oedema will occur locally.

4. A wound which has been left completely open, and packed with gauze, may safely be enclosed in plaster without a window (closed plaster method). The wound is usually exposed after 5 days in these circumstances so that secondary suture may be undertaken or whatever other procedure appears to be appropriate. Winnet Orr used the closed plaster technique extensively during the First World War when faced with massive evacuations of injured troops. Their wounds were treated by early excision, left open and a closed plaster was applied. This treatment met with considerable success but his technique has been superseded by better stabilisation of open fractures and plastic surgery with early split skin grafting, rotation, transposition or free vascularised flaps from abdomen (rectus), iliac crest, chest wall (latissimus dorsi) — see Figure 1.47 — or forearm.

TREATMENT OF INFECTED WOUNDS

65% to 70% of accidental wounds yield potentially pathogenic organisms when cultures are taken on admission to hospital (Patzakis, 1974). The vast majority of these wounds will not develop infection if appropriately treated. Those wounds that are not associated with severe tissue destruction, flap elevation or avulsion, and which have only a minimal to moderate crushing component, should be associated with an infection rate of less than 2%. More severe injuries with extensive damage to the soft tissues, including muscle, skin and neurovascular structures particularly when accompanied by fracture, will probably have an infection rate of anywhere between 10% and 40%.

Wound infection does not usually appear for 2 or 3 days after injury. Initially when there is cellulitis, and bacteriological cultures reveal a pyogenic organism, strict rest and the administration of high dose antibiotic therapy are appropriate. A certain number of these wounds will not however respond rapidly to this treatment, and other wounds will present late with already established infection.

The management of established infection requires considerable judgement. When it is clear that there is pus present within the wound, early surgical débridement is advisable. Surgery is also indicated when it is suspected that necrotic tissue or slough is retained within the wound, or when there is retained foreign material or debris, though again considerable judgement is required and a vain search should not be made for shotgun pellets, pieces of shrapnel or multiple fragments that are widely dispersed in the tissues. By and large, however, there is an increasing tendency towards early exploration and drainage of the wound and radi-

cal débridement of necrotic tissues, particularly when there is established infection after a compound fracture. In these circumstances bone is treated rather like soft tissue and necrotic or grossly infected bone tends to be excised leaving only healthy tissue behind.

It should be emphasized that the decision to proceed to early radical débridement of an infected wound should be carefully thought out, should not be undertaken overhastily, and is not usually appropriate during the early phase of cellulitis. When there is a fracture present wound débridement is generally more pressing so as to prevent intractable osteomyelitis; in general, simple soft tissue infection tends to be more benign in its behaviour when there is no underlying fracture and there is less urgency in proceeding to early débridement.

When early débridement of a wound is undertaken, the tissues should be packed open and free drainage allowed to occur. The wound is left undisturbed for 24 hours before being inspected and subsequently having regular dressing procedures.

As soon as appropriate cultures and sensitivities have been reported, high dose antibiotic therapy is commenced. The wound should be immobilized, and the patient observes a regime of strict rest. When there is an underlying fracture, it is usually stabilized with a plaster cast or with an external fixation device.

Following débridement of the infected wound, treatment will depend upon the subsequent course of the infection. Usually wound discharge will rapidly diminish as will the surrounding oedema and inflammation. Normally the wound will look clean and relatively uninfected after some 5 days and secondary suture may be contemplated at that time. The wound may however retain slough or necrotic material and this may require excision. It may prove impossible to close the skin and in these circumstances split skin grafting may be necessary after healthy granulation tissue has developed. It is sometimes appropriate to close the wound over irrigation when there is a large cavity and dead space cannot be obliterated. Irrigation should not be used for more than 3 to 5 days.

Débridement of an infected wound
This is the procedure used when it is judged that an established infection will be most appropriately managed by surgical intervention. The wound is opened up usually throughout its length. When there are sinuses present it may not be necessary to open up the entire wound, but the sinus tracks should be exposed, and the sinuses entirely excised including surrounding scar tissue if practicable. Fresher wounds are opened throughout their length and are explored to their depths. Pus is gently swabbed out and any loculi or cavities are opened. Necrotic tissue is identified and is excised with scissors until the wound edges appear

to be healthy. The wound should not be swabbed too vigorously or considerable bleeding will occur. When bone is involved necrotic or infected looking bone is usually excised. The wound is then packed widely open.

Secondary suture

This may be carried out as soon as the infection has been overcome, but is only suitable in a certain number of patients. Appropriate antibiotic cover should be available. The skin edges should be healthy and there should be early ingrowth of epithelium. There should be no residual adherent slough and no infected crevices within the wound. Granulation tissue should look healthy, firm and reddish in colour. Residual discharge should be minimal and nonpurulent.

Techniques

Skin flaps are mobilized by under cutting, with or without excision of the wound margins, and are approximated over the granulating area with interrupted sutures. Tension must be avoided and it is always better to leave part of the wound open than to force it closed with tight stitches. When secondary closure is possible, a drain should be left in the wound to allow any further discharge to escape freely.

Closed irrigation

This is used when an infected wound is closed over dead space, or when considerable bleeding is anticipated. Two tubular surgical drains are placed in the wound through adjacent skin. Saline, or saline containing antibiotics, is run into the wound through a drip giving set and through one of the tubular drains. As the wound is closed the other drain will start to drain first blood and then irrigation fluid. If this does not occur a syringe may be used to suck the irrigation out through the drain. Subsequently this drain is connected to a collecting bag. It is important to run the irrigation through briskly so that blood clots do not occur as these will block the irrigation system. As the effluent irrigation becomes clear the rate of irrigation system may be reduced. Usually this kind of closed irrigation system is retained for no longer than 5 days.

Secondary haemorrhage

Secondary haemorrhage usually occurs as the result of wound sepsis. A small premonitory haemorrhage may occur and suggests that the patient should be kept under careful observation. A significant increase in bleeding requires that the wound is gently opened and the bleeding vessel, normally an artery, is sought and tied off. If no single large vessel can be identified gauze packing may be used alone, and is removed some 3 to 4 days later in the operating theatre.

Severe haemorrhage which threatens to exsanguinate the patient and which cannot be controlled by gauze packing must be treated by proximal ligation. Very occasionally it is necessary to ligature the main vessel of the limb, but this should be undertaken only in exceptional circumstances as it will involve the risk of distal gangrene, especially so in the lower limb. When the procedure is used in order to save life the risk is sometimes justified.

OPERATIVE TREATMENT IN GAS GANGRENE

Prophylaxis

The anaerobic organisms producing gas gangrene infection are saprophytes which flourish in devitalized or necrotic tissue, especially fleshy muscle. Early wound excision is therefore the best preventative measure. If this is contraindicated or is impracticable, débridement should be as thorough as possible. Antibiotics should also be used in high doses from the moment the patient is admitted to hospital, and should be continued intravenously for at least 3 days. It should be stressed however that when conditions are ripe for the development of gas gangrene in the wound, antibiotics will not prevent this dangerous disorder. When there is considered to be a serious risk of gas gangrene, the wound should always be left widely open. Injudicious primary suture of a contaminated wound may well be a determining factor in the development of the disease. A wound which is left open and packed rarely becomes infected. Other factors which predispose to the condition include delay in adequate primary treatment, also any interference with the blood supply to the part, e.g. injury to the main vessel of the limb, tourniquets, tight plasters and compartment syndromes.

Hitchcock has shown that frank necrosis of tissue or muscle is not necessary for gas gangrene to develop. It is sufficient that relative local hypoxia occurs in order that the clostridial spores may be converted to vegetative forms with rapid multiplication.

Gas gangrene is seen most commonly after trauma, and almost half of the patients who present will have an open wound. Some 30% of the patients however will develop gas gangrene after routine surgical operations and a small proportion will have primary gas gangrene without open injury to the skin (Hitchcock, 1982).

Operative diagnosis

Early diagnosis is a matter of life and death, and no hesitation should be felt in exploring the wound at the first suspicion of anaerobic infection. Stitches are removed and the wound margins are retracted. In assessing the nature of the infection a distinction should be drawn between *true gas gangrene* (*Clostridium myositis*) and *anaerobic cellulitis*. True gangrene is essentially an infection of fleshy muscle; it involves previously healthy fibres, and spreads longitudinally within the sheaths, so that a muscle or group of muscles may be involved throughout its entire length. In anaerobic cellulitis the infection is confined to cellular connective tissue within the wound, and to muscle which is already necrotic from trauma or vascular damage. In both conditions collections of malodorous gas may be found in the depths of the wound, or raising blebs on the skin surface, and small areas of necrosis will be found throughout the tissues.

The wound, having been opened up, is enlarged if necessary to permit a thorough examination. A search is made for areas of discolouration, and for gas bubbles in the subcutaneous tissue and in the depths of the wound. Muscle sheaths are opened and the fibres are inspected. In the early stages of anaerobic infection the affected fibres are paler than normal, a lustreless pinkish grey shade being described; later they become deeply congested, slate blue or frankly gangrenous, and bubbles of gas may be seen between them.

Conservative operation

'In the established case of gas gangrene, bold surgery, blood transfusion, and Penicillin are essentials' (Stammers, 1948). The use of antitoxin is somewhat controversial and in a recent review Hitchcock does not believe that its administration affects the course of the disease. If antitoxin is to be given 200 000 units should be given together with a blood transfusion which is repeated as necessary.

The affected region is exposed by a long skin incision which is placed in the long axis of the limb, and has the wound at its centre. The sheaths of the affected muscles are opened up by longitudinal incision until healthy fibres are exposed. All fibres which show even a suspicion of infection are ruthlessly excised until healthy muscle, which bleeds and contracts on section, is revealed. Adjacent muscles are examined and, if

necessary, are treated in the same way. Owing to the longitudinal spread of the infection an entire muscle or group of muscles may require to be removed. Any discoloured areas of skin or fascia are excised too. The wound is dusted liberally with penicillin powder and is kept widely open by means of gauze packing. Penicillin therapy is continued in high dosage by intravenous administration.

In *anaerobic cellulitis* the infection is confined to cellular connective tissue within the wound, and to necrotic muscle fibres. Such tissues alone require to be removed. The excision is therefore much less radical than that required for true gas gangrene.

Hyperbaric oxygen therapy can be used as an adjunct to surgery and may assist to the extent that a more distal amputation can be undertaken when ablative surgery is required (Darke, 1977).

Amputation

The fact that gas gangrene tends to be confined to individual muscles or groups of muscle saves many limbs from amputation. Except when there is massive gangrene, the wound should always be explored before amputation is considered, in the hope that the infection can be eradicated by conservative operation. Indications for amputation are:

1. Massive gangrene, where the infection involves most of the muscles in the injured segment of the limb; here amputation is the only possible lifesaving measure
2. The coexistence of a compound fracture, and extensive disease
3. Serious impairment of blood supply as will occur when the main artery of the limb is damaged.

The amputation must be sufficiently high to allow all infected muscle to be removed but it need not necessarily be above the level of subcutaneous spread. The wound is left widely open and is packed with gauze.

REFERENCES

Darke S G, King A M, Slack W K 1977 Gas gangrene and related infection: classification, clinical features and aetiology, management and mortality. A report of 88 cases. British Journal of Surgery 64: 104–112

Dudley H A F 1973 Some aspects of modern battle surgery. Journal of the Royal College of Surgeons of Edinburgh 18: 67–75

Gustilo R B 1982 The management of open fractures and their complications. W B Saunders, New York

Hitchcock C R 1982 Gas gangrene in the injured extremity. In: Gustilo R B (ed) The management of open fractures and their complications. W B Saunders, New York, p 183

Patzakis M, Harvey J I P, lvler D 1974 The role of antibiotics in the management of open fractures. Journal of Bone and Joint Surgery 56A: 532

Stammers F A R 1948 War supplement. British Journal of Surgery 2: 274

FURTHER READING

Owen-Smith M S 1981. High velocity missile wounds. Arnold, London

8

Hand surgery: tendon and nerve repair

G. HOOPER

GENERAL CONSIDERATIONS

Anaesthesia

Adequate anaesthesia is essential for operations on the hand. The method of obtaining anaesthesia should be compatible with use of the tourniquet (see below).

General anaesthesia or a brachial plexus block are indicated for major and prolonged operations. Bier's block is very suitable for minor operations (such as carpal tunnel release, removal of a ganglion, or decompression of tendon sheaths) but the tourniquet becomes uncomfortable after a while and the technique is unsuitable for procedures lasting more than about 15 minutes.

Local anaesthetic infiltration is not recommended for routine use in hand surgery. Although anaesthesia may be adequate the local anatomy tends to be obscured by oedematous tissue. A digital nerve block is acceptable for operations on the distal part of the finger; 3–4 ml of 1% lignocaine *without adrenalin* is injected into the web spaces on either side of the finger around the dorsal and palmar digital nerves (Fig. 8.1). Subcutaneous infiltration of local anaesthetic in a tense ring around the base of the finger should be avoided as there is a small but real risk of causing mechanical embarrassment to the circulation.

Tourniquet

A tourniquet should be used whenever possible. A bloodless field is a great aid to precise identification and handling of tissue in the hand.

A finger tourniquet has a limited place, in operations on the distal part of the finger. The traditional type of finger tourniquet applied by clipping rubber tubing around the base of the finger is not recommended as the pressure exerted is very variable and it is not possible to exsanguinate the finger; a much more effective device is the finger of a rubber glove (Figs 8.2 & 8.3). If a finger tourniquet is used it should be applied after the digital nerve block has been inserted.

For most operations a pneumatic tourniquet is used. Before inflation the limb is emptied of blood by firstly elevating the arm and then applying a rubber bandage

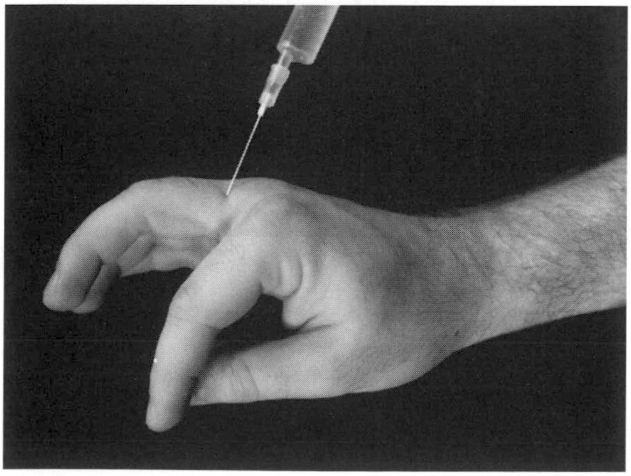

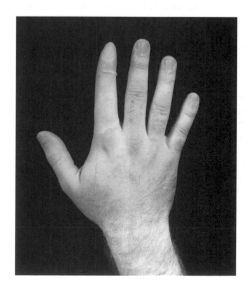

Fig. 8.2 Finger tourniquet. The finger of a rubber glove is placed over the digit

Fig. 8.1 Digital nerve block anaesthesia

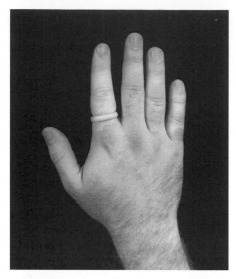

Fig. 8.3 Finger tourniquet. After cutting the end of the finger of the rubber glove it is rolled to the base of the finger

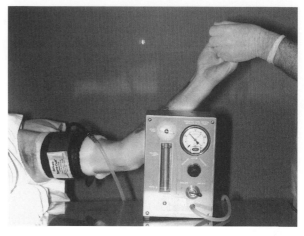

Fig. 8.5 Pneumatic tourniquet. The tourniquet is inflated and the rubber bandage removed

firmly from the fingertips to the upper arm (Figs 8.4 & 8.5). The limb should be kept elevated until the tourniquet is inflated. The inflation pressure is 50 mm of mercury above systolic pressure and it is essential that the pressure is checked regularly during the operation. The tourniquet may be left in place for up to 1½ hours in a fit young patient. Tourniquets should be checked and calibrated regularly during routine theatre maintenance and unreliable or suspect equipment taken out of service immediately. If these simple rules of use are not kept then problems will certainly arise.

The preliminary bandaging must be omitted if the hand is infected as there is a theoretical risk of promot-ing spread of infection proximally. In these circum-stances the arm is elevated for several minutes before the pneumatic tourniquet is inflated in the usual way.

Skin preparation

The hand is painted with an antiseptic such as Betadine, using two sponges in holders; one supports the hand while the other is used for painting (Fig. 8.6). When there is an open wound on the hand, skin preparation is slightly modified (p. 176).

Position of the hand

The hand should rest on a small table and the surgeon and any assistants should be seated comfortably. The forearms of the operator and assistant rest on the table; this aids precise handling of instruments and prevents

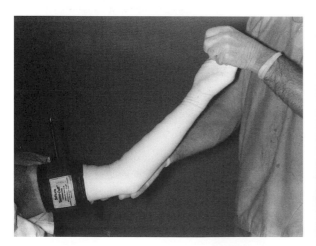

Fig. 8.4 Pneumatic tourniquet. After applying the tourniquet around the upper arm, the arm is exsanguinated by elevating it and wrapping a rubber bandage around it

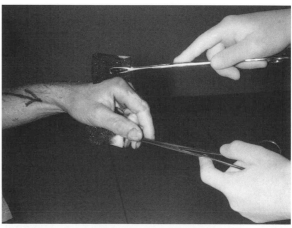

Fig. 8.6 Skin preparation. Note the use of two sponges in holders, one to support the hand and one to paint it

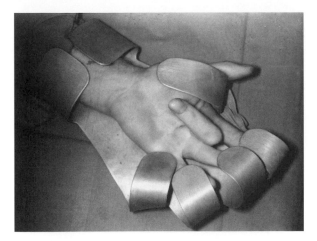

Fig. 8.7 A lead hand in use

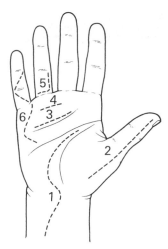

Fig. 8.9 Acceptable incisions on the palmar aspect of the hand:
1. An incision should not cross the wrist at right angles.
2. The 'mid-lateral' incision must lie dorsal to the ends of the flexor creases in the digits.
3. A transverse skin crease incision.
4. A transverse palmar incision.
5. Transverse incisions may be made in the flexor creases of the digits and may be extended by mid-lateral incisions.
6. The useful volar zig-zag incision. The apices of the skin flaps must lie at the end of the flexor skin creases

fatigue. A lead hand (Fig. 8.7) can be used to support the hand in position during the operation if so desired.

Elaborate and specialized instruments are rarely needed in hand surgery but the surgical instruments that are used (scissors, forceps, needle-holders, skin hooks and other retractors) should be of a size appropriate to the delicacy of the procedure and in excellent repair. Bipolar diathermy is preferred.

Magnification is a useful aid. For most purposes suitable magnification is provided by ×2 or ×3 loupes (Fig. 8.8). If higher magnification is needed the operating microscope is used.

Incisions

Incisions in the hand should be planned with care as wrongly placed incisions can damage important structures, or may contract on healing. To avoid scar contractures incisions in the hand should not cross skin creases at a right angle and should be placed to avoid the crease if possible.

Short incisions in a finger should be placed transversely and on the palmer surface they should, if possible, lie in a flexion crease. A longer exposure can be made through a 'mid-lateral' incision, well behind the digital vessels and nerves; unless the incision lies posterior to the ends of the flexor creases it is prone to migrate to the flexor aspect of the finger and heal with contraction. A volar zig-zag incision (Fig. 8.9) avoids this problem.

In the palm, transverse incisions in the flexion creases should be used whenever possible. Zig-zag incisions meeting the flexion creases at 45° are acceptable alternatives (Fig. 8.9). At the wrist, incisions should lie transversely or meet the flexor crease at 45° (Fig. 8.9). For wide exposure at the wrist a transverse incision can be extended by proximal and distal extensions at either end (Fig. 8.10).

In circumstances where a longitudinal incision has been made at right angles across a skin crease the incision can usually be broken up by Z-plasties (p. 15) to avoid scar contractures. Many surgeons favour this technique for dealing with Dupuytren's contracture in the hand (p. 203).

Position of immobilization

If it is necessary to immobilize the hand for any time

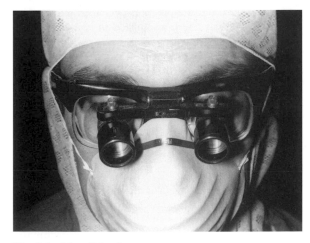

Fig. 8.8 Magnifying loupes

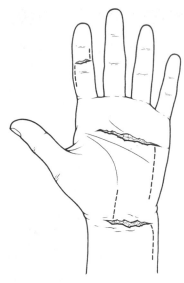

Fig. 8.10 Extending a transverse incision or traumatic wound. Incisions should never cross skin creases at right angles

after surgery or injury, care must be taken to avoid secondary contractures of the interphalangeal (IP) and metacarpophalangeal (MCP) joints. Anatomical studies have shown that the relevant capsular structures are at their maximum length when the IP joints are extended, the MCP joints are flexed to 90° and the thumb is fully abducted from the palm (Fig. 8.11). It is

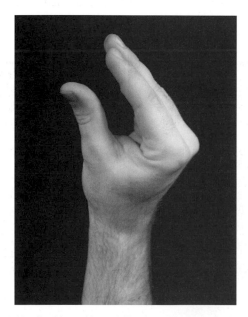

Fig. 8.11 Position of immobilization. The wrist is slightly dorsiflexed, the interphalangeal joints are extended and the metacarpophalangeal joints are flexed. The thumb lies parallel to the fingers

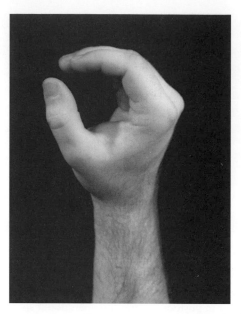

Fig. 8.12 Position of function. If the hand becomes stiff in this position it will still be of some functional use. For reasons discussed in the text, it is *not* the correct position for immobilization of the hand

necessary to hold the wrist in about 15° of dorsiflexion to maintain this position with comfort. This is the 'position of immobilization' and it differs from the so-called 'position of function' (Fig. 8.12). The 'position of function' is the posture in which a stiff hand will be of most functional use; the 'position of immobilization' is the position which will prevent or minimize stiffness.

The position of immobilization can be maintained by a correctly applied boxing glove dressing, reinforced with a plaster back slab to prevent flexion of the wrist (Fig. 8.13). If it is necessary to splint only part of the hand, for example a broken finger, the joints of the part should be placed in the position described above. The thumb must always be immobilized in abduction relative to the palm, to prevent a contracture of the first web space. A stiff thumb that lies in the plane of the palm is useless because it cannot be opposed to the fingers (Fig. 8.14).

It cannot be too strongly emphasized that one of the most common causes of hand dysfunction after surgery or injury, and one that is entirely preventable, is incorrect splintage.

Avoidance of swelling
Oedema is an inevitable accompaniment of trauma and infection but its devastating effects on the hand can be prevented by simple measures. Swelling is prevented, and treated, by elevating the hand and encouraging the patient to exercise it if the primary condition allows.

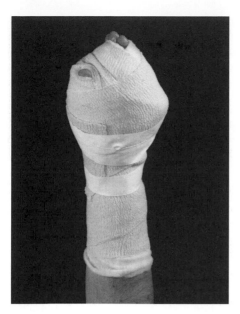

Fig. 8.13 A boxing glove dressing. This will hold the hand in the position of immobilization. A plaster back slab should be applied to keep the wrist dorsiflexed

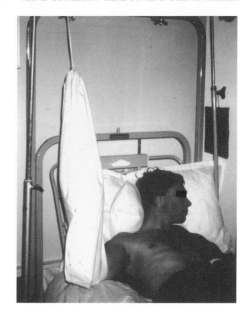

Fig. 8.15 Elevation of the hand

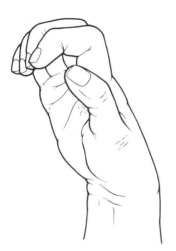

Fig. 8.14 A hand with multiple contractures. This type of crippling hand deformity is still, unfortunately, most often the result of failure to splint the hand in the correct position, to elevate the swollen hand or to supervise the rehabilitation of the patient

Swelling of any severity is an indication for admission to hospital — it cannot be controlled by outpatient supervision. The hand may be kept elevated in a roller towel (Fig. 8.15) or similar support. Elevation is routine after every operation on the hand, and must be maintained until the patient is able to demonstrate that he is able to walk about with the hand held up and exercise it (if it is not splinted). Broad arm slings encourage dependency of the hand and are never needed

after surgery or injury. The patient should be warned against their use.

When the hand is swollen the MCP joints tend to straighten, the IP joints to flex and the thumb to adduct — in other words the hand is held in the very position in which secondary joint contractures are most likely to occur (Fig. 8.16). It is therefore imperative that the swollen hand, in addition to being elevated, is splinted in the position of immobilization until the swelling is under control.

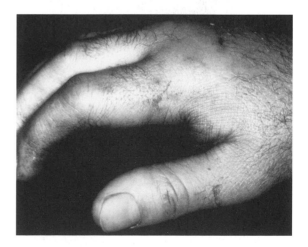

Fig. 8.16 When the hand is even slightly swollen it assumes an undesirable position. The metacarpophalangeal joints are extended, the interphalangeal joints are flexed and the thumb is adducted. Unless the swelling is reduced by elevation and the hand is splinted in the correct position (Fig. 8.11), secondary contractures will occur (Fig. 8.14)

Rehabilitation

The hand does not get better by itself after surgery or injury. All patients, and some more than others, need supervision and instruction in appropriate use of the hand. In most patients who have had minor operations this will consist of reassurance that no damage can be done by putting the hand through a full range of movements, and ensuring that exercises are being done regularly. At the other extreme a few patients will need prolonged inpatient and outpatient treatment by physiotherapy and occupational therapy to restore mobility and function after severe injury or extensive reconstructive surgery. This type of supervision is a vital part of the overall management of the patient undergoing hand surgery and must never be neglected.

WOUNDS OF THE HAND

It is the *initial* assessment and treatment of hand injuries which determines the final result. A trivial injury that is mismanaged can result in permanent disability — disability that might never have occurred had the patient not sought medical attention. It follows that:

1. New patients should be dealt with by a surgeon who has some training and experience in the management of hand injuries.
2. Full surgical technique (i.e. aseptic precautions in a properly equipped operating theatre) is essential in managing wounds.
3. Appropriate anaesthesia must be provided.
4. All except the most trivial wounds must be carefully explored so that all foreign matter may be removed and the full extent of the injury determined. A tourniquet is essential.
5. Primary closure of the skin and repair of other structures is carried out *only if conditions permit.*

Skin preparation

Dirt should be removed from the skin of the hand using an appropriate preparation; soap and water is usually suitable but a solvent may be needed for greasy dirt. Skin preparation is completed by painting around the wound with an antiseptic. It is most important that antiseptic solutions are not allowed to enter the wound as they may damage tissues in the hand. Instead the wound should be irrigated with normal saline solution.

Wound excision

All wounds are contaminated with bacteria to a varying degree. Bacterial proliferation will cause clinical infection which must be prevented by removing contaminated and dead tissue. Any ragged, devitalized or grossly contaminated skin edges are excised to leave the wound edges as healthy as possible. It is better to accept a slight deficiency of skin rather than leave doubtful skin that is almost certain to become infected. Subcutaneous fatty tissue which often prolapses through the skin on the palmar surface should also be excised.

The wound is thoroughly explored to ensure the removal of any foreign material and all devitalized tissue, and to identify possible damage to the deeper structures. If the wound must be enlarged any incision used for this purpose should conform with the principles given on page 173. Thorough irrigation using normal saline in a syringe will clear blood clot and superficial debris from the wound and allow more precise exploration.

Bleeding points should be coagulated with bipolar diathermy.

Wound closure

Primary suture is permissible if:

1. the wound is recent — not more than 4-6 hours old
2. contamination has been minimal
3. the skin edges can be brought together without tension.

If these conditions do not pertain *the skin should not be sutured.* There are three main options if a wound has not been primarily sutured:

1. Adequate closure can often be obtained by pressure of dressing alone, any parts which remain unclosed being allowed to heal by granulation. With such treatment healing of small wounds may be expected to occur without infection and with the formation of a supple scar, a result far superior to that obtained when primary suture has been followed by even a mild degree of sepsis.
2. A wound with skin loss may be left open and the hand splinted and elevated. After 2–3 days the wound is inspected in the operating theatre and the wound is closed by some form of skin grafting, or a decision is made to allow the wound to close by granulation. This form of management has relatively little place in the care of hand wounds and is definitely not indicated if tendons, bones and joints are exposed, when treatment should be as in (3) below.
3. The wound is covered by an appropriate form of skin graft at the time of the original excision.

The indications for these various methods are best illustrated by discussing the management of some common types of wound of the hand.

Linear cuts and lacerations

The wound should be carefully explored but excision of tissue is seldom needed. Recent wounds may be closed primarily.

Bursting injuries

These are the result of severe compression such as may occur when the hand is trapped in rollers. The skin may literally burst open, exposing tendons, bones and joints. Because of the swelling it is impossible, and in any case it is undesirable, to close the wound primarily. All dead and contaminated tissue is carefully removed. A few loose stitches may be necessary to secure a covering for exposed tendon and bone. The hand is splinted in the position of immobilization and elevated. Further inspection is carried out 48 hours later when the swelling will be much less. Wounds with edges lying in contact may be left to heal; gaping wounds or areas of skin loss should be closed by an appropriate skin grafting procedure.

Wounds with raised skin flaps

The displaced skin is thoroughly cleaned with saline; ragged edges and obviously devitalized parts are excised. The viability of the flap can be assessed by deflating the tourniquet cuff and examining the flap for return of colour and arterial bleeding. If the flap is considered viable it is secured in position with a few stitches without tension, and the hand is splinted and elevated. Firm dressings prevent the accumulation of blood under the flap. In practice it is seldom that such a flap is found to have an intact circulation and as a general rule the skin flap with a distal base is always suspect. It is advisable to remove doubtfully viable skin during the initial surgical procedure rather than take a chance and be presented with an area of necrotic skin and surrounding infection at a subsequent wound inspection. The gliding structures of the hand underlying such a flap may be irrevocably damaged.

If partial or complete excision of a flap has been decided upon the skin defect is dealt with as described in the next section.

Wounds with skin loss

All loss of skin in the hands and fingers should be made good by skin grafting as soon as practicable. This not only hastens healing, but by preventing infection it avoids fibrosis and contracture, and preserves the function of deep tissue that would otherwise be exposed.

Partial thickness grafts as a method of skin replacement in the hand are less satisfactory on the palmer than on the dorsal surface because the grafted skin is relatively easily traumatised. Full thickness grafts of some variety are generally indicated when there has been loss of skin from the palmar surface of the hand. Free full thickness grafts have good wearing characteristics, but have the disadvantage of lack of sensation and inability to take over exposed tendon and bone.

A skin flap is necessary to cover exposed tendon and bone. Such flaps should be planned and executed by a surgeon with special training in the techniques of plastic surgery; an ill-designed flap can create more problems than it solves. General guidance on the types of flap available are given on page 14. Suffice it to say here that, depending on the defect, it may be possible to use locally based pedicle grafts from the hand or it may be necessary to raise a flap from more distant sites such as the groin or deltopectoral areas. In some circumstances a free flap transfer with microvascular anastomosis may be required. Wherever the flap is obtained it is of the utmost importance that, in so far as is possible, swelling of the hand due to dependency is avoided and secondary stiffness due to joint contracture is prevented.

Occasionally the skin of an injured finger that must be amputated can be preserved with its blood supply intact and used to cover a defect in the hand.

One special type of injury associated with skin loss that should be mentioned is the *ring avulsion*. In this injury, fortunately uncommon, the patient's ring is accidentally torn from the finger, removing the skin as a sleeve of tissue. The injury often occurs when, in jumping from the back of a truck, the ring is caught on some projection on the tailboard. Tempting though it is to replace the skin on the finger this should not be done as the digital vessels are almost always either avulsed or thrombosed and death of the skin is inevitable. Immediate amputation is indicated unless circulation is definitely present in the skin or can be restored by microvascular reconstruction.

Wounds with division of nerves

These are dealt with below on pages 188–189 and specific features of injuries to the median, ulnar and radial nerves are described on pages 190–195. It need only be emphasised here that when there is a wound overlying a nerve it should be assumed that the nerve is damaged and the wound should be explored in circumstances that will allow primary repair if division is confirmed. Formal testing of motor and sensory function cannot be relied on in the recently injured patient.

Wounds with division of tendons

The techniques of tendon repair and management of specific tendon injuries in the hand are dealt with below (pages 181–185). Once again it must be emphasised that a wound overlying a tendon may be associated with damage to the tendon. Although formal testing of the action of the tendon may not be reliable in the acutely injured patient, much may be learned from noting the position of the digits relative to each other. If there is any doubt about the action of the tendons the wound must be explored in conditions that allow appropriate repair or reconstruction to be carried out.

Finger tip injuries

A *subungual haematoma* is usually caused by a crushing injury to the finger tip. A collection of blood forms under tension below the nail. The blood is easily evacuated by drilling the nail with an unwound paper clip that has been brought to red heat in a flame.

Traumatic amputations of the finger tip are common injuries. If soft tissue alone has been lost the wound will usually close rapidly if protected by dressings. If bone is exposed it should be trimmed back to allow primary closure of the skin, using local advancement flaps if necessary (p. 14). Finger length should not be conserved if the result is a tight tender scar adherent to bone. There is little place for partial or full thickness free grafts in finger tip injuries; the former lacks stability to hard use and the latter lacks sensation: the result of using either type of graft is often a finger that is overprotected by its owner.

Injuries involving the nail bed require careful repair with fine absorbable sutures if abnormal nail growth is to be avoided.

Bites

All wounds sustained from contact with teeth are potentially serious, because of the risk of infection. Except in countries where rabies is endemic, human bites are much more dangerous than dog bites because of the virulence of the organisms involved.

Bites of all descriptions, and any wound sustained from an adversary's teeth, should be treated with great respect. Exploration and excision should be particularly thorough and should be carried out with adequate anaesthesia. *It is safer if no stitches are inserted in the wound.* Often a tooth will penetrate a metacarpophalangeal joint when the fist is clenched; when the MCP joint is extended the puncture wound becomes sealed by the extensor hood. The patient may present some days after the incident with an early septic arthritis of the MCP joint. The joint should be explored, thoroughly irrigated with saline and the wound left open. The hand is immobilized in the optimum position. Pending identification of the bacteria involved a broad spectrum antibiotic is prescribed and should be combined with an antibiotic effective against anaerobic organisms. Careful supervision of the patient is essential if stiffness is to be avoided (see also page 174).

Foreign bodies in the hand

Unless the foreign body can be identified easily by palpation its removal is likely to be much more difficult than would appear. Many inert foreign bodies can be left in situ. If exploration is indicated it must be performed under adequate anaesthesia with tourniquet control. A radio-opaque body should be identified on radiographs taken in two planes immediately before operation. To assist in location a paper clip may be taped to the skin and after taking the radiograph a corresponding mark is made on the skin surface. If a needle or similar elongated object is being sought the incision should be made across the long axis, provided this does not conflict with the principles laid down on page 173.

Wooden foreign bodies may be contaminated, so the wound should not be stitched after their removal.

Splinter below the nail. As a rule, attempts have already been made to extract the splinter which has become broken off well below the nail bed. Under a local anaesthetic, a V-shaped portion of nail overlying the splinter is removed with scissors. This allows the splinter to be lifted out and provides drainage should infection supervene (Fig. 8.17).

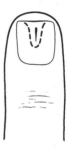

Fig. 8.17   Removal of a splinter below the nail

Injection injuries. Material may be injected under very high pressure from industrial grease guns and paint sprays. The usual history is that the nozzle blocked and then cleared suddenly as the user was testing it against his finger. The entry wound may be a quite innocent-looking puncture but the injected material has often penetrated for a considerable distance into the hand. If left, the extensive tissue damage becomes manifest over a few days and amputation is usually necessary. Treatment consists of early recognition of the severity of the injury and immediate exploration, which may be extensive. As much as possible of the injected material is removed, together with all obviously devitalized tissue and the incision is left open.

Traumatic amputation of the hand

Crushing or mangling injuries of the hand must be treated by adequate excision of dead and contaminated tissue according to the principles outlined already. All viable tissue must be conserved for use in any secondary reconstructive procedure, and skin loss should be made good as soon as possible.

Elective amputations are dealt with in Chapter 9.

Replantation

When part of the hand has been amputated by a clean cut without severe crushing, surgical replantation using microsurgical techniques may be feasible. The indications for replantation vary somewhat among surgeons, but the following are general guidelines:

- *Unsuitable*
    — patient with significant medical or psychological problems
    — heavily contaminated, crushed or improperly preserved parts
    — single fingers
    — amputations at or distal to the interphalangeal joint
- *Suitable*
    — thumb amputations
    — multiple amputations of fingers (not all parts are necessarily replanted)
    — transmetacarpal, transcarpal and distal forearm amputations

Preservation of parts. The amputated part is placed in a sterile polythene bag which is sealed and placed on ice. Ice, saline, antiseptics and preservatives should not be placed in the bag with the part. An occlusive dressing is placed on the stump and the patient and the part are transferred to a centre where microsurgical skills are available, and where a final decision can be made about the feasibility of replantation. Because of the limited amount of soft tissue in the hand, and especially in the fingers, replantation may be a possibility for up to 24 hours after injury.

Technique of replantation. Two surgical teams are initially needed, one to identify structures in the amputated part and the other to identify structures in the stump. Because of the length of the operation further surgical help may be needed during the procedure; replantation is a team effort, not a 'one-man show'.

The part is reattached by internal fixation of the bones, after first shortening them. Unless skeletal shortening is carried out the microvascular repair will be under tension and will surely fail. In the fingers the sequence of repair is:

1. Repair tendons.
2. Repair vessels under the microscope using 10/0 sutures; as a general rule at least two veins must be repaired for each artery. Vein grafts are often needed to reconstruct the vessels.
3. Finally the digital nerves are repaired.

Obviously this sequence may require some modification when amputations at other levels are dealt with.

After operation a close watch must be kept on the circulation, and reoperation to inspect the anastomoses may be necessary if there is suspicion of thrombosis. Reconstruction using vein grafts is usually needed if a segment of thrombosed vessel has to be removed.

FRACTURES IN THE HAND

Fractures of the metacarpal bones and phalanges are extremely common. Like all injuries in the hand, they can cause long term disability if mismanaged. Many fractures need little or no treatment beyond encouragement in normal use of the hand; overtreatment, in the form of unnecessary splints and plasters, must be avoided. Other fractures, particularly displaced fractures, those involving joint surfaces or those associated with soft tissue damage may require very careful attention.

The main factor governing management is the stability of the fracture. Stability can usually be gauged from the clinical and radiographic appearance of the injury. Some common patterns are:

Stable

Isolated fractures of the metacarpal bones, undisplaced fractures of the phalanges.

Unstable

Multiple fractures of the metacarpal bones, fractures of the base of the thumb metacarpal involving the trapezio-metacarpal joint (Bennett's fracture), transverse and oblique fractures of the phalanges with displacement, fractures involving the condyles of the phalanges.

Stable undisplaced fractures do not need to be immobilized. Active use of the hand is advised. Taping an injured finger to an adjacent one (Fig. 8.18) will often give the patient some confidence in using the hand.

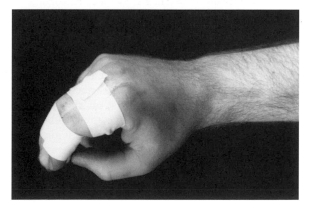

Fig. 8.18   Garter strapping for stable fractures of the phalanges. The interphalangeal joints must be left free. Some absorbent material should be placed between the fingers to prevent pressure sores over bony prominences

Unstable fractures must be reduced and held in position. If there are several fractures in the hand the whole hand should be splinted in the position of immobilization using a boxing glove dressing supported by a plaster slab. The hand must be elevated to control oedema. If there is only one fracture of a phalanx it can be splinted with a strip of metal covered with foam rubber (Fig. 8.19); uninjured digits are left free of splintage. The splint keeps the metacarpophalangeal joint flexed to a right angle and the interphalangeal joints straight. The surface marking of the MCP joint, and hence the position for placing the bend in the splint, is the distal palmar skin crease. Particular care should be taken to avoid rotational deformities in fractures of the proximal phalanges by ensuring that the palmar part of the splint points to the tuberosity of the scaphoid at the base of the thenar eminence.

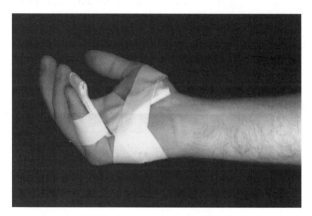

Fig. 8.19 Splintage for unstable fractures of the phalanges. Note that: 1. The splint is well covered with tape to prevent scratching from the edges of the metal. 2. The bend in the splint lies at the distal palmar skin crease. 3. The palmar part of the splint points to the tuberosity of the scaphoid, to prevent malrotation of the finger. 4. It is unnecessary for the splint to extend proximal to the wrist

Some fractures cannot be stabilised easily by external splintage and internal fixation should be considered for them. Common examples are Bennett's fracture, fractures involving the condyles of the proximal phalanges and multiple displaced fractures of the hand. Internal fixation should also be considered in displaced open fractures with significant soft tissue damage (see below).

Adequate internal fixation of most fractures can be obtained by the use of fine (0.035″ or 0.045″) Kirschner wires driven by a power drill. It is usually possible to reduce the fracture closed and then introduce the wire percutaneously (Figs 8.20 & 8.21). A check radiograph is then obtained. (It is not good practice to introduce the wire under image intensifier

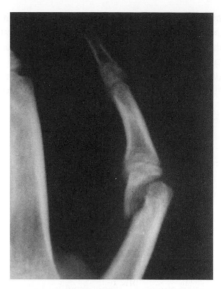

Fig. 8.20 X-ray of a typical unstable fracture. Fractures of the condyles of the proximal phalanges are often displaced, resulting in significant deformity of the finger

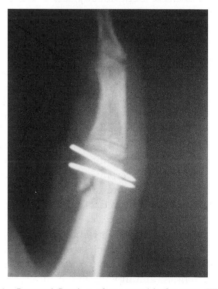

Fig. 8.21 Internal fixation of an unstable fracture. When the fracture has been reduced it is often possible to insert the Kirschner wires percutaneously on a power drill

screening as the surgeon's hands may be exposed to an unacceptable level of radiation over the course of several such procedures.) Open reduction is sometimes needed if the fracture cannot be reduced accurately. Wires can be cut short or left protruding through the skin according to choice. Protruding wires do not cause infection and the wire is of course easier to remove; however the exposed wire can injure adjacent fingers and may be inadvertently withdrawn if the end catches on some object such as clothing. Protruding wires may be removed from bone 3–4 weeks after fixation as the fracture is usually stable by this time. It should be mentioned that fractures of the phalanges remain visible for many weeks on radiographs, so that assessment of healing is made clinically, not radiographically.

Compound fractures

Open fractures of the fingers pose special problems, because the combination of a fracture and damage to the gliding tissues such as tendons can result in a stiff, largely useless digit which interferes with the function of the other fingers. This problem is likely to arise when either the proximal or intermediate phalanges have been broken, since the tendons pass over them. Loss of movement is not a problem in compound fractures of the terminal phalanges and treatment is directed towards obtaining a stable finger tip that will stand up to heavy work; since bone healing is seldom a problem, appropriate management of the wound is the priority.

In all open fractures careful débridement is necessary. Damage to soft tissue structures should be identified and a decision made about primary reconstruction. Associated damage to tendons, vessels or nerves is an indication for internal fixation with Kirschner wires to allow accurate repair of the soft tissues. Extensor tendons should be repaired with fine nonabsorbable mattress sutures. The results of primary repair of flexor tendons are not good when there is an open fracture at the same level. However, if primary repair is not done and a decision is taken to conserve the finger and carry out secondary flexor tendon grafting when the fracture has healed, the patient and surgeon are committed to a programme of management lasting several months with a very uncertain outcome. Primary amputation should be therefore considered when an open fracture of a single finger is associated with considerable damage to soft tissue. There is little point in 'saving' a finger if the result is a stiff, painful and useless part. This is particularly so in the case of the manual worker to whom an early return to work and settlement of any compensation claim are of great economic importance.

Multiple open fractures in the hand should be stabilized with multiple Kirschner wires for 3–4 weeks, until soft tissue healing allows mobilization of the hand. In this type of injury some degree of functional impairment is almost inevitable but it should be minimized by treatment. A minimum of Kirschner wire should be used, placed so that the hand can be brought into the position of immobilization. If at all possible the wires should avoid transfixing tendons.

Primary arthrodesis of an interphalangeal joint (p. 204) is indicated when an open intra-articular fracture is complicated by damage to tendons, but circulation and sensation in the finger are unimpaired. An arthrodesis of a metacarpophalangeal joint of a finger should never be done, as function of the other, normal, fingers may be impaired. Fusion of the MCP joint of the thumb is permissible.

TENDON INJURIES

Anatomy

A tendon is composed of longitudinal bundles of collagen fibres, loosely bound together. When it is cut or torn, the ends become frayed by separation of the collagen bundles, so that longitudinal sutures tend to cut out.

Where a tendon pulls round a curve or bend, it is enclosed within a synovial sheath which contains synovial fluid. Sheaths surround the extensor tendons where they pass beneath the extensor retinaculum on the dorsum of the wrist. The anatomy of the synovial sheath around the flexor tendons is described on page 198.

The flexor tendons are retained in position as the fingers flex by the fibrous flexor sheaths which extend from the level of the metacarpal joints to the intermediate phalanx. The sheaths are not continuous, otherwise the finger would not be able to flex. There are several complete annular pulleys lying between which are cruciate pulleys, which allow the flexor sheath to shorten considerably as the finger is flexed.

On the back of the hand the extensor tendons are covered with paratenon, which is a specialized form of loose fat containing elastic fibres.

General considerations

Tendon healing

When a tendon is severed in a synovial sheath, considerable retraction may occur to a distance equal to the amplitude of movement of the tendon. Its ends become smoothly rounded over making no attempt to proliferate. Cut ends may remain loose within the sheath or they may become stuck down to the surrounding tissues, particularly if there has been any element of infection. When severed in paratenon, the tendon shows less retraction. New vascular connective tissue invades the gap between the tendon ends, which become linked by fibrous tissue. Initially the fibrous union has a loose and disorganized appearance but rapidly the fibres become orientated in the line of the tendon pull and the eventual scar closely resembles normal tendon. With subsequent use, the vascular adhesions associated with the repair break down and function is restored. This healing process will occur naturally in all situations except within the synovial sheath but, unless the tendon ends are approximated, either by surgical repair or external splintage, the tendon will heal with elongation and consequent impairment of function. Prognosis in tendon suture, therefore, depends on the type of tendon and the situation in which it has been divided: tendons surrounded by paratenon in the forearm or dorsum of hand usually heal well and satisfactory function is usually restored; the poorest results of tendon repair are seen in the flexor tendons of the fingers, where they lie within the fibrous flexor sheath, since dense and permanent adhesions may form. Such adhesions may be minimized by atraumatic technique, the use of a nonirritant suture material and healing of the wound in conditions of absolute asepsis. Tendon suture, therefore, must not be regarded as a minor operation but should be carried out only in a fully equipped operating theatre with adequate assistance.

Clinical examination

Although clinical examination is important it is seldom possible to accurately diagnose the nature and extent of tendon damage in the hand. The patient is usually in pain and may be unable or unwilling to co-operate. It is a safe rule to assume that in any wound of the hand underlying structures have been cut until proved otherwise by surgical exploration. However, the diagnosis of a divided tendon may sometimes be deduced by the posture of the part (Fig. 8.22). General or regional anaesthesia may be used and a pneumatic tourniquet is essential.

Associated injuries. Fractures associated with tendon divisions are best stabilised by internal fixation. Nerves and important vessels divided at the level of the tendon injury can also be repaired at the same time.

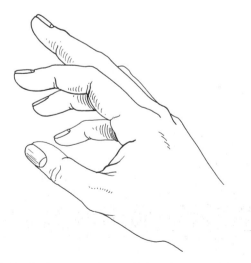

Fig. 8.22 In the unconscious patient or unco-operative patient posture of the fingers may indicate tendon damage. In this case the flexors of the long finger have been divided

Tendon suture

Materials for tendon suture. These must be nonreactive in the tissues otherwise adhesions will form. Stainless steel wire, monofilament nylon, Prolene or Mersilene mounted on atraumatic needles are appropriate.

Technique. The method of suturing employed should hold the cut ends of the tendon in firm apposition until healing is complete. It is necessary to obtain some sort of 'splicing' effect into the tendon ends, since simple longitudinal stitches will cut out between the fibres. To reduce the likelihood of adhesions to surrounding structures, the suture material should be buried as far as possible within the tendon. Figure 8.23 illustrates two of the techniques which may be used to join tendon ends of equal size. The tendon ends, if ragged, are cut cleanly across and the suture material mounted on a fine, straight needle is passed through the tendon in a manner indicated in the diagrams.

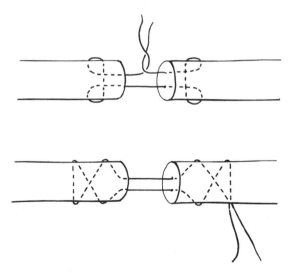

Fig. 8.23 Two methods of suture of tendons of equal diameter.
Top the Kessler stitch. *Bottom* the Bunnell stitch

Following tendon repair, it is necessary to protect the suture line from stress by appropriate splintage.

Secondary tendon repair

The same techniques may be applied to secondary tendon repair but it is essential that the suture line should lie in healthy tissues. If the tendon is repaired in a scarred bed, it will become stuck down to the surrounding scar. Thus it may sometimes be necessary to carry out a plastic procedure in the overlying skin, or, if the deep tissues are scarred, it may be preferable to bypass the area by means of a tendon graft and thus avoid a suture line within the scar tissue.

Tendon grafting

Tendon grafting is carried out when a gap exists between the tendon ends or where it is necessary to avoid a repair in scar tissue, or in the case of flexor tendon injuries in the finger within the fibrous flexor sheath, where a delayed direct repair is likely to be associated with adhesion formation. The operation is almost invariably performed as a secondary procedure after skin healing. The tendons of palmaris longus and plantaris are most commonly used. A toe extensor may be used if other tendons are not available. The palmaris tendon is best mobilized through a series of 3 or 4 short transverse incisions placed along the course of the tendon. Palmaris is sometimes absent — it is important to confirm its presence prior to anaesthesia. The plantaris, which gives an excellent length of strong, slender graft, is approached through a short incision in the medial aspect of the tendo Achilles near its insertion. The tendon is then removed using a tendon stripper. A tendon graft is usually of a smaller diameter than the tendon to which it is being attached and therefore end to end suture is rarely possible and the technique illustrated in Figure 8.24 can be used.

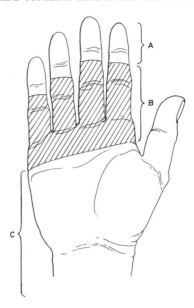

Fig. 8.25 Flexor tendon zones. Primary suture is permitted in Zone A, for a tenodesis at this level gives a good result. Within Zone B primary repair should be carried out only by the experienced. Tendon adhesions at this level would lead to stiffness and poor function. Within Zone C primary suture is satisfactory

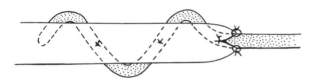

Fig. 8.24 The Pulvertaft suture for tendons of unequal size

In using a tendon graft, it is important to obtain correct tension otherwise the motor unit will not function properly. In the case of a finger flexor, the correct tension may be judged by comparison with the degree of flexion in the other fingers in the resting state.

Flexor tendon injuries

Tendon injuries occur most frequently in the hands because the hands are so exposed to risk of industrial or domestic injury. The particular problems of divisions within the fibrous flexor sheath have been referred to earlier and it is this structure which dictates the technique of repair (Fig. 8.25). Outside the fibrous flexor sheath, primary tendon repair may be carried out by one of the methods illustrated in Figure 8.23.

Within the fibrous flexor sheath, if the superficial tendon alone is divided, the disability is negligible and it should not be repaired. Division of the profundus alone, distal to the superficialis tendon, may be repaired primarily even though it lies within the flexor sheath, for, although adhesions may form, a strong tenodesis at this level gives satisfactory function.

It is the treatment of divisions of both tendons within the flexor sheath that is difficult and controversial. The standard teaching has been that a delayed flexor tendon graft should be performed when the skin has healed and passive movements in the finger are full. This is still safe advice, especially for an inexperienced surgeon dealing with the primary injury. However there has been a return to the practice of primary flexor tendon repair in 'no man's land' (the previously prohibited area of the fibrous flexor sheath) by many experienced hand surgeons, with results that are equal to those obtained by delayed tendon grafting. The technique is demanding on both patient and surgeon (as indeed is flexor tendon grafting) and is totally contraindicated if the patient is likely to be uncooperative, or in any tendon injury other than a straightforward clean cut. If possible both tendons should be repaired using a buried Kessler suture of wire or nylon. A running 6/0 Prolene suture is inserted around the circumference of the tendon junction. The flexor sheath is repaired and the skin is closed. Elastic band traction is attached to the finger nail (Figs 8.26 & 8.27), allowing active extension of the finger but only passive flexion; with this arrangement there is no stress across the tendon repair. Passive movement of the tendon within the sheath lessens the tethering effect of the inevitable adhesions that form around the healing tendon. The traction is maintained for a minimum of 4–6 weeks and requires daily supervision.

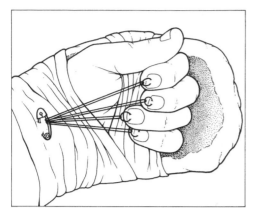

Fig. 8.26 Finger traction after primary tendon repair. Elastic bands are attached to sutures passed through the nails of the involved fingers and keep the fingers passively flexed

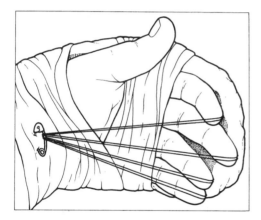

Fig. 8.27 Finger traction after primary tendon repair. The patient is encouraged to extend the fingers actively, against the tension in the elastic bands. Passive overdistraction of the tendon repair is prevented by the back slab which keeps the wrist and metacarpophalangeal joints flexed by about 30°

Flexor tendon graft in the finger
Either a midlateral or volar zigzag incision (Fig. 8.9) may be used with appropriate extensions to the palm. The fibrous flexor sheath is then excised leaving three intact pulleys to prevent bow stringing of the graft. The superficialis tendon is excised and the profundus is resected proximally to midpalm and distally to leave a short stump. The palmaris or plantaris graft is then drawn through the pulleys, extreme care being taken to avoid damage to its surface that would increase the risk of adhesion formation. The graft is then attached to the distal stump of profundus or to an osteoperiosteal flap elevated from the distal phalanx, using the pullout stitch shown in Figure 8.28. At this stage of the operation the incision in the finger may be closed. The proximal junction with the cut end of the profundus tendon

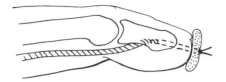

Fig. 8.28 Technique of attachment of the flexor tendon to the distal phalanx. The pullout stitch is fastened over a button at the finger tip and is withdrawn at 3 to 4 weeks when healing will have occurred. This technique can be adapted to attach tendon to bone in other situations

is made using the technique illustrated in Figure 8.24, and is covered, if possible, with lumbrical muscle.

After the operation, the fingers are bandaged in semiflexion for 3 weeks. Thereafter active exercises are instituted, at first gently, and then with increasing vigour until maximum recovery is achieved, which may take several months.

Two-stage grafting using sialastic rod. When there is heavy scarring it is unlikely that a flexor tendon graft will be successful. A silastic rod may be used to maintain the patency of the fibrous flexor sheath and to promote the formation of a new synovial sheath within it. At the first stage, the divided tendons are excised to midpalm and a silastic rod of suitable calibre is placed within the flexor sheath, which is left intact except for a limited resection at the site of the original injury. The rod is anchored distally by means of a single stitch and the proximal end is cut obliquely in the midpalm. The cut ends of the flexor profundus and flexor superficialis are then sutured together in the midpalm. Postoperatively the finger is kept mobile by passive movement. At least 6 weeks later the palmer and distal extremities of the old incision are reopened and a separate incision is made at the distal aspect of the forearm through which the superficialis tendon is identified and divided. It is mobilized carefully and brought out in the palmar wound. The suture line to profundus is freed from adhesions. The two ends of the silastic rod are then identified. The distal end of the superficialis graft is attached to the rod by suture and the rod is withdrawn at its distal end, drawing the tendon through the sheath. The tendon is then fixed as described above for the free tendon graft.

Repair of flexor pollicis longus
The tendon should be repaired primarily in clean cut wounds. Even if adhesions should form the function is usually very satisfactory as the thumb is stable in gripping. Arthrodesis of the interphalangeal joint should be considered as a simple alternative to grafting in late injuries. Since the thenar muscles are still working the function of the thumb is excellent after this procedure.

Extensor tendon injuries

Because the extensor tendons of the hand and wrist are surrounded by paratenon, their management is much easier and the end result generally more satisfactory than obtains with flexor tendon repairs. Primary suture is the treatment of choice and presents no particular problems except for difficulty in identifying individual tendons in multiple divisions and the possibility of adhesion formation beneath the extensor retinaculum.

Mallet finger

This is caused by an acute flexion injury of the terminal segment, which either disrupts the extensor tendon or avulses it from its insertion with a fragment of bone. Surgical repair is not necessary. Satisfactory healing can be obtained by immobilizing the terminal joint of the finger in full extension for 6 weeks. The splint is illustrated in Figure 8.29.

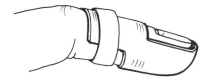

Fig. 8.29   Plastic finger splint used for mallet finger

Boutonnière deformity

This results from division or rupture of the central slip of the extensor expansion at the level of the proximal interphalangeal joint. It is very liable to be missed at the time of the initial injury since no immediate disability is apparent. With time, however, the 2 lateral slips of the extensor tendon slide forward around the sides of the joint and come to act as flexors leading to progressive flexion deformity of this joint with hyper-extension of the distal interphalangeal joint. In open injuries over the proximal interphalangeal joint it should be assumed that the central slip has been cut. The wound should be explored formally and the slip repaired. In closed injuries splintage of the proximal interphalangeal joint in extension for 6 weeks using a splint such as is illustrated in Figure 8.30, is successful, if commenced early. The results of surgery to correct the late deformity are by no means good and are bound to fail if the finger has become stiff.

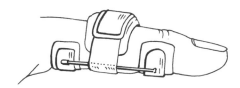

Fig. 8.30   Splint for boutonnière deformity

Rupture of the extensor pollicis longus tendon

This usually occurs a few weeks after an undisplaced fracture of the distal radius. The rupture of this or indeed any of the extensor tendons of the fingers may also be complications of rheumatoid arthritis. The disability from rupture of the extensor pollicis longus tendon is not always great but, if it gives rise to handi-cap, surgical treatment is desirable. Direct suture is not possible because there is a large gap between the tendon ends and the most useful procedure is a tendon transfer using extensor indicis proprius as the motor tendon. This is divided through a short incision at the level of the neck of the second metacarpal; the extensor indicis proprius tendon is on the ulnar side of the extensor digitorum communis tendon of the index. Through a separate incision, it is joined to the distal part of the extensor pollicis longus tendon using the technique shown in Figure 8.31. The thumb is splinted in extension for 4 weeks.

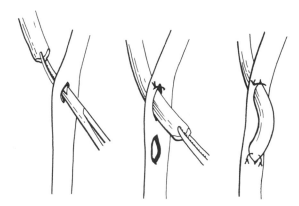

Fig. 8.31   Technique for linking two tendons

Tendon transfer

Tendon transfers are used either to restore active movement, where this has been lost as a result of neurological disease or damage to muscle and tendon, or to correct imbalance of muscle which might lead to deformity. In order for a tendon transfer to succeed, the following principles must be observed:

1. any fixed deformity must first be corrected either by soft tissue release or osteotomy;
2. the muscle must be strong enough to perform the new task required of it — transfer of a tendon always weakens the muscle slightly;
3. the muscle must have sufficient amplitude of motion to perform its new role;
4. the transferred muscle should ideally have an allied or synergistic action to the muscle which it is replacing although, perhaps surprisingly, this is of less importance in the hand than it is in the lower limb;

5. a straight line pull is desirable;
6. it is of absolute importance that the transferred muscle can be spared from its original function.

Tendon transfers may be attached to an existing tendon or to bone (Figs 8.31 & 8.32). Details of the very many tendon transfers used for restoration of function in the hand are to be found in more specialized texts. Some examples are listed below.

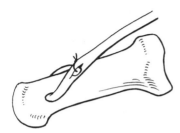

Fig. 8.32   Method for attaching a tendon to bone

1. Extensor indicis to extensor pollicis longus, as described on page 185.
2. Triple transfer for radial nerve paralysis. In this condition there is drop-wrist with loss of extension in the fingers and thumb. The following tendon transfers may be carried out:
   a. pronator teres to extensor carpi radialis brevis;
   b. flexor carpi ulnaris or flexor carpi radialis to the extensors of the fingers;
   c. palmaris longus to extensor pollicis longus.
3. Restoration of opposition of the thumb in median nerve palsy, using the superficialis tendon from the ring finger looped through a pulley in flexor carpi ulnaris. The extensor indicis proprius may also be transferred around the ulnar side of the forearm and across the palm to provide the same function.

NERVE INJURIES

General considerations

Structure of a peripheral nerve
A major peripheral nerve is made up of a large number of fibres — there may be as many as 50 000 in the median nerve of the forearm. Each fibre consists of an *axon* and its cellular coverings. The axon is the process of a nerve cell lying within the central nervous system or a ganglion of the autonomic nervous systems and links this cell with an appropriate end-plate, the structural unit being called a *neurone*. The peripheral nerves carry, to a varying degree, fibres concerned with motor, sensory and sympathetic functions. Two main fibre types occur — the *myelinated* and *unmyelinated*. In the

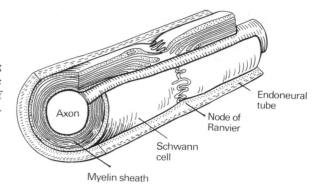

Fig. 8.33   Details of myelinated nerve

former, the Schwann cell sheath, which invests all peripheral nerve fibres, is wrapped around the axon in many layers, which contain the myelin, a complex lipoprotein (Fig. 8.33). At intervals along its length, the myelin sheath is interrupted at the nodes of Ranvier. In unmyelinated fibres, the Schwann cell layer contains no myelin.

Myelinated fibres conduct more rapidly than unmyelinated fibres and transmit the efferent impulses to skeletal muscle and the afferent impulses from some sensory endings concerned with pain and light touch. The majority of sensory fibres are, however, unmyelinated as are those of the sympathetic nervous system.

Groups of nerve fibres are aggregated into bundles or fascicles which are surrounded by a thin, but well organized layer of connective tissue, the *perineurium*. Usually a number of fascicles are bound together as a group, called a fascicular bundle, surrounded by internal *epineurium*. There is a strong and distinct layer of epineurium surrounding the fascicles that make up a nerve trunk (Fig. 8.34). Fascicles tend to branch and regroup along the length of the nerve forming as it were an intraneural plexus so that the cross-section arrangement of bundles varies from point to point along the course of the nerve.

The connective tissues of a peripheral nerve are surprisingly strong so that it is not uncommon to find

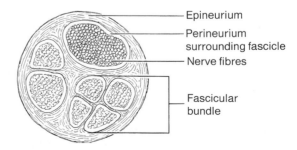

Fig. 8.34   Diagrammatic cross-section of a peripheral nerve

the major nerves as the only intact structures in a severely injured limb. The peripheral nerves are supplied by many small nutrient arteries which communicate freely within the nerve. It is possible, therefore, to mobilize quite long lengths of nerve without damaging the blood supply.

Classification of nerve injuries

Nerve injuries may be divided into three degrees of severity. In first degree nerve injuries (*neurapraxia*), axons are not disrupted but nerve conductivity is temporarily lost, probably as a result of local dispersal of the myelin sheath. Many pressure palsies are of this type. In second degree nerve injuries (*axonotmesis*), greater violence produces disruption of the axons but the supporting connective tissues of the nerve remain in continuity. In third degree injuries (*neurotmesis*), the nerve is completely divided.

Following division of a nerve, elastic traction causes the ends to separate and spontaneous recovery never takes place. At the proximal stump a traumatic neuroma forms which consists of numerous fibrils sprouting from the cut end of the severed axons together with proliferation of the supporting tissues within the nerve. In the distal stump a bulbous end forms consisting of the supporting elements only.

Recovery following nerve injury

Since neurapraxia and axonotmesis are lesions in continuity, complete and perfect recovery may be anticipated. In neurapraxia this may take place within hours or days of the injury. In axonotmesis the recovery time depends on the distance between the level of injury and the end organ supplied by the nerve, axonal regeneration occurring at the rate of about 1 mm per day. In neurotmesis recovery does not take place unless surgical repair of the divided nerve is carried out. Even then, recovery is usually imperfect for it depends on the success with which axons reconnect with distal Schwann cell sheaths (which will guide them to the periphery) and also whether motor axons reach motor end-plates and sensory axons reach sensory end organs.

Factors which influence recovery include age of the patient, the younger having the better prognosis; the level of the lesion, the more proximal having poorer prognosis; the violence which produces the original injury, the more severe the violence the poorer the prognosis. Mixed nerves, which carry both motor and sensory functions, such as the median or ulnar nerve, have a poorer prognosis than for example the radial nerve, which is largely a motor nerve and usually recovers well. A large gap between the nerve ends at the time of repair militates against recovery for the gap must be closed by extensive mobilization with possible damage to its blood supply, or a nerve graft, which seldom succeeds as well as a direct suture.

Clinical features

It must be emphasized here that when there is a wound overlying a nerve it is mandatory to test the appropriate motor and sensory functions and, if there is any doubt whatsoever about nerve function, the wound should be explored in circumstances that will allow primary repair if indicated. It should be appreciated that the classical signs of nerve injury — flaccid paralysis and sensory loss — are difficult to elicit and interpret after recent trauma when the patient is upset and in pain.

As a working rule, a closed injury is usually either a neurapraxia or an axonotmesis whereas neurotmesis is usually associated with an open wound. With open wounds, it is possible to establish with certainty if the nerve has been divided during the course of the wound excision. In practice, then, nerve injuries in the absence of open wounds are treated conservatively until a reasonable period has elapsed to allow for spontaneous recovery and the nerve is explored surgically only if the anticipated recovery does not take place. A reasonable recovery interval may be estimated from the fact that axonal regeneration takes place at about 1 mm a day. By measuring the distance from the site of injury to the first muscle or area of skin supplied by the nerve, an estimate of the likely rate of recovery can be calculated. An advancing Tinel sign, that is, a point of sensitivity on the course of the injured nerve, is also a useful guide to the progress of recovery and gives an indication that at least part of the nerve is in continuity.

Difficulties in the assessment of nerve injuries can arise when several degrees of nerve injury are present at the same time. Thus in traction injuries of the brachial plexus, it is not uncommon to have all three degrees of nerve injury involving different nerve roots. In such circumstances surgical exploration may be necessary to establish the severity of injury and plan treatment.

Electrophysiological assessment of nerve injuries

Changes in the conductivity of nerves and in the electrical activity of muscles can be used to aid clinical diagnosis of nerve injury and give an objective measure of recovery.

Nerve conductivity. Peripheral nerves may be stimulated by surface electrodes placed along their course and the resultant response in a peripheral muscle is picked up by electrodes placed over the muscle. Likewise afferent sensory potentials may be detected in a nerve in response to peripheral sensory stimulation within the nerve territory. Both motor and sensory conduction tests give an indication of the integrity of the nerve and the conduction velocity can be assessed by measuring the distance between stimulus and recording electrode and the time taken for the stimulus to reach that point. Conduction velocity is frequently delayed in neurapraxia and is particularly characteristic of compression lesions of peripheral nerves. The level of injury may be localized by identifying a segment of the nerve in which maximum delay occurs. In axonotmesis and neurotmesis no conductivity takes place after Wallerian degeneration is established (i.e. by the end of the second week). The return of measurable conductivity may precede the clinical signs of recovery.

Electromyography. When a needle electrode is placed in a normally innervated resting muscle no electrical activity is detected, whereas in denervated muscle small 'fibrillation' potentials can be detected firing at irregular intervals. Fibrillation potentials do not occur in neurapraxia.

MANAGEMENT OF NERVE INJURIES

Whatever the degree of nerve injury, it is important that the tissues supplied by the nerve should be maintained in healthy condition pending recovery. The patient must be advised of the need to protect anaesthetic skin from accidental injury and he must be shown how to retain by passive movement the mobility of joints whose muscles are paralysed. It may be necessary to provide some form of splintage to maintain function and prevent contractures during the recovery period.

Surgical repair of divided nerves

Should nerves be repaired at the time of primary wound treatment or as a delayed procedure when the wound has healed? The argument in favour of a primary repair is that it spares the patient a further operation. However, if the wound is extensive and the result of considerable violence, definitive nerve repair is best done as a delayed procedure, because it would add considerably to the length of the initial wound treatment and also because it is difficult to identify the extent of nerve damage and therefore the amount of nerve which must be resected. It is sound practice to restrict primary nerve repair to clean, incised wounds of limited extent where the surgeon has the necessary experience, instruments and time at his disposal. In all other circumstances the cut ends of the divided nerve should be identified at the time of primary wound treatment, and approximated with two or three inert sutures carefully placed so that the correct rotation of the nerve is maintained. It is often easier to match the cut ends of the nerve at this stage than at a secondary procedure. Isolating the site of nerve division with a silastic tube is useful in preventing adhesion of the nerve to the surrounding muscles or tendons, which may also have been damaged at the same level.

Primary nerve repair

Magnification, by loupes or the operating microscope, is essential to prevent further damage to the nerve by clumsy dissection and to ensure accurate orientation of the nerve and placement of sutures. Sutures must be of relatively inert material such as nylon and prolene and should be size 8/0 or less, although larger size sutures may be used as temporary stays. Silk sutures and absorbable sutures have no place in nerve surgery as they always provoke an inflammatory response that will cause further damage to the nerve. Tension at the site of the repair must be avoided as it provokes a fibrotic reaction.

The standard repair is by *epineural suture.* Minimal trimming of the nerve ends is carried out with an extremely sharp blade with the nerve resting on a firm surface, care being taken not to crush it. It is usually necessary to remove only 1–2 mm in a cleanly cut nerve. The ends are drawn together by stay sutures inserted in the circumferential epineurium. Correct orientation of the nerve is facilitated by noting the arrangement of the fascicular bundles within the nerve and the presence of any blood vessels on the surface. A minimum number of 8/0 nylon sutures are used to pick up the epineurium — for example about 6–8 in the median nerve and 2 or 3 in a digital nerve.

Secondary nerve repair

Secondary nerve repair is carried out after an interval of several weeks when associated muscle and tendon injuries have healed and the possibility of infection has been eliminated. It is difficult and unwise to try and identify the nerve within scar tissue at the site of injury. The incision should be long enough so that the nerve may be identified in healthy tissues proximal and distal to the level of injury and it is then easy to dissect to the injured site. Having identified the point of division, the neuroma is resected with a fresh scalpel blade or razor beyond the limit of scar tissue, which can be recognized when the nerve bundles pout separately from the cut surface (Fig. 8.35). The epineurium at this stage has proliferated and is easy to suture. Two lateral sutures are first placed in the epineurium joining the nerve ends in their correct orientation, which is of paramount importance. This will have been facilitated by the correct placement of sutures at the time of the primary approximation and can be helped by matching small blood vessels or nerve bundles. It is obvious that the quality of recovery in a mixed nerve will depend largely on the correct matching of the nerve ends. Using the 2 lateral sutures as stay sutures, the nerve may be rotated to allow further sutures to be placed around the periphery on the superficial and deep aspects of the nerve (Fig. 8.35).

It is important that the suture line should not be

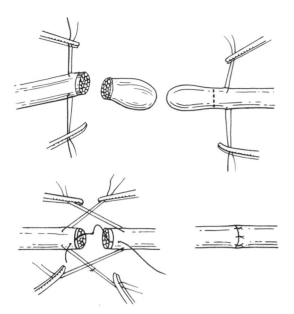

Fig. 8.35 Secondary nerve suture. Note the guide suture inserted into the epineurium at corresponding points on the circumference and held with dissimilar pair of forceps. These help to maintain correct orientation of the nerve ends throughout the repair

under tension, which means that gaps greater than 2 or 3 cm cannot be repaired by direct suture unless length can be gained by some device such as anterior transposition of the ulnar nerve at the elbow or by flexing joints over which the nerve passes. Larger defects can only be repaired by means of a nerve graft. A nerve, which can be spared, such as the sural or saphenous, is used and a sufficient length is obtained to allow enough segments to match the diameter of the nerve which is being bridged. The epineurium of each graft is then sutured to the internal epineurium around the fascicular bundles of the recipient nerve using the operating microscope and microsurgical technique (Fig. 8.36).

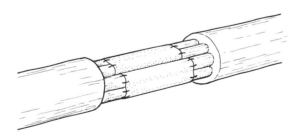

Fig. 8.36 Nerve grafting. Multiple lengths of a smaller expendable nerve may be used to bridge a gap in a larger nerve. Sutures are placed in the epineurium of the graft and the epineurium of the fascicular bundles. As few sutures as possible should be used and care taken to stagger suture lines across the nerve to minimize local fibrosis. Microsurgical technique is essential

Recovery following nerve grafting is always imperfect and the quality of the result reflects the skill and experience of the operator.

Partial nerve division

If a partial nerve division is noted at the initial exploration of the wound then primary epineural repair should be carried out. However it is often the case that adequate exploration is not done and only later does it become apparent that there is a neurological deficit which requires exploration of the nerve at the site of injury. It is rarely possible to carry out resection of a lateral neuroma and repair by loop suture as illustrated in Figure 8.37. If there is a larger defect after resection of the neuroma, as is almost invariably the case, an inlaid cable graft is required.

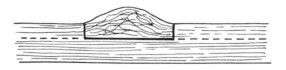

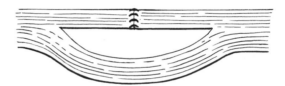

Fig. 8.37 Loop suture used to repair partial division of a nerve. The intact and damaged fascicles are carefully separated and the damaged portion resected and repaired as shown. Inlay grafting is often preferable to this technique

Postsurgical management

Following surgical repair by any of the foregoing techniques, it is necessary to protect the suture line from tension for 3 weeks. This requires immobilizing the limb, usually with the joints over which the nerve passes in a position of flexion, by means of a plaster cast which is removed at the end of 3 weeks and gentle mobilization of the limb commenced. If acute flexion of any joint has been necessary in order to overcome shortening of a nerve, then mobilization of the joint must be gradual and may be achieved by either serial changes of the plaster cast producing progressively lesser flexion or else by means of a turnbuckle plaster, in which a hinge with a series of graduated stops allows gradual extension of the limb over a period of 3 or 4 weeks.

The brachial plexus

The commonest injuries to the brachial plexus are the result of traction. This may occur at birth but in adult life it is frequently the result of motor cycle injuries, the head and shoulder being forced apart by the violence resulting from contact with the ground.

Anatomy

The brachial plexus lies partly in the antero-inferior corner of the posterior triangle of the neck, partly behind the clavicle, and partly in the axilla. It consists of trunks, divisions, cords and branches. The *upper trunk* arises from the anterior rami of C5 and 6; the *middle trunk* from C7; and the *lower trunk* from C8 and T1. Behind the clavicle the trunks divide into anterior and posterior divisions. The upper 2 anterior divisions unite to form the *lateral cord*; the lower anterior division forms the *medial cord*; all 3 posterior divisions unite to form the *posterior cord*.

Main branches of the cords. The *median nerve* is formed by the union of a branch of the lateral cord and a branch of the medial cord. The *ulnar nerve* is the main continuation of the medial cord; the *radial nerve,* of the posterior cord. Other branches are the *musculo-cutaneous* (lateral cord); the *medial cutaneous nerves of arm and forearm* (medial cord); the *circumflex nerve,* and the *nerve to latissimus dorsi* (posterior cord).

Open injuries

A wound overlying the brachial plexus that is associated with a neurological deficit should be explored and any divided nerves repaired following the principles outlined above. The wound is frequently a result of stabbing and there may be vascular injury. Although vascular repair takes priority, management of the brachial plexus injury is much simpler if nerve repair can be carried out as a primary procedure.

Traction lesions

Traction lesions of the brachial plexus are of three types — *upper,* when roots C4, 5 and 6 are involved; *lower,* when roots C7, 8 and T1 are involved; or *total,* when the entire arm is rendered flaccid and anaesthetic. In management of traction lesions in adult life it is important that a clear prognosis be established at an early stage. Virtually full recovery will occur after neurapraxia or axonotmesis. If the lesion is in continuity but Wallerian degeneration has occurred in the nerve, proximal recovery may occur but the prognosis for the hand is poor. Where a complete avulsion of one or more of the roots has taken place, no recovery can be expected at that level. It should be borne in mind that combinations of different nerve lesions are common in brachial plexus injuries.

Prognostic indicators. Injuries of the upper roots of the plexus tend to do better than complete injuries or injuries of the lower roots. Supraclavicular lesions have a worse prognosis than infraclavicular. Severe pain lasting for more than 6 months carries a poor prognosis. Horner's syndrome is associated with a poor prognosis for lesions of the lower roots.

Nerve root avulsions from the cord do not recover and are irreparable. They can be recognized by early exploration of the brachial plexus. Later when the meninges have healed they can be demonstrated myelographically by the presence of traction meningoceles at the level of avulsion.

Management

In the management of traction injuries of the brachial plexus, as in all other forms of peripheral nerve injury, meticulous attention must be paid to the prevention of contractures by ensuring that all joints are kept mobile by being put through a full passive range of movements regularly. The anaesthetic skin should also be protected and care taken to avoid pressure sores etc.

In lesions with good prognostic indications treatment is conservative and recovery is anticipated. In those with poor prognostic features early surgical exploration is advocated in some centres with a view to establishing the prognosis and, if possible, to carrying out surgical repair. Direct repair of the plexus is rarely possible and repair can only be effected by means of cable grafts using the sural or saphenous nerve. These operations require a high degree of skill and experience and should be performed only in specialized centres. Even in the best hands, the recovery rate following surgery is poor.

If at a year following a brachial plexus injury, the arm remains totally flail and anaesthetic, the patient may choose to have a shoulder arthrodesis and an above elbow amputation followed by the fitting of a passive prosthesis. In practice a functional prothesis can only be fitted if there is voluntary control of elbow and shoulder. Only a few highly motivated patients achieve functional use of their prosthesis. Amputation of the limb does not relieve painful symptoms and should never be done for this purpose.

Median nerve

The median nerve is the most frequently injured of all the peripheral nerves because of its exposed situation on the flexor aspect of the forearm and hand where incised wounds are common. It is also very vulnerable to compression within the tight confines of the carpal tunnel.

Anatomy

The median nerve originates in 2 roots arising from the medial and lateral cords of the brachial plexus. In the upper arm it descends first along the lateral side of the brachial artery, then crosses it anteriorly to run on its medial side into the cubital fossa. It leaves the fossa between the heads of pronator teres, and descends in the forearm between flexor sublimes and flexor profundus. In the lower third of the forearm it becomes more superficial by emerging at the lateral side of flexor sublimis. About 2.5 cm above the wrist it comes to lie in front of the sublimis tendons, to the ulnar side of flexor carpi radialis, between it and palmaris longus (which may, however, be superficial to it). It then enters the palm of the hand, passing deep to the flexor retinaculum.

Motor distribution. The median nerve supplies all the muscles on the front of the forearm (except flexor carpi ulnaris and the ulnar part of the flexor digitorum profundus). In the palm it supplies the short muscles of the thumb (except the adductor) and the lateral two lumbricals.

Sensory distribution. The skin of the thumb and of the lateral 2½ fingers (except on the dorsum of their proximal segments) is supplied by digital branches of the median nerve. The greater part of the palm is supplied by the palmar branch. The sensory distribution of the median nerve is one of the most important tactile areas of the body and has been aptly called the eyes of the hand.

Median nerve injury

The possibility of a median nerve injury at or above the elbow can be investigated most simply by asking the patient to clench his fist. If the nerve is injured above elbow level, this movement is impossible, since the thumb and the lateral 2 fingers have no power of flexion. Flexion of the medial 2 fingers by flexor profundus is preserved. In the case of wounds about the wrist, the clinical diagnosis of median nerve injury is less easy, since the branches to the long flexor muscles will usually be intact. Paralysis of the thenar muscles will, however, be present, and can be detected from the patient's inability to bring the thumb into opposition. Anaesthesia will be found in the area of sensory distribution of the nerve. When dealing with the common incised wounds on the flexor aspect of the forearm, it is of great importance to make a careful clinical assessment of the extent of the tendon and nerve injury prior to surgery for the divided ends of these tissues may retract and be difficult to find at the time of the wound excision, unless the surgeon knows precisely which structures to look for.

Exposure of the median nerve in the upper arm and cubital fossa is closely related to the brachial artery (Fig. 8.38) and the operation is similar to that described for exposure of the artery (p. 40). Just above wrist level (where injuries are common), the nerve lies on the ulnar side of flexor carpi radialis tendon (Fig. 8.39). Owing to its flattened shape it is easily mistaken for a tendon.

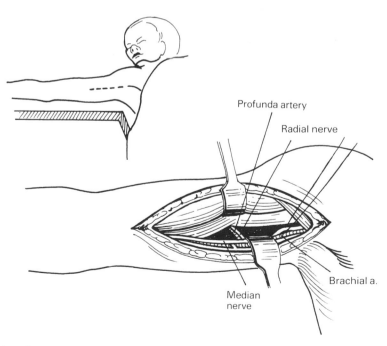

Fig. 8.38 Exposure of median nerve in upper arm. Note that the nerve crosses the brachial vessels from lateral to medial side as it passes distally

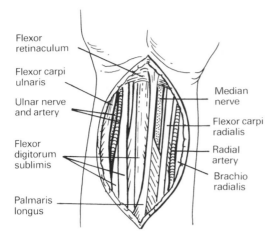

Flexor retinaculum

Flexor carpi ulnaris

Ulnar nerve and artery

Flexor digitorum sublimis

Palmaris longus

Median nerve

Flexor carpi radialis

Radial artery

Brachio radialis

Fig. 8.39   Relationships of the median nerve above the wrist

Following repair of the median nerve the suture line should be protected by immobilization of the arm in an appropriate position. Where the nerve has been injured above or around the elbow, flexion of the elbow will often allow the nerve to be sutured without tension. Where the injury is more distal in the forearm, there is often a temptation to flex the wrist in order to allow closure of the gap but this should be resisted as the nerve will inevitably become adherent to the site of the injury and a traction lesion will result as the flexed wrist is subsequently straightened. Even although the nerve is injured distally in the forearm, any tension at the repair should be relieved by flexion of the elbow.

Considering that the median nerve is mixed, the degree of recovery after suture is better than might be expected. Some 60% of patients regain adequate motor and sensory function.

Carpal tunnel syndrome

The median nerve, in common with most other peripheral nerves, may be subject to compression where it passes through confined anatomical tunnels. Carpal tunnel syndrome is by far the most common of these 'entrapment' neuropathies. It affects usually women around the time of the menopause. They are regularly awakened with pain centred in the median distribution but often radiating diffusely to involve the whole hand and forearm. The patient has to exercise the hand in order to promote venous return and allow the symptoms to subside. During the day, the discomfort may return during activities involving repeated gripping movements with the wrist flexed. Objective neurological changes persist within the median nerve territory only after the syndrome has been present for many months or years. The syndrome has many variations and may less commonly affect men and adults of any

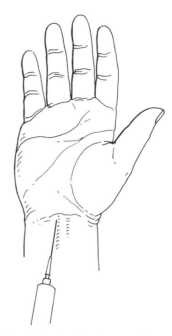

Fig. 8.40   Site of injection into the carpal tunnel to the ulnar side of palmaris longus tendon

age. Some space-occupying condition, such as oedema or synovitis within the carpal tunnel, may be the precipitating factor. Delay in electrical conductivity of the median nerve across the wrist will confirm the diagnosis in cases of doubt.

In mild cases of short duration, conservative measures may be tried. These include the provision of a night splint, which immobilizes the wrist in a neutral position, or an injection of hydrocortisone 25 mg into the carpal tunnel, the site of injection being placed just ulnar to the palmaris longus tendon, between the median and ulnar nerves (Fig. 8.40). If symptoms persist, surgical decompression is necessary. The operation can be satisfactorily done with Bier's regional anaesthesia. The incision curves gently from the ulnar border of the tendon of palmaris longus where it crosses the distal wrist crease and extends to the midpalm (Fig. 8.41). The palmar fascia is incised to expose the transverse carpal ligament, which is then divided vertically at its midpoint (normally on the ulnar side of the median nerve). Care must be taken to avoid injury to the nerve, which may be adherent to the under surface of the ligament; it is wise therefore when the first opening is made in the ligament to pass a dissector underneath it to protect the deeper structures from injury. The ligament must be completely divided, the median nerve inspected and a neurolysis carried out if it is found adherent to the surrounding tissues. The skin only is closed and early mobility of the hand encouraged.

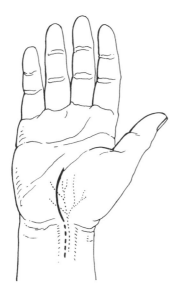

Fig. 8.41 Incision for carpal tunnel decompression is placed slightly towards the ulnar side of the midline to avoid the palmar cutaneous branches of the median nerve

Ulnar nerve

Whereas injuries to the median nerve are particularly important because of the sensory loss which ensues, with ulnar nerve lesions the motor loss of the intrinsic muscles of the hand which control fine skilled finger movements is the main complaint, the ulnar sensory distribution being less critical than that of the median nerve.

Anatomy

The ulnar nerve originates as the main continuation of the medial cord of the brachial plexus. In the upper arm it descends along the medial side of the brachial artery in its proximal half; it then deviates medially, accompanied by the ulnar collateral artery, and pierces the medial intermuscular septum to enter the back of the arm, where it runs down under cover of the medial border of triceps. At the elbow it is closely applied to the back of the medial epicondyle, from which it passes on to the medial ligament of the joint. It enters the forearm deep to the aponeurosis joining the humeral and ulnar heads of flexor carpi ulnaris and runs down under cover of this muscle, lying on flexor digitorum profundus. Approaching the wrist the nerve becomes superficial between flexor carpi ulnaris and flexor digitorum sublimis. It then pierces deep fascia and enters the palm by passing superficial to the flexor retinaculum within Guyon's canal. In the lower third of the forearm, and at the wrist, the nerve is closely related to the ulnar artery which lies on its lateral side.

Motor distribution. In the forearm the ulnar nerve supplies only flexor carpi ulnaris, and the medial half of flexor digitorum profundus. In the hand it supplies most of the short muscles — the hypothenar muscles, all the interossei, the medial two lumbricals, and the adductor pollicis.

Sensory distribution. The medial 1½ fingers and the medial border of the palm are supplied by the ulnar nerve.

Exposure in the upper arm is by an approach similar to that described for the brachial artery (p. 40). The ulnar nerve is identified to the medial side of the vessels in the upper half of the arm. It is then traced downwards as it diverges from the vessels and pierces the medial intermuscular septum, to enter the posterior compartment of the arm.

Exposure at the elbow. A curved incision is made in the line of the nerve, and with its centre just behind the medial epicondyle. By division of the deep fascia the nerve is exposed as it lies in the postcondylar groove. In the distal part of the wound the nerve passes out of sight between the two heads of flexor carpi ulnaris; it is exposed by longitudinal separation of the fibres of the muscle. As the nerve is elevated from its bed, 5 branches may be encountered. An articular twig to the elbow joint can be divided; the other branches are muscular (2 to flexor carpi ulnaris, and 2 to flexor digitorum profundus), and these should be preserved.

Exposure at the wrist requires no special description. The nerve lies between flexor carpi ulnaris and flexor digitorum sublimis, and enters the palm by passing superficial to the flexor retinaculum. The ulnar artery is closely applied to its lateral side.

Ulnar nerve compression

The ulnar nerve is subject to compression at 2 sites where it passes through tight anatomical tunnels: on the medial aspect of the elbow and at the wrist. At the elbow the cubital tunnel is bounded superficially by the aponeurosis which joins the 2 heads of origin of flexor carpi ulnaris and on its deep surface the medial ligament at the elbow joint. This tunnel becomes progressively narrowed as the elbow is flexed. Any encroachment on the tunnel from pathology in the elbow joint, such as chronic arthritis, may compress the ulnar nerve. Tardy ulnar neuritis may occur many years after an elbow fracture, commonly after an injury of the lateral condyle, causing a valgus deformity. At the wrist, the nerve is closely tethered as it passes through Guyon's canal and again is vulnerable at this site to any space-occupying lesion, such as a ganglion.

Unlike median nerve compression, ulnar nerve compression is usually painless but presents a slow and insidious loss of sensation and motor power within its territory. The level of compression can be identified by careful neurological examination — thus, if the sensory impairment involves the dorsal aspect of the hand, the lesion is probably at the elbow for the dorsal cutaneous branch of the ulnar nerve separates from the main trunk above the wrist. If the dorsal sensation is preserved, then the lesion lies probably at the wrist. If all sensation is intact but the ulnar innervated intrinsic muscles are paralysed, then the compression must involve the deep palmar branch of the ulnar nerve after it has separated from the main trunk as it passes deeply into the palm at the level of the piso-hamate ligament. Surgical exploration of the nerve at the site indicated by the clinical examination will then identify the compressing agent and allow the nerve to be released.

Anterior transposition. After any operative treatment (neurolysis or nerve suture) at the level of the elbow, the nerve should never be replaced in its original bed behind the medial epicondyle, but should be transposed to the front of the elbow, so that it may pursue a shorter course, where it will be less subject to stretching and friction. This procedure, which can overcome up to 7–8 cm of shortening, greatly facilitates any form of nerve repair which involves trimming or resection. The operation of anterior transposition (Fig. 8.42) is specific for the conditions of traumatic neuritis and of recurrent dislocation of the nerve. After the nerve has been exposed and freed, its displacement may at first be prevented by the muscular branches; these may be elongated by separating them gently in a proximal direction from the parent trunk. When this has been done, the nerve can usually be brought without difficulty to the front of the medial epicondyle. In the upper part of the wound, the medial intermuscular septum is resected as its presence can result in continuing pressure on the nerve. The common flexor origin is now divided 1 cm distal to the medial epicondyle and the ulnar nerve displaced anteriorly to lie deep to the flexor muscles on the anterior capsule of the elbow joint. The common flexor origin is re-attached by suture and the elbow is subsequently immobilised at 90° of flexion in a plaster splint for three weeks to allow the muscles to heal. Subcutaneous transposition of the ulnar nerve leads to recurring ulnar neuritis and should not be done.

Medial epicondylectomy is an alternative to anterior transposition for ulnar neuritis. After mobilization of the nerve at the elbow the medial epicondyle is exposed subperiosteally and removed with an osteotome. The osteotomy is made in line with the medial surface of

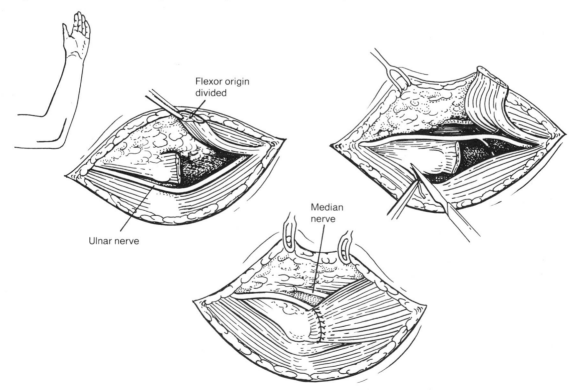

Fig. 8.42 Anterior transposition of the ulnar nerve. The nerve is brought to lie in front of the elbow deep to the flexor muscles and in the same plane as the median nerve
Figures 8.33, 8.40, 8.41, 8.42 are adapted from illustrations in Lamb D W, Hooper G & Kuczynski K (eds) 1989 The practice of hand surgery, 2nd edn. Blackwell, Edinburgh

the shaft of the humerus and care should be taken to remove any remaining bony prominence. The periosteum and the flexor origin are sutured over the bone. Postoperatively the arm is supported in a sling but early mobilization is encouraged.

Radial nerve

Because of its close relationship to the humerus the radial nerve may be injured in fractures of this bone or may be involved in callus formation. The important posterior interosseous branch of the radial nerve may be injured in fractures of the upper third of the radius, to which it is closely related, and is subject to compression during its course through supinator.

Anatomy

The radial nerve begins as the direct continuation of the posterior cord of the brachial plexus, and descends behind the axillary artery. In the upper part of the arm it passes backwards between the long and medial heads of triceps, and then winds round the humerus, under cover of the lateral head and between it and the medial head. In the lower third of the arm it pierces the lateral intermuscular septum, and runs down to the front of the lateral condyle, lying in the cleft between brachialis and brachio-radialis. The profunda artery and veins accompany the nerve in its course around the humerus. At the level of the epicondyle the radial nerve gives off its posterior interosseous branch, and then crosses the capsule of the elbow joint to enter the forearm, where it runs distally under cover of brachio-radialis. In the lower third of the forearm it emerges at the posterior border of brachioradialis and descends over the abductor and extensor tendons of the thumb to supply the skin of the lateral two-thirds of the dorsum of the hand, and part of the dorsum of corresponding digits.

The posterior interosseous nerve passes to the back of the forearm by winding round the lateral side of the upper third of the radius, through the substance of the supinator muscle. It then descends between the superficial and deep muscles, and breaks up into branches supplying them.

Motor distribution. The radial nerve, from its main trunk, supplies triceps, brachioradialis, extensor carpi radialis longus, anconeus, and part of brachialis. Through its posterior interosseous branch it supplies all remaining muscles on the back and radial side of the forearm; these include the dorsiflexors of the wrist (except extensor carpi radialis longus), the extensors of the fingers and thumb, and the long abductor of the thumb.

Sensory distribution is unimportant, since there is considerable overlap from adjacent nerves — the lateral cutaneous of forearm (from musculocutaneous), and the posterior cutaneous (from ulnar).

Radial nerve injury

Injury to the radial nerve occurs most commonly in the distal part of the upper arm, so that its branches to triceps are intact. All other muscles supplied by it (see above) are likely to be weakened or paralysed, and a characteristic *drop wrist* deformity is present. Sensory loss is restricted to a small area on the dorsal aspect of the first web. Lesions of the posterior interosseous nerve are characterised by dropping of the fingers alone for the radial wrist extensors are usually preserved and there is no sensory loss.

Since the radial nerve is mainly motor, repair is more successful than is the case with any other important nerve trunk. Full functional recovery may be expected in 70 to 80% of cases, but, if the lesion has been at a high level, it may not be complete until well over a year from the time of operation. If there is no recovery then tendon transfer to restore function (p. 186) is usually very successful.

Infra-axillary exposure. The radial nerve at first lies posterior to the proximal part of the brachial artery, and the approach to this part is similar to that described for the artery (p. 40).

Exposure in the middle third of the arm. Here, the nerve passes obliquely round the posterior surface of the humerus, lying in the musculospiral groove. An incision is made on the back of the arm in the line of the nerve. The interval between the long and lateral heads of triceps is opened up, and further distally the lateral head is divided in the line of the nerve. The fascial roof of the groove is incised to expose the nerve, which, accompanied by the profunda vessels, lies partly on the bone and partly on the upper fibres of the medial head (Fig. 8.43). Branches of the nerve to the triceps muscle should be carefully preserved.

Exposure in the lower third of the arm is obtained by downward prolongation of the above incision, and by opening up the cleft between the brachialis and brachioradialis muscles.

Exposure of the posterior interosseous branch. Repair of this nerve is unlikely to be practicable but it may be necessary to expose it in operations on the upper part of the radius or in compression lesions of this nerve within the supinator muscle. Its origin from the radial nerve on the front of the lateral epicondyle should first be identified. From there it is traced down to the point where it enters the substance of the supinator deep to the arcade of Frohse. By division of the superficial fibres of this muscle, the nerve is completely displayed.

INFECTIONS OF THE HAND

Severe infections of the hand are fortunately less common than formerly. This is no doubt attributable

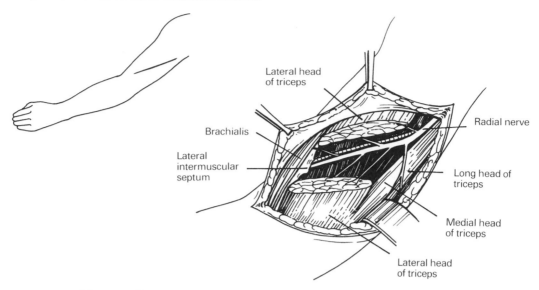

Fig. 8.43   Exposure of the radial nerve on the posterior aspect of the upper arm

to better treatment of wounds and antibiotic treatment of early infections. Nevertheless, when severe infections do occur they can rapidly cripple a hand unless managed correctly. A false sense of security can be engendered by treatment with antibiotics which may suppress but not eradicate infection.

The general principles of management of hand infections are quite straightforward and comprise:

1. rest in the position of immobilization
2. elevation to minimize oedema
3. appropriate antibiotic treatment
4. surgical drainage of localized pus
5. rehabilitation when the infection is under control.

Antibiotics
Most infections are due to penicillin-resistant staphylococci. Until the organism has been cultured and identified it is appropriate to treat the patient with a broad-spectrum antibiotic that is active against penicillinase-producing organisms. Anaerobic bacteria are a particular problem with human bites and an appropriate agent should be added to the antibiotic regime. Antibiotic treatment should be continued until after the patient begins to regain active, pain-free hand movements.

Surgical treatment
If there is a localized abscess it must be drained surgically by the most direct route. Adequate anaesthesia and a bloodless field are both essential for any drainage operation. Without them adequate exploration of the abscess cavity is impossible and there is a distinct risk of overlooking a 'collar stud' extension of the abscess.

Subcuticular infections

Septic blisters
These are common on the palmar surface of the fingers and in the finger webs. The epidermis becomes elevated by a collection of pus within the layers of the skin. The raised epidermis may be shaved off with a scalpel. A careful search must be made for any track leading to a deeper abscess which must be explored and laid open.

Paronychia
This is an infection of the nail fold (Fig. 8.44). Mild

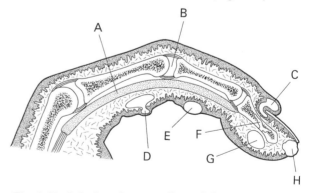

Fig. 8.44   Infections that may affect a digit:
A. Tendon sheath infection
B. Septic arthritis
C. Paronychia
D. Subcuticular abscess with subcutaneous 'collar stud' extension
E. Subcuticular abscess
F. Osteomyelitis
G. Pulp space infection
H. Apical pulp space infection

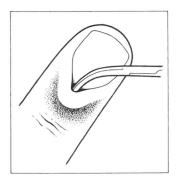

Fig. 8.45   Paronychia. Pus is drained by separating the nail fold from the nail with artery forceps

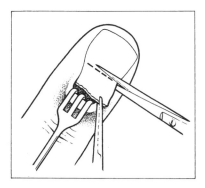

Fig. 8.46   Paronychia. If infection has extended beneath the nail, part of it must be removed to ensure free drainage

cases can be aborted by antibiotic treatment; if this is unsuccessful or too late, pus will collect deep to the nail or spread around it in a horseshoe fashion. Pus under the nail is drained by removing an appropriate amount of the proximal part of the nail (Figs 8.45 & 8.46). Part of the nail fold must be lifted as a flap to gain access.

Carbuncles in the hand

Like carbuncles elsewhere, these result from a staphylococcal infection of hair follicles and therefore occur on the dorsum of the hand or the proximal segments of the fingers. They respond well to antibiotic treatment and surgical intervention should be restricted to the removal of any sloughing tissue.

Subcutaneous infections

Pulp space infections

The three pulp spaces on the flexor aspect of the fingers are separated by the flexor creases where the skin is attached to the underlying fibrous flexor sheath. The fatty tissue in the terminal space is subdivided into 15–20 compartments by fibrous septa between the skin and the periosteum of the terminal phalanx. Infection

in the terminal pulp space therefore does not spread down the finger, but causes a rapid build up of pressure which may be associated with sloughing of the overlying skin and osteomyelitis of the terminal phalanx. Necrosis of the terminal phalanx is not unusual and is probably secondary to bone infection, although thrombosis of vessels due to pressure or bacterial toxins may be involved.

In the early acute phase antibiotic treatment is often successful. If localization of pus occurs, indicated by persistent pain, localized tenderness and perhaps subcuticular pointing of pus, then it should be drained by the shortest route. An 0.5 cm incision is made over the most tender point (Fig. 8.47) and deepened until pus is encountered. Extensive incisions are unnecessary but the original incision may have to be extended to allow thorough exploration and drainage of the cavity. Sloughing tissue may be excised but only obviously dead, sequestrated bone fragments should be removed.

An apical abscess is a special type of pulp infection. Infection is localized to the area under the free margin of the nail, just dorsal to the tip of the phalanx (see Fig. 8.44). Treatment consists of evacuating the pus through a small incision over the most tender point. If there is much pus under the nail a triangular segment

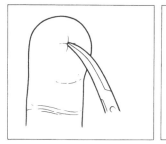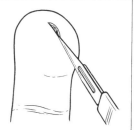

a

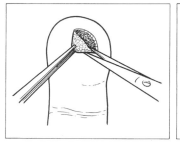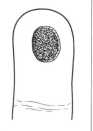

b

Fig. 8.47   Terminal pulp space infection. The point of maximum tenderness is found by clinical examination. An incision is made at this point. The wound may be enlarged by removal of skin to ensure that there is a cavity that can drain freely

should be removed, as in the treatment of a retained splinter beneath the nail (p. 178).

Infection in the middle and proximal pulp spaces is less common than in the terminal space. The spaces are bounded, but not entirely closed, by attachments of the skin creases to the fibrous flexor sheaths and laterally by fascial attachments between the skin and the phalanges; they are not subdivided by fibrous septa. Localized pus, which can track to the web spaces, should be drained by a longitudinal incision over the point of maximum tenderness, or where there is visible pointing.

Web space infections

The space between the bases of the fingers communicates with the dorsum of the hand and proximal pulp spaces of the fingers via loose connective tissue at the side of the fingers. Infection in these areas can spread to the web spaces, or the spaces may become infected directly from an abrasion on the overlying skin.

In the early stages the infection is in the nature of a diffuse cellulitis which may resolve with antibiotic therapy. Later the adjacent fingers are separated by the swollen web, which bulges out both palmwards and dorsally, and adjacent web spaces may become involved.

Any drainage operation should be delayed until the infection is localized, and then the abscess should be drained by the most direct route, usually a short transverse incision on the palmar surface about 1 cm proximal to the web margin (Fig. 8.48). Forceps are inserted and opened to allow the pus to drain. If the incision is kept short it is most unlikely that the digital nerves and vessels will be injured.

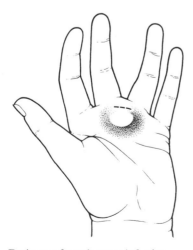

Fig. 8.48 Drainage of a web space infection

Tendon sheath infection

The synovial sheath of the flexor tendon is usually infected by direct puncture wounds, particularly where the skin is in close contact with the sheath at the skin creases, but infection may also spread into it from adjacent lesions.

The synovial sheaths surround the flexor tendons within the fibrous flexor sheaths; those of the index, middle and ring fingers end proximally at about the level of the metacarpophalangeal joints, but the sheath of the thumb is continuous with the radial bursa, and that of the little finger with the ulnar bursa (Fig. 8.49). The ulnar bursa is the name given to the synovial sheath that surrounds all the tendons passing to the fingers in the palms; it extends about 2.5 cm proximal to the wrist joint. There is usually a communication between the radial and ulnar bursae, deep to the flexor retinaculum. There is therefore a potential risk of infections in the tendon sheaths of the little finger and thumb spreading proximally to the palm and forearm.

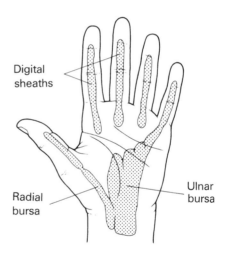

Fig. 8.49 The synovial sheaths in the hand

In an established, untreated tendon sheath infection there is severe, throbbing pain and swelling of the finger which takes up a slightly flexed position. Passive movements cause severe pain. This clinical presentation is considerably modified by antibiotic treatment: swelling is not marked and limited passive and active flexion may be possible without pain. However there is usually localized tenderness along the sheath and passive *extension* of the proximal interphalangeal joint causes pain.

When the ulnar bursa is infected there is swelling of the whole hand, often extending above the wrist. The fingers are characteristically held in a semiflexed position and passive extension causes severe pain.

Compression of the median nerve in the carpal tunnel also contributes to the pain. Infection of the thumb and radial bursa causes swelling of the thumb and thenar eminence, and the thumb is held slightly flexed.

Surgical exploration is indicated for any tendon sheath infection that has not settled completely after 48 hours of adequate antibiotic treatment. The fibrous sheath is exposed through volar incisions placed at the entrance of the sheath and the distal skin crease of the finger (Fig. 8.50). A 1 mm diameter catheter is threaded up the sheath from the proximal incision and the sheath is thoroughly irrigated with normal saline. The hand is splinted in the position of immobilization in a boxing glove dressing, the irrigation is continued and antibiotics are given systemically. If the ulnar bursa is infected it should be explored through a longitudinal incision on the volar aspect of the wrist, care being taken not to cross the wrist at a right angle (Fig. 8.50). The flexor retinaculum is divided, carefully protecting the median nerve, to expose the ulnar bursa which should be opened and irrigated. The radial bursa is approached through an incision on the ulnar border of the tendon of flexor carpi radialis, with careful identification and retraction of the median nerve. The distended radial bursa is identified, opened and an irrigation catheter passed into it.

It is rare now to encounter extensive sloughing of the flexor tendons due to delay in treatment. When it occurs amputation of the finger should be considered because permanent stiffness is inevitable and may well compromise the function of other fingers.

Septic arthritis in the hand

Infection of interphalangeal and metacarpophalangeal joints may be due to extension of infection from surrounding soft tissues, or follow penetrating injuries of the joint (p. 178). Wounds of the knuckle sustained by contact with an adversary's teeth are particularly dangerous.

In the early stages infection is confined to the synovial membrane and splintage, elevation and antibiotic treatment may be sufficient to control it. However, infections are seldom encountered at this early stage and it is safer to recommend exploration of all penetrating injuries under antibiotic cover. The extensor tendon is retracted or, if it has been partially divided, the wound is extended to allow a clear view of the joint. Any fragment of bone and cartilage is lifted out and the joint is thoroughly irrigated with normal saline. The wound is left open and the hand is splinted until the infection has settled. Thereafter active movements are commenced.

Infections of the palmar spaces

The *palmar subaponeurotic space* (or superficial middle palmar space) lies deep to the palmar aponeurosis and superficial to the flexor tendons (Fig. 8.51). It contains the superficial palmar arch and the digital branches of the median and ulnar nerves.

The *ulnar and radial bursae* have already been described.

The *midpalmar space* extends between the little and ring finger metacarpal bones and lies between the interossei and the ulnar bursa (Fig. 8.51). The tendon

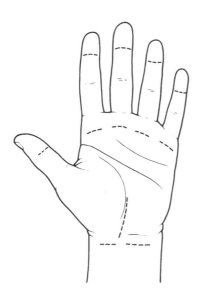

Fig. 8.50 Incisions for drainage of synovial sheaths in the hand

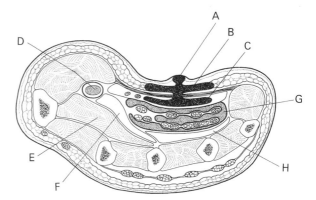

Fig. 8.51 A transverse section through the proximal part of palm:
A. Subcuticular palmar abscess
B. Subcutaneous palmar abscess
C. Subaponeurotic palmar abscess
D. Flexor pollicis longus tendon in radial bursa
E. Adductor pollicis
F. Thenar space
G. Ulnar bursa
H. Deep palmar space

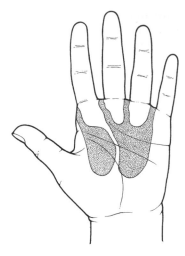

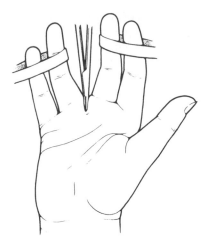

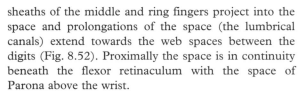

Fig. 8.52   The thenar and middle palmar spaces are extended to the web spaces by the lumbrical canals

Fig. 8.53   Draining the middle palmar space along a lumbrical canal

sheaths of the middle and ring fingers project into the space and prolongations of the space (the lumbrical canals) extend towards the web spaces between the digits (Fig. 8.52). Proximally the space is in continuity beneath the flexor retinaculum with the space of Parona above the wrist.

The *thenar space* lies deep to the thenar muscles and superficial to adductor pollicis (Fig. 8.51). It is separated from the mid-palmar space by a septum which extends from the long finger metacarpal bone. A lumbrical canal extends from the space towards the radial border of the index finger (Fig. 8.52). The tendon sheath of the index finger communicates with the space.

Infection of the palmar subaponeurotic space is not uncommon and is usually secondary to an abrasion or penetrating wound of the palm. When pus is localized in the palm it must be drained and a careful search made for any connection with another, deeper collection since 'collar stud' abscesses are often found in this region (Fig. 8.51). It is now extremely uncommon to encounter infections of the deep palmar spaces. They are usually secondary to spread of infection from appropriate tendon sheaths, or a web space infection tracking down a lumbrical canal. The characteristic sign of deep infection is loss of the normal concavity of the palm, together with swelling of the dorsum of the hand. Passive movements of the fingers are limited and extremely painful. Localization of pus usually becomes evident by tracking to the surface of the palm or one of the webs. The midpalmar space is drained through one of the appropriate lumbrical canals (Fig. 8.53) and the thenar space via the lumbrical canal on the radial border of the index finger; if pus points elsewhere it may be drained directly.

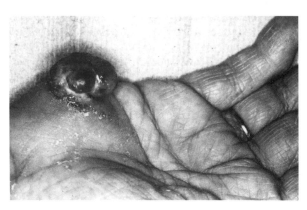

Fig. 8.54   Pyogenic granuloma

Other infections

Cellulitis and lymphangitis. These are usually due to streptococcal infection and are spreading infections that usually do not localize. As there is no local collection of pus, drainage is not needed. Indeed, surgical interference is positively dangerous and may cause further spread of infection. Treatment is by rest, elevation and antibiotics.

Pyogenic granuloma. This lesion is the result of an abnormal response to a minor penetrating injury. An infected mass of granulation tissue appears at the site of the injury (Fig. 8.54). It is painful and bleeds easily. Treatment is by excision, ensuring that any subcutaneous extension of the granuloma is removed.

CONGENITAL ANOMALIES OF THE HAND

Malformations of the hand are not particularly uncommon, occurring in about 1 per 1000 live births.

Many different types of anomalies are seen and, rather than attempting to be comprehensive, this section will deal with the principles of their management. The role of surgical treatment, rather than details of surgical operations, will be described.

Classification

Deformities may be:

1. isolated, affecting only the hand and upper limb
2. associated with other congenital anomalies, perhaps together recognized as a malformation syndrome
3. associated with a generalized skeletal dysplasia.

Many deformities have no genetic basis (e.g. those associated with thalidomide ingestion during pregnancy) but others have a very clear cut inheritance. It is most important for the parents to have advice from a clinical geneticist on the pattern of inheritance, if any, of the congenital deformity affecting the child.

In describing the deformity it is best to keep to a very simple overall classification of types. One such, used by many hand surgeons, is given in Table 8.1, together with examples of some of the many anomalies.

Principles of management

Because of the relative rarity of individual anomalies it is important that children with these conditions are

Table 8.1 Classification of congenital anomalies of the hand

Type	Example
Failure of formation of parts	
i. Transverse	Congenital absence of forearm and hand
ii. Longitudinal	Absence of radius and thumb ('Radial club hand')
Failure of separation of parts	Syndactyly (fused fingers)
Duplication	Polydactyly (extra digits)
Overgrowth	Macrodactyly (isolated overgrowth of a digit)
Congenital constriction band syndrome	Partial amputation or annular grooves
Associated with skeletal dysplasias	Multiple enchondromatosis (Ollier's disease) often affects the hands
	The hand is abnormally shaped in many skeletal disorders, e.g. Marfan's syndrome, achondroplasia
Miscellaneous (conditions not classifiable elsewhere)	Camptodactyly (contractures of the IP joints)
	Clinodactyly (congenital lateral curvature of the little finger)

seen by a surgeon with appropriate special experience, preferably soon after birth. Many congenital anomalies of the hand do not require, or are not amenable to, any form of surgical treatment and in any case the need for surgery is seldom pressing; however it is important to establish an early relationship with the parents and to advise them on the likely programme of management for their child.

The aim of surgical treatment is to improve hand function; surgery to improve appearance is undertaken only if there will be no deterioration in function. The goal of reconstruction is a hand that has active pinch and grasp; good skin sensation is fundamental to this. Prolonged, careful observation of the use the child makes of his limb is necessary before any decision about surgery can be made, and here the help of an occupational therapist with special interest and experience in this field can be invaluable. Children are able to develop extremely useful patterns of function even in the presence of severe anomalies.

Timing of surgery

Soft tissue procedures, such as removing a useless floating extra digit, can be done at an early age but sometimes more complicated soft tissue operations (such as separating a syndactyly) are best left until the hand is larger as this makes any surgery much easier. Bone and joint procedures and tendon transfers (which may be required for example in providing a thumb) should be delayed for the same reason; however, if the proposed surgery is likely to alter the pattern of prehension it should not be long delayed as it is more difficult for the older child to develop a new pattern of prehension. Generally speaking, it is desirable to have all major procedures completed before the child is due to go to school for the first time as by then he has established a pattern of use of the hand and disruption of education should be kept to a minimum.

DUPUYTREN'S CONTRACTURE

Dupuytren's disease is a proliferative disorder of the palmar and digital fascia in the hand, and occasionally affects the planter fascia in the foot. It is extremely common in middle-aged and elderly people in Britain and many other countries where population is of mainly European origin, but rarely affects Chinese, Indian or African people. A fairly strong autosomal dominant pattern of inheritance has been demonstrated in a proportion of patients in several studies. There is probably an association with some other disorders, notably epilepsy, alcoholic cirrhosis and diabetes, but the link is not clear. The disease is equally common in manual and non-manual workers, but injury may occasionally cause progression of the disease in someone who is prone to develop it. Women are affected less often than men.

The characteristic early lesion is a collection of fibroblasts and contractile myofibroblasts in the longitudinal fibres of the fascia, or between the fascia and the skin, forming a nodule. Nodules coalesce to form cords of fibrous tissue extending into the fingers. Shortening of these cords causes contractures of the fingers.

Clinical features

The ulnar part of the hand is most often affected, although thumb involvement is not rare. Early nodules are often uncomfortable and their removal may be requested for this reason. However surgical removal is often followed by rapid recurrence and progression to contracture. It is preferable to inject the lesion with a long-acting corticosteroid preparation, which often relieves the discomfort. The same management is recommended for the fibrofatty pads (Garrod's pads, Fig. 8.55) sometimes seen on the dorsum of the proximal interphalangeal joints in young patients who have a strong likelihood of developing Dupuytren's disease in later life.

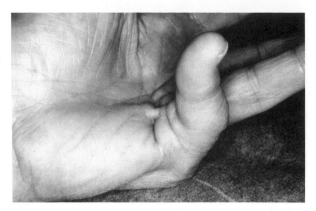

Fig. 8.56 Dupuytren's contracture. There is a 90° flexion contracture of the metacarpophalangeal joint of the little finger

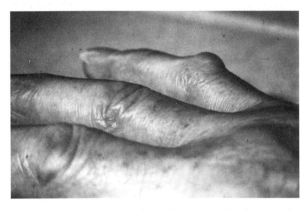

Fig. 8.55 A knuckle pad (Garrod's pad) on the dorsum of the proximal interphalangeal joint of the little finger

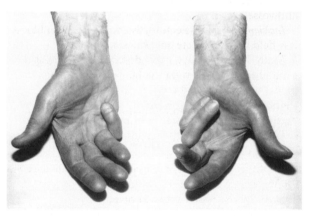

Fig. 8.57 Dupuytren's contracture. Severe contractures of the proximal interphalangeal joints of fingers in both hands

If cords of affected fascia are confined to the palm, finger contractures do not occur. It is only when they pass into the fingers that shortening of the cords is likely to pull the fingers into flexion. If the metacarpophalangeal joint is pulled into flexion (Fig. 8.56) a secondary joint contracture is very unlikely to develop, since the tethering band still allows further active flexion, thus bringing the capsular ligaments of the MCP joint to their full length (see 'Position of Immobilization', p. 173). In contrast if the proximal interphalangeal joints are pulled into flexion by their tethering cords (Fig. 8.57) secondary joint contractures

rapidly occur, for the cord prevents the PIP joint being put in full extension, the position in which the capsular ligaments are at full length. These points are of great importance in predicting the likely results of fasciectomy.

Treatment

The treatment of established Dupuytren's contracture is surgical. The type of operation, and its timing, should be decided on an individual basis.

Timing

The rate of increase of contractures is very variable; in some patients it remains static for many years and in others becomes severe within a few months. Surgery should be carried out before secondary joint contractures have developed. Thus there is no urgency when the MCP joint alone is affected, since secondary contractures do not occur and a good correction can always be obtained, but if the PIP joint is involved surgery should not be long delayed for secondary joint contractures may result in a permanent flexion contracture, even after removal of the involved fascia.

Types of operation

Local fasciectomy is the treatment of choice. Recovery is rapid after this procedure, in which only the affected, abnormal fascia is removed. *Radical fasciectomy,* i.e. removal of all fascia, normal and abnormal, is no longer practised; it is followed by severe swelling and stiffness of the hand and the overall results are poor. *Subcutaneous fasciotomy* is seldom done although it has a small place in the management of elderly unfit patients with a single longitudinal cord causing flexion of the MCP joint. The cord is cut with a tenotomy knife in the palmar region; it is risky to cut the cord in the finger because of the close relationship of the digital nerves and vessels to it.

Incisions. Local fasciectomy is carried out in a bloodless field with adequate anaesthesia.

Many incisions have been described and most surgeons have their own particular favourites. The main points to bear in mind are:

1. The cords of abnormal tissue must be adequately exposed.

2. The principles of siting scars on the hand described on page 173 must be observed.

3. There is no single method of dealing with Dupuytren's contracture because the extent and severity vary so much between patients.

4. Skin flaps must be made as thick as possible, but one should be aware of the fact that the digital nerves and vessels may lie superficial to affected fascia in the finger. Therefore a direct cut down on to the fascia must be avoided and the flaps must be raised from it with due care.

The most frequently used incisions are illustrated in Figure 8.58. A single cord may be dissected out through a longitudinal incision from the palm to the finger, which is closed with Z-plasties. A good, simple exposure is provided by the volar zig-zag incision. Mid-lateral incisions in the fingers are preferred by some, but the exposure is not so good. If a wider exposure of the palmar fascia is needed a transverse incision is placed in the distal palmar crease, and this can be combined with incisions entering the fingers. At the end of the procedure the transverse palmar wound is left open, thus allowing any haematoma to drain freely; recovery is rapid and painfree. The transverse wound closes quickly, leaving a fine scar.

The thickened fascia is readily identified both by vision and touch as the tissue is hard and tough. The affected fascia is defined by combination of sharp and

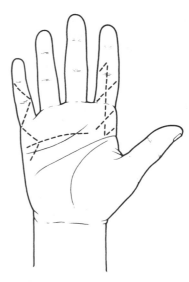

Fig. 8.58 Incisions used for partial fasciectomy. A volar zig-zig incision provides good exposure and may be combined with a transverse palmar incision when a wider exposure of the palmar fascia is needed. Many surgeons use a longitudinal incision to expose the abnormal fascia and then break up the incision with multiple Z-plasties

blunt dissection, care being taken to identify and protect digital vessels and nerves. Following excision of the involved tissue the tourniquet can be released to allow identification and coagulation of any small bleeding vessels. Many surgeons do not release the tourniquet at this point, but rely on careful identification and coagulation of vessels during dissection to ensure haemostasis. The results of both techniques are probably equally good.

Postoperative management

The hand is placed in a boxing glove dressing with a dorsal back slab and kept elevated to minimize swelling. After a few days the dressings are removed and mobilization is started under the supervision of a physiotherapist. A night splint to keep the MCP joints and IP joints extended is worn for several weeks.

Recurrence. Recurrence should be distinguished from extension, which is development of the disease elsewhere in the hand. It is not uncommon, particularly in young patients with a strong diathesis. It is usually apparent within 2 years of operation. Treatment is by further fasciectomy. If the skin is involved, as it usually is, it is necessary to excise the overlying skin and replace it with a full thickness free skin graft taken from the inner aspect of the upper arm. Recurrence under such a graft is uncommon.

Amputation. Amputation of a finger is rarely indicated as a primary treatment but is sometimes requested by a patient who has had several operations for recurrent disease in a finger. Dorsal skin from an amputated finger can be used to replace involved skin in the palm. Recurrence is uncommon beneath the transferred skin.

SURGERY OF THE ARTHRITIC HAND

The hand can be affected by many types of arthritis, the most frequently encountered being osteoarthritis, rheumatoid arthritis and psoriatic arthropathy.

Osteoarthritis

In the hand this typically affects the distal interphalangeal joints and the trapeziometacarpal joint at the base of the thumb.

Distal interphalangeal joints
Osteoarthritic lipping of the distal interphalangeal joints is manifested as Herberden's nodes. Pain is often slight despite advanced arthritic changes on radiographs (Fig. 8.59). If pain is a problem arthrodesis of the affected joint is indicated (see below).

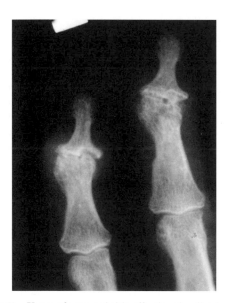

Fig. 8.59 X-ray of osteoarthritis affecting the distal interphalangeal joints

Occasionally a ganglion (or 'mucous cyst') arises from the dorsum of an osteoarthritic interphalangeal joint, and typically lies to one or other side of the extensor tendon. Successful removal is by no means easy and operation is only indicated if the ganglion is very large or otherwise troublesome. The neck of the ganglion must be dissected down to the joint and removed. Abnormally thin skin over the lesion should be

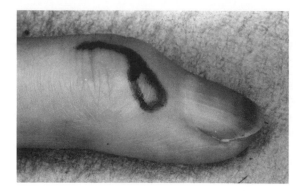

Fig. 8.60 Removal of a mucous cyst. Abnormal skin over the cyst should be removed and the defect closed by advancing a flap of normal skin

excised and a local rotation flap used to close the defect (Fig. 8.60). Unless these precautions are taken recurrence or a synovial fistula can occur. Arthrodesis of the joint may be necessary to control the latter.

Arthrodesis of an IP joint. The use of interosseous wiring is recommended for arthrodesis of the IP joints and the MCP joints of the thumb. (As noted previously, arthrodesis of the MCP joints of fingers is very disabling and should not be done.)

The distal IP joint is approached through an H-shaped incision on the dorsum of the finger, the proximal IP joint through a curved dorsal skin incision with reflection of the extensor tendon. Collateral ligaments are divided to allow complete dislocation of the joints and careful removal of all articular cartilage; the normal configuration of the joint surfaces should be maintained to allow contact of cancellous bone. Using a 0.035″ Kirschner wire on a power drill, two parallel holes are drilled 0.5 cm either side of the joint. A loop

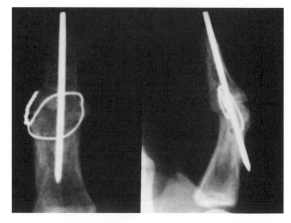

Fig. 8.61 X-ray showing arthrodesis of an interphalangeal joint. Intraosseous wiring is a very reliable method

of No. 0 (BS Gauge 26) monofilament stainless steel wire is passed through the holes. A 0.035″ diameter Kirschner wire is then driven retrograde from the joint and then, whilst holding the bones in contact at the desired angle, back across the joint. The wire loop is then tightened and its twisted end buried in soft tissue. Very stable fixation is obtained with this technique (Fig. 8.61). The longitudinal wire should remain in place for about 6 weeks.

Recommended angles for arthrodesis are shown in Table 8.2.

Table 8.2   Recommended angles for arthrodesis

Thumb	MCPJ	20°	IPJ	10–20°
Index finger	PIPJ	20°	DIPJ	10°
Middle finger	PIPJ	30°	DIPJ	10–20°
Ring finger	PIPJ	40°	DIPJ	15–30°
Little finger	PIPJ	50°	DIPJ	20–40°

Trapeziometacarpal joint of thumb (Fig. 8.62)
Osteoarthritis of this joint most often affects middle-aged women, causing pain and sometimes a progressive adduction deformity of the metacarpal bone of the thumb. Surgical treatment is indicated only if conservative treatment, in the form of anti-inflammatory analgesics, local steroid injections, or rest in plaster, have been unsuccessful. Several different operations are available.

Arthrodesis. This procedure is not recommended. It is technically difficult to obtain a surgical fusion of

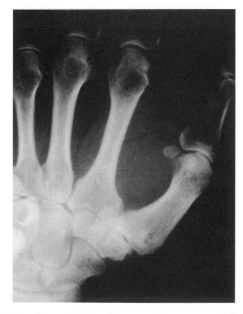

Fig. 8.62   Osteoarthritis of the trapeziometacarpal joint of the thumb

this joint. Even if the joint is fused pain may not be relieved as often adjacent joints are affected by early osteoarthritis which may progress and become symptomatic once the trapeziometacarpal joint is immobilized.

Osteotomy. This is a very simple procedure. A dorsally based wedge of bone is removed from the metacarpal bone about 1 cm from the joint. The osteotomy is closed and held with an intraosseous loop of wire (Fig. 8.63).

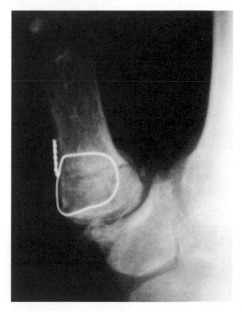

Fig. 8.63   Metacarpal osteotomy for trapeziometacarpal osteoarthritis of the thumb

Arthroplasty. Excision arthroplasty involves removal of the trapezium. Pain relief is good, but the thumb tends to be weak in gripping. The bone is approached by a transverse incision at the base of the metacarpal. It is important to avoid damage to the terminal branches of the radial nerve. The radial artery is identified where it courses across the anatomical snuff-box and is carefully protected. The trapezium should be removed in one piece by sharp division, under direct vision, of the capsular and ligamentous structure attached to it.

The excised trapezium may be replaced by an 'anchovy' of rolled tendon, usually a strip of flexor carpi radialis, or a silicone rubber spacer; these are forms of interposition arthroplasty. Total replacement of the trapeziometacarpal joint with a miniature artificial ball and socket joint has been described but is still under evaluation.

Rheumatoid arthritis

The surgery of the hand affected by rheumatoid arthritis is a highly specialized field which is more properly

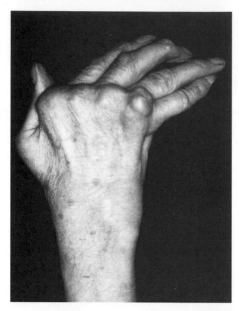

Fig. 8.64 Rheumatoid arthritis. Ulnar deviation of the fingers and subluxation of the metacarpophalangeal joints. (Reproduced with permission from Lamb & Hooper, 1985)

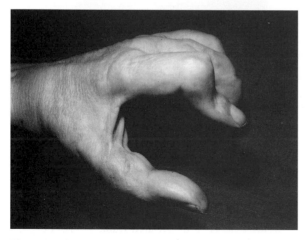

Fig. 8.65 Rheumatoid arthritis. Boutonnière deformity caused by rupture of the central slip of the extensor apparatus over the proximal interphalangeal joint

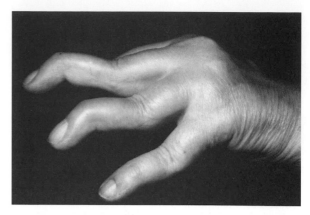

Fig. 8.66 Rheumatoid arthritis. Swan-neck deformity of several fingers

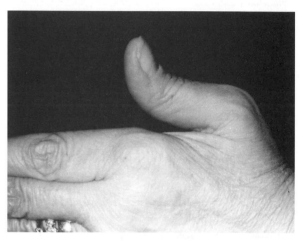

Fig. 8.67 Rheumatoid arthritis. Z-deformity of the thumb. (Reproduced with permission from Lamb & Hooper, 1985)

covered in detailed texts to which the reader is referred (Flatt, 1983; Green, 1982). However, because the condition is so common, some general principles of surgical management are given here.

The aim of surgical treatment of the hand affected by rheumatoid arthritis is to relieve pain and improve function. A deformed hand is not in itself an indication for operation. As with congenital hand anomalies, careful assessment of the patient's capabilities by an occupational therapist with particular experience of the condition is always necessary before embarking on reconstructive surgery. Provision of simple aids for everyday activities may achieve far more than any surgical operation.

The common problems associated with the rheumatoid hand and their surgical treatments are listed in Table 8.3. Several procedures may be needed in the same hand and careful planning is necessary. It is preferable to carry out several small procedures, rather than combine them as one major hand reconstruction. If multiple operations are needed they should commence with simple, usually highly successful procedures, rather than complex ones requiring a lot of effort and determination on the part of the patient in the rehabilitation period. The following sequence is recommended:

1. dorsal wrist surgery
2. flexor tendon surgery

Table 8.3 Surgical treatment of rheumatoid arthritis in the hand

Problem	Operation
Wrist	
Synovial proliferation beneath extensor retinaculum	Synovectomy or decompression of extensor compartment
Subluxation of head of ulna	Excision of head of ulna
Rupture of extensor tendons	Reconstruction by tendon transfer, grafting or suture to adjacent tendons
Painful unstable wrist	Arthrodesis
Carpal tunnel syndrome	Decompression of carpal tunnel
Flexor synovitis	Synovectomy
Metacarpophalangeal joints	
Instability and ulnar deviation (Fig. 8.64)	Arthroplasty and realignment of extensor apparatus
Fingers	
Flexor synovitis	Flexor synovectomy
Boutonnière deformity (Fig. 8.65) Swan neck deformity (Fig. 8.66)	Various procedures, depending on type and mobility of deformity
Unstable PIP joint	Arthrodesis
Thumb	
Rupture of extensor pollicis longus tendon	Tendon transfer using extensor indicis proprius
'Z' deformity (Fig. 8.67) Adduction deformity	Various procedures, depending on type and mobility of deformity

3. metacarpophalangeal joint surgery
4. proximal interphalangeal joint surgery and correction of other finger deformities
5. realignment of the thumb in the most useful position relative to the reconstructed fingers.

STENOSING TENOSYNOVITIS

In the condition of stenosing tenosynovitis there is some obstruction to the free movement of a tendon within its sheath, due either to a thickening of the tendon or to fibrosis and constriction in the sheath. The cause is not known, although trigger fingers are common in insulin-dependent diabetic patients. The synovitis, if present, may be secondary to the condition rather than its cause.

Trigger digit

The lesion consists of a swelling of the flexor tendons at the mouth of the fibrous flexor sheath, together with narrowing and thickening of the first (A1) pulley of the sheath. The powerful flexors can pull the thickened tendon proximal to the area of stenosis but the less powerful extensors are unable to straighten the digit which may lock in a position of acute flexion. The patient may have to straighten the digit passively, or it may straighten with a painful jerk, the discomfort often being felt at the proximal interphalangeal joint. A thickened and tender nodule can sometimes be palpated in the tendon.

The condition will often respond to an injection of cortisone and local anaesthetic into the sheath. The needle should be inserted from the lateral aspect of the digit at the level of the proximal phalanx and care should be taken not to inject into the tendon itself. Surgical decompression is indicated if the problem recurs or does not respond to injection and is carried out through a short transverse incision just distal to the distal transverse palmar skin crease. If the thumb flexor tendon is affected the incision is sited at the proximal flexor crease. Care is taken to identify and protect the digital nerves — this is particularly important in the case of trigger thumb in which the radial digital nerve crosses the sheath and is particularly vulnerable. The proximal pulley of the fibrous sheath is then incised longitudinally.

Congenital trigger thumb

This is a similar condition which occurs in infants. The child is noted to have a flexion deformity of the thumb and usually a large nodule is palpable in the flexor tendon. The condition may improve spontaneously or with splintage but if it does not, surgical release should be carried out at the age of 2–3 years.

De Quervain's syndrome

The first dorsal compartment of the extensor retinaculum, containing the extensor pollicis brevis and abductor pollicis longus tendons, is affected at the level of the radial styloid. The patient experiences localized pain at this site during movement of the thumb or when the wrist is ulnar deviated while the hand is gripping a heavy object, for example when pouring out tea. There is local tenderness and usually a swelling at the site of the lesion. Injection of hydrocortisone 25 mg into the tendon sheath may relieve a significant proportion of cases and is always worth a trial in the first instance. If this fails, surgical decompression is indicated.

A transverse or sinuous longitudinal incision is made over the lesion with great care being taken to preserve the cutaneous branches of the radial nerve which cross this incision. Injury to these nerves will cause more discomfort than the original condition. The thickened tendon sheath is then incised longitudinally and a strip of sheath is removed (Fig. 8.68). It is important to note that there may be subcompartments and multiple

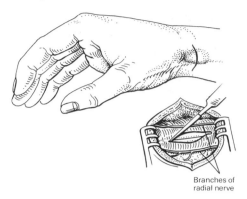

Fig. 8.68 Operation to release a De Quervain's lesion — note the proximity of the terminal branches of the radial nerve

tendons; a careful search must be made to ensure that decompression is complete.

TUMOURS IN THE HAND

Many of the common tumours found in the hand are not neoplastic in nature.

Ganglia

The pathogenesis of ganglia is unclear but they may be due to herniation of synovial tissue from joints or local degeneration of connective tissue. Common sites are the wrist on the dorsomedial and occasionally volar aspects. In the fingers pea-sized ganglia may be found attached to the proximal part of the fibrous flexor sheath.

Surgical treatment is recommended only if the lesion is large and unsightly or if its nature is uncertain, since most will disappear spontaneously and recurrence after excision is extremely common. An alternative to surgical removal is aspiration and multiple puncture with a wide-bore hypodermic needle and syringe, after local infiltration anaesthesia.

Ganglia should be excised in a bloodless field with adequate anaesthesia. The incision (usually a transverse one at the wrist) should be large enough to allow good exposure of the ganglion; cutaneous nerves must be protected when the skin is cut. It is important to trace the connection of the ganglion down to the wrist joint, to excise it and to leave the joint capsule open. Failure to remove the communication with the joint is followed by rapid recurrence.

Pigmented villonodular synovitis

This lesion, also known as 'giant cell tumour of the tendon sheath' is usually found in the middle-aged. It presents as a painless swelling on the flexor or extensor

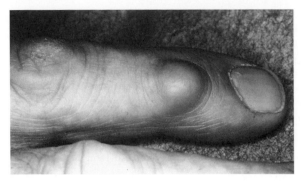

Fig. 8.69 Villonodular synovitis arising from the distal interphalangeal joint

aspect of the finger (Fig. 8.69). Sometimes erosion of the bone is seen on radiographs. The lesion is yellowish in colour and loosely encapsulated. Treatment is by excision which should be complete to prevent local recurrence.

Implantation dermoid

This cystic lesion contains solid material. It develops after the implantation of skin into subcutaneous tissue by minor trauma, and is common on the flexor aspects of the hand or fingers where the skin is heavily keratinized (Fig. 8.70). Removal of an implantation dermoid through a suitably placed incision presents no difficulty but care should be taken to remove the entire wall of the cyst.

Glomus tumour

This tumour arises from the glomus body and the most common site is in the terminal segment of the finger, often at the base of the nail. It is usually only a few millimetres in diameter and well encapsulated. The patient complains of pain, cold sensitivity and exquisite

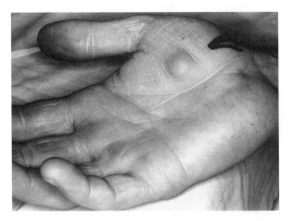

Fig. 8.70 Implantation dermoid

tenderness when the lesion is touched, to such an extent that examination of the finger may be refused. A subungual tumour may be visible as a purplish lesion under the nail but often the only clue to its presence is a distortion of the lunula. Exploration and complete excision is necessary and general anaesthesia is advisable. If the tumour is subungual, part of the nail must be removed to allow access.

Enchondroma

This is the most common bone tumour found in the hand and is usually asymptomatic. It may come to light because a pathological fracture occurs through the tumour. The fracture should be treated in the usual way and it is not uncommon for the lesion to heal completely thereafter. If it does not, or a further fracture occurs, the enchondroma should be thoroughly scraped out with a curette. Bone grafting is usually unnecessary (Figs 8.71 & 8.72).

Squamous carcinoma

The back of the hand is not an uncommon site for this tumour, especially in those exposed to sunlight or industrial irritants. Management is discussed on page 9.

Malignant melanoma

The hand is a relatively rare site for this tumour but when it does occur the thumb is most often involved and the lesion is usually subungual. It may fungate around the nail fold and then be mistaken for a chronic

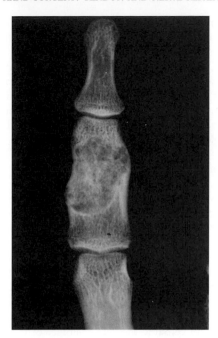

Fig. 8.72   After curettage the lesion has healed

nail bed infection and be treated inappropriately. The management is discussed on page 9.

MAJOR COMPLICATIONS IN HAND SURGERY

Even the simplest operation can end with major loss of hand function due to complications which are largely preventable.

Stiffness and joint contractures

These are almost invariably due to one or more of the following factors:

1. failure to control swelling of the hand (p. 174)
2. incorrect splintage (p. 173)
3. inadequate supervision or lack of patient co-operation during rehabilitation.

Reflex sympathetic dystrophy

This condition (also termed Sudeck's atrophy) is well known as a complication of fractures at the distal end of the radius, but it is not always realised that it can occur after any hand injury or operation. The cause is obscure although an abnormal response of the sympathetic nervous system to a painful stimulus has been suggested. A similar condition, usually termed *causalgia,* can occur after nerve injuries.

Clinical features

This condition is twice as common in women.

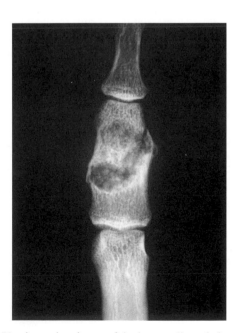

Fig. 8.71   An enchondroma of the intermediate phalanx. Note the fracture

Following operation the patient suffers from uncharacteristically severe pain and within a few days the hand becomes stiff. There are often skin changes with a glossy, puffy appearance to the hand which may have a blue or red colour. Any attempt to move the hand, whether actively or passively, causes further pain and is resisted. Untreated, the condition results in permanent stiffness, although there is a tendency to slow and incomplete improvement over many months.

Prevention

Careful post-operative supervision is essential. Patients who have undue pain after operation with no apparent cause are definitely at risk and their progress should be watched closely. Patients who are over-protective of their hand and reluctant to carry out mobilization exercises are another high-risk group. It must be emphasised that RSD occurs frequently after so-called 'minor' procedures, such as carpal tunnel decompression or release of trigger digits, that are usually done as out patient procedures. A patient who has had such a procedure remains the responsibility of the surgeon until the wound has healed and the hand is fully mobile.

Treatment

It is most important to recognize the condition early before the hand has become stiff. At this stage it is often possible to prevent the full-blown condition provided the patient can be encouraged to mobilize the hand. Admission to hospital is mandatory so that pain can be controlled with non-addictive analgesics and supervised physiotherapy commenced. Stellate ganglion blocks and guanethidine regional intravenous blocks are extremely useful in controlling pain.

Compartment syndrome

A compartment syndrome occurs when increased pressure within a limited tissue space impairs the circulation to tissues within the space. The tissue space is usually a fascial compartment of a limb, containing muscles, blood vessels and nerves. In the upper limb the flexor compartment of the forearm is most often involved, but the intrinsic muscles of the hand can also be affected. Muscles and nerves will be irreversibly damaged within a few hours unless circulation is restored. Late fibrosis of the forearm muscles causes the characteristic deformity of *Volkmann's ischaemic contracture* (Fig. 8.73).

Pressure within a compartment can be increased by external causes, such as crushing injuries, tight plaster casts or dressings, or by an increase in volume of tissue within the compartment. The latter may occur after trauma which causes tissue damage or bleeding within the compartment or following reperfusion after a

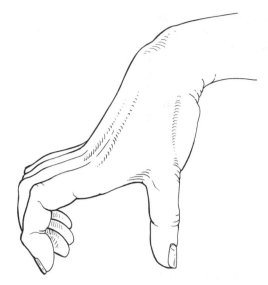

Fig. 8.73 Volkmann's contracture of the flexor muscles of the forearm is the late result of untreated compartment syndrome. There are permanent flexion contractures of the wrist and interphalangeal joints and inability to grip

period of ischaemia, for example when circulation is restored after arterial repair or removal of a tourniquet. Once the pressure rises sufficiently to occlude the microcirculation there will be further ischaemia and swelling, promoting a vicious circle of rising intra-compartmental pressure and tissue damage.

It is important to realise that a compartment syndrome can occur even though the peripheral pulses are intact. The microcirculation is occluded by a relatively small increase in pressure whereas the major vessels running through a compartment are not occluded until the compartmental pressure exceeds systolic pressure.

Clinical features

The main symptom is severe, increasing pain which is resistant to analgesics. Active movements are avoided and passive movements, for example extending the fingers when the flexor compartment is involved, results in severe pain. The affected muscles may be clinically swollen and have a firm, 'woody' feel to touch. Loss of pain associated with paralysis of involved muscles is an ominous sign, usually indicating severe ischaemic damage to nerves and muscle necrosis.

Treatment

If there is the slightest suspicion of a compartment syndrome all dressings must be divided down to skin immediately. Unless there is complete relief of symptoms within a few minutes the skin and fascia over the compartment should be divided as a matter of urgency. In cases of doubt it is always safer to do a fasciotomy than to 'wait and see'.

To decompress the flexor aspect of the forearm a long incision is made from above the elbow, over the forearm in a curve and extending into the palm of the hand in the usual fashion for carpal tunnel decompression. The deep fascia and the carpal tunnel are divided. At this point the swollen muscles bulge from the wound and, provided the operation has been done in time, their colour rapidly returns to normal. No attempt should be made to close skin or fascia. The wound is simply dressed. A few days later the limb is inspected under general anaesthesia when it will be found that the muscle swelling has dramatically decreased. The wound can then be closed by a combination of suture and split skin grafting.

Compartment syndrome is much less common in the hand itself. Intrinsic muscles may be decompressed by direct incisions over the muscle compartments.

REFERENCES

Flatt A E 1983 Care of the arthritic hand, 4th edn. C V Mosby, St. Louis

Green D P 1982 Operative hand surgery. 2nd edn. Churchill Livingstone, New York

FURTHER READING

Flatt A E 1977 The care of congenital hand anomalies. C V Mosby, St. Louis

Flatt A E 1983 Care of the arthritic hand, 4th edn. C V Mosby, St. Louis

Green D P 1982 Operative hand surgery. 2nd edn. Churchill Livingstone, New York

Lamb D W, Hooper G 1985 Colour aids to hand conditions. Churchill Livingstone, Edinburgh

Lamb D W, Hooper G, Kuczynski K 1981 The practice of hand surgery, 2nd edn. Blackwell, Oxford

Lister G 1984 The hand. Diagnosis and indications, 2nd edn. Churchill Livingstone, Edinburgh

McFarlane R M 1987 Unsatisfactory results in hand surgery. Churchill Livingstone, Edinburgh

McFarlane R M, McGrouther D A, Flint M H 1990 Dupuytren's disease. Churchill Livingstone, Edinburgh

Spinner M 1978 Injuries to the major branches of the peripheral nerves of the forearm, 2nd edn. Saunders, Philadelphia

9

Amputations

J. CHRISTIE

INDICATIONS FOR AMPUTATIONS

Amputation of a limb or part of a limb is required when the vitality of the part is destroyed by injury or disease or when the life of the patient is threatened by the spread of a local condition. Amputation may also be desirable in patients with deformity or paralysis, where it is considered that the patient would be better served by an artificial limb. The decision to proceed to amputation is usually taken after careful consideration. Other alternatives may be available and many factors must be taken together in determining the most suitable management for the individual patient. Assessment on an inpatient basis is often helpful and the opinion of a specialist in some other field of endeavour may be invaluable. In considering the indications for amputation it is necessary to make a clear distinction between the upper and lower extremities. It is important to preserve stability and length in the lower limb and if these cannot be restored, the patient may well be better off with an artificial limb. Stability is not essential to useful function of the upper limb and even a grossly deformed or shortened arm may be preferable to a replacement prosthesis (Figs 9.1–9.3).

The majority of patients who come to amputation in Britain have vascular disease and of these some 20% have diabetes. Some 10% of patients lose a limb as a result of some other cause, most commonly injury. The majority require amputation of the lower extremity; a small and important group have loss of the upper extremity, occasionally bilateral. The amputation rate is 1 to 1.5 per 10 000 of population; 75% of the patients are aged 60 years or more.

Wounds and injuries

Amputation surgery is sometimes required after injury to a limb. This is usually only considered after the most serious kind of crushing force or when there is traumatic amputation with irretrievable damage to the blood vessels or to the nerve supply of the extremity. Occasionally massive loss of soft tissues or a combina-

tion of injury to bone and soft tissue may preclude limb salvage. Techniques of vessel and nerve repair in combination with planned reconstructive surgery to the bone and soft tissues allows the extremity to be saved except after the most mutilating of injuries. Re-attachment of the totally severed limb is now possible and should be practised when it is probable that the outcome will be superior to that offered by an artificial limb. In general, when there is sharp traumatic amputation, reattachment may be an entirely worthwhile procedure. This is particularly true in the upper extremity when amputation has occurred through the forearm or hand. Traumatic avulsion of a limb usually causes extensive soft tissue and nerve injury and reattachment is likely to be unrewarding.

Microsurgical techniques are also available: these allow small distal vessels to be anastomosed enabling the digits to be reattached after traumatic amputation. When there is significant crushing this is not likely to be successful but it is frequently well worth attempting to resuture the thumb or one or more of the fingers after sharp traumatic amputation particularly at a proximal level.

There are of course certain risks in attempting to preserve a severely mangled limb, particularly of infection — occasionally gas gangrene. Antibiotics given prophylactically will diminish the danger, although when devitalized tissue is present serious infection may still occur. Immunization against the anaerobic organisms is essential in these circumstances.

Vascular disease

The majority of patients who require amputation in Northern Europe and America have vascular disease. Many of these have widespread disease of the vascular tree with major vessel involvement. A relatively small number of patients, particularly those with diabetes, have peripheral arteriolar disease and consequently relatively localized peripheral ischaemic changes. In these circumstances it is often possible to contemplate one of the more conservative amputations.

Figs 9.1–9.3   Showing that the first metacarpal and little finger may allow a competent grip. This man returned to work as a miner after amputation during the First World War. Note the hypertrophy of the little finger (Redrawn from a patient of Mr James A Ross)

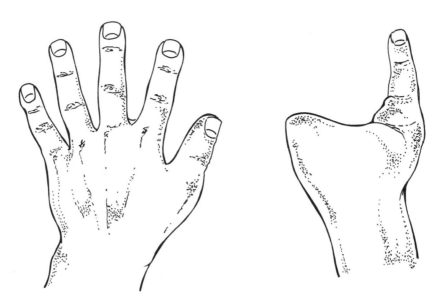

Fig. 9.1   Both hands for comparison following recovery from extensive injury on the right

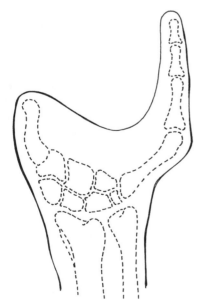

Fig. 9.2   Drawing from X-ray of right hand

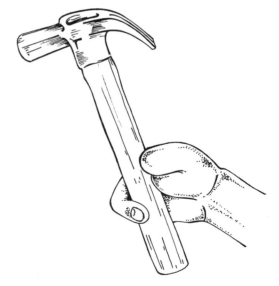

Fig. 9.3   Showing useful function

Infections

Acute infection

Certain acute infections such as gas gangrene can sometimes lead to the need for amputation surgery. Gas gangrene may occur after serious injury or open fracture particularly when there has been severe crush-ing and devitalization of the soft tissues. Gas gangrene also occurs occasionally after surgery to a limb that is severely affected by vascular disease.

Other fulminating infections, for instance severe in-fection in the finger, may occasionally cause extensive damage and require amputation of the digit.

Chronic infection

Chronic infection particularly of bone and joints may lead to amputation, especially if there is progressive deterioration in the general health or a threat of amyloid, both of which may occur as the result of prolonged suppuration. In the lower limbs the loss of function resulting from osteomyelitis or septic arthritis may be such that the patient would be better served by an artificial limb.

Malignant tumours

Certain tumours of the extremities may be treated most suitably by amputation in an attempt to achieve cure or in an attempt to relieve severe local symptoms. Carcinoma arising in the soft parts of the limb may sometimes necessitate amputation, especially if it has infiltrated so as to involve bone. The decision to amputate in the presence of malignant disease should be carefully taken and other available alternatives such as prosthetic skeletal replacement should be considered. (Some tumours such as osteosarcoma may sometimes be managed with reconstructive surgery, rather than by amputation. There is evidence now that the results of irradiation and chemotherapy in the management of Ewing's sarcoma may produce results that are not worse than those achieved after amputation surgery, irradiation and chemotherapy p. 145.)

Deformity

Deformity may be congenital or acquired. Acquired deformity is frequently the result of some underlying neurological disease such as cerebral palsy, myelomeningocele or infantile paralysis. Reconstructive surgery can achieve surprisingly good results in many conditions of this nature which were formally treated by amputation. Shortened bones may be lengthened, malalignment corrected and flail joints stabilized. Amputation is however appropriate if the patient is likely to be better served by an artificial limb. This is seldom true in congenital deformity of the upper extremity where reconstructive surgery is almost always preferable but in the lower limb amputation may be entirely appropriate when deformity is severe.

Congenital limb deficiency

Congenital absence of a limb or part of a limb may lead to the need for amputation or corrective surgery and prosthetic fitting. Congenital absence of the forearm and hand is the commonest deficiency of the upper limb requiring the provision of an artificial limb. Congenital amputation through the upper arm is less common and bilateral absence of the upper extremities is rare now that *Thalidomide* is no longer prescribed.

The focal femoral deficiencies, congenital absence of the fibula and more rarely absence of the tibia may lead to the need for amputation surgery in the lower limb. Congenital ring constriction also occurs and sometimes leads to amputation.

Gangrene

Gangrene occurs usually as the result of ischaemic disease of a limb or of serious infection. Massive gangrene is, of course, an absolute indication for amputation. In *dry gangrene*, which is usually the result of vascular disease, amputation may with advantage be delayed until a line of demarcation has formed. It may be found that the extent of gangrene is less than was suggested by the area of skin involvement, and by skin grafting methods it may be possible to conserve a little extra length of stump. In *moist gangrene*, which is usually infective in nature, especially the serious type known as gas gangrene, amputation is often a matter of considerable urgency (p. 170).

OPTIMUM LEVELS FOR AMPUTATION

The level at which an amputation should be carried out does not entirely depend upon the extent of the injury or disease. Consideration must be given also to the function desired in the remaining stump. This differs very markedly in the upper and in the lower limb. Even the most fragmentary portion of a hand is of much greater value to the patient than the best prosthesis, and every effort must be made to conserve as much tissue as possible. On the other hand, zealous attempts to preserve a seriously diseased foot may be misguided and amputation at an appropriate level is often to be preferred.

The great majority of patients who suffer amputation above the level of the wrist or ankle joint will eventually be fitted with an artificial limb, and their future activity and wellbeing depends largely upon the efficiency with which that limb can function. It is necessary therefore for the surgeon to work in close cooperation with the prosthetist in fashioning a stump to which the best possible prosthetic socket can be fitted. Many patients who come to amputation are old and will require amputation of the lower limb. It is important when possible to preserve the knee joint as very much less energy expenditure is required to walk with a below knee prosthesis than with amputation at the above knee level.

Up to a certain point a longer stump is preferable but too long a stump may be an encumbrance leaving a bony tip that is poorly protected by soft tissues. The prosthetist may also find it difficult to accommodate the longer stump and, in the lower limb, length discrepancy may be impossible to avoid. An amputation at

Table 9.1 Guidelines

Forearm	Optimum length of stump is 20 cm as measured from tip of olecranon. An 8 cm stump is the minimum for useful function. Between these levels as much bone as possible should be saved.
Upper arm	Optimum length of stump is 20 cm as measured from acromion. Above this level as much bone as possible should be saved.
Lower leg	*Syme's amputation.* The tibia and fibula are divided at or immediately above the level of the ankle joint. *Site of election.* Length of tibial stump is 14 cm. An 8 cm stump is the minimum for useful function (see p. 236). Between these levels as much bone as possible should be saved.
Thigh	Optimum length of stump is 25–30 cm, as measured from tip of trochanter. Above this level as much bone as possible should be saved.

the appropriate level on the other hand will provide a stump that is suitable for patient and prosthetist alike.

Certain optimum levels shown in Table 9.1 have been advocated though these should not be accepted too rigidly. Amputations at other levels may be appropriate and when necessary prosthetic design can be varied to accommodate most levels of amputation. A golden rule is that too low a level of amputation can be remedied; too high removal of a limb is beyond repair. Sometimes in older patients who have no prospect of walking a higher amputation usually at the above knee level is chosen to achieve rapid healing and an early return to the wheelchair. Amputation surgery may also be modified in underdeveloped countries to adapt to local circumstances, where only the most simple type of prosthesis is likely to be available.

Choice of level in vascular disease and diabetes

Vascular disease

The mortality rate after amputation for peripheral vascular disease is between 10 and 25%, and is higher with advancing age. One third of these patients will be dead after two years and two thirds will have died after five years (Warren, 1968). About 10% of the patients surviving each year after amputation will lose the remaining limb, slightly more during the first year after amputation. Of below knee amputees, 60% will make good use of their artificial limb compared with 40% of patients who have amputation at the above knee level. Walking metabolic expenditure after above knee amputation is some two times greater than that of a normal individual (Peizer, 1969). This compares with an increase in walking metabolic expenditure of about 20% after below knee amputation. It is hence abundantly clear that, wherever possible, below knee amputation is preferable to the above knee level. Ghormley (1947) described below knee amputation using a long

posterior flap. This has become popular recently and, partly because of its success, there has been an increasing tendency to attempt below knee amputation wherever possible. Some 75% of patients who come to amputation for vascular disease now have successful surgery at the below knee level.

Arteriography, thermography, Doppler instrumentation and dye attenuation studies as well as transcutaneous pO_2 measurements and clinical examination can be helpful in determining the level at which amputation will be successful.

Diabetes

Patients with diabetic gangrene of the lower limb or intractable infection frequently do not have extensive major vessel disease and a relatively conservative excision may be possible. A diabetic ulcer with underlying osteomyelitis may require local resection only. Amputation of one or more toes or ray resection in the fore part of the foot may be sufficient. When there is more extensive involvement transmetatarsal amputation or amputation of the toes may be indicated. Amputation through the midfoot level or Syme's amputation may also be appropriate.

When there is absence of peripheral pulses in diabetes, reconstructive vascular surgery may prevent the need for a more radical amputation, or may precede a relatively conservative operation in the foot.

Clinical examination of the peripheral pulses, skin viability, tissue turgor, nail growth, hair growth and distal sensation are all important in determining the level at which amputation will succeed in diabetes.

Choice of level in neoplastic disease

Occasionally a benign tumour causing great deformity may require amputation surgery. Large lymphatic malformations or angiomatous tumours fall into this category. When malignant disease is suspected, biopsy should be carefully interpreted before embarking upon definitive surgery. It is usually better to wait for paraffin sections than to rely on frozen section particularly when bone is involved. Since the site of the biopsy should not interfere with subsequent surgery, preliminary investigations such as CT scanning are essential.

Low grade tumours may require local ablation or block resection. Aggressive tumours such as osteosarcomata may require more radical removal. Advice from an oncologist may be useful. Secondary deposits can be effectively sought using isotope studies and CT scans.

Choice of level in children

Children usually require amputation as a result of trauma, malignant disease, congenital abnormalities or limb shortening. Growth of a limb after amputation in the child will be affected. After above knee amputation the major growing epiphysis of the femur is removed and very little increase in length will occur. It is therefore essential that as much length as possible is preserved, and if at all possible a through knee amputation is to be preferred. Growth in length of the stump is also diminished after below knee amputation as the proximal tibial epiphysis fails to contribute the expected amount of growth. It is therefore essential that 13 cm of tibia should be preserved if at all possible and the tibia may easily be shortened later if necessary. Proportionate amputation is therefore not appropriate in the child.

Bony overgrowth also occurs in the immature stump, such as the appositional new growth beyond the site of section of the tibia, fibula or femur. This bony overgrowth does not increase stump length significantly but periosteal spikes of new bone form beneath the tip of the stump and cause discomfort. Overgrowth is more common in the younger patient and frequently requires revisional surgery.

Syme's amputation is preferable to below knee amputation in children as the distal growing epiphysis of the tibia is preserved.

Site of amputation in the presence of skin loss

Occasionally there is extensive skin loss or degloving of skin after a severe crushing injury. It is important to realize that full thickness skin cover is not necessary over the entire stump area, and length may be preserved, even though it is necessary to contemplate skin grafting over some of the stump. This may be undertaken as a secondary procedure. Such a stump may prove to be remarkably durable despite fairly large areas of split skin graft cover.

Choice of level in the presence of sensory deficiency

Sensory deficiency of the foot frequently leads to indolent penetrating ulcers and metatarsal osteomyelitis. When intractable lesions of this nature are present amputation may be necessary. Syme's amputation may prove to be very successful despite sensory deficiency of the heel (Srinavasan, 1973). Stump care must however be meticulous. Midfoot amputation may also succeed in these circumstances provided that the heel skin is good and stump care is appropriate.

METHODS AND TECHNIQUE OF AMPUTATION

The stump

The optimum length for amputation stumps in different situations has already been discussed. The stump should be firm and smoothly rounded, and it should be conical in shape, tapering distally. Opposing groups of muscles should be fixed together over the end of the sectioned bone so that vascularity and muscular control of the stump may be maintained. Suture of the muscles over the divided bone in this way is known as *myoplasty* (Fig. 9.4). The opposing muscle groups may also be anchored to the divided bone by sutures passed through their substance and fixed through drill holes into the bone end (*myodesis*). Any muscle placed over the bone end is converted into fibrous tissue, but this serves as an effective cushion which protects the skin from pressure against the bone. The joint proximal to the amputation should have a full range of movement and contractures should be avoided if at all possible. The skin should be neatly cut and sutured without too much tension; there should be no folds or puckering and 'dogears' should be avoided. Skin should be freely moveable both on the bone and on the subcutaneous tissue. A terminal scar is satisfactory in the upper limb. It is less desirable in the lower limb though does not cause the patient much discomfort in a well manufactured socket.

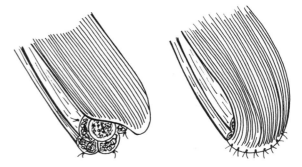

Fig. 9.4   Showing above knee myoplasty before and after suture

Bone should be sectioned carefully and rounded off so that there are no sharp edges. A bone file should be used for this purpose. The tip of the sectioned bone should be covered with a periosteal or osteoperiosteal flap to enhance the vascularity and weight bearing properties of the stump.

Methods of amputating

All amputations (except the guillotine method) are designed to provide the bone stump with an adequate covering of skin and soft tissues.

Guillotine amputation

This is the most primitive type of amputation. All tissues of the limb are divided at the same level, and the bone end is left exposed on the cut surface. This method is useful when the distal part of the limb is trapped (as by machinery or in mining accidents), and an amputation has to be carried out on the spot. It may be employed also in the presence of gross sepsis. As a rule reamputation must be performed at a higher level in order that the bone end may be covered with soft parts. The operation is now generally regarded as unsatisfactory, because, unless special precautions are taken, considerable retraction of the soft parts occurs and the exposed bone is very liable to secondary infection. Skin traction may be used in an attempt to prevent this.

Circular amputation

This should not be confused with the guillotine method. The skin and muscles are divided circularly, but at a lower level than the bone, so that they provide a covering for the bone stump. The proposed level of bone section is first determined and the circular skin incision is made at a distance below this equal to the diameter of the limb. When skin and subcutaneous tissues have been incised they are allowed to retract upwards, and then at the new level of the skin edge the muscles are divided down to the bone. A large scalpel or amputation knife is employed for division of the soft parts; it should be used with a sweeping circular motion, the blade being kept perpendicular to the surface of the bone. Retraction of the cut muscles then takes place, and is assisted by stripping the bone with an elevator until the level for section is exposed. The circular method is most suited to a cylindrical segment of a limb, e.g. the upper arm.

Amputation using a racquet incision

In this method a straight incision is carried proximally from a circular or elliptical incision. The method is used especially for disarticulation at the metacarpo or metatarsophalangeal joint, and is applicable also to a disarticulation at the shoulder and hip.

Amputation using flaps

This is the most widely used method of amputation. Either two flaps cut from opposite sides of the limb or a single flap may be used. In order that the bone may be adequately covered it is essential that the combined length of the two flaps, or the total length of a single flap, should be equal to 1½ times the diameter of the limb at the level of bone section. Each flap should be cut to a semicircular rather than a rectangular shape, since a conical and not a cylindrical stump is desired. Amputation at the below knee level in vascular disease is most suitably undertaken with a single long posterior flap or with a 'skewed' posterior flap. This provides a better blood supply than an anterior flap and its use appears to offer improved wound healing. When there is normal vascularity equal anterior and posterior flaps may be used or a long posterior flap to avoid terminal scarring.

When unequal flaps are used the shorter flap should be rather broader than the longer flap so that the skin edges to be sutured are of equal length. A good blood supply to the flaps must be assured particularly when a single long flap is employed. When the flaps have been marked out by the skin incision, they are dissected upwards until the level of bone section is reached. The distal part of the flap should consist of skin and deep fascia alone, but the proximal part should contain sufficient muscle to cover the bone end. As the flap is dissected upwards, the knife is gradually made to cut more deeply until at the level of bone section all muscles have been divided. It is better to cut the flaps over generously (and to trim off redundant skin later if required) than to end up short.

Choice of method

In succeeding sections of the chapter certain classical amputations are described, and the method which is most suited to each is detailed. These operations, however, are not universally applicable, and in a number of patients the operation is modified by the extent of injury or disease.

The most appropriate operation may be one which will allow as much as possible of the limb to be saved. This is particularly true when the injury or disease extends up to or beyond the optimum level for amputation (see Table 9.1). Difficulty always arises when there has been crushing injury with marked destruction of the soft parts. Enough bone should be removed to allow the bony stump to be adequately covered, but length should be preserved by using whatever viable tissue is available from whatever aspect of the limb. It is sometimes reasonable to cover the bone end with muscle and to contemplate split skin grafting at a later date in order to preserve length, though extensive areas of skin grafting should probably best be avoided. When there is extensive mangling, the skin on one side of the limb may be uninjured, and the use of this as a single flap will avoid unnecessary sacrifice of bone (Figs 9.5–9.7). If the skin is destroyed up to the same level around the greater part of the limb circumference the circular method of amputation may be most appropriate.

Management of the soft tissues

Skin

The skin should be handled carefully during amputation surgery. Skin flaps should be neatly cut; although dogears will disappear, a poorly formed stump will delay limb fitting often for some weeks after amputation. On the rare occasions when a guillotine amputation is used, elastoplast traction to the leg may be applied in order to draw the skin and tissues distally. When there has been a severe crushing injury the limb must be carefully inspected for degloving. When this

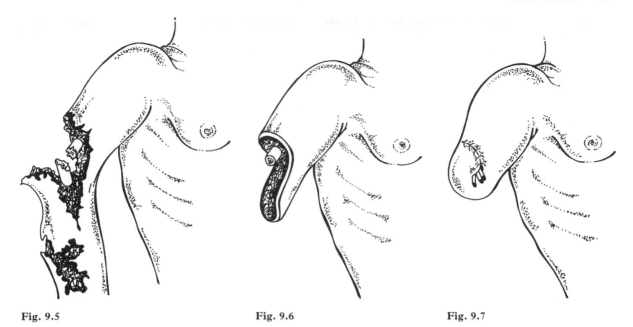

Fig. 9.5   **Fig. 9.6**   **Fig. 9.7**

Figs 9.5–9.7   Injury often dictates the most appropriate skin closure. In order to preserve length, a single medial flap has been used.

occurs the skin is sheared from its blood and nerve supply and will become necrotic. This is best appreciated by pinching the cuticle between the thumb and index finger. The fact that the skin has sheared off from the underlying tissues can usually be easily felt. The availability of skin flaps is frequently determined by the injury and in certain circumstances it may be necessary to consider skin grafting. Skin should be closed using a subcuticular absorbable suture.

Muscle

Some form of myoplasty should be performed as a routine. Diederich described careful closure of opposing muscle groups over the bone end. Younger patients should also have the muscles anchored to the bony stump by sutures passed through drill holes. Opposing muscle groups are then closed over the bone end.

Patients with peripheral vascular disease normally have the Dederich type of myoplasty (1963) though a few surgeons also anchor the muscles to the bony tip in ischaemic disease. It is important to judge the amount of muscle that is to be left behind fairly accurately and to avoid too floppy a stump on the one hand and too bony a stump on the other. When there is vascular disease present, skin and muscle should be raised as one flap in an attempt to preserve blood supply.

Nerves

The major nerves are usually divided cleanly with a knife. The nerve is pulled down before division and allowed to retract into the soft tissues. The sciatic nerve is ligatured first to prevent bleeding. A fine suture is used.

Tingling and phantom feeling is commonplace after amputation, and this is more severe after loss of an upper extremity. A feeling of paraesthesia in the absent foot or arm is almost invariable but this is frequently a relatively minor symptom. More severe phantom discomfort and pain can occur, particularly when there has been delay in wound healing or after severe traction injury, and may be difficult to treat.

Bone division

After division of the bone during amputation, all sharp edges and prominences should be carefully rounded off with a bone file (Fig. 9.8). Various authors including Loon (1962), Ertl (1949) and Mondray (1952) have described techniques of osteoplasty. In the younger and

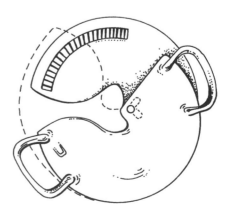

Fig. 9.8   Retractor for use in thigh amputation. It protects the tissues while bone is being sawn

more active patient it is usually wise to raise up a sleeve of periosteum before the bone is divided. This is closed over the bony stump and is said to provide a more comfortable stump. During below knee amputation in the younger patient it may be helpful to create a bony bridge between the divided tibia and fibula. To do this osteoperiosteal flaps are raised from the tibia (before it is divided) using a small osteotome. Periosteum is lifted off with flakes of cortical bone. After division of the tibia and fibula at approximately the same level the periosteal flaps are swung across to be sutured to the periosteum on the fibula (Figs 9.9–9.13). With time

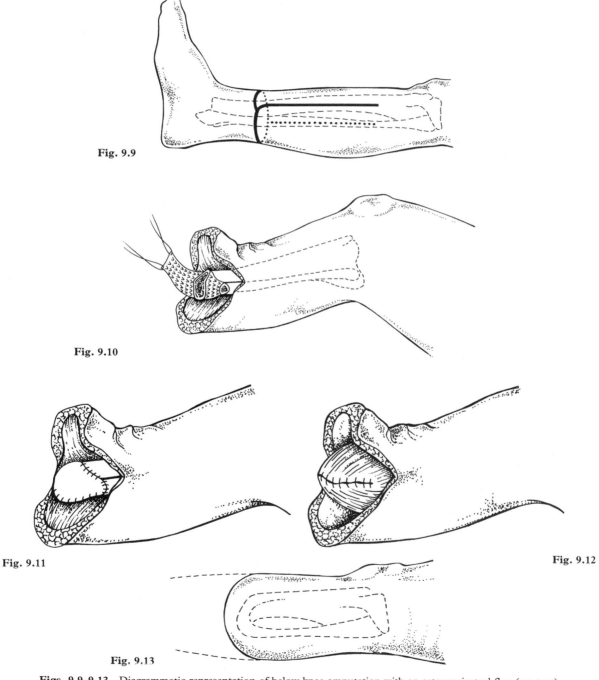

Fig. 9.9

Fig. 9.10

Fig. 9.11

Fig. 9.12

Fig. 9.13

Figs. 9.9–9.13 Diagrammatic representation of below knee amputation with an osteoperiosteal flap (see text)

a bony bridge should form between the two bones. The advantage of this technique is that a more stable and non-compressible below knee stump is formed.

Swanson (1964) in America has developed silastic implants in the shape of a champagne cork to plug the end of the bony stump. The technique is not widely used in Britain but is likely to be an area in which there will be further research.

Postoperative management

Immediate postoperative fitting

Berlamont of Berkplage was probably the first to introduce immediate postoperative fitting. Normally a plaster is applied to the stump and a prosthetic extension is fixed to the plaster in order to allow partial weight bearing immediately after surgery (Fig. 9.14). In a prospective study, Mooney (1971) found that there were less complications of wound healing if plaster over a soft dressing only was applied. The addition of weightbearing through a prosthetic extension increased healing complications considerably. In their series the use of a simple elastocrepe bandage was associated with highest incidence of problems.

Immediate postoperative fitting is not used extensively in Britain at present and the provision of a prosthetic device is usually delayed until the wound appears to be healing, though not necessarily healed.

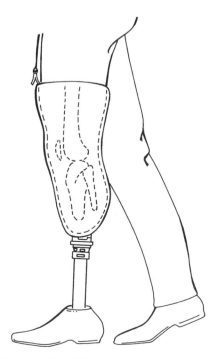

Fig. 9.14   An early walking plaster pylon

Controlled environment

Controlled environment treatment is a form of post-surgical dressing applied to the stump (Redhead, 1978). A polyvinyl chloride sleeve is placed over the amputation stump and seals proximally. A consul is attached distally to the sleeve and pumps sterile air into the sleeve at constant pressure and humidity. This dressing may be used for some days after amputation and intermittent positive pressure can be applied. It is unlikely to be adopted as routine management in the postamputation period in most centres and will be reserved for specialized problems.

Postoperative dressing

A fluffed gauze and wool dressing may be used after below knee amputation, after which the leg is usually encased in a plaster cylinder (see Fig. 9.46). This is retained for 10 days unless there appears to be an indication for inspecting the wound in which case the plaster is cut off. After above knee amputation some surgeons prefer to use a plaster cast though many still use an elastocrepe bandage.

It is usually the surgeon's intention to provide the patient with an artificial limb as soon as the wound appears to be healing favourably. The wound need not be entirely healed though should in other respects be reasonably stable. It is often perfectly appropriate to commence limb fitting and walking training some 9 or 10 days after the amputation. A simple temporary device such as the Little pneumatic walking aid, or a plaster with a prosthetic extension, may be used to commence walking training; alternatively an artificial limb may be made up, the socket normally being manufactured from a cast of the amputation stump. After surgery every effort should be made to keep the patient mobile and to prevent flexion contractures occurring in the joints.

AMPUTATION IN THE PRESENCE OF SEPSIS

Amputation in the presence of sepsis presents two main problems. It is necessary to decide at which level amputation is likely to succeed and also which method of surgery is most appropriate.

There is always a risk of infection occurring at the site of amputation and the wound should usually be left open. It is sometimes justifiable to close the wound primarily in the presence of distal infection but in these circumstances free drainage should be allowed from the wound through a drain site, or irrigation may be used. It is to be stressed however that in the presence of severe infection the wound should only be closed in exceptional circumstances.

Sometimes the surgeon may prefer to plan the amputation in two stages. The first stage then represents a preliminary amputation to remove the infected part. Subsequently a secondary procedure is planned in order to provide a satisfactory stump.

Method of amputating

There are various techniques available to the surgeon when frank infection is present in a limb that requires amputation. Frequently the leg is amputated at its definitive level and flaps are raised in the usual manner but at the end of the operation the wound is left open and the flaps are closed gently over gauze packing. This may be removed after 5 days and the flaps closed in the normal way. Alternatively the surgeon may decide simply to excise the distal infected part, using a guillotine type of amputation if necessary, and proceeding to definitive amputation at the site of election when it is clear that the infection has settled.

Level of amputation

When a first stage of provisional amputation is undertaken this should usually be as low as possible in order to preserve enough tissue to allow a satisfactory definitive amputation at some later stage. The procedure should of course be carried out through viable tissues but need not necessarily be above the level of infection provided that free drainage is ensured. In this way maximum length can be conserved. Even when it is hoped that the amputation will be definitive it should if possible be carried out below the optimum level in case further bone resection is required later.

AMPUTATIONS IN THE FINGERS AND HAND

Anatomy

For the performance of amputations in the hand, the surgeon should know the exact position of the various joints and the arrangement of the tendons to the different digits.

Surface marking of joints (Fig. 9.15)

The distal interphalangeal joint is at a level 6 mm distal to the crease on the palmer surface: on the dorsum it is 3 mm distal to the knuckle prominence when the finger is flexed. *The proximal interphalangeal joint* is opposite the distal of the 2 creases which are seen close together on the palmar surface; on the dorsum it is 6 mm distal to the knuckle prominence. *The metacarpophalangeal joint*: the level of this joint is 18 mm proximal to the crease at the finger web; on the dorsum the joint level is 12 mm distal to the knuckle. *The wrist joint* is opposite the proximal of the 2 main creases on the anterior surface of the wrist.

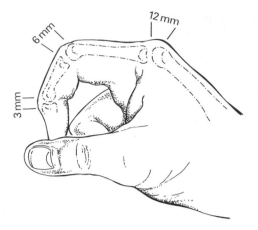

Fig. 9.15 Surface markings of the finger joints. The measurements given indicate the distance of each joint distal to the angle of the knuckle

Tendons

Each digit has at least 4 tendons, or sets of tendons; those required for the movements of flexion, extension, abduction and adduction.

In the fingers flexor profundus is inserted into the base of the terminal phalanx, and the flexor sublimis by slips into the middle phalanx. The extensor tendon, by means of its tripartite expansion, is inserted into both middle and distal phalanges. The interossei are inserted into the extensor hood; each of the 4 lumbrical muscles, arising from the tendons of flexor profundus in the palm, passes on the radial side of the metacarpophalangeal joint, also to join the extensor expansion on the dorsum of the proximal phalanx.

In the thumb the long flexor and the long extensor tendons insert into the base of the distal phalanx. The remaining tendons insert into the base of the proximal phalanx, except abductor pollicis longus, which extends only as far as the base of the metacarpal.

Structures of metacarpophalangeal and interphalangeal joints

The capsule of these joints is greatly strengthened in front by the tough *volar plate*, which has a firm distal attachment to the base of the phalanx.

Posteriorly, the capsule merges with the expanded extensor tendon. The joints are opened from the dorsum, therefore, when this tendon has been divided.

Arteries

The 4 *palmar digital arteries* arise from the superficial palmar arch. The 3 medial ones run towards the webs, and each divides into two branches which supply contiguous sides of the fingers; the fourth runs to the ulnar side of the 5th finger. The *radialis indicis* runs along the lateral side of the index finger, and the *prin-*

ceps pollicis supplies a branch to each side of the thumb; both of these arise directly from the radial artery.

Indications

Amputations in the fingers and hand are required most commonly after injury. Amputation of a finger may be required also when there is serious infection, to prevent spread of the infection to the palm, or because a stiff or deformed finger has resulted. Occasionally amputation may be required for neoplastic disease.

Principles of amputation in the hand

The surgeon should usually conserve as much tissue as possible though certain principles will act as a guide in establishing the optimum level for amputation, particularly in the fingers. The extent and nature of injury will determine the availability of skin and soft tissues, and will allow the surgeon to judge the most suitable method of closure. Skin closure should not be under tension and soft tissue cover over the bony stump is desirable, otherwise an adherent and painful scar will result. It is of course preferable to cover the bony stump with volar skin and soft tissue though this is not always practicable. Where possible amputation through the middle or distal phalanx is preferable to disarticulation at the interphalangeal joint since the attachment of flexor and extensor tendons is thereby preserved. At a level proximal to the insertion of the tendons to the middle phalanx, some surgeons prefer to preserve a stump of the proximal phalanx which will be actively flexed by residual intrinsic attachment, and to some extent will assist the power grip. Disarticulation of the long or ring fingers at the metacarpophalangeal joint has the disadvantage of allowing coins and small objects to pass through the hand and is less popular than section through the proximal phalanx. When the index or little finger requires shortening proximal to the sublimis insertion, the surgeon must decide whether a stump of the proximal phalanx should be left. Some surgeons argue that a proximal phalangeal stump may be useful to the manual worker as it enhances power grip and preserves the width of the hand and metacarpal arch. The long finger however largely takes over the function of the index finger in these circumstances and is used for pinch grip and fine work. Disarticulation of the index or little finger at the metacarpophalangeal joint leaves a somewhat ugly hand, and most surgeons prefer to remove the finger through the metacarpal head by oblique section. This will produce a more acceptable cosmetic result and in the index should be distal enough to preserve the attachments of the deep transverse ligament of the palm.

Formal amputations are rarely possible after injury and flaps should be obtained from residual undamaged skin. Removal of bone is reduced to the minimum which is compatible with adequate cover of the stump. It is important to provide adequate skin cover over the bone as any tension will leave a tender and adherent scar. The scar should be placed dorsally if possible using a longer volar flap.

It is sometimes possible to devise a skin flap from a seriously injured finger in order to cover a skin defect in the palm of the hand. The finger is split longitudinally and the bones and nail bed are removed. The skin is then opened out and sutured into the defect in the palm after being trimmed as required (Figs 9.16 & 9.17).

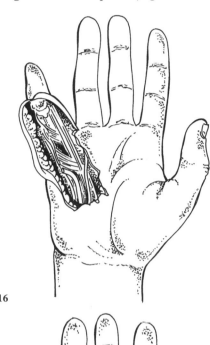

Fig. 9.16

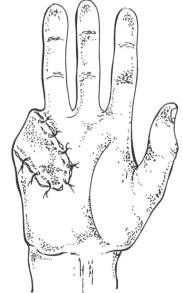

Fig. 9.17

Figs 9.16 & 9.17 Skin from a finger used to replace a defect in the palm

The digital nerves should be drawn out and sectioned carefully and should be allowed to retract into the soft tissues. There is evidence that cauterization of the nerve trunk using diathermy may prevent at least to some extent the occurrence of painful digital neuromata which are not uncommon after digital amputation and which may be extremely troublesome.

Amputation of the terminal phalanx of a finger
Most traumatic amputations occur at the tip of the digit. It is important that good quality skin should be used to cover the bone and this should not be allowed to become adherent. As elsewhere in the hand volar flaps are most suitable. An effort should be made to preserve the base of the phalanx in order to preserve the tendon insertions to the stump. When this is not possible amputation through the middle phalanx may be preferred.

It is sometimes possible to preserve the tip of the finger by using local advancement flaps as described by Kutler (see p. 14). In general, split skin cover over the tip of a digit is unsatisfactory since it lacks sensation and often becomes adherent in the region of the bony stump. In small children there are remarkable powers of tissue regeneration and simple cleaning and dressing of the digit may be all that is required. Skin grafts should not be considered.

Formal amputation of the terminal phalanx (Fig. 9.18)
When the situation allows, a formal procedure should be undertaken. A transverse incision is made on the dorsal surface of the digit about 6 mm distal to the knuckle; it is continued as far as the lateral border of the finger on each side and is deepened down to the base of the phalanx. A long palmer flap is then cut; this should extend almost to the tip of the finger and must be rectangular and not pointed in shape. It is carefully dissected, the knife being kept close to the phalanx. The bone is then divided with bone shears close to its base, after which the flap is folded back and secured with 3 or 4 interrupted sutures. As a rule there are no vessels which require ligature.

The incision for *disarticulation* through the terminal joint is made a little more proximally and the joint is opened by division of the flattened extensor tendon. The volar flap is then carefully fashioned, the terminal phalanx removed along with the nail bed, and the flap is sutured over the intermediate phalanx.

Many surgeons prefer amputation through the distal third of the intermediate phalanx rather than disarticulation at the interphalangeal joint, since the latter may leave a somewhat expanded or drumstick appearance. Alternatively, the condyles of the intermediate phalanx may be trimmed.

Amputation through the middle or proximal phalanx
Unequal anteroposterior flaps (the longer being on the palm side), or a single long palmar flap, are employed. The digital vessels may require to be ligatured. As much as possible of the 2nd phalanx should be preserved for the sake of its tendon insertions. If these can not be preserved amputation through the proximal phalanx, at the base of the finger or obliquely through the metacarpal head, is preferable.

In the index or fifth fingers, unless half of the middle phalanx can be preserved, most surgeons feel that the finger should be shortened obliquely through the metacarpal head. The middle finger will then acquire the important functions of the index. A few surgeons prefer to preserve a stump of the proximal phalanx (Fig. 9.19) and believe that this contributes to power grip, particularly in manual workers. The long and ring fingers are probably best shortened through the proximal phalanx unless the tendons inserted into the middle phalanx can be preserved (Fig. 9.20).

Amputation through the base of the proximal phalanx
Amputation of the long or ring fingers may be best undertaken through the base of the proximal phalanx.

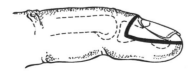

Fig. 9.18 Incision for formal amputation of terminal phalanx of finger

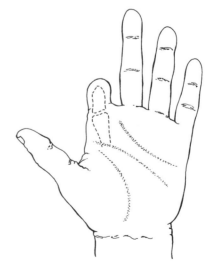

Fig. 9.19 A stump of the index or little finger proximal phalanx should rarely be left

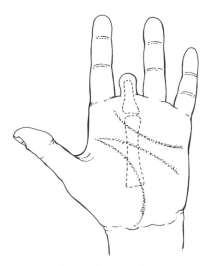

Fig. 9.20 Amputation at the base of the long or ring fingers should preserve a stump of the proximal phalanx

The attachment of the interosseous muscles to the proximal phalanx are preserved and the palmar ligaments supporting the metacarpal arch are also retained. Scarring in the web is kept to a minimum and there is no fear of injuring the lumbricals and interossei to the adjacent fingers. The need for dissection towards the palm is avoided in infection and this helps to limit spread of disease.

The *operation* is very simply performed. Two lateral flaps are cut by an incision which begins over the dorsum of the metacarpophalangeal joint and passes round each side of the finger a little distal to the web (Fig. 9.21). The digital arteries are secured and the flexor and extensor tendons are divided. The proximal

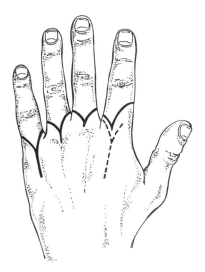

Fig. 9.21 Incisions for basal amputations of the fingers

phalanx is then cleared as far as its base, which is divided cleanly with an osteotome or bone shears. The skin flaps fall naturally together and are secured by 2 or 3 stitches. The retention of the base of the phalanx causes no undue projection.

Disarticulation at the metacarpophalangeal joint
This classical operation is less often employed than previously as it has certain disadvantages as already outlined. Disarticulation of the index or little fingers leaves a somewhat ugly hand; disarticulation of the long or ring finger allows small coins to drop through and it is preferable to leave the base of the proximal phalanx.

The *incision* is similar to that described for amputation through the base of the proximal phalanx, except that it begins more proximally over the metacarpal neck and so becomes racquet shaped. The flexor tendon is first divided, and the dissection is carried proximally until the joint is exposed. The digital arteries are secured. Disarticulation is most easily performed from the palmar aspect, the strong palmar ligament being divided. The collateral ligaments with the interosseous tendons are then cut and the disarticulation is completed by division of the expanded extensor tendon. No attempt should be made to anchor the tendons in any way. When it is the index or 5th finger that requires to be removed it is an advantage to make a longer flap on the marginal side so that the scar falls towards the middle of the hand and is less subject to pressure.

Removal of a metacarpal head?
The deformity resulting from disarticulation of the index or little finger through the metacarpophalangeal joint is somewhat conspicuous. The hand has a very much better cosmetic appearance if the metacarpal head is sectioned obliquely, preserving the attachment of the metacarpal ligament, and the metacarpal arch. After oblique removal of the metacarpal head the stump of the metacarpal should be covered by interosseous muscle (Figs 9.22–9.24).

Amputations in the thumb
Every effort must be made to preserve as much of the thumb as circumstances will allow, as it is of preeminent importance in the hand. Reconstructive procedures should be employed whenever practicable in order to avoid loss of length. Replantation surgery may also be used in certain circumstances. Even a stump composed of the metacarpal alone or of part of the metacarpal is of great value. No formal amputations need to be described. Flaps are obtained from available skin, and the minimum amount of bone is removed.

When there is skin avulsion from the thumb leaving part of a phalanx exposed, it may be possible to achieve

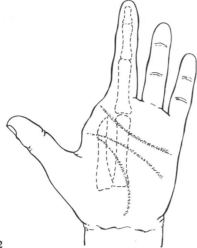

Fig. 9.22

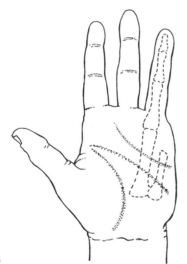

Fig. 9.23

Figs. 9.22 & 9.23 Amputation at the base of the index or little finger should normally be through the metacarpal head by oblique section

skin cover using grafting procedures so as to avoid sacrificing the segment of bone which could not otherwise be covered.

Amputations in the hand

No formal amputations require to be described, for it is essential that as much of the hand as possible should be saved. When fingers and metacarpal heads are lost, the remaining parts of the metacarpals form a most useful pad against which the thumb can be opposed. Even a stump composed of the carpal bones alone is of value especially if the thumb or part of the thumb can be saved also.

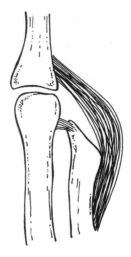

Fig. 9.24 Showing use of the first dorsal interosseous muscle to cover the stump

DISARTICULATION AT THE WRIST JOINT

This operation is rarely practicable, owing to the difficulty of obtaining flaps sufficiently long to cover the expanded ends of the forearm bones. Preservation of the inferior radio-ulnar joint allows the power of pronation and supination to be retained but these movements cannot be transmitted to an artificial hand. The circumference of the forearm changes in rotation, and the artificial socket is either too tight to permit the change of shape or too loose to secure a firm hold on the stump. The operation has, therefore, little to commend it, and an amputation through the lower third of the forearm is usually to be preferred.

AMPUTATION THROUGH THE FOREARM

Anatomy

Muscles

Anterior surface. The superficial muscles are pronator teres, flexor carpi radialis, palmaris longus, flexor digitorum sublimis and flexor carpi ulnaris. Pronator teres passes obliquely laterally to gain insertion into the middle of the lateral surface of the radius. The other muscles run down to the wrist keeping the above relationship from lateral to medial side, although flexor sublimis is on a somewhat deeper plane. The deep muscles are flexor digitorum profundus, which clothes the anterior and medial surfaces of the ulna in its upper three-fourths, flexor pollicis longus which covers the anterior surface of the radius to a similar extent, and pronator quadratus which covers the anterior surface of both bones in the lower fourth.

Lateral border and dorsum. The superficial muscles are brachioradialis, extensor carpi radialis longus, extensor carpi radialis brevis, extensor digitorum communis, extensor digiti minimi and extensor carpi ulnaris. The deep muscles are abductor pollicis longus, extensor pollicis brevis, extensor pollicis longus and extensor indicis; these all become superficial in the lower third of the forearm, the 3 tendons of the thumb crossing to the radial side.

Vessels

The radial artery in the upper two-thirds of the forearm is overlapped by brachioradialis; in the lower third it lies superficially between brachioradialis and flexor carpi radialis. *The ulnar artery* runs a deeper course lying on the surface of flexor profundus; it becomes superficial towards the wrist and passes anterior to the flexor retinaculum. *The anterior interosseous artery* runs down on the front of the interosseous membrane; *the posterior interosseous artery* is found between the superficial and deep muscles of the dorsum.

Nerves

The median nerve is at first deep to flexor sublimes, but appears on its radial side just above the wrist. *The ulnar nerve* lies on flexor profundus on the medial side of the ulnar artery; with the artery it becomes superficial at the wrist. *The radial nerve* accompanies the radial artery in the middle third of its course in the forearm; it then turns dorsally and breaks up into its terminal sensory branches. Its more important *posterior interosseous* branch runs a deep course among the dorsal muscles, breaking up into branches which supply them.

Operation

For the fitting of an artificial hand the optimum length of the forearm stump is 16–20 cm measured from the olecranon. A stump measuring less than 8 cm is useless for transmitting movement to an artificial elbow joint, so that, if this amount of bone cannot be conserved, an amputation through the upper arm may be preferred. Between these levels as much of the limb as possible should, of course, be saved.

Usually volar and dorsal flaps are raised but a circular incision may be used in the lower third of the forearm which is roughly cylindrical. In cases of injury flaps will be obtained from whatever skin is available. Vessels and nerves are identified during the division of the muscles and are dealt with in the usual manner (p. 219). When the muscles have been divided the knife is entered between the two bones in order to divide the interosseous membrane and the muscular

fibres arising from it. Both bones are then cleared for a short distance with an elevator, so as to expose bare bone to the saw. The radius being the more movable bone is divided first. Muscles which have a humeral attachment should be sutured over the bone ends, so that all possible mobility of the elbow joint may be retained.

Krukenberg amputation

The Krukenberg amputation is used infrequently in patients with bilateral loss of the arms through the forearm. The operation separates radius and ulna, so allowing pincer function and providing relatively crude grasp. Usually the operation is used on one side only, though bilateral Krukenberg procedures have been discussed. Those requiring more detailed information are referred to an article by Mathur (1981).

DISARTICULATION AT THE ELBOW JOINT

Disarticulation at the elbow is not a popular operation. The stump is club-shaped and unsightly, and the artificial limb cannot be fitted with a mechanical elbow joint at the correct level. In cases of injury there are unlikely to be sufficient soft parts available to cover the expanded end of the humerus. The one advantage of the operation is that the artificial limb, which must be fitted by means of a lacing leather, or a plastic, socket secures a very firm hold on the stump and does not tend to rotate.

Technique

For a formal operation all the various methods of amputating have been individually recommended using circular, racquet, or flap incisions. The choice will depend upon the conditions present. It should be noted that large flaps are required, owing to the relatively large size of the lower end of the humerus.

Muscles and tendons are divided just below the joint level. *The brachial artery* is identified in the middle of the cubital fossa on the medial side of the biceps tendon, and *the median nerve* lies just medial to the artery. *The ulnar nerve* is found between the medial epicondyle and the olecranon, in company with branches of the ulnar collateral and supratrochlear arteries. *The radial nerve* runs in front of the radio-humeral joint, and is accompanied by the profunda artery. These vessels and nerves are dealt with in the usual manner. It is recommended that the disarticulation should be commenced from the lateral side, the knife being entered between the head of the radius and the capitellum.

AMPUTATION THROUGH THE UPPER ARM

Anatomy

Muscles

Biceps lies superficially on the anteromedial aspect of the arm and is easily identified. *Coracobrachialis*, which is posteromedial to biceps, extends only as far as the middle of the humerus. *Brachialis* is closely applied to the front of the humerus in its lower two-thirds. Triceps forms the muscular mass on the posterior aspect.

Vessels

The brachial artery runs a fairly superficial course, being overlapped by the medial border of biceps. Its main branches are the *profunda* which accompanies the redial nerve, and the *ulnar collateral* which accompanies the ulnar nerve. *The cephalic vein* ascends in the superficial fascia at the lateral border of biceps.

Nerves

The median nerve is at first lateral to the brachial artery, but crosses anteriorly in the middle of the arm to reach its medial side. *The ulnar nerve* deviates medially from the artery, and passes posteriorly through the medial intermuscular septum to reach the back of the medial epicondyle. *The radial nerve* runs a spiral course round the back of the humerus under cover of triceps. It pierces the lateral intermuscular septum to reach the front of the lateral condyle, where it lies between the brachioradialis and brachialis. *The musculocutaneous nerve* pierces coracobrachialis and runs down between biceps and brachialis. It pierces deep fascia a little above the elbow to become the lateral cutaneous nerve of the forearm. *The medial cutaneous nerve* of the forearm pierces deep fascia in the middle of the arm and runs superficially over the medial side of the elbow.

Operation

Amputation should not be carried out through the lower 7–8 cm of the humerus since the stump is then too long to allow the fitting of a prosthetic elbow joint at the correct level. A stump measuring 20 cm from the acromion is regarded by prosthetists as ideal. Above this level as much of the limb as possible should be conserved. It should be noted that a stump which is much shorter than this is incapable of transmitting movement to an artificial limb, but is of the greatest value in preserving the normal contour of the shoulder (Figs 9.25 & 9.26).

Either flap or circular incisions are employed, the choice depending upon the conditions present. If flap are fashioned these should be made lateral and medial rather than anterior and posterior. The vessels and nerves are identified during division of the muscles and are dealt with in the customary manner.

AMPUTATION AT THE SHOULDER

Anatomy

Muscles related to the shoulder joint

On three sides the joint is strongly supported by muscles, the insertions of which are fused with the capsule: *anteriorly*, subscapularis; *superiorly*, supraspinatus and infraspinatus; *posteriorly*, teres minor. *Inferiorly*, the joint is related to the long head of triceps, but this is in contact with the capsule only when the arm is abducted. The long head of biceps passes through the joint cavity over the head of the humerus. More remote

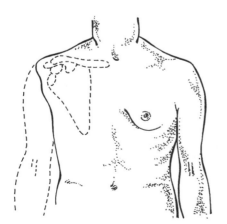

Fig. 9.25

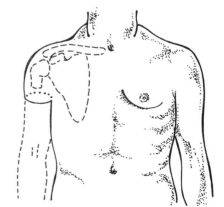

Fig. 9.26

Figs 9.25 & 9.26 Disarticulation through the shoulder joint results in unsightly angular deformity. Amputation through the upper end of the humerus preserves the contours of the shoulder, although the stump is useless

relations are: *anteriorly*, short head of biceps and cora-cobrachialis, which lie on subscapularis and are in turn covered by pectoralis major and by the anterior fibres of deltoid; *superiorly*, the main part of deltoid arising from the acromion arch; *posteriorly*, the posterior fibres of deltoid.

Vessels

The axillary artery lies anteromedial to the joint, separated from it by subscapularis. When the arm is abducted to a right angle its course is indicated by a straight line drawn from the mid point of the clavicle to the junction of the arm with the posterior axillary fold; when the arm is by the side this line is curved. Its *posterior humeral circumflex* branch, which may be encountered in amputations at the shoulder, runs round the surgical neck of the humerus under cover of deltoid. *The axillary vein* is on the medial side of the artery. *The cephalic vein* ascends in the groove between pectoralis major and deltoid.

Nerves

At the level of the shoulder joint the brachial plexus has evolved into the main nerve trunks of the limb. These lie grouped around the axillary artery. The *median* and *musculocutaneous nerves* are lateral, the *ulnar nerve* is medial, the *medial cutaneous nerve of the forearm* is anterior, and the *radial* and *circumflex nerves* are posterior. The *medial cutaneous nerve of the arm* lies on the medial side of the vein.

In amputations at the shoulder the head and tuberosities of the humerus should always if possible be preserved. If a disarticulation through the joint is performed the acromion process alone remains to form the prominence of the shoulder; the normal rounded contour is lost, and an angular and unsightly shoulder results (Fig. 9.25). Disarticulation may, however, be necessitated by certain injuries, or be considered advisable in cases of malignant disease of the humerus.

Disarticulation at the shoulder joint

The classical method of carrying out this operation was first described by Spence in 1856, and, with no more than slight modifications, it is still employed at the present time.

The approach to the joint is by the racquet method. With the arm held slightly abducted and rotated laterally the incision is made as shown in Figure 9.27. It begins just lateral to the tip of the coracoid process and extends downwards in the line of the humerus; at the level of the axillary folds it splits to encircle the limb. The vertical part of the incision is deepened, and the clavicular fibres of the deltoid and the pectoralis major tendon are divided. The knife is now swept round the lateral and posterior sides of the incision, and is made

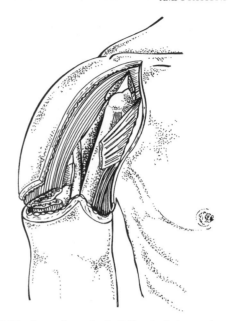

Fig. 9.27 Spence's method of disarticulation at the shoulder joint

to cut deeply to the bone, so that the deltoid muscle is divided cleanly a little above its insertion. The large lateral flap containing the deltoid is turned upwards, care being taken to avoid injury to the posterior humeral circumflex which enters its deep surface. The tuberosities of the humerus and the shoulder joint are now exposed. By cutting against the superior and anterior surfaces of the anatomical neck of humerus the capsule of the joint, together with the capsular muscles and the long head of biceps are divided. The limb is rotated first medially and then laterally to allow this part of the operation to be carried out. The head of the humerus is then dislocated forwards, and the disarticulation is completed. The knife is now inserted between the humerus and the soft parts on the medial side and is made to cut downwards to the bone. The remaining muscles, together with the brachial vessels and the nerve trunks, are divided above the lower level of the skin incision on the medial side. In Spence's original technique, division of the medial flap was completed in one sweep by bringing the knife sharply through the tissues from within outwards into the skin incision already made. It was the duty of the assistant to grasp the partially formed flap, following the track of the knife, and to secure the vessels by pressure between the finger and thumb. After the flap had been divided the vessels were picked up and ligatured. In modern practice it is customary to identify and ligature the vessels before the division is carried out. The flaps are trimmed if necessary and are sutured. Drainage of the wound for 24 to 48 hours is advisable.

Amputation through the upper end of the humerus

In cases where it is found possible to conserve the upper end of the humerus, the first stages of the operation are very similar to those described for disarticulation. The deltoid flap is not reflected so far upwards, and the capsular muscles are not, of course, divided. For section of the bone an electric or Gigli saw is recommended. Longer flaps may be required, depending upon the amount of humerus which it is possible to retain.

INTER-SCAPULO-THORACIC AMPUTATION

This operation is sometimes necessary for malignant growths involving the scapula or the upper end of the humerus. It consists in removal of the upper limb altogether with the scapula and the lateral two-thirds of the clavicle. The incision is shown in Fig. 9.28. Its horizontal part is used to expose the clavicle which is cleared and divided with a Gigli saw near its medial end. The lateral or main part of the bone is elevated, and its middle third is removed. Through the access thus afforded the subclavian vessels are divided between ligatures, and the trunks of the brachial plexus are treated by simple section at a higher level. In the anterior part of the racquet incision pectoralis major and minor are divided close to the chest wall. From the posterior part of the incision the medial flap is raised as far as the vertebral border of the scapula. Removal

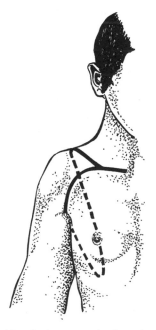

Fig. 9.28 Incision for inter-scapulo-thoracic amputation

of the forequarter is then completed by division of the muscles which attach the scapula to the trunk—trapezius, levator scapulae, the rhomboids, serratus anterior and latissimus dorsi. All haemorrhage is arrested, and the flaps are sutured with drainage.

AMPUTATION OF THE TOES

Anatomy

Metatarsophalangeal and interphalangeal joints
The metatarsophalangeal joints are situated 2.5 cm proximal to the free border of the web. In the lateral 4 toes, the proximal and distal interphalangeal joints are respectively 6 mm and 3 mm distal to the joint prominence on the dorsum. In the great toe the interphalangeal joint is at a level midway between the base of the nail fold and the joint prominence.

The capsule of these joints is greatly strengthened below by the tough *plantar ligament,* which is firmly attached to the base of the phalanx. In the first metatarsophalangeal joint this ligament is replaced by the 2 sesamoid bones. Dorsally the capsule is deficient, its place taken by the expanded extensor tendon.

The toes
Each toe, provided that it is not deformed, takes at least a proportion of the weight borne by the forefoot; it relieves the pressure on the head of its metatarsal, and contributes largely to the normally resilient gait. The little toe is of less value than the others in this respect, but its removal leaves the head of the 5th metatarsal forming a prominence on the side of the foot, over which a painful corn is very liable to develop. Amputation of any toe, therefore, should not be undertaken lightly, nor should it be performed for conditions such as hammer toe, which can be corrected by other measures (p. 139). It is necessitated as a rule by crushing injuries, or for deformities which are incapable of correction.

The great toe has, of course, much greater functional importance than all the others, and should be conserved whenever possible. If partial amputation is unavoidable every effort should be made to obtain a stump which will be mobile and capable of weight-bearing.

Partial amputation of the great toe

Amputation of the terminal phalanx
If a functionally useful stump is to be obtained, it is essential to preserve the base of the terminal phalanx, into which the long flexor and extensor tendons are inserted. In cases of injury, flaps are obtained from whatever skin is available. Preference should, if possible, be given to a longer flap on the plantar aspect,

so that the scar will not be subjected to pressure. The incision for a formal amputation is shown in Figure 9.29. The long plantar flap is reflected back, the knife being kept close to the bone, in order to avoid injury to the planter digital arteries which provide the blood supply to the flap. The bone is divided with bone shears or with a sharp osteotome just distal to its base. If a *disarticulation* is necessary the joint is best opened from the plantar surface. The flap is folded over the end of the stump and is secured with a few interrupted sutures.

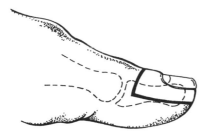

Fig. 9.29   Incision for amputation of terminal phalanx of great toe

Amputation through the proximal phalanx
A stump comprising less than one complete phalanx is of little or no value for weight-bearing; it tends to become dorsiflexed and in the way. No more than the base of the phalanx should therefore be preserved.

Amputation of the great toe at its base
The base of the proximal phalanx should always if possible be retained, for thereby the insertions of the short muscles of the toe remain intact. These muscles are of value in giving support to the head of the metatarsal and ensure a better stump.

The formal operation is carried out by the racquet method. The incision is shown in Figure 9.30. It

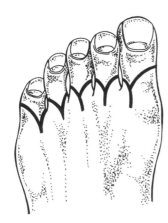

Fig. 9.30   Incisions for basal amputations in the toes

should be noted that the handle of the racquet is placed well to the lateral side of the dorsum, in order that pressure on the scar will be avoided; it extends proximally as far as the head of the metatarsal. The blade of the racquet encircles the toe obliquely so that the medial flap extends almost as far distally as the interphalangeal joint. The flaps are dissected back and the digital arteries are secured and ligatured. The long tendons are divided. The first phalanx is cleared and divided with an osteotome just distal to its base. The flaps fall naturally together and are opposed with a few interrupted sutures.

Disarticulation at the metatarsophalangeal joint
The incision is similar to that described above, except that the straight part extends proximally as far as the neck of the metatarsal, and a shorter flap on the medial side will suffice. The flaps are reflected back to expose the joint, and the digital arteries are secured. The long tendons are divided. The joint is opened from the plantar surface, the insertions of the short muscles being divided along with the capsule against the base of the proximal phalanx, so that the sesamoid bones are preserved. When the disarticulation has been completed the capsular structures are sutured together over the exposed metatarsal head in order to support it and to prevent retraction of the short muscles.

Disarticulation of the lateral four toes
Disarticulation at the metatarsophalangeal joint should be carried out in cases of injury where the base of the phalanx cannot be preserved. It is indicated also in the relatively common deformity in which one toe has become displaced backwards on the others, and is pressed upon by the shoe; such a toe is useless, both for weightbearing and as a spreader to the other toes.

As in the case of the great toe the racquet approach is employed. The incisions for the different toes are shown in Figure 9.30, and the operation follows the lines already described. The inexperienced operator should note that the metatarsophalangeal joints are situated much further proximally than would be anticipated.

Amputation of all of the toes
Amputation of all of the toes is usually indicated where there is fixed clawing or dislocation of the metatarsophalangeal joints leading to gross deformity. This frequency occurs in rheumatoid arthritis, and amputation of the toes may sometimes be preferred to forefoot arthroplasty.

Flint and Sweetnam reported their experience of the procedure in 1960, and Green discussed the technique in 1985. Dorsal and volar incisions run across the toes sweeping into the web spaces as they pass across the foot. The toes are disarticulated at the metatarso-phalangeal joint, the arteries are secured, and the long tendons and nerves are divided and allowed to retract.

AMPUTATIONS IN THE FOOT

Amputations through the foot, particularly through its midpart, have had a relatively poor reputation over many years. Warren (1968) and Pederson (1954) described the use of the transmetatarsal amputation which now has an established place in surgical practise particularly in patients with diabetes and relatively localised peripheral vascular disease of the toes.

Recently there has been increasing interest in amputations more proximally in the foot. Amputation through the metatarsal bases or disarticulation at the tarsometatarsal joints (described by William Hey of Leeds (1810) and by Lisfranc (1815)) may be ex-tremely useful after trauma, particularly crushing inju-ries of the forefoot. This type of amputation may also be used in the diabetic foot.

Chopart's amputation or disarticulation through the midtarsal joints (the talonavicular joint on the medial side of the foot and the calcaneocuboid joint on the lateral side of the foot) has generally been considered to be an unsatisfactory procedure. Bingham, writing in Murdoch's textbook (1970), stated that with suitable tibialis anterior transplant a satisfactory stump may be achieved. This is particularly so after injury but the procedure has yet to establish its place in the diabetic foot. It is particularly important to note that unless a satisfactory tibialis anterior transfer to the neck of the talus can be achieved the procedure is likely to fail.

In undertaking amputation through the foot a long volar flap should be used when at all possible. When a junctional scar, that is a scar between volar and dorsal skin, is placed in a weight-bearing area considerable discomfort is likely to ensue. One of the conspicuous advantages of amputation through the foot is that an ordinary shoe or surgically made boot may be adequate footwear and a formal artificial limb is usually not necessary.

Transmetatarsal amputation

There are several series which have been published to show that transmetatarsal amputation, performed for peripheral vascular disease, particularly in diabetes, is attended by a large percentage of successful results. The absence of palpable pulsation below the femoral artery is not an absolute contra-indication to the opera-tion provided that the skin on the dorsum of the foot is warm and well nourished and there is no spreading infection.

Technique

The amputation is undertaken using of a long plantar flap, which extends to a level just proximal to the flexion crease at the base of the toes; the dorsal part of the incision crosses the necks of the metatarsals, at which level these bones are divided. Since primary healing is always in some doubt, the flaps must be handled with great gentleness and not held with dis-secting forceps; they should be trimmed as required and sutured accurately, so that the skin is neither redundant nor under tension (Figs 9.31 & 9.32). It is advised that the stitches should be left in place for 14 days.

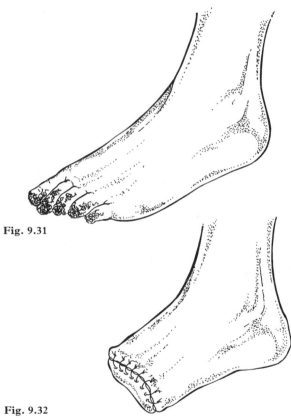

Fig. 9.31

Fig. 9.32

Figs 9.31 & 9.32 Transmetatarsal amputation for dry gangrene of the toes. A long plantar flap is employed, and the metatarsals are divided at the levels of their necks

Tarsometatarsal amputation

A long volar flap is used if possible. The foot is shortened through the bases of the metatarsals or by disarticulation at the tarsometatarsal joint. The long toe flexors and extensors should be anchored to the soft tissues of the foot. After closure of the wound a padded dressing is applied.

Midtarsal or Chopart's amputation

A long volar flap and a shorter dorsal flap are raised from the skeleton of the foot provided suitable skin is available. The midtarsal joints are exposed and disarticulation of the foot is completed through the talonavicular joint on the medial side of the foot and through the calcaneocuboid joint on the lateral side. The tibialis anterior is identified and is sutured into a drill hole through the neck of the talus. The remaining long extensor muscles and long flexors are anchored to soft tissues particularly to the remains of the midtarsal capsule. The long volar flap is swung over the divided foot and sutured on the dorsum. A padded dressing and a below knee plaster are applied in order to maintain the ankle in the neutral position. The plaster should be retained for 6 weeks in order to allow the tibialis anterior muscle to anchor in the neck of the talus.

SYME'S AMPUTATION

Anatomy

Structure of the ankle joint
The capsule is attached on all sides to the margins of the articular surfaces, and is arbitrarily divided into *anterior, posterior, medial and lateral ligaments.* The medial (*deltoid*) ligament is fanshaped and very strong. Its apex is attached to the malleolus; its base to bony points over a wide area on the medial side of the foot.

Anterior relations of ankle joint
The following structures are in contact with the anterior ligament, from medial to lateral side: tibialis anterior, extensor hallucis longus, anterior tibial vessels, anterior tibial nerve, extensor digitorum longus and peroneus tertius. In the superficial fascia, the long saphenous vein is found anterior to the medial malleolus, and terminal branches of the musculocutaneous nerve lie lateral to the midline.

Structures between medial malleolus and heel
The following structures enter the sole of the foot behind and below the medial malleolus and are bound down by the flexor retinaculum: tibialis posterior, flexor digitorum longus, posterior tibial vessels, posterior tibial nerve and flexor hallucis longus. They lie in that order in the line between the malleolus and the heel. At this level the posterior tibial artery and nerve both divide into medial and lateral plantar branches.

Structures between lateral malleolus and heel
Peroneus longus and brevis lie in contact with the lateral ligaments of the ankle joint. The short saphenous vein lies in the superficial fascia behind the malleolus.

Posterior relations of the ankle joint
The joint is separated from the tendocalcanei by a wide interval filled with fat. The posterior tibial vessels and nerves and the flexor group of tendons are in contact with the medial part of the posterior ligament before they pass below the medial malleolus. The peroneal artery and the peroneal tendons lie behind the lateral part of the ligament.

Aims of Syme's operation

This operation, first described by Syme in 1842, is the classical amputation in the region of the ankle. The tibia and fibula are divided at or immediately above the level of the joint, and their ends are covered with a single flap obtained from the skin of the heel. The end of the stump is at a height of about 6-8 cm from the ground.

Syme's amputation has established itself as a procedure that will provide a durable stump which may be entirely satisfactory. Some 50% of patients are able to walk on the stump without a prosthesis (which may prove to be useful at night), and many become involved in strenuous work. It is difficult to provide a woman with an attractive prosthesis and occasionally the Syme's stump tends to migrate sideways. This amputation is particularly suitable in young men who have a crushing injury of the foot, but the unsightliness of the prosthesis is a drawback in the female although it does not entirely preclude the operation.

Recently the Syme's amputation has been used in patients with diabetes. Wagner (1977) presented a large series of successful Syme's procedures in diabetic patients using a somewhat modified technique and Srinavasan (1973) has shown that the amputation may be used successfully in the sensory deficient foot. There can be no question that Syme's amputation is of special value to patients who do not have access to modern artificial limbs, for they can be fitted with a simple appliance known as the 'Elephant boot'. This is inexpensive to manufacture and gives lasting service (Fig. 9.33).

Technique

The surgeon stands at the end of the table facing the foot, which either overhangs the table or is raised by a sandbag placed under the lower third of the leg. The incision is shown in Figure 9.34. The knife is entered below the tip of the lateral malleolus and is drawn across the sole to a point 2 cm below the medial malleolus. The two ends of the incision are then joined by the shortest route across the front of the ankle joint. Throughout the incision all structures are divided

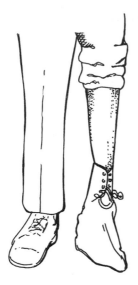

Fig. 9.33 Primitive 'elephant boot' prosthesis that can be used after Syme's amputation

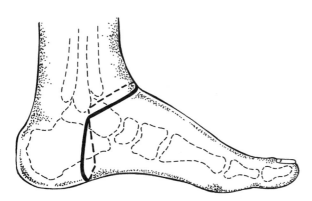

Fig. 9.34 Incision for Syme's amputation

down to bone. On the anterior surface these include the extensor group of tendons and the anterior tibial vessels and nerve. On the medial side, below the malleolus, the incision divides the flexor group of tendons and the plantar vessels and nerves. Laterally, the peroneal tendons are cut. The ankle joint is then opened by division of its anterior ligament; the lateral ligaments are cut from within outwards, and the foot is dislocated in a plantar direction to expose the back of the joint.

The next part of the operation is the most important and the most difficult. It consists in the division of the posterior ligaments of the joint, the detachment of the insertion of the tendocalcaneus and the dissection of the calcaneum out of the heel flap. During these stages of the operation the plantar dislocation of the foot is steadily increased (Figs 9.35–9.39). There is

great danger of injuring the posterior tibial and peroneal arteries when the posterior ligament is cut, for both arteries are closely applied to the back of the ligament. Their branches which supply the skin of the heel are also in danger when the calcaneum is being dissected out of the flap. To avoid such accidents, which may result in sloughing of the flap, *the knife is kept closely applied to the bone throughout these stages of the operation.*

The anterior tibial artery, the medial and lateral plantar arteries, and the two saphenous veins are the main vessels which require ligature. As the stump is to be an end-bearing one, particular attention should be paid to the shortening of nerve trunks, so that these do not become involved in scar tissue at the end of the stump. Anterior tibial and musculocutaneous nerves are identified, and cut short. The medial and lateral plantar nerves should be dissected upwards out of the heel flap to their point of origin from the posterior tibial nerve; this trunk is then divided well above the ankle region.

If the articular surface of the tibia and fibula are healthy, the malleoli alone are removed. Otherwise the bones are divided immediately above the level of the ankle joint. The saw is applied exactly at right angles to the axis of the leg. The heel flap is folded over the bone ends, and after being trimmed as required is sutured in position. Drainage may be provided by a strip of corrugated plastic brought out at one corner of the wound; this is removed within 48 hours.

Syme's amputation in diabetes
When Syme's amputation is undertaken in the diabetic patient several modifications must be considered. In the first place it is probably wise to cut the heel flap slightly larger. The incision usually starts about 1 cm in front of the medial malleolus and passes across the front of the ankle joint to 1 cm in front of the lateral malleolus and then by the shortest route across the sole of the foot.

Wagner (1977) prefers a two-stage amputation. During the first stage the heel is enucleated in the usual way but the medial and lateral malleoli are not removed. The wound is closed and when it is soundly healed some 5 or 6 weeks later, the malleoli are removed through small incisions at a second stage procedure. Some surgeons however prefer to remove the malleoli during the first operation but most leave the distal articular surface of the tibia and do not section the tibia as previously described.

When there is significant infection in the foot as is often the case in diabetes it may be wise to close the Syme's amputation over irrigation. Two tubular drains may be left in the cavity of the stump. Saline, con-

Figs 9.35–9.39   Stages in a Syme's amputation

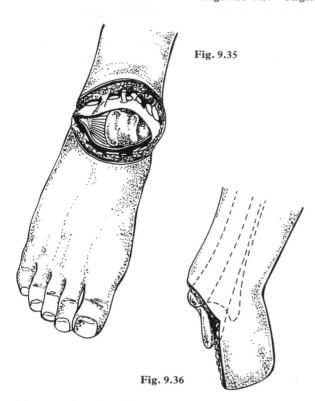

Fig. 9.35

Fig. 9.36

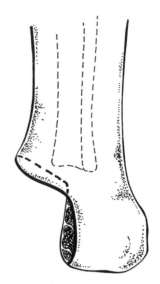

Fig. 9.38   Showing the heel flap prior to closure

Fig. 9.35   Division of the anterior structures and opening of the ankle joint
Fig. 9.36   Division of medial and posterior ligaments of ankle joint, prior to dissection of the calcaneum out of the heel flap

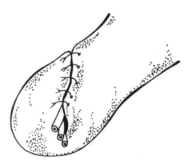

Fig. 9.39   Operation completed

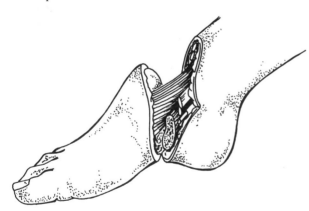

Fig. 9.37   Bones about to be divided

taining an appropriate antibiotic, runs into the cavity through one of the drains, and escapes into a urinary bag through the other. The irrigations may be run fast enough to keep the effluent fluid relatively clear. The drains may be retained for up to 10 days.

OTHER AMPUTATIONS AT THE ANKLE

Modified Syme's amputation
Many modifications of Syme's original amputation have been described, with variations of the incision and of soft tissue and bony procedures. In general the original technique has outlived all of these variations. Figure 9.40 shows Syme's amputation using an elliptical incision and with division of the tibia and fibula slightly higher than usual. It is doubtful whether this operation has anything to commend it and it has not won widespread approval.

Pirogoff's amputation (Fig. 9.41)
This is similar to Syme's amputation except that the posterior part of the calcaneum is retained in the heel flap, and is opposed to the sawn surface of the tibia

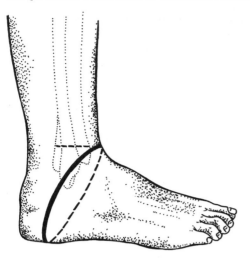

Fig. 9.40   Modified Syme's incision

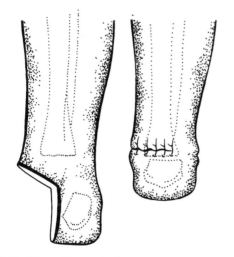

Fig. 9.41   Pirogoff's amputation

by sutures which take up the periosteum or are passed through drill holes in the bones. It provides a longer stump than does Syme's amputation, and one which is even better suited to end-bearing, but in view of the difficulty of fitting an artificial foot with an ankle joint at the correct level, it is seldom employed nowadays except in developing countries.

AMPUTATION THROUGH THE LEG AT THE BELOW KNEE LEVEL

Anatomy

Muscles

Anterior group. Tibialis anterior lies immediately lateral to the tibia in the upper two-thirds of the leg.

Extensor digitorum longus is lateral to tibialis anterior and in front of the fibula. Extensor hallucis longus lies between tibialis anterior and extensor digitorum, and partly hidden by them. In the lower third these muscles pass on to the front of the tibia, where they are joined by peroneus tertius.

Lateral group. Peroneus longus and brevis cover the lateral surface of the fibula, brevis being anterior and on a deeper plane. In the lower third both muscles incline backwards to pass behind the lateral malleolus.

Posterior group. The muscular mass of the calf is composed of gastrocnemius superficially and soleus which is immediately deep to it. These muscles (together with the unimportant plantaris tendon) combine to form the tendo calcaneus. The deep muscles are popliteus (which does not extend below the upper third of the leg), flexor digitorum longus, flexor hallucis longus and tibialis posterior. Flexor digitorum longus is closely applied to the back of the tibia, and flexor hallucis longus to the back of the fibula. Tibialis posterior lies between them on the interosseous membrane, and is on a still deeper plane.

Vessels and nerves

The *anterior tibial artery* enters the anterior compartment of the leg by piercing the upper part of the interosseous membrane. In the upper two-thirds it runs a deep course on the anterior surface of the membrane; in the lower third it lies on the front of the tibia. The *posterior tibial artery* runs for the greater part of its course between soleus and the fascia covering tibialis posterior; distally it is directly behind the ankle joint. The *posterior tibial nerve* accompanies the artery on its lateral side. The *peroneal artery* is found on the back of the interosseous membrane, close to the fibula. The *long saphenous vein* ascends in the superficial fascia on the medial surface of the leg; the *short saphenous vein* on the posterior surface.

Objectives of amputation

Amputation at the below knee level through the middle third of the leg is the operation of choice when it is not possible to preserve the foot or the heel. The ideal length of tibial stump is 14 cm. A stump that is shorter than 8 cm tends to slip out of the socket of an artificial limb and is very difficult to accommodate comfortably and effectively in the patellar tendon bearing prosthesis. When it is not possible to save at least 8 cm of the tibia the patient may be better served by knee disarticulation or amputation through the thigh.

A distinction should be made between those amputations that are undertaken as a direct result or consequences of peripheral vascular disease and amputations in which vascular disease is not a problem. Ghormley described below knee amputation using a long posterior flap in 1947. Burgess (1981) has been largely responsible for popularising this technique and it is probably now the most commonly used method of below knee amputation in patients with vascular impairment. Recently amputation at the below knee level using a long posteromedial flap using an elliptical incision has been described, but only the conventional long posterior flap technique will be described here.

Patients who do not have ischaemic disease in the limb, particularly younger patients, are probably better served by amputation at the below knee level with careful myoplasty and osteoplasty. In these patients equal or unequal skin flaps may be used. Unequal flaps have the advantage that the scar is not terminal and may be placed away from the sectioned tibia, though this is not particularly important if the patient is to be provided with a patellar tendon bearing prosthesis.

Myoplasty is designed to anchor the opposing muscle groups firmly around and over the sectioned bone. When osteoplasty is used a periosteal sleeve may either be closed over the sectioned bone (and is thought to provide a more comfortable stump) or periosteal strips raised from the tibia are sutured across to the fibula in the hope that bony union between the sectioned tibia and sectioned fibula may occur. This provides the patient with a firmer stump.

Conventional below knee amputation
(Figs 9.42–45)

The proposed level of bone section is marked by a scratch on the skin, and the flaps are marked out. The combined length of the two flaps should be equal to 1½ times the diameter of the limb at the level of bone section. The skin is incised and the long saphenous vein will be encountered at the medial corner of the anterior flap, and the short saphenous vein at the middle of the posterior flap. The flaps are dissected back in the usual way. The periosteum covering the subcutaneous surface of the tibia should be raised (in lieu of deep fascia in this area) along with the anterior flap; the posterior flap may contain some muscle at its base. Division of the muscles is completed at the level of bone section. The posterior tibial vessels and nerve are encountered between the soleus and tibialis posterior in or near the midline. The knife is introduced between the bones, and the interosseous membrane along with any remaining muscle fibres is divided. The anterior tibial vessels and nerve and the peroneal vessels lie on opposite sides of the membrane, the latter being close to the fibula. Vessels and nerves are dealt with in the usual manner.

The fibula is divided first — a little higher than the tibia, so that its end will not press on the skin; it is an

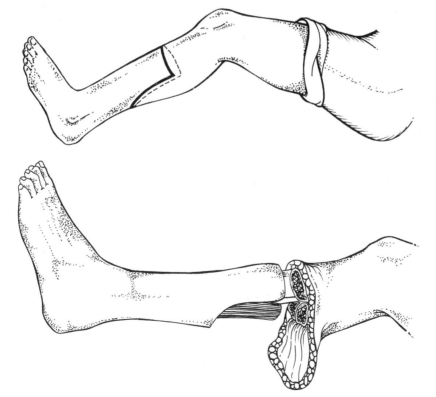

Fig. 9.42

Fig. 9.43

Fig. 9.42 & 9.43   Captions see overleaf.

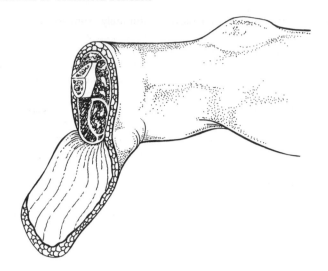

Fig. 9.44

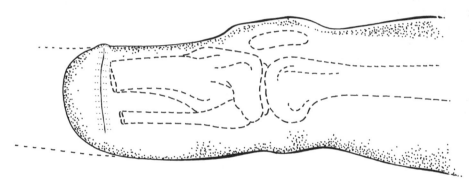

Fig. 9.45

Fig. 9.42–9.45   Below knee amputation using a long posterior flap

additional advantage if the saw cut is made obliquely. The tibial stump is bevelled anteriorly, also to avoid pressure on the skin by the bone edge (see Fig. 9.44); this is conveniently done before the main saw cut. The posterior muscles are sutured across the bone end to the periosteum that has been raised with the anterior flap. If haemostasis is assured and dead space avoided, drainage is probably unnecessary but does no harm, provided that the drain is removed within 48 hours.

In patients where less than 14 cm of tibia can be preserved, flaps should be cut in any manner which will entail least sacrifice of bone. Removal of the fibula in these patients may allow the use of flaps which would otherwise be too small.

Amputation with a periosteal bridge

Whatever form of amputation is used at the below knee level, myoplasty (suture of the opposing muscle groups over the end of the tibia) should be used. Many surgeons prefer a slightly more complex procedure in those patients not affected by vascular disease. The

operation is designed to fashion a secure myoplasty, and also fashion a periosteal bridge between the tibia and the fibula which will ultimately form a bony bar between the two bones (see Fig. 9.10). The technique described here is derived from descriptions by Loon (1962), Ertl (1949) and Mondray (1952), and has been recommended by Murdoch (1968).

Anterolateral and posteromedial vertical incisions are made on the leg from a point about 2.5 cm above the proposed level of bone section. These incisions are taken distally so as to allow 8 to 10 cm of the tibia to be exposed beyond the proposed level of section. The incisions are then joined circularly around the leg. The anteromedial and posterolateral skin flaps formed in this way are dissected proximally from the deep fascia. The anterior group of muscles including the extensors and the peroneals are now divided transversely at the same level as the distal skin incision. The entire group of muscles is raised from its bed on the tibia and the fibula, leaving periosteum undamaged. The posterior group of muscles is dealt with in the same way being raised from the posterior aspect of the tibia and fibula, once again leaving periosteum and interosseus membrane undamaged.

The fibula is divided at the level of proposed tibial section and is removed with the interosseous membrane. Two osteoperiosteal flaps are now raised from the intact tibia, one on its medial aspect and one on its lateral aspect. Periosteum is raised with an osteotome and small flakes of cortical bone are also lifted from the tibia. When both osteoperiosteal flaps are completed to the level of proposed tibial section, the tibia is divided and prepared. The lateral osteoperiosteal flap is now sutured to the deep surface of the fibula and the medial tibial osteoperiosteal flap is drawn across the divided end of the tibia and is sutured to the lateral side of the fibula, thus creating a bridge between the two bones (see Fig. 9.11).

The major vessels are isolated and ligatured, and the posterior tibial nerve is divided and allowed to retract. The muscle groups are sutured under light tension over the tibia and fibula after suitable tailoring. Usually most of the soleus and deep posterior muscles must be removed. It is necessary to secure both groups of muscles by anchoring sutures to the periosteum of the tibia at the base of the osteoperiosteal bridge to prevent lateral dislocation of the muscle groups.

The skin flaps are now tailored and sutured over a Redivac drain.

Below knee amputation in vascular disease (see Figs 9.42–9.45)

Below knee amputation in the presence of vascular disease is undertaken normally without a tourniquet. The below knee stump should not be shorter than 8 cm but is frequently cut slightly shorter than when the tissues are otherwise healthy. A short anterior flap is marked out and will cross the leg transversely no more than 1 cm distal to the proposed site of tibial section. A long and somewhat square posterior flap is marked out and will be almost 1½ times the diameter of the leg in length, or approximately 12 cm. The anterior or transverse incision is made through skin and deep fascia and divides the anterolateral group of muscles transversely. The tibia is exposed on its subcutaneous and lateral surfaces. The short anterior flap fashioned in this way is raised from the tibia proximally for approximately 1 cm. The anterolateral muscles are also raised from the interosseous membrane and the fibula. The anterior tibial vessels are ligatured and the nerve is divided and allowed to retract. The tibia is now divided, most conveniently with a Gigli saw. The peroneal muscles and musculocutaneous nerve are divided over the fibula which is sectioned with large bone cutters or a Gigli saw, 0.5 cm proximal to the site of tibial section.

Attention is now turned to the posterior flap. Skin is incised and the posterior muscle groups are divided obliquely from the tibia to the skin incision. This is conveniently done using an amputation knife. The posterior tibial nerve is divided and allowed to retract and the posterior tibial vessels are divided and ligatured.

The posterior mass of muscles including the gastrocnemius, the soleus and the deep posterior muscles should be tailored carefully so that the posterior flap is not too bulky. Virtually all of the deep posterior muscles will require to be removed and much of the soleus will also be removed. The gastrocnemius is tapered to the tip of the flap. Bone ends are prepared in the usual way and carefully rounded off. The wound is closed, suturing the posterior muscles to the periosteum overlying the tibia and to the deep fascia overlying the anterior group of muscles. The skin is closed over a suction drain.

Postoperative management after below knee amputation
Whatever technique of below knee amputation is used it is probably wise to apply a padded wool and gauze dressing which is encased in plaster of Paris to the midthigh level. A window may be cut over the patella for inspection (Fig. 9.46). The immediate postoperative fitting of a prosthetic extension is popular with some surgeons but is not widely used.

AMPUTATION THROUGH THE LEG IN THE UPPER THIRD

It has already been stated that, in patients to whom modern artificial limbs are available, this is not a good amputation, and that if at least 8 cm of tibia cannot be conserved, it may be preferable to amputate at or above the knee.

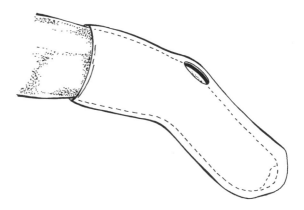

Fig. 9.46 Plaster of Paris dressing after below knee amputation. A wool and gauze dressing is applied to the stump before the plaster is wrapped. A window is cut over the patella to allow inspection

Rarely however and in communities in which modern artificial limbs are not available this can prove to be an excellent amputation as it adapts to the simplest type of artificial limb: the historical 'peg-leg'. On this the patient *kneels*, and the weight is borne, therefore, on a surface which is well accustomed to pressure. With such an appliance a 5 cm stump of tibia is ideal, and a longer stump is only an encumbrance. Flaps should be fashioned so that the scar does not lie on the kneeling surface. It should be emphasized, however, that this amputation is rarely used now.

DISARTICULATION AT THE KNEE JOINT

Through knee amputation provides a stump with some inherent advantages. The femoral condyles are expanded and allow for satisfactory suspension of an artificial limb. There is a large end bearing surface which is extremely comfortable within the socket of an artificial limb. There are however certain disadvantages: the stump is long and it is difficult to level the knee centre of a prosthetic extension with that of the natural knee of the normal leg. The knee therefore looks ugly. The amputation is very suitable for young and active men but tends to be less popular in young women with unilateral loss of a leg. It has been recommended for use in vascular disease but is no substitute for below the knee amputation when this is possible. Some patients who require through knee amputation in ischaemic disease develop discomfort over the lateral femoral condyle because of ischaemic changes in the skin at that site. For this reason it is not an amputation that can be wholeheartedly recommended in vascular disease and the author's preference is for above knee amputation when there are significant ischaemic changes in the leg, when the below knee level is not likely to succeed. Through knee amputation is always to be preferred to above knee amputation in the child as it preserves the distal growing epiphysis of the femur.

Technique

The operation is carried out with the patient lying on his face. Unequal anterior and posterior flaps may be used or medial and lateral flaps as described by Smith in 1852. If a long anterior flap is used this will extend to a level 2.5 cm below the tibial tubercle and is completed after flexing the knee. The shorter posterior flap should be about half the length of the anterior flap. Equal anterior and posterior flaps, or a circular incision are infrequently used. When medial and lateral flaps are used, the lateral flap is marked out from 2.5 cm below the tip of the patella vertically downwards to the upper border of the tibial tubercle and then curves

laterally to the midline of the posterior popliteal crease at the back 2.5 cm above the joint line. The lateral flap should extend to at least 2.5 cm beneath the upper border of the tibial tubercle and should be approximately half of the AP diameter of the leg in length. The medial flap should be approximately 4 cm longer than the outer flap in order to provide ample skin over the stump. Once the skin flaps have been prepared the popliteal fossa is opened and its contents defined. The popliteal vessels are divided between ligatures, below any branches that might supply the flaps (Fig. 9.47). The popliteal nerves are sectioned cleanly at the upper limit of the fossa. All muscles bounding the fossa, together with the posterior capsule lining its floor, are divided and the joint cavity is laid open. The knee is now flexed to a right angle, the capsule of the knee joint is exposed and the ligamentum patellae is divided at the front, and is turned upwards. The capsule of the knee joint is divided, the menisci removed and the cruciate ligaments are also divided. The patella is left in situ and the ligamentum patellae is sutured to the cruciate ligaments and the remains of the posterior capsule of the joint. The skin flaps are closed after trimming and a suction drain is left in the knee joint. The scar will lie either posteriorly when a long anterior flap is used or in the intercondylar area when medial and lateral flaps are used.

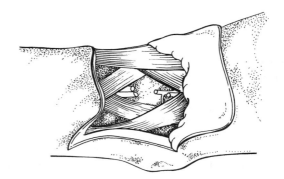

Fig. 9.47 Posterior approach to the knee in disarticulation

After through knee amputation there is frequently a synovial discharge from the wound for some days, but this resolves spontaneously.

AMPUTATION THROUGH THE THIGH

Anatomy

Muscles

The anterolateral group consists of sartorius and quadriceps femoris. Sartorius runs obliquely down the thigh from lateral to medial side. The quadriceps is formed by rectus femoris and the 3 vasti, which combine to form the patellar tendon. The vasti clothe the shaft of the femur on its lateral, anterior and medial surfaces.

The medial group consists of gracilis and the 3 adductors. Gracilis runs down superficially. Adductor magnus, by far the bulkiest muscle of the group, extends down as far as the adductor tubercle. Adductors longus and brevis have high insertions into the femur, and are encountered only in amputations above the middle of the bone.

Posterior group ('hamstrings') are biceps, semitendinosus and semi-membranosus. Biceps is inserted into the head of the fibula. The other two muscles both pass to the medial side of the upper end of the tibia.

Vessels
The *femoral artery* lies along the upper two-thirds of a line drawn from the midinguinal point to the adductor tubercle (when the thigh is slightly flexed, abducted and rotated laterally). In the upper third of the thigh the artery is medial to sartorius; in the subsartorial canal in the middle third, it is posterolateral. At the junctions of middle and lower thirds it passes through the opening in adductor magnus to become the *popliteal artery*, which is closely applied to the femur. The *femoral vein* in its lower part is posterior or posteromedial to its artery; in its upper part it is medial. The *profunda vessels* lie deeply on the anterior surface of adductor magnus. The *long saphenous vein* ascends in the superficial fascia on the medial side.

Nerves
The *femoral nerve* breaks up into branches immediately below the inguinal ligament; the only one requiring to be recognized in an amputation is the saphenous nerve, which accompanies the femoral artery as far as the opening in adductor magnus.

The *sciatic nerve* divides at a varying level in the thigh into *medial* and *lateral popliteal nerves*; these nerves lie on the posterior surface of adductor magnus, the lateral popliteal nerve passing under cover of biceps.

Objectives of amputation
The patient with amputation through the lower or middle-third of the thigh is fitted with an artificial limb which is usually in total contact with the stump and which will allow at least some weight to be taken by the ischial tuberosity against the upper and posterior rim of the socket. The femoral stump acts as a lever and moves the artificial limb. Its ideal length is 25–30 cm as measured from the tip of the trochanter or some 70% the length of the femur. The bone should be divided 8–10 cm above the knee joint. When the amputation is at the above knee level in children as much

length as possible should be preserved as the distal growing epiphysis of the femur is lost.

The through knee level in children is used if at all possible in order to preserve this epiphysis. When no more than 15 cm of the femur can be preserved in the adult, the thigh tends to slip out of the socket of the artificial limb and is not efficient as a lever. When disease or injury is so severe that no more than 10 cm of the femur can be preserved, disarticulation through the hip joint is probably preferable so that a Canadian No 1 prosthesis may be fitted. A tourniquet may be used during above knee amputation but must be applied on the thigh. It has the advantage of returning to the body blood which could otherwise have been lost with the discarded limb.

When through thigh amputation is used, opposing muscle groups are sutured together over the bone end so that muscle action on the stump remains balanced. Otherwise unopposed flexors of the hip and adductors of the thigh will tend to pull the stump into flexion and adduction.

Amputation through the lower third of the thigh
An appropriate method of amputating at this level is by unequal anteroposterior flaps, the longer flap being placed anteriorly. The extremity of the anterior flap is in the neighbourhood of the proximal border of the patella; the posterior flap is half the length of the anterior. The quadriceps tendon is divided at the level of anterior incision, and is raised in the flap (Figs 9.48 & 9.49). The hamstrings are cut at the level of the posterior incision. The femoral vessels are identified as they pass through the opening in adductor magnus. The medial and lateral popliteal nerves are found on the back of this muscle, the latter under cover of biceps. The lower tendinous fibres of the adductor are divided, and the vessels and nerves are dealt with in the usual way. The femur is sawn transversely, 8–12 cm above its lower end. The quadriceps tendon is turned back over the bone stump, and is sutured to the hamstrings. The flaps are approximated and sutured. Drainage for 48 hours may be advisable as a precautionary measure, but if all bleeding points are ligatured it is not necessary, since the section is made through tendinous muscle, and oozing is minimal.

Myoplasty
Younger and more active patients who do not have vascular disease are probably better served by a technique of myoplasty with myodesis that anchors the vastus lateralis, adductors and hamstrings to the femur by sutures passed through drill holes in the bone. Murdoch (1968) has recommended that these muscles are divided at the level of bony section, and that the quadriceps expansion is left long, is drawn over the

Fig. 9.48

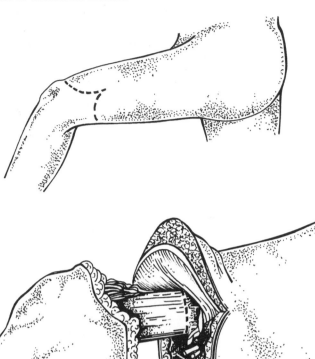

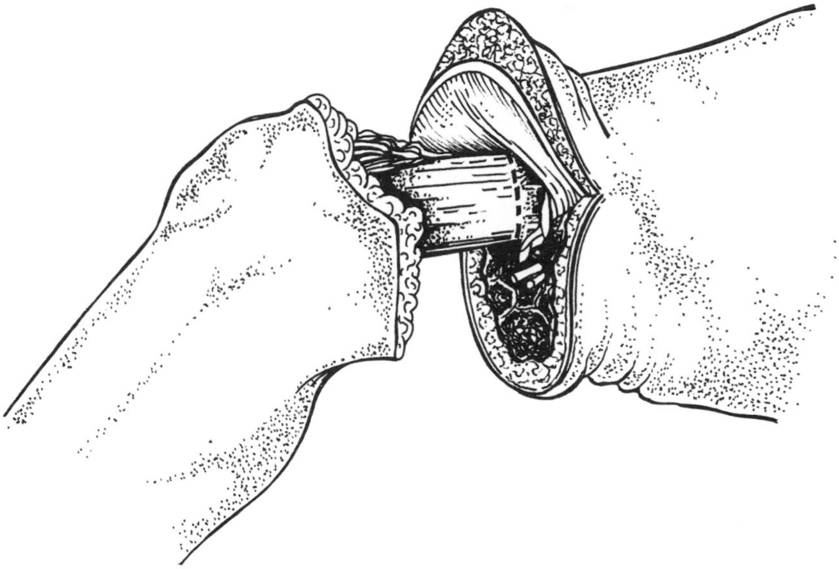

Fig. 9.49

Figs 9.48 & 9.49 Amputation through the lower third of the thigh

end of the divided bone and sutured to the anchored hamstrings posteriorly (see Fig. 9.4).

Amputation through the middle third (Figs 9.50 & 9.51)

At this level the flaps may be placed *anterolaterally* and *posteromedially*, to avoid the risk of splitting the femoral artery longitudinally, but their exact position will, of course, depend upon the amount of bone which can be preserved. The flaps are reflected proximally, the knife being made to cut more and more deeply, so that at the level of bone section all muscles have been divided. The femoral and profunda arteries, and the medial and lateral popliteal nerves (or the sciatic nerve) are dealt with in the usual manner. The flaps are trimmed as required, and are sutured. Drainage for 48 hours is essential, owing to the large area of cut muscle from which considerable oozing may occur.

Amputation through the upper third

When more than 10 cm of the femur, measured from the tip of the greater trochanter, cannot be preserved disarticulation through the hip joint is probably appropriate. When 10 cm of the stump or more can be retained the skin flaps will be fashioned as available and muscle will be trimmed as required. It is usually possible to provide a patient with a short stump of this nature with some form of suitable artificial limb.

Supracondylar amputations

Supracondylar amputations are mentioned simply to dismiss them as being of little value to the patient. There is little purpose in performing the Gritti-Stokes amputation in which the patella is anchored to the divided femur after its articular surface has been removed. This procedure risks non-union between the patella and the femur.

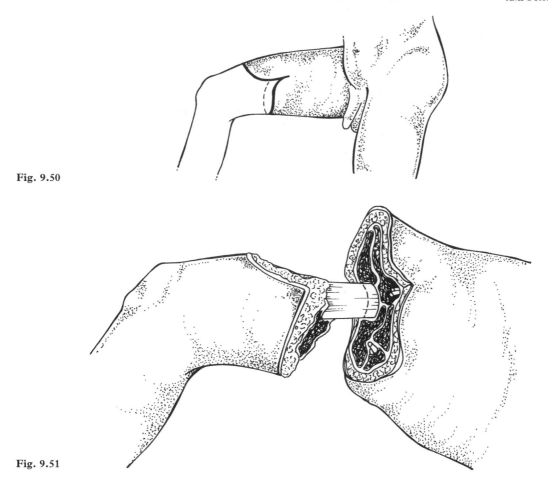

Fig. 9.50

Fig. 9.51

Figs 9.50 & 9.51   Amputation through the middle third of the thigh

Amputation through the distal femur does not allow the prosthetist enough room to place a prosthetic knee device beneath the socket in such a way that the prosthetic knee centre will level with that of the remaining normal knee. It is suggested therefore that these amputations should no longer be used.

AMPUTATION AT THE HIP

Anatomy

Muscles related to the hip joint
On all sides the joint is covered with muscle which is partly fused with the capsule. *Anteriorly* there are rectus femoris, iliopsoas and pectineus, in that order from lateral to medial side; more remote anterior relations are sartorius and tensor fasciae latae. *Posteriorly* lie piriformis, obturator internus (with the gemelli) and quadratus femoris; covering these is gluteus maximus. *Inferiorly* — obturator externus.

Vessels and nerves
The *femoral artery* enters the thigh behind the mid-inguinal point, lying on the psoas muscle. The *femoral vein* is on its medial side, and the *femoral nerve* lies laterally. The *sciatic nerve* lies on the posterior surface of obturator internus and quadratus femoris, under cover of gluteus maximus.

When more than 10 cm of the femur, measured from the tip of the greater trochanter, cannot be preserved, disarticulation through the hip joint is the amputation of choice and allows the patient to be fitted with the Canadian No 1 prosthesis (Fig. 9.52). This has a large socket which encloses the amputation stump and encircles the patient at his waist. It is a comfortable socket which allows the patient remarkably good function. Disarticulation is usually required after certain injuries or in some patients with sarcoma involving the upper part of the femur.

Disarticulation at the hip joint
Two classical methods have been described: the

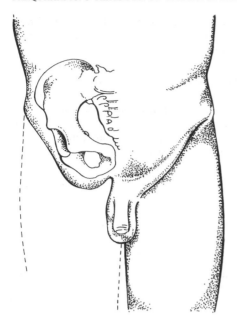

Fig. 9.52 Disarticulation of the hip joint. The proximal femur should be removed entirely

method of the anterior racquet, and that of the single posterior flap. The second method is to be preferred from the point of view of limb fitting, as it yields a firmer and more compact stump, but the choice will necessarily depend upon the conditions present. The incisions for the two methods are shown in Figure 9.53. The handle of the racquet is placed in the line of the femoral vessels, and the medial flap is the longer,

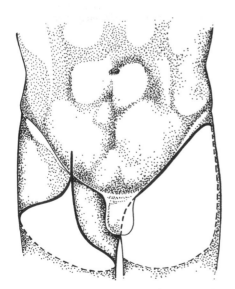

Fig. 9.53 Incisions that may be used for amputation at the hip

so that the scar will fall away from the perineum. In the alternative method the original length of the single posterior flap should be 1½ times the anteroposterior diameter of the limb at the level of the hip joint; the anterior part of the incision is 2.5 cm below and parallel to the inguinal ligament. In each method the first part of the operation consists in exposure and ligation of the femoral vessels. The anterior muscles are divided in the line of the incision, and the joint is opened from the front. The adductors, the hamstrings and gluteus maximus are cut so that portions of them remain in the flaps. The sciatic nerve is found lying deep to gluteus maximus, and is cut short. Disarticulation is completed by division of the capsule and of the remaining short muscles which are inserted into the trochanteric area. The flaps and muscle stumps are trimmed as required to prevent flabbiness of the stump. (In the method of the single posterior flap, all muscles are cut close to the pelvis, with the exception of those required to give reasonable bulk to the flap.)

INTER-INNOMINO-ABDOMINAL AMPUTATION

This operation may be undertaken for the removal of malignant growths of the pelvic bones or upper end of femur, or of the related soft tissues. Gordon-Taylor published in 1959 a personal series of 108 cases, with no deaths in the last 50. He urged that this amputation should always be preceded by a biopsy, since metastases in the pelvic bones from an unsuspected renal carcinoma may present an X-ray picture very suggestive of primary sarcoma.

Technique
An elliptical incision is advocated, its lateral part overlying the iliac crest and its medial part crossing the medial side of the limb a little below the perineum, but this may be varied according to the situation and extent of the tumour. The abdominal muscles attached to the iliac crest are divided close to the bone, and the peritoneum is stripped medially. The common iliac vessels are ligatured in continuity. The inguinal ligament is divided at each end; the conjoined tendon and rectus muscle are severed close to the pubis, and the spermatic cord is displaced medially. The pubic bone is cleared on its anterior and posterior surfaces, and the symphysis is divided with a strong knife or with a chisel. The posterior part of the ilium is cleared, the greater sciatic notch is identified, and with the aid of curved forceps a Gigli saw is passed through its apex. The ilium is then divided upwards and outwards towards the back of the iliac crest.

The innominate bone, together with the lower limb,

can now be drawn away to expose the lumbosacral trunk, and the first and second sacral and obturator nerves; these are injected with local anaesthetic and are divided. The external iliac, obturator, gluteal and pudendal vessels are divided, but should be ligatured first, since, although the common iliac vessels have already been tied, fairly brisk bleeding may still occur. Separation of the hindquarter is completed by the division of psoas, piriformis and levator ani, and by the detachment of ischiocavernosus and the crus penis

from the ischiopubic ramus. The stumps of muscles are sutured together to give as much support as possible to the peritoneum.

Recently there have been minor modifications to Gordon-Taylor's technique. Sir G. Gordon-Taylor himself later replaced ligature of the common iliac artery by individual ligations of the external iliac artery, and internal iliac artery beyond the origin of the superior gluteal vessel. This safeguards the blood supply to the large posterior flap.

REFERENCES

Burgess E M, Matsen F A 1981 Determining amputation levels in peripheral vascular disease. Journal of Bone and Joint Surgery 63A: 1493

Dederich R 1963 Plastic treatment of the muscles and bone in amputation surgery. Journal of Bone and Joint Surgery 45B: 90

Ertl J 1949 Amputations stumpf. Chirurgie 20: 218

Flint M, Sweetnam R 1960 Amputation of all toes. Journal of Bone and Joint Surgery 42B: 90

Ghormley R K 1947 Amputation in occlusion vascular disease in peripheral vascular disease. W H Saunders & Co., Philadelphia

Green R M, Rob C G 1985 Amputation of all the toes. In: Dudley H, Carter D C (eds). Rob and Smith's operative surgery, 4th edn. Butterworths, London, p 402

Hey W 1810 Practical observations in surgery, 2nd edn. Cader and Davies, London

Lisfranc J 1815 Nouvelle methode operation pour l'amputation patient du pied dans son articulation tarso metatarsiennei. Gabon, Paris

Loon H E 1962 Below knee osteomyoplasty. Artificial Limbs 6(2): 86

Mathur B P, Nardang I C, Piplani C L, Majid M A 1981 Rehabilitation of the bilateral elbow amputee by the Krukenberg procedure. The Journal of the International Society for Prosthetics and Orthotics 5: 3

Mondray F 1952 Der muskepkrafige oberations. Unfterschenketstumpf. Chirurgie 23: 517

Mooney V, Harvey J P, McBride E, Snelson R 1971 Comparison of postoperative stump management: plaster vs. soft dressings. Journal of Bone and Joint Surgery 53A: 241

Murdoch G 1968 Myoplastic techniques. Bulletin of Prosthetic Research 10–9: 4

Murdoch G (ed.) 1970 Prosthetic and orthotic practice. Arnold, London, p 141

Pederson H E, Day A J 1954 The transmetatarsal amputation in peripheral vascular disease. Journal of Bone and Joint Surgery 36A: 119

Peizer E, Wright D W, Mason C 1969 Human locomotion. Bulletin Prosthetic Research 10: 12

Redhead R G, Snowdon C 1978 A new approach to the management of wounds of the extremities — controlled environment treatment and its derivatives. Prosthetic and Orthotic International 2: 148

Srinavasan J 1973 Syme's amputation in insensitive feet. Journal of Bone and Joint Surgery 55A: 558

Swanson A B 1964 The Krukenberg procedure in the juvenile amputee. Journal of Bone and Joint Surgery 46A: 1540

Wagner F W Jr 1977 Amputations of the foot and ankle: lumbar status. Clinical Orthopaedics 122: 62

Warren R, Kilm R B 1968 A survey of lower extremity amputations for arterial insufficiency. J and A Churchill Ltd, London

OPERATIONS ON THE SCALP

Anatomy

The various layers of the scalp are shown diagrammatically in Figure 10.1.

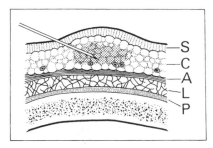

Fig. 10.1 Drawing to show the layers of the scalp and the depth at which local anaesthetic should be injected

Skin is thick and dense, and contains many sebaceous glands.

Connective tissue binds down the skin to the galea aponeurotica, so that these three layers of the scalp move as one. It consists of a dense network of fibrous tissue containing only small lobules of fat, and forms the main thickness of the scalp; within it lie the vessels and nerves.

Aponeurosis. The *galea aponeurotica* is a thin but dense aponeurosis, into which are inserted the frontal and occipital muscles. Its lateral margins blend with the strong temporal fascia.

Loose areolar tissue occupies the space between the galea and the pericranium. This space is limited by the origins of the frontal and occipital muscles, and on each side by the attachment of the galea to the temporal fascia. It is traversed by emissary veins which connect the dural sinuses with veins of the scalp. It constitutes the 'dangerous layer' of the scalp, since within this space blood or pus may collect, and may spread over the entire dome of the skull. Infection within the space may extend via the emissary veins to the dural sinuses.

Pericranium may be regarded as the periosteum on the external surface of the skull. It is continuous with the outer layer of the dura at the foremen magnum, and is attached to it at the sutures. Unlike periosteum elsewhere, it is easily stripped off the bone, and has little share in providing its blood supply.

Local anaesthesia in the scalp

Lignocaine 2% is commonly used with adrenaline 1 : 200 000. For injections of amounts greater than 20 ml it is usual to dilute the adrenalin to 1 : 400 000 but lignocaine without adrenalin can be used. Approximately 10 ml of fluid should be injected for each 3 cm of incision. It is important to avoid subgaleal injections because the nerves lie in the connective tissue layer into which the anaesthetic solution should be injected. Because the layer is dense injection into it requires considerable pressure. If there is little resistance it implies that the solution is diffusing into the subaponeurotic space and satisfactory anaesthesia will not be obtained.

Arrest of haemorrhage in the scalp

Whenever possible operative incisions should be made vertically in line with the main vessels. When long incisions are required they should be made in short sections whilst the cut edges are compressed against the skull by the assistant's finger tips (Fig. 10.2). Before the pressure is relaxed curved artery forceps are applied to the cut edge of the galea at 1 cm intervals and then pulled back so that the galea is drawn over the cut surface, stretching and occluding the bleeding vessels. A more efficient method is by the application of Raney clamps over skin and galea. These methods are necessary because the scalp vessels are enmeshed in the fibrofatty layer and cannot be picked up with forceps in the customary manner.

Wounds of the scalp

The smallest scalp wound is potentially serious because infection may result in a troublesome and prolonged cellulitis of the scalp or osteomyelitis of the skull. It is particularly dangerous if the wound overlies a

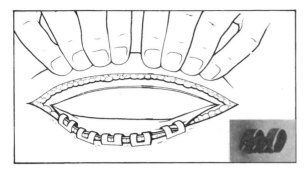

Fig. 10.2 Method of arresting haemorrhage in an operative incision in the scalp – first by pressure with the assistant's finger tips, and later by drawing the cut edge of the aponeurosis over the wound margins. Inset shows a Raney clip used in neurosurgical practice

depressed fracture, below which the dura may be torn, because then there is the risk of the development of a cerebral abscess. The extent and severity of the wound is determined by careful examination and by skull radiographs. This preliminary procedure may suggest that, after simple first-aid treatment, the patient should be transferred to a neurosurgical centre.

Shaving of the hair. In simple scalp wounds without gross contamination it is usually sufficient to shave the hair for a distance of 5 cm around the wound. Before doing so the selected area should be cut as short as possible with scissors and then thoroughly washed with soap and water. A safety razor has advantages over a 'cut-throat' since a supply of new blades can be made readily available although the 'cut-throat' razor does not clog so readily.

Débridement. In simple cases débridement (as contrasted with complete excision of the wound) is adequate and where necessary a local anaesthetic is infiltrated *through clean undamaged skin* in order to avoid the spread of infection. Under a good light the scalp edges are retracted and the wound is carefully examined, bleeding being temporarily arrested by gauze packing and scalp compression. Tags of devitalized tissue (skin, galea or pericranium) and any foreign material are removed and the wound is thoroughly washed out with saline. If the wound is grossly contaminated antibiotic can be applied locally.

Excision of the wound is essential when gross contamination is present, or if an underlying fracture has been detected. Local or general anaesthesia will be required depending on the extent of the damage and the age of the patient and a large area of the surrounding scalp (the whole scalp in large wounds) should be shaved. The wound edges and all devitalized tissue are meticulously excised but excision should be limited to only a few millimetres since there is a considerable risk

of producing a scalp defect which will require special procedures to close.

Methods of suturing the scalp

In simple scalp wounds, where excision has not been necessary, the cut edges are brought together loosely but accurately with a minimum number of interrupted sutures. A two-layer closure should always be done in wounds more than 3 or 4 cm in length (Fig. 10.3).

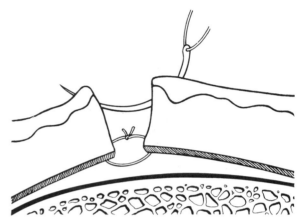

Fig. 10.3 Scalp suture in two layers — the deeper suture has not yet been tightened

Operative incisions and traumatic wounds *after excision* should always be repaired in two layers. First, the galea is approximated by interrupted sutures of fine silk, or preferably absorbable material, placed about 1 cm apart which take the main strain of the suture line and ensures sound healing. The skin edges are then brought accurately together by a further layer of stitching, interrupted or continuous. Rarely bleeding from a scalp vessel continues after wound suture but can be controlled by pressure or additional skin sutures. Very large lacerations, especially if there are flaps permitting collections of blood should, whenever possible, be drained by suction for 24 hours but if this is not available it is safer to leave the wound undrained.

Repair of defects. Every effort should be made to bring the scalp edges together. Because of the excellent blood supply, some wound tension is permissible although healing is then very dependent upon complete absence of infection and, despite the additional loss of tissue, careful débridement and wound excision should be performed. By undercutting, the scalp edges can usually be approximated by one of the plastic procedures illustrated (Figs 10.4 & 10.5) a two-layer closure always being performed. These are not minor procedures, however, and should not be attempted by the inexperienced.

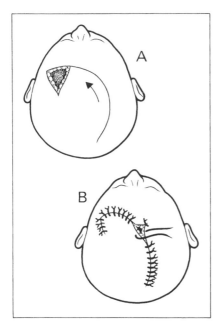

Fig. 10.4   Repair of scalp defect by a single rotational flap

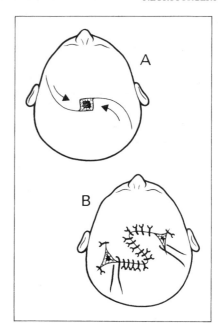

Fig. 10.5   Repair of scalp defect by double rotational flaps

OPEN WOUNDS OF THE SKULL AND BRAIN

Transfer to a neurosurgical centre

There is no reason why patients requiring neuro-surgical treatment should not be transferred to a specialist hospital equipped for neurosurgical work but before considering this it is very important to ensure that there are no other injuries such as rupture of the abdominal viscera which may require treatment in situ. Occasionally a neurosurgical team will travel to the hospital in such cases but in general the need for the neurosurgical team to be available for the reception of casualties from a wide area implies that the neuro-surgeon is reluctant to move from his base for a single case. Doubts as to the best procedure can usually be resolved by telephone consultation with the neuro-surgical centre.

Whenever possible, skull X-rays should be carried out on the patient's admission to hospital since these may reveal an unsuspected fracture or one more extensive than first diagnosed, thus altering the entire plan of treatment. Patients with head injuries, however, are very often extremely restless and X-rays of good quality cannot be obtained. In these situations it is often better to defer further radiographs until the patient's condition has stabilised or simply to proceed as a matter of urgency in dealing with the fractures already shown.

If the scalp wound is found in association with an underlying skull or brain injury and when transfer to a neurosurgical centre has been decided upon, the initial treatment should be confined to simple first-aid measures. The scalp should not be shaved for fear of introducing further infection and the wound should not be disturbed or probed. Gauze dressing with crepe bandage should be applied although if there is brisk bleeding from the scalp it is permissible to control this with loose sutures.

A general surgeon is unwise to operate on any scalp wound until he has excluded a fracture by radiography. 'Probing' the wound by finger or instrument to detect fractures is unreliable and quite unacceptable. Nevertheless there is an undeniable need for the general surgeon to be able to deal with head injured patients for whom it may be impossible in the circumstances which exist to obtain more expert care. Most of the surgery of head injuries is not beyond the scope of one well grounded in general surgery.

Treatment of a large scalp wound

To reduce the risks of infection and facilitate the operation, the entire scalp should be shaved. A local anaesthetic is usually quite satisfactory, the solution being injected into the scalp a few centimetres from the wound margin on each side. This enables all operative procedures to be carried out painlessly since the skull and brain are insensitive and the dura contains few nerves. In a restless and uncooperative patient and with extensive scalp laceration a general anaesthetic is recommended. It has the additional advantage that a clear airway is assured and the anaesthetist becomes a valuable member of the team keeping constant watch on the patient's respiratory state and attending to resuscitative measures. A meticulous excision of the wound is performed but wide removal of healthy tissue should be avoided so as to leave as little denuded skull as possible. When the wound is a small one it is frequently necessary to obtain better access — either for the purpose of thorough excision or in order to deal effectively with an underlying fracture. In the latter case general anaesthesia is preferable to local anaesthesia. The wound may be enlarged by extending the extremities into an 's' shaped wound. Alternatively a small laceration can be excised and sutured and then a '∩' shaped flap of scalp (which includes the sutured wound) is cut and reflected, haemorrhage being controlled by the methods described earlier.

Treatment of underlying ('compound') fractures

Linear (i.e not depressed) fractures

If the fracture is a clean linear one, without displacement, then no special treatment is required and the scalp wound, after excision, is carefully sutured. When a fracture is comminuted all small bone fragments should be removed but larger fragments, especially in cosmetic areas, can be washed in antibiotic solution and replaced.

Depressed fractures

Having exposed the whole extent of the depression, a small burr hole is made through undamaged bone

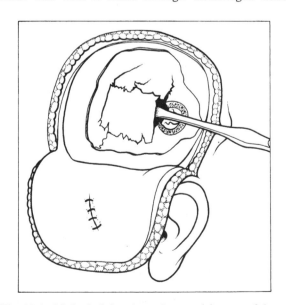

Fig. 10.6   Method of elevating a depressed fracture of the skull through an opening made with burr or trephine in undamaged bone adjoining the defect. In compound fractures all bone fragments which are contaminated should be removed

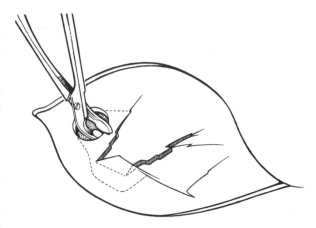

Fig. 10.7   Rongeur of depressed and comminuted fragment

at the periphery of the depression through which an elevator is introduced and used as a lever to raise the depressed fragments (Fig. 10.6). Only the most minor depressions can be dealt with in this way and it may be safer for the inexperienced operator to refer this procedure to a neurosurgical centre as he may do more harm than good. Grossly depressed and comminuted fragments should not be dealt with in this way but the bone edges rongeured away to allow the loose fragments to be carefully removed (Fig. 10.7). Fragments in the region of a venous sinus should not be elevated by a general surgeon. Any resultant defect in the skull is unlikely to cause symptoms but if necessary can easily be repaired at a later date (*Cranial defects*, p. 262).

Treatment of the dura

The dura is often intact in compound fractures and in such cases should never be opened unless from its bulging and plum coloured appearance there is strong reason to suspect a subdural haematoma. When a dural tear is present its whole extent should be exposed by removal of bone as required. Small pieces of felt with attached thread (patties) should be placed beneath the tear to protect the usually swollen underlying brain. Ragged dural edges should be sparingly excised but the tear should not be enlarged unless the underlying brain requires inspection. The dural tear should be carefully sutured with interrupted sutures of fine absorbable material, but if, as is often the case, the dura has retracted, then small tears may be covered with gelfoam and larger defects covered with a transplant of pericranium or fascia lata. If the patient's condition does not permit this a large sheet of gelfoam is applied over the surface of the brain and dural repair left for a later operation. No attempt should be made to close the dura if there is swollen brain.

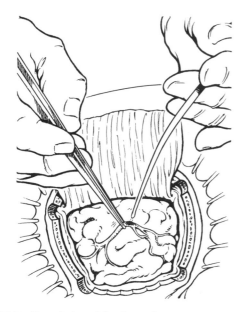

Fig. 10.8 Coagulation of dural vessels

Arrest of haemorrhage from dural vessels
All dural vessels are best sealed by the coagulating diathermy current (Fig. 10.8), applied to the vessels with sharp-pointed dissecting forceps. Use the smallest effective current to avoid damaging the underlying brain. Bleeding from the surface of the dura can be controlled by the application of muscle grafts taken from the temporalis muscle; when hammered or crushed to a thin sheet they adhere firmly to any tissue against which they are pressed. Gelatine haemostatic foam is also effective.

Tearing of dural sinus
Repair is best left to the expert but haemorrhage may be controlled by elevating the patient's head and applying a muscle graft or gelatine foam. Very large tears may be closed by a running silk ligature over which a muscle stamp or gelatine foam is pressed until bleeding ceases. If the tear cannot be repaired then the sinus must be under-run with a ligature or plugged with a muscle graft accepting the very considerable risk that the interruption of major venous drainage from the brain may well result in severe cerebral oedema.

Treatment of brain injury
Penetrating wounds of the brain are usually due to indriven fragments of bone but it is common for these to be embedded at any depth within the brain. Operation is designed to remove all devitalized cerebral tissue, extravasated blood, bone fragments and any accessible foreign bodies; in addition all haemorrhage must be arrested. A complete débridement of this na-

ture is dependent upon adequate exposure and direct vision. It is usually necessary, therefore, to perform a small craniotomy or enlarge the opening of the skull with rongeur forceps. Penetrating wounds of the brain are best dealt with by neurosurgeons.

Removal of damaged brain tissue
Damaged cerebral tissue can be removed by irrigation and suction. A gentle jet of warm saline is directed into the wound from a syringe and weak suction (25–30 cm Hg) through a finebore nozzle (3 mm lumen) is used to remove all devitalized brain matter and blood clot but leaving healthy brain matter alone. Suction is continued until the cavity is surrounded by healthy, undamaged brain tissue during which procedure any indriven bone fragments are discovered and removed with forceps. The utmost gentleness must be observed since any kind of rough handling will lead to destruction of valuable brain tissue or to interference with blood supply. The most meticulous attention must be paid to the arrest of haemorrhage for otherwise a postoperative clot is likely to form and to compress the brain. Bleeding points are controlled by diathermy coagulation.

Gunshot wounds of the brain
The wound of entry is often small and may be overlooked or treated as a simple scalp wound. The inner table is invariably more extensively fractured than the outer table and indrawn bone fragments are usually present. The missile may still be within the brain. Operative treatment is carried out as described above and the wound track in the brain followed and cleared of all damaged tissue. In the case of through-and-through wounds both entrance and exit wounds should be similarly treated. The question of whether a missile or other foreign body embedded in the brain should be removed depends upon its accessibility. When it lies within the track of brain destruction it will naturally be removed as part of the débridement. When it lies very deep in the brain the last portion of its track is often invisible. Attempts to follow and extract it can result only in further damage to healthy brain tissue. A deeply embedded foreign body may cause no symptoms when left in situ provided the area of more gross destruction in the superficial part of its track has received adequate attention. Attempts to remove deeply embedded foreign bodies are best left to neurosurgeons. The treatment described is effective for gunshot wounds due to low velocity missiles but many modern high velocity missiles unfortunately produce considerable brain pulping at a distance from the track.

Fractures involving the paranasal air sinuses
Frontal fractures or those involving the thin floor of the

anterior fossa often extend into the frontal or ethmoidal air sinuses and constitute a potential danger of pneumatocele, meningitis or brain abscess. The diagnosis is made from the radiographs or from the observation of cerebrospinal fluid rhinorrhoea but alternatively the condition may be found during wound exploration. If, during the exploration of an open wound, a fracture is found to extend into an air sinus, most commonly the frontal, dural tears in the vicinity should be carefully repaired. If there is a large defect in the sinus wall then it is usual to remove the mucous lining on the grounds that the risk of infection is reduced and a muscle graft should be placed in the sinus.

Cerebrospinal fluid rhinorrhoea
Provided adequate antibiotic treatment is continued for several weeks the risk of meningitis or brain abscess is small but if there is a profuse CSF rhinorrhoea or if a pneumatocele develops a dural graft should be applied as soon as the patient's condition permits.

EXTRADURAL AND SUBDURAL HAEMORRHAGE

Extradural haemorrhage is due most commonly to traumatic rupture of the middle meningeal vessels and occasionally tears of the dural veins or sinuses. Subdural haemorrhage may result from rupture of veins passing to the superior longitudinal sinus or the lateral sinuses and also from cerebral laceration. It is unnecessary to know the detailed course of the middle meningeal artery other than to appreciate that it enters the scalp through the foremen spinosum in the temporal fossa and then divides into an anterior and posterior branch embedded in the outer layer of dura.

Extradural or subdural haemorrhage although uncommon are very important closed head injuries since active surgical intervention is necessary and the results of energetic intervention are most gratifying. A massive haemorrhage not only produces local compression of the brain but also dangerous displacements which block cerebrospinal fluid pathways producing a rapid rise in intracranial pressure. Surgery consists of the evacuation of the clot and arrest of bleeding.

Operation is justified on the *suspicion* of extradural or subdural haemorrhage but if practicable the patient should be referred to a neurosurgical centre or if doubt exists advice by telephone should be sought. If, however, such facilities are not available the operation, which is, or can be, a relatively simple one, is well within the scope of a general surgeon and should not be withheld merely because expert aid is not available. Mortality after such operations is rarely due to the operative trauma. Death is frequently attributed to

concurrent brain injury but failure of diagnosis or hesitancy to operate in the early stages of clot formation is certainly a factor of equal importance. Exploration through a burr hole in the skull is a simple matter to determine whether a surface haemorrhage has occurred. Performed under local anaesthesia it entails so little risk yet is more than justified, even when negative findings are obtained. If an extradural or subdural haemorrhage is present simple enlargement of the exploratory opening is often all that is required to provide the access necessary for treatment of the condition.

Diagnosis
Extradural haemorrhage is relatively uncommon, forming about 2% of all head injuries admitted to hospital. The classical picture of a latent or 'lucid' interval following the injury, lasting for a few minutes to several hours, is the exception rather than the rule. Where it does occur it is followed by headache, giddiness and drowsiness, deepening into a coma but extradural haemorrhage should always be suspected when after some degree of recovery from the initial concussion the patient's condition deteriorates. As restlessness and drowsiness develop the pulse rate falls and blood pressure rises. Minor pupillary inequalities are not generally helpful and it is the *trend* of the changes in the signs which is so important in the diagnosis. A fixed, dilated pupil almost always means raised intracranial pressure — usually an expanding mass on the same side, very likely an extradural or subdural clot, although it can be due to cerebral oedema or intracerebral haematoma. A late sign of grave prognostic import, it usually indicates stretching of the third nerve with associated compression of the midbrain and downward displacement of the brainstem.

Subdural haemorrhage is more common than extradural haemorrhage. If presenting acutely, it is usually associated with major brain injury so a true 'lucid interval' is rare. In the *acute* form deterioration in consciousness may appear within a few hours of injury but in the *subacute* form several days may elapse before deterioration is evident. A *chronic* form may not manifest itself for several weeks or months. *Acute* subdural haematomas usually accompany severe brain laceration and oedema: the primary brain damage rather than brain compression by the clot often accounts for the clinical features when a patient with subdural haematoma presents acutely.

Localising signs
These are of great assistance in diagnosis especially in extradural haemorrhage where the bleeding is relatively confined. A deterioration in the conscious level nearly always precedes other clinical changes. An expanding lesion, especially if an extradural clot, is usually on the

same side as the first pupil to be dilated and/or fixed and, less reliably, contralateral to the first signs of limb weakness. Many intracranial clots are unaccompanied by skull fracturing but if present (radiologically or clinically) this increases the likelihood of an intracranial haematoma and is a good indicator of the site of an extradural clot that may be present.

Special investigations

For acute trauma, *computed axial tomography* (CAT scanning, Fig. 10.9 and page 256) is the best single radiological investigation, certainly better than Magnetic Resonance Imaging (MRI scanning, page 256), especially for showing and distinguishing brain swelling (oedema) and haematomas. On CAT scans extra-cerebral haematomas are seen as high density shadows producing ventricular distortion/displacement. In the absence of CAT scanning echo-encephalography or carotid angiography may reveal displacement of the brain's midline. However one must not delay for radiological studies if the patient's clinical condition demands urgent surgery to look for an intracranial blood clot. Patients may have to be assessed clinically, and exploratory burr holes performed.

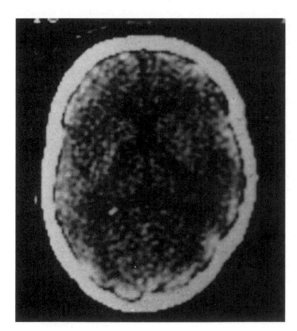

Fig. 10.9 CAT scan

Burr hole exploration

Extradural bleeding will usually have occurred deep to the external evidence of injury manifested in the form of an abrasion or bruising or a boggy swelling of the scalp. Urgent exploration, without guidance from CAT scans, is best performed at the site of the external injury

and it must be recognized that this may indicate the presence of a fracture running into the temporal region. If a fracture is seen on X-ray at another site the burr hole can be made at this site. Without this guidance, or to extend the search beyond these sites, make burr holes at standard sites ipsilateral to the side of initial pupillary dilatation/fixity (failing that, contralateral to initial limb weakness): a temporal burr hole immediately above the mid point of the zygomatic arch, a frontal burr hole (just in front of the coronal suture, i.e. just behind the hairline, in the parasagittal plane of the pupil), and a burr hole at the parietal eminence. If no haematoma is found on one side of the head a similar exploration should be performed on the opposite at once.

Preparation and position of patient

For an urgent procedure preparation may be minimal but whenever possible the entire scalp should be shaved since both sides may require exploration. A special

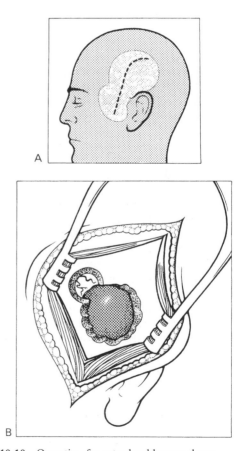

Fig. 10.10 Operation for extradural haemorrhage. (A) shows area to be infiltrated with local anaesthetic and the incision employed. (B) the initial opening in the skull is made with a burr or trephine, and is then enlarged with rongeur forceps to allow adequate access to the clot

head rest is not essential and the head can be placed on a soft sand bag or pillow. The head is elevated and turned to the opposite side, the surgeon and assistant standing at either side of the patient's head. Towels are applied to shut off the operation area (if possible over an overhead table) leaving an area beneath which the anaesthetist will have free access to the nose and mouth.

Anaesthesia

Either local or general anaesthesia may be employed. Endotracheal intubation ensures a good airway. Muscle relaxants and controlled ventilation prevent straining and increase of intracranial pressure. Light anaesthesia is sufficient if the line of the incision is infiltrated with local anaesthesia.

Access

For a temporal burr hole the incision begins at the lower border of the zygoma halfway between the eyebrow and meatus and runs upwards and slightly backwards for about 5 cm (Fig. 10.10). Haemorrhage is controlled by digital pressure and a self-retaining retractor placed in the superficial part of the wound. The superficial temporal artery is often severed and should be controlled by diathermy coagulation. In the lower part of the wound the temporalis muscle, covered by fascia, is incised and the muscle split down to the bone. A strong self-retaining retractor is placed in the split

down to the bone to hold the muscle fibres apart. The burr hole is made immediately above the midpoint of the zygomatic arch, using a perforator on a Hudson's brace (Fig. 10.11). The perforator should be turned rapidly with *gentle* downward pressure to prevent sudden perforation of the bone. When the inner table is penetrated a characteristic rocking or juddering sensation is produced. The perforator should then be replaced with a burr and the hole enlarged. Because the burr tapers and cuts a funnel-shaped hole it is very safe to use but the surgeon should still be careful not to plunge the instrument intracranially, especially through the thin bone of the temporal fossa. If an extradural haemorrhage has occurred the clot will now be seen presenting in the burr hole, or alternatively, the dura may be plum coloured and bulging due to the presence of subdural haemorrhage. In either case the burr hole should be enlarged by the rongeur. If the dura appears normal in colour (pinkish white shade) but is tense it is probable that cerebral oedema is present but if the dura is slack the exploration should be regarded as negative.

Treatment of extradural haematoma

The first essential is to enlarge the wound of access, for not only must the blood clot be removed but, if possible, the site of the bleeding should be identified and secured. The skin incision is extended upwards and backwards and the split in the temporalis muscle also extended. If necessary the temporal fascia is in-

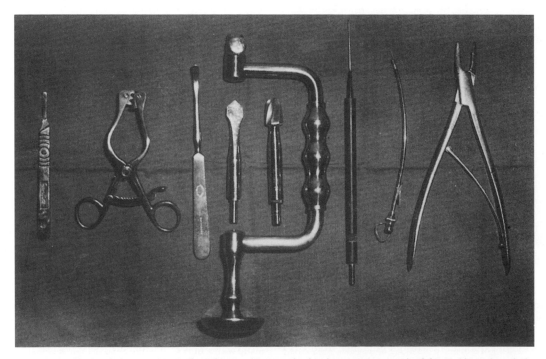

Fig. 10.11   Hudson's brace with skull perforator, burrs and other instruments required for making a burr hole

cised transversely along the temporal line and the muscle fibres on each side of the split scraped from their origin. By strong retraction a much wider skull exposure can now be obtained. The burr hole is then enlarged in the direction indicated by the situation of the clot, usually towards the skull base. The clot is evacuated by suction and displacement with a smooth instrument or blunt probe and washed away with a stream of saline. As the clot is removed the ruptured meningeal vessel may come into view but its identification may be difficult on account of continued haemorrhage. A clear field in the depths of the wound can be obtained by irrigating with warm saline but the essential feature is to have good suction. Haemostasis is achieved by diathermy coagulation or the application of a silver clip. If the artery is ruptured at the base of the skull at the foramen spinosum, and diathermy coagulation fails to control the haemorrhage a small plug of cotton wool or bone wax may be inserted into the foramen.

Frequently the site of the haemorrhage is not visible and it is unnecessary to search for it. The wound should be drained, ideally by vacuum drainage, the end of the drain being placed extradurally. If the clot is extensive and passes posteriorly the skin incision may be extended into a ∩-shaped flap and either a formal craniotomy performed or further bone removed by rongeur. Dural haemorrhage may be difficult to control after the vessels have been stripped off from the deep surface of the skull. It is helpful in these circumstances to put small pieces of gelfoam or muscle between the dura and undersurface of the bone and to stitch the dura to the pericranium over the bone edges (Fig. 10.12).

Treatment of acute subdural haemorrhage

Such haemorrhages are usually due to rupture of the cortical veins, sometimes in the region of the lesser wing of the sphenoid, (i.e. on the inferior surface of the frontal lobe or around the temporal pole), sometimes in the fronto-parietal region. In the subdural plane blood

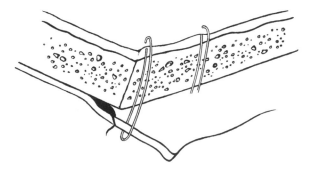

Fig. 10.12   Hitch stitches for control of an extradural blood vessel

spreads easily. Subdural clots may be well shown by CAT scanning or by cerebral angiography. Without this guidance subdural haematomas may be met during the search by burr holes (described above) for extradural clots. Suspect subdural haematoma if the dura is dark in colour and bulging. The dura should be carefully incised and the incision extended in a cruciate manner, whilst the underlying brain is protected by a retractor or small felt patty. The haematoma is now aspirated as completely as possible by suction, aided by flushing with warm saline. If bleeding continues the burr hole and dural incision can be enlarged in the direction from which the haemorrhage appears to come, so that the bleeding vessel can be located and sealed by diathermy coagulation. If the surgeon is satisfied that all bleeding has been arrested the wound may be closed, but otherwise it should be drained without a vacuum. If no clot, extradural or subdural, is found at the first burr hole further burr holes may be made as described above for extradural haematomas. If on the first exploration the underlying brain is slack then it is unlikely that there is any large increase of intracranial pressure and further explorations are unnecessary. On the other hand, whether or not an extradural clot has been removed, if the brain is tight but no subdural blood found on one side, although the commonest cause is cerebral oedema, there may be an acute subdural haematoma on the opposite side of the head. Acute subdural haematomas are commonly associated with severe cerebral laceration and intracerebral haemorrhage, especially in the temporal lobe, and to deal with this a large area of brain must be exposed and devitalized brain tissue and intracerebral clot removed by a combination of irrigation and suction.

The wound is closed by approximating the split temporalis muscle with 2 or 3 interrupted sutures and the scalp sutured in two layers. (Chronic subdural haematomas are considered later on page 261.)

Cerebral oedema is commonly associated with extra- and subdural haemorrhage. Treatment is by the intravenous administration of hypertonic solutions such as mannitol, which by its osmotic action causes fluid to be withdrawn from the swollen brain into the general circulation. One gram per kilogram body weight is given rapidly as a 20% solution and thereafter continued as a 20% solution at a rate of approximately 100 ml per hour. Levels above 310 milliOsmoles per litre of serum osmolality should be avoided.

At present it is widely believed that steroids do not significantly reduce brain oedema caused by trauma although they may reduce cerebral damage caused by post-operative cerebral hypoxia or ischaemia. Ventilation may be necessary to maintain arterial oxygenation but the value of controlled hyperventilation just to reduce $PaCO_2$ is questionable.

SIMPLE (i.e. non-compound) DEPRESSED FRACTURES

Compound fractures of the calvarium should be explored (see page 249 — *Open Wounds of skull and brain*).

Simple fractures are frequently unassociated with brain damage, and in the absence of neurological signs it is often unnecessary and indeed may be dangerous to elevate them. If, however, the fragment is depressed for more than the whole thickness of the skull, or if it is lying end-on, or is obviously spiculated, operation is generally advocated. The depressed area of bone is exposed by turning down a '∩' shaped scalp flap and the fracture is elevated by the method described on p. 250. The dura should not be opened unless it is already torn or there is evidence of underlying injury and unattached bone fragments should not be removed for they will readily consolidate as healing occurs.

Indentation of the skull, without true fracture, may occur in infants. When the depression is sharply incurved, operation is indicated. Through a curved incision a small opening is made at the margin of the depression and a smooth periosteal-elevator inserted and used to elevate the depressed area of bone.

SPECIAL DIAGNOSTIC PROCEDURES IN CRANIAL NEUROSURGERY

Computed Axial Tomography (CAT scanning — Figs 10.9 & 10.13)

X-rays are passed through the head as an X-ray tube rotates around it; the rays are detected, stored and computed to produce images of the skull and brain in different planes. Intravenous contrast media can reveal regions of increased vascularity or of breakdown of the blood-brain barrier. CAT scans show intracranial ventricles and other CSF-spaces, intracranial masses including neoplasms, brain abscesses and other brain lesions. Currently, CAT scans are much better than MRI scans for showing acute intracranial problems, especially acute haemorrhage (spontaneous or traumatic), in the neurosurgical field.

Magnetic Resonance Imaging (MRI scanning)

A large magnet and an introduced radiowave make the body's protons resonate and emit electromagnetic waves which are detected to enable a computer to produce images in different planes.

MRI scanning is unique in showing regions of demyelination. Like CAT scanning it shows CSF-spaces, intracranial masses such as neoplasms and other brain lesions, but MRI-scanning has advantages in showing tumours such as pituitary tumours and acoustic neuromas that are closely adjacent to the skull base.

Cerebral Isotope Scanning (Fig. 10.14)

This is useful if CAT- or MRI-scanning are not available. A short-life radioactive isotope is injected intravenously and the radioactive emission from the head measured by a scanning gamma camera which produces a picture of radioactive densities within the skull. Vascular lesions such as tumours and abscesses appear as regions of increased density.

Angiography

Displacement of cerebral vessels can show the site of intracranial masses including haematomas and neo-

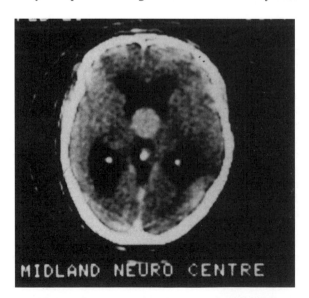

Fig. 10.13 CAT scan showing choroid cyst of the third ventricle

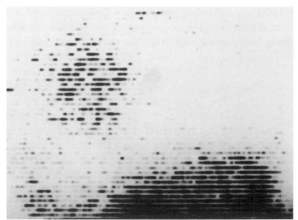

Fig. 10.14 Cerebral isotope scan showing increased uptake in the high posterior parietal region caused by a meningioma

plasms. The nature of some neoplasms may be diagnosed from characteristic patterns of their blood supply. However, the particular application of angiography is to show abnormalities (e.g. aneurysms or vascular malformations) of the cerebral vessels themselves (Fig. 10.15).

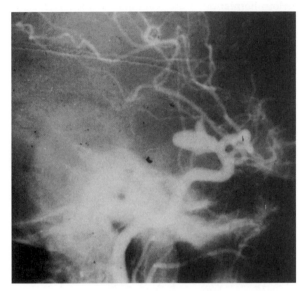

Fig. 10.15 Carotid angiogram showing aneurysm of the intracranial carotid artery

Angiography uses iodinated contrast media, ionic e.g. *meglumine diatrizoate* or non-ionic (better but more expensive) e.g. *iopamidole.*

Angiography is performed in the X-ray department, usually under local anaesthesia, often with sedation. The contrast agent is usually injected through a catheter introduced through the femoral artery and advanced under X-ray control into the chosen carotid or vertebral artery in the neck; contrast is injected and many serial X-rays are taken with an automatic film changer as the contrast passes through the head.

In an emergency the contrast may be injected by *direct puncture*. Common carotid injection is simplest. The patient lies on his back with the neck slightly extended. Local anaesthetic is injected at a site in front of the sternomastoid and deep to the carotid. An arterial cannula, or even an 18 gauge needle, is inserted through the carotid and then withdrawn until arterial blood spurts out. A large syringe containing contrast medium is attached through fluid-filled tubing to the needle. Taking care not to inject any air, one injects approximately 10 ml of contrast medium rapidly under pressure. An immediate exposure (*arteriogram*) is made followed by a quick change of film and a second expo-

sure (*venogram*) 2–3 seconds later. Usually the lateral projections are taken first and then the same procedure followed to obtain an antero-posterior view. For bilateral carotid angiography, no more than 50 ml of ionic contrast medium should be injected, more if the contrast is non-ionic.

Ventriculography (Fig. 10.16) – *Ventricular Puncture*
Contrast medium introduced into the cerebral ventricles is visualised on plain skull X-rays. In the absence of CAT- or MRI-scanning, ventriculography (separately or in conjunction with cerebral angiography) may show hydrocephalus or the presence and site of a space-occupying lesion e.g. neoplasm.

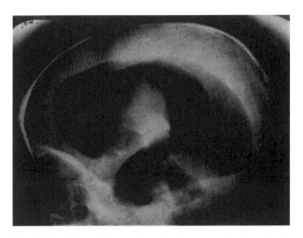

Fig. 10.16 Air ventriculogram showing gross hydrocephalus

Ventricular puncture is performed under local anaesthetic. A frontal burr hole on one side or on both is made immediately in front of the coronal suture, just behind the hairline, in the parasagittal plane of the pupil. A ventricular cannula is introduced through such a burr hole (aiming from the front to the nasion, from the side to the external meatus) until the frontal horn is penetrated, usually 5–6 cm deep to the cerebral surface. Successful entry into the ventricle is shown by the release of cerebrospinal fluid (CSF) from the cannula when the stylet is removed. A similar cannula is inserted on the second side. CSF is withdrawn, 5–10 ml at a time, and replaced by a slightly smaller quantity of air. Ventriculography can be performed through a single burr hole especially if, instead of air, water-soluble contrast (e.g. 5 ml of a 300 mg/100 ml solution of *iopamidole*) is introduced to give better visualization.

The interpretation of ventriculograms depends on abnormalities of the ventricles including inequalities in size, displacements and filling defects.

METHODS OF ACCESS IN BRAIN OPERATIONS

The osteoplastic flap

This method is now universally adopted for the exposure of any part of the cerebral hemispheres. A flap may be made in the frontoparietal, parietal or parieto-occipital regions of the skull, according to the estimated position of the cerebral lesion and must be of sufficient size to give the access which is required. The increasing use of the microscope in neurosurgery has encouraged the use of much smaller exposures than formerly.

The true osteoplastic flap (Fig. 10.17), where the bone flap is cut and turned down with the scalp adherent to it, is rarely, if ever, performed nowadays.

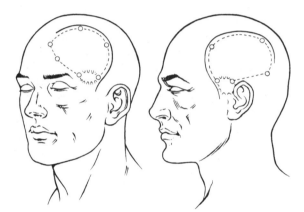

Fig. 10.17 The position of osteoplastic flaps for exposure in the frontoparietal and parietal areas. Dotted lines are shown between burr holes

The scalp incision is '∩'-shaped, the base of the flap being sufficiently broad for an adequate blood supply and scalp haemorrhage arrested by the methods described on p. 247. Four or five burr holes are made along the periphery of the exposed skull, the two holes at the base of the flap being placed considerably nearer than are the ends of the scalp incisions so that the narrow base can be rongeured more easily. The hand operated Hudson's brace, used in conjunction with a burr, is used for making the burr holes. The dura is separated from the skull with a curved dissector insinuated through the burr holes. By means of a special guide a Gigli saw is passed between adjacent holes and the intervening bone is divided — with an outward bevel so that the freed portion of skull, when replaced, will not sink below its normal level. Haemorrhage from the diploë of the skull is arrested by rubbing in bone wax, and meningeal haemorrhage by diathermy coagulation. Bleeding from the dural sinus may be controlled by applying a muscle graft.

Incision of the dura (Fig. 10.18)

It is usual to employ a 'U' shaped incision with its base towards the nearest venous sinus. If the dura appears tense it is advisable to give intravenous *Frusemide* 40–80 mg and/or intravenous *Mannitol* (1 gm/Kg body weight) as 20% solution very rapidly to reduce brain volume before opening the dura widely, as otherwise serious herniation of the brain may occur.

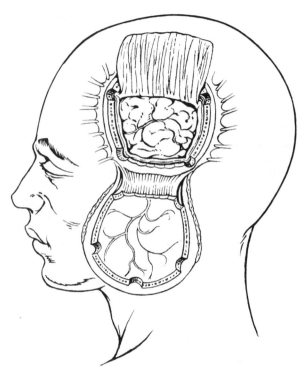

Fig. 10.18 Method of turning down a flap based on the temporalis muscle. The skin flap has been reflected along with the skull flap and the dura opened as a U-shaped flap

Replacement of the flap

At the end of the operation, after suture of the dura, the portion of skull is replaced in position, secured by absorbable pericranial stitches, and the scalp repaired in two layers.

Posterior fossa approaches

The operation may be done with the patient in the three-quarter prone position, the head firmly held in a head holder. The prone position, with the neck flexed, is easier to achieve but great care should be taken to avoid pressure on the eyes and, by the interposition of appropriately placed sand bags, on the abdomen and chest. The sitting-up position, whilst reducing intracranial tension and facilitating exposure, has very considerable danger of air embolus and with good anaesthesia is no longer necessary.

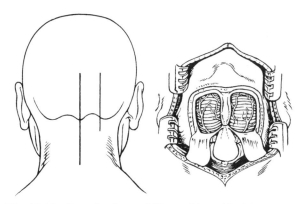

Fig. 10.19 Posterior fossa midline and lateral incision

A skin incision (Fig. 10.19) may be made either vertically in the midline or paramedially, extending up the head in a curvilinear fashion if more lateral exposure is required. Self-retaining superficial retractors are inserted and the nuchal muscles separated by cutting diathermy in the midline down to the occipital bone in the arch of the atlas. A larger, deeper, self-retaining retractor is then inserted. A burr hole is made in the occipital bone on each side of the midline and, after separating the dura, the bone is nibbled away with rongeur forceps downwards to include the posterior margin of the foramen magnum, upwards as far as the transverse sinus and laterally to the mastoid process. The posterior arch of the atlas may also be removed.

BRAIN TUMOURS

Brain tumours are either extrinsic, such as meningiomas, acoustic neuromas and pituitary tumours, or intrinsic, such as metastatic tumours and gliomas.

Meningiomas
These arise usually in the neighbourhood of dural sinuses, compressing the cerebral cortex and often invading the overlying bone. Meningiomas commonly arise from the falx, the lateral angle of the sagittal sinus (parasagittal meningiomas), the sphenoidal ridge and over the brain's convexities. *Parasagittal* meningiomas are exposed by craniotomy extending to or over the midline. For the occasional operator the safest method of removal is to gut the tumour with diathermy loop and then dissect out the shell, displacing it towards the tumour's central cavity. If the tumour lies on the *convexity* the dura can be incised around the margin and removed with the tumour. *Parasagittal* meningiomas are treated similarly but they often invade the sagittal sinus, and again the occasional operator should confine himself to removing the tumour and to diathermying the involved dura of the venous sinus. *Sphenoidal wing* meningiomas are closely related to the middle cerebral artery and complete removal is difficult.

Acoustic neuromas
These are situated in the cerebellopontine angle on the posterior aspect of the petrous temporal bone. A paramedian posterior fossa craniectomy is performed and the cerebellum on the affected side retracted medially or partially excised to expose the tumour. If possible the tumour is completely removed otherwise it is incised and its contents evacuated.

Pituitary tumours
These may compress the optic nerves and distort the carotid. *Frontal craniotomy* is performed and the frontal lobe elevated to reveal the optic nerve and tumour. An incision is made into the capsule and the contents aspirated or curetted away.

Small or entirely intrasella pituitary tumours are best removed through a *transphenoidal* approach. In the transphenoidal route (Fig. 10.20) the upper lip is everted and an incision made in the gingivolabial sulcus. The mucoperiosteum is displaced upwards until the floor of the nose and nasal septum are exposed, the submucous resection of the septum is carried backwards along the vomer to the roof of the nasopharynx, and the anterior wall of the sphenoidal air sinus is removed with punch forceps to expose the dura of the pituitary fossa. This is penetrated and the tumour removed piecemeal. An alternative approach to the sphenoid sinus is through the medial wall of the orbit and the ethmoidal air sinus.

Metastatic tumours of the brain
These are often well demarcated and, if sufficiently large, can be well localized and removed through an incision in the overlying brain.

Gliomas
These are infiltrating tumours, poorly demarcated from the surrounding brain. As a rule total removal is not feasible. The patient's condition can sometimes be dramatically improved by puncture of a neoplastic cyst or by the partial removal of the tumour by incising the cortex (in an area which is functionally unimportant) and then removing the tumour piecemeal by suction and forceps (the so-called internal decompression).

BRAIN ABSCESS

Brain abscesses occur following implantation through compound skull fractures, blood-borne spread from anywhere in the body, and spread from infections of

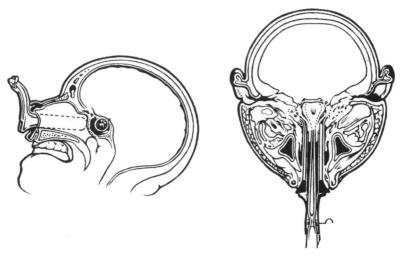

Fig. 10.20 Transphenoidal hypophysectomy

the fronto-ethmoidal or mastoid sinuses. From sinus infection abscesses occur in the frontal and temporal lobes and in the cerebellum, the latter two in association with middle ear disease. In the early stages of cellulitis antibiotics may prevent progression into a definite abscess cavity. If an abscess forms, however, it constitutes a surgical emergency and drainage should be provided as a matter of urgency. The site of the abscess can be diagnosed from the source of the infection and from the physical signs. Frontal abscesses often present with lethargy and confusion, temporal lobe abscesses may present very acutely with deepening coma and a contralateral hemiplegia, cerebellar abscesses may show nystagmus and inco-ordination. In all three there may be papilloedema, rapidly progressing coma, and death. Abscesses are shown best by CAT-scanning (with i.v. contrast), also by isotope-scanning, sometimes by angiography.

Frontal and temporal lobe abscesses (Fig. 10.21) are best drained by making a frontal or temporal burr hole, opening the dura in a cruciate fashion to reveal the bulging brain and inserting a ventricular cannula directly through the brain into the abscess. The wall of the abscess, which is often encapsulated, is felt as a characteristic resistance and when this is penetrated pus oozes out under pressure through the needle. The needle should be carefully retained in position and antibiotics instilled. If a CAT scan is not available for subsequent examination of the progress of the abscess, a small quantity of air may be introduced into the abscess cavity together with the antibiotic. The air can be shown subsequently by plain x-rays. After removal of the pus, small abscesses rapidly shrink, a process that can be observed radiologically. Large chronic abscesses which have developed a firm capsule will require more

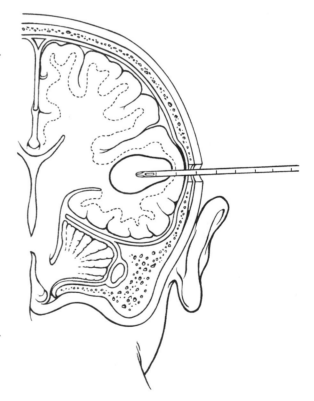

Fig. 10.21 Tapping of cerebral abscess

than one aspiration of pus. Such large abscesses, however, frequently require formal craniotomy and excision as they are unlikely to heal satisfactorily by simple aspiration.

Sub-dural empyema

The formation of pus in the subdural space may result from the same sources as brain abscesses but especially from air sinus infections. Patients are often toxic and present focal signs such as hemiplegia or epilepsy due to inflammation in the underlying cortex and veins. The pus should be evacuated and antibiotics instilled as soon as possible. Burr holes are made bifrontally and biparietally to allow the removal of the usually small amount of pus and the placement of two to three small catheters in each burr hole for the administration of antibiotic. Some surgeons, however, favour a wide craniotomy with removal of the pus and placement of a few catheters in the space. Epilepsy is common in this condition and all patients should be treated with prophylactic anticonvulsants.

OPERATIONS FOR TRIGEMINAL NEURALGIA

If drug treatment becomes ineffective in relieving trigeminal neuralgia, an operation on the nerve is indicated. The most common is glycerol or radiofrequency destruction of the trigeminal ganglion. This is performed under local anaesthesia with sedation or general anaesthesia, the needle being inserted about 2.5 cm from the corner of the mouth and directed towards the pupil (as seen from the front) and the middle of the zygoma (as seen from the side). The needle enters the cave of Meckel and cerebrospinal fluid can often be aspirated, confirming the position of the needle, which is further confirmed by A-P and lateral radiographs. 0.1 to 0.4 ml of glycerol is then injected with the patient sitting or a current passed through an insulated needle.

In some cases, especially in patients younger than 50 years or when pain involves the first trigeminal division, some neurosurgeons favour a bigger procedure, posterior fossa *craniectomy* under general anaesthesia, to treat trigeminal neuralgia by displacing a compressing vascular loop away from the sensory root of the trigeminal or by partial division of the sensory root.

INTRACRANIAL ANEURYSMS AND SUBARACHNOID HAEMORRHAGE

Intracranial aneurysms are largely confined to the circle of Willis (Fig. 10.22) and the middle cerebral artery at its first primary branching in the stem of the lateral fissure. The patient complains of sudden onset of severe headache and neck stiffness, sometimes with temporary loss of consciousness. CAT scanning shows subarachnoid blood. Lumbar puncture shows evenly blood stained CSF with xanthochromic supernatant. If the patient survives this initial haemorrhage he is at

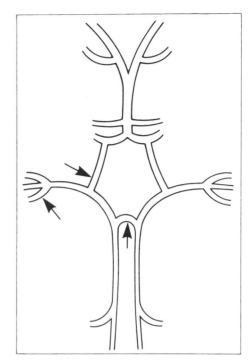

Fig. 10.22 Diagram of the circle of Willis. Arrows indicate the commonest sites for an intracranial aneurysm

grave risk of further haemorrhage which is often more serious. Angiography confirms the existence of an aneurysm and its site. If the patient's condition is satisfactory operation is performed at the earliest opportunity. The operative treatment depends upon the site of the aneurysm. The ideal treatment is occlusion of the neck of the aneurysm with a clip, so that it is excluded from the cerebral circulation; if this is not possible the aneurysm sac may be strengthened by fibrous reaction induced by gauze wrapping. Aneurysms of the intracranial part of the internal carotid artery can be dealt with by common carotid ligation but before this is performed a good cross circulation must be demonstrated by angiography.

CHRONIC SUBDURAL HAEMATOMA

This condition may occur after an apparently trivial injury and manifest itself a considerable time later. Characteristically the patient has a fluctuating course of lethargy or coma and there may be a contralateral or ipsilateral hemiparesis. Diagnosis and treatment can be made by burr holes (Fig. 10.23). These are made under local anaesthesia in the midpupillary line at the coronal suture and parietal eminences. If at one or more of the openings the dura is found to be dark in colour it is incised and the underlying haematoma,

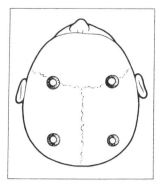

Fig. 10.23 The 'four burr hole' method of diagnosis and treatment of subdural haematoma

which is usually fluid, is evacuated by irrigation and suction. Unless there is radiological evidence to the contrary the procedure should be repeated on the opposite side since bilateral collections are common.

CRANIAL DEFECTS

These may be due to the removal of bone fragments in comminuted or depressed fractures, and less frequently are the result of exploratory or decompression operations. Repair of the defect may be desirable for cosmetic or psychological reasons or to protect the brain from possible injury at work or play. It is advisable to wait at least 6 months after the wound has been soundly healed to ensure the absence of infection. The defect may be filled with autogenous bone graft taken from the ribs or ilium, by the implantation of a titanium plate or more conveniently by acrylic plastic.

STEREOTACTIC SURGERY

Stereotactic methods are used to place an instrument, usually a metal probe, cannula or electrode, very accurately within the brain. There are many stereotactic instruments available but in general all follow the same principles of securing a rigid frame to the head, the taking of CAT scans to show the brain (or X-rays to show ventricular contours outlined by radio-opaque dye) and the establishment of their relationship to the stereotactic frame which usually has radio-opaque rulers and scales engraved. The stereotactic instrument directs an instrument, often through a burr hole, to the desired target. Tumours may be biopsied and abscesses tapped very accurately. Stereotactic probes can destroy a focus of brain tissue by freezing or by heat coagulation using a radiofrequency current and in this way may treat symptoms of movement disorders, mental disorder, and chronic pain. With guidance from stereotactic frames highly-focused radiotherapy can be concentrated on intracranial targets to treat certain neoplasms and vascular malformations (*stereotactic radiosurgery*).

DIAGNOSTIC PROCEDURES ON THE SPINAL CORD AND ROOTS

Lumbar puncture

Lumbar puncture is undertaken for a wide variety of diagnostic and therapeutic purposes. It provides an opportunity to detect purulent or blood stained c.s.f. and to obtain cerebrospinal fluid for laboratory measurements, including cell count, gram stain, culture and antibiotic sensitivity. In addition, protein, glucose and immune globulins and serology may be measured.

In difficult cases or sometimes in very obese patients, the procedure is facilitated by having the patient seated and the spine bent forwards but it is more usual to perform the procedure with the patient lying on his side. In either case, the spine must be flexed as much as possible in order to open out the interspinous spaces through one of which the puncture is made. Spinal flexion is achieved by having the patient with knees flexed and drawn up to the chest and the neck flexed. This position can be steadied by an assistant. A fine calibre spinal needle is preferable because it produces only a small tear in the dura and minimizes the risk of post puncture headache. It should be very sharp with a short bevel into which the stylet fits accurately. A line joining the highest points of the two iliac crests crosses the interval between the fourth and fifth lumbar spines (Fig. 10.24) and the puncture may be made in this space or one above or below.

After cleansing the skin a local anaesthetic is injected into the skin and subcutaneous tissues and the lumbar puncture needle then inserted midway between the

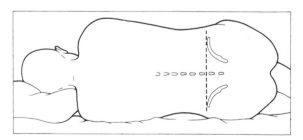

Fig. 10.24 Left lateral position for lumbar puncture. Line joining iliac crests indicates 4th/5th interspace — the usual site for insertion of needle

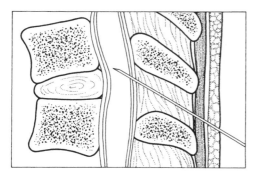

Fig. 10.25   Lumbar puncture needle introduced between the spinous processes

spinous processes (Fig. 10.25). It should be advanced strictly in a sagittal plane with the point directed slightly towards the head. Immediately after the skin is pierced the resistance of the tough supraspinous ligament is encountered and overcome. At a further depth of about 4 cm the lesser resistance of the ligamentum flavum and of the dura mater is felt. Thereafter entry of the needle point into the spinal canal is denoted by a sudden sensation of decreased resistance. As soon as this is felt the stylet is withdrawn and cerebrospinal fluid should escape in drops. When the needle appears to have been introduced to the required depth but no fluid appears it has probably deviated laterally and the needle should be withdrawn and reinserted. Normal cerebrospinal fluid is colourless and crystal clear.

Cisternal puncture
This is rarely necessary and is a dangerous procedure, best left in the hands of the expert. It may be required if lumbar puncture fails to tap the cerebrospinal fluid or for myelography in patients with multiple spinal blocks. The procedure is best done with the patient sitting with the neck strongly flexed. The puncture site is exactly in the midline above the spine of the axis in the plane of the two mastoid processes and the needle is directed upwards and forwards in the sagittal plane to strike the under surface of the occipital bone. The point of the needle is then directed lower until the needle is felt to penetrate the posterior occipito-atlantal ligament immediately below the posterior margin of foramen magnum. This is encountered at approximately 5 cm depth and cerebrospinal fluid should escape when the stylet is withdrawn.

Spinal manometry
Lumbar fluid pressure is a reasonably accurate measurement of intracranial pressure provided that the head and vertebral column are in the same strictly horizontal plane. Apart from diagnosing benign intracranial

hypertension (after an intracranial space occupying lesion has been excluded) there is no indication for spinal manometry in patients with increased intracranial pressure and its use in patients with mass lesions in the spinal canal may well precipitate or intensify compression of the spinal cord and nerve roots.

Myelography
The spinal cord and canal can be shown by the introduction of contrast medium into the spinal subarachnoid space. The medium is usually introduced by lumbar puncture after the removal of 5 ml of cerebrospinal fluid for laboratory studies. When a small amount of contrast medium has been injected, X-rays can confirm that it is in the subarachnoid space. If this is satisfactory the remaining contrast medium is injected and, with the patient prone and tilted head-down, X-rays are taken to visualize the flow of contrast medium. If it is arrested or displaced by any obstruction within the spinal canal the level is accurately determined.

Lesions such as spinal neoplasms and intervertebral disc protrusions cause characteristic displacement, distortion or obstruction of the CSF pathway shown by the contrast. A study showing the spinal cord is *myelography*, one limited to the levels of the cauda equina, *radiculography*.

As contrast medium, Myodil (an oily liquid which may lead to arachnoiditis) has been replaced by non-ionic iodinated water-soluble agents such as *iopamidole* or *iohexol* (5–10 ml may be used — but not more than a total of 3 gm of iodide).

Isotope scan
The spine may be scanned in a similar fashion to cerebral isotope scan (Fig. 10.14) following the intravenous injection of a different (bone-seeking) intravenous isotope. This may show multiple spinal lesions, e.g. vertebral infections or neoplasms.

Computed Axial Tomography (CAT scanning)
This procedure (see p. 256) shows the spine and its contents in transverse sections and, after computer reconstructions, in coronal and sagittal planes also. It is especially valuable for showing disorders of vertebral bone including spondylosis, tumours, trauma and deformity. Many believe that CT-myelography, i.e. CAT scanning performed within a few hours after myelography, is the best single investigation for complex spinal problems.

Magnetic Resonance Imaging (MRI scanning)
MRI scanning shows the spine and its contents in slices in sagittal, coronal and transverse planes. Currently it is the best single radiological study for myelopathy.

SPINA BIFIDA

Spina bifida is a congenital defect in the bony wall of the spinal canal through which the canal contents may protrude. It is almost invariably posterior, usually in the lumbosacral region, less often in the cervical and most rarely in the thoracic region.

Meningocoele

This is saccular protrusion of dura mater often covered completely or incompletely with skin and containing cerebrospinal fluid. The cord is normal and not displaced but spinal nerve roots may be caught up in the wall of the sac: if so, patients may have flaccid paralysis of leg muscles and sphincters, in which case the result of surgical repair is poor. Repair is done to treat ulceration of the sac and to prevent its rupture and infection. A transverse elliptical incision is made along the sides of the sac and the surrounding skin undermined. The sac is then opened about 3 cm from the base and inspected to see if there are any nerve roots within it. If possible these are freed and replaced in the canal. The redundant part of the sac is either cut away and the remaining portion repaired with fine sutures or, after tapping, the sac is inverted into the defect and the fascia and skin closed in layers over it. The muscles are approximated in the midline, so as to give a strong repair, but rotation flaps may be needed to ensure adequate skin cover.

Myelomeningocoele

In myelomeningocoele the cord is within the sac, the dura of the sac may be deficient, and invariably there are serious neurological disabilities. Excision of the sac is usually not possible but it can be emptied by tapping, the open dural layer stitched closed, the sac replaced in the bony defect, and the muscle and fascia closed over it as for simple meningocoele.

Hydrocephalus

Commonly myelomeningcoele is associated with hydrocephalus which may require separate treatment by ventricular shunting. This is done by inserting a catheter into one of the dilated lateral ventricles of the brain and connecting the catheter, usually via some flushing device with a valve to regulate CSF flow, to another silicon catheter which may be passed down the jugular vein into the heart (*ventriculo-atrial shunt*) or passed down over the chest wall into the peritoneum (*ventriculo-peritoneal shunt*).

SPINAL INJURIES

Operation may be indicated in dislocations and fracture/dislocations of the vertebral column, especially when these are associated with neural damage or where there is gross instability with the risk of increasing the neurological deficit. Such interventions are designed to (i) stabilize unstable fractures or (ii) remove compressions, such as prolapsed disc fragments or vertebral fragments. The neurological signs may be due to injury to cord or nerve roots or a combination and these may be partial or complete. Careful neurological examination is mandatory and X-rays should be taken in both anteroposterior and lateral planes to reveal fractures or displacements. CAT scanning of the spine gives valuable detail of bony injury.

In general lesions above the tenth thoracic vertebra can be considered as causing predominantly cord lesions. If the transection is complete, as is unfortunately commonly the case in thoracic lesions, then no recovery can be expected since central nervous system fibre injury does not regenerate. On the other hand injuries below that level, even complete motor and sensory paralysis, may be due mainly or entirely to root lesions which are potentially recoverable. After cord injury there is an immediate loss of function below the level of the transection. This may last for several weeks before the return of reflex activity but without the return of voluntary power or sensation.

It is reasonable to take the view that complete loss of power and sensation below the level of the cord injury does indeed imply that cord damage is complete and irrecoverable but, if neurological loss is partial or the injury predominantly affects the roots, immediate measures should be taken to ensure that no further injury occurs. This is particularly important in cervical spine injuries where often unstable fracture/dislocations are unrecognised before serious damage occurs. In all suspected cases of cervical spine injury the neck should be immobilized with a simple collar and if an unstable fracture is demonstrated cervical traction should be instituted.

Cervical spine injury — skull traction

There are various types of skull traction apparatus available but the simplest is the Gardner tongs which can be applied very simply under local anaesthesia. The penetrating points are applied about 6 cm above the ear, just in front of the parietal eminence.

In fracture/dislocations of the cervical spine steady traction may reduce a partial dislocation. In any case it should be used to immobilize and stabilize cervical fractures. Cervical traction is best used on the Stryker frame so that the patient can be turned without interfering with the traction. Unstable cervical fractures should be stabilized permanently by posterior fixation or by anterior fusion. In both cases grafts are taken from the superior iliac crests. In the posterior approach the spines and vertebrae of the cervical spine are exposed. Split portions of iliac crest are laid on either side of the cervical spines across the unstable segment and wired in place. The patient must be maintained in traction until consolidation is achieved. Anterior fusion produces more immediate fixation (see p. 266) and traction can often be dispensed with, providing a secure collar is used. Locked fracture/dislocations at the cervical level are difficult and dangerous to reduce. Usually, a part or whole of the locked articular facet must be removed and such patients are best dealt with in a neurosurgical centre.

Thoracic and lumbar spine

In thoracic and lumbar injuries with complete transection, reduction of the dislocation prevents gross angulation (a cause of bed sores), and stabilization of the spine facilitates rehabilitation.

In the lumbar spine, where the damage is entirely root damage, exploration may be indicated if myelography or CAT scanning reveals any evidence of compression.

In *missile* wounds of the spinal column the cord may be compressed by in-driven fragments of bone or retained missile and, if radiological examination suggests this, a laminectomy should be performed without delay. After removal of the lamina and exposure of the dura, a search should be made for the displaced fragments and foreign bodies.

Stability depends on whether the ligaments are divided or not. Wedge fractures and compression fractures are usually associated with intact ligaments and are stable but dislocations and fracture/dislocations invariably have ligamentous rupture and are unstable.

Recovery

Attention should be predominantly directed, however, to the prevention of complications which endanger life or render it intolerable (urinary infections, bed sores and contractures). This can be achieved by correct nursing and careful attention to bladder drainage until reflex control of micturition is established. Immobilization of the patient on a Stryker frame reduces the risk of these complications and facilitates nursing. Later, physiotherapy, education in the use of supportive apparatus and general rehabilitation may restore the paraplegic patient to a useful role in society.

LAMINECTOMY

Laminectomy or excision of the spinal lamina can be performed at cervical, thoracic or lumbar levels and provides a wide exposure of the spinal dura and under-

lying cord or nerves. The procedure is essentially the same at each level.

The patient is usually positioned prone with the spine flexed by placing pillows or sand bags under the upper part of the chest and hips or placing the head in a head holder so that the neck may be flexed. It is important to ensure that the abdomen is unobstructed and that respiration is not impeded. The skin and muscles are infiltrated over the full extent of the midline incision which should extend at least one vertebral level above and below the desired lamina exposure. The skin is incised and held apart by self-retaining retractors and the fibromuscular attachments to the spinous processes are separated by sharp dissection down to the bone. The incision is continued down to the base of the spinous process on each side and an osteotome is used to scrape periosteum and muscles away from the spinous processes and laminae. Further self retaining retractors are inserted to hold the muscles laterally. After haemostasis has been achieved, the spinous processes are removed using rongeurs and then the laminae until the dura is exposed. Particular care should be taken that the under blade of the rongeurs does not push on cord or roots beneath the laminae especially if there is a mass displacing the dura. Extradural masses such as metastases or discs are cautiously removed piecemeal using pituitary rongeurs; intradural masses are exposed by carefully incising the dura and retracting the edges by sutures attached to the sides of the wound. In closure the dura is sutured with a continuous fine suture and the muscles opposed by strong sutures, closing the gap left by the bony excision. Extradural drainage is rarely required.

INTERVERTEBRAL DISC PROTRUSION

This can occur at any level but is most common in the lower lumbar discs. In the cervical region acute disc prolapse is rare.

Lumbar disc compression

Most cases of severe and persistent sciatica and many cases of severe low back pain are caused by a protrusion of an intervertebral lumbar disc. The protrusion occurs backwards and usually to one side into the vertebral canal where it presses on the nerve roots. The most common sites are between L5 and S1, and L4 and L5. The primary treatment is immobilization by strict bed rest but if there is motor deficit and especially evidence of bladder involvement there is urgent need for removal of the disc protrusion. It is usual to confirm the diagnosis by myelography/radiculography, CAT-scanning or MRI-scanning. A limited laminectomy, with the removal of the whole of the fifth and the

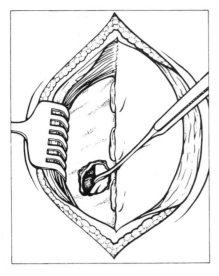

Fig. 10.26 The fenestration operation for intervertebral disc protrusion. The ligamentum flavum and the contiguous margins of the two laminae have been removed on the affected side. The nerve root and the main theca have been retracted to expose the protrusion

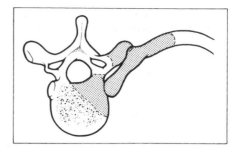

Fig. 10.27 Anterolateral decompression. Drawing to show extent of bone removal

x-ray films), paraspinal muscles are elevated medially from the transverse processes and laminae, the transverse processes rongeured down to their bases on the pedicles, with removal of the medial end of the rib articulating across the disc lesion and also of the rib above. One works medially through the intravertebral foramen anterior to the dura (theca) to remove the disc protrusion and adjacent vertebral bone with rongeurs, bone punch or high-speed drill. More extensive exposure of the thoracic spine is achieved through a thoracotomy giving an antero-lateral approach to deal with disc and vertebral body lesions (Fig. 10.27).

Cervical disc compression
Chronic degenerative changes in the disc are frequently seen: a combination of ligamentous hypertrophy and osteophytic formation produces cord or root compression. Acute disc prolapse is uncommon, occurs in the younger age groups, and may produce a sudden quadriparesis or quadriplegia. An emergency laminectomy will decompress the cord and cautious retraction of the root will allow removal of the prolapsed fragment. Safer procedures for acute or chronic disc lesions involve anterior cervical decompression and intervertebral fusions as described by Smith-Robinson or Cloward. The disc is approached from the front by an incision in the neck. The carotid sheath is retracted laterally and the larynx, trachea and oesophagus medially to reveal the anterior aspect of the cervical column. The affected disc is identified by lateral X-ray using a marker thrust into the anterior aspect of one of the discs. Thereafter the affected disc and a portion of the upper and lower vertebrae around it are reamed and drilled out down to the dura. The disc fragments are removed en route and a careful search made for any loose fragment. The defect in the bone is filled with a plug of bone taken from the iliac crest.

lower half of the fourth lumbar laminae, gives good access to the lower two intervertebral discs although a neurosurgeon would generally prefer the *fenestration* procedure (Fig. 10.26) in which access is gained through an interlaminar space. The ligamentum flavum bridging the space is excised and the margins of the contiguous laminae are nibbled away to reveal the nerve root. The theca and nerve root are gently retracted which brings the protruded disc into view. The annulus fibrosis covering the protrusion is excised, the interior of the disc curetted, and all degenerated and readily detachable tissue removed. Specially angled scoops and pituitary rongeur forceps are useful. This lateral approach is sufficient for the common unilateral disc protrusion but if there is a large central disc it is safer to perform a partial laminectomy. Spinal fusion is unnecessary after this procedure.

Thoracic disc compression
Thoracic disc protrusions are rare, difficult and dangerous. Commonly they press back into the spinal cord. Operation to remove the protrusion has a high morbidity rate. It should not be performed by the inexperienced.

A posterior approach by laminectomy is especially likely to cause unacceptable damage to the spinal cord: in general for thoracic disc problems and other lesions anterior to the dural tube (theca) it is much better to make an approach more laterally, e.g. by costotransversectomy (Fig. 10.27). In this procedure, through a paramedial incision centred at the level of the disc lesion (vertebral levels are checked on intraoperative

SPINAL COLUMN INFECTION

Bacterial infection, blood-borne or extending from a local source, may reach the extradural space primarily or after first involving the vertebrae. Infected extradural material may be granulomatous or relatively liquid pus. There is severe spinal pain, frequently exquisite local spinal tenderness. Patients may be acutely ill with fever. Myelography demonstrates an extradural compression. A decompressive laminectomy should be performed as soon as possible and the pus aspirated and antibiotic solution instilled. It is unnecessary and unwise to open the dura to see if the infection has spread but tubes may be inserted into the extradural space for the subsequent administration of antibiotics. Systemic antibiotics therapy is essential.

TUBERCULOSIS OF THE SPINE

Tuberculous infection of the spine (Pott's disease) is a local manifestation of a generalised disease: it is essential to deal with the primary focus of infection. If recognised early tuberculous spondylitis and extradural abscesses may be managed by chemotherapy without surgery.

Operative treatment in spinal tuberculosis attempts: (1) to provide drainage of abscesses; (2) to remove necrotic material including sequestra, and also tuberculous granulation tissue; (3) to remove any source of spinal cord compression either by necrotic debris or bony deformity and (4) to stabilize the spine to encourage healing or prevent further deformity.

When abscesses must be drained in spinal tuberculosis aspiration is ideal but often the pus is too thick to be evacuated in this way. Drainage is then by open operation under antibiotic control to prevent secondary infection. At the time of drainage an attempt should be made to eradicate the local focus, local chemotherapy applied, and a full course of systemic antituberculous therapy continued postoperatively. Cervical abscesses are approached through an incision behind the sterno-mastoid, avoiding the accessory nerve. Thoracic abscesses are drained by costotransversectomy or antero-lateral decompression and lumbar abscesses through a nephrectomy incision. Patients with spinal tuberculosis may become paralysed because of cord compression by abscess or debris, sometimes from a sequestrum or a bony deformity. If any paresis does not improve under conservative treatment or becomes worse then operation is indicated.

In tuberculous spondylitis the disease is anterior to the posterior longitudinal ligament, i.e. anterior to the theca. Posterior approaches through laminectomies are ill-conceived and may greatly increase spinal instability and deformity. Usually it is better to approach these lesions more laterally by costotransversectomy or, for more extensive exposure, by an anterolateral approach through a thoracotomy (Fig. 10.27).

Pus, necrotic debris, sequestra and bone compressing the cord anteriorly are removed. If bone loss is considerable, bone grafting to fill the vertebral cavity is often necessary. Vertebral fusion, e.g. posteriorly (Fig. 10.28), may be used to stop progressive spinal deformity or to stabilize the spine after surgery. Postoperatively the spine must be immobilized until spinal stability, with consolidation of bone grafts, has been achieved.

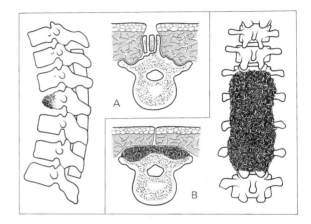

Fig. 10.28 Two methods of spinal fusion. In Albee's operation (A) a compact graft is placed between the split spinous processes. In Brittain's operation (B) cancellous bone chips are packed against the posterior surfaces of the vertebrae, which have been denuded of cortical bone

SPINAL NEOPLASMS

Spinal tumours are either extradural, such as secondary deposits in vertebrae, or intradural. Intradural tumours may be intramedullary, i.e. within the cord itself (astrocytomas, ependymomas), but most are extramedullary, arising from the meninges (meningiomas) or from nerve roots (schwannomas). Although extramedullary, these tumours frequently embed themselves in the cord. Diagnosis is made by clinical examination and confirmed by myelography or CAT- or MRI-scanning. Operation should be carried out promptly because of the risk of developing paraplegia. Having used a radio-opaque marker to identify the site of the tumour, the spines and laminae of the affected levels are removed.

Extradural metastatic tumours usually strip readily from the dura. They may be removed with pituitary rongeurs. No attempt should be made to remove the entire tumour: attempts to remove the tumour from in front of the cord may cause considerable cord damage. One should be content with removing the posterior and lateral portions of the tumour. Radiotherapy can be given subsequently.

The presence of an intradural tumour is often revealed by swelling of the dural tube. If the tumour has obstructed the CSF, dural pulsation is often absent below that level. Small tumours may be located only after the dura has been opened. Meningiomas are removed along with the involved area of dura. Schwannomas usually require sacrifice of the involved root (usually a sensory root). Intramedullary tumours are rarely amenable to radical surgery.

ANALGESIC SPINAL SURGERY

Certain severe intractable pains, such as those due to cancer, can be relieved by sectioning the posterior nerve roots or spinothalamic tract.

Posterior rhizotomy

Because of the considerable overlap it is insufficient to sever a single posterior (i.e. sensory) root for one dermatomal or sclerotomal involvement and it is usual to plan for the section of two roots above and below, as well as the affected root, to achieve satisfactory anaesthesia. Roots are exposed by complete laminectomy and identified as they emerge through the intervertebral foremen. They are severed halfway between the exit foramina and the cord, after being carefully separated from the anterior root.

Spinothalamic tractotomy or cordotomy

This is a very effective analgesic operation and can be performed in the thoracic or cervical region. Most neurosurgeons prefer the cervical level because of the more uniform distribution of fibres, less limited space and less need to rotate the cord. The operation is performed in the prone or lateral position and a midline incision made over the occipital bone and upper three cervical vertebrae. The incision is deepened in the midline to the arch of the atlas which is removed and the dura opened. The dentate ligament is identified and severed at its attachment to the lateral wall and heavy artery forceps clamped on it up to its insertion into the cord. A pointed scalpel blade is inserted 3 mm into the cord and brought round circumferentially to the anterior root. The technique of this operation is not standardized and some operators will prefer to use the older thoracic exposure. Sphincter disorder, transient paresis and skin injury due to unnoticed trauma are well recognized but small risks of the procedure. Many cordotomies are performed percutaneously by inserting a needle laterally into the spinal theca and then passing a fine electrode through the needle into the spinothalamic tract where a lesion is made by radiofrequency current. It has the advantage that the procedure can be done under local anaesthesia which is useful for patients when general anaesthesia is dangerous.

FURTHER READING

Apuzzo M L J 1993 (ed) Brain surgery. Churchill Livingstone, New York

Findlay G, Owen R 1992 (eds) Surgery of the spine. Blackwell, London

Hitchcock E, Teixeira M, Pinto J 1983 Percutaneous trigeminal radio-frequency rhizotomy. Journal of the Royal College of Surgeons of Edinburgh 28: 74–79

Schmidek H H, Sweet W H (eds) 1988 Operative neurosurgical techniques, 2nd edn. Grune and Stratton, New York

Smith R R 1980 Essentials of neurosurgery. J B Lippincott, Philadelphia

Symon L, Thomas D G T, Clarke K 1989 Neurosurgery. In: Dudley H, Carter D and Russell R C G (eds) Rob and Smith's Operative Surgery, 4th edn. Butterworth, London

Torrens M J, Dickson R A 1991 (eds) Operative spinal surgery. Churchill Livingstone, Edinburgh

11

Face, mouth and jaws

A. C. H. WATSON & J. A. WILSON

WOUNDS

The chief aim in the treatment of all facial wounds is to reduce disfigurement to the minimum. Minor injuries can be dealt with by the casualty officer or general surgeon according to the principles laid down in Chapter 1. Most cases of extensive injury will require the attention of a skilled plastic surgeon who should, if possible, carry out the initial repair. However, if specialist help is not immediately available it is the responsibility of the surgeon carrying out the initial repair to do nothing which will make later reconstruction more difficult. The main concern should be to avoid unnecessary scar formation by careful cleansing of the wound, débridement and accurate repair of the tissues in layers with fine sutures.

Because of the great vascularity of the face, primary suture is usually a safe procedure, even for such injuries as dog bites, when combined with modern antibiotics and tetanus prophylaxis. Irregular lacerated wounds should be trimmed with a sharp knife or fine scissors. Formal excision of a wound is usually unnecessary and could result in unjustifiable sacrifice of healthy tissue. It is important however to remove all ingrained dirt and gravel rash by scrubbing with a brush under general anaesthesia, even if the wound is a partial thickness abrasion. Only in this way can one avoid leaving disfiguring pigmented scars which are difficult to remove adequately later. Bleeding is usually controlled by pressure, forceps and ligation of vessels with the finest available material or diathermy, preferably with the bipolar coagulator.

Wounds with skin loss

Since the facial skin is so elastic, skin loss is often more apparent than real, the wound gaping in a frightening manner due to muscle retraction and oedema. Often it will be found at operation that there is little or no tissue missing once the 'jigsaw' puzzle has been completed. If skin, muscle or vermilion border is missing, it may be possible to rearrange the local tissues and achieve a reasonable closure of the wound, but in most instances the help of the plastic surgeon should be sought. Flap repairs should not be attempted as a primary procedure in a recent facial injury. Even skin grafts need careful choice, planning and design and are best left to the expert. Where the whole thickness of the lip, cheek or nose is missing, skin should be united to mucous membrane around the margins of the defect (the so-called 'skin to mucosa' suture). This procedure, by avoiding a raw area, allows rapid healing with minimal distortion of the remaining tissues and facilitates the formal definitive repair that can be carried out later.

Methods of skin suture (Figs 11.1 & 11.2)
To minimize scarring, needles and suture materials to close the skin should be of the finest available (6/0 nylon, prolene or dexon), inserted without tension.

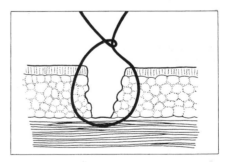

Fig. 11.1

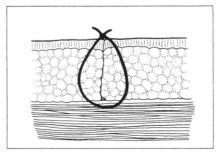

Fig. 11.2

Figs 11.1 & 11.2 Method of suturing the skin of the face; designed to cause the minimum amount of scarring

Subcutaneous sutures (of 5/0 chromic catgut or dexon) should only be used where essential and should not be placed closer than 5 mm to the skin surface. Each suture should be tied without strangulation of the tissues and the knots placed to one side of the wound so that their removal is simple. In clean straight cuts a single subcuticular running suture of 4/0 or 5/0 prolene can be inserted and removed 7–10 days later. A small 'twist nylon' drain can be inserted at one end of the wound and removed within 24–36 hours. No dressings are usually required, but the suture line must be kept free of crusts as these will encourage local sepsis and ugly stitch marks. Regular application of an antiseptic ointment or vaseline can be of help. The wound edges may be supported by strips of adhesive tape once the skin has been cleaned and dried with a swab soaked in ether.

Skin sutures are usually removed on the 3rd–5th day, subcuticular sutures after 7–10 days. All sutures must be removed with the patient lying flat, occasionally sedated or even anaesthetized and in a good light, with the right instruments and by a competent person.

In the case of wounds involving the whole thickness of the lip or cheek, the mucous membrane, muscles and skin should be sutured separately. In wounds of the eyelid, the tarsal plate must be identified and sutured to reduce the risk of distorting the margin of the eyelids. Careful attention should be paid to the possibility of damage to the canthal ligaments and the nasolacrimal ducts in wounds near the inner canthus, and expert help sought if necessary. Vision in the injured eye must be checked and, if there is any possibility of damage to the globe, an ophthalmologist called. Damage to the parotid duct and facial nerve branches may be found in wounds of the cheek and these structures should be identified at the initial operation and repaired by someone who is practised in the use of the operating microscope. It may be impossible to identify and repair fine and complex structures at the secondary operation, and one cannot overstress the importance of calling on experienced specialist help at the beginning.

FRACTURES OF THE MANDIBLE, MAXILLA, ZYGOMA AND NASAL BONES

Fractures of the mandible

Most fractures of the mandible are compound into the mouth even if they are not compound externally. Because of this, a low grade infection in the wound is not unusual particularly if dental hygiene is poor. A considerable degree of displacement is frequently encountered especially with bilateral fractures. The muscles that close the jaw, being attached posterior to the fracture line, cannot control the anterior fragment of the mandible which is pulled downwards and backwards by the muscles of the floor of the mouth and the effects of gravity. This distorts the dental occlusion, is painful and makes eating difficult. The fracture must be reduced accurately to allow bony union in good position, restore the dental occlusion and enable the patient to eat normally. The danger with bilateral fractures is obstruction of the airway caused by the tongue falling backwards, and by increasing oedema of the floor of the mouth. This is particularly liable to happen if the patient is unconscious and is allowed to lie supine. Conscious patients can be nursed sitting up or prone or lying on their side. If unconscious, they *must* be nursed prone or on their side. Only rarely will an urgent tracheostomy be required: often an endotracheal tube will be a safer and better alternative.

The reduction and fixation of mandibular fractures is usually carried out by the maxillofacial surgeon. If the upper jaw is intact, it acts as a point of fixation to which the lower jaw can be supported and splinted. Indeed in some cases of fracture of the lower jaw all that may be needed for definitive treatment is a simple barrel-bandage support (Fig. 11.3).

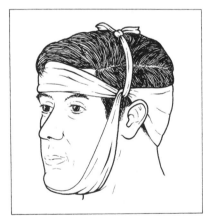

Fig. 11.3 Method of bandaging to support a fractured mandible

Other methods of fixing mandibular fractures include:

1. *Interdental 'eyelet' wiring* — this can be used if there are healthy teeth in the adjacent upper jaw. Stainless steel wire (gauge 26–32) is used to make eyelet wires that are twisted around teeth and then linked by another set of wires inserted through the eyelets (Fig. 11.4). By tightening this last set of wires the jaws are fixed together by 'intermaxillary fixation' (IMF). The linking wires can be cut in an emergency and a pair of wire cutters should be kept by to the patient's bed for use in an emergency.

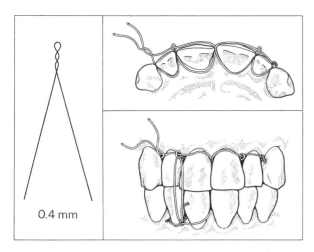

Fig. 11.4 The 'eyelet' method of interdental wiring for fractured mandible

2. *Arch bars* — these are slender bars of malleable metal, which can be bent to fit against the outer surfaces of the teeth, to which they are secured by wiring. In this way only the actual fracture is immobilized and a certain amount of jaw movement is possible.

3. *Open reduction and direct wiring* of the fractured bone (Fig. 11.5).

4. *Open reduction and plating* of the fracture. Some surgeons use compression (AO) plates (see p. 149).

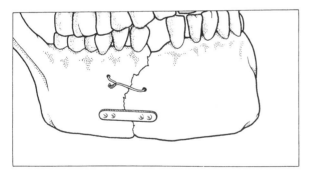

Fig. 11.5 Illustrating two methods of mandibular fracture fixation-wiring and plating

Fractures of the ramus or condylar part of the mandible are seldom associated with much displacement. Mastication is encouraged, since this preserves mobility and helps to restore normal occlusion. If serious malalignment of the teeth is present, the mandible should be splinted by one of the methods described. Some condylar fractures are followed by joint stiffness and it may then be necessary to excise the condyle, in order to obtain a false but more mobile joint.

Fractures of the mandible with soft-tissue damage

Such injuries result from gunshot wounds and from the more serious road accidents. There may be widespread destruction both of soft tissue and of bone.

The main danger in such fractures is asphyxia. This may be due to aspiration of blood into the respiratory passages, or to mechanical blockage from falling back of the tongue which is deprived of its normal anterior support.

Whenever possible such cases should be sent to a *faciomaxillary* centre, where treatment is carried out jointly by the maxillo-facial and plastic surgeon. The general surgeon must, however, be familiar with the principles of plastic repair, for in most cases he will be responsible for the initial treatment, and on this much depends. His main aims should be to arrest haemorrhage and to guard against the complication of asphyxia during transit by ensuring a good airway and by aspirating secretions as required. In general, he should be careful to do nothing which may jeopardize the chances of a good final result in more expert hands.

Exploration and excision of the wound is carried out as soon as possible. Endotracheal anaesthesia should always be employed and the pharynx packed-off around the tube to prevent aspiration of blood into the respiratory passages. In certain cases tracheostomy may be required. The wound is carefully explored, foreign bodies, loose teeth and completely detached fragments of bone being removed. Soft-tissue loss is dealt with by stitching mucous membrane to skin around the margin of the defect. Fixation of the mandibular fragments may be effected by interdental wiring, direct wiring, plating or external pin fixation. Defects in the bone can be made good by bone grafting at a later date.

Fractures of the maxilla

Injuries involving the alveolar segment of the maxilla (le Fort 1 fractures) are relatively simple to treat and malalignment of the alveolus and teeth can be corrected in the same way as mandibular fractures by interdental wiring, or a variety of dental splints. Those fractures occurring as part of a complicated middle third facial fracture may be associated with damage to adjacent structures such as the orbit, the nasolacrimal apparatus, the nose and the ethmoidal region. An associated fracture of the anterior cranial fossa may be complicated by CSF rhinorrhoea. These injuries need co-operation between oral and maxillo-facial surgeon, the plastic surgeon, ophthalmologist and often the neurosurgeon, and are not operations to be embarked upon by ill-trained surgeons with poor facilities in the accident unit. The repair of these injuries must observe two cardinal principles:

1. adequate exposure in ideal surroundings
2. recognition that the bony fragments must be reduced and stabilized by wiring, pinning or plating before any soft tissue reconstruction begins.

Fractures of the zygomatic bone

These may be easily missed if the soft tissues are badly bruised or oedematous. The zygomatic bone is usually separated from its normal attachments and displaced forwards, downwards and inwards. A palpable 'step' deformity in the infra-orbital margin, facial flattening, diplopia, anaesthesia in the distribution of the infra-orbital nerve, epistaxis and difficulty in opening the jaw fully are symptoms that should suggest a displaced fracture of the zygoma. Occipito-mental x-ray views will confirm the extent of the fracture and its degree of comminution.

The Gillies approach is normally used to correct the displacement. Under general anaesthesia, a small incision is made in the temporal region inside the hairline and carried down through the temporalis fascia to display the temporalis muscle fibres. A lever (Bristow elevator or even a screwdriver) is then inserted through the incision and directed downwards beneath the zygomatic arch. Using a rolled up swab as a fulcrum, the zygoma is then levered into its normal position usually with an audible click. If the fracture cannot be reduced or is unstable, an open reduction with exploration of the orbital floor and direct wiring at several sites may be needed.

Fractures of the nasal bones

Damage to the nasal bones depends on the extent and the direction of the force applied. Frontal injuries are more likely to damage the septal cartilage; lateral injuries are more likely to depress the thin nasal bones. Lateral displacement of the nasal bones is usually associated with a C-shaped fracture of the cartilage which runs down through the perpendicular plate of the ethmoid and through the vomer. Diagnosis of nasal fracture is clinical. If there is massive swelling of the nose then a fracture has almost certainly occurred. X-rays may be negative in the presence of a fracture and conversely vascular markings on non-fractured nasal bones may be mistaken for bone injury. It is sometimes worth taking a facial view, however, to look for associated fractures — for example of the malar bone. A nasal fracture with gross nasal displacement should be manipulated into place within 3 weeks of the injury (preferably within the first 2 weeks) since some nasal fractures become fixed quite soon. It is advisable to manipulate nasal fractures in children where gross displacement leads to subsequent growth deformities. Nasal manipulation in adults can satisfactorily be undertaken under local anaesthesia. The nose may be generally infiltrated from the external route. Nasal manipulation is successful, however, in only about two-thirds of patients. The remaining one-third will require some form of septal correction procedure or formal rhinoplasty. The success of nasal manipulation has been shown not to be influenced by the presence or absence of packing or external nasal splintage and to be independent of the type of anaesthesia and the grade of surgeon performing the procedure.

INFECTIONS

Infections of dental origin

Alveolar abscess is caused by suppuration spreading from the tooth pulp, through the root canals to the periodontal ligament. It usually subsides rapidly after extraction of the offending tooth.

Sub-periosteal abscess may follow an alveolar abscess which is untreated; it may appear either on the internal or external surface of the bone. The abscess should be drained into the mouth by an incision in the muco-periosteum parallel to the alveolar margin. Drainage from the skin surface should always be avoided.

Ludwig's angina represents usually a further spread of the infection, resulting in a cellulitis within the submental and submandibular triangles. Its treatment is considered on page 290.

Osteomyelitis of the jaws

This may be due to spread of some local condition such as dental sepsis or infection of the maxillary sinus. Most cases subside under prolonged antibiotic therapy. Operation is indicated if a fluctuating abscess forms, and is then limited to incision and drainage. This may be carried out either from the mouth or from the skin surface, according to the conditions present. If necrosis of bone occurs sequestrectomy may be required.

Parapharyngeal abscess

Parapharyngeal abscess may complicate tonsillitis and is considered on page 289.

BENIGN CONDITIONS

Protruding ears — otoplasty

This operation is performed for protruding ears. There are many variations in technique but the one described here does not involve cutting cartilage.

Operation (Figs 11.6 & 11.7)
The protruding ear is bent so that the missing antehelical curve becomes visible. It is marked with methylene blue and then divided into four equal sec-

surface of the ear. It is touched with methylene blue and pulled back on each occasion so that the cartilage is tattooed. An elliptical incision is made on the posterior surface of the ear and the skin discarded. The cartilage is exposed and the tattooed dots identified. Using 2/0 white silk (so that it is not seen under the skin of the lateral surface of the ear) horizontal mattress sutures are inserted in each of the groups of 4 dots. When these are tied the curve of the antihelix is formed. The skin edges of the ellipse are brought closer together and can be stitched without tension with 3/0 silk.

A pressure dressing is put on and left for a week, at which time the stitches are removed. Care has to be taken not to pull the ear forwards for at least 3 months after the operation lest the stitches are torn through the cartilage.

Haematoma of the auricle

If a haematoma is not aspirated almost immediately, it will organise, resulting in the so-called wrestler's or cauliflower ear. The skin which is normally very adherent to the cartilage is pulled away and in a remarkably short time cartilage is resorbed by the pressure of a haematoma.

If the haematoma does not evacuate with a large bore needle, multiple incisions must be made with strict asepsis to prevent perichondritis. Once all the clot has been removed, preferably under general anaesthesia, a pressure dressing is applied using wet cotton wool to fill all the contours of the ear. The ear must be examined daily because further accumulations of fluid will occur for many days.

Rhinophyma

This is a hypertrophic condition of the nasal skin due to a diffuse adenomatosis of the sebaceous glands. Operative treatment is to shave off the redundant masses with a sharp knife until the normal shape of the nose is restored. Great care is taken not to open into the nasal cavity by keeping a finger within the nostril during the procedure. Haemorrhage is controlled by hot packs. Healing occurs with surprising rapidity, epithelium spreading from the retained parts of the glands.

Dermoid cysts (see also congenital cysts, p. 284)

The result of the incorporation of ectoderm at the time of closure of embryonic fissures during the third and fourth weeks in utero, *facial dermoids* occur commonly in the superciliary region (*external angular dermoid*), or at the root of the nose. Not infrequently they are attached to the bone, and may even have fibrous connections through bone diploë with dura mater, so that their removal may present some difficulty. A cyst lateral

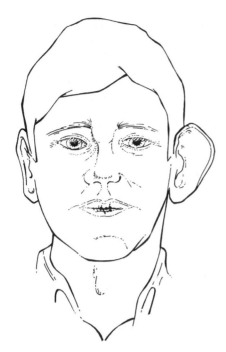

Fig. 11.6 Bat-car showing loss of antihelical fold

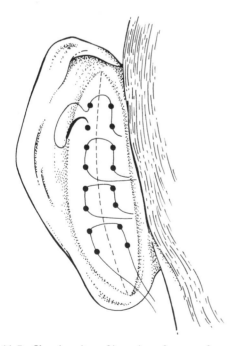

Fig. 11.7 Showing sites of insertion of sutures for otoplasty

tions. Four points are marked in each section 7 mm from the line of the antihelix and 4 mm apart. A needle is passed through each of the points (8 in each side of the antihelix) so that it appears through the posterior

to the nasal ala is a nasoalveolar cyst which arises from an epithelial rest at the junction of the frontonasal and maxillary processes.

Sublingual dermoids protrude either submentally or, if located above geniohyoid, upwards in the floor of the mouth. They should be excised through a horizontal incision in the submental region. The mylohyoid is divided in the line of the incision to expose the cyst, which can usually be enucleated with surprising ease. If not, a finger placed within the cyst cavity acts as a useful guide to its extent and connections. It is distinguished from a thyroglossal cyst by its suprahyoid position. No sign of a duct is seen and there is no need to remove the hyoid bone.

Removal of leukoplakia

Leukoplakia, from the Greek 'white patch', is malignant in 5% of cases and must be biopsied.

From the lip (Figs 11.8–11.10)

The condition, when it affects the lip (usually the lower), is called actinic cheilitis. To remove this requires replacement of the vermilion of the lip or else an ugly deformity results. The incision is made along the mucocutaneous junction and the vermilion dissected free of the underlying orbicularis oris. The dissection is continued down into the gingivo labial sulcus. The mucosa can then be pulled forwards and the leukoplakic edge excised. The clean mucosa is then stitched to the skin at the excision site with multiple sutures of 5/0 prolene. The lip swells greatly after a lip shave but with the help of ice-packs it should look reasonably normal within 2 weeks.

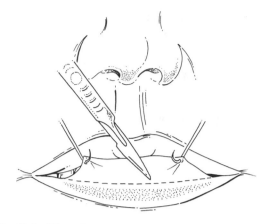

Fig. 11.9   Dissection

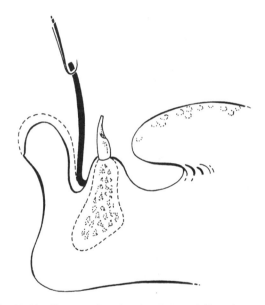

Fig. 11.10   Cross-section showing extent of dissection

From the buccal mucosa

Leukoplakia, or any small lesion here, should be removed in the transverse axis as closure is easier and contraction less. If available, laser excision is a useful alternative with good functional results.

From the tongue

Under general anaesthesia, the tongue is pulled forwards with a tongue clip and the leukoplakia excised. It is nearly always possible to close the area primarily with chromic catgut sutures.

Excision of ranula

Any cyst on the floor of the mouth appears blue domed and tense resembling a frog's belly and so can be called a ranula. A mucous retention cyst is excised locally

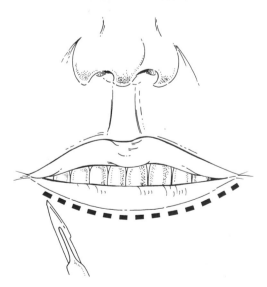

Fig. 11.8   Incision for vermilion advancement

after incising over the dome and dissecting it out taking care not to damage the submandibular duct. Each oral cyst should be sent to the pathology department however because tumours of minor salivary glands, half of which have a malignant potential, present in this way.

Ranulas which are lymphangiomas present a greater problem. It is impossible to excise them completely and so residual lymphangiomas can recur shortly after excision. It is for this reason that marsupialization is occasionally performed. Excision of a lymphangioma can be fairly complete from the oral route, however, provided its form (a central body with peripheral pseudopodia) is kept in mind during the dissection. Obviously not all of the pseudopodia can be removed because some will travel deep into the neck and possibly as far as the axilla. A fairly complete dissection is performed and the mucosa of the floor of the mouth closed with chromic catgut after taking care not to include the submandibular duct in any stitch.

Thyroglossal cysts

Lingual varieties of these, situated in the posterior part of the tongue, may bulge upwards into the mouth. They can be enucleated through a median longitudinal incision, the tongue being drawn forward as far as possible. Haemorrhage is likely to be profuse and the operation is not an easy one. The treatment of thyroglossal cysts presenting in the neck is considered on page 293.

Papillomata

Papillomata of the lips, palate, tongue or mucous surface of the cheek should be excised, since they usually increase in size, and it is impossible to exclude the possibility of malignant change.

Submandibular calculus

A stone impacted in the submandibular duct should be removed through an incision in the floor of the mouth. Catgut stay sutures are used to elevate the duct and to prevent the calculus slipping back into the gland. Intraglandular calculi require submandibular gland removal (p. 319).

Affections of the mandibular joint

'Clicking' jaw

This occurs usually in young women. The cause is obscure, but it probably lies in some irregularity or laxity of the disc. Indications for operation are pain and persistent locking which are greatly relieved by meniscectomy. The superficial temporal vessels may be encountered and require ligature. The posterior part of the masseter is detached from the zygomatic arch, and the joint is opened by division of the lateral liga-

ment in the line of its fibres. The articular disc is drawn laterally with a fine hook or forceps, and is removed in its entirety. Care is taken to avoid injury to the upper branches of the facial nerve. The auriculotemporal nerve, which runs laterally behind the joint, between it and the parotid gland, is usually not endangered.

Painful joint disorders

Degenerative changes occur as a result of malocclusion due to overclosure or loss of permanent teeth. Treatment is by dental splintage or low dose antidepressant therapy, or by high condylectomy if these fail.

Recurrent dislocation

This may be associated with a torn disc, and can be treated effectively by meniscectomy, since this allows the mandibular head to sink more deeply into the articular fossa.

Ankylosis of the joint

This may be a sequel to intra- or periarticular infections or to osteo- or rheumatoid arthritis. Intra-articular ankylosis is treated by excision of the head and neck of the mandible (Rowe, 1982) although some success has been reported using bovine cartilage grafts. Periarticular ankylosis can be treated by the excision of a wedge-shaped segment of mandible just in front of the angle, so that a false joint is formed.

MALIGNANT DISEASE

General considerations in treatment

The advent of high energy irradiation has greatly improved the prospects of curing the primary condition while major advances in reconstruction have also made radical excision more acceptable. Small squamous carcinomas respond equally well to radiotherapy or surgery. Large tumours require combination therapy, since salvage irradiation and salvage surgery after failure of primary therapy are equally disappointing. The initial use of radiotherapy may preclude certain techniques of mandibular conservation and may obscure the original tumour margins resulting in inadequate resection. Most surgeons, therefore, advocate treatment by radical surgery, followed by radiotherapy as soon as healing has taken place. For certain radio-resistant tumours (e.g. minor salivary gland tumours, malignant melanomas) surgery is the treatment of choice. Patients with acquired immune deficiency syndrome (AIDS) can develop Kaposi sarcoma lesions of the facial skin and oral mucosa. These respond well to local irradiation, as do malignant lymphomas. An adequate pretreatment biopsy, from the growing margin of the tumour, is of course mandatory. Cisplatinum and methotrexate are the two most widely used single agents, although the toxicity of the former limits its capacity for true palliation in some patients. Methotrexate is used in some centres in combination with primary radiotherapy but can provoke severe mucositis. The development of radiosensitisers may, in the future, limit such cytotoxic damage. No single agent or combination chemotherapy regime has any place in primary treatment of head and neck epithelial tumours. Certain drugs have a limited role in palliation of advanced or recurrent disease.

Lip tumours

Wedge excision

Up to one third of the lower lip can be excised with this procedure and primary closure is accompanied by no deformity and minimal scarring provided that the limbs of the 'V' are of equal length (Fig. 11.11). The margins of excision are marked at least 0.5 cm from each edge of the tumour. The vermilion edge is marked with a needle and methylene blue. From these marks a V is drawn on the inner and outer surfaces. The sides of the V are curved in order to avoid a decrease in the depth of the lip after suture (Fig. 11.12). The excision is performed along these lines in a through and through manner and the inferior labial artery is clamped and tied. Closure is begun by opposing the orbicularis oris and when this is completed the oral mucosa is stitched with interrupted sutures of 3/0 chromic catgut. The skin and vermilion are closed with 4/0 prolene taking care to appose accurately the vermilion edges.

Buccal mucosa

Small tumours superficial to the buccinator muscle (Fig. 11.13) can be removed with a good margin pre-

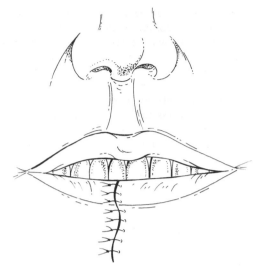

Fig. 11.12 Lip closure

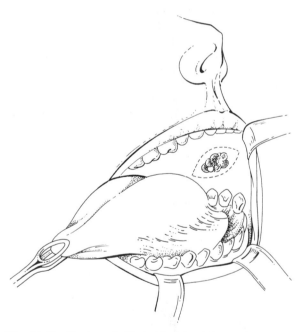

Fig. 11.13 Horizontal elliptical incision is better than vertical for removal of small tumours of the buccal mucosa

serving the facial skin. Consideration should be given to the stripping off most of the buccal mucosa where wide field changes in the epithelium are suspected. A split thickness skin graft from the thigh is sewn into place using the quilting technique. This is to ensure a good take because intraoral skin grafts are prone to displacement and haematoma formation due to normal movements. The quilting technique involves placing multiple sutures 1 cm apart stitching the graft to the underlying muscle, the end result resembles a quilt.

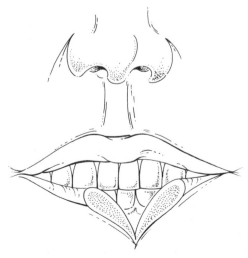

Fig. 11.11 Wedge excision

Alternatively, the graft can be supported by two bolsters of flavine wool on the inner and lateral surface of the cheek. The two are attached by through and through sutures so that the skin graft is sandwiched. Split skin grafting is less suitable for the repair of large defects because of the risk of trismus.

If the tumour is placed more posteriorly, then it is difficult to gain access unless a cheek flap is elevated via a Weber Fergusson incision (p. 280). When this is extended intraorally in the gingivo buccal sulcus it allows the cheek to be reflected back off the maxilla. Access to posteriorly placed tumours is then more direct and a quilted skin graft is applied as before. Where a neck dissection has been performed, the submandibular approach forms a natural extension and with good exposure.

Large tumours

These require a through-and-through excision of buccal skin. It is difficult to achieve closure of this defect with a pectoralis myocutaneous flap and so either a lined forehead flap (Fig. 11.14) is used or, if the patient has not had a radical neck dissection, a sternomastoid myocutaneous flap. One alternative is to raise a bilobed temporal flap: the forehead lobe is used to line the cheek defect, and the lobe from the parietal scalp, in the territory of the posterior branch of the superficial temporal artery, provides skin cover. The forehead flap or nasolabial flap can also be used to line the cheek where a deltopectoral flap has been used for skin cover. Where facilities for microvascular anastomosis are

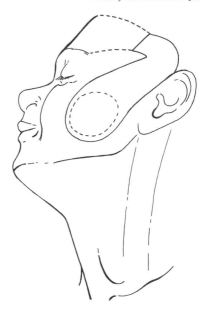

Fig. 11.15 Lined forehead flap covering cheek defect

available, free flaps such as the fasciocutaneous flap based on the radial artery give good intraoral repair.

If a lined forehead flap (Fig. 11.15) is required it should be prepared two weeks prior to the cheek excision. The end of the forehead flap is lifted and a split thickness skin graft is stitched to its undersurface. The flap is then resutured into place in order to give the split skin time to attach. The flap is lifted when required after the through-and-through excision and the split skin is sewn to the remaining buccal mucosa and the forehead skin to the facial skin.

After three weeks the pedicle is divided, the upper part of the defect is sewn into place and the remaining forehead skin is returned to its original site, removing the split thickness skin which was used as a temporary cover for the aponeurosis. Only a small defect remains at one side of the forehead lined with split thickness skin.

Tongue

In operating on the tongue for tumour, several principles must be borne in mind.

1. Due to the spaces created by the intrinsic tongue muscles and also the milking action of the tongue movement, cancer can spread widely particularly in a posterior direction and in general terms at least a 2 cm excision margin is required.

2. As long as 1 cm of floor of mouth mucosa can be preserved, the tongue will retain a lot of mobility and dentures can be worn or teeth preserved which will help articulation.

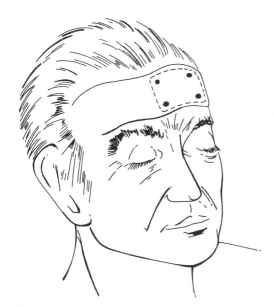

Fig. 11.14 Preparation of lined forehead flap. The split thickness skin graft is sewn onto the under surface of the forehead skin and held for seven days by buttons

3. Free skin grafts are difficult to place in the oral cavity and should be used only after intra-oral resection of tongue tumours. Their use after a mandibulotomy can result in fistula formation.

4. If more than half of the tongue is removed soft tissue should be replaced otherwise the oral cavity will be crippled, and the patient will suffer air escape during speech in addition to dysphagia.

Partial glossectomy

A radical or a partial neck dissection is performed and the pedicle is left attached to the submandibular region. The tongue can be approached either from the oral cavity or by splitting the ramus of the mandible. For the occasional mouth surgeon the former route is preferable but the latter gives much superior exposure.

In order not to disseminate tumour into fresh tissue the exophytic or ulcerative surface is coagulated with diathermy (Fig. 11.16). The margin of excision is tattooed with methylene blue and the tattoo marks are embedded deeply into the tongue so that they will be visible during excision. An accurate assessment of spread of the tumour is therefore essential. The actual excision along these marks is done with cutting diathermy. The lingual artery will be divided and requires ligation. When the excision line is cut it is deepened towards the neck dissection space and the whole mass is removed in continuity. A pectoralis major flap is used if any appreciable amount of tongue tissue is removed (Fig. 11.17). It is passed under the neck flaps and sutured to the tongue muscle and also to the tongue mucosa taking care to create as good a sulcus as possible because, if the patient can wear teeth after surgery, morbidity is minimal (Fig. 11.18). A common mistake is to insert too large a flap. This becomes apparent when anaesthesia wears off and tongue muscle tone is

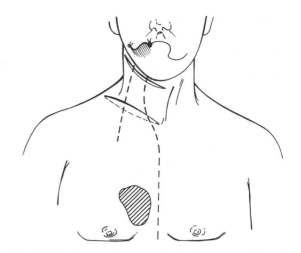

Fig. 11.17 A pectoralis major flap has been passed into the mouth to cover the defect following excision of tongue tumour and neck glands

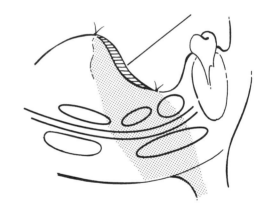

Fig. 11.18 Cross-section showing pectoralis major flap in position following the excision indicated in Fig. 11.16

restored. The flap should, therefore, be two thirds of the length of the tongue remnant with correspondingly shorter intersuture distance on the flap side.

A nasogastric tube is passed and is held in place for 10 days at which time it should be obvious whether or not the pedicle flap has taken. If it has, then normal feeding can be resumed. If the flap begins to necrose then it will continue to do so for up to 10 days. The necrotic tissue should be removed but it is unnecessary to remove and replace the flap (as it would be if a forehead or delto pectoral flap were used) because the muscle should scar and provide bulk and also a surface which can later epithelialize. If it is kept free of necrotic debris with frequent débridement then maximal saving of muscle tissue is possible.

Total glossectomy

This operation may on rare occasions be necessary

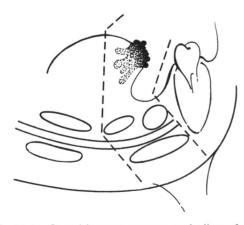

Fig. 11.16 In excising a tongue tumour the lines of excision should not be wedge shaped or else deep tumour will be left. Dotted lines show incisions for removal of tongue tumour in continuity with neck glands

for tumours of the central tongue base that have not responded to radiation. It is on its own a difficult operation with which to obtain cancer clearance since tumours at the base of the tongue spread around the hyoid and via the vallecula into the pre-epiglottic space of the larynx. Thus the more logical procedure is a total glossolaryngectomy but, since this leaves the patient with absolutely no possibility of communication, even the hardiest quail at the prospect.

The actual excision of a whole tongue is simply performed with cutting diathermy going around the floor of the mouth and through the vallecula. The body of the hyoid must be removed to get some access to the pre-epiglottic space even if the larynx is left. The operation should be accompanied by at least an upper neck dissection so access is combined from the mouth and neck.

The large hole remaining in the mouth is closed with a pectoralis myocutaneous flap. This is not mobile but its bulk makes it superior to other flaps and swallowing is not too difficult. Speaking on the other hand is difficult since it takes a great deal of skill to learn new tricks of articulation.

The flap is stitched to the remaining mucosa of the floor of the mouth and to the vallecular remnant. The nasogastric tube can be removed usually at the 10th day and normal swallowing commenced.

Tumours of the floor of the mouth

The surgical treatment of tumours of the lateral floor of mouth (or lateral oropharynx) should include a therapeutic or elective neck dissection, as adequate access disrupts the tissue planes of the submandibular triangle. The nodes in this drainage area have a greater chance of being cleared by a combined cervical and intra-oral approach. The continuity of the mandibular arch should be preserved if at all possible. If only the lingual plate of the mandible is involved by tumour, and a cortical shave is not adequate to remove it, then any remaining teeth in the involved area are removed and a sagittal split along the socket-line is performed. Where the occlusal surface of an edentulous mandible is involved, horizontal bone removal, with or without the contents of the alveolar canal may be possible, provided that the bone is not excessively atrophic. Any procedure on an irradiated mandible may fail due to osteoradionecrosis.

If a full thickness segment of the mandibular ramus requires excision, retention of a posterior strut will assist reconstruction. Full thickness resection of the anterior arch should be avoided if at all possible because of the ugly cosmetic and disastrous functional results — with oral incontinence of food and saliva, dysarthria and dysphagia. If such a resection is necessary a free bone graft is unlikely to take. A wide range of composite, vascularised bone grafts is now, however, available — e.g. spine of scapula on a lateral trapezius myocutaneous flap, rib on a pectoralis major myocutaneous flap or a radial forearm flap. Use of a sternomastoid and clavicle flap is best avoided as it may compromise the clearance of upper deep jugular nodes at radical neck dissection. An alternative is to perform secondary bone grafting e.g. of an iliac crest strut after a few weeks' use of an intraoral spacer to separate the bone ends.

With regard to soft tissue replacement, the aims are to produce a mobile tongue remnant and a sulcus so that dentures can be fitted. Split skin grafts can be used in anterior floor of mouth reconstruction, provided that the inevitable contracture will not over-restrict mobility of the tongue tip. If bone is exposed here, bilateral nasolabial flaps, based lateral to the angle of the mouth and extending along the nasolabial fold to the bony nasal pyramid, can be tunnelled into the mouth and sewn together to cover the defect. The pedicles are divided at 3 weeks. Larger anterior defects require a pectoralis major or lateral trapezius myocutaneous flap, or a free radial forearm fasciocutaneous flap. If a lateral floor of mouth defect is too large for primary suture, a single nasolabial flap or a split skin graft may also be used, particularly if the mandible is intact and the bulk of a myocutaneous flap might impede tongue mobility. Split skin grafts probably allow the optimum formation of a lateral sulcus.

Removal of floor of mouth tumour

A neck dissection will have been performed and the specimen left attached to the submandibular region. The tumour is fulgurated and a safe margin marked and tattooed. If the tumour has begun to involve the mandible then a partial mandibulectomy with remnant of the lingual plate is planned. The excision is performed intraorally and it is joined on to the neck dissection. This leaves everything pedicled on the mandible. The limits of mandibular resection are determined by dissecting the soft tissue upwards off the medial side of the mandible and performing a mandibular osteotomy between the symphysis and the mental foramen, carefully preserving the soft tissues attached to the ramus. Using a fissure burr the mandible is divided vertically a safe distance in front of and behind the tumour. Finally it is split vertically between the inner and outer plates so that the two vertical incisions are joined and the specimen can be removed. The appropriate repair is determined by the considerations outlined above.

Palate

Tumours related to minor salivary glands are usually pleomorphic adenomas. Adenoid cystic and mucoepidermoid tumours are the most common malignant salivary tumours at this site. Squamous cell carcinoma is rarely primary on the hard palate and more usually represents spread from the nose and sinuses.

Removal of benign tumours

These present as smooth palatal swellings. They should be excised as pleomorphic adenomas and this includes the overlying mucosa. A bare area is left on the palate which is covered in the first instance with gauze impregnated with Whitehead's varnish. This is removed at 10 days, and the area left to epithelialise on its own.

Removal of malignant tumours

In a small tumour, where the extent of nasoantral involvement is in doubt, the area of involved mucosa is removed in continuity with the underlying palatal bone, by demarcating the line of bony removal with an osteotome and then using a chisel in the thickest area to lever off the fragment. If the underlying mucosa is healthy and can be retained intact, a split skin graft can be applied directly. Although liable to contracture, mucosa stripped from the soft palate should also be grafted as the long term functional results are superior to those where the soft palate is allowed to cicatrise without a graft. In malignant tumours of the palate with extensive nasoantral involvement the antrum must be removed but the orbit can be preserved.

Incisions. A Weber Fergusson incision is made (Fig. 11.19), starting at one of the creases lateral to the orbit and continuing for 4 cm below the lower eyelashes to the medial canthus. The incision should be 2–3 mm from the lid margin to prevent postoperative lymphoedema. It then goes down in the nasojugal crease to the nasal ala. From here it goes under the nostril to the philtrum of the lip down which it turns

to split the lip just to one side of the midline. It is completed by incising the gingivobuccal sulcus back to the tuberosity of the maxilla. The flap is dissected from the face of the maxilla with cutting diathermy because the facial muscles are very vascular. Dissection is continued backwards to the maxillary tuberosity.

Excision. The first step is to pass a Gigli saw through the nose into the nasopharynx. It is grasped here with a right angled artery forceps and drawn into the mouth. Keeping to one side of the tumour with a good margin the hard palate and alveolus are split. Using a chisel the nasal process of the frontal bone is split up to the frontonasal suture line which is at the level of the anterior cranial fossa (Fig. 11.20). The chisel is turned at right angles here, and cuts through the ethmoids are made. The zygomatic arch is cut with a Gigli saw and the maxillary process of the zygoma is divided similarly through the inferior orbital fissure. Finally, using a 5 cm osteotome in the pterygomaxillary fissure followed by division of the remaining soft tissues with heavy scissors, the maxilla is freed and removed. The bleeding from the maxillary artery is easily controlled by ligature or diathermy and bleeding from the pterygoid plexus of veins is stopped by packing. The eye position is preserved if the lateral canthus, the periosteum of the orbital floor and the medial canthus are preserved.

Closure. It is better to have a prosthodontist present to fit a denture and obturator immediately, but failing this the whole cavity can be packed with gauze soaked in Whitehead's varnish. The cheek flap is grafted with a split thickness graft to stop contraction and is returned to its original position. If an obturator is not fitted im-

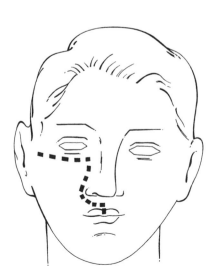

Fig. 11.19 Weber Fergusson incision

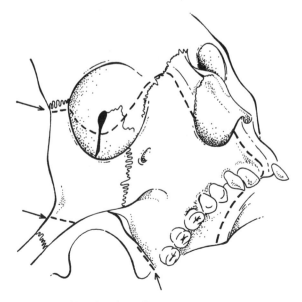

Fig. 11.20 Showing sites of bone cuts in maxillectomy

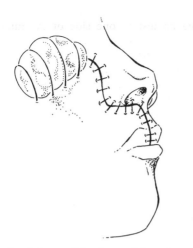

Fig. 11.21 Final closure following excision of maxillary tumour with pack in orbital cavity

mediately it must be applied when the pack is removed at 2–3 weeks (Fig. 11.21).

Tumours of the external ear

Radiotherapy is the primary treatment of tumours of the auricle but small lesions of the helix can be removed by wedge excision. The V-shaped incision is easy to close provided a little more cartilage than skin is excised. The skin is repaired with 3/0 Prolene (Figs 11.22 & 11.23).

If the tumour is in the concha of the ear then primary closure is impossible without severely deforming the ear. A full thickness skin graft is necessary to fill the defect. This is best taken from the post auricular skin crease and primary closure in this site is very easy even after a large amount of skin is excised. The skin graft is

stitched into the conchal defect with multiple 5/0 silk sutures and tied over a bolster of acriflavine wool which is left for one week.

CONGENITAL ANOMALIES

Cleft lip and palate

The embryological watershed that separates clefts of lip and palate is the incisive foramen. Clefts anterior to this (the 'primary palate') may be complete or incomplete, and may or may not be associated with posterior clefts (the 'secondary palate'). Cleft palate may occur in isolation. Clefts are complex deformities which can cause a variety of problems throughout childhood and beyond, and should only be treated by a specialist surgeon working closely with a team of colleagues in other specialities, e.g speech therapist, orthodontist and ENT surgeon.

Cleft lip

This deformity is usually unilateral, sometimes bilateral and very rarely median. It is due to failure of fusion between the maxillary process of one or both sides (the 'lateral elements') and the medial nasal process, which forms the central area or prolabium. In addition to the cleft, there is displacement and distortion of structures, in particular the nose.

Closure of the cleft lip

The general aims are to restore the normal symmetry of the upper lip, to provide a mobile lip, a symmetrical nose tip, to close the nasal floor and anterior palate and correct any distortion of the alveolar arch.

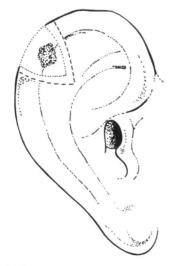
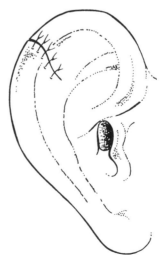

Figs 11.22 & 11.23 Wedge excision of ear tumour. Broken line indicates limit of cartilage excision

Timing of the operation

Most surgeons prefer to delay repair of the cleft lip until the age of about 3 months when the child is obviously thriving, gaining weight and has a haemoglobin level of at least 10 gm %. The intervening period allows one to exclude or treat other serious congenital malformations that could be a threat to life, i.e. oesophageal or intestinal atresia, heart defects, imperforate anus etc. The time interval also allows the orthodontist the opportunity to carry out any presurgical oral orthopaedic treatment to narrow the cleft which can make the surgical closure more simple and give a better result. A few surgeons carry out immediate repair of the cleft lip in the newly born infant, which is of psychological advantage to the parents, but most are waiting to see if the long term results are as good as later repair. Surgery should be postponed if there is any doubt about the child's condition and if oral or nasal swabs show the presence of pathogens such as group A β-haemolytic streptococci. Surgery is best done under general anaesthesia with an oral endotracheal tube in place and the pharynx carefully packed.

Principles of lip repair

Various operations are currently in use but they all entail paring the edges of the cleft, lengthening the cleft side of the lip to bring the cupid's bow into a horizontal position, and identification and dissection of the abnormally placed fibres of the orbicularis muscle. These fibres on each side of the cleft will be found sweeping upwards and gaining an attachment to the alar base laterally and the base of the columella medially. These bundles must be detached, brought down to a more horizontal position and sutured across the lip to form a new orbicularis oris sphincter. The most commonly used technique is that of Millard (1958) in which a medial flap of skin and muscle is rotated downwards, and orbicularis and skin advanced

from the lateral element to fill the resulting gap below the nose (Figs 11.24–11.26). Freeing of the alar base from the piriform margin to allow its advancement medially may be associated with wider dissection of the alar and septal cartilages to improve symmetry. Bilateral clefts of the lip may be closed one side at a time or both at once.

The mucosal layers of the lip and anterior palate are closed with 4/0 or 5/0 chromic catgut, the muscle in the lip with 5/0 vicryl and the skin with interrupted 6/0 nylon sutures. At the end of the operation it is prudent to apply splints to the elbows to prevent the child from placing his or her fingers in mouth and normal bottle or breast feeding is resumed as soon as possible. The sutures from the skin are removed under basal sedation or intravenous ketamine anaesthesia in 5–7 days time.

Cleft palate

Clefts of the secondary palate are due to failure of the palatal processes of the maxilla to fuse with each other and with the premaxilla which is developed from the medial nasal process and which carries the 4 upper incisor teeth. The anterior (primary) palate, extending through the alveolus to the incisive foramen, is usually closed at the same time as the lip repair. The secondary palate which may be cleft from the uvula as far forwards as the incisive foramen is usually closed in one stage, most often between the ages of 6 to 12 months. The aim of this operation is to provide an intact roof to the mouth and a mobile soft palate capable of providing competent velopharyngeal closure that will allow the child to speak well. If this function is not achieved, speech will develop the characteristic cleft palate quality.

Principles of surgery

Numerous operations have been employed over the years to close palatal defects. The principles of surgical closure were laid down as the result of observations

Figs 11.24–11.26   *Millard's rotation-advancement cleft lip repair*

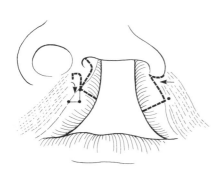

Fig. 11.24   Markings

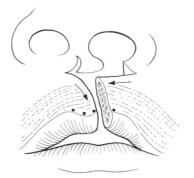

Fig. 11.25   Flaps cut

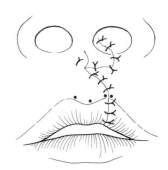

Fig. 11.26   Incisions sutured

meticulously recorded by Veau (1931). He showed that not only must the palatal repair involve accurate suture of the nasal and oral mucosal lining to reduce scarring and prevent fistula formation but the palatal muscles must be sutured accurately across the midline after detaching their abnormal insertion into the posterior margin of the hard palate. Only in this way can the levator muscle sling act properly and move the soft palate backwards and upwards to provide adequate velopharyngeal closure. Most operations begin with paring of the edges of the cleft and this is followed then by mobilization of mucoperiosteal flaps raised from the oral surface of the palate on each side of the cleft with the help of relaxation incisions so that they can be slid medially to meet in the midline without tension.

Surgical technique

The baby is positioned with a pad under the shoulders and the neck extended. A tongue stitch is inserted. A Dott or Kilner gag is used to hold the mouth open and keep the endotracheal tube out of the way. 1/200 000 adrenaline in 0.25% Marcaine is injected into the palatal shelves.

Variations of Veau's technique are still used by many surgeons. Mucoperiosteal flaps are raised and peeled back off the bony surface of the hard palate (Figs 11.27 & 11.28). This allows the surgeon to identify the posterior palatine arteries and carry out a careful dissection in each lateral recess, freeing the muscle attachment from the pterygoid plates and if need be fracturing the hamular process to release tension. With this kind of approach it is simple to detach the soft palate muscles from their abnormal attachment to the posterior border of the hard palate and bring the muscle ends across the midline where they can be sutured together with 4/0 vicryl (Figs 11.29 & 11.30). The nasal lining is then closed with interrupted sutures of 4/0 vicryl and the oral mucosal layer is enclosed with interrupted 4/0 vicryl or chromic catgut sutures. After this operation the child's arms should be splinted to prevent the infant from inserting objects into the mouth and disturbing the palate. Oral feeding should be restarted as soon as possible, taking care after each feed to give the child plenty of water to wash out the palate and prevent food lodging in each lateral recess.

The aim of cleft lip and palate surgery is, as Professor Kilner used to stress, to make the child 'look well, eat well and speak well'. Many of these children may require secondary operations in later childhood and adult life to improve the appearance of the lip and nose, to bone graft the alveolar cleft, to deal with any fistulae which cause trouble and to carry out secondary operations if velopharyngeal closure is incomplete. Hearing problems may make it necessary to insert grommets to aerate the middle ears, and problems of dental occlusion and normal dental care require the attention of our dental colleagues. A team approach is essential and it must be organized with care and compassion.

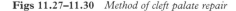

Figs 11.27–11.30 *Method of cleft palate repair*

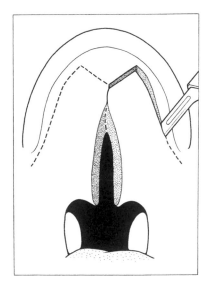

Fig. 11.27 Skin flaps are raised from the hard palate

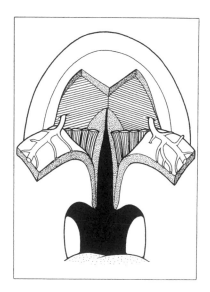

Fig. 11.28 The posterior palatine arteries have been preserved and the levator palate muscles detached

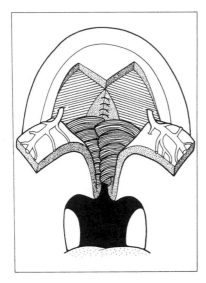

Fig. 11.29 Muscle ends sutured together across the midline

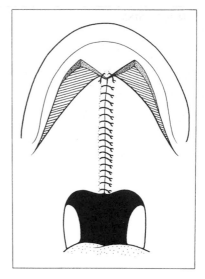

Fig. 11.30 Oral mucosal layer sutured in the midline

OTHER DEFORMITIES

Major craniofacial deformities

There are several types of severe deformity of the cranium — due to premature fusion of sutures — which may also involve the skull base and facial bones. Examples are the deformities of Crouzon's syndrome (cranio-facial dysostosis), Apert's syndrome (acrocephaly — syndactly) and Hypertelorism. These grossly disfiguring deformities can now be treated successfully in specialist cranio-facial centres. The operations involve complex osteotomies and rearrangement of the deformed cranial and facial bones with correction of the associated soft tissue deformities.

Congenital cysts, fistulae and sinuses of the head and neck

There are numerous sites where, due to a failure of embryological fusion lines, cysts, fistulae and sinuses can persist. The most important point about these is to recognise that chronic enlarging cysts and persistent recurrently infected sinuses may be congenital in origin, even in adolescents and adults. If so, ablative surgery is likely to need to be much more extensive than first appears necessary. Dermoid cysts and sinuses may be in the midline of the face, particularly the nose, where they may separate the halves of the nasal septum and even communicate with a defect in the skull base. External angular dermoids at the outer corner of the eyebrow or eye lie in a depression in the bone. Pre-auricular sinuses may extend deeply along the external auditory meatus. Branchial fistulae pass upwards and medially between the internal and external carotid arteries to reach the pharynx, and thyroglossal fistulae can be traced through the hyoid bone to the base of the tongue.

The best chance of removing these lesions completely is at the first operation. Unfortunately many of them appear superficial and trivial at first sight, and excision is attempted on a minor out-patient operation list. As a result it is likely to be incomplete, condemning the patient to what may be many years of trouble and repeated surgery.

Correct pre-operative diagnosis will ensure that the operation is carried out with a full knowledge of the anatomy and likely extent of the lesion. CT scans may be of value, and injection of methylene blue is often of help in defining sinuses and fistulae during operation.

REFERENCES

Millard D R 1958 A radical rotation in a single harelip. American Journal of Surgery 95: 318
Rowe N L 1982 Ankylosis of the temporo-mandibular joint.
Journal of the Royal College of Surgeons of Edinburgh 27: 67
Veau V 1931 Division Palatine. Masson Cie, Paris

FURTHER READING

Bull T R 1974 A colour Atlas of ENT Diagnosis. Wolfe Medical, London

Cummings C W 1986 Otolaryngology head and neck surgery. Mosby, St. Louis

Edwards M, Watson A C H 1980 Advances in the management of cleft palate. Churchill Livingstone, Edinburgh

Goldman J L 1987 The principles and practice of rhinology: A text on the diseases and surgery of the nose and paranasal sinuses. Churchill Livingstone, New York

Maisels D O 1974 The influence of presurgical orthodontic treatment upon the surgery of cleft lip and palate. British Journal of Orthodontics 1: 15

Maran A G D 1988 Logan Turner's diseases of the throat, nose and ear, 10th edn. Wright, London

Maran A G D, Lund V J 1990 Clinical rhinology. Thieme Verlag, Stuttgart

McGregor I A 1989 The fundamental techniques of plastic surgery, 8th edn. Churchill Livingstone, Edinburgh

Rowe N L, Williams J L 1985 Maxillo-facial injuries. Churchill Livingstone, Edinburgh

12

Neck, mastoid and salivary glands

J. M. S. JOHNSTONE, J. A. WILSON & R. F. RINTOUL

GENERAL TECHNIQUE

Anaesthesia

This is maintained by tracheal intubation and has special advantages in cervical operations. It obviates the necessity for a face mask, the harness of which may encroach upon the operation field. It allows the anaesthetist full control from a distance, and ensures an adequate airway whatever the position of the head.

Preparation and draping of the part

All hair below the level of the ear on the affected side should be shaved off if it is likely to interfere with the operation. Sterile towels must be applied according to a planned technique, by which it is virtually impossible for them to slip, and by which the patient's face and the anaesthetic apparatus are completely excluded from the field of operation. A satisfactory method of draping is shown in Figures 12.1 and 12.2.

Avoidance of disfigurement

Unless they are planned correctly and are sutured with care, incisions in the neck are liable to heal with widely stretched unsightly scars. Such scars especially in female patients, may constitute a serious disfigurement. The measures necessary to minimize scarring do not normally detract from the efficacy of the operation; they involve the expenditure of a little more time and trouble on the part of the surgeon, but will be most gratefully appreciated by the patient.

Incisions

Unless wide access is of paramount importance (as in the case of operations of the air passages or for the removal of malignant glands), all incisions should be made transversely so that they lie in the natural creases or cleavage lines (Langer's lines) of the skin (Figs 12.3 & 12.4). These represent the direction in which the skin splits, if punctured with a round instrument. The

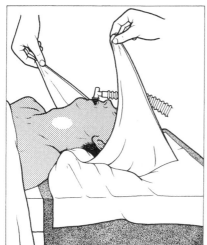

Fig. 12.1

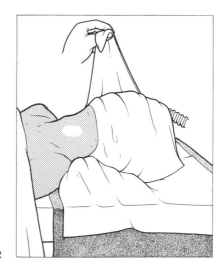

Fig. 12.2

Figs 12.1 & 12.2 Method of draping for operations on the neck. A sterile waterproof sheet and two sterile towels are laid beneath the head and neck. The uppermost towel is then folded across over the point of the chin, to cover the face and the anaesthetic tube

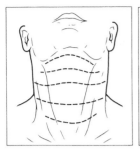 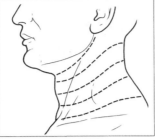

Fig. 12.3   **Fig. 12.4**

Figs 12.3 & 12.4   Lines of the natural creases (Langer's lines) in the skin of the neck. All skin incisions should, if possible, be made parallel to these lines

disposition of skin tension is such that, when an incision is made in the cleavage lines, there is little tendency for the wound edges to separate, so that the scar may become almost invisible. If a single transverse incision gives insufficient access, two such incisions at different levels may be employed (p. 305). Skin and superficial fascia are reflected to expose the underlying platysma, which is then divided in the same line, preferably at a slightly different level. Identification of the platysma as a separate layer is facilitated if the fibres overlying the sternomastoid are divided first.

Closure of the wound
The platysma is sutured as a separate layer. Fine needles and suture material are selected, and interrupted sutures are employed throughout. Each skin stitch is made to traverse the surface close to the wound, and is tied with only sufficient tightness to bring the edges into apposition. Michel or alternative skin clips (see Chapter 1) are especially suitable for neck operations unless a subcuticular suture is used. Clips should be removed on the 3rd or 4th day.

Avoidance of haematoma formation
This is most essential, since a haematoma, besides predisposing to infection, may result in a disfiguring scar due to subcutaneous fibrosis. All haemorrhage should therefore be arrested by ligature or diathermy coagulation, and as an additional safeguard the wound should usually be drained for 24–48 hours. Suction drainage is especially useful in neck operations.

WOUNDS

Cut-throat
This is due most commonly to attempted suicide. Since the head is thrown back at the time of wounding, the great vessels usually escape injury. In most wounds of any depth, however, the air passages are opened, either

the thyrohyoid membrane or the thyroid cartilage itself being divided. Homicidal cut-throat is usually in the lower part of the neck, and, if it is of any depth, it is likely to be fatal, because of injury to the great vessels.

Operative repair should be carried out as soon as the patient has been resuscitated. Where there has been extensive damage to the larynx, a tracheostomy should be performed in order to ensure that post-traumatic oedema will not obstruct the airway. If possible the tracheostomy is performed through an incision separate from the main wound as the first step in the operation and anaesthesia can then be maintained by way of the tracheostomy tube. The skin wound is enlarged sufficiently for adequate access. Bleeding vessels (usually branches of the superior thyroid and lingual arteries) are secured. If the internal jugular vein has been damaged it should be ligatured above and below the site of injury. General débridement is carried out, and the severed structures, which may include the thyroid cartilage, are repaired as accurately as possible with interrupted sutures. The skin wound is closed by suture, a small drain or gauze pack being left in position to allow the escape of serum.

In wounds of greater depth, especially those above the thyroid cartilage, the cavity of the pharynx is sometimes opened. The pharyngeal wall should then be closed as accurately as possible with interrupted sutures. If the epiglottis is severed it is repaired in a similar manner. Because of the risk of infection, the superficial part of the wound (skin and platysma) may be left open and packed with gauze; it can then be closed by delayed primary suture after 2 or 3 days. In cases of gross damage, a nasogastric tube is passed into the stomach for feeding.

Other wounds
When vital structures escape immediate damage, the main danger is that of infection in the tissue spaces of the neck. The treatment is according to general surgical principles. Careful débridement is carried out, adequate access being obtained by enlargement of the wound, and by division of sternomastoid if necessary.

INFECTIONS

Abscesses can occur in any of the fascial spaces of the neck. Up to 27 fascial spaces have been described but there are only three important spaces in the neck where infections occur. These are the retropharyngeal space, the parapharyngeal space and the submandibular space.

Retropharyngeal abscess
The retropharyngeal space lies between the pharynx

and the posterior layer of the deep fascia which bounds the prevertebral space. It separates the pharynx from the vertebral column and extends from the base of the skull to the posterior mediastinum as far as the bifurcation of the trachea. Anteriorly it connects with the pretracheal space so that infections can spread via this latter space to the anterior mediastinum. In infants, the abscess is due to lymphadenitis secondary to an upper respiratory tract infection and in the adult usually signifies a tuberculous infection of the cervical spine.

Operation

In the child the abscess is best incised per orum. The child is placed in the supine position with the head extended and, using a tonsil gag with a tongue plate, the bulging posterior pharyngeal wall is easily seen. A vertical incision is made in the midline and the pus is evacuated. Using finger dissection, the space is opened up so that any loculated areas are drained. *In the adult* the space is best approached from the lateral direction. A horizontal incision is made, one finger breadth below the angle of the jaw. The tail of the parotid gland is dissected from the sternomastoid and this latter structure is retracted. The carotid sheath is identified and retracted posteriorly. The superior constrictor is then identified and, by passing a finger lateral and posterior to the pharynx, the retropharyngeal space can be entered. The loculated area is broken down with blunt finger dissection and the pus evacuated. A drain is inserted into the space and brought out through the lateral side of the neck. The drain is gradually shortened over a period of 3 or 4 days. When confirmation has been received of the tuberculous origin, the appropriate chemotherapy should be commenced.

Parapharyngeal abscess

The parapharyngeal space lies lateral to the pharynx connecting with the retropharyngeal space posteriorly. Laterally, it is bounded by the lateral pterygoid muscle and the parotid gland. It extends from the base of the skull to the level of the hyoid bone where it is limited by the fascia over the submandibular gland. Posteriorly is the carotid sheath. The origin of the infection should be identified and dealt with prior to drainage of the space. Some 60% of patients have an associated tonsillitis and so the tonsil should be removed. The remainder of the patients have an infected lower third molar tooth which should be extracted.

Operation

A horizontal incision is made on the anterior border of the sternomastoid muscle (Figs 12.5–12.7) and the muscle is retracted posteriorly. The deep cervical fascia is usually found to be thickened due to the infection

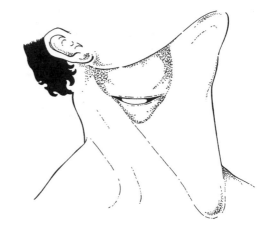

Fig. 12.5 Incision for parapharyngeal abscess

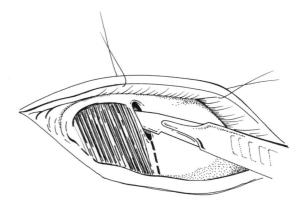

Fig. 12.6 Incising the fascia at the anterior border of sternomastoid

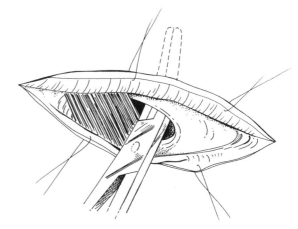

Fig. 12.7 Opening into parapharyngeal space

and this must be broken down in order to gain access to the space, between the carotid sheath and the cervical viscera. Once the pus is evacuated blunt finger dissection should open the space widely from the base of the skull to the hyoid. A drain is inserted and the appropriate chemotherapy commenced. The drain is shortened over a period of 3 or 4 days and, once the tonsil or tooth has been dealt with, recurrence is unlikely.

Acute mastoiditis

Because of the availability of antibiotics for acute otitis media, acute mastoiditis is now rare. When infection does occur it is usually well controlled by chemotherapy whilst pus tends to track superficially to form a subperiosteal abscess requiring only simple drainage and with little risk of intracranial complications. The classical cortical mastoid operation of Schwartze is sometimes indicated, however, in more chronic stages of otitis media when profuse purulent otorrhoea, pulsating and increasing in amount, together with pyrexia and mastoid tenderness persist after adequate antibiotic treatment. If an acute mastoiditis fails to respond to parenterally administered antibiotic within 48 hours, the mastoid should be exposed surgically in the acute stage. In established mastoiditis, there is a risk of facial nerve paralysis, labyrinthitis, sigmoid sinus thrombosis, meningitis, otitic hydrocephalus and intracranial sepsis. The presence of an extradural, subdural or brain abscess should be suspected if headache, malaise, drowsiness, swinging pyrexia, changes in mood or localising signs are detected.

Operation
With the patient's head turned to the side on a sandbag, a postauricular incision is made 2 cm from the post aural crease right on to the bone of the mastoid. It extends from the anterior attachment of the pinna to the mastoid tip. In young children with no mastoid tip, a high posterior incision will avoid facial nerve damage. The periosteum of the mastoid is elevated anteriorly to the external auditory canal and superiorly. The triangle bounded by the junction of the mastoid bone with the tympanic ring, the supra meatal crest and the posterosuperior meatus is called Macewen's triangle and is the surface marking of the antrum which lies 1.5 cm deep in the adult (Fig. 12.8). Entry into the mastoid should be at this point to avoid the facial nerve and dura. Once the mastoid antrum is found, the mastoid air cells are drilled out (or chiselled if no drill is available). The middle fossa dura and sigmoid sinus are protected by smooth bone and should be approached with great care.

If *extradural infection* is present the exposed dura is thickened and oedematous with granulations and in such cases all the affected bone should be removed until healthy dura is exposed. The lateral sinus should not be opened. The wound is then irrigated with antibiotic solution and the upper part of the wound closed

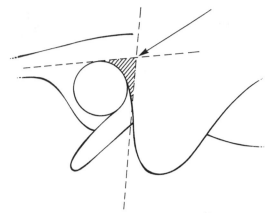

Fig. 12.8 Site for drilling in mastoid infection (Macewen's triangle). Triangle marked by two tangents and margin of auditory meatus

with interrupted sutures. A thin rubber dam drain is stitched into the lower part of the wound and pus removed from the external ear into which a small pack is inserted. A pressure dressing is applied.

A general surgeon should perform this surgery only in an emergency when simple decompression of pus and drainage of abscess suffice. After this the patient should be referred on to an otolaryngologist for specific management of the ear condition. It is dangerous for an inexperienced operator to attempt formal mastoidectomy. The facial nerve may be transected or the incus dislocated, and if the dura is inadvertently opened in the presence of infection the resulting complications may be serious.

Submandibular space infections (Ludwig's angina)

The submandibular space is bounded above by the mucous membrane of the floor of the mouth and tongue and below by the deep fascia, and extends from the hyoid to the mandible. The space superior to the mylohyoid muscle is called the sublingual space and contains the sublingual gland; the space inferior to the muscle is the submaxillary space. The submandibular gland, which is wrapped around the mylohyoid muscle, extends into both spaces. Anteriorly lies the submental space between the two anterior bellies of digastric.

Operation (Figs 12.9 & 12.10)
The vast majority of infections of this space are of dental origin. The offending tooth should be identified and removed. Incision of the space is not usually rewarded by evacuation of much pus. There is generally cellulitis of the floor of the mouth and submandibular space but, by merely opening the space after removal of the tooth and the administration of the appropriate antibiotic, resolution is usually rapid. In severe cases,

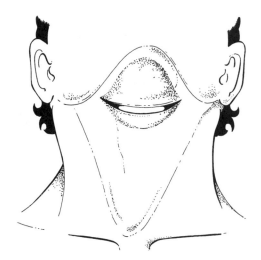

Fig. 12.9 Incision for submandibular space abscess

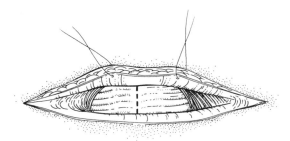

Fig. 12.10 Midline vertical incision in mylohyoid

however, the tongue may be pushed posteriorly by the oedema of the floor of the mouth and tracheostomy may be required.

CONGENITAL ABNORMALITIES

Congenital torticollis

This is regarded as being due to a birth injury, causing either rupture of fibres of sternomastoid or the vessels supplying it. Degeneration of the affected fibres occurs, and is followed by fibrous tissue replacement which results in contracture (or failure of normal growth) of the muscle. If the condition is untreated the other muscles of the affected side and the deep fascia become shortened as well. An alternative view is that the condition is due to a developmental aplasia of the muscles and other soft tissue structures on the affected side of the neck.

The condition is normally recognised soon after birth when a 'sternomastoid tumour' may be present. In most babies, the condition resolves spontaneously. Passive manipulation is widely practised and may be helpful. Persistent shortening will eventually interfere

with growth of the face on the affected side. This will result in hemihyperplasia and is judged an indication for operation.

Operation

A horizontal incision 5 cm in length is made with its centre over the lower part of sternomastoid 2.5 cm above the clavicle. Under direct vision, both heads of the muscle are then divided together with the deep cervical fascia and are allowed to retract. If scalenus anterior is shortened and is found to be preventing correction of the deformity, it also is divided together with the carotid sheath if necessary. The platysma and skin are then sutured and a small drain may be left in the wound.

After treatment is most essential in order to prevent recurrence of the deformity. Physiotherapy is started 2 or 3 days after operation with suitable analgesia. This involves manipulating the head and neck through a full range of movements 4 times a day.

Branchial cyst

A branchial cyst is derived from the second branchial pouch. An alternative aetiological theory is that the cysts originate from squamous cell rests within lymphoid tissue, as they can arise anywhere in the neck without any pharyngeal communication. The cyst is lined by stratified squamous or non-ciliated columnar epithelium and gradually accumulates a cholesterol rich fluid. It most commonly presents in early adult life as a painless, globular swelling at the anterior border of sternomastoid roughly one third of the distance between the mastoid process and sternum.

The diagnosis can readily be confirmed by fine needle aspiration cytology. Treatment is by excision unless the lesion is secondarily infected in which case incision and drainage may be necessary.

Operation

The patient is placed supine, with the head and the neck slightly extended and the chin rotated to the opposite side (Fig. 12.11). A skin crease incision is made over the swelling at least 2 cm below the angle of the jaw (so as to avoid the cervical branch of the facial nerve) and carried deep through platysma. The deep cervical fascia is incised along the anterior border of the sternomastoid and the muscle is retracted posteriorly. The cyst can then be enucleated with ease but care should be taken on the deep surface which may lie between the internal and external carotid arteries (Fig. 12.12), and posterosuperiorly where the cyst may be close to the accessory nerve. Occasionally, a track passes between these two vessels and can be traced up to the base of the tonsil, although there is no necessity to open into the pharynx.

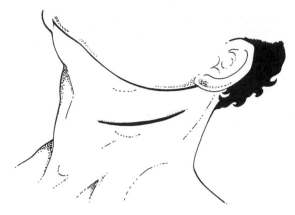

Fig. 12.11   Incision for branchial cyst

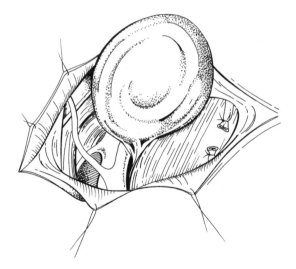

Fig. 12.12   Branchial cyst extending deeply between the internal and external carotid arteries

Branchial fistula and sinus

A branchial fistula is probably derived from incomplete obliteration of the precervical sinus, an epithelial lined space formed by downgrowth of the second branchial arch over the second, third and fourth branchial clefts to fuse with the fifth arch. The small opening of the fistula lies over the lower third of the anterior border of the sternomastoid and the tract, if complete, runs upwards to the pharyngeal wall at the level of the palatine tonsil. The fistula lies between structures derived from the second and third branchial cleft and therefore passes between the internal and external carotid arteries. More often however the tract is a sinus of variable length with a blind ending. Occasionally the fistula is derived from the first branchial cleft; the opening then lies over the anterior border of the upper third of sternomastoid and runs towards the external auditory meatus in close relation to the facial nerve.

The small opening of the branchial fistula intermittently discharges a glairy, mucinous substance and may be recurrently inflamed. The extent of the lesion may be demonstrated by a sinogram using lipiodol. Treatment is by excision of the fistula and this must be complete so as to avoid recurrence.

Operation

The patient is positioned as for excision of a branchial cyst. Methylene blue is injected into the fistula as this will be seen if the tract is inadvertently divided during dissection. Two skin crease incisions may be used (Fig. 12.13); the first is an elliptical incision around the opening of the fistula and the second is made above the upper border of the thyroid cartilage. Through the first incision the tract is traced deep through the

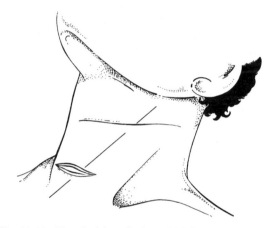

Fig. 12.13   Two incisions for branchial fistula (see text)

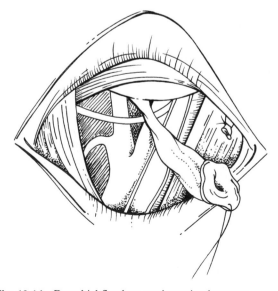

Fig. 12.14   Branchial fistulous track passing between internal and external carotid arteries

cervical fascia at the anterior border of sternomastoid and it is then traced upwards towards the carotid bifurcation. The fistula is then passed up from the first to the second incision for the remaining part of the dissection between the internal and external carotid arteries (Fig. 12.14) and between the hypoglossal and glossopharyngeal nerves. It is divided flush with the pharyngeal wall. A finger introduced into the mouth and pushed against the inside of the pharyngeal wall aids the last stage of dissection. Finally a drain should be laid along the length of the wound and the tissues closed in layers.

Thyroglossal cyst and fistula

The thyroid gland develops from the caudal end of a diverticulum known as the thyroglossal duct. The duct grows downwards in the midline from the foramen caecum and is closely related to the posterior aspect of the hyoid cartilage (Fig. 12.15). Incomplete regression of the duct may result in a thyroglossal cyst or fistula.

A cyst may lie above or, more commonly, below the hyoid bone and is found in the midline unless pushed to one side by the thyroid cartilage. The lesion is spherical, tense, sometimes inflamed and moves with swallowing or protrusion of the tongue. It may resemble ectopic thyroid and, if necessary, must be differentiated by a thyroid scan. A fistula probably forms after spontaneous discharge or drainage of an infected thyroglossal cyst. The opening lies in the midline and intermittently discharges a glairy mucinous substance.

Treatment of both cyst and fistula is by excision. To prevent recurrence the remnant of the thyroglossal duct must be traced back to the foramen caecum at the junction of the middle and posterior third of the tongue.

Operation

An endotracheal tube should be passed and the patient is placed supine with a sandbag under the shoulders and the head on a ring. A skin crease incision 4 cm long is made over the prominence of the cyst and carried deep through platysma. The deep cervical fascia is divided longitudinally in the midline to expose the cyst which can then be mobilized by blunt dissection. It must be assumed that a connection persists between the cyst and the foramen caecum. A core of tissue from the deeper aspect of the cyst is therefore traced to the inferior border of the hyoid bone (Fig. 12.16), the middle 1 cm of the bone is carefully mobilized from the underlying thyrohyoid membrane and excised with bone nibblers. The core with the adherent excised segment of bone can then be traced towards the foramen caecum (Fig. 12.17). A finger introduced into the mouth to push the posterior part of the tongue downwards and forwards aids the last part of the dissection. The wound should be closed with a drain in place.

Dissection of the thyroglossal fistula may be carried out through two small skin crease incisions both for convenience of access and improved cosmetic appearance. First, the fistulous opening is excised with a

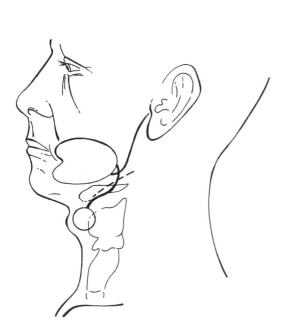

Fig. 12.15 Thyroglossal cyst and tract in relation to hyoid cartilage and tongue

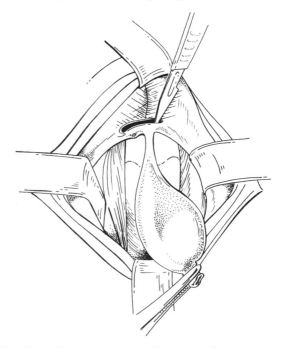

Fig. 12.16 Thyroglossal cyst and tract traced to lower border of hyoid

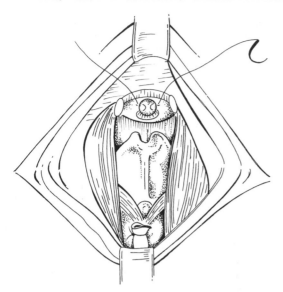

Fig. 12.17   Tract deep to hyoid passing towards foramen caecum

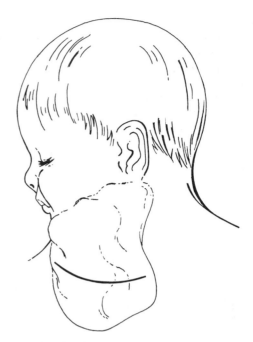

Fig. 12.18   Incision for cystic hygroma

transverse elliptical incision and the tract followed proximally through the deep fascia towards the inferior border of the hyoid bone. A second incision is then made at the level of the hyoid and the dissected tract.

Lymphangioma

Lymphangiomas or tumours of lymph vessels, are of three clinical types: simple lymph cysts, cavernous lymphangiomas and cystic lymphangiomas. The latter (known as cystic hygromas) are extremely rare but quite dramatic on presentation in the newborn child. Very large lesions with upper airway obstruction require urgent surgery with a temporary tracheostomy. There is a place, however, for observation of smaller lesions, some of which may regress during the first 1 to 2 years of life. Magnetic resonance imaging (Jacobson, 1988), which avoids exposure of the child to irradiation, may be useful in assessing the extent of the lesion. Before treatment is commenced, a chest X-ray should be taken to make sure that there is no mediastinal extension which could complicate the anaesthetic. The parents should be warned that reoperation may be necessary before final eradication of the cyst is accomplished. The main structures at risk during the operation are the facial nerve, the internal jugular vein and, to a lesser extent, the carotid artery. A nerve stimulator, if available, is useful intraoperatively as the hypoglossal, accessory and vagus nerves may also be at risk.

Operation

In a large cystic hygroma, an incision is made in the skin crease lines over the maximum convexity of the cyst (Fig. 12.18). The skin is dissected very care-

fully off the thin walled cyst and, at the end of the operation, redundant skin is excised. The sternomastoid is elevated from the lesion and supported by tapes once the accessory nerve is identified. Inferiorly, once the omohyoid muscle has been elevated, it is usually necessary to open the carotid sheath to dissect the lesion off the internal jugular vein. It may also be adherent to the subclavian vein in the root of the neck. A child's mastoid is not well developed and the facial nerve is not protected by the mastoid in the newborn. Dissection should therefore stop 2.5 cm inferior to the mastoid. A formal superficial parotidectomy is necessary to identify and preserve the branches of the facial nerve. Extensions of the cyst can go into the floor of the mouth, the axilla, the pectoral region, the retropharyngeal space and the parapharyngeal space. Not all of these can be excised at the initial operation. There is little point in injecting sclerosing fluid into the remnant because the cyst is multilocular and the sclerosant will have little effect.

Laryngocoele

Lower animals often have air sacs to enable them to submerge for long periods. The remnant of these air sacs in the human are the ventricle and saccule of the larynx (Amin, 1988). Cystic enlargement of the saccule causes hoarseness, while external extension through the thyrohyoid membrane creates an airsac in the neck. This diagnosis must be kept in mind for any neck cyst which shows air on plain X-ray.

Operation

An incision is made over the air sac at the level of the thyrohyoid membrane. Skin flaps are elevated and the sac is always seen anterior to the sternomastoid muscles. The sac is mobilized to the thyrohyoid membrane where it will have a very broad base. If it is merely excised at this point in the operation, recurrence will be inevitable because a large portion of the sac will remain within the larynx. The upper half of the thyroid ala is therefore removed (Fig. 12.19) and the narrow neck of the sac entering the ventricle of the larynx is seen. It can be transected and ligated at this point and the sac removed. The ligated point can be reinforced by stitching the strap muscles to the remnants of the thyrohyoid membrane. A drain is inserted and the wound is closed in two layers.

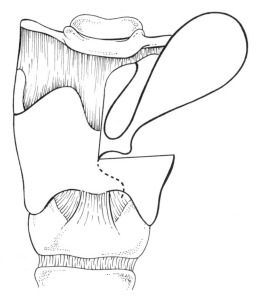

Fig. 12.19 Removal of upper half of thyroid cartilage allows laryngocoele to be removed at its neck

Cervical rib and the 'scalenous syndrome'

The mechanism by which a cervical rib can give rise to vascular or neuritic manifestations in the upper limb is in considerable dispute. The usual explanation is that stretching and friction occurs as the lower trunk of the brachial plexus arches over the cervical rib, or over the fibrous band extending forwards from an incomplete rib. Identical symptoms can occur, however, in the absence of any demonstrable bony abnormality. In such cases it is thought that the nerve trunk or artery may be irritated by hypertrophy, spasm or abnormal insertion of one of the scalene muscles (scalenus anterior or scalenus medius). Postfixation of the brachial plexus has also been held responsible.

Resection of a cervical rib or scalenotomy if no bony abnormality is present are indicated in patients whose symptoms are sufficient to incapacitate them, and who are unrelieved by exercises and physiotherapy (Roos, 1982).

Excision of a cervical rib

A sandbag is placed between the patient's shoulders, and the arm is drawn strongly downwards. The incision extends laterally from the clavicular attachment of sternomastoid to the anterior border of trapezius at the junction of its middle and lower thirds. The lateral border of sternomastoid is then retracted medially. When the phrenic nerve has been exposed, it is elevated from the surface of scalenus anterior, which is then divided at its insertion into the first or cervical rib. The knife edge is kept against the bone, so that the subclavian artery and the thyrocervical trunk are not endangered. The supra-scapular nerve is then sought and is used as a guide to identification of the trunks of the brachial plexus (p. 190). The plexus is retracted gently downwards and forwards; the posterior (or lateral) border of scalenus medius is defined, and the fibres of this muscle inserted into the cervical rib (and possibly burying it from sight), are erased from it. The rib is next disarticulated at its attachment to the seventh cervical vertebra, or is divided as far posteriorly as possible, and is then removed.

Scalenotomy

Division of scalenus anterior alone may be successful in relieving symptoms by allowing the subclavian artery and brachial plexus to slide forwards to a lower level on the first rib. Stretching, compression, or friction are thereby abolished. The operation should comprise more, however, than simple division of the scalenus anterior. The subclavian artery and the lower trunk of the brachial plexus should be carefully freed. If the nerve trunks appear to be stretched over the medial tendinous fibres of scalenus medius, these fibres also should be divided.

THE PHARYNX

Nasopharynx

The nasopharynx lies behind the nose and extends from the base of the skull to the level of the soft palate.

Adenoidectomy

Excision of the nasopharyngeal tonsils (adenoids) is indicated when chronic infection leads to obstruction and persistent mouth breathing.

Operation. After orotracheal intubation the child's head is extended. A gag is inserted in the mouth and the adenoid pad is pushed into the midline as far as possible. A Laforce adenotome is inserted behind the palate and the adenoids are pushed into the cup. On closing the blade the adenoids are removed and the bleeding is easily controlled with gauze swabs until haemostasis occurs. The swab count is of paramount importance and should be checked by the surgeon.

Removal of angiofibroma of the naso-pharynx
The diagnosis is made by angiography and the radiologist may be able to embolize the main feeding vessels (Davis, 1987). If this facility does not exist then the maxillary artery should be clipped. The approach to this vessel is through the anterior wall of the maxillary sinus via an incision in the gingivolabial sulcus. The posterior wall of the sinus is removed and the fat of the pterygomaxillary fossa is dissected until the tortuous artery is seen. A clip ligature can be applied to it at this point.

A transpalatal approach is made by an incision medial to the course of the palatine arteries anteriorly and behind the greater palatine foramen posteriorly (Figs 12.20 & 12.21). The flap is dissected from the hard palate and, at the posterior end of the hard palate, the nasopharynx is entered. The tumour then usually bulges down into the wound and it is removed by finger dissection. When dissection is commenced there usually is copious bleeding. Attempts to stop this bleeding will fail. The only way to stop the bleeding is to remove the tumour as quickly as possible and to pack the nasopharynx (Bremer, 1986; Harrison, 1987).

When bleeding is controlled a postnasal pack is inserted and the palate replaced and sewn in place with

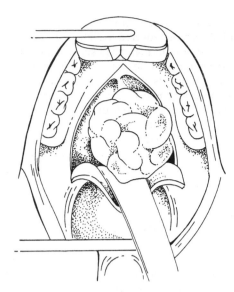

Fig. 12.21   Angiofibroma seen through transpalatal incision

chromic catgut. The postnasal pack is removed after 72 hours.

Oropharynx
The oropharynx extends from the level of the soft palate to the hyoid bone, communicating freely with the oral cavity at the anterior faucial pillars.

Tonsillectomy
The indications are tonsillitis uncontrolled by antibiotics, history of quinsy, suspected tonsillar lymphoma or to obtain histology of a tonsil when there is a malignant neck node with no discernible primary as small squamous carcinomas of the tonsil can present with cervical metastases.

Operation. The patient is anaesthetized with a nasal endotracheal tube and placed supine with the head extended. The tonsil is grasped with Lucs forceps and pulled towards the midline. The mucosa is incised from the superior to the inferior pole. Using dissection scissors, the peritonsillar plane is opened up between the tonsil capsule and the superior constrictor. Bleeding is controlled by diathermy or linen ties and dissection is continued down until a tonsil pedicle is established at the base of the tongue. This is snared and then removed.

Removal of the lateral wall of the oropharynx for carcinoma
This operation is performed for carcinoma invading the tonsil, palate or lateral base of tongue (the so-called 'retromolar trigone'), and is always combined with a radial neck dissection. The name Commando Operation — a combined excision of mandible and oro-

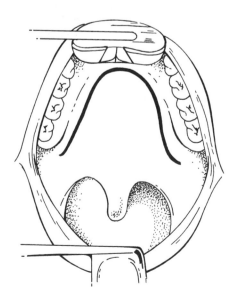

Fig. 12.20   Transpalatal incision for angiofibroma of nasopharynx

pharynx — is not always justified. For smaller tumours the mandible can be reflected laterally but not resected.

Incision. Access to the oropharynx and mandible via the upper neck incision (p. 305) is improved by continuing it forwards and splitting the lip. The neck dissection specimen is pedicled on to the angle of the mandible and the upper flap is dissected over the angle and up to the interdental line. The masseter is divided from its insertion onto the mandible and, using a periosteal elevator, all the soft tissue (masseter and parotid) is elevated subperiosteally up to the coronoid process, the notch and the neck of the condyle. Anteriorly a similar elevation is performed up to the mental foramen.

Excision. The temporalis muscle is divided from the coronoid process with Mayo scissors. The neck of the mandible is divided with a Gigli saw (Fig. 12.22). No attempt should be made to remove the head of the mandible which causes troublesome bleeding from the pterygoid plexus of veins. With a Gigli saw the horizontal ramus of the mandible is divided posterior to the mental foramen.

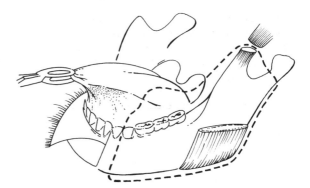

Fig. 12.23 Showing the extent of tissue removal in Commando Operation

difficulty in swallowing (Logemann, 1979). Reconstruction using the pectoralis major musculocutaneous flap is favoured. Only if a posterior strip of mandibular ramus has been preserved is bone replacement feasible.

In order to cut the flap a line is drawn from the acromion to the xiphisternum. A perpendicular from this line to the midpoint of the clavicle (Fig. 12.24) marks the course of the thoraco-acromial artery which supplies the flap. The lower end of this line approximates to the lower edge of pectoralis major. Here, below and medial to the nipple at about the level of the 6th rib an island flap of skin the required size is incised. A plane is made deep to pectoralis major and the pectoralis major is incised. A thin muscle pedicle following the line of the artery is created and dissected subcutaneously up to the clavicle: adequate exposure of the muscle pedicle is achieved either by cutting down on it or by elevating the skin in the line of a deltopectoral flap. The muscle pedicle with the attached myocutaneous island is passed under the neck skin and it is sewn in place using 2/0 Vicryl two layers.

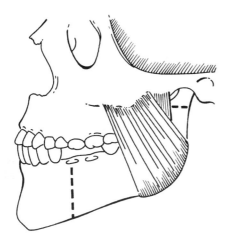

Fig. 12.22 Showing sites on bone cuts for excision of mandible

The oral cavity is entered at this point and the mandible is swung laterally. Using cutting diathermy, the tongue is incised 2 cm from the tumour margin. Once the lateral edge and base of the tongue have been incised, the diathermy incision continues up the posterolateral wall and finally the soft palate, always staying 2 cm away from the tumour edge. This leaves the specimen pedicled on to the parapharyngeal space (Fig. 12.23). With a finger protecting the carotid artery in this space the specimen is finally removed, in continuity with the neck dissection.

Closure. While the wound can be closed primarily this is not advised since it cripples the oral cavity and causes

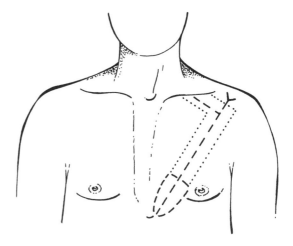

Fig. 12.24 Markings for pectoralis major myocutaneous flap

Two suction drains are inserted and the neck wound is closed as for a radical neck dissection (p. 307). The gap in the chest wall from which the flap was taken can be closed primarily by undercutting and approximating the edges with tension sutures.

After care and complications. Nasogastric feeding is commenced when bowel sounds are heard. It is removed a week after it has been established that fluid can be drunk with no fistula being apparent. If a fistula is noted the nasogastric tube is left in place until the fistula closes. Fistulae are rare because of the bulk and vascularity of myocutaneous flap that is brought in and also because of the excellent blood supply. If a large fistula develops it should be left for about a month and then closed using local skin to supply inner lining and a pectoral flap for outer lining.

Hypopharynx

The hypopharynx extends from the hyoid level to the cricopharyngeus muscle. It consists of a posterior wall, the piriform sinus and the post cricoid region. Tumours in these sites are treated with radiation unless a neck gland is palpable when primary surgery is the treatment of choice. Tumours of the piriform sinus and post cricoid regions comprise 90% of tumours, and although some of the former can be dealt with by laryngectomy and partial pharyngectomy, the majority require a total laryngopharyngectomy or laryngo-pharyngo-oesophagectomy.

Laryngopharyngectomy

Incision. If the patient has had an initial radical neck dissection the head is turned back into the midline and extended. A tracheostomy is performed between the second and third rings after dividing the thyroid isthmus. A number 12 tracheostomy tube is inserted and general anaesthesia continued via this route.

Excision. The sternomastoid on the unoperated side is retracted laterally and a plane is developed medial to the carotid sheath down to the prevertebral fascia. From this plane it is easy to free the laryngopharynx from base of tongue to the oesophagus. The strap muscles are divided at the lower end and the lobe of the thyroid on the affected side is left attached to the specimen. The other lobe is freed from the specimen and retracted laterally with the inferior thyroid artery intact.

The upper end of the specimen is divided above the hyoid bone and the base of the tongue is transected through the vallecula. The transection is completed through the posterior pharyngeal wall. The specimen is swung downwards and the oesophagus is transected at least 3 cm distal to the tumour (Fig. 12.25). Resection is completed by cutting the posterior wall of the trachea at the level of the tracheostome.

Closure. The tracheostome is brought out through

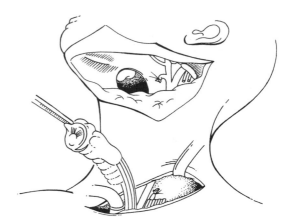

Fig. 12.25   The larynx has been freed leaving an orostome. Oesophagus is transected in the upper third

the lower skin flap and stitched in place as described on page 302. The gap between the tongue and the oesophagus is best filled with a deltopectoral flap (p. 16). The upper end is sutured to the tongue and posterior pharyngeal wall in two layers with 2/0 Vicryl (Figs 12.26–12.28). The flap is tubed, skin surface in, with the same material making sure the edges of the skin are inverted into the tube. The lower end is stitched end-to-side to the oesophageal remnant. A nasogastric tube is passed and the skin is closed in two layers. The chest wound is skin grafted and, after 3 weeks, the tube is divided and the remnant returned to the chest wall.

After care and complication. If the blood supply remains intact then the nasogastric tube can be withdrawn about the 10th day. Nearly always there is a small leak from the lower anastomosis but this will self heal in about a week.

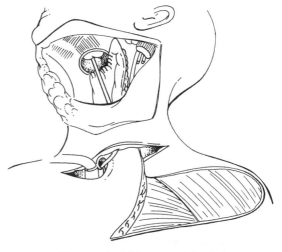

Fig. 12.26   Upper end of deltopectoral flap being sewn to posterior pharyngeal wall

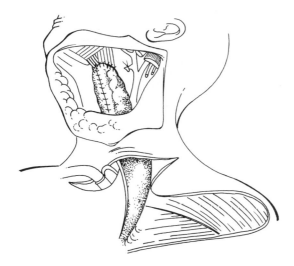

Fig. 12.27   Deltopectoral flap being tubed

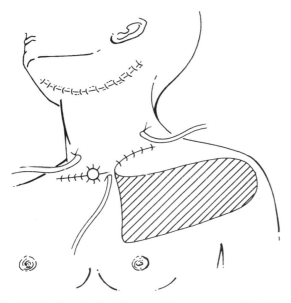

Fig. 12.28   Completion of laryngopharyngectomy. Split skin graft is applied to the chest wound

After two weeks the tracheostomy tube can be removed. A silastic stoma button may be required. It is rare to establish oesophageal speech after this operation but good communication can be achieved by the patient's articulating on the vibrating column of air generated by an oral or cervical vibrating device.

Total laryngopharyngo-oesophagectomy
If the tumour extends more than 3 cm below the post cricoid area then a total oesophagectomy is required. Reconstruction is by a viscus such as colon, stomach or revascularised jejunum. Since transposing the stomach only involves one anastomosis, i.e. in the neck, this is

preferred to colon transposition (p. 107). If it is possible to resect only the cervical oesophagus, however, and still allow several centimetres of clearance below the macroscopic lower limit of the tumour, then use of a free jejunal interposition graft obviates the need for extensive intrathoracic dissection and carries a much lower postoperative morbidity (Coleman, 1987; Ujiki, 1987).

After the pharynx has been transected at the base of the tongue and the larynx divided from the trachea, the specimen is pedicled on the oesophagus. This can be dissected with a finger down as far as the aortic arch; via a midline abdominal incision the stomach is pedicled on the right gastric artery and the first part of the duodenum is freed. The vagi are transected and the oesophagus is dissected up to the arch. The stomach can then be pulled up into the neck through the posterior mediastinum. The oesophagus is divided from the stomach and the cardia is closed in two layers. The fundus is opened to the appropriate size and this is sewn in layers to the posterior pharyngeal wall and tongue base. The prolonged postoperative ileus which follows this procedure may require parenteral nutrition for about 5 days. Thereafter, nasogastric feeding is instituted and feeding by mouth can usually be started by the 10th day.

Removal of a pharyngeal pouch
A pharyngeal pouch is a posterior, midline, pulsion diverticulum of the mucosa of the hypopharynx through the weakest part of the wall between thyro- and cricopharyngeus (Maran, 1986). Food passes into it more readily than into the oesophagus causing dysphagia, aspiration, cough and choking episodes.

As a preliminary to the operation the pouch, the oesophagus and the intervening bar are visualised by a wide oesophagoscope. The pouch is then packed with gauze soaked in acriflavine to facilitate dissection. The gauze pack is brought out through the mouth so that it can be pulled out when the pouch is excised. A nasogastric tube and oesophageal bougie are inserted into the oesophagus.

Excision. A horizontal incision is made at the level of the cricoid cartilage (Fig. 12.29). The sternomastoid is retracted and the carotid sheath is identified. The middle thyroid vein should be ligated and divided to open the access. The pouch is often firmly attached to the oesophagus but a plane must be found to dissect the pouch up to its pedicle. The pack is removed, the pedicle is transected and stay sutures placed at each end of the opening into the pharynx.

A cricopharyngeal myotomy is an essential part of this operation. A finger is inserted into the oesophagus in between the sutures and passed through the cricopharyngeus. As far posteriorly as possible in order

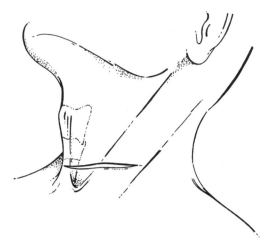

Fig. 12.29 Incision for removal of pharyngeal pouch.

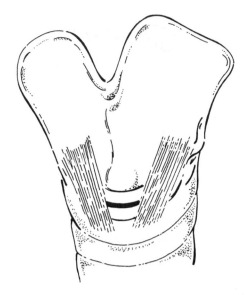

Fig. 12.30 Incision for laryngotomy

to avoid damaging the recurrent laryngeal nerve, the criopharyngeus is incised with a number 11 blade down to the mucosa. In order to accomplish a good myotomy it must be at least 4 cm long. The opening in the pharynx is then closed with inverting sutures to the mucosa using 3/0 chromic catgut. The muscle layer is sutured with 3/0 dexon. A suction drain is inserted and the wound closed in layers. The nasogastric tube can be removed in 5 days provided the wound is airtight, and feeding commenced.

Alternative operations for pharyngeal pouch

Dohlman's electrocoagulation. This requires special instruments including a Dohlman's endoscope with 2 beaks, one of which fits into the pouch while the other enters the mouth of the oesophagus. The bar between the two is first coagulated and then incised using special diathermy forceps.

Diverticulopexy. This is a satisfactory method provided a myotomy is also performed. The pouch is dissected and the fundus stitched as high as possible so that the neck is directed downwards. A preliminary endoscopy is mandatory to exclude the rare complicating carcinoma within a pharyngeal pouch.

THE LARYNX

Laryngotomy

Since tracheostomy is a difficult operation for the inexperienced, or when suitable methods of haemostasis are not available, acute airway obstruction is best dealt with by a laryngotomy. The midline of the cricothyroid membrane is just below the skin surface, well superior to the thyroid, and may be palpated easily.

The head is extended and an incision is made with a number 10 scalpel blade above the upper border of the

cricoid cartilage (Fig. 12.30). This is deepened into the cricothyroid membrane and an airway is established. The blade is then turned through 45°. Only a temporary tube should be inserted into this slit because of the risk of laryngeal stenosis but it allows time for arrangements to be made for a tracheostomy or intubation.

Laryngectomy

A number of partial laryngectomy operations have been devised to preserve or reconstruct enough of the larynx to provide voice and to avoid the need for a tracheostomy. Also a number of variants of the total laryngectomy create a fistula between the trachea and oesophagus so that voice may be produced. All these operations are, however, very specialized and only total laryngectomy is considered here. This is the operation for salvage following failed radiotherapy and is also the primary treatment in T3 and T4 laryngeal tumours with palpable neck nodes, when it is performed with a radical neck dissection.

Incision (Fig. 12.31)

A nasogastric tube is passed and a horizontal incision is made at the level of the thyroid prominence. If a neck dissection is performed then a half-H incision (p. 305) is used. In the suprasternal notch, the midline site of the permanent tracheostomy is marked.

Excision

The strap muscles are divided at their lower end and the thyroid isthmus identified and divided so that the lobe of the thyroid gland on the side of the tumour can be excised. The sternomastoid muscle on each side is

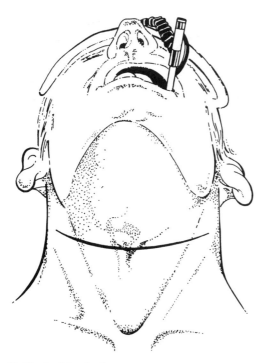

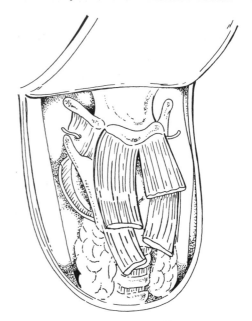

Fig. 12.32 Dissection completed showing horns of hyoid and thyroid

Fig. 12.31 Incision for laryngectomy

retracted and a plane created between the carotid sheath and the larynx. The suprahyoid muscles are divided from the body of the hyoid. The latter is grasped with Allis forceps and drawn forwards so that the lesser horns can be dissected out. The stylohyoid ligament is cut on each side and the hyoglossus is divided from the greater horn on each side. The thyrohyoid ligament is then divided to display the tip of the greater horn (Figs 12.32 & 12.33). The muscles are carefully dissected in the midline until the outline of the epiglottis is seen. This is grasped with Allis forceps and pulled forwards. Entry into the pharynx is made through the vallecula so that the tip of the epiglottis is exposed.

Cuts are made with dissecting scissors from the tip of the epiglottis to the tip of the greater horn of the hyoid on each side. The second cuts are from this point to the tip of the superior cornu of the thyroid cartilage, identifying and ligating the superior laryngeal artery as it crosses the cornu. At this point, the tumour can be seen and assessed by pulling the larynx forwards. The constrictor muscles are next divided from the posterior lamina of the thyroid cartilage and this also divides the mucosa of the pyriform fossa.

The level for the permanent tracheostomy can now be established and the trachea is transected. The endotracheal tube is withdrawn and general anaesthesia continued via a tracheostomy tube. This allows the larynx to be drawn further forwards and the post cricoid mucosa is divided below the arytenoid cartilages. From

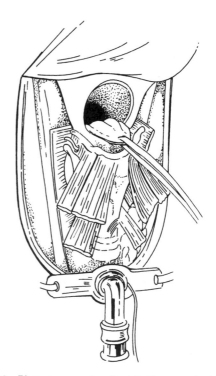

Fig. 12.33 Pharynx opened and epiglottis grasped with Allis forceps

here the trachea is dissected from the oesophagus to the site of the tracheostomy. The lobe of the thyroid to be saved is dissected from the specimen, and, on the side to be removed, the inferior and superior thyroid vessels and the middle thyroid veins are ligated and divided. The specimen can now be removed by transecting the posterior tracheal wall slightly higher than the anterior level since it is to be turned forwards.

Closure and tracheostomy

The pharynx is reconstructed round the nasogastric tube with an inverting Connell suture (p. 344) of 3/0 chromic catgut. The closure is reinforced by two more layers of submucosa and constrictor muscle, sutured with 3/0 Vicryl. An ellipse of skin of a size to admit an index finger is excised from the previously marked midline site. The trachea is brought out through this hole and the first layer of sutures (3/0 chromic catgut) joins the fascia around the trachea to the subcutaneous tissue. The second layer of 3/0 silk or Prolene joins the mucosa to the skin. Two suction drains are inserted and the wound closed with catgut to the subcutaneous layer and clips to skin.

After care and complications. Feeding is commenced via the nasogastric tube when bowel sounds return. If there is no leakage on ingestion of coloured food dye, or on a gastrografin swallow, oral feeding is commenced at 10 days. A fistula of less than 2 cm in diameter which persists for a month can be closed with local skin flaps, while one over 2 cm will probably require to be closed with a pectoralis myocutaneous flap (Weingrad, 1983).

Speech therapy is started when the nasogastric tube is removed. About half the patients learn useful oesophageal speech.

THE TRACHEA

Tracheostomy

Indications

Tracheostomy assists respiration in the following ways: (1) it relieves any upper airway obstruction; (2) it reduces the dead space; (3) it affords direct access to the tracheobronchial tree and enables this to be readily cleared by aspiration of secretions; (4) with the aid of a cuffed tube, it allows positive pressure respiration to be maintained for a prolonged period. These objectives can be achieved, to some extent, by the use of an endotracheal tube in the first instance (p. 90). Tracheostomy is thus reserved for those occasions where access to the bronchial tree is required for more than a few days or where endotracheal tube cannot be passed.

Anatomy

The trachea begins as a continuation of the larynx at the lower border of the cricoid cartilage. As it descends it becomes more deeply placed so that at the base of the neck it lies 2–4 cm from the skin. This means that the inexperienced operator is forced upwards and may do an incorrect high operation. Superficial relations are: skin; superficial fascia; the investing layer of deep fascia splitting above the sternum to enclose the suprasternal space; sternohyoid and sternothyroid muscles; pretracheal fascia and the isthmus of the thyroid gland, which overlies its 2nd, 3rd and 4th rings. Veins which lie superficial to the trachea are (a) anastomosing veins connecting the two anterior jugulars; (b) an anastomosing vein connecting the two superior thyroids, above the thyroid isthmus; (c) the inferior thyroid veins descending vertically from the isthmus. In children the trachea is more superficial than in adults, but it is also smaller and more mobile, so that it may be more difficult to locate. The innominate artery and left innominate vein may be anterior relations of the trachea in the neck, as may the thymus gland.

Operation

Tracheostomy is not an easy operation and, performed wrongly, leads to chronic stenosis of the upper airway. The only complete ring in the upper respiratory tract is the cricoid and, since it is cartilage, it has an inherent elasticity. When damaged, the cricoid strives to maintain its ring and stenoses. The loss of integrity can be due to surgical excision of the cricoid or absorbtion following perichondritis as a result of an adjacent tracheostomy through the first tracheal ring. Cricoid stenosis may not cause stridor but the reduction in air flow can cause recurrent lower respiratory tract infections whose cause may appear obscure.

Incision (Fig. 12.34)

A horizontal skin incision at the level of the 3rd tracheal ring often heals better than a vertical one. Small skin flaps are elevated and the strap muscles separated in the midline.

Approach

The strap muscles are retracted and the trachea is palpated under the pretracheal fascia along with the isthmus of the thyroid gland. Ligation of the isthmus (Fig. 12.35) adds to the complexity of the procedure, but if it is pushed upwards then it can slip down and cause difficulty in changing the tube. Occasionally thyroid veins are seen coming down from the isthmus and these must be tied meticulously or blood wells up behind the sternum. The isthmus is freed from the trachea by blunt dissection and divided between clamps. The ends are oversewn with 3/0 chromic catgut.

The cricoid and first ring are identified. A vertical midline incision is made from the space below the second ring to the space below the fourth ring. At this

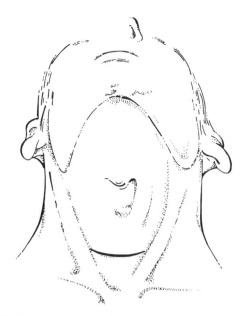

Fig. 12.34   Incision for tracheostomy

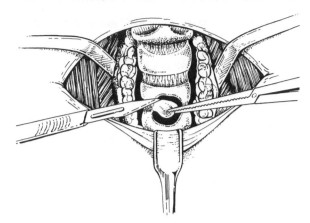

Fig. 12.36   Excision of tracheal rings

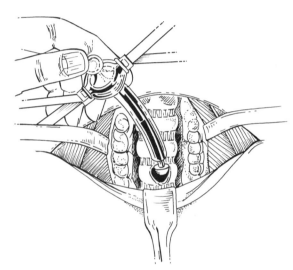

Fig. 12.37   Insertion of tracheostomy tube

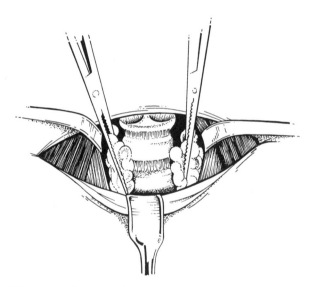

Fig. 12.35   Strap muscles retracted and thyroid isthmus divided

Closure (Fig. 12.38)

This should be loose, as tight suture of the wound causes surgical emphysema at the first cough. The tracheostomy tube is sutured in place until the first change at 48 or 72 hours as prior replacement of the tube is difficult if no tract is established.

After care

Humidification. The trachea is lined by columnar epithelium and is used to receiving warm humidified air from the upper respiratory tract. A tracheostomy bypasses this and, until the epithelium metaplases or becomes adjusted to the new airflow, crusting is a danger, both within the trachea and the tube. Humidification is therefore essential. It is best done via a tank humidifier from which warm wet oxygenated air is blown over the stoma via a cup fitting over the tube.

If this is not available, an excellent and well tried method is to put 5 ml of normal saline down the tube

point the anaesthetist is advised to withdraw his endotracheal tube (if the procedure is being performed under general anaesthesia) to the level above this cut. If the tracheal cartilages are not calcified then semicircles can be excised on either side of the vertical split with a scalpel (Fig. 12.36). If they are calcified it may be easier to make horizontal cuts above and below the third ring to the space below the fourth ring. The anaesthetist withdraws his endotracheal tube, and blood is sucked from the lumen. The tracheostomy tube is inserted (Fig. 12.37) and retractors withdrawn.

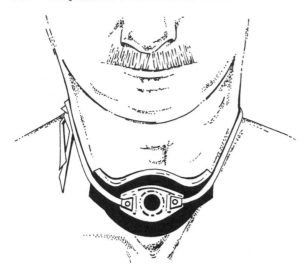

Fig. 12.38 Tracheostomy tube in position with tapes round the patient's neck

via a syringe, to suck out the secretions and then to instil another 5 ml of saline which is left. This should be repeated every 2 hours for the first 48 hours and 4-hourly for the next 5 days.

Clearance of secretions. This is an essential step and should be done as often as outlined above. The nurse should wear a mask and gloves when the tracheostomy is new. A sterile tube is attached to the lower end of Y-connection and suction to one of the upper limbs. The tube is inserted as far down the trachea as possible and when a finger is placed over the open end of the Y this creates the suction. The tube is then withdrawn over a period of 3 seconds. On no account should the tube be inserted with suction on because it will be sucked on to the tracheal wall causing abrasions and coughing.

Replacement of tube. This should be done by a doctor at about 3 days. The danger especially in a fat person, whose trachea is far from the surface, is that the tube is placed anterior to the trachea where it may cause fatal erosion of the brachiocephalic artery. Even if the tube is in a false passage, some air will appear to be emitted from it during expiration since the stoma is open to the surrounding tissue. A good airflow, therefore, must be apparent if the tube is in the correct place.

Thereafter the tube should be replaced daily.

Care of cuff. Modern low pressure cuffs can be used for prolonged periods without risk of tracheal stenosis provided the tube is well splinted to minimise movement. If these are not available, other cuffs should be let down 5 minutes every hour. This is to protect the cartilages. Ischaemic mucosa will re-epithelialize after the tube is withdrawn but cartilage necrosis causes tracheal collapse or stenosis.

MALIGNANT GLANDS OF THE NECK

One in 5 patients with a head and neck cancer will present with a lymph node on one side of the neck. One in 20 will have bilateral lymph nodes and one in 20 will have a fixed lymph node. The radical neck dissection operation is designed to remove *en bloc* all of the 80 lymph nodes which are normally present on one side of the neck. The prognostic significance of bilateral neck glands in the presence of a head and neck primary is so grave that the results of bilateral neck dissection make the operation hardly worth performing. If a gland is fixed to the mandible, the skin or the external carotid artery then removal along with one of these structures presents little problem. If, however, it is fixed to the prevertebral fascia, the brachial plexus, the common carotid artery or the base of the skull, then removal by surgery is often impossible and the operation should not be attempted.

Partial neck dissection is not recommended except for thyroid carcinoma (p. 313). If the aim of the operation is to remove the entire lymph draining field on one side of the neck then to cut through it compromises the clearance and is not advocated. The so-called functional neck dissection which preserves the sternomastoid muscle, the internal jugular vein and the accessory nerve, requires special expertise if the clearance of the metastatic lymph nodes is to be complete. The operation described here is the classical, radical neck dissection first described by Crile in 1921.

Biopsy
When several glands are enlarged, a single discrete gland may be subjected to excisional biopsy. Incisional biopsy of a fixed swelling may lead to fungation of the tumour on the skin surface. In this situation fine needle aspiration cytology is preferable (Wilson, 1987).

Radical neck dissection

Preparation
Following endotracheal intubation, the patient is laid supine with the head extended and turned to the opposite shoulder. A flat pillow is placed under the ipsilateral shoulder to make dissection of the posterior triangle easier. It is advisable to stitch or tape the skin towels in place because it is difficult to isolate the area posterior to the trapezius muscle by using towel clips alone.

Incisions
An incision for neck operations must fulfil the following conditions:

1. It must provide adequate access.

2. It must be capable of extension during the operation or in the event of further disease.

3. It must not damage vital structures in or beneath the skin.

4. It must always heal well producing a scar that is cosmetically acceptable.

The blood supply to the skin of the neck comes down from the face, up from the chest, around from the trapezius and also from the contralateral external carotid. The most poorly vascularised area in the neck (Fig. 12.39) is in the middle over the common carotid artery. A poorly designed incision placed vertically in this area is liable to break down especially if the patient has been irradiated. This means that the carotid artery becomes exposed after surgery with a risk of carotid artery rupture. It is best, therefore, to avoid 3 point junctions and vertical incisions in the centre of the neck.

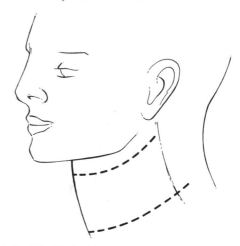

Fig. 12.40 MacFee incision

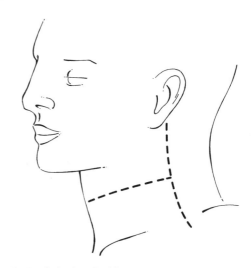

Fig. 12.41 Schechter incision

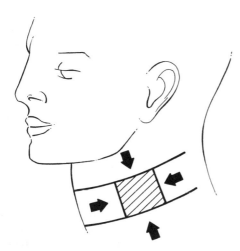

Fig. 12.39 Showing the area of the neck most prone to ischaemic necrosis

The incisions recommended for radical neck dissection are firstly the *MacFee incision* (Fig. 12.40) which consists of 2 horizontal limbs. The first begins over the mastoid process, curving down to the hyoid bone and up again to the point of the chin. The second lies about 2 cm above the clavicle, starts laterally at the anterior border of the trapezius and ends medially at the midline. The second type is a half-H incision described by *Schechter* (Fig. 12.41). The vertical limb runs down the anterior border of the trapezius from the mastoid process to the clavicle. Exactly half way down this line a horizontal incision is marked to reach the prominence of the thyroid cartilage.

The skin flaps are elevated to include the platysma which preserves the blood supply and also increases the strength of the skin flaps by up to 10%. In the submandibular area, in order to preserve the cervical branch of the facial nerve, the plane of elevation is deepened onto the body of the submandibular gland and the fascia over the gland is included in the flap.

Dissection of the inferior margin

The sternal and clavicular heads of the sternomastoid muscle are divided with a knife — no vessels need to be ligated at this point. The carotid sheath is now visible and the dissection is continued down to the wall of the internal jugular vein. In order to isolate the internal jugular vein to ligate it, it is important to go as close to the wall as possible. Non-toothed dissecting forceps and Metzenbaum scissors are used. Before passing any instruments around the vein the vagus nerve should be identified and protected. Mixter forceps are eased around the vein and 3 strands of 2/0 silk are used to ligate the vein in continuity, two at the lower end.

These are tied from above downwards, and a further suture ligature added at the lower end. The vein is then divided. If the vein is torn during these manoeuvres there is a risk of air embolus. The hole should be occluded and the vein dissected above and below the hole so that it may be ligated safely.

The omohyoid muscle is then identified and divided. The fat pad lying between the internal jugular vein and the omohyoid is dissected and pushed upwards. Underneath the prevertebral fascia the phrenic nerve runs medially downwards on the scalenus anterior. When this is identified the dissection can proceed laterally superficial to prevertebral fascia on the brachial plexus to the anterior border of the trapezius. The external jugular vein must be divided in the dissection of this fat pad. Lying between the prevertebral fascia and the fat pad are the transverse cervical vessels which should be preserved if possible.

Dissection of the posterior margin

The transverse cervical artery gives a vertical branch which runs up anterior to the anterior border of the trapezius. This can cause troublesome bleeding and so it should first be divided and ligated. Again, using blunt dissection, a tunnel can be made up the anterior border of the trapezius and the fat dissected off (Fig. 12.42). The upper third of the trapezius is crossed by the sternomastoid muscle whose fibres are divided with a scalpel to the lateral surface of the mastoid bone. During this dissection the accessory nerve is divided as it enters trapezius at the junction of its middle and lower thirds.

Dissection of the anterior margin

The omohyoid is followed up to its insertion into the hyoid bone. This forms the anterior part of the dissection. By making a tunnel along the omohyoid, this dissection can be done very quickly. The muscle is then divided from the hyoid bone, and the submental fat

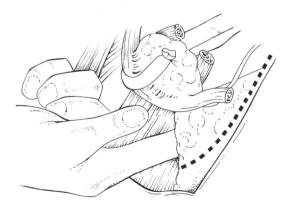

Fig. 12.42   Blunt dissection up anterior border of trapezius to create a tissue plane

pad is divided in the midline until the anterior belly of the digastric muscle is identified.

Deep dissection

The posterior margin of the dissection is grasped in Allis forceps and turned forwards The fat pad is dissected from the prevertebral fascia and the underlying muscles, the levator scapulae and the scalenes. It is tethered down by the three cutaneous branches of the cervical plexus, namely the anterior cutaneous nerve of neck, the great auricular nerve and the lesser occipital nerve. These neurovascular bundles are identified and divided and ligated well away from the phrenic nerve. This allows the specimen to be swung forward and the internal jugular vein is once again identified. Following this superiorly using Metzenbaum scissors, the carotid sheath is divided up to the jugular foramen. It is important to identify the transverse process of the atlas and, just above this, the posterior belly of digastric will be found. This is retracted upwards and the upper end of the jugular vein is then seen. It is freed of its fascial connections and Mixter forceps are passed round it. Three 2/0 silk sutures are passed around the vein and tied and an additional suture ligature is applied at the upper end. The vein is then divided and the rest of the sternomastoid can be cut. It is important to cut this muscle in a line extending from the tip of the mastoid process to the angle of the jaw. If one goes above this level then the facial nerve is at risk. As the jugular vein is dissected out of the carotid sheath the vagus nerve will be seen closely applied to the common carotid artery. It must be preserved throughout the dissection. Once the upper end of the jugular vein has been divided the hypoglossal nerve can be seen coming inferiorly from the hypoglossal foramen, crossing the occipital, external carotid and lingual arteries. It is crossed by three pharyngeal veins which join the pharyngeal plexus to the internal jugular vein. These must be ligated and divided (Fig. 12.43) because if they are torn they tend to slip underneath the hypoglossal nerve, putting this at risk during the subsequent attempt at haemostasis.

Dissection of the superior margin

The anterior edge of the submandibular gland is intermingled with the submental fat and the submental artery can cause troublesome bleeding if it is not identified and ligated. The edge of the gland is dissected posteriorly from the lateral surface of the mylohyoid muscle. When the posterior edge of the mylohyoid muscle is seen it is retracted forwards and, if the submandibular gland is pulled inferiorly at this point, the lingual nerve will be seen. It is freed from the gland and the submandibular duct can be ligated safely. The facial vessels entering the gland superiorly, one finger's

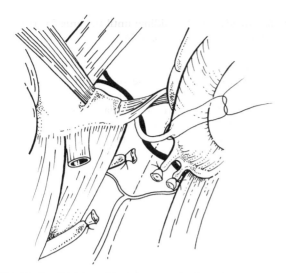

Fig. 12.43 Division of 3rd pharyngeal vein as it passes under the hypoglossal nerve

breadth anterior to the angle of the mandible, are divided. The cervical branch of the facial nerve has already been protected by inclusion in the initial dissection of the submandibular fascia. The lower end of the facial artery can be seen entering the inferior border of the submandibular gland just above the posterior belly of the digastric. When this is divided the specimen can be removed. Two suction drains are inserted and the incision is sutured in two layers.

Complications

Immediate complications. Bleeding may require re-exploration for identification of the bleeding point. A suspected *pneumothorax* is confirmed radiologically and under water seal drainage may be necessary. *Raised intracranial pressure* is prevented by avoiding dressings around the neck, by preventing hyperextension of the neck, and by sitting the patient up as soon as possible after the operation. If it occurs then the patient should be given 200 ml of 25% mannitol intravenously as quickly as possible.

Intermediate complications. Chylous fistula occurs following unrecognized operative injury to the thoracic duct. It may not manifest itself until the patient is being given tube feeds. At this time the suction drainage increases dramatically in amount and may reach 500 ml a day, the drainage consisting of thick white fluid resembling milk. The patient must be returned to theatre and the injured duct should be oversewn with 4/0 silk. *Seroma,* or a collection of serum under the neck flaps, can be prevented by using suction drainage for at least five days. The seroma should be aspirated and a pressure dressing applied to avoid failure of skin healing. *Carotid artery rupture* is usually the combination of

several complications, namely wound breakdown, infection, stripping of the adventitia of the artery and drying of the artery (Maran, 1989). If the skin breaks down, complete débridement should be carried out and the carotid artery covered with a skin flap at the earliest opportunity. Until this is possible the artery should be kept moist with soaks. Ligation of the common carotid artery for rupture is followed by a 20% mortality and a 50% morbidity rate.

Late complications. Frozen shoulder is a common complication after a radical neck dissection since the accessory nerve is always cut. The reason for the shoulder stiffness is that the shoulder girdle falls forward and it becomes impossible for the patient to abduct the arm in the usual fashion. This causes adhesions in the capsule of the shoulder joint and a subsequent frozen shoulder. It should be prevented by starting shoulder exercises as soon as possible after the operation. Hypertrophic scar formation may occur if a vertical incision is used in the middle of the neck. The scar should be excised and the tension removed by a z-plasty repair.

Reticuloses and primary lymphatic tumours
These are not as a rule amenable to surgery, but open biopsy may be required to establish nodal architecture and to allow immunohistochemical typing of lymphocyte populations.

TUBERCULOUS CERVICAL ADENITIS

This condition is not common in Europe but is still common in Asia and Africa. The bacillus, most often the bovine variety, reaches the lymph nodes by direct drainage, usually from the tonsil. It is very rare for patients with tuberculous cervical adenitis to have an associated pulmonary tuberculosis. Some 20% of cases have discharging sinuses, 10% a cold abscess and 10% are adherent to skin. The vast majority are unilateral and 90% involve only one gland group, the commonest being the deep jugular chain, followed by the nodes in the submandibular region, and then those in the posterior triangle.

Operation
Diagnosis usually necessitates removal of the glands especially when chemotherapy has been ineffective or is unavailable. If the glands are very large and matted, local removal is dangerous since they are often attached to the wall of the internal jugular vein and indeed can sometimes form the wall of the vein. If this is borne in mind, then removal of the gland is straightforward through a horizontal neck incision. If bleeding from the internal jugular vein is encountered, it can be stopped with finger pressure while the vein is dissected above

and below the matted glands so that it can be ligated and the segment of vein excised with the glands.

In cases where the whole neck is full of glands and the vein is extensively involved, a functional neck dissection is performed. This involves removal of the fat with the associated lymph nodes in the posterior and anterior triangles of the neck, preserving the sternomastoid muscle, and the accessory nerve and, as far as possible, the internal jugular vein.

If removal is not followed immediately by appropriate chemotherapy, sinuses can form with persistent drainage and unsightly scars. Since it is almost certain that infection has spread from the ipsilateral tonsil, this should be removed either at the same operation or later.

THE THYROID AND PARATHYROID GLANDS

Anatomy

The thyroid gland
This lies in the lower part of the front of the neck, clasping the trachea and overlapping the sides of the larynx. It consists of a right and a left lobe united across the front of the trachea by the isthmus. Each lobe is piriform in shape with its apex upwards; it extends above to the level of the middle of the thyroid cartilage, and below almost to the clavicle. The isthmus, which is about 2 cm deep, overlies the 2nd, 3rd and 4th rings of the trachea. The gland is enclosed in a sheath of pretracheal fascia, so that it moves up and down with swallowing. Between the gland and its sheath are networks of anastomosing blood vessels.

Relations. The gland is covered superficially by sternohyoid, sternothyroid, and the upper part of omohyoid, and is overlapped in its lower part by sternomastoid. Medially, it is related to cricoid cartilage and inferior constrictor above and to trachea and oesophagus below. Posteriorly, it lies on the carotid sheath and the prevertebral muscles.

Blood supply. The superior thyroid artery arises as the first branch of the external carotid; it passes under cover of the infrahyoid muscles and enters the upper pole of the thyroid lobe. *The inferior thyroid artery* arises from the thyrocervical trunk, a branch of the subclavian. It ascends along the medial border of scalenus anterior as far as the level of the 6th cervical vertebra. It then turns medially behind the carotid sheath to reach the middle of the back of the thyroid, and runs down alongside the gland for a short distance before entering its substance. *The superior thyroid vein* emerges from the upper pole of the lobe and runs backwards across the carotid arteries to enter the internal jugular vein. *The middle thyroid vein* emerges from the lower part of the lateral border of the lobe and crosses the common carotid artery, to join the jugular. *The inferior thyroid veins* emerge from the isthmus or lower medial part of the lobe, and descend in front of the trachea to end in the left innominate vein.

Associated nerves. The external laryngeal nerve, which is a terminal division of the superior laryngeal branch of the vagus, runs downwards on the inferior constrictor, to end by supplying the cricothyroid muscle. Near its termination it is in fairly close proximity to the superior thyroid artery, and is liable to injury when this vessel is secured.

The recurrent laryngeal nerve supplies all the intrinsic muscles of the larynx. It arises from the vagus — on the right side as it crosses the subclavian artery, and on the left side as it crosses the aorta. It hooks round the artery, and ascends into the neck in the groove between trachea and oesophagus. Just before it enters the larynx below the lower border of the inferior constrictor, it lies against the posterior surface of the thyroid gland, within its sheath and closely related to the termination of the inferior thyroid artery; it is therefore liable to be injured during the ligation of this vessel.

The parathyroid glands
These are two pairs of reddish brown glands each about the size of a small pea and ellipsoid in shape. They are situated usually in relation to the posterior aspect of the thyroid lobes.

The superior gland is fairly constant in position, lying behind the upper third of the lobe and related to the lateral surface of the trachea. It is stated to lie invariably between the true capsule of the gland and its fascial sheath. It may, however, be placed relatively far forwards, in which case it is liable to be accidentally removed in the operation of subtotal thyroidectomy.

The inferior gland is situated usually behind the lower part of the lobe, either above or below the inferior thyroid artery as it enters the thyroid substance. Considerable variations, however, exist. The gland may be found behind the oesophagus, either in the neck or in the posterior mediastinum, or it may lie in the anterior mediastinum in relation to the thymus. Occasionally it may be situated within the thyroid substance.

Indications for operation

Simple diffuse goitre
Patients with this condition seek operation for cosmetic reasons or to relieve pressure symptoms related to adjacent structures. Such pressure affects usually the trachea, the oesophagus or the large veins at the root of the neck. These mechanical effects are always more evident when there is a retrosternal prolongation of the goitre, since there is then less room for expansion. It should be noted that simple diffuse enlargement of the thyroid in young adolescents (*pubertal goitre*) usually resolves spontaneously without treatment.

Simple nodular goitre

In this type of goitre there are additional and much stronger reasons for advising operation, for in the course of time such goitres not infrequently become toxic, and are always liable to undergo malignant change. The estimated risk of malignancy in nodular goitre is about 5%. In a young patient, this adds to the indications for operation since a carcinoma diagnosed only by histological examination after thyroidectomy has an incomparably better prognosis than when it is diagnosed by the clinician before operation. In women in the older age groups — especially in the goitrous districts where nodularity of the thyroid is relatively common — operation may be reserved for cases where hardness of the nodules, fixation, or recent increase in size is suggestive of malignant change.

Solitary thyroid nodules

An isolated thyroid nodule in a man is more likely to be malignant than in a woman but many nodules which seem to be isolated on clinical examination are, in fact, part of a multinodular goitre. *Ultra sound scanning,* in skilled hands, can determine whether a nodule is indeed isolated and can give some indication of its size and the likely pathological process involved. When this examination clearly demonstrates a simple cyst, this will allow the surgeon to defer operation or to evacuate the contents with a hollow needle (Sykes, 1981). In most other cases, however, it is a sound policy to advise exploration of any isolated thyroid swelling, even when it is not causing symptoms, since malignancy can only be detected by histological examination of the excised thyroid lobe. Some clinics now carry out *fine needle aspiration* (FNA) or *drill biopsy* of all solitary nodules for preoperative cytological or histological diagnosis but this procedure requires the help of an experienced pathologist (Wade, 1983). *The uptake of radioactive iodine* by a nodule has been suggested as a method of excluding malignancy since increased uptake (known as a 'hot nodule') is seldom malignant whereas a 'cold nodule' may or may not be malignant. However, this is of no practical benefit in the euthyroid patient (Wheeler, 1988) since it does not influence the decision in favour of operation.

Toxic diffuse goitre (primary toxic goitre)

Thyrotoxicosis, diagnosed clinically and confirmed biochemically, may be associated with no enlargement of the thyroid gland or with a diffuse goitre. Treatment may be carried out by antithyroid drugs, by surgery or by radioactive iodine, and these may be employed separately or in combination. The antithyroid drugs act by inhibiting the synthesis of thyroxine. The drug most commonly used in the United Kingdom at present is *carbimazole* (neomercazole), propylthiouracil being reserved for patients who have a sensitivity reaction to

carbimazole. *Propranolol* may be added to or used on its own although this drug merely acts on the target organs to control symptoms resulting from excess circulating thyroid hormones. In many patients complete remission of thyrotoxic symptoms can be obtained with drugs, avoiding the need for surgery. The younger the patient, the more likely the response to antithyroid drugs, but if this fails, and symptoms recur after completion of a year's treatment, operation should be advised. The realization that some patients with thyrotoxicosis also have auto immune thyroiditis (as indicated by raised antibody titres) will influence the surgeon in withholding operation. In these cases, destruction of functioning tissue by the immune process will lead eventually to control of the toxic state but operation should not be withheld on these grounds alone. Young adults (between 18 and 40 years) with diffuse hyperplasia of the gland often respond well to antithyroid medication, but are likely to be impatient for cure, and may find the prolonged treatment tedious and unacceptable. Sometimes they develop further gland enlargement while under such treatment due to the increased TSH output by the pituitary which follows reduction in circulating thyroid hormones. Older people respond less readily, but they are likely to be more tolerant of prolonged treatment. All cases of thyrotoxicosis should be regarded as a combined medicosurgical problem, and should be assessed by a physician before operation is considered. All should receive medical treatment in the first instance, whether this be employed in the expectation that by itself it will be curative, or merely as a preoperative measure to make the patient safe for surgery. It is obvious that the decision will depend upon a number of factors, including the initial response obtained. Indications for operation are (1) lack of response to antithyroid therapy; (2) toxic effects of the drug; (3) relapse after apparent cure; (4) a gland which is large and cosmetically disfiguring, or which is causing pressure symptoms, especially if these are due to a retrosternal prolongation. Operation is contra-indicated when there has been a failure of response to preoperative treatment, and when the patient has a cardiac problem.

Treatment by radioactive sodium iodide solution (*radioiodine*) is very effective in controlling thyrotoxicosis and there are some who believe that it is a reasonable first treatment at all ages (Halnan, 1983). Its use in UK is generally restricted because of possible carcinogenic effects although there are a number of reports of its use in children in USA (Hayek, 1970). In the majority of centres this form of therapy is used only in cases selected from the following groups: (1) patients over 45 years of age, or those whose life expectancy, because of associated disease, does not exceed 20 to 25 years; (2) patients of any age who have not reacted to antithyroid drugs, and who are either bad surgical risks or have refused operation; (3) all patients who have relapsed after thyroidectomy.

Toxic nodular goitre (secondary toxic goitre)
This shows little response to antithyroid drugs, although good results have been claimed in some centres by the use of radio-iodine. Most surgeons will have little hesitation in advising operation, especially in the coarsely nodular types of goitre, or if a single localized nodule appears to be present, for such goitres are likely to be resistant to any form of conservative treatment, and to develop a high degree of toxicity. Medical treatment is advised, therefore, only as a preliminary to operation, and in patients who are bad surgical risks. In preparation for operation, a radioactive isotope scan is occasionally of value in detecting excessive activity in one part of the gland thus allowing the surgeon to concentrate his efforts on removing the affected lobe.

Preoperative treatment
Adequate preparation by medical treatment is essential before surgery on any toxic thyroid. Many surgeons advise routine laryngoscopy to assess vocal cord function — in case the patient complains of a hoarse voice postoperatively — but the report by Jarhult (1991) suggests that this is probably not necessary since the surgeon's assessment of the patient's voice is generally reliable.

When the thyrotoxicosis is moderate, adequate preparation can usually be achieved by the administration of iodine, which stimulates colloid storage, so that activity and vascularity of the gland is diminished. Aqueous iodine solution (Lugol's solution) 0.3 ml three times daily is generally used. Propranolol alone, 40 mg 3 times daily, may be used for rapid preoperative preparation (Yawhan, 1983) although this is not recommended in the severely thyrotoxic patient (Feely, 1981).

In patients with severe thyrotoxicosis, antithyroid drugs should be given either as definitive treatment or as part of the preparation for surgery. Carbimazole may be started as a single daily dosage of 30 to 60 mg — depending upon the severity of the thyrotoxicosis — and maintained at this dose until the patient's thyroid function tests are normal. The dose is then progressively reduced to between 5 and 15 mg daily. In the final 10 days prior to surgery, iodine is also given since it is credited with reducing the vascularity of the gland (Marigold, 1985).

Subtotal thyroidectomy (Fig. 12.44)
This implies the removal of the greater part of the enlarged gland, the operation being a bilateral one, leaving an equal and symmetrical amount of gland tissue on each side. The proportion of gland to be re-

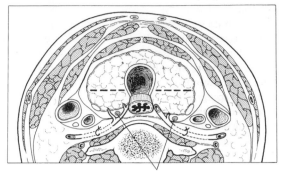

Recurrent laryngeal nerves

Fig. 12.44   Transverse section of neck to illustrate the amount of gland left in situ at the operation of subtotal thyroidectomy. The inferior thyroid arteries, the recurrent laryngeal nerves and the parathyroid glands are shown in their relationship to the remaining gland segment

moved depends upon the condition present. *In simple goitre* it is advisable (because of the risk of myxoedema) to leave an amount of gland on each side equal at least to a normal lobe. *In toxic goitre* there is a general tendency to leave very little thyroid tissue since the risk of recurrent thyrotoxicosis is greater than that of myxoedema. The amount suggested is 3–4 g on each side (assessed by volume) depending partly on preoperative antibody levels. When the gland is greatly enlarged, as much as 7/8 of it may therefore be removed. This is often best achieved by removing the whole of one lobe and leaving a single remnant on the opposite side. It is safer to err on the side of leaving too little rather than too much, since recurrent thyrotoxicosis is a less desirable and less easily managed complication than myxoedema. The latter may recover without medication (Noguchi, 1981) while recurrent hyperthyroidism can be troublesome unless there is an element of thyroiditis. The part of the gland left in situ is a strip of the posterior surface of the lobe. This surface is closely related to the recurrent laryngeal nerve and (usually) to the parathyroid glands, and if it is left undisturbed these structures are unlikely to be injured.

Premedication and anaesthesia
In all toxic cases effective premedication is most important, in view of the effect of emotional stress on thyroid activity. The patient should have had a good night's sleep prior to operation and reach the operating theatre in a calm state of mind. General anaesthesia is normally favoured in this country. Endotracheal intubation, advisable in all cases, is essential when deviation or constriction of the trachea has been produced since the ensured airway reduces venous congestion. The neck veins can be further emptied by tilting the operation table and patient some 15° head up.

Technique

A small pillow or sandbag is placed between the shoulders so that the neck is extended and rotation of the head is avoided if the patient's head is supported on a ring. The skin incision can be marked by pressing a length of thread onto the skin just before using the scalpel, keeping in the line of the skin creases, 2–3 cm above the sternum. The 'collar' incision is then made, extending to the lateral borders of the two sterno-mastoid muscles. (With larger goitres the incision is made a little higher so as to provide better access to the superior thyroid pole). In order to give a neater scar, the platysma is divided at a slightly higher lever than the skin. The flaps of skin, superficial fascia and platysma are then reflected upwards to the level of the thyroid cartilage, and downwards to the sternum. Prior injection of saline, containing 1 in 300 000 parts of adrenaline, is useful in reducing blood loss and in opening up this plane. The anterior jugular veins are divided between ligatures. The investing layer of deep fascia is incised vertically in the mid line, any anastomosing veins being secured, and the interval between the infrahyoid muscles is opened up to expose the sheath of pretracheal fascia covering the gland (Fig. 12.45). The sheath is now incised, and a finger is passed over the front of each lobe to ascertain its size and extent. As a rule the larger lobe is dealt with first, and by retraction of the infrahyoid muscles the greater part of its anterior surface is exposed. This is facilitated if the surgeon stands on the opposite side to the lobe being

Figs 12.45–12.50 Subtotal thyroidectomy

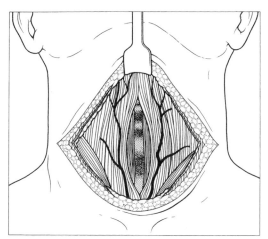

Fig. 12.45 Incision of deep fascia in the midline

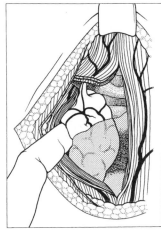

Fig. 12.46 Mobilization of the right lobe

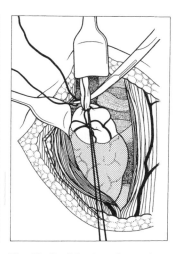

Fig. 12.47 Ligating of superior thyroid vessels

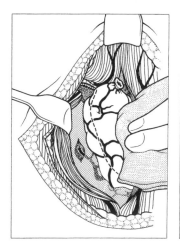

Fig. 12.48 Exposure of the inferior thyroid artery

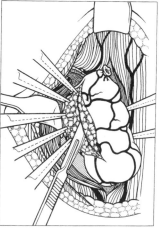

Fig. 12.49 Division of the gland

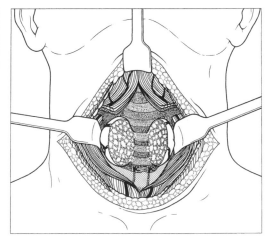

Fig. 12.50 Appearances after the subtotal removal

mobilized. If necessary, the sternomastoid muscle is mobilized laterally by division of the fascia along its medial border. Improved access can be then obtained by division of the infrahyoid muscles (high up, so as to cause the minimum damage to their nerve supply). The lateral surface of the lobe is cleared by the finger (Fig. 12.46), during which procedure the middle thyroid vein, if present, is divided between ligatures. The muscles are retracted strongly in an upward and lateral direction, and the upper pole of the gland is delivered at the wound, when the vascular pedicle comprising the superior thyroid vessels becomes apparent. These vessels are divided between ligatures, the lower being tied first (Fig. 12.47) so as to provide countertraction for accurate placing of the upper ligature. If possible, a double ligature should be applied to the upper stump. The lobe is drawn forwards and medially, and search is made behind it for the inferior thyroid artery and recurrent laryngeal nerve. The artery should be identified at a safe distance from the gland within the fascial sheath, which is carefully incised at the level of the cricoid cartilage where the artery emerges from behind the common carotid (Fig. 12.48). At this point a ligature is applied to the inferior thyroid artery in continuity. Unfortunately, this does not guarantee the avoidance of damage to an anomalous recurrent laryngeal nerve on the right side and it is preferable to identify and safeguard the nerve in all cases. A finger is then swept round the lower pole of the lobe which is delivered forwards, and the inferior thyroid and other veins are secured.

A flat dissector is now insinuated between the isthmus of the gland and the trachea, and these structures are gently separated. The decision having been made as to the amount of gland tissue to be left behind (p. 310) several pairs of forceps are applied to the capsule of the lobe on its posterolateral aspect along the line of proposed section. These serve to steady the gland and to arrest haemorrhage. The lobe is then sectioned from lateral to medial side (Fig. 12.49), in a plane towards the front of the trachea. An ordinary scalpel should be used in preference to the diathermy knife, in view of possible injury to the trachea or to the recurrent laryngeal nerve. When both thyroid arteries have been ligatured there is surprisingly little bleeding from the flat cut surface of the gland, and what little there is can usually be controlled by ligatures.

The opposite lobe of the gland is then treated in a similar manner, an equal amount of gland tissue being left behind. All haemorrhage is arrested, either by fine ligatures or by diathermy coagulation (Fig. 12.50). If the infrahyoid muscles have been divided they are repaired by suture. The wound is then closed, drainage being provided by Redivac suction (p. 345) for 24–48 hours.

Removal of retrosternal goitre

The diagnosis will usually have been made or at least suspected before operation — either from the severity of dyspnoea or from radiological examination. Fortunately the retrosternal prolongation of the gland seldom has any vascular connections within the thorax so that its blood supply is readily controlled from above. The cervical part of the gland is mobilized as far as possible, the superior thyroid vessels and middle thyroid vein being secured. A finger is then insinuated downwards behind the intrathoracic extension, and is used to free it from surrounding structures. By pressure from the finger below, aided by slight traction from above, the retrosternal part of the gland can usually be delivered upwards into the wound. The cavity is packed with gauze while the inferior thyroid artery is secured and the customary resection carried out. The gauze packing is now withdrawn and is replaced by a drain, after which the wound is closed.

Postoperative treatment

With adequate preoperative preparation, thyroid crisis after thyroidectomy for toxic thyroid should not occur. It does no harm, however, to keep the patient in a quiet room, well sedated with morphine or allied drugs, and to continue the preoperative drugs for a few days.

Hemithyroidectomy (lobectomy)

The lobe of thyroid to be resected is mobilized as in the first stage of the subtotal operation. It is particularly important to trace the recurrent laryngeal nerve throughout its visible course and to divide branches of the inferior thyroid artery without damaging the nerve. Ligature of the artery in continuity is not essential but it may help in the avoidance of damage to the nerve by reducing haemorrhage as branches of the artery are divided close to the nerve. The parathyroids are preserved, preferably with their blood supply. The entire thyroid lobe is then removed together with the isthmus and a thin slice from the front of the opposite lobe to give a better cosmetic result.

Total thyroidectomy

The technique of this procedure is essentially a bilateral version of the hemithyroidectomy already described. If it is not possible to preserve the parathyroid glands intact, it is preferable to reimplant them within the sternomastoid muscle rather than to remove them completely. Total thyroidectomy may be successful in effecting cure of a carcinoma, and should be advocated in those cases where the growth is sufficiently mobile or if tumour is found in one of the lymph nodes outside the thyroid (Hargreaves, 1981). If the tumour is of papillary type and is confined to one lobe, lobectomy with removal of the isthmus is usually sufficient. Dissection of lymph nodes need only be carried out when they are involved by tumour. The discovery of isolated lymph node metastases from a carcinoma of the thyroid which is undetectable clinically (lateral 'aberrant' thyroid) requires total or near total thyroidectomy combined with removal of all laterally placed nodes — especially in the younger patient (Frankenthaler, 1990).

Excision of isthmus

Excision of thyroid isthmus and medial part of each lobe may be required for the relief of pressure on the trachea caused by carcinoma or chronic thyroiditis. Operation is also of value in obtaining tissue for histological diagnosis in the hope that radiotherapy (in the form of radioactive iodine) may help to control a growth if it is not amenable to surgical excision. Autoimmune thyroiditis (lymphadenoid goitre or Hashimoto's disease) should not be confused with carcinoma clinically since antibodies are detectable in the serum, whereas chronic thyroiditis (Riedel's Struma) is indistinguishable from carcinoma without biopsy and is not associated with serum antibodies.

Complications of thyroid surgery

With adequate preoperative treatment and a careful operative technique, immediate complications are rare but later problems arise.

Haemorrhage. Excess bleeding, which does not pass along the drainage tube, may result in accumulation beneath the infrahyoid muscles and may lead to serious dyspnoea from pressure on the trachea or on the recurrent laryngeal nerves. It should be noted that the neck may show no obvious swelling on clinical examination. Instruments should be available at the patient's bedside so that the wound can be opened up. The patient is returned to theatre for evacuation of clot and securing of the bleeding vessel. If carbimazole has been given preoperatively, it may be responsible for a tendency to bleeding; this can be counteracted by the administration of vitamin K (Holl-Allen, 1967).

Respiratory obstruction. Laryngeal oedema may follow tension haematoma and result in obstruction of the airway. The obstruction may be further aggravated if one or both vocal cords has been paralysed by damage to the recurrent laryngeal nerve. Passage of an endotracheal tube should be placed in the hands of one skilled in this procedure.

Recurrent laryngeal nerve paralysis. This may result from pressure on the nerve by blood clot or by oedema in which case recovery can be anticipated. Provided that the nerve has been seen and avoided at operation, any paralysis can be considered as temporary. The prognosis as regards recovery of function after organic injury is poor.

Hypothyroidism. This is encountered after operations for simple goitre or for thyrotoxicosis but rarely after hemithyroidectomy where there may be hypertrophy of the residual lobe. Treatment consists in the administration of the synthetic L-thyroxine, using thyroid function tests to control the dosage.

Recurrent thyrotoxicosis. This is due either to inadequate removal of thyroid tissue or to subsequent hyperplasia of the tissue that has been left. It is not uncommon in primary toxic goitre, but very rare in the secondary form of the disease. In cases where there is autoimmune thyroiditis, recovery can be expected after a course of antithyroid drugs. Further operation should be avoided if possible and the administration of radioiodine may be considered as an alternative to antithyroid drugs.

Postoperative hypoparathyroidism. This may be caused by removal of or injury to the parathyroid glands, with resultant lowering of the serum calcium. Frank *tetany* is uncommon and usually transient. It is treated by the intravenous administration of 20 ml of 20% calcium gluconate. Some degree of parathyroid deficiency may persist permanently, and may lead to a variety of indefinite symptoms. Treatment consists in the administration of pharmacological doses of vitamin D.

Parathyroidectomy

Overactivity of one or more of the parathyroid glands, a solitary adenoma or multiglandular hyperplasia, gives rise to the condition of hyperparathyroidism. This, by increasing the metabolism of calcium, may be the responsible factor in the development of skeletal decalcification (osteitis fibrosa), or in the formation of calculi in the urinary tract (Barnes, 1984). Patients may also present with gastrointestinal symptoms or psychiatric problems. Exploration is indicated when the provisional diagnosis of parathyroid tumour is confirmed by the combination of persistent hypercalcaemia and low serum phosphate. Parathormone (PTH) assay, when available, will show an elevated level to indicate the cause of the deranged calcium metabolism. Removal of the affected gland or glands will normally bring about a complete cure of the condition but it is only rarely that any swelling can be detected on clinical examination.

Clinics which specialize in parathyroid surgery may use a variety of *localization techniques* although Serpell (1991) did not find that this reduced the operating time for an experienced surgeon. Technetium and thallium subtraction scanning accurately locates adenomas weighing more than 1 g (Carlson, 1990) and may be accompanied by high-resolution ultrasonography and computed tomography. Selective venous catheterization of the neck veins is used to obtain blood samples at various sites draining the thyroid gland. Parathormone levels in each sample are then assessed to determine the site of a parathyroid tumour (Hsu, 1983). As an operative aid to location of the parathyroids, methylene blue may be used to stain the glands: a dilute solution containing 5 to 7.5 mg/kg lean body weight is injected intravenously one hour preoperatively.

If these facilities are not available, the entire thyroid gland should be exposed by a surgeon experienced in this type of operation. To ensure unrestricted access, the infrahyoid muscles are usually divided. Both lobes of the gland are then mobilized sufficiently to allow exploration of their posterior surfaces, and a thorough search is made in all the normal situations of the parathyroid glands. A tumour of the superior parathyroid is as a rule easily located, since this gland is fairly constant in its position, behind the upper third of the thyroid lobe, and within the fascial sheath. The best way to locate the inferior parathyroid (if this is in its normal position) is to identify the inferior thyroid artery as it approaches the back of the lobe, and then to follow it downwards, when the gland should be found, crossed by its branches. The recurrent laryngeal nerve should be identified and safeguarded.

If no tumour is found in the normal situations for the parathyroid glands, the surgeon should be prepared to extend his search into the upper part of the thorax, splitting the sternum if necessary. Both the retrosternal space and the retro-oesophageal space should be explored. Approach to the latter is obtained by incising the deep fascia above the inferior thyroid artery, and by inserting a finger downwards and medially, behind the oesophagus. If it is possible to identify a branch of the inferior thyroid artery running downwards into the thorax this may point the way to a parathyroid tumour. Parathyroid glands may even be found in or adjacent to thymic tissue according to Wang (1976) who has made a detailed study of their anatomy.

When the enlarged gland has been found it can be removed without difficulty, after small vessels supplying it have been secured. Normal glands are left undisturbed.

THE SALIVARY GLANDS

Anatomy

The parotid gland
This fits into the space behind the mandible, below the external ear and in front of the mastoid process. It overlies the posterior belly of digastric below, and deeply it is applied to the styloid process and its muscles. It is enclosed by a sheath which is derived from the deep cervical fascia, and which sends processes into the gland substance dividing it into lobules. Its *upper pole* lies just below the zygomatic arch, and is wedged between the meatus and the mandibular joint. The superficial temporal vessels, temporal branches of the facial nerve, and the auriculotemporal nerve are found

entering or leaving the gland near the upper pole. The cervical branch of the facial nerve, and the two divisions of the retromandibular vein emerge from its *lower pole*. Its *anterior border* overlies the masseter; from it emerge the parotid duct and the zygomatic, buccal and mandibular branches of the facial nerve.

The external carotid artery grooves the deep surface of the gland, and may pass through its substance; it terminates behind the neck of the mandible by dividing into maxillary and superficial temporal arteries.

The facial nerve, is intimately related to the parotid gland. The main trunk, after emerging from the stylomastoid foramen, almost immediately enters the posteromedial surface of the gland and splits up into its two main sub-divisions: the *temporo-zygomatic* and the *cervico-facial*, from which the terminal branches arise. The branches lie with remarkable constancy in the plane superficial to the *retromandibular vein*. This vein is formed within the substance of the gland by the continuation of the superficial temporal vein joined by the maxillary veins from the pterygoid plexus. The plane in which the vein and the branches of the facial nerve lie has been designated by Patey (1957) the *faciovenous plane*.

The parotid duct emerges from the anterior border of the gland, runs horizontally across the masseter, and pierces the buccinator to open on the mucous membrane of the mouth opposite the second upper molar tooth.

The submandibular gland
This is situated partly below the mandible and partly deep to it. The body of the gland overlaps both bellies of digastric inferiorly. It is enclosed in a loose sheath of deep cervical fascia. The *superficial surface* is covered only by platysma and deep fascia. The *medial surface* lies on mylohyoid, hyoglossus and pharyngeal wall from before backwards. Between the gland and hyoglossus are the lingual nerve, the submandibular ganglion and the hypoglossal nerve. The *deep part* of the gland is a prolongation extending from its medial surface under cover of mylohyoid. It is accompanied by the *submandibular duct* which opens into the mouth on the sublingual papilla at the side of the frenulum of the tongue.

The facial artery ascends in a deep groove on the posterior end of the gland, and then turns downwards and laterally between the gland and the mandible to enter the face at the anterior border of masseter.

Indications for operation

Acute suppurative parotitis (parotid abscess)
This is still occasionally seen as a postoperative complication in debilitated patients with inadequate oral

hygiene. It frequently responds to antistaphylococcal antibiotic therapy, warm packs and rehydration. Incision and drainage should be carried out if the infection does not subside within 48 hours. Fluctuation should not be awaited, since it is masked by the tense parotid fascia. Delay in providing drainage may lead to spread of the infection to the deep tissue planes of the neck.

A small incision is made over the most prominent part of the swelling. Pus is located by sinus forceps, and a small drain is inserted.

Simple tumours of the parotid

The most common is the pleomorphic adenoma or 'mixed' tumour, which, although essentially benign and enclosed within a well formed capsule of compressed parotid tissue, tends to recur after local removal. This is because the growth not infrequently permeates the capsule, giving rise to 'island' tumours in the surrounding gland. Local removal of the tumour by *enucleation* carries a considerable risk of recurrence. The preferred operation is *conservative parotidectomy,* which is defined as partial or total removal of the parotid gland with preservation of the facial nerve. This can only be achieved by identifying and exposing the nerve and its branches throughout the gland (Hobsley, 1981). The operation is made possible by the realization that the gland can be split sagitally, in the plane of the facial nerve, into superficial and deep parts which can be removed separately, while the intervening nerve and its branches are preserved intact. The great majority of 'mixed' tumours are situated in the superficial part of the gland, and can be removed very adequately by superficial parotidectomy. The monomorphic adenoma or Warthin's tumour is a cystic lesion, usually in the tail of the gland, often in older male subjects and occasionally bilateral. Although this lesion may be dealt with adequately by local excision, it is usually diagnosed only postoperatively and, therefore, superficial parotidectomy is the operation of choice for benign lesions.

Chronic parotitis (parotid sialectasis)

This is due most commonly to infection or duct obstruction, or to a combination of the two. In the event of failure of conservative treatment, which may include duct irrigation and radiotherapy, removal of the affected gland by conservative total parotidectomy is advocated. Superficial parotidectomy is not advocated as the residual sialectatic deep lobe can produce a troublesome postoperative salivary fistula.

Carcinoma of parotid

Malignancy of the parotid gland may be adenocarcinoma, carcinoma expleomorphic adenoma, mucoepidermoid carcinoma, which has a variable biological behaviour and tumour grading, or adenoid cyst carcinoma, which has a propensity for perineural spread. Total conservative parotidectomy may be practicable in carcinoma of the gland, if some at least of the branches of the facial nerve are free of the growth and can be preserved. When removal of the tumour necessitates sacrifice of the entire facial nerve, this necessity should be weighed against the certainty that nerve function will eventually be destroyed by the tumour. Partial excision combined with radiotherapy gives the best prospect of palliation in unresectable lesions.

Uncommon parotid conditions

Parotid calculi are much less common than submandibular gland calculi. Since the symptoms are more suggestive of infection, and because of their small size, they are frequently missed. They may become impacted either at the hilum of the gland or at the bend of the duct at the anterior border of the masseter. If a calculus is palpable from the mouth, it may be removed by an incision made directly upon it through the mucous membrane. An approach from the skin surface may be necessary, but carries the risk of causing an external fistula.

Parotid fistula. A *gland fistula* is an uncommon sequel to operation on the gland or to rupture of an abscess. It usually closes spontaneously.

A *duct fistula* results most commonly from injury to the duct. If the injury is recognized at the time, immediate end-to-end suture of the duct should be carried out over a nylon thread, which is left projecting into the mouth. More often the condition is not recognized until a chronic fistula has formed. It is then unlikely to be cured by anything less than a superficial parotidectomy.

Enucleation

Removal of a parotid lump by enucleation is not recommended since the proximity of the growth to the facial nerve cannot be determined and its malignant potential is unknown i.e. there is risk of injury to the nerve and of incomplete tumour removal. After local excision of a 'mixed' tumour, postoperative radiotherapy is probably advisable in all cases, and is regarded as essential if the capsule has ruptured during the dissection.

Superficial parotidectomy

It is an advantage if the anaesthetist can provide hypotensive anaesthesia and also elevate the head of the table to reduce venous congestion. If a nerve stimulator is to be used (and it is advised for the less experienced surgeon) then the whole side of the face up to the profile line must be seen. A transparent adhesive drape is therefore preferable and is easy to use.

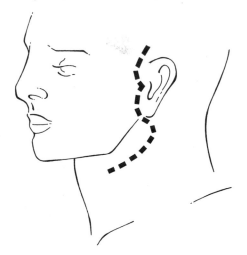

Fig. 12.51   Incision for parotidectomy

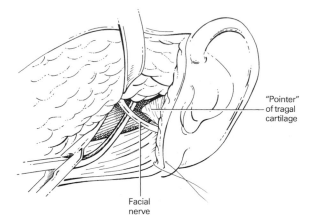

Fig. 12.52   Showing position of the facial nerve in relation to the tip ('pointer') of the tragal cartilage

Incision

Many incisions have been described but these vary mostly in their course at the ear lobe. The skin overlying and just anterior to the mastoid process is very thin and is devoid of underlying muscle which brings its main blood supply. Three point junctions and loops are to be avoided here to prevent ischaemic necrosis. The incision advised is shown in Figure 12.51. It starts at the top of the helix and dips into the tragal notch. It then proceeds inferiorly immediately in front of the ear and turns back gently under the ear lobe to 1 cm inferior to the tip of the mastoid bone. From there it goes down to the tip of the greater horn of the hyoid bone, following the line of the skin creases.

Excision

The skin flap is dissected off the parotid gland as far forwards as the anterior border of masseter muscle, taking care not to damage the peripheral branches of the facial nerve. The tail of the parotid is lifted off the surface of the sternomastoid muscle. The great auricular nerve is found entering the gland at the anterior border of sternomastoid. It is divided as close to the gland as possible so as to hasten recovery of sensation in the area. The sternomastoid is then retracted and a search is made for the posterior belly of digastric muscle. This is followed upwards to the mastoid bone. The facial nerve bisects the angle made by the digastric muscle and the tympanic plate.

The next landmark of the facial nerve to be sought is the point of the tragal cartilage. The dissection is carried deeply along the perichondrium of the tragal cartilage and parotid tissue is separated from it. The cartilage ends in a pointer which points to the facial nerve, 1 cm medially and inferiorly (Fig. 12.52). Once the pointer is found and the digastric dissection com-

pleted, a bridge of parotid tissue will be seen overlying the facial nerve. This bridge can confidently be elevated down to the level of the digastric muscle. Precise haemostasis is secured using pledgets, bipolar diathermy and 3/0 silk ligatures. Unipolar diathermy may cause thermal injury to the nerve. Once the nerve is found, it is followed forwards but it runs rapidly to the surface and account has to be taken of this in the dissection. After about 2 cm it divides into an upper and lower division. The upper division is dissected out first and, using small artery forceps passed along the line of the nerve (Fig. 12.53), the parotid tissue is cut away from the nerve. The most superior branch is followed first and will be found to cross the mid point of the zygoma. It then divides into its terminal branches to the fore-

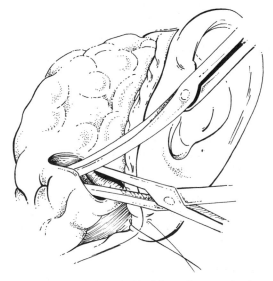

Fig. 12.53   Parotid tissue is lifted from the nerve by the opened blades of mosquito forceps and cut with fine scissors

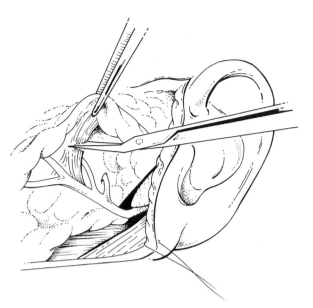

Fig. 12.54 Between each branch of the nerve a bridge of parotid tissue passing between the superficial layer and the deep layer is being divided

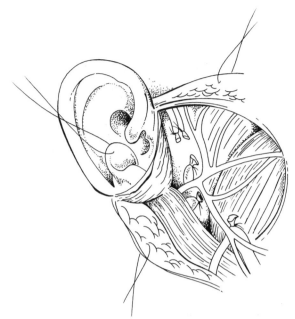

Fig. 12.55 Facial nerve displayed after removal of parotid gland

head and eyebrow. The parotid is swung down and the branch to the corner of the eye is dissected. The next branch is to the lower lid and then a major branch is found running parallel to the duct. This is the buccal branch which supplies the nose, upper lip and lower eyelid. It usually arises from the upper division but can arise from the lower one. At this stage half of the gland should have been dissected from the nerve and turned downwards (Fig. 12.54). The lower division of the nerve is dissected in the same way and branches to the upper lip, corner of mouth and lower lip must be identified and dissected. The superficial lobe can then be removed leaving the facial nerve exposed on the masseter and retromandibular portion of the gland (Fig. 12.55). If a stimulator is available to demonstrate that all the branches are intact, then in the event of postoperative paralysis the patient can be reassured that function will eventually return.

If hypotension has been induced, this is reversed to a systolic blood pressure of at least 100 mmHg before final haemostasis. Adrenalin soaks are useful and in this way multiple ties can be avoided. Diathermy should not be used for haemostasis unless it is the bipolar type. Unipolar diathermy spreads and so heat injury to the nerve is possible. Finally, the skin wound is sutured in two layers with one or possibly two suction drains. Having the drains over the exposed nerve does not seem to increase the risk of facial paralysis.

Complications

The main complication is *facial nerve paralysis*. Partial weakness of the facial muscles is quite common and is recoverable if the facial nerve has been identified and preserved at operation. In a total paralysis, if the nerve stimulation test at the end of operation was satisfactory, the lesion is neurapraxia and no treatment is indicated. Without the test, the wound must be reopened and the nerve examined. If a division is found it should be repaired by primary suture using 10/0 silk under the microscope. There is no immediate treatment for a partial facial paralysis; function ought to return if some movement is present after the operation. *Bleeding* is rare and is usually venous from the retromandibular vein. It can be easily recognized and re-ligated. A not infrequent late complication (after a month) is *Frey's Syndrome*. When the parotid is removed, the secreto-motor fibres are divided and they subsequently grow back into the skin, blood vessels and sebaceous glands. When smell and taste are stimulated vasodilatation and sweating occur. Most cases resolve spontaneously over a period of 6 months and only 10% require treatment. The latter is designed to interrupt the parasympathetic reflex arc and is best done by turning back the ear drum and dividing Jacobsen's nerve which runs over the promontory of the middle ear (tympanitic neurectomy).

Total parotidectomy with preservation of the facial nerve

This is necessary for tumours extending to the retromandibular portion of the parotid gland which lies in the parapharyngeal space. The operation proceeds as above (p. 315) until the extension between superficial and deep lobes becomes apparent. This can be between the upper and lower divisions of the facial nerve or below the lower division. If the attachment is between the two main divisions, then the dissection of the superficial lobe from the facial nerve should be performed from below upwards so that the superficial lobe is pedicled on the tumour. At this point using blunt pointed scissors the main trunk, upper and lower divisions and distal branches of the nerve are dissected from the underlying tissue. This allows access between the two main divisions which can be retracted. If the tumour presents inferior to the lower division of the nerve, the superficial lobe dissection can be continued down to this point and only the lower division with its distal branches needs to be dissected to allow access to the parapharyngeal space. It can then be retracted upwards. The parapharyngeal space contains much loose areolar tissue which allows easy finger dissection. The retromandibular vein always requires to be ligated and divided but the external carotid artery has usually been pushed deeply into the space by the tumour and rarely presents any problems.

Total parotidectomy with sacrifice of the nerve and nerve graft

This is usually the procedure required for the excision of malignant disease of the parotid. For adenoid cystic carcinoma, wide removal of the nerve is required. Depending on the position of the tumour and its extent, consideration may have to be given to removal of the temporomandibular joint, the external auditory meatus, the zygoma or mastoid bone and skin overlying the growth.

Details of nerve grafting lie beyond the scope of this book but the following principles should be observed:

1. The best suited graft is the great auricular nerve: it is easily accessible; up to 8 cm can be removed; it has two branches of suitable diameter to anastomose to the upper and lower divisions.

2. There should be no tension at the anastomosis.

3. No scar tissue should intrude at the anastomosis and so the sheath should be cut back and only a minimal number of sutures used. Research has shown that the type of suture used and the method of fixation of the junctions do not influence functional outcome.

4. The use of the operating microscope is advisable to allow interfascicular repair.

Removal of calculi from the submandibular duct

If calculi can be felt in the duct, intraoral removal is possible, using local anaesthetic infiltration or a dental block. In order to prevent the calculi from sliding back into the gland as a result of the manipulations, a silk suture is passed round the duct behind the stone and retracted upwards (Fig. 12.56). With a

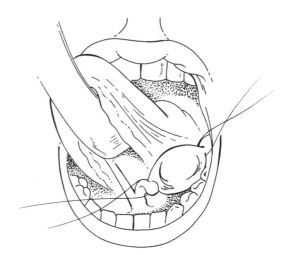

Fig. 12.56   Isolation of calculus in submandibular duct

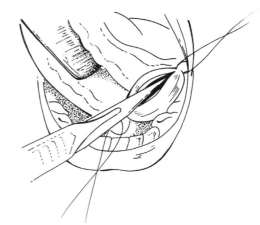

Fig. 12.57   Incision of submandibular duct

number 11 blade, the duct is incised directly over the stone (Fig. 12.57). The tissue is thicker than normal due to the irritation caused by the stone and often up to 1 cm of soft tissue must be incised before the stone is found and removed. No attempt to suture the duct is necessary.

Removal of the submandibular gland for calculi

This is advised when the gland is chronically inflamed or is the site of stone formation. Tumours of the gland itself are comparatively rare, but secondary carcinoma of the related lymph glands is commonly encountered. Many of these lymph glands are inseparable by dissection from the salivary gland, and in any operation for their removal the salivary gland must be included in the excision.

Incision

The area is prepared and draped so that the corner of

the mouth and angle of jaw are visible as well as the upper half of the neck. A horizontal skin crease incision is made two finger breadths below the ramus of the mandible. The incision should be deepened to the body of the submandibular gland before raising skin flaps. The aim is to avoid damaging the cervical branch of the facial nerve which lies in the plane between the platysma and the investing fascia of the neck 2 cm below the horizontal ramus of the mandible. As the tissues superficial to the investing fascia are lifted off the body of the gland in the formation of a flap, so is the nerve protected. This flap is developed up to the ramus of the mandible and is then gently retracted by an assistant.

Excision

2.5 cm anterior to the angle of the mandible, the bone is grooved by the facial vessels. These are also crossed by the cervical branch of the facial nerve and so to tie the vessels prior to the development of the fascial flap is to put the nerve at risk. The nerve can also be damaged by over-use of diathermy. Although the facial artery can be dissected out of its groove on the gland, it is simpler to divide and ligate each end. Once the artery and vein have been divided at the upper end, the gland is dissected bluntly off the ramus into the submental area. The submental vessels are tied and the submental fat pad and the anterior part of the gland are then dissected backwards off the surfaces of the anterior belly of digastric and the mylohyoid muscle. At the posterior border of mylohyoid a Langenbeck retractor is used to pull the muscle forwards. This reveals the duct, the hypoglossal nerve running along just above the greater horn of the hyoid and, when the gland is pulled posteroinferiorly, the lingual nerve (Fig. 12.58). With this manoeuvre the lingual nerve is pulled down in a U-shape and is attached to the gland by the submandibular ganglion. A small vessel accompanying the ganglionic attachment must be clamped carefully to

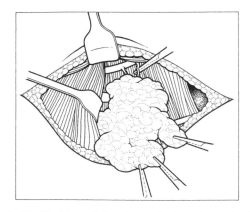

Fig. 12.58 Excision of left submandibular salivary gland

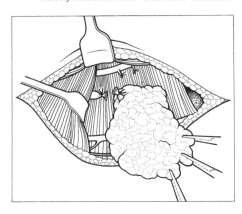

Fig. 12.59 The lingual nerve and hypoglossal nerves are displayed deep to the gland. The submandibular duct has been divided

free the gland from the nerve. The duct is then tied with catgut and divided (Fig. 12.59). If the operation is being performed for calculi within the gland, make sure that the duct is removed as far forwards as possible or else stones dislodged into the duct from the operative manipulation may pass into the patient's mouth several days after the operation. (Explanations for this are apt to be confusing and embarrassing.) The only attachment of the gland now is the proximal end of the facial artery entering its posteroinferior margin just at the superior border of the posterior belly of digastric. The artery should be identified and suture ligatured with silk, after which it is divided and the gland removed. One suction drain is usually sufficient and it is tucked up underneath the mandible. Since a stab wound leaves an ugly mark in a very visible part of the neck if brought out underneath the incision, it is best brought out as far posteriorly as possible (Wilson, 1991).

Complications

Arterial haemorrhage is unlikely if the proximal end of the facial artery has been suture ligatured. The drain is removed after 72 hours but it is best then to apply a pressure dressing for 24 hours because the operative site is essentially a dependent area and seroma collection is not infrequent. If it occurs it should be aspirated daily and pressure dressings applied until its ceases. If the cervical branch of the facial nerve has been contused or cut the mouth will be pulled to the opposite side by the normal muscle tone. This is an ugly deformity and is made worse by voluntary movement such as smiling and talking. If the nerve has only been bruised, the mouth will probably be straight in the resting position. If it has been divided, the mouth will be squint even at rest. Whatever the deformity, 6–9 months should elapse prior to offering further treatment. This quite simply aims to equalize tone on the lower lip by cutting the equivalent branch on the other side. No functional defect results.

If the lingual or hypoglossal nerves are damaged little disability results and there is no specific treatment, but every effort should be made to avoid such injury (Milton, 1986).

Removal of the submandibular gland for tumour

Most benign tumours of the submandibular gland are pleomorphic adenomas and provided one keeps as far from the surface of the tumour as possible, the operation described above is quite suitable. There is no place for enucleation. Malignant tumours are more common in the submandibular than the parotid gland and may require a radical neck dissection or at least an upper neck dissection or a suprahyoid dissection. This is described on p. 304, but involves the additional removal of the digastric muscle and the associated fat and lymph nodes up to the mastoid process and including the tail of the parotid gland. Malignant tumours of the submandibular gland involving the mandible are usually secondary metastatic nodes and should be recognized as such. A search for the primary tumour is necessary so that the tumour can be treated as a whole. Metastatic nodes attached to the mandible in this site will necessitate a partial mandibulectomy in order to obtain adequate removal.

Other conditions and operations

Ectopic salivary tumours
These tumours are rare and between 80 and 90% occur within the oral cavity, the commonest site being the hard palate. Some 60% are cylindromata, this being a designation referring to the unique histological pattern. These tumours are locally invasive and may also metastasise; they therefore carry a grave prognosis, although not so grave as that for squamous carcinoma in similar sites (Harrison, 1956). About 40% of ectopic salivary tumours are of the 'mixed' type similar in behaviour to those arising in the parotid gland.

Preliminary biopsy is advised in order to establish the diagnosis. The treatment of choice in cylindromata is radical diathermy excision, including a wide margin of healthy tissue, if this is practicable. In the case of palatal tumours an obturator will usually be required to occlude the defect produced by the excision. For surgically inaccessible tumours irradiation probably offers the best palliation. In the case of 'mixed' tumours, simple enucleation is usually adequate.

REFERENCES

Amin M, Maran A G D 1988 The aetiology of laryngocoele. Clinical Otolaryngology 13: 276–272

Barnes A D 1984 The changing face of parathyroid surgery. Annals of the Royal College of Surgeons of England 66: 77–80

Bremer J W, Neel H B, DeSanto L W, Jones G C 1986 Angiofibroma: treatment trends in 150 patients during 40 years. Laryngoscope 96: 1321–1329

Carlson G L, Farndon J R, Clayton B, Rose P G 1990 Thallium isotope scintigraphy and ultrasonography: comparative studies in localisation techniques in primary hyperparathyroidism. British Journal of Surgery 77: 327–329

Coleman J J, Searles J M, Hester R et al 1987 Ten years' experience with the free jejunal autograft. American Journal of Surgery 154: 394–398

Davis K R 1987 Embolisation of epistaxis and juvenile nasopharyngeal angiofibromas. American Journal of Roentgenology 148: 209–218

Feely J, Crooks J, Forrest A L, Hamilton W F, Gunn A 1981 Propranolol in the surgical treatment of hyperthyroidism including severely thyrotoxic patients. British Journal of Surgery 68: 865–869

Frankenthaler R A, Sellin R V, Cangir A, Goepfert H 1990 Lymph node metastasis from papillary-follicular thyroid carcinoma in young patients. American Journal of Surgery 160: 341–343

Halnan K E 1983 Leading article. British Medical Journal 287: 1821–1822

Hargreaves A W 1981 Surgical aspects of carcinoma of the thyroid gland. Annals of the Royal College of Surgeons of England 63: 322–324

Harrison D F N 1987 The natural history, pathogenesis and treatment of juvenile angiofibroma. Archives of Otolaryngology, Head and Neck Surgery 113: 936–942

Harrison K 1956 A study of ectopic mixed salivary tumours. Annals of the Royal College of Surgeons of England 18: 99

Hayek A, Chapman E M, Crawford J D 1970 Long-term results of treatment of thyrotoxicosis in children and adolescents with radioactive iodine. The New England Journal of Medicine 283: 949

Hobsley 1981 Surgery of the parotid salivary gland. Annals of the Royal College of Surgeons of England 63: 264–269

Holl-Allen R T J 1967 Haemorrhage following thyroidectomy for thyrotoxicosis. British Journal of Surgery 54: 703

Hsu F S F, Clark O H, Serata T Y, Nissenson R A 1983 Rapid localisation of parathyroid tumours by selective venous catheterisation and parathyroid hormone bioassay. Surgery 94: 873

Jacobson H G 1988 Magnetic resonance imaging of the head and neck region. Present status and future potential. Journal of the American Medical Association 260: 3313–3326

Jarhult J, Lindestad P-A, Nordenstrom J, Perbeck L 1991 Routine examination of the vocal cords before and after thyroid and parathyroid surgery. British Journal of Surgery 78: 1116–1117

Logemann J A, Bytell D E 1979 Swallowing disorders in three types of head and neck surgical patients. Cancer 44: 1095–1105

Maran A G D, Wilson J A, Al Muhanna A H 1986 Pharyngeal diverticula. Clinical Otolaryngology 11: 219–225

Maran A G D, Amin M, Wilson J A 1989 Radical neck dissection: a 19 year experience. Journal of Laryngology and Otology 103: 760–764

Marigold J H, Morgan A K, Earle D J, Young A E, Croft D N 1985 Lugol's iodine: its effect on thyroid blood flow in patients with thyrotoxicosis. British Journal of Surgery 72: 45–47

Milton C M, Thomas B M, Bickerton R C 1986 Morbidity study of submandibular gland excision. Annals of the Royal College of Surgeons of England 68: 148–157

Noguchi S, Murakami N, Noguchi A 1981 Surgical treatment for Graves' disease: A long-term follow up of 325 patients. British Journal of Surgery 68: 105–108

Patey D H, Ranger I 1957 Some points in the surgical anatomy of the parotid gland. British Journal of Surgery 45: 250

Roos D B 1982 The place of scalenectomy and first rib resection in thoracic outlet syndrome. Surgery 92: 1077

Serpell J W, Campbell P R, Young A E 1991 Preoperative localization of parathyroid tumours does not reduce operating time. British Journal of Surgery 78: 589–590

Sykes D 1981 Solitary thyroid nodule. British Journal of Surgery 68: 510–512

Ujiki G J, Pearl G J, Poticha S, Sisson G A, Shields T W 1987 Mortality and morbidity of gastric 'pull-up' for replacement of the pharyngoesophagus. Archives of Surgery 122: 644–647

Wade J S H 1983 The management of malignant thyroid tumours. British Journal of Surgery. 70: 253–258

Wang C A 1976 The anatomic basis of parathyroid surgery, Annals of Surgery 183: 271–275

Weingrad D N, Spiro R H 1983 Complications after laryngectomy. American Journal of Surgery 146: 517–520

Wheeler M H 1988 Investigation of the thyroid. Surgery 62: 1477–1479

Wilson J A, McIntyre M A, Haacke N P, Maran A G D 1987 Fine needle aspiration biopsy and the otolaryngologist. Journal of Laryngology and Otology 101: 595–600

Wilson J A 1991 Excision of the submandibular gland. Current Practice in Surgery 3: 34–37

Yawhan L, Gyi K M, Paw K, Brang L, Oo M, Myint H 1983 Propranolol in the surgical treatment of thyrotoxicosis. Journal of the Royal College of Surgeons of Edinburgh 28: 365–368

FURTHER READING

Edels Y 1983 Laryngectomy: diagnosis to rehabilitation. Croam Helm, London

Kleinsasser O 1988 Tumours of the larynx and hypopharynx. Thieme Verlag, Stuttgart

Tucker H M 1987 The larynx. Thieme Verlag, New York

Wright D 1987 Scott-Browns otolaryngology. Butterworths, London

13

Breast surgery

R. F. RINTOUL & A. C. H. WATSON

Anatomy

Extent

The breast lies embedded in the superficial fascia of the chest wall. It extends vertically between the 2nd and the 6th costal cartilages, and horizontally from the edge of the sternum nearly to the mid-axillary line. A process of the breast, known as the *axillary tail,* extends upwards and laterally along the lower border of pectoralis major into the axilla, where it reaches as high as the 3rd rib; this process, unlike the rest of the breast, lies below the deep fascia. The breast lies upon three muscles — pectoralis major, serratus anterior and external oblique, but is separated from these by deep fascia.

Structure

The secretory acini of the gland are embedded in a fairly dense fibrous stroma, and are grouped in *lobules.* Aggregations of lobules form the *lobes* of the breast (15–20 in number), which are arranged in a radiating manner. Each lobe is drained by a single duct, which is formed by coalescence of the ducts of the component lobules; these ducts converge to open on the summit of the nipple. There is no fascial capsule to the gland as a whole. The lobes are partly separated from each other by irregular and incomplete fibrous septa which are continuous with the gland stroma. Bands of fibrous tissue pass from the stroma both to the skin (ligaments of Cooper) and to the deep fascia. These fascial bands are accompanied by lymphatics which are of importance in the spread of carcinoma.

Blood supply

Arteries supplying the breast are the lateral thoracic (from the 2nd part of the axillary artery), perforating branches of the internal mammary artery, and lateral branches of the 2nd, 3rd and 4th intercostal arteries. The *veins,* which form a plexus beneath the areola drain mainly to the axillary and internal mammary veins.

Lymphatic vessels

The glandular acini are surrounded by plexuses of small lymphatic vessels. These communicate by vessels accompanying the ducts with the *subareolar plexus,* and also by vessels passing deeply with the plexus on the deep fascia underlying the breast. Cutaneous lymphatics draining the skin surface communicate directly with the subareolar plexus, and, by means of vessels accompanying the ligaments of Cooper, with the lymphatics of the gland stroma. From both superficial and deep plexuses channels pass to the regional lymph glands.

Axillary lymph glands

Lymph glands abound in the axilla, and they all directly or indirectly receive lymph from the breast. Their arrangement is irregular, but they may be divided arbitrarily into five chains or groups.

The *anterior chain* lies under cover of the pectoral muscles, forming the anterior wall of the axilla. The *posterior chain* lies on the posterior wall of the axilla alongside the subscapular vessels. The *lateral chain* lies along the upper part of the humerus on the medial side of the axillary vessels. Glands of the anterior chain (*pectoral nodes* — Level 1) are usually the first to become involved in breast cancer; they are in actual contact with the axillary tail of the gland and may become involved by direct infiltration. The posterior and lateral chains drain respectively the scapular region and the upper limb, but they have numerous connections with the anterior chain, and are potential sites of spread in carcinoma.

The *central group* of glands (Level 2) lies embedded in the fat in the central part of the axilla, and receives afferents from all three chains. The *apical group* (Level 3) is found at the extreme apex of the axilla, in the space between pectoralis minor and the clavicle, and is covered by the clavipectoral fascia. Afferents reach these glands from all three chains and from the central group. Some vessels come directly from the breast, so these glands may be the first to become involved in carcinoma. Afferents from the apical glands drain mainly to the blood stream at the origin of the innominate veins, but some pass to the supraclavicular glands.

Other associated lymph glands

The *supraclavicular glands* lie in the lower part of the posterior triangle, and belong to the lower group of deep cervical glands. They receive afferents from the apical glands, and also from the internal mammary glands.

The *internal mammary glands (anterior mediastinal or parasternal glands)* lie alongside the artery of the same name, one or two small glands being found deeply placed in each of the upper three or four intercostal spaces close to the sternum. They receive afferent vessels which originate in the lymphatic plexus of the deep fascia, and which pass deeply along the course of the perforating branches of the internal mammary artery. Their efferents pass mainly to the innominate vein, but communicate also with the cervical glands.

CARCINOMA OF THE BREAST

General considerations

Mode of spread of carcinoma

The long and widely held concept that breast carcinoma spreads in an orderly fashion from a recognisable primary tumour to lymphatics and hence to the blood stream is no longer acceptable. Many clinical trials and the observations of surgeons and radiotherapists over the past 25 years have led to the conclusion that, at the time of diagnosis, breast carcinoma is often a systemic disease with small non-detectable secondary growths (*micrometastases*) already present elsewhere in the body. Involved axillary lymph nodes need not necessarily be detected clinically and there may be no evidence of local lymphatic spread within the breast. Alternatively, there may be widespread changes in the vicinity of the primary growth without any distant metastases.

Spread of the tumour within the breast itself may be by direct infiltration or by permeation along the periacinar and periductal lymphatics. The involvement of surrounding structures — the skin or pectoral muscles — occurs either by direct extension of the growth, or by permeation along lymphatic channels. Such permeation occurs along the vessels which accompany the ligaments of Cooper towards the skin surface; contraction of these growth processes leads to fixation or actual dimpling of the overlying skin, and later to the development of cutaneous nodules. Permeation towards the pectoral fascia results in fixation of the tumour on its deep aspect. At any stage, extension to the regional lymph glands by embolism or by permeation may occur in an unpredictable fashion. This is mainly to the axilla but lymphatic spread occurs also to the internal mammary glands or to the peritoneal cavity, and both thoracic and abdominal organs may become involved.

Clinical staging

It is usually considered essential to have some clinical method of classifying the stage to which the disease has progressed in order to make comparisons between various methods of treatment and to judge the patient's progress. Such methods of classification are based upon clinical findings alone, although these may be assisted by radiological and other preoperative investigations. Findings obtained at operation or by histological examination are not included.

The most commonly used classification is that proposed by the International Union against Cancer in 1960 (Table 13.1) The Manchester Classification has four similar stages. The TNM system is based on clinical and radiological evidence related to tumour (T), regional lymph node (N) and distant metastases (M) (Table 13.2).

Unfortunately, experience has shown that individual patients do not pass from one stage to the next as their disease progresses although any method of staging suggests that this should be the case. In addition to the

Table 13.1   International Union against Cancer Classification

Stage I
Tumours less than 5 cm in greatest diameter. Skin fixation absent or incomplete. No fixation to underlying muscles. Axillary nodes not palpable.

Stage II
As for Stage I, but with palpable mobile nodes in the homolateral axilla.

Stage III
Tumours more than 5 cm in greatest diameter.
or skin fixation complete
or skin involvement wide of the tumour
or peau d'orange
or fixation to underlying muscles
or palpable and immobile nodes in axilla
or palpable supraclavicular nodes
or oedema of arm.

Stage IV
Distant metastases present, regardless of condition of primary tumour and regional lymph nodes.

Table 13.2   T N M Classification

T	Size of *T*umour (maximal diameter)	
	T1	2 cm or less
	T2	2 to 5 cm
	T3	Over 5 cm
	T4	Involving chest wall or skin
N	Lymph *N*ode status	
	N0	No metastases
	N1	Mobile involved nodes
	N2	Fixed involved nodes
M	Distant *M*etastases	
	M0	None
	M1	Distant metastases

unpredictable nature of the disease, there are considerable limitations in the methods of clinical assessment. Lymph nodes may be enlarged because of hyperplasia rather than tumour involvement and the presence of lymph nodes may be disputed even between experienced clinicians. Clinical examination also ignores possible spread to the internal mammary glands. Evidence for lymph node hyperplasia comes from histological examination of palpable nodes and from the regression of axillary lymph nodes in patients who, as part of a multicentre trial arranged by King's College Hospital, London (Edwards, 1972), had simple mastectomy without radiotherapy. It was suggested that regional lymph nodes played an important part in the patient's resistance to the tumour (Baum, 1973) and it is now accepted that host reaction, in the form of hyperplasia of regional lymph nodes, indicates a relatively favourable prognosis (Forrest, 1981).

In all methods of clinical staging the accuracy of the axillary examination is important. In particular, differentiation between Stages I and II depends upon the examiner's impressions regarding the presence of palpable axillary lymph nodes and McNair (1960) cast very grave doubts about the validity of any such assessment. Their conclusions have remained unchallenged for over 30 years. In a carefully devised study, five senior clinicians (surgeons and radiotherapists) were asked to examine the axillae of 10 patients whose breasts were concealed. In 6 of these the breasts were normal, and there was no reason for expecting the axillary glands to be enlarged; 3 of the remaining 4 suffered from breast carcinoma, and 1 from a breast abscess. Thus 100 axillary examinations (10 patients, 20 axillae, 5 examiners) were available for study. In the patients without breast pathology, positive findings were recorded in 48% of the examinations (20% by one examiner, 73% by another). In the patients with breast pathology, the findings were almost identical — again 48% of positive findings, and a range of 20–80% between the different examiners. These figures indicate that staging by clinical impressions of palpable axillary glands is both valueless and misleading.

Recent methods of investigation have not solved the difficulty in staging. While *mammography* is helpful in the early detection of a previously unsuspected cancer, *bone scanning,* using a radio-isotope, has resulted in early detection of skeletal metastases. *Magnetic resonance imaging* may detect unsuspected metastases but the low detection rate does not justify its use even in the high risk patient (Jones, 1990). Isotope bone scanning also lacks sensitivity and thus, patients initially considered to have an early tumour may, in fact, already be in Stage IV. The *biochemical 'marker'* CA15–3 — an abnormal serum protein — is proving of great value in the detection of metastatic bone

disease (O'Brien, 1992) so that use of isotope bone scanning can be restricted to patients with a persistently elevated level following primary surgery.

Prognostic factors
One of the major advances in breast cancer during the last two decades has been the realisation that some tumours, when grown in tissue culture, will take up the hormone oestradiol. The test, available in specialised centres, estimates the oestrogen receptor (ER) status of the patient and hence the likelihood of any residual tumour to respond to hormone manipulation (Hawkins, 1980). However, many tumours have a mixed cell population, hence the estimation of the number of receptor sites (measured as concentration) does not take into account the number of tumour cells which are *not* hormone dependent. In general, ER positive tumours have a better prognosis than those which are ER negative (Forrest, 1981) but the mixed cell population detracts from the reliability of the test as an indication of hormone responsiveness. The histological state of the axillary lymph nodes is, at present, the best indicator of likely metastatic spread (Forrest, 1979; Baum, 1980) and hence an indicator of prognosis. Hyperplasia of the regional nodes is favourable whereas the involvement of lymph glands by growth indicates an increasing risk of tumour recurrence as the number of affected glands increases. Assessment by isotope scans of liver and bone, CT brain scans and biochemical tests did not contribute further to the definition of those with a bad prognosis in almost 200 patients attending the Edinburgh clinic of Forrest (1979) over a 4 year period.

Choice of treatment
The apparently unending controversy as to the best treatment of breast cancer — and the widely varying procedures adopted in different clinics — takes on a new perspective when it is appreciated that the value of surgery to the breast area is limited to local control of the disease. In the 1930s the standard treatment was the classical radical operation of Halsted which included careful clearance of the axilla. This operation was subsequently extended by Dahl-Iversen (1963) to include removal of the parasternal and supraclavicular lymph nodes but the results did not show any advantage over more conservative procedures. During the past 25 years, there has been a trend away from the radical forms of mastectomy. The removal *en bloc* of internal mammary nodes has been practised in America although there has been no evidence of improved clinical outcome (Haagensen, 1986). No longer does radical surgery entail removal of all pectoralis muscle (Hayward, 1980) and studies have shown that radical surgery is not required if radical radiotherapy follows simple surgery (Forrest, 1980). In fact, some surgeons

are content to carry out wide tumour excision and to follow this with radiotherapy (Barr, 1989). To a large extent, radiotherapy offers the same prospect of disease control as excisional surgery with the additional benefit that irradiation can reach the parasternal and supraclavicular nodes with less morbidity than surgery. The move away from radical surgery towards conservative surgery has been accompanied by systemic adjuvant therapy (p. 326), and it is anticipated that indicators of an individual patient's prognosis will allow this to be used selectively.

It is difficult, therefore, to lay down any firm principles for guidance in the treatment of breast carcinoma, but the following method of correlating the treatment with the clinical stage of the disease has found fairly general acceptance, and may be taken as representing the majority view at the present time. To a large extent, the treatment of breast cancer is a highly individual matter (Burn, 1980) and it is important that treatment should be *for the patient* rather than *of the disease*.

In Stage I and II cases, complete removal of breast tissue — total mastectomy — is advisable in the great majority of patients, together with exploration of the axilla. The extent of axillary dissection depends on the surgeon's preference and may involve simple excision of a pectoral node for histological examination or complete clearance of the axillary contents in the form of a modified radical mastectomy. In the more conservative surgical approach, the state of the axillary glands is assessed during the operation and a decision to refer the patient for radiotherapy is reinforced in the light of histological evidence of involved axillary nodes. In addition, some surgeons chose to obtain lymph glands from the internal mammary chain for histological examination so as to help in determining the prognosis of the disease.

In Stage III cases, total mastectomy is advised provided that this will result in complete removal of the breast tumour (and involved underlying muscles) and allow for adequate skin closure. The extent of axillary dissection will depend more on the disease than the surgeon's preference and the operation will most likely be followed by radiotherapy if the excision has been inadequate. In the *more extensive Stage III case*, irradiation may precede surgery, the aim being to prevent fungation of the tumour and provide local control of the disease.

In Stage IV cases, treatment can be no more than palliative. Mastectomy may be advised in order to deal with or to prevent fungation. Radiotherapy is often effective in relieving the pain of isolated metastases in bone or, when there is fungation of the growth, radiotherapy may reduce the offensive discharge and allow the ulcer to heal. Pleural effusions are dealt with by aspiration. Progress of the disease may be controlled by hormone therapy, by ovarian ablation, by the administration of antimitotic drugs, or by a combination of these methods.

Adjuvant therapy. In the management of 'early' breast cancer, the survival rates and disease-free interval can be improved by the use of cytotoxic or anti-oestrogenic drugs *at the time of the initial surgery.* Chemotherapy is of value in the pre-menopausal patient with axillary node involvement and routine *Tamoxifen* should be prescribed for both pre- and post-menopausal patients (Baum, 1992). The basis for this treatment lies in the fact that micrometastases may be undetected and are likely to be destroyed by chemotherapy or controlled by an anti-oestrogenic drug. Recent evidence suggests that adjuvant chemotherapy in early breast cancer may also protect against the development of new primary tumours in the first 10 years of follow-up (Arriagada,1991). The choice of drugs is largely dependent on the surgeon's desire to minimise side effects while effectively acting on residual tumour cells. The optimum duration of *Tamoxifen* therapy has not yet been determined but should be for a minimum of two years (Preece, 1991).

Diagnosis of malignancy

It is often impossible to differentiate with certainty on clinical evidence between a simple swelling and an early malignant one. A period of observation is then unjustifiable, since the delay in treatment may allow the disease to spread. Investigation by mammography — sometimes with the addition of ultrasound (Warwick, 1988) — and fine-needle aspiration cytology are essential investigations before proceeding with excision biopsy.

Needle puncture is of value in solitary swellings thought to be cystic when aspiration of fluid confirms the diagnosis. Cytological examination of the aspirate for malignant cells is helpful but not essential since refilling of a cyst which has been evacuated, or persistence of a lump following aspiration, will alert the surgeon to the need for biopsy.

Fine-needle aspiration biopsy. This term (FNA) implies the microscopic examination of cellular material removed from a solid lump through an aspirating needle — possibly under mammographic guidance to assure accurate sampling (Masood, 1990). Its value depends on the availability of a skilled cytologist to interpret films made and stained at the time of aspiration.

Needle biopsy. A core of tissue can be removed with a Tru-cut needle under local anaesthetic but the accuracy is less than 75% (Owen, 1980). Unfortunately, needle biopsy is of least value in the small doubtful tumour where it may be impossible to obtain representative tissue for the histologist. The use of ultrasonic guidance, where available, allows the radiologist to place the needle with more accuracy and obtain a worthwhile sample.

Localization biopsy. Mammographic screening — the radiological examination of the breasts of symptomless women — allows for the detection of small impalpable areas of disease within the breast. Since the absence of malignancy cannot be ascertained without histological examination, a method of localizing the abnormality has been devised for the guidance of surgeons. Under mammographic control, a hollow needle is placed within the lesion which is to be excised. Through the needle a fine wire, incorporating a 'hook', is placed at the needle tip and brought out through the overlying skin by removing the hollow needle (Chaudary, 1990; Aitken, 1991). Alternatively, a coloured dye is injected through the needle which is then withdrawn. Following the later method, the surgeon excises the breast tissue marked by the dye and submits it to histological examination. Where the wire method has been used, the relevant tissue is excised without displacing the wire. The tissue, including the wire, is then X-rayed to check that the area of abnormality detected on mammography has been satisfactorily marked and excised — 'specimen radiology'. In cases where the accuracy of the excision is in doubt, the specimen is marked with ligaclips to allow for orientation in relation to the remaining breast. If necessary, further tissue can then be excised from the appropriate area (Nedelman, 1992).

Excision biopsy for histological examination (paraffin sections) may be the only method of confirming malignancy and has the advantage of minimizing the delay before reaching a diagnosis. Some patients prefer this approach particularly where wide excision may be the definitive surgery. It is important that the skin incision for *any* excision biopsy should lie *within* the ellipse required for mastectomy, should this later become necessary, so that the mastectomy incision does not encroach on the biopsy site. In the event of mastectomy being required after excision biopsy, the patient is fully aware of the diagnosis and of the surgery to which she has agreed. There is no evidence that the delay between the two operations affects the eventual outcome.

Diagnostic incision. To make an incision directly into the substance of the swelling, and to reach a diagnosis from the character of its cut surface is an entirely rational procedure. Occasionally an experienced surgeon may be required to use this method unless a pathologist skilled in frozen section histology is available. On section with the knife a carcinoma feels hard and gritty 'like an unripe pear'. Its cut surface is seen to merge imperceptibly into the surrounding fat; it has a striated appearance, and becomes concave owing to retraction of fibrous tissue. An area of fibrocystic dysplasia, or a fibroadenoma, has a more rubbery consistence and becomes convex on section; the former may show areas of cystic formation, while the latter is clearly encapsulated. Small swellings should be completely excised with a good margin of healthy breast tissue, before being cut into. In the case of large swellings, it is better to make an incision through the overlying skin, and to deepen it so as to cut directly into the centre of the tumour in situ. (If excision is carried out, a large cavity is left and may well contain cancer cells; this cavity may be opened and the cells dispersed over the wound, if the local excision is followed by mastectomy.) Should the naked-eye appearance and frozen section — if available — indicate malignancy, the exploratory wound is closed and, after gloves and towels have been changed, the appropriate elective treatment is at once carried out. This approach assumes that the patient would prefer to have mastectomy rather than wide excision should malignancy be confirmed. The use of diagnostic incision is now rarely required in view of the available alternatives.

Operative staging

During mastectomy for breast carcinoma, the axillary content can be more accurately examined than was possible before the operation (Table 13.3) and nodes are removed for histological examination. Unless the surgeon is confident that he has cleared all nodes from the axilla, the finding of involved glands will necessitate radiotherapy. Thus, the patient may be put in operative *stage A* if local surgery is all that is required, *stage B* if local surgery must be supplemented by radiotherapy because of massive local tumour or positive nodes (indicating high risk malignancy), or *stage C* where treatment is of a general and palliative nature for widespread disease.

Table 13.3   Levels of axillary glands

Level 1	Low axilla — lateral to lateral border of pectoralis major
Level 2	Mid axilla — around pectoralis minor muscle
Level 3	Apical — adjacent to axillary vein

Local excision and 'quandrantectomy'

The ideal treatment for breast cancer is to have breast conservation and cure of the disease. Local excision of a tumour, with a clear margin of uninvolved breast tissue, is now acceptable for the *younger patient* provided the operation is followed by radiotherapy. Spitalier (1986) has reported a 25 year experience of this method for operable carcinoma. Wide local excision is also suitable for the *elderly patient* in order to minimise her stay in hospital and avoid the risk of poor wound healing which follows more extensive surgery. Radiotherapy is not usually necessary in the elderly but *Tamoxifen* should be given as a routine. In fact, many elderly patients can benefit from *Tamoxifen alone*, surgery being reserved for those tumours which are unresponsive (Bates, 1991).

In addition to the patient's consent, wide local excision requires a single focus of tumour — as determined clinically or mammographically — plus a situation where an adequately shaped residual breast can be constructed. '*Quandrantectomy*' implies excision of the whole of the involved duct system with a clearance of at least 2 cm and is thus only applicable to a small tumour.

Simple (total) mastectomy and axillary sampling

Treatment of the primary disease is important for adequate local control and for staging of carcinoma. Removal of the breast as a whole may also be advised when the gland is the seat of a simple tumour of large size, such as an intracanalicular fibroadenoma, or of widespread fibrocystic disease. It is the operation of choice in Paget's disease of the nipple (Dixon, 1991) and in multiple duct papillomas where the site of the tumour cannot be determined and where the risk of undetected malignancy exists. When it is performed in the treatment of carcinoma, and is to be followed by radiotherapy, the following points in the technique are important:

1. Iodine should not be used for preparation of the skin, nor should adhesive strapping be applied postoperatively, since any irritation produced lowers the skin tolerance to irradiation.

2. While the skin of the nipple and areola and that overlying the tumour must be excised, the total amount of skin removed should be as limited as possible. Tightly stretched skin, and areas which have healed by granulation or grafting do not tolerate irradiation well. If such conditions are present, the dosage may require to be reduced.

3. In order that the irradiation may be concentrated on as small an area as possible, undermining of skin flaps and opening-up of tissue planes around the breast are reduced to a minimum.

4. The pectoral fascia, unless the growth is adherent to it, should not be removed. Retention of the fascia lessens the risk of post-irradiation fibrosis in the muscles, and allows the maximum dose of therapy to be employed.

5. Drainage, if not of the 'vacuum' type (p. 345), should be carried out through one end of the main wound, rather than through a stab-wound placed below it. In this way the operative field and the area consequently requiring irradiation, are more confined.

6. In Stage III cases, where the tumour is fixed to the pectoral muscle, part of the muscle should be removed along with the breast.

Technique of operation

During the operation the arm is placed on a rest or is supported by an assistant in the abducted position. It is an advantage to have the head of the table elevated 15–30 degrees to reduce venous congestion.

Incision. In the incision generally employed the central part is made in the form of an ellipse, which includes both the nipple and the skin overlying the tumour. The axis of the ellipse depends, therefore, on the relationship of the tumour to the nipple. Whenever possible, the axis of the ellipse should be transverse so that no part of the scar is visible above normal clothing (Fig. 13.1). The extent of the ellipse will vary with the size of the breast. The skin flaps should be just adequate for covering the chest wall after the gland has been removed. Any upper extension of the incision should not lie too close to the margin of the axillary fold, or a 'bridle' scar may result.

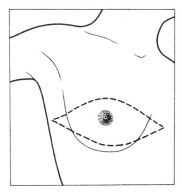

Fig. 13.1   Transverse incision for simple (total) mastectomy

Excision. The skin is raised from the breast substance and is reflected back on each side. There is no clear plane between skin and breast, but prior infiltration of a 1 in 300 000 adrenalin solution serves as a guide during dissection and also diminishes blood loss. The thickness of the skin flaps is increased as the dissection progresses. It is usually desirable that the entire breast (and not only the visible protuberant part) should be removed. For this the flaps must be reflected sufficiently to expose the full anatomical extent of the gland and the axillary tail (Fig. 13.2). When these limits have been defined, the breast is freed by sharp dissection from the underlying pectoral fascia starting just below the clavicle. Bleeding occurs from perforating branches of the internal mammary and intercostal arteries. Most of these vessels require ligature or diathermy coagulation, since haemostasis must be as complete as possible. When the breast has been freed from the anterior surface of the pectoralis major muscle, the axillary tail can be clearly defined and traced upwards to allow

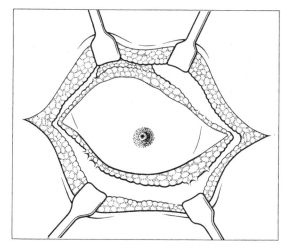

Fig. 13.2 The breast about to be dissected off the pectoral fascia and the axillary tail defined

lymph gland sampling — *level 1 dissection* — and full examination of the axilla. Branches of the lateral thoracic vessels require to be secured as axillary contents are freed and removed along with the breast. (It is helpful to mark this area of the specimen with a suture so as to assist the pathologist in his search for lymph nodes.) Removal of a piece of tumour for oestrogen receptor assay can now be done before the excised breast is sent to the pathologist. The skin wound is sutured, drainage being provided by a small strip of plastic or by two Redivac tubes (Fig. 13.3).

Modified radical mastectomy

Objectives
This operation, pioneered by Patey (Handley, 1975), is used by many surgeons for primary treatment of breast cancer as an alternative to postoperative radiotherapy for involved axillary glands. It can also be used in clin-

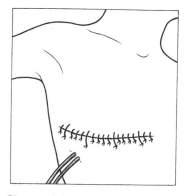

Fig. 13.3 Closure of the wound. It is preferable to use a subcuticular suture

ics where adequate radiotherapy is not available. The pectoralis major is widely retracted and the pectoralis minor removed. This gives adequate exposure for a *level 3 axillary dissection* so as to allow the lymph glands to be cleared as completely as in the Halsted operation. Its main advantage over radical mastectomy is cosmetic, in that the axillary fold is maintained and there is no hollowing below the clavicle. It also gives a stronger and more useful arm.

Technique
The incision employed is an elliptical one as for simple (total) mastectomy (Fig. 13.4). The breast, together with the deep fascia, is dissected laterally off the pectoralis major (Figs 13.5 & 13.6). This muscle is now made to relax by an assistant raising the arm so that the elbow points towards the ceiling; its lower margin is cleared, and a retractor is placed against its deep surface. When this is drawn forwards, it enables the dissection to be carried upwards in the plane between the two pectoral muscles. Pectoralis minor and the clavipectoral fascia are now exposed. This muscle is divided at its insertion and is reflected medially; a branch of the thoraco-acromial artery and the lateral thoracic artery, which run respectively along its upper and lower borders, require to be secured. The pectoralis minor can then be drawn downwards and erased from its costal origin. The axilla is now uncovered, and the dissection of its contents can be commenced. The fascial sheath of the axillary vessels is incised from the clavicle to the lower border of latissimus dorsi. The lower leaf of this fascia, and all fatty and glandular structures which lie below and medial to the vein, are stripped downwards by gauze dissection, i.e. by using the finger covered with several thicknesses of gauze. The apical glands, which lie in the fat at the medial side of the axillary vein just below the clavicle, are removed in this way, as also are the lateral chain of glands which are medial to the vein at a lower level (Fig. 13.7). The stripping process is continued downwards until the muscles of the posterior axillary wall (subscapularis, teres major and latissimus dorsi), and the serratus anterior (forming the medial wall) are completely cleared of all fascial, fatty and glandular tissue. In this part of the dissection, the nerve to latissimus dorsi on the posterior wall, and the nerve to serratus anterior on the medial wall, are identified and carefully preserved. The upper branches of the axillary artery and their companion veins are usually sacrificed; the subscapular vessels are preserved only if the surrounding fatty tissue which harbours the posterior chain of glands can be cleared without difficulty. The intercostobrachial nerve is divided as it emerges from the second rib space.

Figs 13.4–13.7 *Modified radical mastectomy*

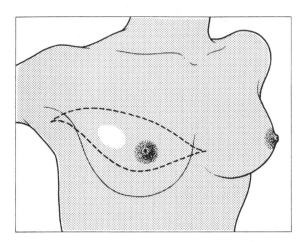

Fig. 13.4   Elliptical incision including nipple and skin overlying the tumour

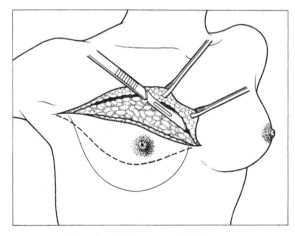

Fig. 13.5   Dissection of the upper skin flap

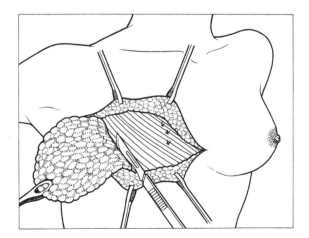

Fig. 13.6   The breast is dissected laterally off the pectoralis major

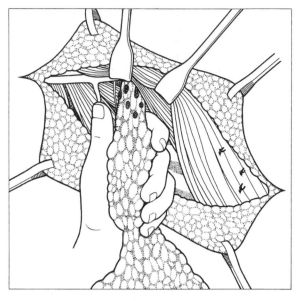

Fig. 13.7   Mobilization of apical glands and axillary tail using the breast for traction. It is not always necessary to sacrifice the pectoralis minor muscle as in this case

Radical mastectomy (Fig. 13.8)

The classical operation of radical mastectomy (Halsted) was designed to remove the breast containing a tumour and the entire system of lymphatic glands *en bloc* which involved sacrifice of at least part of pectoralis major and the whole of pectoralis minor muscles in addition to other structures. The assumption that such a radical procedure would remove all possible tumour cells is no longer accepted and it has no advantages over the other procedures already described.

Hormone manipulation for progressive disease. In spite of intensive research over many years, no reliable

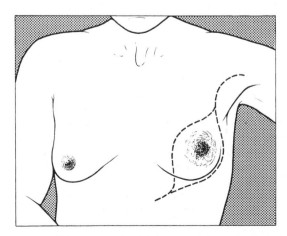

Fig. 13.8   The extent of incision required for radical mastectomy

method of determining which patients are most likely to respond to endocrine therapy has yet been established but measurement of the ER (oestrogen receptor) content of breast tumour tissue provides some indication of response. The collected results of studies throughout the world provide clear evidence that receptor analysis is of value in the management of advanced disease (Griffiths, 1981). More than 94% of all patients with ER negative tumours failed to respond to endocrine therapy whereas more than half of those with ER positive tumours responded. The most striking effects are relief of pain, improvement in nutrition, and regression of local lesions. Thus, osteolytic lesions may calcify and pathological fractures heal. The effects, however, are only temporary, since, after a varying interval, the tumour cells lose their hormone dependence, and thereafter the disease progresses rapidly. No claims for permanent cure have been recorded, nor are they at present anticipated although remission may last for several years in some cases.

In pre-menopausal patients, whose tumours are ER positive, removal of the ovaries will frequently delay progress of the disease, and such patients may be advised to submit to oophorectomy at the first sign of recurrence. Ovarian irradiation is an alternative to this operation and success is now reported (Dixon, 1990) with the LH/RH agonist goserelin (Zoladex). Remission of the disease following these procedures implies that the tumour is sensitive to hormone deprivation but failure of response suggests that further endocrine therapy is unlikely to be rewarding.

In post-menopausal patients, the anti-oestrogen drug *Tamoxifen* is of proven value. It binds to the oestrogen receptor in tumour cells but has very little oestrogenic activity and very low toxicity. Use of the drug gives rise to good objective remission in about 30–40% of patients with metastatic breast cancer. When used in premenopausal patients — where it is equally effective — amenorrhoea may result and appropriate advice should be offered regarding the avoidance of pregnancy. *Aminoglutethimide,* an agent which inhibits steroid (especially oestrogen) synthesis by the adrenal and other tissues, will give rise to similar objective remissions in post-menopausal women with acceptable toxicity.

Adrenalectomy and hypophysectomy were introduced about 1953 as a method of obtaining hormone deprivation but their value has been superseded by the use of anti-oestrogen drugs since oestrogens can still be detected in the serum after adrenalectomy but not after *Tamoxifen.* Both operations are major procedures, associated with a considerable mortality and morbidity, and are no longer required for breast cancer.

Combination cytotoxic chemotherapy. The use of three or more potent drugs, aimed at reducing the bulk of tumour tissue, is used for the patient with recurrent breast cancer who is unresponsive to endocrine manipulation or whose tumour is ER negative. A number of drug regimes have been devised, mainly in the form of intermittent or 'pulsed' doses involving one intravenous injection each 2–4 weeks. Although many useful remissions have been obtained, the result is, at best, temporary and side effects may be unpleasant.

BENIGN BREAST DISEASE

It is now realised that many breast lumps are not pathological but simply reflect variations (or aberrations) in the normal pattern of cyclical development and involution of breast tissue. The descriptive term 'aberrations of normal development and involution' (ANDI) includes many conditions which were previously considered as pathological. This classification allows the younger patient to be reassured that a fibroadenoma, for example, in non-pathological and that surgery can be safely avoided. Many patients, however, prefer to be reassured by removal of their lump and insist on an operation. In these circumstances, it is important to realise that normal tissue immediately adjacent to the healed biopsy site may later take on the characteristics of a new lump (Hughes, 1989) and add to the patient's anxiety.

Many simple lesions of the breast which are causing pain or anxiety are dealt with adequately by local excision. This is carried out usually through an incision over the swelling, and in a line radiating from the nipple, because of the supposed risk of dividing the lactiferous ducts. Some surgeons prefer to place their incisions transversely to the radial line, pointing out that no harm results from possible division of the ducts, and that the cosmetic result is much better. A much more important consideration, however, is that the incision should be *within the ellipse* required for subsequent mastectomy should this unexpectedly become necessary.

Breast cysts
Many isolated breast swellings, which do not at first appear to be cystic, prove to contain fluid when aspiration is attempted. This should be the initial form of investigation of an isolated breast lump and allows for FNA (see page 326) if the lump is solid. Repeated aspiration of breast cysts is a safe procedure provided that the lump disappears completely.

Fibrocystic disease
Operation is indicated when discomfort or anxiety persist after reassurance, or when malignancy cannot absolutely be excluded. A cyst or a localised area of fibroadenosis is too adherent to be shelled out like a fibroadenoma; as a rule it should be removed along

with surrounding normal tissue. Haematoma formation should be avoided by reconstruction of the breast tissue by sutures, or by suction drainage for 24–48 hours.

Fibroadenoma

This 'tumour', which is usually small and encapsulated, can be enucleated without injury to the surrounding breast tissue. To enable this to be done, the incision must be carried through the capsule. It is impossible to enucleate cleanly round the capsule, since this is firmly attached to the fibrous stroma of the gland. With a giant fibroadenoma occupying the greater part of the breast, simple mastectomy may be the best procedure.

Duct papilloma

This condition, which is situated usually in one of the larger ducts deep to the areola, should be suspected when there is serous or sanguineous discharge from the nipple. Multiple duct papillomas — usually situated peripherally — may become malignant but a solitary intraduct papilloma is not usually considered to be premalignant. The tumour may be felt beneath the areola, or its presence may be determined at a point where local pressure produces the discharge. When its site can be identified, local excision is the treatment of choice in all cases. At operation the dilated duct is located by introducing the blunt end of a fine straight needle, which should then pass into the cavity containing the papilloma (Fig. 13.9). The affected duct system is now excised through an incision extending around the margin of the areola, while the needle is held in position (Atkins, 1964). The excised tissue is submitted to histological examination so that mastectomy can be performed if malignant change is detected.

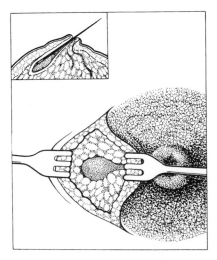

Fig. 13.9 Local excision of a duct papilloma. Inset shows needle in duct used as a guide to the location of the tumour

Gaillard Thomas's method

This method is advised in young women who desire an inconspicuous scar. It is also used in young men who request excision of gynaecomastia involving the whole breast tissue. (Gynaecomastia underlying the nipple is removed through a circumareolar incision). An incision is made round the circumference of the inferolateral quadrant of the breast following the submammary sulcus. The deep surface of the gland is freed by dissection from the pectoral fascia, and the breast as a whole is turned upwards (Fig. 13.10). The tumour is then identified, and dealt with from the deep aspect, after which the breast is allowed to fall back and the incision is sutured. Drainage for 24 hours should always be employed.

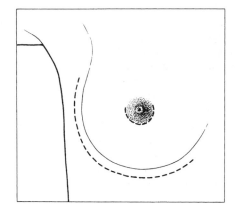

Fig. 13.10 The Gaillard Thomas approach for the removal of simple lesions of the breast. Para-areolar incision for a localised excision is also shown

The approach described is applicable to tumours in any part of the breast, and not, as is frequently stated, only to those in the lower half. Indeed, the method is perhaps most useful in the case of tumours in the superomedial quadrant, where the scar of a direct approach might be visible during the wearing of evening dress. There is no difficulty in throwing up the mamma sufficiently for the necessary access to be obtained.

BREAST ABSCESS

Acute inflammation of the breast (acute mastitis) occurs during lactation, the infection entering through a crack in the nipple or it may occur without obvious explanation. A broad spectrum antibiotic is advisable at the stage of cellulitis since the causative staphylococcus is liable to be resistant to penicillin, but the formation of pus must be anticipated. Unless the inflammation settles quickly, drainage of pus should be considered so as to avoid tissue necrosis due to local pressure. Abscess in the non-lactational breast is due to mammary duct ectasia and mainly occurs in the periareolar region. In many cases, repeated aspiration is sufficient and avoids the need for prolonged dressing which follows open drainage (Dixon, 1992).

In patients with inflammation involving a major part of the breast, operation should not be delayed until there is fluctuation, for this sign will be elicited only when the abscess has become superficial, and by that time the breast may have suffered irreparable damage. If, after two or three days of antibiotic therapy, tenderness, induration or other signs of inflammation show no signs of subsiding, it is almost certain that deep-seated pus is present, and the surgeon should proceed to an operation for drainage.

Technique

The incision, which should lie over the area of maximum tenderness, may be placed radially or transversely according to preference. When pus is encountered the gloved finger is introduced and the abscess cavity is explored. This is usually partially loculated from the presence of permeated and softened fibrous septa. Such septa, which are nonresistant to the finger, are gently broken down so that the loculi communicate freely. Any loculus which cannot be laid open in this way must be drained by a separate incision. If the abscess appears to be pre-mammary, i.e. situated in the subcutaneous tissue, a communicating loculus within the breast substance should be sought.

If the abscess cavity extends deeply into the gland, counterdrainage or dependent drainage is advisable. A pair of forceps is introduced into the cavity, and is gently pushed towards the nearest point on the periphery of the breast (Fig. 13.11). The second incision is

made by cutting down on the point of the forceps. A strip of corrugated plastic is then passed between the two openings (Fig. 13.12). Alternatively, if drainage through the second incision is considered to be adequate, the primary incision may be sutured.

Retromammary abscess occurs in the cellular tissue between the breast and the deep fascia. The gland itself is usually not involved but is pushed forward by the swelling. An incision is made along the submammary sulcus, and sinus forceps are introduced. After pus has been evacuated, a search is made for any intramammary prolongation of the abscess, or for a focus of infection in the sternum or ribs. Such abscesses may be tuberculous, in which case the skin incision should be closed, and appropriate chemotherapy instituted.

Chronic subareolar suppuration

Such suppuration occurs most commonly in one or more of the major ducts (Fig. 13.13) and is likely to result from blockage of the duct orifice by inspissated secretion, or from involutionary changes leading to chronic dilatation (*duct ectasia*). It may be the cause of persistent or intermittent discharge from the nipple; alternatively, by pointing on the skin of the para-areolar region, it may give rise to a *mammillary duct fistula*.

Operations for drainage, or local excision of the affected duct, are apt to be unsatisfactory, and Thomas (1982) advises excision of the nipple and major ducts as an alternative. In the presence of a fistula, excision of the fistula must be combined with excision of the involved duct or total duct excision under antibiotic cover (Dixon, 1991).

Hadfield's (1969) operation aims to excise the entire major duct system, while preserving the nipple, with little or no reduction in the size of the breast.

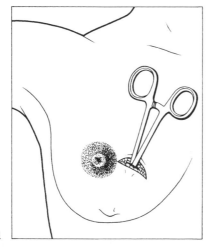 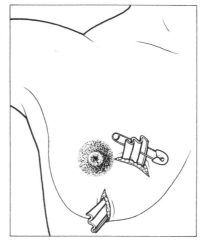

Fig. 13.11   **Fig. 13.12**

Figs 13.11 & 13.12   Method of draining a breast abscess

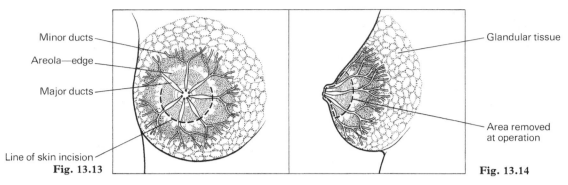

Minor ducts

Areola—edge

Major ducts

Line of skin incision

Fig. 13.13

Glandular tissue

Area removed
at operation

Fig. 13.14

Figs 13.13 & 13.14   Schematic drawings to show the anatomy of the major lactiferous ducts of the breast, and the extent of an operation for their removal (After Hadfield)

Technique of excision of major duct system

An incision is made along the lower half of the areolar margin, and any sinus present is excised. The areolar flap is reflected upwards from the underlying breast tissue, the lactiferous ducts being divided as they enter the nipple. The block of tissue containing the major ducts can then be excised as a roughly conical mass, with long axis of 2.5–4 cm and with a base (lying deeply) of approximately the same diameter as that of the areola (Fig. 13.14). Any obvious ducts entering the mass are closed by ligature or by diathermic coagulation as they are divided, and the cavity in the breast substance is obliterated by deep sutures. The nipple, if previously indrawn, is everted by a purse-string suture applied round the deep surface of its base. The areolar flap is then sutured back in position. The breast is kept well supported by strapping or by a firm brassiere during healing of the wound.

According to Hadfield, future pregnancies cause no undue disturbance in a breast which has been subjected to this operation — except possibly for a little local tenderness if the pregnancy occurs within 12 months of surgery.

PLASTIC OPERATIONS ON THE BREAST

Inverted nipples

Correction of indrawn nipples is often requested in order to permit breast feeding; occasionally it may be sought on aesthetic grounds or because of recurrent infection. Operations that do not divide the shortened ducts beneath the nipple frequently fail, and division of the ducts obviously makes breast feeding impossible. The wise surgeon is therefore very cautious before offering to operate for this indication. If the patient accepts that she will not be able to breast feed, then the ducts can be divided, freeing the nipple and allowing it to be pulled out. The resulting defect deep to the nipple is closed by advancing adjacent breast tissue. The ducts can be approached through a periareolar incision or by splitting the nipple (Morris, 1980).

Reconstruction of pendulous and hypertrophic breasts

Operation may afford great relief to patients who suffer physically from excessively heavy breasts, or who are socially or economically embarrassed by their condition.

Meticulous planning of the operation is essential. Detailed measurements must be taken in order that smoothly contoured and symmetrical breasts may be obtained, and special precautions are necessary to ensure that the blood supply to the nipple and skin flaps is preserved. The operation, therefore, is one of some magnitude and should not normally be undertaken by those without special training or experience in plastic surgery. The patient must be made aware, before committing herself to an operation, that there will be significant scarring, possible loss of sensation to nipples or breasts, possible delayed healing and, at worst, loss of part or all of the nipple. Symmetry cannot be guaranteed.

Operation

A number of different operations have been described. Of these, the following two have proved satisfactory:

1. The nipple may be transplanted at the apex of a pedicle of breast tissue. This is cut in such a way that the nipple remains attached to its lactiferous ducts and its blood supply is maintained.

2. When the breasts are very large, the nipple and areola may be more safely transplanted as a free graft. No attempt is made to conserve the function of the breast, and the operation is indicated therefore in women who are approaching the menopause, or who have very pendulous (and probably functionless) breasts.

Firstly, the nipple and areola are excised in the manner employed for raising a free full-thickness skin graft (p. 13). A large wedge of the lower part of the breast is amputated and the remainder is trimmed suitably and sutured to form a new prominence. Finally, the nipple and areola are grafted on to a circular bed prepared in the appropriate position.

In the inferior pedicle technique (Robbins, 1977) the skin overlying a wedge of the lower half of the breast is de-epithelialised, bearing the nipple at its apex. Breast tissue and excess skin is then excised from medially, laterally and above the nipple, according to the pre-operative planning, and the nipple sutured into its new position at a higher level. Medial and lateral flaps of skin and breast tissue are then sutured over the de-epithelialised pedicle, giving a scar which runs from the nipple vertically down to the submammary crease, where it joins a long scar running in the crease.

Reconstruction following mastectomy

Immediate reconstruction is carried out in some clinics where the patient has available the combined skills of a cancer specialist and a plastic surgeon. Most *general* surgeons will select, for secondary referral to the plastic surgeon, patients who particularly request the operation and who have survived at least two years since mastectomy. The objectives of re-construction are volume replacement, maintenance of a cleavage between the breasts, absence of scars visible with normal clothing and unrestricted arm mobility.

Most techniques involve the insertion of a *silicone prosthesis*. Extra skin can be gained, either by tissue expansion in a plane deep to the pectoralis major and serratus anterior muscles, or by the use of a flap. A *latissimus dorsi musculo-cutaneous flap* uses skin overlying this muscle to replace the skin deficiency following mastectomy, and the muscle itself to cover and protect the implant. The flap is based on the thoracodorsal artery, which must be carefully preserved at the time of mastectomy if reconstruction is considered a possibility.

The results of reconstruction using silicone implants are often compromised by capsular contracture around the prostheses, and recent questions raised about the safety of implanted silicone have increased the indication for reconstructive techniques which avoid the use of implants. They involve more major operations and have hitherto been held in reserve by most reconstructive surgeons for use if simpler methods have failed. The best of these techniques is the *Transverse Rectus Abdominis Musculocutaneous (TRAM) flap*. A transverse ellipse of skin and fat is raised from the lower abdomen, pedicled on branches from the superior epigastric vessels which run in relation to the rectus abdominis muscle. The muscle on the opposite side from the mastectomy is usually used for the pedicle, and the part of the flap further from the pedicle must be discarded, as its blood supply is tenuous. The flap is transposed through a tunnel to the breast site where it is folded, trimmed and de-epithelialized appropriately to form a breast mound.

Loss of rectus muscle and anterior rectus sheath can cause weakness in the lower abdominal wall. This can usually be prevented by preserving a strip of sheath and innervated muscle and repairing the defect, but sometimes reinforcement with a synthetic patch of, e.g. *Goretex* is advisable.

The viability of the distal part of the pedicled TRAM flap can be uncertain, and vascularity can be improved by microvascular suturing of the divided inferior epigastric vessels (which are considerably larger than the superior epigastrics) to vessels in the axilla. This can be done to augment the superior pedicle or to replace it. In the latter case — the *Free TRAM Flap* — the greater part of the rectus muscle can be preserved in its place. This is becoming the technique of choice where facilities are available, but it is a time-consuming and expensive procedure.

REFERENCES

Aitken R J, Chetty U 1991 Non-palpable mammographic abnormalities. Journal of the Royal College of Surgeons of Edinburgh 36: 362–371

Arriagada R, Rutqvist L E 1991 Adjuvant chemotherapy in early breast cancer and the incidence of new primary malignancies. Lancet 338: 535–538

Atkins H, Wolff B 1964 Discharges from the nipple. British Journal of Surgery 51: 602–606

Barr L C, Brunt A M, Goodman A G, Drury A, Phillips R H, Ellis H 1989 The primary management of breast cancer: is breast conservation feasible for all patients? Annals of the Royal College of Surgeons of England 71: 390–393

Bates T, Riley D L, Houghton J, Fallowfield L, Baum M 1991 Breast cancer in elderly women: Cancer Research Campaign trial comparing treatment with tamoxifen and optimal surgery with tamoxifen alone. British Journal of Surgery 78: 591–594

Baum M 1973 Immunological considerations. Journal of the Royal College of Surgeons of Edinburgh 18: 351–356

Baum M 1980 Carcinoma of breast. Annals of the Royal College of Surgeons of England 62: 35–38

Baum M, Houghton J, Riley D 1992 Results of the Cancer Research Campaign Adjuvant Trial for perioperative cyclophosphamide and long-term Tamoxifen in early breast cancer reported at the tenth year follow up. Acta Oncologica 31: 251–257

Burn I 1980 Selective policy in the treatment of early breast cancer. Annals of the Royal College of Surgeons of England 62: 49–51

Chaudary M A, Reidy J F, Chaudhuri R, Millis R R, Hayward J L, Fentiman I S 1990 Localization of impalpable breast lesions: a new device. British Journal of Surgery 77: 1191–1192

Dahl-Iverson E 1963 An extended radical operation for carcinoma of the breast. Journal of the Royal College of Surgeons of Edinburgh 8: 81–90

Dixon A R, Robertson J F R, Jackson L, Nicholson R I, Walker K J, Blamey R W 1990 Goserelin (Zoladex) in premenopausal advanced breast cancer: duration of response and survival. British Journal of Cancer 62: 868–870

Dixon A R, Galea M H, Ellis I O, Elston C W, Blamey, R W 1991 Paget's disease of the nipple. British Journal of Surgery 78: 722–723

Dixon J M, Thompson A M 1991 Effective surgical treatment for mammary duct fistula. British Journal of Surgery 78: 1185–1186

Dixon J M 1992 Outpatient treatment of non-lactational breast abscesses. British Journal of Surgery 79: 56–57

Edwards M H, Baum M, Magerey C J 1972 Regression of axillary lymph nodes in cancer of the breast. British Journal of Surgery 59: 776

Forrest A P M et al 1979 Is the investigation of patients with breast cancer for occult metastatic disease worthwhile? British Journal of Surgery 66: 749–751

Forrest A P M 1980 Conservative management of breast cancer. Annals of the Royal College of Surgeons of England 62: 41–43

Forrest A P M 1981 Primary management of breast cancer In: Breast cancer. Update, London, p 14

Griffiths K, Nicholson R I 1981 Steroid receptors In: Breast cancer. Update, London, p 33

Haagensen C D, 1986 Diseases of the Breast, 3rd edn. Philadelphia, W B Saunders Company, p 939–941

Hadfield G J 1969 The pathological lesions underlying discharges from the nipple in women. Annals of the Royal College of Surgeons of England 44: 323–333

Handley R S 1975 Carcinoma of the breast. Annals of the Royal College of Surgeons of England 57: 59–66

Hawkins R A, Roberts M, Forrest A P M 1980 Oestrogen receptors and breast cancer: Current status. British Journal of Surgery 67: 153–169

Hayward J L 1980 Radical breast surgery. Annals of the Royal College of Surgeons of England 62: 43–45

Hughes L E, Mansel R E, Webster D J T 1989 Benign disorders and diseases of the breast. Bailliere Tindall, London, p 45

Jones A L, Williams M P, Powles T J et al 1990 Magnetic resonance imaging in the detection of skeletal metastases in patients with breast cancer. British Journal of Cancer 62: 296–298

McNair T J, Dudley H A F 1960 Axillary lymph nodes in patients without breast carcinoma. Lancet 1: 713

Masood S, Frykberg E R, McLellan G L et al 1990 Radiologically directed fine-needle aspiration biopsy of non-palpable breast lesions. Cancer 66: 1480–1487

Morris A M, Lamont P M 1980 A method for correcting the inverted nipple. British Journal of Plastic Surgery, 33: 41

Nedelman R, Dixon J M 1992 Marking of specimens in patients undergoing stereotactic wide local excision for breast cancer. British Journal of Surgery 79: 55

O'Brien D P, Horgan P G, Gough D B, Skehill R, Grimes H, Given H F 1992 CA15-3: a reliable indicator of metastatic bone disease in breast cancer patients. Annals of the Royal College of Surgeons of England 74: 9–12

Owen A W M C, Anderson T J, Forrest A P M 1980 Closed biopsy for breast cancer. Journal of the Royal College of Surgeons of Edinburgh 25: 237–241

Preece P E 1991 What's new in breast disease? Journal of the Royal College of Surgeons of Edinburgh 36: 145–146

Robbins T H 1977 A reduction mammaplasty with areolar-nipple based on an inferior dermal pedicle. Plastic & Reconstructive Surgery, 59: 64

Spitalier J M, Gambarelli J, Brandone H et al 1986 Breast-conserving surgery with radiation therapy for operable mammary carcinoma: a 25 year experience. World Journal of Surgery 10: 1014–1020

Thomas W G, Williamson R C N, Davies J D, Webb A J 1982 The clinical syndrome of mammary duct ectasia. British Journal of Surgery 69: 423–425

Warwick D J, Smallwood J A, Guyer P B, Dewbury K C, Taylor I 1988 Ultrasound mammography in the management of breast cancer. British Journal of Surgery 75: 243–245

FURTHER READING

Baum M 1980 The management of advanced breast cancer. British Journal of Hospital Medicine 23: 32

Bonadonna G 1980 Adjuvant chemotherapy in breast cancer. British Journal of Hospital Medicine 23: 40

Cooperman A M, Esselstyn C B (eds) 1978 Symposium on breast cancer. Surgical Clinics of North America 58: No. 4. Saunders, Philadelphia

Forrest A P M, Roberts M 1980 Screening for breast cancer. British Journal of Hospital Medicine 23: 8

Hadfield G J 1981 Cancer of the breast: retrospect, circumspect and prospect. In: Hadfield J, Hobsley M (eds) Current surgical practice, vol. 3. Arnold, London, ch 19

Hughes L E, Webster D J T 1980 The treatment of early breast cancer. British Journal of Hospital Medicine 23: 22

Ward C M 1981 Breast reconstruction after cancer — aesthetic triumph or surgical disaster. British Journal of Plastic Surgery 34: 124

14

Abdominal surgery: access and procedures

J. M. S. JOHNSTONE & R. F. RINTOUL

Position for operation

For most abdominal operations the patient is placed in the supine position. The arms may be laid alongside the body and anchored by the simple apparatus shown in Figure 14.1. The hands should not be placed beneath the buttocks since damage to the circulation or nerve supply of the fingers may result. For lower abdominal operations the arms may be folded across the chest and secured by the safety-pinned bed-jacket.

Operations on retroperitoneal structures such as the kidney and ureter, are performed usually with the patient in the lateral position.

Trendelenburg position. Downward tilting of the head-end of the table is used frequently in operations on the pelvic organs. Its effect is to cause the more mobile organs to gravitate towards the diaphragm so that a less obstructed view of the pelvis can be obtained. The rubber mattress supplied with the modern operating table prevents the patient from sliding headwards (Fig. 14.2).

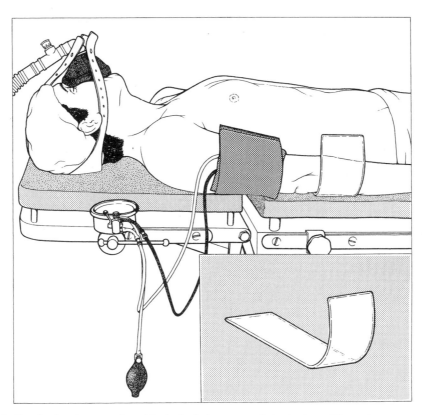

Fig. 14.1 Method of anchoring the arms alongside the body by means of plastic plates. These plates (one shown in inset) are introduced transversely between the patient and the mattress, where they are firmly secured by the patient's weight. Sphygmomanometer is shown in position for the purpose of blood pressure recording during the operation

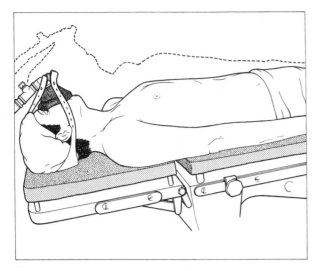

Fig. 14.2 The Trendelenburg position

ABDOMINAL INCISIONS

Anatomy of abdominal wall

Muscles

The muscles of the anterior abdominal wall are external oblique, internal oblique, transversus abdominis and rectus abdominis. (The pyramidales muscles are frequently absent and are of no surgical importance.) In general the first three of these arise at the side of the trunk — from the lower ribs, lumbar fascia or iliac crest. As they traverse the front of the abdomen they become aponeurotic, and are inserted mainly into the *linea alba*, a band of fibrous tissue extending in the mid line from the xiphoid process to the pubis. Before they reach the linea alba they combine to form a sheath for the rectus muscle. Above the umbilicus the linea alba is 1–2 cm wide, but in its lower part it is much narrower.

External oblique runs mainly downwards, forwards, and medially, but its upper fibres are nearly horizontal, its lower ones (inserting into the iliac crest) nearly vertical. Its lower free border forms the *inguinal ligament* which stretches from the anterior superior spine to the pubic tubercle.

Internal oblique runs mainly in a slightly upward direction but its lower fibres, which descend to the pubis, are nearly vertical.

Transversus abdominis runs mainly horizontally, but its lowest fibres run downwards along with those of internal oblique. Its deep surface is lined by transversalis fascia; between this and the peritoneum there is a layer of extraperitoneal fat of variable thickness.

Rectus abdominis lies alongside the linea alba, stretching from the front of the pubis to the xiphoid process and to the 5th, 6th and 7th costal cartilages. Its sub-stance is traversed by three horizontal *tendinous intersections* one opposite the umbilicus, another near the xiphoid, and a third midway between these.

Rectus sheath

This is formed by the aponeuroses of external oblique, internal oblique and transversus, the last two of which are arranged in a somewhat complicated manner.

The *anterior sheath* is complete from rib margin to pubis. In its upper three-fourths it is formed by external oblique and by the anterior lamina of internal oblique. In the lower one-fourth it is formed by all three aponeuroses. It is adherent to the tendinous intersections of the rectus muscle.

The *posterior sheath* is complete only as far down as a point midway between umbilicus and pubis, where it ends as a free border, the *linea semicircularis*. Below this level the sheath is deficient, the rectus being separated from the peritoneum by transversalis fascia alone. It is formed by the posterior lamina of internal oblique fused with transversus. Some fleshy fibres of transversus appear in the upper part of the posterior sheath.

Vessels

The *inferior epigastric vessels* are the only ones of surgical importance. The artery, arising from the external iliac, runs upwards and medially from just above the midinguinal point; it then passes under cover of the lateral margin of the rectus and enters its sheath. The companion veins join the external iliac vein.

Nerves

The nerves of the abdominal wall are the *lower five intercostal*, the *subcostal*, the *iliohypogastric* and *the ilioinguinal.* These run an oblique course in the abdominal wall, lying mainly between transversus and internal oblique. All except the last two enter the rectus sheath and pierce rectus to end as cutaneous branches.

All incisions should be planned to give adequate access to the operative field, but at the same time to inflict the minimum of damage to the abdominal wall, so that a strong and durable scar will result. Provided that the necessary access can be obtained, splitting of a muscle in the line of its fibres (fleshy or aponeurotic) is preferable to division. Healing then occurs much more readily, there is no tendency to disruption of the scar, and subsequent function is unimpaired. In children, the skin incision should conform to Langer's lines (p. 287), otherwise the scar becomes increasingly unsightly with age. With few exceptions, a transverse skin incision can be used for all abdominal surgery in children.

The midline incision

It is no longer necessary to restrict the use of a midline

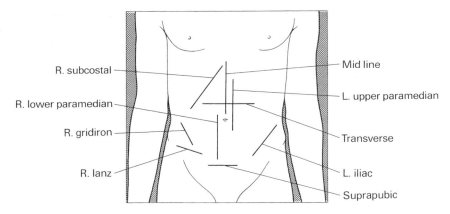

Fig. 14.3 Abdominal incisions

incision to the upper abdomen (Fig. 14.3) since mono-filament sutures which retain their strength until heal-ing is complete, provide for satisfactory wound closure. The incision traverses the linea alba, which is practi-cally avascular, so that the abdomen can be both quickly opened and quickly closed during an emer-gency operation. It is particularly useful in the presence of peritoneal contamination since tissue exposed to the infection is minimized.

The incision is sited in relation to the anticipated pathology but can be readily enlarged if required. Major exposure for aorto-iliac reconstruction may be obtained by a midline incision from the xiphisternum to pubis. At the umbilicus, the incision may be carried through or around it as preferred by the surgeon.

After the skin has been incised the linca alba is divided to expose the peritoneum, which is covered by the thin transversalis fascia. These are usually divided as one layer. In the upper abdomen this division should be made a little to one side of the midline, or the knife may pass between the layers of the falciform ligament. Below the umbilicus, care is taken at the lowest part of the incision to avoid damage to the bladder.

Closure of the incision is effected by a single layer of sutures as a 'mass closure' technique followed by skin suture. Interrupted or continuous sutures of monofila-ment nylon are used, inserting the needle at least 1 cm from the edge of the incision (Bucknall, 1983) and 1 cm from the adjacent suture. If it is possible to ap-proximate the peritoneum (together with transversalis fascia) and the linea alba as separate layers, this should only be attempted if the linea alba can be repaired as already described under 'mass closure'. Prior to skin suture, infiltration with 0.25% *Marcain* (with adrena-line 1 in 400 000 solution) will provide postoperative pain relief.

The paramedian incision
This widely used incision is applicable to both the

upper and the lower abdomen. Its chief advantage lies in the exceptionally strong scar which results although it cannot be readily extended and it is vulnerable to infection in septic cases.

The incision is made parallel to the midline, and at a distance of 2–3 cm from it. The anterior rectus sheath is divided in the line of the skin incision. Forceps are placed on the medial cut margin, which is retracted to expose the medial edge of the rectus muscle. In the upper abdomen the anterior sheath must be freed by sharp dissection, since it is adherent to the tendinous intersections which transverse the muscle. The rectus is then displaced laterally (Fig. 14.4) to expose the poste-rior sheath, which in the upper part shows fleshy fibres of the transversus. The posterior sheath is incised in the line of the skin incision, together with transversalis fascia and peritoneum.

Closure. The incision is sutured in three layers — firstly peritoneum and posterior sheath as one layer,

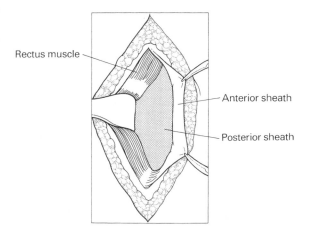

Fig. 14.4 Paramedian incision. The rectus muscle has been retracted laterally to expose the posterior sheath, which is then incised together with the peritoneum

secondly anterior sheath, and thirdly skin. Tension sutures are unnecessary if adequate sutures and a good suturing technique are available. The strength of the repair lies in the fact that the intact rectus muscle covers and gives support to the incisions into the anterior and posterior sheaths (Fig. 14.5).

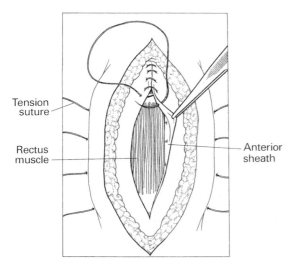

Fig. 14.5 Closure of paramedian incision. The rectus muscle covers the suture line in the posterior sheath. The anterior sheath is being repaired by a continuous suture. (Tension sutures are shown but are rarely needed — see Burst abdomen)

The gridiron incision

This is the incision most commonly used for removal of the appendix. It gives only limited access, but can readily be enlarged by the method described below.

The incision, 7–10 cm in length, lies at right angles to the line joining the anterior superior spine and the umbilicus. Classically its centre should be placed at McBurney's point, i.e. at the junction of the lateral and middle thirds of that line. It is the normal practice, however, to vary the position of the incision according to the supposed situation of the appendix, as judged from the site of maximum tenderness or muscle guarding.

External oblique aponeurosis is split in the line of its fibres (which is the same as that of the skin incision). If the incision is high or laterally placed, fleshy fibres of the muscle are encountered and are split along with the aponeurosis. Both margins of the split are held aside with haemostats or with small retractors, leaving exposed the fleshy fibres of internal oblique running transversely and slightly upwards. This muscle, together with transversus, the fibres of which run in approximately the same line, is then split by blunt dissection. The closed end of a Mayo's scissors or the handle of a scalpel is used for the initial separation, and the split is widened by stretching it between the two forefingers. The fingers are then replaced by small retractors (Fig. 14.6), after which transversalis fascia and peritoneum are picked up as one layer and are incised.

Closure. The peritoneal incision being small can be closed effectively with a running suture, the ends of which are tied together. The split fibres of transversus and internal oblique are very loosely approximated by one or two stitches which pick up both muscles (Fig. 14.7). Alternatively, each muscle split may be closed by suture of the overlying fascia. The external oblique aponeurosis is then sutured, and finally the skin.

Enlarging the gridiron incision. If more access is required in a medial direction the split in internal oblique and transversus is extended into the rectus sheath. If extension is required in an upward or downward

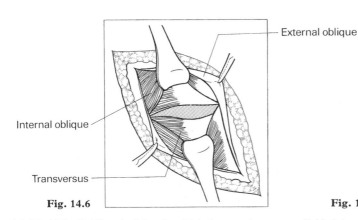

Fig. 14.6

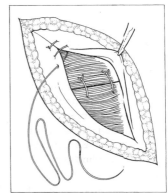

Fig. 14.7

Figs 14.6 & 14.7 Gridiron incision, in which the muscles are not divided, but are split in the line of their fibres — external oblique in the line of the skin incision, internal oblique and transversus in a more or less transverse direction. The muscles are held apart by retractors, to expose transversalis fascia and peritoneum, which are then incised as one layer. The method of closing the incision is shown

direction, these muscles may be divided at right angles to their fibres. The muscles cut in this manner are repaired without difficulty with interrupted stitches. No special liability to postoperative hernia has been recorded.

The Lanz incision is a minor modification of the gridiron. The skin incision is made more or less transversely and lies in the interspinous crease. Thereafter the muscles are divided as in the classical gridiron approach. The method has a definite cosmetic value in producing an almost invisible scar, but difficulties are encountered if the incision requires to be enlarged.

Muscle-cutting iliac incision

This incision is employed for exposure of retroperitoneal structures such as the ureter or external iliac vessels. The skin incision is placed at the appropriate site and all muscles are cut in the same line.

Closure. The cut muscles are sutured in layers. If this is carefully done there is no tendency to hernia.

Subcostal incisions are most useful in operations on the gall bladder or spleen. They are also favoured for operations on the adrenal glands (when bilateral exposure is required) or for major operations on the liver.

Kocher's incision begins in the midline below the xiphoid process, and runs downwards and laterally 2.5 cm below and parallel to the costal margin. All muscles, including the rectus, are divided in the same line. The 8th, 9th and 10th intercostal nerves are found running downwards and medially between internal oblique and transversus. Not more than one of these nerves should be divided: the others are carefully retracted and preserved.

Closure is effected in three layers. The first layer comprises peritoneum, posterior rectus sheath and (more laterally) internal oblique and transversus. The anterior rectus sheath and the external oblique are now repaired, and, finally, the skin. No attempt is made to suture the rectus muscle itself — see below.

Transverse incisions may be employed in both upper and lower abdomen. Two distinct types of such incision can be described.

Transverse division of all layers. Both anterior and posterior rectus sheaths are divided transversely — in the line of their fibres. The recti also are divided transversely, so that excellent access is obtained (Fig. 14.8). Division of the recti in this manner causes no interference with their nerve supply, which has a segmental distribution. The method is most suitable for use in the upper abdomen where the rectus is adherent at its tendinous intersections to the anterior sheath. For this reason the cut rectus muscle does not retract, and accurate suture of its sheath is all that is required in the way of repair. The incision may be used for cholecystectomy (p. 427) or pancreatic operations (p. 441).

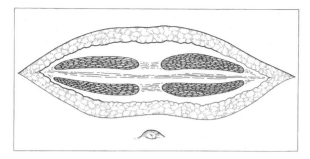

Fig. 14.8 Upper abdominal transverse incision, with division of rectus muscles. Note that the cut muscles do not retract, and that accurate suture of their sheaths is all that is required in the way of repair

With vertical separation of the recti (Pfannenstiel). This method is more suited to the subumbilical region, where the recti have no tendinous intersections and are more mobile within their sheaths. The skin and anterior rectus sheaths are incised transversely. The anterior sheaths are elevated from the underlying recti both upwards and downwards by sharp dissection. The recti are widely separated and held apart by retractors (Fig. 14.9), and transversalis fascia and peritoneum are then incised in a vertical direction. For bladder exposure, these layers are swept upwards and the prevesical fascia is divided.

The lower abdominal transverse incision, placed close to the pubis, is popular for gynaecological operations where limited access is required and a good cosmetic result is considered important. An incision 2 cm above the pubis is favoured by many urologists and provides adequate exposure of the bladder.

The low pararectal incision is described in the section on femoral hernia where access to the peritoneal cavity and to the femoral canal may be required.

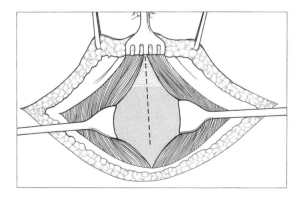

Fig. 14.9 Lower abdominal transverse incision with vertical separation of the recti. The incision is curved so as to lie in the skin creases. After the anterior sheaths have been incised, and the superior flap elevated upwards, the recti are separated and held apart by retractors. Transversalis fascia and peritoneum are then incised in a vertical direction

Transverse incisions in children

In all children transverse abdominal incisions give good access, heal well with minimal scarring and should be used where possible (Fig. 14.10). Muscle layers should be closed in one or two layers according to preference with a slowly absorbable material such as 2/0 or 3/0 Vicryl; the skin should be closed with a fine absorbable suture such as 4/0 plain catgut. In infants, a transverse upper abdominal incision can be used to gain access to the entire peritoneal cavity and is suitable for all operations other than those on the distal large bowel and bladder. Blood loss is critical and can be reduced by cutting with diathermy (Fig. 14.11).

Upper abdominal. A transverse skin incision is made across the width of the rectus abdominis at a level one third of the distance from the umbilicus to the xiphisternum. Subcutaneous fat and anterior rectus sheath are divided in the line of the incision. Muscle fibres are lifted from the posterior rectus sheath with artery forceps and the fibres can then be safely cut with diathermy between the open blades (Fig. 14.11). Posterior rectus sheath and peritoneum are gripped with two artery forceps and a fold is lifted clear of underlying structures. A small incision is made in the fold with a scalpel and extended under direct vision with scissors along the full length of the wound. In the newborn, the umbilical vein lying in the free margin of the falciform ligament must be identified and divided between ligatures.

Lower abdominal. A transverse lower abdominal incision started in the right iliac fossa and extended towards the left (Fig. 14.10B) gives access to the distal half of the ileum, the caecum and ascending colon and a similar incision in the left iliac fossa extended to the right (Fig. 14.10C) gives access to the sigmoid colon and rectum. However, in the older child, when extensive mobilisation of the colon is anticipated, a transverse incision may be inadequate and the midline approach is preferred.

A *right-sided transverse lower abdominal incision* is made high in the right iliac fossa. The skin incision is started on the right side of the abdomen and extended towards the mid-line, crossing a point one third of the distance from the umbilicus to the superior iliac spine. The external oblique aponeuroses is divided obliquely in the line of the incision and the muscle fibres of internal oblique and transversus split by blunt dissection towards the lateral margin of the rectus sheath. The fascia transversalis and peritoneum are then divided transversely to give access to the peritoneal cavity. The incision can be extended with ease across the midline by dividing the rectus muscle with cutting diathermy (Fig. 14.12).

A *left-sided transverse lower abdominal incision* is placed low in the iliac fossa so as to cross a point two thirds of

Figs 14.10–14.12 *Abdominal incisions in children*

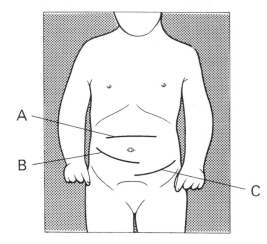

Fig. 14.10 A, transverse upper; B, right transverse lower placed high in the iliac fossa; C, left transverse lower placed low in the iliac fossa

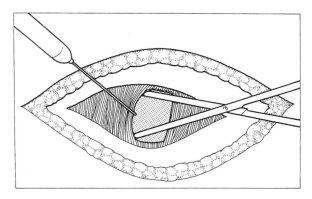

Fig. 14.11 Muscle fibres lifted by artery forceps and cut with diathermy

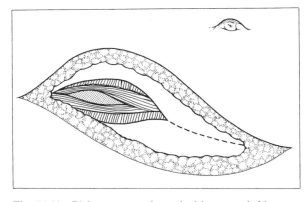

Fig. 14.12 Right transverse lower incision extended by dividing the rectus

the distance from the umbilicus to the superior iliac spine. In other respects the incision is identical to the approach from the right side. In the newborn it must be remembered that the bladder extends up towards the umbilicus, the apex being tethered by the urachus flanked on either side by an umbilical artery.

In renal surgery, the kidney is approached through a right or left transverse abdominal incision which starts laterally in line with the tip of the twelfth rib and runs medially towards the midline. The external and internal oblique and the transversus abdominis muscles are split or divided in the line of the wound. An extra-peritoneal approach is gained by sweeping the peritoneum medially. The renal fascia is identified and divided longitudinally and the kidney is found lying deep to the perinephric fat. For access to the distal ureter and bladder a Pfannenstiel incision is used.

GENERAL TECHNIQUE

Screening of the skin
The skin around the incision should be covered with side towels. This is not only a part of the customary aseptic ritual; in addition it prevents irritation of the delicate serous surface of the bowel from contact with the iodine or other antiseptic which has been used for skin preparation.

Opening of the peritoneum
The utmost care must be taken to ensure that no underlying viscus is wounded during incision of the peritoneum. When the peritoneum has been exposed a small bite is taken with dissecting or artery forceps, and is lifted forwards. It is an advantage to do this during a period of expiration, when the viscera tend to fall away from the abdominal wall. The fold which is lifted up may be given a gentle shake to dislodge any adherent structure, or it may be pinched between finger and thumb so that its thickness can be estimated. A second pair of artery forceps is then applied alongside the first, and the fold is carefully incised (Fig. 14.13). If an opening into the peritoneal cavity is not immediately apparent the forceps should be taken off and reapplied.

When the initial opening has been made, it is enlarged upwards — usually by cutting with scissors under direct vision. It is enlarged downwards by cutting with a knife against two fingers of the left hand which protect the bowel (Fig. 14.14).

Gentle handling and care of the bowel
Gentle handling is an essential part of all abdominal operations. Forcible traction on the gut or on its mesentery is never permissible. If the incision gives insufficient access it must be enlarged or a fresh incision

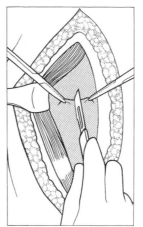 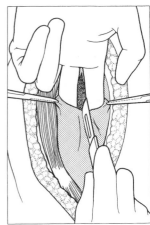

Fig. 14.13   **Fig. 14.14**

Figs 14.13 & 14.14   Method of opening the peritoneum. Injury to the underlying viscera is avoided by the technique depicted

employed. Bowel is slippery to hold, and a firm grasp is most easily obtained with the aid of a large swab; this should be wrung out in hot saline, for dry gauze may abrade the delicate serous surface.

Bowel is very readily damaged by *chilling* or *drying*, and no more than is necessary should be brought out of the wound. If a coil of bowel has to be retained on the surface for even a short time, it should be covered with a hot moist towel which is renewed frequently.

Separation of adhesions
All adhesions should be separated as far as possible under direct vision. For the most filmy adhesions, the finger covered with a moist swab may be used as a blunt dissector. Stronger adhesions should be cleanly divided with fine curved dissecting scissors, the curve being directed away from the structure which is more likely to suffer from damage. If there are widespread adhesions, as may occur after a previous operation, they should not be disturbed more than is necessary, for they are likely to reform — possibly over a wider area. Separation is carried out only in those adhesions which may give rise to trouble (e.g. by kinking of the gut), or which prevent the necessary access from being obtained. Any area in the bowel which has been damaged may be invaginated by means of continuous or interrupted Lembert sutures (see Fig. 14.16).

Prevention of soiling of peritoneal cavity
In operations for any condition of localised intra-peritoneal sepsis, one of the first cares of the surgeon is to prevent the infection spreading to other parts of the peritoneal cavity. Whenever a mass is encountered, and there is even a suspicion that it is inflammatory in

origin, the rest of the peritoneal cavity should be care-fully *packed-off* before the mass is disturbed. This necessitates the insertion of large abdominal swabs or packs placed in such a manner as to surround the mass, so that any septic exudate will be diverted to the surface or will be absorbed by the gauze, before it can permeate to other parts of the peritoneal cavity. This careful technique applies even when peritoneal lavage and broad spectrum antibiotics are available.

Any operation which entails opening the lumen of the gut carries a risk of contaminating the peritoneal cavity. This risk is minimized: (1) by bringing the gut outside the abdomen while it is being opened; (2) by completely surrounding it with gauze packs, so that no septic material can enter the wound; (3) by the use of a clamp which will prevent the escape of intestinal con-tents; (4) by careful suturing of the gut afterwards, and (5) by discarding all instruments, packs, etc., which have become potentially contaminated, and by using clean gloves and towels for subsequent stages of the operation.

Danger of retained swabs
Abdominal packs should have tapes sewn on to them. Forceps are attached to these tapes, and also to any swabs which are introduced into the wound or placed in its vicinity. All swabs put out for an abdominal operation should be of large size. Any swab used for mopping is not left lying near the wound, but is imme-diately discarded. In most operating theatres the sister is responsible for knowing the exact number of swabs that have been issued, and for checking these at the end of the operation. *Raytex* swabs, which are radio-opaque, may be used as routine; they can be demon-strated on X-ray examination if there is a discrepancy in the swab-count. These, however, should be no more than *additional* safeguards; the surgeon should aim at a technique which will make it almost impossible for a swab to be retained within the abdomen.

Methods of suturing gut
It is customary for any incision which opens the lumen of the small bowel to be repaired by two layers of su-tures. The deeper sutures are *through-and-through* ones transfixing all coats. (As they are effective in arresting haemorrhage from the gut wall they are also called *hae-mostatic* sutures.) They may be either continuous or interrupted. A special variety of through-and-through suture is known as the 'loop on the mucosa' (*Connell*) suture; in this the needle is passed twice in succession through each cut edge (first from without-inwards and then from within-outwards). It is effective in preventing eversion of the mucous membrane. A simpler and equally effective inverting suture is shown in Figure 14.15. This continuous suture is started within the lumen and finishes at the same point (after apposition of the two bowel ends) so that the knot disappears into the lumen. The anterior layer of the anastomosis is treated as an extension of the posterior layer, the needle being passed from one lumen to the other before tight-ening the thread. By any method the sutures, since they penetrate the lumen of the gut, are potentially infected, and should be covered over. This is done by the inser-tion of a second row of sutures which invaginate the first suture line by bringing together over it the bowel wall on each side. These sutures, which are known as *Lembert* sutures, take up the serous and muscular coats on each side of the deep suture line and about 5 mm

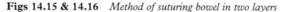

Figs 14.15 & 14.16   *Method of suturing bowel in two layers*

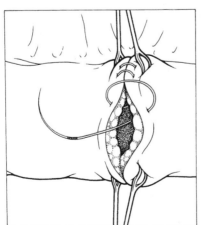 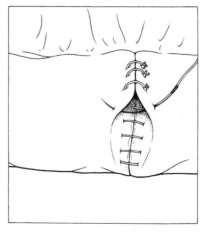

Fig. 14.15   Fig. 14.16

Fig. 14.15   Through-and-through stitches transfixing all coats and inverting the mucosa
Fig. 14.16   *Lembert* or seromuscular sutures which do not penetrate the mucosa. They are used to invaginate the previous suture line, and to bring serous surfaces into firm and even contact

distant from it, but do not penetrate the mucous membrane (Fig. 14.16). The serous surfaces thus brought into contact are gummed together by lymph exudate, and the junction rapidly becomes organized and watertight. For incisions of any length a continuous Lembert suture may be employed.

Needles

Fine round-bodied needles are used throughout — straight or curved according to individual preference. *Atraumatic* needles have a tubular end instead of an eye, and into this the suture material is suaged by the manufacturers. They inflict the minimum of trauma on the bowel wall, and make for smooth suturing.

Suture materials

Fine absorbable sutures — such as catgut, dexon, polydioxanone (PDS) and vicryl — are suitable for through-and-through sutures, since the persistence of an unabsorbable suture on the mucous surface may predispose to ulceration. For Lembert sutures either catgut, linen or silk may be used. Alternatively, a slowly absorbed material (dexon, PDS or vicryl) provides a useful alternative which can be used for both layers.

Reposition of viscera and repair of incision

The edges of the peritoneal incision are grasped with forceps and are lifted away from the patient. Provided that there is no distension and the abdominal wall is relaxed the viscera should fall back into the abdomen almost of their own accord. Should a distended coil of bowel fail to go back easily it should be gently compressed to empty it of gas. If the intestines or omentum interfere with suture of the peritoneum they may be covered with a moist abdominal pack which is held down with a spatula or with a special depressor. When the suture line is nearly complete the pack and depressor are withdrawn. If the suturing is being carried out under tension, and the stitches tend to cut out, the needle may be made to pick up muscular fibres along with the peritoneum, or each bite may be taken from the inner surface of the peritoneum, parallel to the cut edge. Alternatively, a continuous mattress suture may be used, placing several sutures before tightening up and approximating the edges of the wound. When the tension is due to incomplete anaesthesia the surgeon should cover the wound with a towel, and wait until the necessary relaxation is obtained. Whatever method of suturing is preferred, it is essential to insert the needle at least 1 cm from the wound edge and place the loops of suture about 1 cm apart.

Suture materials

Catgut, dexon or PDS, which are absorbed by the body, are commonly employed for sutures which approximate peritoneum and the adjacent layer of abdominal wall. Catgut is also satisfactory for the muscular or aponeurotic layers in small wounds particularly in a thin, young, well nourished patient where difficulty in wound healing is not anticipated. Nonabsorbable material such as linen, silk or monofilament nylon is essential for repair of the linea alba in midline incisions and may also be used in the superficial layers of the abdominal wall in elderly patients, the obese or those liable to put strain on the wound postoperatively as a result of coughing.

Drainage of the peritoneal cavity is unnecessary following a 'clean' operation but is essential in cases of severe peritoneal sepsis. When the source of infection has been dealt with by resection or aspiration, antibiotic lavage should be carried out to cleanse the most contaminated area and then the entire peritoneal cavity (Stewart, 1980). The purpose of drainage is to allow the escape of inflammatory exudate or of pus which forms *after* completion of the operation.

Suction drainage

The *Redivac* or alternative closed drainage system is now generally available and can be used to advantage in any part of the abdominal cavity. Unless pus is viscid, it will pass through the larger size of tube. Suction is applied from the 'vacuum' bottle or suction device to numerous side-holes in the tube within the patient. The side-holes are essential since suction applied to a single tube drain will draw bowel and omentum against the tube, with resultant damage and cessation of drainage. For thick exudate, 'sump' drainage is instituted by inserting one tube within the other (Figs 14.17 & 14.18). The outer tube projects for

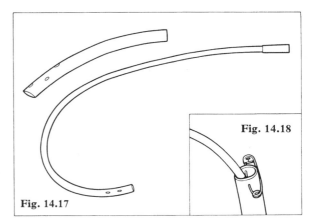

Fig. 14.18

Fig. 14.17

Figs 14.17 & 14.18 Two plastic tubes, the narrower placed within the wider, for 'sump' drainage by suction to the inner tube. Fig. 14.18 shows method of securing the inner tube. The safety-pin compresses slightly but does not transfix the inner tube

Figs 14.19 & 14.20   *Double-tube suction drainage (sump drainage) applied to the peritoneal cavity*

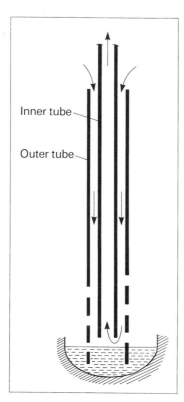

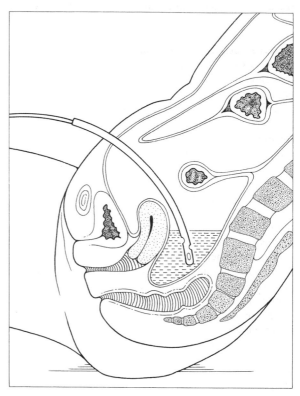

Fig. 14.19   Diagram to illustrate the mechanics of the method. A continual current of air, activated by the suction, passes down through the outer tube and up through the inner tube. Any fluid collecting in the outer tube is immediately sucked away, but no suction occurs at the openings in this tube. For the sake of clarity the internal end of the inner tube is shown at a slightly higher level than that of the outer tube, but it may be difficult to maintain the tubes in this position. A similar effect is obtained by introducing both tubes to the same depth and by cutting a single hole in the inner tube 1–2 cm from its end

Fig. 14.20   Diagram to show the method in use for drainage of fluid from the recto-uterine pouch, the patient being nursed in the propped-up position

Drainage of the wound

The wound in the abdominal parietes is less resistant to infection than is the peritoneal cavity, and wound sepsis is a common cause, not only of prolonged convalescence, but also of postoperative hernia. The risks of wound infection are present in all cases of peritoneal sepsis or potential sepsis (e.g. in the presence of an inflammatory exudate). Such risks may be reduced by systemic chemotherapy, antibiotic lavage or local antibiotic spray. In cases of severe sepsis, a narrow strip of corrugated plastic may be placed in the wound down to the abdominal wall suture, the superficial layers of the wound being closed loosely around it.

ANASTOMOSIS OF GUT

Anastomosis between segments of gut may be required in order to short-circuit some obstructive or other lesion, or to re-establish continuity after resection has been carried out.

The junction may be effected in one of two ways — *lateral anastomosis, or end-to-end anastomosis.* The latter method is applicable mainly to the intestines, and is

2–3 cm outside the wound; the inner tube is longer and is connected to suction. A number of holes are cut in the lower part of the outer tube, and the inner tube has a single hole cut in it close to its end, as shown in Figure 14.19. A continual current of air, activated by the suction, passes down through the outer tube and up through the inner tube. Any fluid collecting in the outer tube is immediately sucked away. No suction occurs at the openings in the outer tube, so that the surrounding tissues are not drawn against it. This method of suction drainage may be applied to any part of the peritoneal cavity where it is thought that fluid may collect — below the diaphragm, in Morison's pouch or in the pelvis. For drainage from the pelvis the patient should be nursed in the propped-up position (Fig. 14.20).

dealt with in a later chapter (pp. 471–472). The first method has a wider application, and will be described here.

Lateral (side-to-side) anastomosis

Most surgeons use clamps for this operation, in order to steady the gut, to control haemorrhage and to prevent escape of contents, but others prefer to rely on a skilled assistant. The clamps must be of the *light occlusion* type, which will cause the minimum of trauma to the gut. The blades may be protected by rubber tubing, but if they are sufficiently light this is unnecessary.

For a *gastrojejunostomy* a segment of each viscus 8–9 cm in length is included in the clamp; for an *enteroanastomosis* about half this length will suffice. A long swab is laid between in order to absorb any escaping contents, and the clamps are approximated. They are secured either by a locking device (Fig. 14.21) or by tying together. Adjacent loops of bowel are returned to the peritoneal cavity, and gauze packs are placed around the clamps, so that no escaping intestinal contents can enter the wound.

The anastomosis is carried out usually by a relatively standardised technique which employs four layers of sutures, as follows.

Posterior serous suture

This is a continuous Lembert suture which unites the adjacent surfaces of the two loops of gut. A short end is retained in forceps at the start of the layer (Fig. 14.21), and the suture is tied when the first layer has been completed.

The lumen of each segment is now opened, within the limits of the posterior serous suture, by an incision parallel to the suture line and approximately 5 mm from it. In the first instance the incision should be made through serous and muscular coats only; the mucosa is then picked up with forceps and incised separately. This limits soiling of the cut edges. As soon as the lumen has been opened intestinal contents are carefully mopped away with small gauze pledgets held in forceps. For a gastrojejunostomy the length of each opening should be 5–6 cm.

Posterior all-layers suture

Catgut, dexon, PDS or vicryl may be used. The suture begins at one extremity of the incision and unites the posterior cut edges, traversing all coats of the gut. The short end is held in forceps. An ordinary overhand continuous suture is employed, but, after every five or six stitches, a lock stitch is inserted to prevent a possible purse-string effect being produced. When the other extremity of the incision is reached, the suture is carried round the corner and is continued in the reverse direction as the anterior all-layers suture (Fig. 14.22).

Anterior all-layers suture

This begins as a continuation of the posterior layer, the needle passing from one lumen to the other as before excepting that the wall of each gut edge must be traversed separately. As the suture is tightened towards the start of the suture (held in forceps), the mucosa is inverted by the loop of thread which has just been inserted. The suture is continued in this manner, to complete the junction between the cut edges of gut, and is tied to its own end.

The anastomosis should now be water-tight, and the clamps are removed so that any bleeding points can be identified. These are dealt with by the insertion of additional interrupted sutures.

Anterior serous suture

This is required to cover the previous suture line which is potentially infected, and to bury any tags of mucous membrane which may be pouting between the stitches. A continuous Lembert suture is employed; during its application the bowel is held taut between the ends of the posterior serous suture, which have been retained in forceps (Fig. 14.23).

It should be noted that there are numerous minor variations from the technique described above. Some surgeons prefer a simple over-and-over suture for the third layer but, although taking a shorter time to complete, this method is much more likely to result in eversion of mucosa with a consequently greater risk of leakage. In cases where difficulty in suturing the corners is anticipated, it has been recommended that the all-layers suture should be threaded with a needle at each end, and that a start should be made in the middle of the posterior cut edges; the needles are then made to sew in opposite directions until they meet again anteriorly.

AFTER TREATMENT IN ABDOMINAL OPERATIONS — SEQUELAE AND COMPLICATIONS

General measures

Careful case selection and preoperative preparation will forestall later problems but good postoperative care is an essential adjunct to abdominal surgery if unpleasant sequelae and complications are to be minimised.

Position in bed

When returned to bed after operation the patient should be placed in the semi-prone position, in order to obviate the risk of vomitus being inhaled into the respiratory passages. As soon as consciousness returns he may be turned on to his back, and this position is maintained until normal circulation has returned and hypotension, if present, is corrected; if necessary the foot

Figs 14.21–14.23 *Technique of lateral anastomosis by four layers of sutures.*

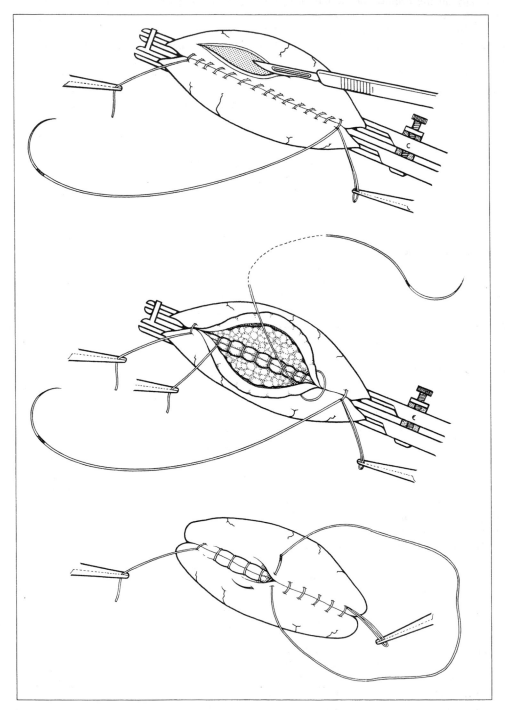

Fig. 14.21   Posterior serous suture completed. Bowel wall being incised — serous and muscular coats only in the first instance.

Fig. 14.22   Posterior through-and-through suture completed. Anterior through-and-through suture in progress.

Fig. 14.23   Anterior serous suture (the final layer) nearing completion

of the bed is raised on blocks. When the condition permits, and usually on the evening of the day of operation, the patient may be allowed to adopt any position which he finds most comfortable. As soon as is practicable, he should be propped up in order to allow of maximum pulmonary ventilation. This is particularly important in the elderly and in those who have undergone a major operative procedure.

Sedation
With modern anaesthetics, skilfully administered, patients may pass imperceptibly from the state of anaesthesia to that of sleep, and may awake several hours after operation, feeling little the worse for their experience. In many cases, however, this happy ideal is not attained; the patient becomes conscious or semiconscious soon after his return to bed, and pain and restlessness develop. Such cases may be treated effectively by intravenous injection of morphine 10 mg or heroin 5 mg or alternative synthetic analgesic. The dose can be titrated to meet the patient's needs by diluting the drug to 10 ml and injecting slowly until the desired effect is achieved (Justins, 1992). A similar dose, or a slightly larger one (morphine 15 mg or heroin 10 mg), is usually given intramuscularly on the first and second nights after operation and may be repeated if necessary. Thereafter restful nights can usually be obtained by use of a hypnotic combined with a milder analgesic. Continued administration of morphine or heroin should be avoided if possible, unless actual pain is present, since, by diminishing the cough reflex, it favours the development of pulmonary complications.

Diet and fluid intake
Even after operations on the stomach and duodenum the necessity for withholding fluids by mouth is no longer accepted. Sips of water can be given as soon as bowel sounds return, provided that the patient does not vomit. In most major cases intravenous infusion is given as routine, in order to replace fluid lost during the operation and to supply the daily fluid requirement. When intravenous infusion has been instituted preoperatively for the correction of fluid and electrolyte deficiency, it will usually be continued during and after operation. Balanced saline solution, plasma expanders or blood transfusion may be given according to the needs of the patient, noting all fluids on a balance chart so that the patient receives the correct type *and* volume of fluid for his requirements (p. 23). Intravenous infusion is continued until an adequate oral intake of fluid has been achieved. Diet is then gradually increased through the stages of fluid and semisolids until a normal diet is attained. Any protein or vitamin deficiency (p. 24) should be corrected at the same time. Dietary

progress then follows the needs and reactions of the patient, rather than any arbitrary rules.

Bowel action
One of the benefits of early ambulation (see below) and early feeding is that the normal bowel function may be attained within 2 or 3 days of operation without the necessity for aperients. A mild aperient may, however, be prescribed on the second or third night after operation, but in the case of major operations or those involving the lower bowel, it may be delayed for several days longer. Colicky pains, due to flatulent distension of the bowel, are a frequent source of discomfort during the first 2 or 3 postoperative days. Relief from these can usually be obtained with the help of suppositories.

Exercises and period of bed rest
Early ambulation is now accepted as routine and many patients can return to the comfort of their own home on the same day as operation. After many 'minor' abdominal operations (appendicectomy, herniorrhaphy, etc.) the patient may be encouraged to get up for a little while on the evening of operation, and, if possible, to walk to the toilet. In most major cases he can be helped into a chair by the first or second postoperative day. The benefits of such early activity are considerable. Cardiac, respiratory and excretory functions are stimulated, and there is less time for muscular weakness to develop. Complications such as atelectasis, respiratory infection and retention of urine have become much less frequent. Young patients recovering from some simple operation such as an uncomplicated appendicectomy will often appreciate being allowed to return home on the third or fourth postoperative day with their stitches in situ. Indeed, if their bowels have moved, and if there has been no rise of temperature or pulse rate, there would seem to be no reason why they should not do so. In major cases or where ambulation is likely to be delayed, deep breathing exercises should be commenced as soon as possible after operation. The patient should be encouraged and helped to change his position in bed at frequent intervals, and active exercises for the abdominal and limb muscles should be carried out. Such treatment should, if possible, be under the instructions and supervision of a trained physiotherapist.

Complications

Vomiting
After modern anaesthesia vomiting does not normally occur or is no more than transient. Persistent vomiting may indicate the threat of some serious complication such as paralytic ileus or acute dilatation of the stomach, a condition which requires prompt gastric decompression. In nervous patients, however, vomiting may

persist for no detectable reason. Anti-emetic or sedative drugs are usually effective.

Retention of urine

Difficulty in initiating the act of micturition occurs chiefly in older men, especially after operations on the pelvic organs. It frequently responds to simple remedies which include reassurance and allowing the patient to sit or stand at the side of the bed, while attempting to urinate. Suppositories are often effective in stimulating both bowel and bladder. The injection of a parasympathetic stimulant such as *Carbachol* should only be used if bladder outflow obstruction is not suspected. Catheterization is necessary if all other methods fail and if obvious distension of the bladder is present, and should be retained until the patient is fully ambulant. Even then, he may be unable to pass urine when the catheter is removed. If the patient can be induced to pass water naturally he seldom has any further trouble unless some organic cause for the obstruction exists. When the operation is of such a nature that difficulty with micturition may be anticipated — e.g. excision of the rectum — a urethral catheter may be left in situ for 2 or 3 days.

Abdominal distension

In its mild form this may be regarded as a sequel to abdominal operation, rather than as a complication, since some temporary inhibition of peristalsis is inevitable. It is rarely of any serious significance, but should not be ignored lest it prove to be a warning of some serious complication such as acute dilatation of the stomach or paralytic ileus. Treatment is by gastric aspiration, either intermittent or continuous. This is effective in relieving distension, not only of the stomach, but also of the greater part of the small bowel, since intestinal peristalsis is inhibited by gastric distension, and is restored when this is relieved. The tube should normally be retained until there is evidence of peristaltic activity as shown by bowel sounds on auscultation or by the passage of flatus per rectum. Distension after lower abdominal operations is due often to colonic stasis, and can usually be relieved by suppositories or enemata. The treatment of true ileus is described on page 464.

Pulmonary complications

These include conditions such as bronchitis, pneumonia and pulmonary atelectasis. They are most liable to occur after upper abdominal operations in older patients, but are infrequent with modern methods of anaesthesia and with insistence on deep breathing exercises early in the postoperative period. In general, treatment is on medical lines including physiotherapy, but bronchoscopy may be employed to remove liquid secretions or plugs of mucus from the bronchi: endotracheal intubation, possibly with artificial ventilation, is indicated in cases where severe respiratory embarrassment exists, and may be a lifesaving measure (p. 302). Pulmonary embolism is a major complication of any operation and may occur without warning from phlebothrombosis in the veins of the lower limb or of the pelvis.

Phlebothrombosis (DVT) is a relatively common complication after abdominal operations. Its apparently increased incidence is due probably to the fact that it is now more frequently recognized. It occurs usually in the deep veins of the calf (posterior tibial veins), and less commonly in the femoral and iliac veins. Its significance lies in the danger that pulmonary embolism may result from detached fragments of clot entering the circulation. It becomes manifest usually between the third and tenth day after hospital admission. Routine examination daily, or the occurrence of minor elevations of temperature or pulse rate, will lead to early diagnosis. Various measures used in the prevention of phlebothrombosis include graduated compression stockings, subcutaneous heparin 5000 I.U. subcutaneously two or three times daily (starting before operation and continuing until the patients is ambulatory), intermittent compression of the legs during operation, protection of the leg veins from pressure during and after surgery, intravenous dextran and by exercises in the postoperative period. When phlebothrombosis or pulmonary embolism has actually occurred, the best treatment is by a combination of rest, elevation of the limb and anticoagulant therapy (p. 48). Ligation of the femoral or iliac veins, or even of the inferior vena cava, has been practised in some clinics, to limit access of emboli to the lungs, but the value of such procedures has not been established. Percutaneous insertion of a transluminal filter (p. 63) into the inferior vena cava offers a simpler alternative, provided an experienced operator is available. When the condition is quiescent and the patient is about to become ambulant, the limb should be provided with support, by an elastic stocking or by bandaging, in order to prevent recurrent swelling.

Postoperative peritonitis

This term is usually restricted to peritonitis which develops unexpectedly after operation. It may be due to accidental contamination during the operation; more frequently, it results at a later stage from leakage of bowel content at a suture line due to bowel ischaemia. The onset is insidious and the diagnosis difficult, for the classical signs of peritonitis (pain and muscular rigidity) are lacking, and little abnormal may be found on examination, except for some elevation of temperature and pulse rate. Later, the clinical picture may become that of paralytic ileus (p. 462), when there is progressive distension of the abdomen with profuse vomiting. The prognosis must then be guarded for the patient's condition may steadily deteriorate. Treatment is that of the paralytic ileus (p. 464), combined with intensive chemotherapy. Operative intervention is often necessary in order to inspect the anastomosis and drain collections of pus. However, this should be preceded by ultrasound scanning since any localised collection — e.g. subphrenic or pelvic abscess — may thus be detected and drained (Lucarotti, 1991).

Postoperative renal failure

This very serious complication has a mortality of about 50% (Linton, 1988). It may follow severe sepsis or prolonged hypotension such as may be associated with extensive injury or operations on the cardiovascular system. 50 ml of 25% mannitol given intravenously over 3–5 minutes may rapidly increase the urinary output but if renal failure persists, the fluid intake should be restricted so as to maintain the daily fluid balance (pp. 23 & 591). Haemodialysis or peritoneal dialysis may then need to be considered.

Burst abdomen

Disruption of the abdominal wound is unusual with correct suturing technique and materials but may occur in elderly or debilitated subjects, especially if they are suffering from advanced malignant disease, protein or vitamin C deficiency or uraemia, and also in those who have been treated by corticosteroids. Persistent cough, vomiting or abdominal distension may be contributing causes. The disruption is most likely to occur about a week or 10 days after operation. As a rule it develops suddenly, in which case the patient complains that 'something has given way,' and the surgeon is summoned hastily because one or more coils of intestine are seen to have prolapsed on to the abdominal wall. In many cases there is no warning of the catastrophe, but sometimes the patient may have complained of some discomfort in the wound, and a serosanguineous discharge may have been noted. Immediate operative repair is advisable. First-aid treatment, while the theatre is being prepared, consists in covering the parts with sterile towels wrung out of warm saline; these in turn are covered with abundant cotton wool and a firm binder is applied. The patient is warned to avoid coughing if at all possible. At operation the protruding abdominal contents are wrapped in fresh packs wrung out of warm saline, and are carefully protected while the wound surfaces and surrounding skin are cleansed and disinfected; after the skin has been towelled-off,

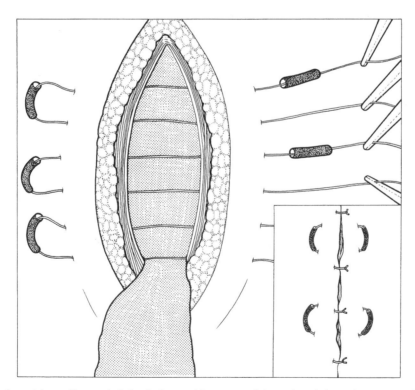

Fig. 14.24   Method repairing a disrupted abdominal wound by means of through-and-through mattress stitches of strong silk, stainless steel wire or nylon. The stitches are made to pass through all layers of the abdominal wall about 2.5 cm from the wound edge, and are passed through pieces of rubber tubing to prevent them from cutting into the skin. A few additional sutures are inserted to coapt aponeuroses and skin

they are washed gently with saline, and are returned to the abdomen, where they are retained by the introduction of a moist pack into the wound. Repair of the wound is carried out by the use of through-and-through stitches of thick silk, monofilament nylon or stainless steel wire, which are made to traverse all layers of the abdominal wall from skin to peritoneum about 2–3 cm from the wound edge. Mattress sutures are used as giving the most secure closure; they may be tied over small swabs or rubber tubing (Fig. 14.24) so that they cannot cut through the skin. Care must be taken that bowel is not trapped in the wound as these sutures are tightened. To avoid such an accident the retaining pack is left in position until the last stitch is about to be tied. Additional sutures may be inserted to draw together the aponeurosis and skin, but accurate co-aptation of these layers should not be attempted lest drainage from the wound be impeded.

REFERENCES

Bucknall T E 1983 Factors influencing wound complications: a clinical and experimental study. Annals of the Royal College of Surgeons of England 65: 71–77

Justins D M 1992 Postoperative pain: a continuing challenge. Annals of the Royal College of Surgeons of England 74: 78–79

Linton A 1988 In: Ledingham I McA, MacKay C (eds) Jamieson and Kay's textbook of surgical physiology, 4th edn. Churchill Livingstone, Edinburgh, p 403

Lucarotti M E, Virjee J, Thomas W E G, Leaper D J 1991 Intra-abdominal abscesses. Surgery 98: 2335–2341

Stewart D J 1980 Generalised peritonitis. Journal of the Royal College of Surgeons of Edinburgh 25: 80–90

FURTHER READING

Fleck A, Ledington I McA 1988 Fluid and electrolyte balance. In: Ledingham I McA, MacKay C (eds) Jamieson and Kay's textbook of surgical physiology, 4th edn. Churchill Livingstone, Edinburgh, Ch 3

Maingot R 1985 Abdominal operations, 8th edn. Appleton-Century-Crofts, New York, Ch 9

15

Minimal access surgery

J. H. SAUNDERS

LAPAROSCOPIC SURGERY FOR GENERAL SURGEONS

The appearance of laparoscopic cholecystectomy on the surgical scene in 1987, developed simultaneously in Europe and the United States, has started a revolution in general surgical techniques never before witnessed. Prior to this, the laparoscope had been the almost exclusive domain of the gynaecologist or for those few surgeons who conducted diagnostic abdominal laparoscopy. It was reports in the European literature in the early eighties of laparoscopic appendicectomy and repair of inguinal hernia that led to the formal development of laparoscopic cholecystectomy.

Now, some 7 years later, the appearance of departments of minimal access surgery are testimony to the arrival of the new speciality. The procedures themselves are separating naturally into *basic*, e.g. cholecystectomy and appendicectomy and *advanced*, such as inguinal herniorrhaphy, fundoplication and colon resection. This chapter will concentrate on the practice of laparoscopic cholecystectomy.

The surgical revolution continues unabated to this day, the publicity surrounding it being fuelled by many different interests.

1. Patient pressure

A laparoscopic operation is a photogenic event and the patients have been very well informed by the mass media and business advertising mechanisms. Laparoscopic surgery in general is now seen as a major improvement upon traditional methods and their demands, rightly or wrongly, have forced the pace of development and availability.

2. Commercial pressures

This has always been, and will continue to be, a major driving force in laparoscopic surgery development. Laparoscopic surgery requires sophisticated technology for TV imaging and pressure monitoring, together with a new range of specialized instrumentation in the form

of safety trocars and the laparoscopic equivalents of diathermy tools, scissors, dissectors, staplers, ligators, etc.

Major business interests were guilty in the early days of forcing the commercial pace ahead of the natural professional surgical development in their attempts to achieve market domination. Also, their marketing has continued to emphasize the benefits of single use instrumentation (and therefore sales) in preference to developing robust cleanable re-usable products.

3. Private practice

The ability to offer 'state of the art' laparoscopic surgical procedures was initially seen as the ideal marketing tool to boost private practice. Competition is such now that it has become essential to offer it just to prevent patients seeking treatment elsewhere. It can only be hoped that these professional commercial pressures will not compromise the best interests of the patient when exposed to new, relatively untested, procedures.

The early consequences

The consequences of these pressures initially meant that the appropriate training was lacking and that surgical ego and over-enthusiasm was difficult to control. Under-estimation of the necessary skill required, combined with a lack of discipline by both the new surgeons and the supporting companies resulted in some avoidable clinical problems and unnecessary negative publicity. Thankfully, the situation is now much better regulated with every surgeon understanding the need for, and having ready access to, specific good quality training with the instrument companies playing a central supporting role.

However, it remains the duty of every surgeon to mould the commercial zeal he is subject to towards solely supporting the best interests of the patient.

The training requirements

Stage 1 (see p. 687)
Training should start at the side of your gynaecological

colleagues to do 40–50 diagnostic laparoscopies under expert supervision. Unfortunately, the first hurdle of being able to establish a pneumoperitoneum safely in all types of abdomen and then carry out a diagnostic laparoscopy is all but forgotten about in the eagerness to do the actual operation.

Stage 2
Ideally, book a specific training course that offers not only simulator work but experience in the clinical setting with the opportunity to watch and assist the expert teacher. The greater the clinical exposure the better it should aim to be involved in a minimum of 5–6 patients.

Stage 3
When ready to commence in your own hospital, try and get help from colleagues with more experience to supervise and guide your early efforts.

LAPAROSCOPIC CHOLECYSTECTOMY

Patient selection
Biliary colic, severe biliary dyspepsia or acute cholecystitis remain the usual indications for cholecystectomy. Removing asymptomatic gall-stones found incidentally will always be a source of argument but there is no new logic that such a gall-bladder should be removed laparoscopically simply because it is a lesser trauma to the patient.

Patient satisfaction studies for the new operation of around 75–80% are similar to the open procedure, suggesting that the criteria for selection still need to improve independent of the method of surgery.

If there is a suspicion that the patient may be suffering from common bile duct stones based upon the usual criteria of clinical history, examination, ultrasound size of the bile duct, disturbed liver function etc., then that patient should undergo an ERCP with a view to papillotomy prior to any proposed surgery. Some surgeons prefer to perform intravenous cholangiography on all patients on the day prior to surgery as a screening process. It can be argued that the investigation is not risk free and that as a very large proportion will be negative, the overall effort and expense is not justified.

Having completed basic training in the new procedure, and ideally getting expert help for the first few sessions, the laparoscopic surgeon should carefully select the initial patients to maximize the chances of success and the building of confidence i.e. he should choose thin, female patients with small stones in a thin-walled non-obstructed gall-bladder and with no previous abdominal surgery. It is a high quality ultrasound

examination that provides this information and working closely with the radiologist is essential to get the best results. It is an excellent judgmental exercise to try and predict the anticipated difficulty of the operation based upon the ultrasound findings. The patient presenting with acute cholecystitis should not be attempted until experience has been gained with at least 40–50 procedures.

Patient management
One hour prior to surgery, the patient empties the urinary bladder, starts primary pain relief with a suitable NSAID (unless contra-indicated), usually Voltarol 100 mgs by suppository, and receives pre-medication. In theatre, there is no need for routine urethral catheterization or nasogastric intubation. They are used only very selectively and based upon individual patient circumstances. There are no special anaesthetic requirements, apart from a preference to use short-acting opiates. However, with the increasing emphasis on day care and short stay surgery even for laparoscopic cholecystectomy, there is a major swing towards a total intravenous approach to anaesthesia with the benefit of rapid recovery and minimal side-effects.

Postoperatively, a second Voltarol is given. The aim is to have the patient fully alert, mobile and drinking on the evening of surgery. Opiates may be strictly reserved to control the occasional severe referred diaphragmatic pain that occurs in 5–10% of patients.

Dissection technique
Gall-bladder retraction, correct tissue tension and the ability to rotate Calot's triangle to work both anteriorly and posteriorly are the keys to good dissection technique. The basic choice lies between the American and French approach. For the American approach, the patient is placed supine, both the fundus of the gall-bladder and neck of gall-bladder are fixed and retracted and the main working port is in the epigastrium (Fig. 15.1).

In the French approach, the patient is in the Llyod Davies position with surgeon operating from between the legs. The fundus of the gall-bladder lies free while retraction is upon the neck of the gall-bladder with countertraction on the porta hepatis (Fig. 15.2). Most surgeons prefer the American approach from the simplicity of set-up and the ease of retraction but all surgeons have encountered times when the French approach is more appropriate, e.g. when the liver is fixed to the diaphragm such that fundal retraction is not possible or when the gall-bladder is so thickened that fundal retraction is inappropriate.

The patient will normally be kept supine. However, repositioning may have to be used — a head-up/feet down position may be the only way to see Calot's triangle in

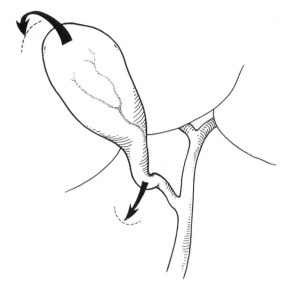

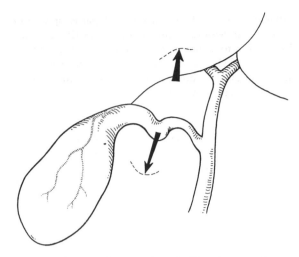

Fig. 15.2 Gall-bladder retraction: the French approach. The fundus lies free. The neck is retracted toward the mid-clavicular port. The porta hepatis is gently lifted to provide countertraction.

Fig. 15.1 Gall-bladder retraction: the American approach. The fundus is retracted both above the liver and laterally. The neck is retracted toward the mid-clavicular port.

an obese patient with a large omentum while rotation of the patient to the left will allow a large left lobe of the liver to drop away. It should be remembered that the risks of deep vein thrombosis (DVT) are likely to be substantially increased by the combination of positive abdominal pressure and decreased venous return in the head-up position.

Rules of dissection — the Edinburgh method
These aim to maximize the safety of the procedure in their active prevention of potential complications. The techniques described have come to be known as the Edinburgh method, developed, tried and tested on over 300 surgeons undergoing training in laparoscopic cholecystectomy. It must be remembered that the rules can be applied only after preparation for dissection by

the correct amount of gall-bladder retraction and tissue tension.

Of all the dissection tools appraised, the Dubois hook (Richard Wolf) has proven to be the most versatile, neatest and safest in general use. It has the combined functions of coagulation diathermy, pledget, retractor and examiner of tissue, and with only a little practice offers quick, safe, precise and bloodless dissection.

Rule 1. Initial display of the biliary anatomy
The gall-bladder is held above the liver and the omentum and duodenum retracted caudally to define the neck of the gall-bladder, Calot's triangle and the common bile duct or lateral margin of the portal triad. An atraumatic retractor is applied to the neck of the gall-bladder to rotate and display the anterior and posterior

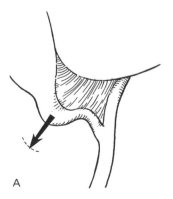

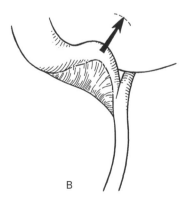

Fig. 15.3 Display of Calot's triangle. The grasper is applied to the neck of the gall-bladder to allow angulation and viewing of the anterior (A) and posterior (B) aspects

aspects of the triangle (Fig. 15.3). The landmarks are viewed, interpreted (the picture orientation MUST be correct) and the initial dissection point defined, i.e. exactly midway between the neck of the gall-bladder and the junction of cystic duct with the common bile duct. Failure to 'roadmap' obsessively and regularly puts the common bile duct at grave risk, particularly when it has a small calibre and dissection is occurring at too low a level i.e. on the portal triad itself (Fig. 15.6).

Rule 2. Skeletalization (Fig. 15.4)

The microsurgical TV system allows progressive dissection of the layers i.e. the anterior and posterior peritoneal covering of Calot's triangle, followed by the adventitial strands around the duct and artery. Skeletal-ization of the proximal halves of these structures mobi-lizes the neck of the gall-bladder into the beginning of the gall-bladder plane and opens up Calot's triangle. Skeletalization is always performed towards the gall-bladder, i.e. by moving the dissection hook away from the essential structures to prevent injury. Also, skeletalization does not go near the cystic duct junc-tion. This must be left intact to prevent potential dia-thermy injury to the common bile duct or tenting when clips are being applied to the cystic duct. The only reasons for dissecting at the junction itself are to get below a stone impacted in the cystic duct or much more rarely, when the cystic duct is very short.

Rule 3. Final display of biliary anatomy

After skeletalization, the surgeon can normally be en-tirely sure that he has mobilized only the cystic duct and has excluded, BY SURGICAL DISSECTION, the presence of the biliary anomaly that causes all sur-geons the most anxiety, i.e. an extra-hepatic right he-patic duct (Fig. 15.5) that has an incidence of 1 in 200 patients. Only then are the duct and artery clipped/ divided and the gall-bladder dissection proceeded with.

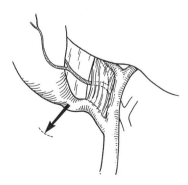

Fig. 15.4 Skeletalization. The duct and artery are cleared to display the lateral half of Calot's triangle, the neck of the gall-bladder is totally freed and the gall-bladder/liver plane entered into

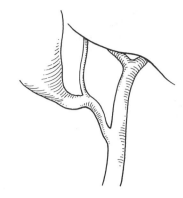

Fig. 15.5 Extrahepatic right hepatic duct. It is essential in each and every laparoscopic cholecystectomy to search for, identify and protect this anomaly by the technique of skeletalization

Rule 4. Controlled response to bleeding

Careful dissection in a layered fashion will minimize significant haemorrhage. Any bleeding looks magnified and therefore initially frightening. Hurried attempts at diathermy, clipping, etc., particularly early in dissec-tion, may injure an essential structure and lead to the need for rapid intervention by open surgery. The usual advice is to let it stop spontaneously. If the bleeding is occurring posteriorly in Calot's triangle, then simply continue dissection anteriorly for a few minutes or vice versa.

Rule 5. Stay out of the liver

If the plane between the gall-bladder and the liver is fibrosed and difficult or impossible to develop, then the back wall of the gall-bladder should simply be left in situ and the remainder of the gall-bladder excised. Attempting to remove the whole gall-bladder in this situation may well result in liver haemorrhage that is impossible to control.

Rule 6. Know when to stop

The patient will have given consent for both open and laparoscopic surgery but many surgeons wrongly feel that resorting to an open procedure is an admission of failure. Continuing a laparoscopic dissection in the face of mounting difficulties and no progress is a recipe for injuring essential structures. It is a good rule to open a patient if no real progress is being made after a maximum of one hour of laparoscopic dissection, i.e. with failure of skeletalization to display Calot's triangle.

What about operative cholangiography?

Surgeons experienced in open cholecystectomy already have a policy. Logic would dictate that that policy should be applied to laparoscopic surgery but in real life, the technical difficulties of the procedure have meant that there is a tendency to do less and less

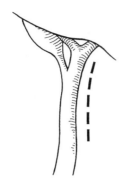

Fig. 15.6 The 'small' common bile duct is in grave risk of injury when mistaken for a standard-sized cystic duct if inaccurate dissection takes place at the wrong level or if premature cannulation is attempted

routine operative cholangiography. Correct use of the skeletalization technique described above means that operative cholangiography is not necessary to define the cystic duct and biliary tree. If a cholangiogram is attempted early in the dissection phase, then occasionally the catheter is found to have been inserted into a small calibre common bile duct (Fig. 15.6) or into an anomalous right hepatic duct as found in a series published from the United States. If the cystic duct has been surgically defined, it follows that the only reason for an operative cholangiogram is to exclude the possibility of common bile duct stones. In practice, our decision for cholangiography tends to be based upon the actual size of the cystic duct, i.e. the larger it is the more likely to proceed to X-rays as a precaution.

Nevertheless, it is important for every laparoscopic biliary surgeon to carry out cholangiography competently as required and he should attempt this procedure routinely as part of his learning experience. Of the multiplicity of choices and techniques available, the steps that we have found best are:-

1. Clip and divide the cystic artery. This elongates the cystic duct to its maximum length.
2. Clip the cystic duct at the junction with the neck of the gall-bladder.
3. Resite the retractor from the neck of the gall-bladder through the epigastric port to alter the angle of the cystic duct to receive the catheter.
4. Make an incision in the cystic duct using sharp hook scissors to nick the anterior wall.
5. Using a Reddick Olsen cholangiogram clamp, insert a 5FG urinary catheter or equivalent into the cystic duct, clamp over it and proceed with the X-rays.

Experience indicates that there is a preferential filling of the distal common bile duct and it is not always possible to display the whole biliary tree.

What about endoscopic common bile duct exploration?

This is currently being developed in the United States and elsewhere with the choice of transcystic duct exploration or open duct exploration. Where ERCP and papillotomy support is available, it is difficult to justify peroperative common bile duct exploration. ERCP and papillotomy have excellent figures in terms of morbidity and mortality. With transcystic duct exploration, it can be technically impossible to get into the upper biliary tree and confirm clearance. Equally, the small stones that may be there are well recognised to have the capacity to pass spontaneously and therefore justification for exploration is a relative one. Finally, the traditional mortality of biliary surgery relates to common duct exploration with postoperative biliary leakage and it seems logical in the closed procedure to try and avoid this potential circumstance.

Complications and their prevention

Every surgeon's laparoscopic technique is developed with prevention in mind. His morbidity statistics should be minimized.

Prevention of bleeding

The key points are a precise layered dissection to expose a duct and artery, a carefully controlled response to any bleeding that does occur, expectation that there might be ANY vascular arrangement around the cystic duct, and staying out of the liver during the gall-bladder dissection.

Prevention of biliary leakage

There are four main sources of biliary leakage leading on to biliary peritonitis and its dangerous consequences.

1. *Common bile duct injury.* The high risk situation is where a small calibre common bile duct is mistaken for a cystic duct and accordingly clamped, catheterized or excised. Initial definition of the biliary anatomy with correct orientation should define Calot's triangle clearly. Using skeletalization rather than cholangiography will prevent a narrow common bile duct being unnecessarily injured.

2. *Leakage from cystic duct stump.* If the cystic duct is of larger than usual calibre, up to a centimetre or more, then use of the routine titanium clips for closure is inappropriate. Such a duct is better ligated with an endoloop or equivalent suture technique. Failure to define the Calot's triangle clearly may lead to dissection of the cystic duct upon the neck of the gall-bladder with the risk again of loss of clips and subsequent leakage.

3. *Injury to an extra-hepatic right hepatic duct.* One of the prime benefits of skeletalization is to identify such a

duct before there is a chance to injure it by distal clipping of a presumed cystic duct. Our experience indicates that skeletalization is the safest way of defining such a biliary anomaly and preventing injury.

4. *Leakage from a bile canaliculus.* Approximately 1% of patients will have a bile canaliculus seen as a firm, whiteish tube some 1–2 mm in diameter connecting directly between the liver and the gall-bladder itself, usually near the neck of the gall-bladder. These canaliculi should be routinely looked for early in the mobilization of the gall-bladder itself and are clipped to prevent biliary leakage. Our experience indicates that diathermy across these structures is insufficient to prevent leakage.

THE ROLE OF ERCP IN THE SUPPORT OF LAPAROSCOPIC CHOLECYSTECTOMY

Apart from the pre-operative investigation of patients with suspected common duct stones, it has been found that ERCP plays an essential role in the definition of postoperative biliary leakage (Fig. 15.4). With this accuracy, it has been possible to explore such problem patients using the laparoscope again to deal with cystic duct leakage and siting of drains to control canalicular problems. Its also defines the type of surgery necessary if reconstruction of a common bile duct or right hepatic duct is required.

Clinically, biliary leakage and peritonitis should be suspected in any patient who is not showing the expected return to normal eating and full mobility by the third day and complains of persistent pain, often initially in the right upper quadrant but latterly in a more generalized area. Such patients should be investigated by abdominal ultrasound, liver function studies and ERCP within 4–5 days of surgery so that corrective action can be taken promptly.

THE PRESENT STATE OF LAPAROSCOPIC PROCEDURES

Laparoscopic appendicectomy
This is being practised on a relatively wide scale, despite the fact that it is difficult to define the clinical benefits of laparoscopic appendix removal. It tends to occupy more theatre time, costs more in instrumentation and has no real superiority in patient recovery, time to discharge, etc.

There appear to be three main reasons for this:-

Diagnosis
A diagnostic laparoscopy assists in the differential diagnosis of suspected acute appendicitis, possible pelvic conditions and acute non-specific abdominal pain, particularly in female patients. Management is clarified, unnecessary surgery avoided, and early discharge can take place.

Training
If appendicitis is confirmed, a laparoscopic removal allows practical experience for the young surgeon in training in a relatively safe area.

Frustration
Young surgeons are being excluded from responsibilities for cholecystectomy and inguinal hernia surgery, their traditional training operations, as the seniors practice their laparoscopic techniques. The only practical outlet for young surgeons is diagnostic laparoscopy, laparoscopic appendicectomy and possibly closure of duodenal ulcer perforation.

Laparoscopic inguinal hernia repair
This is rightly regarded, despite the simplicity of the clinical condition and the traditional surgical repair, as an advanced laparoscopic procedure. Of the various laparoscopic methods proposed or tested, at the present time there appears to be an overall preference for the intraperitoneal placement of a prosthetic patch after division and reflection of the peritoneum along the whole length of the inguinal ligament, isolation of the indirect sac within the spermatic cord and fixation of the prosthesis along the inguinal ligament using custom designed staplers. The proponents of this type of surgery argue that there is a negligible recurrence rate, an immediate return to full mobility and activity and therefore that it is superior to traditional techniques. Arguments raised against this form of surgery are that it makes an external repair into an intraperitoneal operation with its attendant new risks, that it involves high cost instrumentation specifically designed for the procedure and that traditional well designed surgery, in particular the Shouldice repair, offer equivalent negligible recurrence rates. In addition, many surgeons have philosophical problems with the placement of a prosthetic patch in this manner. Furthermore, it could be anticipated that whatever method the surgeon used, his results would be a negligible recurrence rate. It follows therefore that in inguinal hernia in particular, there are many pros and cons still active and only time will tell whether laparoscopic repair becomes routine. A selective approach, restricted to recurrent or bilateral herniae, is also being advocated by some surgeons.

Colo-rectal surgery

Benign disease
Geriatric patients recover quickly following minimal access surgery and in rectal prolapse good results are being achieved by a combination of recto-sigmoid mobilization and end-to-end internal circular stapling.

Excision of sigmoid volvulus by internal clipping of the mesentery followed by exteriorization and external end-to-end anastomosis is also a practical process. However, initial experience indicates that there is a long learning curve involved in resection surgery which will naturally and quite rightly restrict widespread adoption of a laparoscopic approach.

Malignant disease

All forms of resection, abdomino-peritoneal, hemicolectomy, total colectomy, etc., are currently being tried and developed into regular procedures. It usually takes the form of what is termed 'laparoscopic assisted' i.e. the mobilization of the segment is carried out initially followed by exteriorization of the lesion and external anastomosis. It follows therefore that a large tumour to be exteriorized needs a large incision and so raises the question of whether it should not have been made in the first place. It is practical to suggest that small mobile tumours may be ideal technically for laparoscopic removal in preference to larger ones.

The extremely important question of course relates to the adequacy or not of cancer clearance. Proponents of laparoscopic removal cite the fact that the pathologists are able to find lymph nodes in the regional drainage as evidence of adequacy. This assertion is undoubtedly true but is countered by the broader argument that no surgeon at the present time is satisfied with the results of colo-rectal cancer surgery, averaging 30% survival at 5 years by open methods. It follows that resorting to laparoscopic means can only increase the potential for a more limited clearance, for local spillage and contamination of the abdomen and the wound itself. Evidence is accumulating of seedling metastatic problems at trocar puncture sites. Only time will tell what will be declared a regular procedure in 5 years time.

Gastric surgery

With the virtual disappearance of peptic ulcer surgery following the remarkable success of H2 therapy, Nissen fundoplication is becoming perhaps the commonest gastric procedure for benign disease. Reports in the European literature of experience of several hundred laparoscopic procedures testify to the feasibility of the operation. However, surgical debate should still be at the stage of reconciling the widely differing operation rates and selection criteria rather than extolling the technical virtues of a laparoscopic fundoplication.

Other procedures being carried out relate to the bypassing of obstructions. Palliative cholecystojejunostomy for malignant biliary and pancreatic disease looks a feasible operation in the absence of ERCP and stenting support or in the failure of such a procedure. Anterior gastrojejunostomy has also been described to bypass pyloric stenosis or duodenal obstruction. It is well recognized that a posterior gastrojejunostmy per-

forms much better than an anterior one and this represents one of the compromises that laparoscopic surgery currently forces upon surgeons.

Duodenal ulcer perforation

This acute condition would seem to be ideal for a laparoscopic approach to effect a simple stitch closure and omental patch over the perforation, conduct peritoneal toilet and to allow such usually compromised patients to recover more quickly in the absence of a full laparotomy incision. Small studies have reported good results. Laparoscopic ulcer perforation closure performed under expert supervision, represents an ideal practical procedure for young surgeons in training.

Cervical sympathectomy

This represents an excellent use of the laparoscope to conduct a percutaneous transthoracic division of the lower cervical sympathetic chain in the management of axillary hyperhidrosis. It bypasses the complexities of a transthoracic approach, gives a clear magnified anatomical definition of the cervical sympathetic chain and allows precise microdissection and injury to the appropriate portion.

CONCLUSION

A whole array of procedures is being developed at present as more and more surgeons gain practical laparoscopic experience and wish to develop that skill. It remains difficult to predict what the range of recognized routine laparoscopic procedures will be in 5 years time. Each procedure, in order to achieve that status, will have to meet several general criteria. The majority of surgeons will have to be satisfied that:

1. It is measurably superior to the traditional equivalent operation.

2. A laparoscopic cancer operation does not give poorer results.

3. It does not require an extraordinary degree of laparoscopic skill and expertise.

4. It is achieved within a reasonable timescale i.e. that it meets the constraints of access to theatre, that it does not produce excessive surgeon fatigue, that there are no knock-on effects of increased waiting list, etc.

5. It is economically acceptable, i.e. that it is not excessively expensive in terms of manpower, training, instrumentation, etc.

Laparoscopic cholecystectomy quickly established itself as the gold standard for laparoscopic surgery. All similar procedures need to be measured against this standard to judge their true value to our patients. Only time will tell which ones will meet the expectations.

FURTHER READING

BOOKS

Cushieri A, Berci G 1992 Laparoscopic biliary surgery. 2nd edn. Blackwell Scientific, Oxford.

Dagnini G 1989 Laparoscopy and Imaging Techniques. Springer–Verlag.

Zucker K A (ed) 1991 Surgical laparoscopy. Quality Medical Publishing, Baltimore, Maryland

PAPERS

Gotz et al 1990 Modified laparoscopic appendiectomy in Surgery. Surgical Endoscopy 4: 6–9

Katkouda N, Mouiel J 1991 A new technique of surgical treatment of chronic duodenal ulcer without laparotomy by videocoelioscopy. American Journal of Surgery 161: 361–364

Leader 1991 Cholecystectomy practice transformed. Lancet 338: 789–790

Nathanson L et al 1990 Laparoscopic repair/peritoneal toilet of perforated duodenal ulcer. Surgical Endoscopy 4: 232–233

O'Rourke N A, Askew A R, Cowan A E 1993 The role of ERCP and endoscopic sphincterotomy in the era of laparoscopic cholecystectomy. Australian and New Zealand Journal of Surgery 63: 307

Reddick E J et al 1991 Safe performance of difficult laparoscopic cholecystectomies. American Journal of Surgery 166: 377–381

Russell R C G 1993 Minimally invasive surgery: biliary surgery. British Medical Journal 307: 1266–1269

Sackier J A, Berci G, Phillips E 1991 The role of cholangiography in laparoscopic cholecystectomy. Archives of Surgery 126: 1621–1626

Schirmer B D et al 1992 Incorporation of laparoscopy into a surgical endoscopy training program. American Journal of Surgery 163: 46–52

Scott-Coombes D, Thompson J N 1991 Bile duct stones and laparoscopic cholecystectomy. British Medical Journal 303: 1281–1282

Stoke M E, Vose J, O'Mara P 1991 Laparoscopic cholecystectomy – a clinical and financial analysis of 288 operations. American Journal of Surgery 161: 355–360

The Southern Surgical Club 1991 A prospective analysis of 1518 laparoscopic cholecystectomies. New England Journal of Medicine 324: 1073–1078

Wickham J E A 1994 Minimally invasive surgery: future developments. British Medical Journal 308: 193–196

Wilson R G et al 1992 Laparoscopic cholecystectomy: a safe and effective treatment for severe acute cholecystitis. British Medical Journal 305: 394–396

Laparotomy for injury or peritonitis

R. F. RINTOUL

An exploratory laparotomy is carried out in conditions where the need for operation is recognized, but where a definite diagnosis cannot be made until the abdomen has been opened. Such conditions arise most characteristically in cases of suspected intraperitoneal injury, whether this is due to crushing or bruising of the abdomen or to a penetrating wound. An accurate preoperative diagnosis is usually impossible although investigation by peritoneal lavage, ultrasound scanning or CT scanning may be helpful. If the evidence suggests that any intraperitoneal viscus has been injured the abdomen must as a rule be explored.

Exploratory laparotomy may be required also in the various emergencies which constitute the 'acute abdomen.' Whenever possible, an attempt should be made to arrive at an accurate diagnosis before the operation is commenced, since this allows preoperative treatment to be planned. In many cases, however, it may be impossible to reach any diagnosis other than that of 'acute abdomen' and the surgeon must proceed to exploratory laparotomy. Where doubt exists, an attempt should be made to decide whether the incision should be commenced in the upper or the lower abdomen. Palpation of the relaxed abdomen, once the patient has been anaesthetized, may reveal a mass which was not previously apparent and help the surgeon in his approach to the problem.

If a diagnosis of acute appendicitis can be made with some confidence, the abdomen is opened by a grid-iron incision in the right iliac fossa. Should it be found that the peritonitis has been caused by an alternative pathological process, it will be preferable to close the incision and to reopen the abdomen in the optimum situation.

LAPAROTOMY FOR INTRAPERITONEAL INJURIES

In *bruising* and *crushing* injuries of the abdomen any intraperitoneal organ may be ruptured without the association of superficial trauma. All *penetrating* wounds of the peritoneal cavity are likely to cause internal damage (Donaldson, 1981). The external wound is not necessarily situated in the anterior abdominal wall — it may be in the thorax, the loin, the buttock or the perineum.

The clinical picture in cases of intraperitoneal injury varies considerably, and may even be misleading when multiple injuries are present, particularly if these include the head or chest. It is advisable to explore the abdomen in doubtful cases unless injury can be excluded with reasonable certainty. Paracentesis, carried out in the four quadrants of the abdomen, may help in this decision (Powell, 1982). *Abdominal lavage* is an alternative diagnostic test; through a cannula inserted just below the umbilicus, 500 ml of saline is run into the peritoneal cavity and returned from the patient by lowering the container below the level of the abdomen. The detection of free gas or fluid (usually blood) in the peritoneal cavity is diagnostic of injury. In the presence of a damaged viscus, shock is usually present and is likely to be severe; it is not in itself a sign of diagnostic value, but if it persists after resuscitative treatment it is strong evidence of internal injury. Another sign of even greater importance is a rising pulse rate. Pain, tenderness and rigidity are present in varying degree but are unreliable in reaching a diagnosis of internal injury. Injuries to the urinary tract, which are most likely to be extraperitoneal, can usually be excluded by the passage of a catheter.

The prognosis in cases of intraperitoneal injury depends very largely on the length of time that is allowed to elapse before operation is carried out. The patient must first, however, receive adequate intravenous therapy, which will often include blood transfusion. The aim of resuscitation is to make the patient fit for anaesthesia and full blood replacement should not be attempted until the start of operation.

Late cases. When the patient comes to treatment 24 hours or longer after the injury, laparotomy may not necessarily be indicated. If the patient has survived in reasonable condition for that time, it is likely that haemorrhage has been arrested spontaneously, and that ruptured viscera have become sealed off by adhesions.

Laparotomy should, however, be performed if there are signs of general peritonitis, or of continued or recurrent intraperitoneal haemorrhage. This is particularly applicable to a patient who fails to stabilize following recovery from a head injury or fixation of major limb fractures.

Technique of exploration

In the absence of any localizing signs it is usual to open the abdomen through a midline incision above and below the umbilicus; through this most of the abdominal organs can be investigated. The incision may be enlarged either upwards or downwards, or by cutting across one rectus muscle. When a wound is present in the anterior abdominal wall, it is a good practice to excise the wound and to use that approach to the peritoneal cavity — at least for the preliminary exploration. A stab wound, the depth of which is unknown, is best explored through a separate incision so that inspection of the damaged area is unimpeded by blood escaping from the laparotomy wound.

If any viscus has been injured there will usually be a certain amount of haemorrhage in the peritoneal cavity. A large collection of blood suggests damage to a solid viscus — spleen, liver, mesentery and omentum being the structures which are most commonly injured. These are, therefore, investigated first in order that the source of bleeding may be located and dealt with.

If the gut has been ruptured, turbid or bile-stained fluid, or (in the case of the colon) faecal matter may be present in the peritoneal cavity. In small perforations, however, owing to the sealing effect of pouting mucous membrane, little or no escape of contents may occur. A 'clean' peritoneal cavity in no way excludes such injuries.

The *small intestine* is injured more commonly than all the other hollow viscera, and it must be systematically examined throughout its entire length. The examination may be commenced either at the duodeno-jejunal flexure or at the caecum. No more than one loop should be withdrawn from the wound at one time; it is examined carefully from both sides, and as soon as it has been passed as being intact it is returned by the assistant to the abdomen. If a perforation of the gut is discovered it is closed with a clamp or with light tissue forceps. The affected loop is retained on the surface, covered with a moist towel, while the rest of the gut is examined. It is most important, especially in penetrating wounds where there may be multiple intestinal injuries, to ascertain the full extent of the damage before undertaking the repair of any single lesion, for the discovery of further injuries will often determine the treatment which is to be adopted, e.g. it may be necessary to resect a segment of bowel.

The *stomach and duodenum* are brought into view by gentle traction on the omentum and are examined both visually and by palpation.

The *transverse colon* is examined at the same time as the stomach. By suitable retraction and by packing off of coils of small bowel, the other parts of the colon are then investigated in turn. The presence of a retroperitoneal haematoma in relation to the fixed vertical parts of the colon suggests a rupture in its posterior wall. Examination of the suspected area should be delayed until full assessment of other injuries has been made, since a resection of colon may be required (see below); this can only be achieved if the surgeon has the necessary experience otherwise the damaged colon should be approached retroperitoneally through an incision in the flank so as to avoid peritoneal contamination.

Injuries of the spleen

The spleen is very commonly ruptured as the result of crushing injuries or of blows on the flank. Suture of the rent may occasionally be possible but *splenectomy* (p. 405) is usually required to control bleeding. If blood for transfusion is not available, unclotted blood from within the peritoneal cavity, after being filtered through gauze and citrated, may be returned to a vein (p. 29).

Injuries of the liver

Penetrating wounds of the liver may be treated on conservative lines, provided that the surgeon feels secure in his belief that no other organ has been damaged. Liver wounds as a whole, however, are usually associated with severe intraperitoneal haemorrhage, and it is on this account that laparotomy is likely to be required. In centres where CT scanning is available, this will already have been done and the findings will be taken into consideration when advising laparotomy. When the abdomen has been opened, both upper and lower surfaces of the liver should be carefully examined. If the operation field is obscured by profuse haemorrhage, this may be arrested by temporary compression of the hepatic artery as it lies in the free border of the lesser omentum — either with a light bowel clamp or digitally (*Pringle's manoeuvre*). Wounds involving the upper or posterior aspects of the liver may be inaccessible from an abdominal approach. They are then best exposed transdiaphragmatically through a right thoracotomy, the chest being opened in the 8th or 9th intercostal space. Wounds which are recognized preoperatively to be thoracoabdominal should as a general rule be explored, in the first instance, through the chest (p. 91). When the tear has been identified it should be gently but firmly packed with gauze, which is left in situ for 2 or 3 minutes. After removal of the gauze, spouting vessels in the liver substance may be picked up and coagulated, or occluded by suture (Kingsnorth, 1992).

Tears are best repaired with deeply placed stitches of thick catgut or other absorbable material carried on a round-bodied needle. If the stitches tend to cut out, they may be supported by a flap of falciform ligament or by a free transplant from the rectus sheath, which is laid on the liver surface. In extensive injuries, devitalised liver tissue should be removed as resectional debridement (Blumgart, 1988) rather than as a more formal hepatic lobectomy. Drainage to the exterior should always be provided using corrugated plastic or suction, as there is likely to be leakage of bile. In some cases, packing of the liver for up to 48 hours may be a life saving measure (Krige, 1992).

Injuries of mesentery

If spleen and liver are intact, laceration of the mesentery is the next most likely cause of haemorrhage. This is a serious injury since the blood supply of the related segment of bowel may be endangered, especially if the tear lies parallel and in close proximity to the gut (Fig. 16.1). Smaller tears and those placed radially to the gut are not so serious, and can as a rule be treated effectively by simple suture; the production of further haemorrhage is avoided if the needle, threaded in the usual way, is passed *eye first* through the mesenteric tissue. The operator must be satisfied that the blood supply of the gut has not been interfered with; either pallor, cyanosis or oedema is a dangerous sign, and may demand resection.

Haematoma of the mesentery results when a vessel is ruptured without laceration of the peritoneal layers. The blood should be evacuated through a small inci-

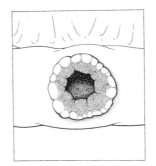
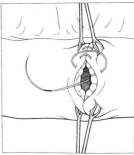

Fig. 16.2　　　　　**Fig. 16.3**

Figs 16.2 & 16.3 Wound of small bowel, such as may be caused either by a penetrating missile or by a crushing injury. The method of repair in the transverse axis is shown

sion, and if necessary the bleeding vessel is ligatured. The related segment of bowel should be examined carefully to ensure that its blood supply is adequate.

Injuries of the small intestine

The systematic examination of the small intestine has already been described.

Simple suture of wounds should be carried out whenever possible. Very small perforations can be closed by a single purse-string suture of Lembert type. Larger wounds are repaired by two layers of sutures. If the edges of the tear are ragged or bruised they may be excised. It is an advantage to stitch up the tear *transversely* (Fig. 16.3), in order that narrowing of the lumen will be prevented. It is probable, however, that the dangers of narrowing have been exaggerated; since the contents of the small intestine are fluid, it is unlikely that obstruction will occur unless the narrowing amounts almost to complete occlusion. If the patency of the gut is in doubt the affected segment may be short-circuited by a lateral anastomosis, or, alternatively, resection may be performed. Areas of bruising on the gut wall (without perforation) should be infolded by Lembert suture.

Resection with anastomosis (p. 471) may be advisable when there are multiple injuries confined to one segment of the gut, or when laceration or bruising is extensive; it is essential if the blood supply of the gut has been destroyed or seriously endangered by associated mesenteric injury.

In most cases of intestinal rupture, drainage of the peritoneal cavity should be provided unless thorough cleansing of the peritoneal cavity has been achieved with antibiotic lavage.

Injuries of the colon

Rupture of the colon as the result of crushing or bruising injuries is not uncommon. When caused by a pen-

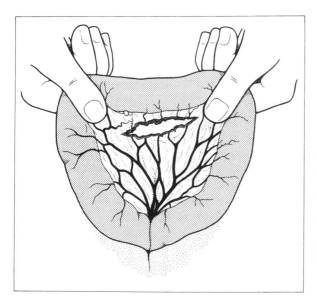

Fig. 16.1 A tear of the mesentery lying parallel and in close proximity to the bowel makes resection imperative, since the blood supply of the gut is seriously endangered

etrating wound it is usually associated with injuries of other viscera. Sometimes there is no more than bruising of the gut wall, but secondary perforation is a likely sequel. Bruised areas should, therefore, be infolded carefully or covered with omentum. Severely injured colon should always be excised (Parks, 1991).

Intraperitoneal ruptures should as a rule be treated by resection. When, however, the perforation is clean-cut and the bowel wall little damaged, as may occur with stab wounds or traversing bullet wounds, careful suture of the tear may be performed. Tetracycline 0.1% solution is used for intraperitoneal lavage — using 1–3 litres of solution — but a drain should be left in position against the sutured bowel, so that any escape of contents will take place towards the surface.

Retroperitoneal rupture is more likely to occur in the fixed vertical parts of the colon. It is more serious than intraperitoneal rupture if it remains undetected, due to the anaerobic organisms which escape into the retroperitoneal tissues. If this type of injury is suspected at laparotomy, the colon is mobilized to allow for thorough inspection, resection and cleansing of the area. The experience of the surgeon and available facilities will determine whether bowel continuity is reestablished or the bowel ends are exteriorized. If a wound is present in the flank it should be explored to assess damage and contamination, and may be drained if necessary. Following repair or resection of colon, the advisability of a proximal colostomy should be considered. This is essential in unfavourable circumstances but otherwise it delays the patient's recovery (Naraynsingh, 1991). When the colonic suture requires protection, a caecostomy may suffice in some cases but a proximal colostomy of *defunctioning type* (p. 475) is a better safeguard against leakage and subsequent infection.

Injuries of the stomach and duodenum are uncommon except in penetrating wounds, when they are usually associated with damage to other viscera.

Both surfaces of the stomach should be examined — the posterior, through an opening made into the lesser sac, either through the anterior layers of the greater omentum or through the transverse mesocolon. Repair is effected by two layers of suture. Wounds of the curvatures of the stomach are accompanied by profuse haemorrhage, and the divided vessels require to be ligatured.

Wounds of the duodenum are likely to implicate surrounding structures such as the pancreas, the common bile duct, the portal vein or the hilum of the kidney, or they may give rise to extensive retroperitoneal extravasation. They are, therefore, usually fatal.

Injuries of the pancreas
Tears in the pancreas should be repaired accurately by suture, access being obtained to the lesser sac via the gastro-colic omentum. Sometimes, in association with a ruptured spleen, the tail of the pancreas is torn completely across. The severed portion should then be removed. Prophylactic broad spectrum antibiotics should be administered; drainage is advisable in all cases (Wilson, 1991).

Injuries of the gall bladder and bile ducts
These will be suspected if there is a large collection of bile in the peritoneal cavity. A ruptured gall bladder or cystic duct is best treated by cholecystectomy. A torn common bile duct may be repaired by suture over a T-tube (p. 437).

Injuries of the kidney
Renal damage is confirmed by intravenous pyelography which demonstrates delay in function or leakage of dye on one side. The associated retroperitoneal haemorrhage may, by sympathetic stimulation, result in an ileus which, unfortunately, adds to the difficulty of interpreting the abdominal signs. Operations for renal injuries are discussed on page 598.

Intraperitoneal rupture of the bladder
The tear, which is necessarily situated on the peritoneal surface of the bladder, is repaired by two layers of suture. The peritoneum, after careful suction and lavage, may be closed. The bladder is kept empty by an indwelling urethral catheter (see also pp. 555 & 623).

LAPAROTOMY FOR PERITONITIS

The necessarily incomplete diagnosis of 'acute abdomen' will be made when the clinical evidence suggests no more than the existence of peritonitis. If there is any reason to believe that the peritonitis has resulted from perforation of the gut, e.g. from a gangrenous appendix or from a perforated peptic or typhoid ulcer, laparotomy is imperative. When advanced generalized peritonitis is present, and when the pulse is rapid and thready, it is always advisable to delay operation for 2 or 3 hours, while the patient's general condition is improved by intravenous infusion, antibiotics and gastric aspiration. A broad spectrum antibiotic is appropriate in all cases, with the addition of a drug active against anaerobic organisms if bowel pathology is suspected.

Principles of operative treatment
Unless the appendix has previously been removed it usually will be suspect. If this is the case it is a good plan to open the abdomen through a right gridiron incision. Should the appendix be healthy it will often be possible through this incision to determine the cause or nature of the peritonitis. If no operative treatment other

than peritoneal drainage is indicated, the incision is utilised to guide a drainage tube, introduced through an appropriate stab wound, down to the rectovesical pouch. If further access is required the gridiron incision can be enlarged so as to allow inspection of the uterine adnexa. Alternatively, if a second incision is indicated the gridiron is easily and rapidly closed. When the appendix is not immediately suspected as the cause of peritonitis, a long midline incision centred over the area of suspected pathology will as a rule be employed.

The priority in all cases of peritonitis is rapid evacuation of toxic exudate by suction. The surgeon may then concentrate his attention on the source of the infection and carry out appropriate definitive treatment such as removal of a gangrenous appendix. Antibiotic peritoneal lavage, using 1–3 litres of tetracycline solution (1 g per litre), is useful in dealing with residual infection (Stewart, 1980). The fluid is directed into the recesses of the abdomen by the exploring hand and trapped debris is aspirated.

Nature of the peritoneal exudate. Brownish-coloured fluid with the putrid smell of bowel organisms is almost diagnostic of a perforated appendix, or a perforated diverticulitis. Milky fluid with flakes of lymph — often bilestained — suggests a gastric or intestinal perforation. In pneumococcal peritonitis the exudate is characteristic; it is greenish-yellow in colour, creamy and odourless. In streptococcal peritonitis the fluid is turbid and sometimes blood-stained. A tuberculous effusion is clear and straw-coloured. In all cases, a specimen of the peritoneal fluid is taken for culture so as to confirm the causative organism and its antibiotic sensitivity.

Pneumococcal peritonitis is usually a primary infection. It occurs most commonly in female children under the age of 10, when it may be associated with a pneumococcal vaginitis.

Conservative treatment may be employed, provided that other causes of peritonitis can be excluded with reasonable certainly. It is usually safer, however, to open the abdomen — even if only to verify the diagnosis, since the risks of missing a gangrenous appendix with general peritonitis greatly outweigh those of operation.

The approach should be through a small gridiron incision. The diagnosis will be made usually from the character of the exudate, and from the failure to find any primary focus of infection within the abdomen. As much as possible of the exudate is removed by suction following antibiotic lavage and the abdomen is closed.

Streptococcal peritonitis is treated on similar lines to those described for pneumococcal peritonitis, but, since the exudate is more toxic, drainage is advisable in all cases.

Peritonitis due to salpingitis

As a rule the peritonitis is localised to the pelvis. Laparotomy is contraindicated, but sometimes the diagnosis is not made until the abdomen has been opened. It is usually advised that the inflamed tube should be left in situ (p. 689). Occasionally, however, there is a tubo-ovarian abscess which requires removal rather than drainage. This should not lead to regret on the part of the surgeon since the function of the tube will have already been destroyed by the severity of the infection. Ruptured ectopic pregnancy is discussed on page 686.

Tuberculous peritonitis

The acute type is uncommon; it occurs usually as a flare-up of a previously unsuspected chronic condition, and is unlikely to be diagnosed before the abdomen has been opened. The condition is then apparent from the presence of clear straw-coloured exudate and of tubercles. As much fluid as possible is removed; a sample is sent for bacteriological examination, and one or more peritoneal nodules are removed for histology (Hodgson, 1988). The abdomen is then closed *without drainage*. If the condition is suspected prior to laparotomy, the diagnosis may be confirmed by laparoscopy, biopsy or culture of peritoneal fluid (Reeve, 1992).

Chronic tuberculous peritonitis. In the *fibrous* or *adhesive* type of tuberculous peritonitis, laparotomy may be carried out in order to establish the diagnosis, or to deal with intestinal obstruction.

REFERENCES

Blumgart L H 1988 Surgery of the liver and biliary tract. Churchill Livingstone, Edinburgh, p. 1045

Donaldson L A, Findlay I G, Smith A 1981 A retrospective view of 89 stab wounds to the abdomen and chest. British Journal of Surgery 68: 793–796

Hodgson T J, Duncan J L, Rogers K 1988 Tuberculosis: a surgical viewpoint. Annals of the Royal College of Surgeons of England 70: 117–119

Kingsnorth A N, Gilmore I T 1992 Traumatic and Iatrogenic emergencies. In: I T Gilmore, Shields R (eds) Gastrointestinal emergencies. W B Saunders, London

Krige J E J, Bornman P C, Terblanche J 1992 Therapeutic perihepatic packing in complex liver trauma. British Journal of Surgery 79: 43–46

Naraynsingh V, Ariyanayagam D, Pooran S 1991 Primary repair of colon injuries in a developing country. British Journal of Surgery 78: 319–320

Parks T G 1991 Abdominal Injuries. In: O'Higgins N J, Chisholm G D, Williamson R C N (eds) Surgical management. Butterworth Heinemann, Oxford, p. 277

Powell D C, Bivins B A, Bell R M 1982 Diagnostic peritoneal lavage. Surgery Gynaecology and Obstetrics 155: 257–264

Reeve P A 1992 Ascites: a guide to diagnosis in the district
    hospital. Tropical Doctor 22: 52–56
Stewart D J 1980 Generalised peritonitis. Journal of the
    Royal College of Surgeons of Edinburgh 25: 80–90

Wilson R H, Moorehead R J 1991 Current management of
    trauma to the pancreas. British Journal of Surgery
    78: 1196–1202

FURTHER READING

Maingot R 1985 Abdominal operations, 8th edn. Appleton-
    Century-Crofts, New York, Ch 13–15 and 21

Trunkey D 1980 Massive abdominal injury; In: Hardy J D
    (ed.) Critical surgical illness, 2nd edn. Saunders,
    Philadelphia, ch 8

17

Stomach and duodenum

I. M. C. MACINTYRE & J. M. S. JOHNSTONE

In recent years there has been a dramatic reduction in the numbers of patients undergoing elective surgery for peptic ulcer disease. The world wide reduction in the incidence of duodenal ulcer combined with the introduction of potent acid-reducing agents has resulted in a decline in the number of patients referred for surgical treatment. Advances in endoscopic treatment of bleed-ing peptic ulcer have led to fewer operations for bleed-ing peptic ulcer. The mortality from gastric cancer has declined throughout the world yet the number of op-erations performed for gastric cancer appears to have declined at the same rate. There has been increasing appreciation that a combination of early diagnosis and radical lymphadenectomy can result in cure.

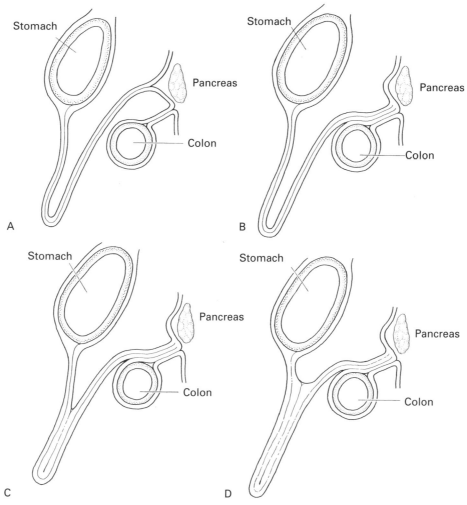

Fig. 17.1 Lateral view showing formation of greater omentum (similar to Nyhus and Westell, p. 42)

Embryology

The stomach originates as a dilatation of the foregut, a simple tube with a dorsal and a ventral mesentery. The dorsal aspect of the stomach grows more rapidly than the ventral aspect forcing the distal stomach and duodenum upwards and to the right. Thus the ventral mesentery becomes the lesser omentum and the dorsal mesentery the greater omentum. The greater omentum is formed by the fusion of the posterior wall of the lesser sac to the transverse colon and mesocolon (Fig. 17.1).

The fusion of the anterior and posterior walls of the omental bursa results in the formation of the gastrocolic omentum which thus has four layers, an important consideration in the operation of radical gastrectomy.

Anatomy

The stomach is divided into three major zones (Fig. 17.2) — fundus, body and antrum. The area around the gastro-oesophageal junction is known as the cardia. The *fundus* is that part of the stomach which lies above the gastro-oesophageal junction; the *body* is limited distally by the incisura angularis where it becomes the *antrum,* which extends to the pylorus.

The inferior 5 cm or so of the oesophagus lie within the abdomen and thus the oesophagus enters the lesser curve of the stomach well below the fundus. Gastro-oesophageal reflux is prevented by a functional lower oesophageal sphincter which results from a combination of pressure difference across the diaphragm, the sling action of the right crus of the diaphragm, the rosette of gastric mucosa which acts as a flap valve and the angle at which the oesophagus enters the stomach. The fundus and proximal body of the stomach are compliant to permit storage of ingested food. This adaptive relaxation is mediated through the vagus and loss of this adaptation following highly selective vagotomy gives rise to the very common feeling of bloating following this operation. The lower body and antrum on the other hand has greater motor activity, acting as a mechanical mill to mix ingested food and deliver it in liquid form (*chyme*) through the pylorus. The nerve fibres which control this motor activity pass along the nerve of Latarjet.

The pyloric sphincter is a well defined ring of circular muscle dividing stomach from duodenum. This sphincter regulates the rate of delivery of chyme into the duodenum and prevents duodeno-gastric reflux although the mechanisms controlling this are not well understood. The duodenum (Fig. 17.2) is divided into four parts. The first part of the duodenum consists of the duodenal bulb or cap, the site of over 90% of duodenal ulcers. The *first part* of the duodenum extends laterally and posteriorly for some 5 cm; the *second part* descends vertically for 10 cm, intimately associated with the head of the pancreas receiving the common bile duct and the pancreatic duct on its concave medial wall. The *third part* of the duodenum passes horizontally and is crossed by the superior mesenteric vessels. The *fourth part* of the duodenum ascends to the left of the aorta to become the duodeno-jejunal flexure.

A cross section through the wall of the stomach (Fig. 17.3) shows that it consists of mucosa, submucosa, a muscle layer (outer longitudinal, middle circular and inner oblique) which for surgical purposes can be regarded as a single layer. The mucosa in the fundus and body of the stomach contains parietal cells

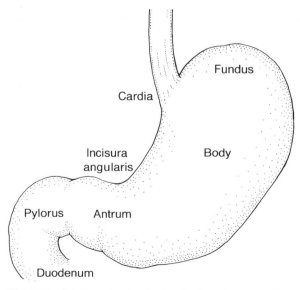

Fig. 17.2 Diagram showing fundus, body, antrum, cardia and duodenum

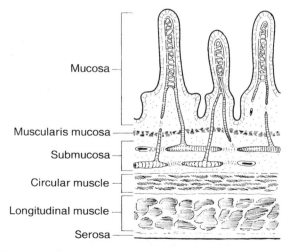

Fig. 17.3 Cross-section through wall of stomach

which secrete acid and chief cells secreting pepsin. The mucosa in this region is thrown into rugal folds while that of the antrum is smooth. Proximally the columnar mucosa lining the stomach may extend up into the lower oesophagus, a phenomenon associated with gastro-oesophageal reflux, which may progress to Barret's oesophagus.

The stomach is completely covered by peritoneum (apart from a small area just below the gastro-oesophageal junction posteriorly). The peritoneum covering the anterior and posterior walls of the stomach meet at the lesser curve and pass upwards as the *lesser omentum* to the porta hepatis.

At the greater curvature, the peritoneal layers meet to form the *greater omentum,* the *gastrosplenic* (lieno-gastric) *ligament,* and the *gastrophrenic ligament.* The greater omentum arises from the greater curvature of the antrum and lower portion of the body of stomach, and extends downwards in front of the transverse colon (Fig. 17.4). As the greater omentum returns over the transverse colon its posterior surface fuses with the anterior surface of the transverse mesocolon.

The lesser sac lies behind the caudate lobe of the liver, lesser omentum and stomach. It extends for a variable distance into the greater omentum in front

of the transverse colon but in most adults this part of the lesser sac is obliterated (Fig. 17.4). The surgeon can gain access to the lesser sac by creating a window in the lesser omentum, transverse mesocolon or gastro-colic portion of the greater omentum. Although the lesser omentum is avascular close to the liver, generous access to the lesser sac is prevented by the structures in the free edge of the lesser omentum (hepatic artery, portal vein and bile duct). Exposure through the mesocolon is limited by the middle colic artery. When wide exposure of the lesser sac is needed, as for example in operations involving the pancreas, the gastro-colic portion of the greater omentum may be widely incised in a line parallel to the greater curvature of the stomach. The incision lies outwith the gastro-epiploic vessels and individual omental vessels are divided between ligatures. Avascular adhesions between the posterior wall of the stomach and front of pancreas have to be divided to allow unrestricted access to the lesser sac.

The *blood supply* to the stomach comes largely from the coeliac axis via its three branches, the hepatic, splenic and left gastric arteries. Arterial arches run along the greater and lesser curvatures between the layers of the omenta. The greater curve arch or arcade is formed from the right gastro-epiploic branch of the

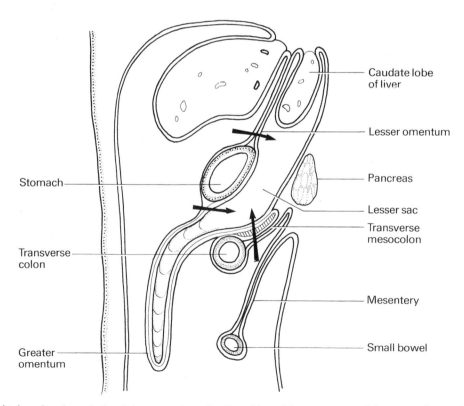

Fig. 17.4 Sagittal section through the abdomen to show the disposition of the omentum and lesser sac. Arrows indicate the means of access to the lesser sac

gastroduodenal artery, and from the left gastro-epiploic branch of the splenic artery. The lesser curve arch is formed from the descending branch of the left gastric artery and the right gastric branch of the common hepatic artery. The blood supply of the greater curve is supplemented by the short gastric branches of the splenic artery which travel in the gastrosplenic ligament to the fundus and upper part of the body of stomach (Fig. 17.5).

The right gastric artery, most commonly a branch of the hepatic, forms an arcade with the left gastric along the lesser curve of the stomach. The gastro-epiploic arcade feeds the greater curvature aspect, the right gastro-epiploic artery deriving from the gastro-duodenal and the left gastro-epiploic from the splenic. In addition the upper part of the greater curvature receives some four or five short gastric arteries from the splenic artery or one of its terminal branches.

The duodenum is supplied by the gastro-duodenal artery, the right gastro-epiploic artery and the superior pancreatico-duodenal artery. The accompanying veins drain into the portal venous system.

The *arteries of the duodenum* are derived from the coeliac and superior mesenteric vessels. The first part of the duodenum receives branches from the right gastric, gastroduodenal and right gastro-epiploic arteries. The superior pancreatico-duodenal artery is one of the two terminal branches of the gastroduodenal (Fig. 17.5) and runs downwards in the concavity of the duodenum to anastomose with the inferior pancreatico-duodenal branch of the superior mesenteric artery. The pancreatico-duodenal vessels form an arcade on the front of the head of pancreas. There is also a posterior pancreatico-duodenal arcade behind the head of the gland. In about 10% of subjects, the superior mesenteric artery gives off a right hepatic branch which ascends behind the pancreas and is usually the sole supply to the right lobe of liver. In 2–3% of individuals, the common hepatic artery arises from the superior mesenteric.

The *veins from the stomach and duodenum* accompany the arteries and drain into the portal system via the splenic or superior mesenteric veins.

Lymphatic drainage. The lymphatics of the stomach anastomose freely in the submucosa, communicate with intermuscular lymphatics, and then drain into a subserosal network. This network drains in turn into large lymphatic vessels which accompany the four main arteries to the lesser and greater curvatures. The submucosal lymphatics of stomach and lower oesophagus communicate freely, facilitating spread of carcinoma between these structures. There is debate as to the degree of communication between antral and duodenal

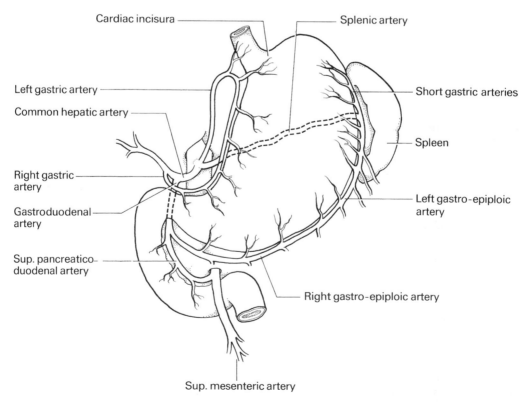

Fig. 17.5 Arterial blood supply to the stomach and proximal duodenum

lymphatics across the pylorus. Material injected into the wall of the stomach spreads evenly in the gastric submucosa but stops abruptly at the pylorus. However, the proximal duodenum occasionally becomes involved by carcinoma arising in the distal stomach, and as direct spread is unusual, retrograde spread from subpyloric nodes may be responsible.

Our understanding of the lymphatic drainage of the stomach has been greatly enhanced by the Japanese concept of 'tiers' of lymph nodes to which gastric cancer may progressively spread. These tiers are known as N1, N2, N3 and N4 and each tier consists of several groups of nodes each of which is numbered (Fig. 17.6). N1 nodes are those lying closest to the stomach and consist of 6 groups:

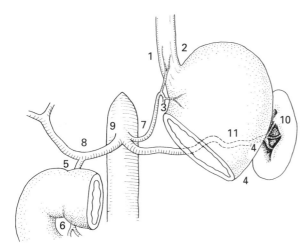

Fig. 17.6   Lymphatic drainage — N1 and N2 nodes

- nodes to right of cardia (No 1)
- nodes to left of cardia (No 2)
- nodes along lesser curve (No 3)
- nodes along greater curve (No 4)
- suprapyloric nodes (No 5)
- infrapyloric nodes (No 6).

The N2 group of nodes are those along the three named branches of the coeliac axis and consists of:

- left gastric artery nodes (No 7)
- common hepatic artery nodes (No 8)
- coeliac artery nodes (No 9)
- splenic hilum nodes (No 10)
- splenic artery nodes (No 11)

The N3 group of nodes are more distant and comprises:

- nodes in the lesser omentum (No 12)
- retropancreatic nodes (No 13)
- nodes in root of small bowel mesentery (No 14)

- nodes along the middle colic artery (No 15)
- para-aortic nodes above left renal vein (No 16)

Knowledge of the lymphatic drainage of the stomach has important implications for the staging and treatment of gastric cancer. The classification of lymph node drainage of the stomach has allowed more precise staging of this disease and thus more precise definition of radical resection known as either R2 or R3 resection. The relevance of the classification of nodes by tiers will become apparent when radical resection for gastric cancer is discussed.

The stomach has both sympathetic and para-sympathetic *innervation*, the latter provided by the *vagus nerve*. Shortly after emerging through the oesophageal hiatus both the anterior vagus and posterior vagus give off hepato-biliary fibres and continue as the anterior and posterior nerves of Latarjet (Fig. 17.7).

The nerves of Latarjet supply branches to the body of the stomach, each branch passing close to a vascular pedicle. These fibres are secretor motor to the parietal cells and are divided in the operation of highly selective vagotomy. The nerve of Latarjet continues towards the antrum to end in a configuration known as the 'crows foot' which innervates the myenteric plexus of the antrum.

INVESTIGATION OF GASTRODUODENAL DISEASE

A detailed history and full physical examination are essential. The following specialized investigations may be helpful when gastroduodenal disease is suspected.

Barium swallow and meal

Barium swallow is used primarily in the investigation of oesophageal disorders whereas barium meal is intended to display the lower oesophagus, oesophagogastric junction, stomach, pylorus and proximal duodenum.

In patients with peptic ulceration, abnormal motility is often apparent during screening. The ulcer crater may be visible 'en face' or in profile, and surrounding oedema and radiating mucosal folds may be seen. In some patients an ulcer crater is not detected but ulceration (past or present) is inferred from scarring and deformity.

In patients with gastric neoplasia the radiological appearances depend upon the type of lesion. Proliferative carcinoma produces a filling defect which encroaches on the gastric lumen while infiltrative lesions produce mucosal irregularity and rigidity of the stomach wall, and ulcerating lesions produce a crater. Radiological discrimination between benign and malignant ulceration can be difficult. Malignant ulcers tend to be large,

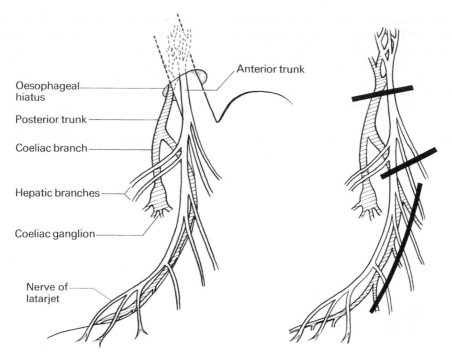

Oesophageal hiatus

Posterior trunk

Coeliac branch

Hepatic branches

Coeliac ganglion

Nerve of latarjet

Anterior trunk

Fig. 17.7 Vagal innervation of the stomach. The three bars indicate the levels of section in truncal vagotomy; selective vagotomy; and highly selective vagotomy

have raised or rolled edges, frequently involve areas outwith the lesser curvature, and do not have mucosal folds radiating from the edge of the ulcer crater. When seen in profile, the ulcer base usually lies within the line of the wall of the stomach. Benign gastric ulcers are often smaller; do not have raised or rolled edges; are particularly common on the lesser curvature; may have radiating mucosal folds; and when seen in profile, the base of the ulcer crater usually projects outwith the line of the wall of the stomach. These guidelines have exceptions so that fibreoptic endoscopy and biopsy is mandatory in all patients found to have a gastric ulcer on barium meal examination.

Fibreoptic endoscopy

As with barium meal examination, accuracy depends on the skill and experience of the individual carrying out the examination. Endoscopy has the advantages that the lesion is seen directly, biopsy or brush cytology is possible, and any source of upper gastrointestinal bleeding can be determined. Either investigation can be used in the diagnosis of duodenal ulcer. Given a firm diagnosis of duodenal ulcer with one technique, there is no need routinely to employ the other. While either investigation can be used to diagnose gastric ulceration, endoscopy allows multiple biopsies of the ulcer and its surroundings and is essential to exclude malignancy. In the event that a gastric ulcer appears benign and medical treatment is employed, vigilance must still be main-

tained with repeat endoscopy after 4 to 6 weeks to confirm ulcer healing. Endoscopy is superior in the diagnosis of erosions and acute and chronic gastritis. Endoscopic biopsy may reveal dysplasia or metaplasia, some varieties of which are potentially premalignant conditions.

Acid secretory testing

Definition of maximal acid output by testing with pentagastrin (or histamine) has little value in the diagnosis of peptic ulceration or gastric cancer. It is true that duodenal ulcer patients often have a high acid output, that patients with gastric ulcer often have a low output, and that gastric cancer is associated with hypochlorhydria or achlorhydria yet there is considerable overlap between the groups. Acid secretory tests were once used to select the type of operation to be performed for duodenal ulcer but are now seldom employed for this purpose. Similarly vagally mediated gastric output may be measured to assess the completeness of a truncal vagotomy. The insulin infusion test has now been replaced by the sham feed test where vagally mediated acid secretion is assessed by asking the patient to chew and subsequently spit out a test meal.

Basal and stimulated serum gastrin

Measurement of fasting serum gastrin levels is used to screen patients in whom the Zollinger-Ellison syndrome (ZES) is suspected. Other conditions associated with hypergastrinaemia include pernicious anaemia, retained antrum after Polya gastrectomy, hyperparathyroidism, and antral G cell hyperplasia. When the ZES is suspected in patients with borderline hypergastrinaemia, a further rise in serum gastrin can be provoked by intravenous secretin injection, intravenous calcium infusion or ingestion of a protein meal. Injection of secretin (2 units/kg. by bolus i.v. injection) is recommended (McGuigan, 1980) and in the ZES provokes a 50% rise in serum gastrin within 10–15 minutes of injection. When the ZES has been confirmed, the tumour may be localized and its resectability assessed by venous sampling from a catheter inserted into the portal venous system by the percutaneous transhepatic technique.

Gastric emptying studies

An isotope labelled test meal may be used to assess the liquid and solid phases of gastric emptying. Impaired emptying of solids may be demonstrated by this technique whereas emptying, as assessed by liquid barium, has shown no abnormality.

PATHOGENESIS OF PEPTIC ULCER AND GASTRIC CANCER

Peptic ulcer

Although much is known about the factors which are associated with the development of peptic ulcer disease, there is much to be learned. Different factors apply in duodenal and gastric ulcer and they are considered as separate entities.

In *duodenal ulcer* disease genetic factors play a role in aetiology with those more aggressive ulcers in particular having a familial tendency. Blood group O is also a risk factor particularly in non-secretors (those unable to secrete blood group substances in a water-soluble form) and again this is most strongly associated in aggressive ulcer disease i.e. disease which is complicated or resistant to treatment. Hyperpepsinogenaemia has also been shown to be a risk factor. Dietary and lifestyle factors such as alcohol intake, smoking and stress have also been implicated.

The balance between acid and pepsin secretion and mucosal resistance has been intensively studied. As a group, patients with duodenal ulcer have a higher acid output probably because of a larger parietal cell mass. Similarly pepsinogens, the precursors of gastric pepsin, are increased in serum of the majority of patients with duodenal ulcer. Much less is known about the other side of the balance: mucosal resistance. The layer of mucus traps the alkaline secretion of the surface epithelium, and prevents back diffusion of acid from the lumen. This barrier may be damaged by bile salts, alcohol and non-steroidal anti-inflammatory agents.

The role of Helicobacter pylori infection remains unclear but it has become established that infection with this organism has become an important, if not the single most important, factor in the aetiology of duodenal ulcer. In the face of persisting infection a duodenal ulcer is unlikely to heal and ulcer recurrence may result from reinfection. The medical treatment of duodenal ulcer now includes agents active against H.pylori such as antibiotics and colloidal bismuth (De-nol).

In *gastric ulcer* acid output plays a less important role while mucosal resistance to acid-pepsin seems relatively more important. Despite this, gastric ulcer has been successfully treated by acid lowering operations.

Gastric cancer

In gastric cancer environmental factors seem more important than genetic, blood group A being a weak risk factor. There is an increased incidence in lower socio-economic groups which may be a reflection of different smoking and dietary habits between the groups. Thus smoking has a positive association while increasing consumption of vegetables and dairy products has a protective effect. There is a strong association between chronic atrophic gastritis and subsequent cancer, some 10% of patients with these changes going on to develop cancer. Mucosal irritants, and nutritional deficits may lead to gastritis as may auto antibodies in pernicious anaemia. Infection with H.pylori may prove to be the single most important factor in the development of chronic gastritis. The progression to intestinal metaplasia, dysplasia and cancer appears to be influenced by N-nitrosamines, powerful carcinogens which derive from dietary nitrites or from the reduction of dietary nitrates by intragastric bacteria. Natural hypoacidity or that induced by peptic ulcer operations may, by altering the bacterial flora, enhance the production of N-nitrosamines.

OPERATIONS FOR PEPTIC ULCER

Elective operations for duodenal ulcer were amongst the commonest procedures performed by the general surgeon in the middle three decades of this century. The decline in elective operations for duodenal ulcer was first noted in the mid 1960s. This decline has continued so that in the 1990s elective operations for duodenal ulcer have become a rarity as more powerful anti-secretory agents have been introduced together with agents which enhance the mucosal barrier and latterly agents active against H. pylori now that its significance has been appreciated. As the role of H. pylori in the aetiology of duodenal ulcer is increasingly understood so the role of acid-reducing operations has become confined to those few cases resistant to medical treatment and to the complications of ulcer disease.

Even here the role of surgery is diminishing as endo-scopic treatment makes an increasing impact on the treatment of bleeding duodenal ulcer.

The surgeon must, however, still be prepared to deal with the long term sequelae of the many patients who have undergone peptic ulcer surgery in previous decades.

INDICATIONS FOR OPERATION FOR PEPTIC ULCER

Duodenal ulcer

Duodenal ulcer is becoming less common in North America and Europe and this decline is likely to be worldwide.

The clinical diagnosis of duodenal ulceration must firstly be confirmed by fibreoptic endoscopy or barium meal examination. The results of 'ulcer surgery' are particularly poor when operation is carried out in the absence of an ulcer or significant scarring. Given a firm diagnosis, the following indications for operations are suggested as guidelines but are by no means universally accepted. Each decision to recommend operation is based on the clinical judgement of the surgeon as applied to the problem of an individual patient.

Chronicity and failure of medical therapy. The classical course of duodenal ulceration is one of periods of relapse interspersed with longer periods of remission. Few surgeons advocate operation unless the patient has experienced symptoms for more than one year and has undergone an adequate course of medical treatment. Measures now available include H2 receptor anta-gonists such as Cimetidine and Ranitidine, the proton pump inhibitor Omeprazole, colloidal bismuth alone or in combination with antibiotics effective against H. pylori. Ulcer healing can be expected after a 6 to 8 week course of an H2 receptor antagonist in about 80% of patients and after a 4 week course of Omeprazole in over 95% of patients. At present, failure of medical therapy may be defined as failure of the ulcer to heal in response to a course of full-dose H2 receptor antago-nist, a subsequent course of Omeprazole; or, relapse after ceasing medical therapy or completing a course of maintenance therapy; or (rarely) development of a complication which precludes continued medical treat-ment. It should be stressed that recurrence of symp-toms does not necessarily indicate ulcer recurrence, and endoscopy should be used to establish the diagno-sis if doubt persists. The decision to advocate surgery is strengthened if the patient has a past history of perfo-ration or haemorrhage and highly selective vagotomy is particularly effective in preventing these complications recurring (Macintyre, 1990). Conversely, the decision to persist with effective medical treatment may be strengthened if the risks of operation are increased by intercurrent disease. Factors influencing the decision include amount of time lost from work, amount of sleep lost, dietary incapacity and the less easily meas-ured factor of impairment of the quality of life.

Development of complications of duodenal ulcer. Emer-gency or urgent surgery may have to be performed on some patients who develop haemorrhage, perforation or pyloric stenosis.

Choice of operation for duodenal ulcer

The original operations described for duodenal ulcer — gastro-enterostomy alone and Billroth I gastrectomy — have no place in the modern surgical treatment of duodenal ulcer. The operations most commonly per-formed are truncal vagotomy with drainage procedure (either pyloroplasty or gastro-enterostomy), truncal vago-tomy with antrectomy, and highly selective vagotomy (also known as proximal gastric vagotomy or parietal cell vagotomy). Polya gastrectomy may occasionally be appropriate. Whilst truncal vagotomy with antrectomy is associated with the lowest recurrent ulcer rates it carries the side effects of both truncal vagotomy and gastric resection. Truncal vagotomy with either form of drainage carries a small but appreciable risk of post vagotomy diarrhoea and dumping. There is little to chose between pyloroplasty and gastroenterostomy in terms of the functional result (Kennedy, 1973). Gastro-enterostomy is arguably easier to reverse especially with modern stapling instruments. Highly selective vagotomy is associated with fewer side effects but a higher recurrent ulcer rate. In the face of powerful anti-secretory agents, recurrent ulcer after highly selective vagotomy will usually respond to medical therapy and for that reason this remains the operation of choice for many surgeons.

Gastric ulcer

The indications for operation in gastric ulcer are:

1. failure of medical therapy
2. development of complications.

The medical treatment of gastric ulcer is similar to that for duodenal ulcer. Endoscopic biopsy to exclude malignancy is essential before starting treatment and again after completing the initial course of treatment to ensure healing. The concern that benign gastric ulcers undergo malignant transformation, although rare, demands that all gastric ulcers should be seen to have healed endoscopically. The problem is complicated by the fact that malignant gastric ulcers have been seen to heal endoscopically.

Gastric ulcers which occur in the pylorus or imme-diate prepyloric area are frequently associated with acid-pepsin hypersecretion and are regarded as a variant of duodenal ulcer from the point of management. The following applies to all other gastric ulcers.

The incidence of gastric ulceration is declining but less sharply than the fall in incidence of duodenal ulcer. A few patients exhibit gastric hypersecretion but the majority have acid-pepsin outputs within or beneath the normal range. A number of factors contribute to this apparent hyposecretion: the functioning parietal cell mass may be reduced by associated gastritis and some secreted acid may leak from the lumen by back-diffusion across a damaged mucosa. Current concepts of pathogenesis add the importance of damage to the gastric mucosa by non-steroidal anti-inflammatory drugs. Acid and pepsin secretion is still essential to exploit the weakened mucosal barrier and cause ulceration. Despite isolated reports of benign gastric ulceration in patients with achlorhydria, the dictum 'no acid no ulcer' is still valid.

The development of complications such as haemorrhage, perforation, gastric stenosis, or malignant transformation is the other principle indication for surgery.

Choice of elective operation for gastric ulcer

The choice of operation for gastric ulcer lies between local excision, gastrectomy, or an acid-reducing operation. A gastric ulcer which persists in the face of modern acid-reducing drugs is, in the author's view, best treated by excision. The increasing safety of modern surgical treatment makes gastrectomy, usually with gastroduodenal anastomosis, the procedure of choice.

DESCRIPTION OF OPERATIONS FOR PEPTIC ULCER

Vagotomy

Truncal vagotomy

Truncal vagotomy is always performed with a drainage procedure because of the risk of gastric stasis and delayed gastric emptying. The abdomen is opened through an upper mid line incision extending some 2 cm below the level of the umbilicus. Access to the abdominal oesophagus can be improved by the use of a self retaining retractor and by head-up tilting of the table by 15–25 degrees. The left lobe of the liver may be either retracted superiorly using a liver retractor or retracted inferiorly after division of the left triangular ligament. A sternal lifting retractor of the Goligher or Walls variety will further enhance exposure and access in this area. With the left hand applying gentle traction to the anterior wall of the stomach the abdominal oesophagus is identified by palpating the naso-gastric tube with the finger and thumb of the right hand. Whilst downward traction is maintained, the peritoneum overlying the abdominal oesophagus is incised

with scissors. Large blood vessels in the peritoneum may be treated by ligation or careful diathermy. With the index and middle fingers of the right hand the surgeon can now carry out gentle finger dissection to mobilise the oesophagus. Continued dissection allows the oesophagus to be encircled and a tape or rubber tube is then placed around it. In over 80% of cases a single anterior and a single posterior vagal trunk are present. Two anterior vagal trunks are present in some 15% of subjects but two posterior vagal trunks occur in only 1%. The anterior vagal nerve trunk or trunks are usually easily visualised at this stage but if not visible they can be readily palpated as taut bands. The posterior vagal trunk usually lies distant from the oesophagus and may be hooked-up as the surgeon's right index finger is swept from left to right behind the oesophagus along the pre-aortic fascia. Finger or pledget dissection can now be used to clean both vagal trunks over a distance of some 6–8 cm. Both are then clipped, with long artery forceps, a 3–4 cm segment of nerve excised for subsequent histological examination and the nerve ends ligated.

At this stage it is important to divide all remaining vagal nerve fibres. This is best done by using a blunt hook to carefully clean the entire abdominal oesophagus of all strands of tissue which will include strands of fascia, and small blood vessels in addition to tiny nerve fibres.

Transthoracic truncal vagotomy

Transthoracic truncal vagotomy is rarely if ever indicated. It is only used when the transabdominal approach is considered contraindicated (e.g. by adhesions from previous gastric surgery). Left thoracotomy is used so that, if necessary, the stomach can be exposed by incising the diaphragm. The patient is placed on his right side, a long incision is made in the 8th or 9th interspace, and the ribs are spread. The lung is collapsed and displaced forwards. The parietal pleura overlying the oesophagus is incised from the aortic arch down to the diaphragm and a soft catheter is passed around the oesophagus for use as a retractor. The two vagus nerves and their plexuses are dissected clear of the oesophageal wall from just below the tracheal bifurcation to the hiatus, and are then resected. The chest is closed with underwater seal drainage.

Selective vagotomy

This operation was introduced in an attempt to reduce the incidence of incomplete gastric vagotomy and avoid some of the sequelae attributed to vagal denervation of other abdominal viscera. The technique entailed sparing the hepatic branch of the anterior vagus and the coeliac branch of the posterior vagus, but as with truncal vagotomy, a gastric drainage procedure was also

performed. The operation is more time-consuming
than truncal vagotomy and showed little or no advantage with regard to the incidence of recurrent
ulceration or other sequelae of surgery. It has been
abandoned in most centres and will not be considered
further.

*Highly selective vagotomy (syn. parietal cell vagotomy,
proximal gastric vagotomy)*

Highly selective vagotomy was developed independently by Johnston and Amdrup in the late 1960s
(Macintyre, 1990). Its object is to denervate the parietal cell mass whilst preserving the vagal supply to the
antrum so avoiding the need for a drainage procedure.
This is done by preserving intact the anterior and
posterior nerves of Latarjet which provide the motor
innervation to the antrum.

Some surgeons prefer to begin the operation by displaying the main anterior and posterior vagal trunks on
the lower oesophagus in the manner described above
for truncal vagotomy. Unless the patient is obese, the
anterior nerve of Latarjet can usually be seen clearly
some 1–2 cm from the lesser curve of the stomach.
As it approaches the antrum it fans out into several
branches. This arrangement has come to be called the
crow's foot (Fig. 17.8). The lesser sac is entered either
through the gastro-colic omentum or through the lesser
omentum. The author's preference is for the former
for three reasons. Firstly opening into the gastro-colic
omentum allows the assistants hand to grasp the
greater curvature and exert the powerful downward
traction necessary to put the nerves and pedicles being
dissected on the stretch. Secondly some vagal fibres
to the parietal cells have been shown to pass into the
greater curve aspect of stomach via the gastro-colic
omentum (Johnson, 1977) and these are divided as the
gastro-colic omentum is cut. Finally those congenital
adhesions in the lesser sac are more easily divided from
below, through an opening through the gastro-colic
omentum.

The peritoneum of the gastro-colic omentum is divided outside the gastro-epiploic arcade and an opening made into the lesser sac. Adjacent vascular pedicles
in this omentum are divided between ligatures to
enlarge the opening. The assistant grasps the greater
curve and draws it down and to the left putting
congenital adhesions between stomach and pancreas
on the stretch. These are divided with scissors. The
anterior leaf of lesser omentum is then divided close to
the lesser curve commencing at a point just above and
to the left of the crow's foot some 7 cm from the pylorus (Fig. 17.8). Rather than leave innervated parietal
cells, the dissection may be extended into the heel of
the crow's foot. This means that only 5–6 cm of antrum remain innervated, but this does not compromise
gastric emptying. Each vessel passing to the lesser curve
is divided between ligatures. Alternatively the vessels
may be doubly clipped with artery forceps prior to division and ligation. Some surgeons use Cushing clips or
Ligaclips but care must be taken to avoid dislodging
the clips by swabbing later in the procedure. The line
of dissection continues upwards alongside the lesser
curve before inclining across the front of the cardia to
the cardiac incisura (Figs 17.9 & 17.10).

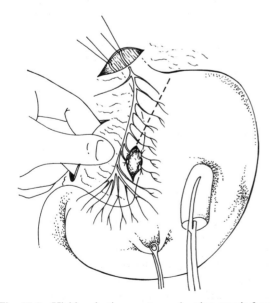

Fig. 17.8 Highly selective vagotomy showing crow's foot
and commencement of division of anterior leaf of lesser
omentum. The dotted line indicates the line of separation to
be used at a higher level (after Figs 6, 8 and 9 in Goligher
J C, British Journal of Surgery, 61: 337)

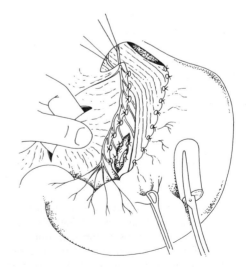

Fig. 17.9 Highly selective vagotomy showing separation of
posterior leaf of lesser omentum and window created into
lesser sac (after Goligher 1974).

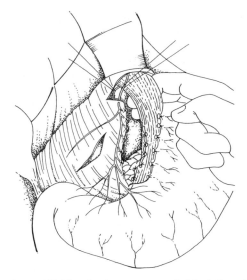

Fig. 17.10 Highly selective vagotomy: finished dissection showing extent of oesophageal clearance (after Goligher 1974)

Before the division of the posterior leaf of the lesser omentum is started, a plane of intermediate loose connective tissue must be divided. This layer contains fine vessels and nerves which must be treated carefully and any temptation to hurry this stage of the operation should be resisted. Attention is then turned to the posterior layer of the lesser omentum which is serially divided by passing a fine pointed instrument (dissecting scissors or artery forceps) backwards through the posterior leaf for them to re-emerge 1–2 cm higher. In this way the leash of vessels in the posterior layer is displayed and can be divided. It may be helpful to begin this dissection from behind through the window in the gastrocolic omentum, by turning the stomach upwards, and dividing the first leash of vessels from within the lesser sac. It is important to keep close to the lesser curve to avoid damage to the posterior nerve of Latarjet. Division of the posterior leaf continues upwards towards the oesophagogastric junction where the bulk of tissue to be divided increases and longer and larger artery forceps are required. Access can be improved by drawing the lower oesophagus forwards and to the left, taking care not to damage either nerve of Latarjet (Fig. 17.10). The clearance must extend for 7–8 cm up the lower oesophagus to ensure that there are no residual vagal fibres passing downwards on the wall of the oesophagus towards the stomach. Failure to complete this part of the dissection is a major cause of incomplete parietal cell vagotomy. When the oesophagus has been cleared the dissection continues towards the fundus as far as the first short gastric vessel dividing all peritoneum passing from fundus to diaphragm, which may contain vagal fibres including the 'criminal' nerve of Grassi.

The operation is completed by checking the amount of distal stomach which remains innervated. As described above, the uppermost branch from the crow's foot is divided if the innervated portion seems too large. Some surgeons cover the bare strip of the lesser curve by suturing the cut edges of peritoneum in the hope of reducing the risk of the rare complication of lesser curve necrosis. A suction drain leading from the region of the oesophageal dissection has been advocated to reduce the chance of post vagotomy dysphagia, a common but almost always transient complication.

Gastric drainage procedures

Pyloroplasty

Pyloroplasty is used as a gastric drainage procedure in conjunction with truncal vagotomy. The operation has the theoretical advantage over gastrojejunostomy that the normal continuity of the gastrointestinal tract is retained. On the other hand if the drainage procedure causes complications and requires to be reversed, taking down a gastro-enterostomy is easier than reconstruction of the pylorus. The procedure is particularly useful when ulceration is complicated by bleeding as the gastroduodenal mucosa can be inspected and the ulcer base transfixed. It is also used in the surgery of perforated duodenal ulcer, the perforation site being incorporated in the incision through the pylorus.

Technique of pyloroplasty. The prelude to any type of pyloroplasty is adequate mobilization of the second part of the duodenum. The peritoneum lateral to the second part of the duodenum is divided and the duodenum is swept toward the mid line. The original Heineke-Mikulicz pyloroplasty consisted of a 5 cm longitudinal incision through all coats of the anterior wall of the pyloro-duodenal region. The incision was closed transversely with multiple rows of interrupted silk sutures but excessive enfolding of tissue frequently narrowed the lumen. Weinberg's modification of the Heineke-Mikulicz technique avoids narrowing by using only one layer which may be continuous or interrupted.

Two stay sutures are inserted deeply 1 cm apart on the anterior aspect of the pyloric ring. The pyloro-duodenal wall midway between these is incised longitudinally to open the lumen for approximately 3.5 cm on the gastric side and 2.5 cm on the duodenal side of the pylorus. If an anterior ulcer is present, the incision is made through it. Ulcer excision should not be attempted. Traction on the stay sutures converts the longitudinal incision to a diamond-shaped opening which is closed transversely (Fig. 17.11) using a single layer of 3/0 polyglycolic acid (Dexon) or polyglycolic/polylactic sutures (Vicryl). All layers of the gastric and duodenal wall should be included. Accurate approximation of the suture line is aided by placing a solitary

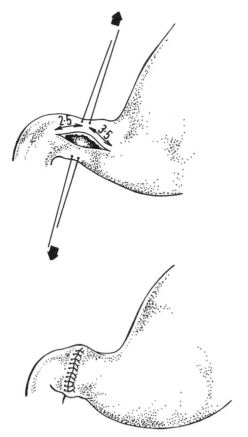

Fig. 17.11 The operation of Heineke–Mikulicz pyloroplasty using one layer of interrupted sutures to close the incision. The stitch for inversion of the mucosa is not essential and may be replaced by a simple through-and-through all coats stitch

central suture to join the ends of the gastro-duodeno-tomy. This closes the diamond and acts as a useful retractor for each half of the suture line closure. No attempt is made to infold the 'dogear' projection at the upper and lower ends of the suture line in case this causes narrowing of the lumen. It is unnecessary to cover the suture line with omentum as leakage is extremely unlikely.

Finney's technique is strictly speaking a gastroduodenostomy rather than a pyloroplasty. It demands more thorough mobilization of the pylorus and first three portions of the duodenum by Kocher's method. The peritoneum and fascia propria on the outer aspect of the duodenum are divided, any adhesions are freed, and the duodenum and pylorus are lifted forwards and toward the midline by gauze or finger dissection. The greater curve of the distal stomach is then applied to the first two parts of the duodenum by three stay sutures (Fig. 17.12) which are knotted and clipped. A posterior continuous Lambert suture of 3/0 Dexon or Vicryl is commenced at the pylorus and extends to just

beyond the furthest stay suture. An inverted U-shaped incision is made through all coats of the stomach, pylorus and duodenum and passing around the suture line (Fig. 17.12). A posterior all coats suture of 3/0 Dexon or Vicryl is then applied, commencing at the divided pylorus. From the lower angle of the incision the suture is carried upwards as a Connell or loop-on-the-mucosa stitch to approximate the anterior walls of the stomach, duodenum and pylorus. The gastroduodenal anastomosis is completed by taking up the posterior seromuscular stitch and continuing it anteriorly to invaginate the all coats layer (Fig. 17.12).

Finney's operation is seldom performed today. The Heineke-Mikulicz pyloroplasty is simpler and less time consuming. If difficulty is anticipated with this form of pyloroplasty, posterior gastrojejunostomy is the alternative of choice.

Gastrojejunostomy (syn. gastroenterostomy)
Gastrojejunostomy involves anastomosis of a loop of proximal jejunum to the stomach. This may be used as a gastric drainage procedure in conjunction with trun-

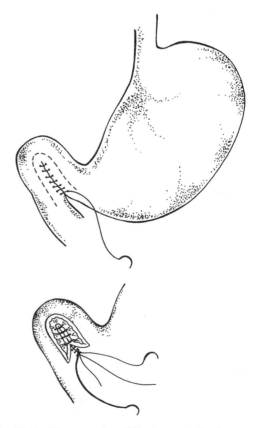

Fig. 17.12 The operation of Finney gastroduodenostomy showing insertion of the posterior seromuscular layer and the start of the posterior all coats layer

cal vagotomy, and occasionally as a bypass in patients with unresectable carcinoma obstructing the distal stomach. Gastrojejunostomy alone was once used to treat duodenal ulcer but, because of the high incidence of recurrent ulceration, is no longer recommended. Retro-colic gastrojejunostomy drains the stomach more effectively and is preferred in ulcer surgery.

Posterior gastrojejunostomy. The greater omentum, transverse colon and lower part of the stomach are brought out of the wound and turned upwards. A hand is passed along the root of the transverse mesocolon to the left of the spine to identify the proximal jejunum as it leaves the duodeno-jejunal flexure. This loop is withdrawn and two pairs of atraumatic tissue forceps (such as Babcock's) are applied to its antimesenteric border at distances of approximately 10 and 20 cm from the duodeno-jejunal flexure.

While the assistant holds up the transverse colon, the surgeon pushes the dependent portion of the distal stomach against the transverse mesocolon which is incised vertically in an avascular area, usually to the left of the middle colic artery. The incision is enlarged with dissecting scissors to a length of about 10 cm and the posterior wall of the dependent portion of gastric antrum is grasped with atraumatic tissue forceps and pulled gently through the window. The most dependent part of the stomach will be used for the anastomosis and the angle of pull should be adjusted until this part lies in the centre of the window. Once sufficient stomach has been made available for anastomosis, the margins of the defect in the mesocolon are sutured to the stomach by interrupted sutures to prevent herniation of the small intestine through the window.

The selected portions of stomach and jejunum are then held up by the tissue forceps, and may be brought into apposition by locking anastomosis clamps such as Lane's, Dott's or Swanson's clamps, and the tissue forceps are removed. The eventual opening in the stomach may lie vertically, obliquely or horizontally and the anastomosis may be isoperistaltic or antiperistaltic. To make an isoperistaltic anastomosis the afferent loop is taken to lie along the distal part of the stomach. There is little to choose between these methods although most surgeons favour an oblique isoperistaltic anastomosis. Regardless of the method employed, the anastomosis is placed in the most dependent part of the stomach to ensure efficient drainage. The transverse colon, omentum and any protruding loops of small bowel are replaced in the peritoneal cavity, and the segments of gut to be anastomosed are surrounded by packs. Side-to-side anastomosis is carried out (p. 347), many surgeons opting to use two layers of continuous absorbable suture such as polyglycolic acid (Dexon) or polyglycolic/polylactic acid (Vicryl).

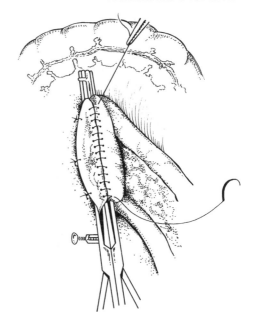

Fig. 17.13 Posterior gastrojejunostomy. A segment of jejunum some 15–20 cm from the duodeno-jejunal flexure has been selected for the anastomosis and the posterior layer of sutures has been inserted

In obese patients with a short thick mesocolon and relatively fixed stomach, a conventional posterior gastroenterostomy may prove difficult. In this event, the gastrocolic omentum is divided between ligatures to gain access to the lesser sac and the selected loop of jejunum is drawn upwards through a window in the transverse mesocolon. Anastomotic clamps can then be applied and the anastomosis performed with relative ease above the transverse colon. On completion, the anastomosis is drawn down through the window in the mesocolon (Fig. 17.14).

Gastro-jejunostomy may also be made using a stapling technique. Both the GIA (Gastro-Intestinal Anastomosis) (Autosuture) and PLC (Proximate Linear Cutter) (Ethicon) are suitable for this purpose. The most dependent part of the stomach is taken through the window in the transverse mesocolon and approximated to the selected jejunal loop, by stay sutures. Light occlusion clamps are placed across the stomach and jejunum.

Stab incisions are made opposite each other in stomach and jejunum using dissecting scissors. The opened GIA or PLC instrument is inserted into the stab incisions placing the larger limb into the gastric side. The instrument is positioned to the hilt of each limb and checked to ensure that position is optimal before closing (Fig. 17.15). The instrument is fired, withdrawn, the staple line checked for bleeding and the conjoined stab incision closed with continuous polyglycolic acid

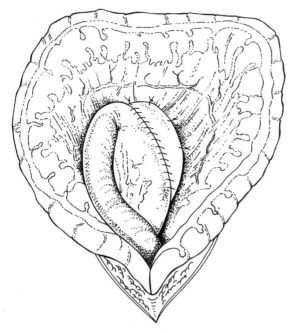

Fig. 17.14 Posterior gastrojejunostomy completed showing the closed window in the transverse mesocolon and an oblique isoperistaltic anastomosis in the mesocolon window, the margins of which are sutured to the stomach with a series of interrupted sutures

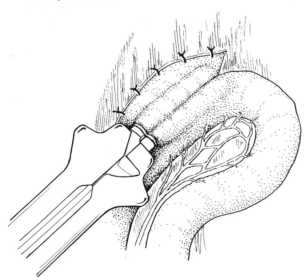

Fig. 17.15 Stapled gastrojejunostomy. Stapling instrument in place

(Dexon) or polyglycolic/polylactic acid suture (Vicryl). The size of the stoma is checked by palpation between finger and thumb.

Partial gastrectomy

Partial gastrectomy is rarely indicated nowadays for

duodenal ulcer but remains the procedure of choice for gastric ulcer. When partial gastrectomy is performed for peptic ulceration the line of proximal transection lies across the body of the stomach, its precise level and angle depending on the size of the organ, the site of any gastric lesion, and the type of anastomosis envisaged. The distal transection line passes through the first part of the duodenum. When operating for duodenal ulcer it is sometimes safer to divide the duodenum proximal to the ulcer, rather than attempt to remove the ulcer-bearing area which may result in subsequent difficulty in closing the duodenal stump and increase the risk of damage to the common bile duct, hepatic artery or pancreas.

Types of gastrectomy

In Billroth's first operation described in 1881, only the pyloric part of the stomach was excised with end-to-end anastomosis between the remaining stomach and duodenum. In the modern gastrectomy more of the stomach is resected, the exact amount depending upon the indication and the site of the gastric ulcer or gastric cancer being resected. The following types of gastrectomy will be described:

- Billroth II (Polya) gastrectomy for proximal gastric ulcer
- Billroth I gastrectomy for gastric ulcer in the antrum
- Billroth II (Polya gastrectomy) for antral carcinoma
- Total gastrectomy for proximal carcinoma.

In the Polya operation (Fig. 17.16) first described in 1911 the duodenal stump is closed and the remaining stomach is anastomosed end-to-side with the jejunum. The modern Polya gastrectomy is a variation of this. The proximal loop of jejunum may be brought through an opening in the transverse mesocolon (retro-colic anastomosis) or in front of the transverse colon (ante-colic anastomosis). A longer loop of jejunum (20–25 cm) is required for an ante-colic anastomosis. The other major variation depends on whether the afferent

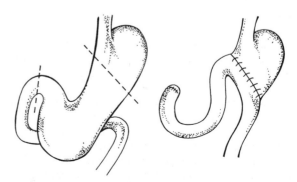

Fig. 17.16 Polya partial gastrectomy

loop of jejunum is brought to the lesser or greater curvature, giving 'isoperistaltic' or 'antiperistaltic' anastomosis respectively. No one method is superior and the choice of technique is dictated by the operative findings and personal preference. It has been suggested that complications are more frequent after antecolic anastomosis because of the longer afferent loop. Although the jejunum is brought through the mesocolon for a retrocolic anastomosis, the stomach should be drawn down through the window on completion and the defect closed around the stomach with interrupted sutures. Failure to close the window may allow jejunum to herniate in the supracolic compartment of the abdomen, or kink and obstruct as it passes through the mesocolon (Stammers' hernia). An ante-colic anastomosis is preferred when there is a small gastric stump or the mesocolon is unusually short or loaded with fat.

A valved anastomosis was introduced by Finsterer in 1913 and several variations have since been described. There is no evidence that a valve improves the functional result and its use cannot be recommended.

Technique of the Polya operation for proximal gastric or for duodenal ulcer
The technique to be described for duodenal ulceration differs from that used for gastric ulcer or gastric carcinoma (see p. 394). After opening the abdomen by a long mid line incision, the duodenum is carefully examined and the mobility of its first part is determined. The stomach is drawn out of the wound and the extent of resection is planned. The mesocolon and first loop of jejunum are examined and a decision is made as to whether a retrocolic or antecolic anastomosis is to be performed.

Mobilization of the stomach. The greater omentum is retracted inferiorly by the assistant putting the tissues being dissected under tension. Starting close to the pylorus it is detached from the stomach, dividing its contained vessels between successive pairs of ligatures. It is not necessary to preserve the main gastro-epiploic arch and it is less tedious to divide the gastrocolic omentum beneath the arch, ligating the main right and left gastro-epiploic vessels at the lower and upper resection lines respectively. The dissection continues from the middle of the first part of the duodenum to the left to the level selected for transection on the greater curve. This usually entails dividing the lower of the short gastric vessels. The stomach is lifted forwards and avascular adhesions between its posterior wall and pancreas are divided with dissecting scissors. The lesser omentum is next incised in its avascular portion. The right gastric artery is identified just above the point where it reaches the upper border of the first part of the duodenum. The right gastric artery may be represented by a leash of vessels rather than a single trunk whereas

the left gastric artery is almost always represented by a single (usually substantial) vessel. The artery is ligated and divided. Division of the lesser omentum continues parallel with the lesser curvature but stops before reaching the left gastric artery as the vessel is dealt with more conveniently at a later stage. The stomach is lifted forwards and the inferior border of the first part of duodenum is separated from the pancreas, carefully dissecting and dividing the small vessels between ligatures. If possible the duodenum is freed for 1 cm beyond the area of ulcer to facilitate subsequent closure of the duodenal stump. Ligation of the gastroduodenal artery is seldom required in elective operations for benign disease and must never be attempted before the common bile duct and hepatic artery have been displayed and safeguarded.

Division of the duodenum and closure of the stump. There are many acceptable methods for carrying out this part of the operation. One traditional method entails placing two straight crushing clamps across the selected transection line (Fig. 17.17) and dividing the bowel with a scalpel. The proximal cut end is covered with a swab and the stomach is turned back over the left side of the wound. The duodenal stump is usually closed in two layers. A continuous seromuscular stitch can be used to pick up the duodenal wall first on one side of the clamp and then on the other, passing over the clamp but not under it. This invaginating stitch is tightened as the clamp is removed and is reinforced by a second continuous or interrupted seromuscular stitch. An alternative method of suture closure uses a

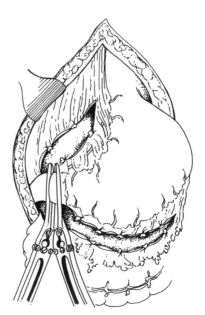

Fig. 17.17 Division of the first part of duodenum between crushing clamps after mobilization

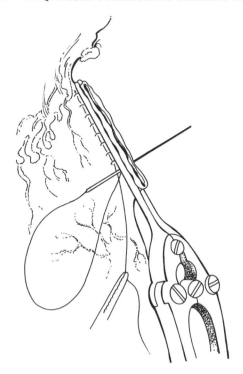

Fig. 17.18 The 'sewing machine' stitch used to close the duodenal stump; a secure method when the stump is short and may be difficult to invaginate

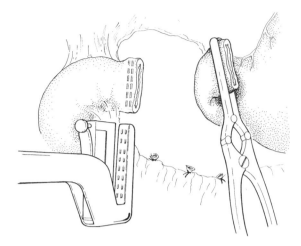

Fig. 17.19 Stapled closure of duodenal stump

'sewing machine' stitch for the first layer (Fig. 17.18). The choice of suture material is a matter of personal preference but many surgeons employ polyglycolic acid (Dexon) or polyglycolic/polylactic acid (Vicryl) for both layers or use non-absorbable material for the outer layer. Many surgeons now use stapling techniques to close the duodenal stump. This can be in the form of a stapler which applies four parallel rows of staples and divides the tissue in the centre (GIA — Autosuture or PLC — Ethicon) (Fig. 17.19). Alternatively the duodenal stump may be closed by a linear stapler (TA30 — Autosuture or RL30 — Ethicon). The row of staples on the duodenal stump may be reinforced by a continuous haemostatic Dexon or Vicryl suture or buried by a layer of interrupted seromuscular stitches of 2/0 Dexon or Vicryl. Leakage from the duodenal stump is one of the major complications of the Polya operation and a drain should be placed down to the stump routinely. Causes of duodenal stump leakage include insertion of sutures under tension which impairs duodenal vascularity. Indeed on the rare occasions in which the tissues are too friable to allow safe closure of the duodenal stump it is preferable to leave a tube drain sutured into the unclosed duodenum and elect to manage a controlled fistula in the postoperative period. Given that there is no distal obstruction to flow down the small intestine this fistula closes readily and the approach exposes the

patient to much less risk than development of stump necrosis and uncontrolled leakage.

Transection of the stomach and retrocolic anastomosis. The stomach is turned back over the left costal margin to identify the left gastric artery as it reaches the lesser curvature just below the oesophago-gastric junction. The vessel is ligated and divided. Both curvatures of the stomach should be entirely bared of omentum at the level selected for anastomosis. The proximal loop of jejunum is brought through the transverse mesocolon and placed alongside the stomach in the position in which it seems to lie most conveniently. Most surgeons prefer to bring the afferent loop to the lesser curvature. The length of afferent loop employed should be such that it is neither too tense nor too lax. Two pairs of Babcock's tissue forceps are applied to the jejunum to mark the points for anastomosis to the lesser and greater curvatures. A light occlusion clamp is placed across the stomach proximal to the level of section and a similar clamp is applied to the selected length of jejunum (Fig. 17.20). Locking twin clamps such as Lane's clamps may facilitate anastomosis. A continuous seromuscular stitch is used to unite the adjacent surfaces of the two viscera and a crushing clamp is then applied to the stomach 1 cm distal to the suture line. The stomach is divided with a scalpel run along the underside of the crushing clamp.

To make a valvular anastomosis, the jejunum is incised for only 3–4 cm opposite the lower part of the cut end of the stomach. The upper part of the open stomach is closed. This may be done using through-and-through sutures like the 'sewing machine' stitch and only the lower 3–4 cm is anastomosed to the open jejunum (Fig. 17.21). The anterior seromuscular layer of sutures is used to anchor the intact jejunum to the upper sutured part of the stomach. The anastomosis is drawn down through the defect in the mesocolon, the margins of which are attached to the stomach wall by interrupted stitches placed about 1 cm above the suture line.

A convenient alternative is to close the gastric remnant with a stapler, a technique which has, surprisingly, been used since about 1910. After ligation of the relevant vascular pedicles, a TA90 (Autosuture) or RL90 (Ethicon) is applied obliquely across. A straight occlusion clamp is placed across the stomach 2 cm distal to and parallel to the stapler. After the stapler is fired the stomach is transected by a scalpel using the stapler as a cutting edge (Fig. 17.22).

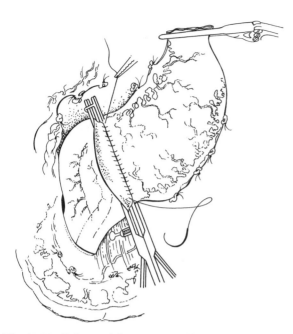

Fig. 17.20 Polya partial gastrectomy. Twin locking clamps have been used in anastomosis and the posterior seromuscular stitch has been inserted

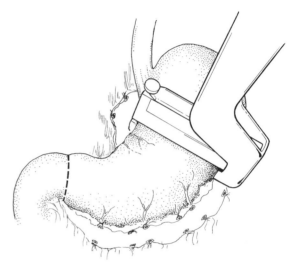

Fig. 17.22 Closure of stomach using linear stapler

The gastro-jejunal anastomosis may be made using a GIA (Autosuture) or PLC (Ethicon) instrument. The selected jejunum is taken through the transverse mesocolon and approximated to the gastric remnant using three interrupted stay sutures. As described for gastro-jejunostomy, stab wounds are made in stomach and duodenum, the limbs of the instrument inserted closed and fired. The resultant single stabs wound is closed with a continuous all-coats layer of Dexon or Vicryl.

Technique of the Billroth I operation
The stomach and first part of the duodenum are mobilized as for the Polya operation. The duodenum beyond the proposed resection line should be healthy and of sufficient calibre for gastro-duodenal anastomosis. The duodenum is divided between clamps as in the Polya operation. Gastric mobilization is completed, and the stomach is transected using two clamps placed at an angle to each other.

The lower clamp encloses a portion of the gastric lumen suitable in size for anastomosis to the duodenum, while the cut-end of stomach held in the upper clamp is closed in two layers to create a new 'lesser

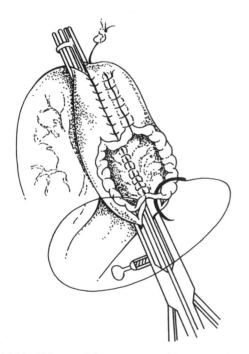

Fig. 17.21 Polya partial gastrectomy with construction of a retrocolic valvular (short stoma) anastomosis. The stomach has been transected and the upper part of the stump has been closed. The lower part only of the cut-end of stomach is being used for the anastomosis

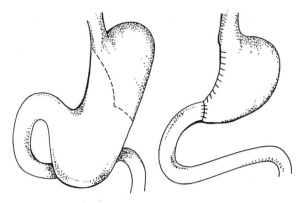

Fig. 17.23   Billroth I partial gastrectomy

curvature' (Fig. 17.23). Alternatively the gastric stump can be closed with a stapling device (TA90 — Autosuture or RL90 — Ethicon) (Fig. 17.24).

Provided that the greater curvature has been mobilized adequately, the gastric remnant can be brought across to the duodenum so that the anastomosis can be performed without tension. If necessary the duodenum can be mobilized by incising the peritoneum along the lateral aspect of its first and second part. The anastomosis is started by placing stay sutures at each end of the tissues to be joined. When a two layer anastomosis is to be made interrupted seromuscular sutures are placed about 1 cm apart. The sutures are gently tightened and knotted after all the sutures have been placed in order to appose the stomach and duodenum. The posterior wall of the anastomosis is completed by an all-coats continuous suture of 3/0 Vicryl or Dexon. This suture is continued forwards as the all-coats layer of the anterior aspect of the anastomosis. The outer layer of the anterior suture line consists of either continuous or interrupted seromuscular sutures. Particular care should be taken over suture placement at the 'angle of sorrow' — the lesser curve aspect of the anastomosis which is especially prone to anastomotic leakage. It is not necessary to leave a drain to the anastomosis but a nasogastric tube in the post operative period is recommended.

Partial gastrectomy for gastric ulcer
When the ulcer lies in the pyloric antrum or lower part of the body of stomach it can be removed as described above with the excised portion of stomach. The Billroth I operation is the procedure of choice but the Polya operation is preferred when the duodenum has been distorted by existing or previous ulceration. On occasion additional manoeuvres may be required and these are described in detail under 'The difficult ulcer' below.

If the gastric ulcer is adherent to the pancreas it can often be pinched off between finger and thumb. If the ulcer has penetrated deeply it is simpler to excise the stomach leaving the ulcer base in situ on the pancreas and cover it with a piece of omentum. A biopsy should be taken from the ulcer and sent for frozen section to ensure that the ulcer is benign.

When the gastric ulcer is situated so high on the

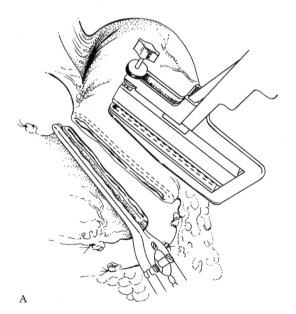

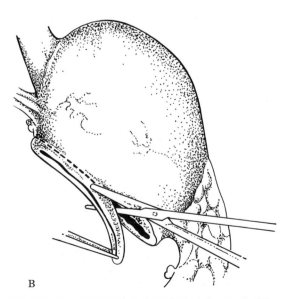

A

B

Fig. 17.24   Billroth I partial gastrectomy. (A) The TA 90 Autosuture device has been used to close the gastric pouch. (B) Excision of a portion of the staple line on the greater curve aspect for anastomosis to the duodenum (courtesy of Autosuture UK Ltd)

lesser curve or posterior wall that clamps cannot be applied easily across the resection line, the Pauchet manoeuvre may be helpful. Two small Payr crushing clamps are applied across the antrum from the greater curvature aspect and the stomach between them is divided with a scalpel. The stomach is held with the Payr clamps so that a tongue-shaped segment of stomach containing the ulcer can be incised with scissors. The walls of the stomach are coapted by a continuous all-coats suture of 3/0 Dexon or Vicryl. Provided that each incised segment is sutured immediately, soiling and bleeding can be kept to a minimum. When the new 'lesser curvature' has been created, the suture line is inverted by continuous or interrupted seromuscular sutures. A gastro-jejunal anastomosis is usually preferred if the gastric stump is small so as to avoid tension on a gastro-duodenal anastomosis.

Postoperative management

Intravenous infusion is used to maintain fluid and electrolyte balance until adequate oral intake is re-established. Opinions vary about the need for a nasogastric tube and the duration of its use. I remove the tube on completion of highly selective vagotomy but retain it for 24–48 hours after truncal vagotomy and drainage or partial gastrectomy. Water by mouth is allowed as soon as bowel sounds return, the amount increasing gradually to permit free fluid intake and ingestion of a light diet by the fourth or fifth day. The tube is reinserted in the uncommon event of abdominal distension, ileus or repeated vomiting.

Complications

Detailed consideration of the complications of ulcer surgery is outwith the scope of this volume, but the management of major specific early and late complications will be outlined. Specific complications in the postoperative period are listed below.

Haemorrhage. Post operative intraperitoneal haemorrhage is rare. It is usually apparent within hours of the initial operation. Where vital signs are affected, immediate re-laparotomy is indicated. Any bleeding from suture or staple lines should be under-run with a suture. Bleeding into the gut lumen is most often due to faulty anastomotic technique and is usually reactionary, becoming manifest in the hours following operation. Aspiration of blood-stained fluid from the nasogastric tube is common after gastric surgery but continued aspiration of frank blood, the onset of haematemesis or melaena, and development of shock reflect significant blood loss into the gut lumen. Morphine is given to relieve anxiety, blood is transfused, a nasogastric tube is inserted if not already in place, and vital signs including hourly urine output and central venous pressure are monitored. Re-operation is indicated if bleeding con-

tinues. When a pyloroplasty has been performed the suture line is opened. It should be remembered that in some cases the duodenal ulcer rather than the suture line is responsible for bleeding. When the patient has a gastrojejunal anastomosis the anterior suture line can be reopened but it may prove simpler to incise the front wall of the stomach so that the suture line can be inspected from above and any bleeding point under-run with a suture ligature.

Obstruction. Obstruction at the site of a pyloroplasty or Billroth I anastomosis usually reflects poor operative technique resulting in narrowing of the lumen by excessive inversion of the suture line, or poor choice of operation if the duodeno-pyloric region was scarred. Obstruction after gastrojejunostomy or Polya partial gastrectomy may be due to faulty anastomotic technique, kinking or volvulus of the jejunal loop, herniation of small intestine through a defect in the mesocolon or behind an antecolic anastomosis, or retrograde jejunogastric intussusception (although this is more often a late complication). Stomal oedema is the most common explanation for persisting early postoperative gastric outlet obstruction. Obstruction which persists for more than 3–5 days after gastric surgery should always be taken seriously. A nasogastric tube is inserted, intravenous fluids are continued, and the patient is investigated by endoscopy and/or radiology in the form of plain abdominal films (erect and supine) and gastrografin meal. If the gastrografin or the endoscope do not pass through the stoma then parenteral nutrition should be started. If the stomal obstruction persists for 3 weeks re-operation is indicated. Obstruction in or around the anastomosis after Polya partial gastrectomy carries added dangers as an obstructed afferent jejunal loop may become grossly distended with resultant necrosis and potentially fatal 'blow-out' of the duodenal stump.

Anastomotic or suture line leakage. Leakage from a gastrojejunal anastomosis, gastroduodenal anastomosis or pyloroplasty is unusual following good operative technique. Leakage from the duodenal stump is a recognised complication of the Polya operation and is prone to occur when there is any obstruction in or around the gastrojejunal anastomosis. Development of duodenal necrosis is often signalled by otherwise unexplained pyrexia or tachycardia, but frank leakage may not become manifest until about the fifth post operative day. The drainage tube down to the duodenal stump should be retained for at least 5 days. Secondary duodenal stump leakage occurs around the tenth postoperative day and is thought to be due to ischaemia. The principles of management are: 1) ensure free external drainage from the leaking stump; 2) protect the surrounding skin; 3) maintain fluid and electrolyte balance; 4) provide parenteral nutrition; 5) stop oral intake; and 6) ensure that there is no distal obstruction that will prevent the fistula from closing spontaneously. Suction sump drainage often aids management and Stomahesive or Baltimore paste can be used to protect the skin. The majority of duodenal fistulae close on conservative management in the absence of distal obstruction.

Late sequelae of ulcer surgery

Recurrent ulceration (see Stabile, 1976). Medical therapy with acid-reducing drugs usually allows ulcer healing. Many recurrent ulcers will heal with H2 receptor antagonists or Omeprazole. Where medical treatment fails gastric resection is usually indicated. The choice of procedure is controversial. When ulceration recurs after highly selective vagotomy or vagotomy and drainage the choice of procedure has been between re-vagotomy, partial gastrectomy and a combination of the two. I always attempt to divide any residual vagal fibres but also resect the distal stomach.

If ulceration recurs after partial gastrectomy, I carry out vagotomy at re-operation and may resect more stomach if there is a substantial gastric remnant. If the recurrent ulcer is in the gastric stump and there is pronounced bile reflux and gastritis at endoscopy, re-anastomosis using a Roux loop of jejunum is advisable.

Entero-gastric reflux (see Alexander-Williams, 1981). The patient frequently complains of post prandial fullness, nausea, pain and vomiting of bitter bile-stained fluid. Enterogastric reflux can be demonstrated on barium meal and quantified by measurement of bile acids in gastric aspirate or scintillation scanning using labelled material (e.g. 99 Tcm HIDA) excreted in bile. Endoscopy reveals an erythematous, hyperaemic mucosa, gastritis being most marked near the stoma. Surgery should not be employed prematurely as many patients improve within 1–2 years. Severe intractable reflux is treated by Roux-en-Y reconstruction if the patient has previously had a Polya gastrectomy or vagotomy and antrectomy. The length of the Roux loop should be at least 50 cm. Interposition of an iso-peristaltic jejunal loop between stomach and small intestine has also been used but has a higher morbidity, the results are less predictable and it is not recommended. In patients with biliary gastritis after vagotomy and gastroenterostomy, simple closure of the gastroenterostomy may be worthwhile if there is no pyloroduodenal narrowing.

Dumping (see Hobsley, 1981). Early dumping occurs within 30 minutes of eating a meal and is distinguished from the syndrome of hypoglycaemia (late dumping) which occurs 60–90 minutes after eating. The features of early dumping are abdominal fullness, nausea, vomiting and diarrhoea, in association with weakness, sweating and palpitation. Symptoms may improve with

time and may be minimised if the patient takes small dry meals and avoids drinking with them. Surgery may be considered if severe dumping persists. This is considered under revisional surgery.

Diarrhoea. Diarrhoea is common after operation involving truncal vagotomy. It may be continuous or episodic but is only severe or explosive in 2–5% of cases. Its aetiology is unknown but is likely to result from parasympathetic denervation of the G.I. tract. The symptoms may improve with time and some patients learn to avoid articles of diet which can precipitate diarrhoea. Simple anti-diarrhoeal agents such as codeine phosphate or loperamide should be tried. Surgery is rarely indicated. When gastric incontinence is thought to be a contributory factor this should be treated by pyloric reconstruction or taking down a gastrojejunal anastomosis. The reversed ileal onlay graft described by Cuschieri (1986) may be helpful in selected patients.

Metabolic upsets and anaemia. Such upsets include malabsorption, weight loss, osteomalacia, and both iron deficiency and megaloblastic anaemia. Although more common after extensive resection, lesser upsets may follow vagotomy and drainage. Management is based on medical treatment.

Gastrojejunocolic fistula. This complication is now extremely rare with the disappearance of gastroenterostomy alone as an ulcer operation, the increased use of operations not involving gastroenterostomy and prompt and efficient management of recurrent ulceration. The fistula develops when an anastomotic or jejunal ulcer following gastroenterostomy or Billroth II gastrectomy erodes the wall of the overlying transverse colon. Severe and intractable diarrhoea results with malabsorption and rapid weight loss. Diarrhoea is not due to passage of food and acid into the colon, but to gastritis, duodenitis and jejunitis caused by faecal organisms entering the upper gastrointestinal tract. The pain of ulceration usually eases with fistula formation possibly because acid secretion falls following the development of severe gastritis.

The diagnosis can sometimes be confirmed by barium meal or endoscopy, but barium enema is much more reliable. After initial nutritional support and bowel preparation a one-stage resection of the affected transverse colon, jejunum and antrum is performed. It may be possible to avoid formal resection of a segment of transverse colon and merely excise a V-shaped margin of colon at the fistula site (Fig. 17.25).

Retrograde jejunogastric intussusception. Retrograde intussusception of one or occasionally both loops of jejunum is a late complication of gastro-enterostomy or Polya partial gastrectomy. There is usually acute epigastric pain and vomiting, visible peristalsis, and a palpable epigastric mass, although the condition can

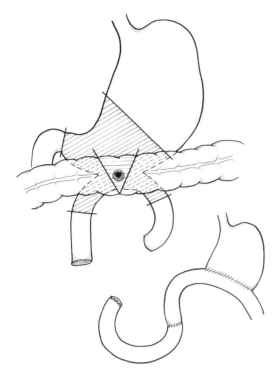

Fig. 17.25   Resection for gastro-jejuno colic fistula

be chronic presenting with intermittent symptoms. Barium meal reveals a gastric filling defect caused by intussuscepted coils of jejunum and endoscopy can be used to clinch the diagnosis. Acute intussusception is treated by immediate operation. Gangrenous jejunum demands resection with revision of the anastomosis. If gangrene is not present the intussusception is reduced and an entero-anastomosis can be performed between the efferent and afferent loops of jejunum. Revision of the anastomosis may also be undertaken but the only guarantee of avoiding recurrence is to carry out a Billroth I conversion.

Gastric cancer. Cancer in the gastric stump occurs slightly more often after gastrectomy than in the general population but only after a lag period of 20 years and may prove to be a complication of vagotomy and drainage. Endoscopy is the mainstay of diagnosis and the cancer is treated by gastric resection, which should be total gastrectomy if a previous gastric resection has been performed.

COMPLICATIONS OF PEPTIC ULCERATION

Perforated gastric or duodenal ulcer

Diagnosis
Perforation of a peptic ulcer usually presents as an acute surgical emergency. Occasionally the perforation

is sealed so rapidly by omentum and adhesions to neighbouring viscera that peritoneal contamination is minimal and localised, with eventual resolution or formation of a chronic abscess. The majority of patients have a preceding history suggestive of chronic ulceration but about one-third have no history of dyspepsia or one which extends for only a week or two. The clinical diagnosis of perforation can be confirmed radiologically in most cases by demonstrating free gas beneath the diaphragm when the patient is erect or sitting. Subdiaphragmatic gas is best seen on erect chest X-ray. If free gas is not apparent perforation may be demonstrated by instilling 50–100 ml of 50% gastrografin down a nasogastric tube or giving the patient gastrografin by mouth.

Principles of operative management
Perforated peptic ulcer is usually treated by operation but may occasionally be managed conservatively.

Preoperative preparation
Mortality can be reduced if precipitate surgery is avoided and 2–3 hours are spent in active resuscitation. Pain and anxiety are relieved by intravenous injection of morphine or pethidine. A nasogastric tube is passed and the stomach is kept empty by nasogastric aspiration. Lavage is contraindicated but a large bore tube should be used if the patient has eaten recently. An intravenous infusion is established to treat dehydration and shock but blood transfusion is not needed unless the patient is grossly anaemic or has the relatively rare combination of ulcer perforation and haemorrhage. Pulse and blood pressure are monitored regularly, a urinary catheter is inserted and hourly urine output is recorded in the presence of shock. Central venous pressure (p. 21) monitoring may be particularly helpful when resuscitating the elderly and patients with cardiovascular disease.

Operative technique
The abdomen is opened by an upper mid line incision if perforation is suspected. If acute appendicitis is thought more likely, it is advisable first to inspect the appendix by a small grid iron or skin crease (Lanz) incision in the right iliac fossa. If the appendix is normal but bile stained free fluid is apparent, the grid iron incision is closed and a separate incision is made in the upper abdomen.

In patients with perforation, gas and turbid bile stained fluid often escape as the peritoneum is incised. Free fluid is aspirated from the peritoneal cavity and the site of the perforation is established. The anterior aspect of the first part of the duodenum and distal stomach are inspected first. A retractor is inserted beneath the liver and the stomach is drawn down, first by gentle traction on the transverse colon and gastrocolic omentum, and then by grasping it with a moist pack (Fig. 17.26). Overlying omentum is gently peeled away by blunt dissection with a pledget or gauze swab. Flakes of creamy fibrin often adhere to the gut near the perforation and are a useful guide to its location. If perforation of the proximal duodenum or distal stomach is not apparent, the remainder of the anterior aspect of the stomach and distal oesophagus is inspected. On rare occasions, the stomach has perforated into the lesser sac and fluid and gas may be seen through the lesser omentum. In this event, the lesser omentum is opened to gain access to the lesser sac. If no perforation is found in the upper G.I. tract the colon, the rectum and the small bowel should be inspected.

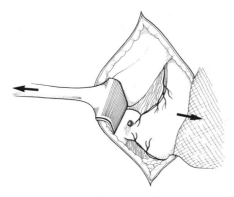

Fig. 17.26 Exposing the first part of the duodenum to reveal possible perforation

Simple closure is the quickest and most appropriate method of dealing with the perforated duodenal ulcer. Retractors are arranged to give the best possible access and any viscera which intrude are packed off. Closure is achieved by inserting 3 or 4 gauge 0 sutures of an absorbable material such as chromic catgut, Vicryl or Dexon which are passed through the entire thickness of the gut wall (Fig. 17.27). The central suture which crosses the perforation is tied last so that it less likely to cut out of the oedematous gut wall. The sutures

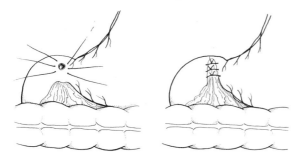

Fig. 17.27 Simple closure of a perforated duodenal ulcer showing insertion of three sutures to close the perforation. The omental tag is secured in place with the same sutures

are inserted in the long axis of the gut to avoid narrowing of the lumen. An additional layer of seromuscular Lambert sutures is not recommended as it merely narrows the lumen of the duodenum. A tag of omentum is used to reinforce closure by tacking it lightly with a suture over the suture line (Fig. 17.28). If scarring makes pyloric or duodenal obstruction inevitable after closure, pyloroplasty or gastro-enterostomy may be unavoidable (see below).

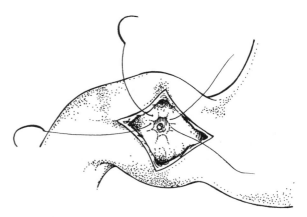

Fig. 17.28 Method of arresting bleeding by underrunning the ulcer during the operation of pyloroplasty.

Where the induration is so marked that sutures tend to cut out, the perforation can be closed with omentum alone. In rare circumstances where the perforation cannot be closed a Portex tube or large Foley catheter may be led through a stab incision to the exterior.

Closure of the perforation is followed by meticulous peritoneal toilet. The subphrenic spaces, paracolic gutters and pelvis are all cleared of fluid by suction and by using large packs. Lavage is advisable and is carried out with warm saline to which tetracycline (1 g/l) may be added if there is purulent peritonitis. The abdomen is closed without drainage unless there is anxiety about the security of perforation closure or frank pus has been present in a specific area of the peritoneal cavity. H2 receptor antagonists should be given for one month starting at the time of operation. Antibiotic therapy is usually reserved for specific indications such as proven bacterial peritonitis or significant chest infection.

Definitive ulcer surgery

The role of emergency definitive ulcer surgery remains controversial. Medical treatment is now so effective that emergency definitive surgery is only indicated for those patients whose ulcer perforates whilst they are taking H2 receptor antagonists or Omeprazole. In such patients, definitive surgery is considered if:

1. anaesthetic and surgical facilities are ideal

2. the surgeon is experienced in carrying out definitive ulcer surgery
3. the patient's general condition is such that the extra time needed for definitive surgery does not impose an unacceptable additional risk
4. purulent peritonitis is not present.

The case for definitive emergency surgery is strengthened:

1. when closure of a stenosed duodenum or pylorus would cause obstruction
2. when the patient has had a previous perforation treated by simple closure
3. when the patient has a perforated gastric ulcer and malignancy is suspected
4. when perforation and bleeding occur together.

The definitive operation usually advocated for a perforated duodenal, pyloric or pre-pyloric ulcer is truncal vagotomy with drainage. The choice between pyloroplasty and gastro-enterostomy is dictated by conditions prevailing in the pyloro-duodenal area. Where possible the perforation is incorporated in a pyloroplasty, but significant stenosis may mean that simple closure with gastro-enterostomy is preferred. Partial gastrectomy is no longer recommended in this context.

Perforation of a gastric ulcer should always raise the suspicion of malignant ulceration, particularly in the elderly. Given favourable circumstances the preferred operation is partial gastrectomy (including the ulcer) with gastroduodenal anastomosis. Given less favourable circumstances it may be wiser to temporise. For example, an elderly patient with perforation of an apparently benign ulcer high on the lesser curve may be better served by excision biopsy of the ulcer margin with simple closure alone.

Non-operative management
The advent of powerful acid suppressing agents has re-awakened interest in the conservative management of perforated peptic ulcer. In the majority of patients operation remains the treatment of choice. In certain situations conservative management should be considered.

Firstly when the risks of a general anaesthetic are considered too great — e.g. the patient who suffers a perforation within hours of an acute myocardial infarction or who has lobar pneumonia.

Secondly when appropriate surgical and anaesthetic skills or equipment are not available.

Patients who at presentation have clinically sealed the perforation, whose signs are localised to the epigastrium and in whom the gastrografin swallow shows no leakage of contrast are being increasingly treated conservatively. Conservative therapy has the disadvantages that the site of perforation usually remains in doubt

and the nature of the underlying condition (benign or malignant) remains uncertain.

Conservative management consists of continued nasogastric aspiration, nil by mouth, intravenous fluids, administration of an H2 receptor antagonist intravenously and appropriate sedation. Antibiotic cover is generally advised. Conservative therapy is abandoned in favour of operation if clinical deterioration suggests continued leakage and worsening peritonitis.

Prognosis
Recognition of the importance of active adequate resuscitation before operation has reduced reported operative mortality from around 25% 50 years ago to 10% today although nearly all of this is accounted for by deaths in the over 65s. This remains a very high operative mortality for any surgical operation. Perforated peptic ulcer thus remains a potentially dangerous condition particularly in the elderly and those ill from intercurrent disease, and mortality rates recorded in the surgical literature may not represent the general experience. The mortality of conservative management is also about 10% or less when corrected selected patients are treated in this way.

Bleeding gastric or duodenal ulcer

Diagnosis and management
The 3 cardinal principles of management of patients with upper gastrointestinal bleeding are:

1. vigorous resuscitation to stabilise the circulation and prevent exsanguination
2. prompt investigation to define the source of bleeding and
3. institution of appropriate measures to arrest bleeding and prevent further haemorrhage.

The great majority of patients bleeding from gastritis, erosions or frank peptic ulcers settle when treated conservatively and it has been traditional to admit all patients to medical rather than surgical wards. In some hospitals these patients are now managed by a 'haematemesis team' of physicians and surgeons, while in other centres all patients are admitted directly to surgical wards. The policy adopted is dictated largely by local circumstances but it is clear that mortality can only be reduced if these patients are managed by experienced clinicians, if resuscitation and investigation are carried out with a sense of urgency, and if an experienced surgeon is involved from the time of admission so that operation can be undertaken if and when appropriate.

Vigorous resuscitation
Blood is grouped and crossmatched so that 4–6 units are available. A wide bore intravenous cannula is estab-

lished to allow rapid transfusion. If peripheral veins are inadequate for this purpose a cannula is placed in a subclavian, jugular or basilic vein. If the patient is shocked, plasma or plasma substitute is used until blood is available; otherwise normal saline is infused in the first instance.

A nasogastric tube (FG16) is passed to try to keep the stomach empty, prevent vomiting, and monitor continued or renewed bleeding. Pulse and blood pressure are monitored every 15 minutes, a urinary catheter is inserted to monitor hourly output if the patient is shocked, temperature is monitored 4-hourly, and haematocrit is checked daily. A separate central venous pressure (CVP) line (p. 21) is an invaluable guide to the rate of fluid replacement in the elderly and those with myocardial insufficiency. Oxygen is given to all shocked patients, unless there are anxieties regarding carbon dioxide retention. Periodic checks on arterial H ion concentration, PO_2 and pCO_2 are used to monitor gas exchange and detect derangement in acid-base balance.

Impaired haemostasis is anticipated in patients needing massive transfusion and in those with deranged liver function. Transfusion of stored blood quickly results in deficiencies of labile factors V and VIII, but these defects can be restored by fresh frozen plasma (FFP) giving one pack for every 3 litres of blood transfused. Regular clotting screens to determine thrombin time, prothrombin time, kaolin-cephalin coagulation time and platelet count are of value in patients with massive bleeding. Vitamin K (5–50 mg IV) is given routinely to all jaundiced patients when prothrombin time is prolonged, but FFP is needed in patients with liver disease who are unresponsive to vitamin K (see p. 25).

Prompt investigation

The patient's history and findings on physical examination provide valuable clues to the source of bleeding but can mislead and should be interpreted with caution. Upper gastro-intestinal endoscopy is the investigation of choice and defines the source of haemorrhage in 80–90% of emergency admissions. Endoscopy should be performed by an experienced endoscopist within 12 hours of admission as the diagnostic yield falls as the interval between admission and endoscopy increases. Ideally, endoscopy is undertaken as soon as the circulatory state has been stabilized, accepting that it may have to be undertaken more urgently in the relatively rare situation where massive continued bleeding threatens exsanguination. Endoscopy is valuable for both diagnosis and therapy. Those patients with no endoscopic abnormality or who have bled from gastritis are unlikely to rebleed. On the other hand patients who have bled from peptic ulcer and have stigmata of recent

haemorrhage, particularly a visible vessel or thrombus in the base of the ulcer, are at high risk of further haemorrhage.

Initial treatment of bleeding peptic ulcer is increasingly endoscopic. The relative merits of laser, heater probe and bipolar coagulation are currently being compared in clinical trials. Injection sclerotherapy which appears to be as effective has the advantage that it is cheap and readily available.

Surgical treatment is indicated for those patients who continue to bleed or who rebleed during or after non-operative treatment.

It must be admitted that the impact of diagnostic endoscopy on mortality has been difficult to define, and much of the reduction in mortality in specialized centres is related to vigorous resuscitation and appropriate timing of surgery by experienced clinicians. Nevertheless, accurate diagnosis of the source of bleeding remains a cornerstone of rational management.

The decision to undertake surgery and time it correctly requires considerable clinical judgement. Operation is obviously indicated as a matter of urgency in patients who are clearly continuing to bleed; the major problem is posed by patients who appear to settle and then have evidence of further haemorrhage. In general, conservative management is indicated in those who have settled clinically and have no endoscopic evidence of continued bleeding. Operation is usually advised when such patients have clinical evidence of re-bleeding, and the indications for operation are stronger in patients over the age of 55 years. It may appear paradoxical to strengthen the recommendation for surgery in older patients but these are the individuals who are least able to withstand the repeated episodes of rebleeding.

Nature of surgery

Once the decision to operate has been taken, active resuscitation is continued. Monitoring of pulse, blood pressure, urine output, central venous pressure continue. Measurement of haemoglobin, haematocrit, arterial blood gases and coagulation studies may also be appropriate. Blood, at first in the form of packed cells, but preferably as fresh whole blood, should be made available in adequate quantities.

The risk of aspirating blood from the stomach into the bronchial tree on induction of anaesthesia is high and an experienced anaesthetist is therefore required.

Before induction of anaesthesia every effort is made to evacuate the stomach through a wide-bore nasogastric tube, and, on induction, a cuffed endotracheal tube is passed quickly to prevent soiling of the bronchial tree.

A laparotomy is performed through an upper mid line incision. The stomach and duodenum are carefully examined for external evidence of ulceration even if endoscopy appears to have defined the source of bleeding. If necessary the lesser sac is opened to inspect the posterior surface of the stomach.

If a gastric ulcer is the cause of bleeding, the alternatives are partial gastrectomy including removal of the ulcer, or gastrotomy with undersewing of the bleeding point, excision biopsy of the ulcer margin (to exclude malignancy) and closure of the gastrotomy followed by truncal vagotomy and a drainage procedure. The risks of failing to appreciate that the ulcer is malignant cannot be over-emphasized, particularly in elderly patients. In general, partial gastrectomy with Billroth I gastroduodenal anastomosis is preferred given that the patient is in good general condition, the lesion is not situated high on the lesser curve requiring an extensive gastrectomy, and the surgeon has the necessary experience.

For bleeding duodenal ulcer the choice lies between (a) under-running the ulcer base with a suture followed by truncal vagotomy and drainage; (b) Polya partial gastrectomy with excision of the ulcer if possible. Although operations involving gastric resection may carry a lower incidence of rebleeding, the lesser procedure of truncal vagotomy and pyloroplasty is now preferred by most surgeons. The ulcer is under-run by two or three sutures of No. 1 Vicryl or Dexon which are inserted deeply through the edges and base of the ulcer before being tied (Fig. 17.28). A 'fish hook' needle is particularly helpful when access to the ulcer is difficult.

If the patient is bleeding from gastritis, duodenitis or erosions operation is necessary only if massive bleeding continues. The interior of the stomach is inspected to confirm that there is no other source of haemorrhage which may have been missed at endoscopy. The choice of operative procedure remains controversial but truncal vagotomy is recommended. The risk of rebleeding is lower if vagotomy is combined with partial gastrectomy and where the patient's condition is satisfactory, an experienced surgeon may prefer resection to vagotomy with drainage procedure.

If the cause of bleeding has not been defined endoscopically and no abnormality is apparent on inspecting the surface of the stomach and duodenum, 'blind' partial gastrectomy should not be performed.

The interior of the stomach and proximal duodenum are inspected to make certain that an ulcer, neoplasm, area of gastritis, Mallory-Weiss tear or varices have not been missed at endoscopy.

Pyloric stenosis
Patients presenting with pyloric stenosis have frequently lost weight, are dehydrated and may have a hypokalaemic, hyponatraemic alkalosis. This is treated by intravenous infusion of normal saline to which potassium chloride is added. A wide-bore nasogastric tube is used to empty the stomach and lavage may be necessary to remove food debris. Where the gastric outlet obstruction is the result of oedema associated with a duodenal or pyloric channel ulcer then treatment with H2 receptor antagonists or Omeprazole may be adequate. Where the narrowing results from fibrosis, however, operative treatment is required.

Before making the decision about definitive management endoscopy is mandatory to exclude malignancy which is now the most common cause of gastric outlet obstruction. Where malignancy has been excluded the operation of choice is usually gastro-jejunostomy with vagotomy as the deformed pyloric channel/duodenum may be difficult to close as a satisfactory pyloroplasty.

THE DIFFICULT PEPTIC ULCER

Some peptic ulcers pose technical problems for the surgeon which may require variations on the basic technique. For the posterior penetrating ulcer the first part of the duodenum should be dissected in the standard way and the right gastric pedicle divided. If the ulcer lies sufficiently proximal it may be dissected free from the first part of the duodenum leaving the ulcer in situ on the pancreas and allowing duodenal closure in the usual way. If the ulcer is too distal or too large to allow safe duodenal closure, a wide-bore drain should be placed into the duodenal stump and the stump closed around this with a purse string suture. The alternative of pre-pyloric division of the stomach retaining a cuff of antrum is not recommended as this retained antrum may produce sufficient gastrin to result in recurrent ulceration.

The high lesser curve gastric ulcer may conveniently be treated by the Pauchet manoeuvre (Fig. 17.29). This involves excising a tongue of lesser curve containing the ulcer and closing this as the new lesser curve. This technique effectively avoids the need for a very radical gastrectomy for a high lesser curve ulcer.

REVISIONAL PEPTIC ULCER SURGERY

With the decline in elective peptic ulcer surgery the need for revisional peptic ulcer surgery has also declined. Few patients develop complications for the first time many years after the original operation.

Taking down of gastroenterostomy
The complications of gastroenterostomy which may result in an indication to take it down are firstly the consequences of gastric incontinence, particularly early dumping syndrome. Where diarrhoea appears to be the result of gastric incontinence more than of the truncal

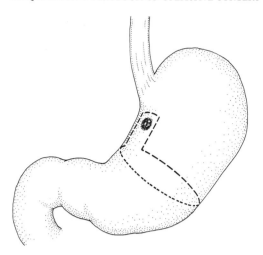 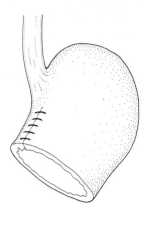

Fig. 17.29   The Pauchet manoeuvre

vagotomy (i.e. the diarrhoea occurs shortly after meals as a component of the dumping syndrome) then taking down the gastroenterostomy may improve the symptoms. Stomal ulceration may occur in relation to a gastroenterostomy many years after its formation and failure of such an ulcer to heal with powerful acid-reducing agents may also be an indication to take down the gastroenterostomy.

The gastroenterostomy is most conveniently taken down using stapling techniques.

The management of these patients requires a detailed history from the patient and observation of the symptoms and signs produced upon eating. Rapid gastric emptying may be confirmed by barium studies and gastric emptying formally assessed by an isotope labelled test meal. Colonization of the small bowel should be excluded by a hydrogen breath test and if present should be treated. Medical treatment of early dumping by Methoxy Pectin should be attempted in the first instance. Revisional surgery should not be attempted until 1–2 years after the original operation as symptoms may improve spontaneously with time.

The operation. The previous upper abdominal scar should be excised. It should be anticipated that there will be multiple adhesions present within the upper abdomen. The gastroenterostomy is located and the afferent and efferent loops defined. If (as is usually the case) a retrocolic gastroenterostomy has been performed, it should first be dissected free from the transverse mesocolon until a finger can be passed behind the gastroenterostomy stoma. The next part of the operation can be greatly facilitated by using a stapling device either the GIA (Autosuture) or the PLC (Ethicon). The limbs of this instrument are placed across the stoma as close to the original suture line as possible. It is important to try to avoid ectopic gastric mucosa on

the jejunal side and equally important to avoid narrowing the stapled jejunal segment. One or more firings of the instrument is performed.

It is advisable to oversew both staple lines with a continuous 2/0 Vicryl or Dexon suture to ensure haemostasis. It is essential to ensure that the lumen of the stapled small bowel segment is of adequate calibre. The defect in the transverse mesocolon is then repaired and the abdomen closed.

Gastric stasis, which might be expected to occur in the vagotomized stomach when the drainage procedure has been reversed, has not proved in practise to be a problem with this procedure provided satisfactory gastric motility has been demonstrated on the preoperative barium and there is no obstruction to the passage of barium through the pylorus or around the duodenal loop.

Reconstruction of pylorus following pyloroplasty

Where history and investigation suggest that the symptoms result from rapid gastric emptying as a result of a pyloroplasty, then reconstruction of the pylorus should be considered. The investigation of such patients is similar to that described above for patients who have post cibal symptoms following gastrojejunostomy. A delay of 1–2 years following the initial operation is recommended to allow for spontaneous improvement in symptoms and conservative treatment with diet and Methoxy Pectin should be attempted in the first instance.

For those patients in whom reconstruction of the pylorus is appropriate the operation should be performed by excising the previous upper abdominal scar. After division of adhesions the pyloroplasty is identified and adhesions along the greater and lesser curve aspects of the pyloric channel and the superior and inferior aspects of the first part of the duodenum are carefully divided. The duodenum is then Kocherized by incising the peritoneum to the right side of the second part of the duodenum which is then drawn forward. By finger palpation the site of the ring of pyloric muscle should be established both above and below the scar of the pyloroplasty. A stay suture is inserted through this ring of pyloric muscle above and below the scar of the pyloroplasty. The anterior wall of the pylorus is then opened between the stay sutures and these stay sutures are then approximated and tied together reconstructing the pyloric ring so that the pyloric ring admits only the tip of one finger. The incision is then closed with continuous Vicryl or Dexon suture and the abdomen closed in the usual way.

Procedures for bile reflux and vomiting
Bile vomiting may occur after any operation for peptic ulcer disease but is most common when a gastro-jejunal anastomosis has been performed. Bile vomiting is usually manifest within a month of the original operation. It is important to exclude stomal oedema and efferent loop occlusion by adhesions or recurrent jejuno-gastric intussusception. This can be done by barium meal and recurrent ulceration should be excluded by endoscopy. Where the bile vomiting continues after Polya gastrectomy and no cause has been established by these investigations then conversion of the Polya gastrectomy to a Roux-en-Y biliary diversion should be considered.

The upper abdomen is opened by excising the previous upper abdominal scar and adhesions are divided. The gastro-jejunal stoma is cleared of adhesions and freed from the transverse mesocolon to enable a finger to be passed behind the gastro-jejunal anastomosis. The afferent loop is dissected free from the stoma for some 5 cm. Its division can be greatly facilitated by the use of a stapling device either the GIA (Autosuture) or the PLC (Ethicon). A small window is made in the mesentery of the afferent loop some 2 cm from the stomach. The mesenteric vessels are then divided between ligatures in a line heading toward the superior mesenteric artery. The afferent loop can then be divided by applying the limbs of the stapling instrument across it (Fig. 17.30).

The divided afferent loop is then anastomosed end-to-side to the efferent loop 50 or 60 cm distal to the stomach. This entero-anastomosis can be performed using either a suturing technique or using a side to side anastomosis with the reloaded GIA or PLC instrument.

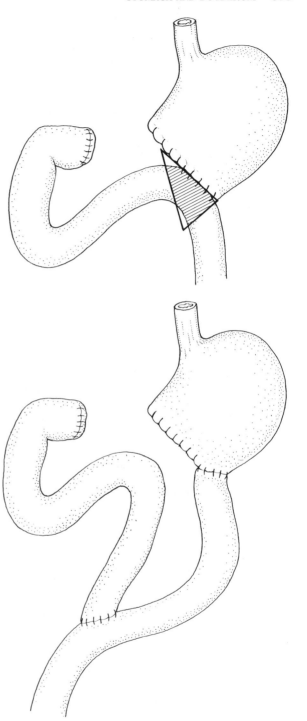

Fig. 17.30 Roux-en-Y diversion for bile vomiting following Polya gastrectomy

OPERATIONS FOR GASTRIC CANCER

Operations for gastric cancer may be classified into curative or palliative. Curative surgery implies sub total gastrectomy for lesions in the distal two-thirds of the stomach and total gastrectomy for lesions in the proximal one-third of the stomach in each case including en bloc removal of greater omentum and draining lymph nodes. Palliative surgery is performed to try to improve the quality of the patient's remaining life by removing a potential source of bleeding, obstruction or pain. In general resection provides better palliation than does mere bypass of the tumour which leaves the patient still vulnerable to the complications of bleeding and of pain through penetration of adjacent structures. Preoperative staging should be carried out in each case. Chest X-ray and liver ultrasound are the basic minimum in terms of imaging investigations to define metastatic spread which would place the tumour beyond cure. CT scanning may be able to define some irresectable cases preoperatively but in practice CT scanning is rarely able to define local inoperability, a decision which is usually made at laparotomy. Laparoscopy has proved useful for assessing metastatic spread to liver and to peritoneum.

Radical sub-total gastrectomy

Laparotomy is performed through a long midline incision. Intraoperative staging begins with the gastric cancer whose size and depth of invasion is noted. Any involvement of adjacent structures such as transverse mesocolon or tail of pancreas may necessitate resection of these structures with the specimen. The presence of hepatic or peritoneal metastases is determined. Radical sub-total gastrectomy is performed for lesions in the distal two-thirds of the stomach.

The procedure begins with division of the omentum to the right of the ascending part of the duodenum to allow Kocherization of the duodenum. Raising the duodenum forward enables assessment of the retro-pancreatic nodes. Clinical suspicion of involvement of these nodes should be confirmed by frozen section and such involvement precludes curative gastrectomy. The greater omentum is then dissected from the transverse colon by sharp dissection through a plane which is bloodless except for some small vessels near the mid line. When the omentum has been cleared from the entire length of transverse colon the anterior layer of transverse mesocolon is incised along its length and stripped up (Fig. 17.31).

This dissection is continued over the anterior surface of the pancreas. The pylorus should now be dissected. The gastrocolic omentum is then divided in line with the first part of the duodenum and the right gastro-epiploic vessels are ligated close to the origin of the right gastro-epiploic artery. The vessels below the first part of the duodenum are divided between ligatures, the gastro-colic omentum is divided close to the porta hepatis and the right gastric artery is divided close to its origin which is usually from the hepatic. The sub-pyloric and supra-pyloric lymph nodes should be included in the resection specimen. The first part of the

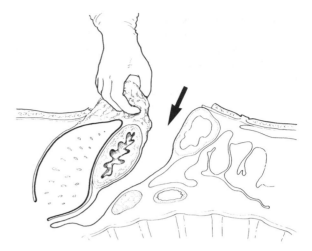

Fig. 17.31 Surgical section showing plane of dissection between anterior and posterior sheets of transverse mesocolon

duodenum, having been bared of tissue, can now be divided. This may be done using either of the techniques described above for resection for peptic ulcer — either using a small crushing clamp (such as a Payr's or Shoemaker) and suturing the duodenal stump by hand or by dividing the duodenal stump using a stapling instrument — the GIA (Autosuture) or PLC (Ethicon) — which will staple both the duodenal and gastric sides of the pylorus prior to division. Alternatively the duodenal stump may be closed using a linear stapler such as the TA30 (Autosuture) or the RL30 (Ethicon). The divided stomach can now be lifted forward to allow dissection of the lymph nodes in the stomach bed. Firstly lymph nodes along the hepatic artery should be dissected out if possible in continuity. The peritoneum forming the anterior leaf of the transverse mesocolon can now be stripped over the pancreas to allow dissection of the lymph nodes along its superior border. The hepatic artery and the splenic artery are followed back to the coeliac axis where the left gastric artery is ligated flush with the coeliac axis and all the left gastric lymph nodes are resected en bloc. The splenic pedicle is then divided between ligatures close to the tail of the pancreas and the peritoneum lateral to the spleen and lateral to the greater curvature and the fundus of the stomach is divided up to the oesophagus. The spleen is thus left attached to the greater curvature by the short gastric vessels. It may be advisable to remove the tip of the tail of the pancreas to ensure that all nodes in the splenic hilum have been removed. The stomach is then transected along an oblique line from just below the cardia to just below the lowest short gastric artery. This may be done conveniently using a TA90 or RL90 stapler. Gastrointestinal continuity is restored by making a Polya type of gastro-jejunal anastomosis which is most conveniently retrocolic.

Radical total gastrectomy

A radical total gastrectomy is indicated for lesions of the upper one-third of the stomach provided the proximal extent of the tumour is such that 5 cm clearance above it can be obtained. The initial steps are carried out exactly as for sub-total gastrectomy. In a total gastrectomy combined resection of the spleen and distal pancreas is performed. Dissection at the cardia can be helped by tilting the patient some 15 degrees into the head-up position and by using a sternal retractor such as the Goligher type. The peritoneum over the oesophageal hiatus is divided and the oesophagus is mobilized by blunt finger dissection. This will allow some 5–8 cm of oesophagus to be drawn into the abdomen. The stomach is then turned upwards so that the posterior wall of the oesophagus can be visualised. The left phrenic artery is then divided between ligatures and the left cardiac nodes are dissected free and included in the resected specimen. Stay sutures are placed on the oesophagus just above the site chosen for transection. The naso-gastric tube is withdrawn by the anaesthetist and the oesophagus transected. Reconstruction is by an oesophago-jejunostomy using a Roux loop of jejunum. The jejunum some 40 cm distal to the duodeno-jejunal flexure is selected and the vessels in its mesentery divided between ligatures using the arcade vessels to ensure sufficient blood supply to the mobilized distal loop. The jejunum is conveniently transected using a GIA or PLC device and the distal divided bowel is brought through a window in the transverse mesocolon to be anastomosed to the oesophagus. This may be done using a suturing technique or a stapling technique. The preferred suturing technique is to use a single layer of all coats interrupted, nonabsorbable, sutures such as Nurolon. An alternative being used increasingly is to use an intra-luminal stapling device such as the EEA (Autosuture) or ILS (Ethicon). Where this is used 6 stay sutures should be placed into the oesophagus each of which should be seen to pass through the oesophageal mucosa which, unless care is taken, may slide proximally. Some surgeons advocate performing a jejunal pouch to act as a reservoir. The simplest of these is the Hunt-Lawrence pouch which consists of a simple J-pouch of jejunum, the limbs of which are conveniently amalgamated using a GIA or PLC stapling device.

Thoraco-abdominal oesophago-gastrectomy

When the lesion is located at or close to the cardia an abdomino-thoracic approach is advised. This may be a one stage procedure performed through a thoraco-abdominal incision or a two stage procedure, the abdominal approach through a midline incision being followed by a right thoracotomy (Ivor Lewis procedure). For the former, when resectability has been con-firmed, the transverse or oblique abdominal incision is extended over the desired intercostal space or rib (usually the ninth) as far back as the edge of the erector spinae muscle (Fig. 17.32).

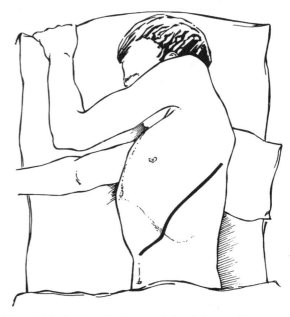

Fig. 17.32   Incision for thoraco-abdominal oesophago-gastrectomy

Incision through an intercostal space usually allows adequate access and the rib above or below the space can be divided to give greater exposure if required. The choice of intercostal space is dictated largely by convenience and the decision to open the seventh, eighth or ninth space is taken while exploring the abdomen. Some surgeons still prefer to enter the chest through the bed of a rib after periosteal elevation and removal of the rib from behind its angle to the costal margin. Division of the overlying muscles may be conveniently done with cutting diathermy and each bleeding point is ligated or coagulated by diathermy. The cartilage of the costal margin is divided and a wedge excised. If rib resection is not employed it is good practice to inject long-acting local anaesthetic (e.g. Marcaine) around the appropriate nerve before closing the incision unless a thoracic epidural catheter has been inserted. The pleural cavity is entered and the wound edges are protected by sterile towels. The intercostal space is opened widely with a large rib spreader as the diaphragm is incised down to the oesophageal hiatus. Diaphragmatic vessels including the inferior phrenic artery require ligation as the diaphragm is divided. Adhesions to the lung base and the lower part of the pulmonary ligament are divided so that the lung can be retracted upwards. The stomach is mobilized as described above and the lower oesophagus is freed through a longitudinal incision in the pleura between aorta and pericardium. There may be one or two small oesophageal arteries passing forward and downwards from the aorta but one should only divide vessels essential for adequate oesophageal mobilization. The oesophagus is encircled by a tape which can be used for retraction. Division of the diaphragm is now completed but a ring of diaphragm may have to be removed if the growth is adherent.

Total gastrectomy with oesophago-jejunal anastomosis is usually performed but some growths of the cardia can be dealt with by anastomosing the oesophagus to the retained distal portion of stomach. Numerous techniques for oesophago-gastric anastomosis are available; it is my own practice to transect the stomach with a stapling device and use one layer of all coats interrupted Nurolon sutures to anastomose the oesophagus to the anterior wall of the gastric pouch. If oesophago-gastric anastomosis is employed it is important to mobilize the duodenum thoroughly and it is advisable to carry out a simple pyloric myotomy (as in the Ramstedt operation) or pyloroplasty to avoid gastric stasis.

The diaphragm is closed with interrupted Vicryl or Dexon. An intercostal drainage catheter is placed in the dependent part of the pleural cavity for subsequent underwater seal drainage and the lung is reinflated. Dexon sutures (gauge 1) can be used to re-approximate the edges of the costal margin.

GASTRIC SARCOMAS AND LYMPHOMAS

Sarcomatous lesions account for only 1–3% of malignant gastric lesions. Most gastric sarcomas arise from lymphoid tissue or smooth muscle (leiomyosarcoma) but rare examples arise from other tissues (e.g. fibrosarcoma, haemangeiopericytoma, neurofibrosarcoma). Gastric sarcomas are also treated by radical excision whenever possible. These neoplasms are usually radioresistant but improved survival has been reported following the use of adjuvant combination chemotherapy.

Lymphoid tumours are more often manifestations of systemic lymphoma than primary localized gastric lymphomas. All patients thought to have gastric lymphoma should undergo laparotomy unless investigation shows diffuse systemic involvement with positive bone marrow biopsy. The gastric lesion is excised radically as described for carcinoma. A full staging laparotomy is also indicated with added wedge biopsy of both lobes of liver, biopsy of glands in the para-aortic and iliac chains, and use of ligaclips to mark the splenic pedicle and gland biopsy sites for subsequent radiographic identification. The patient should be considered for postoperative radiotherapy, particularly in the lymphocyte predominant type of lesion. Chemotherapy is

reserved for patients with diffuse systemic involvement or recurrence after irradiation.

OPERATIONS FOR MORBID OBESITY

Surgical treatment for morbid obesity is indicated in relatively few patients. Surgical treatment should be considered only after the patient has been investigated by a physician, endocrine abnormalities excluded, and conservative treatment under the supervision of a surgeon and dietician has failed to produce sustained weight loss. The surgical management should not be carried out by the surgeon in isolation but in close consultation with physician and dietician both pre- and postoperatively. Indications for the technique vary but only patients with an excess body weight of 45 kilograms or who are 100% above ideal body weight as defined by metropolitan height and weight tables should be considered. Weight loss should be assessed by reduction of mean body mass index (weight in kilograms/height in metres squared) for which the normal range is 15–25 kilograms per metre squared.

A number of surgical approaches to the treatment of obesity have been described including dental occlusion by jaw wiring, the use of intragastric balloon prosthesis placed endoscopically, jejuno-ileal bypass and biliary intestinal or biliary pancreatic bypass. These approaches have been superseded by a variety of gastric operations of which the best appears to be the vertical banded gastroplasty described by Mason (Mason, 1982).

Pre-operative assessment includes measurement of height, weight and calculation of body mass index and correction of commonly associated conditions such as hypertension and diabetes. Rapport between the surgeon and dietician is important and dietetic advice begins preoperatively. Respiratory inefficiency is common in obese patients so that provision should be made for the possibility of postoperative positive pressure ventilation.

After induction of anaesthesia a wide bore orogastric tube (F32) is passed. An upper midline incision extending below the level of the umbilicus is made and a large self retaining retractor inserted. The lower oesophagus is mobilized and encircled with rubber tubing. The lesser sac is opened by widely opening the avascular part of the lesser omentum. A 2 cm length of lesser curve just above the crow's foot is cleared of vascular attachments which are divided between ligatures. The site for the stoma is then selected just to the left of the intra-gastric tube some 10 cm distal to the cardia. The stoma is created by passing the pin of the EEA stapler through both anterior and posterior stomach walls, firing to remove a disc of stomach (Fig. 17.33).

The TA90 bariatric stapler firing four rows of 4.8 mm staples is inserted through the stoma, aligned alongside the intra-gastric tube and positioned to create a proximal pouch of less than 30 ml in volume (Fig. 17.34).

This volume may be assessed by inflating a naso-gastric tube fitted with a balloon. The stoma is now encircled with a strip of Marlex or Gortex 1.5 cm wide and 5.5 cm in length. The length of the strip is critical to the success or failure of the operation. This encircling collar should not be stapled to the stomach and should be covered with omentum to prevent adhesion to small bowel. The 32 gauge tube should be replaced by a naso-gastric tube passed through the pouch to permit postoperative decompression of the stomach.

Post operative care may require initial assisted ventilation and the patient should be nursed from the earliest possible moment in a sitting position. Postoperative diet requires a liquidised 800 calorie diet for the first 4 weeks after operation. Thereafter the patient is able to progress to pureed food and then gradually changes to small amounts of very well chewed food eaten slowly. Regular supervision at the dietetic and surgical clinics should continue for at least 18 months post operatively.

Figs 17.33 & 17.34   *Operation for morbid obesity*

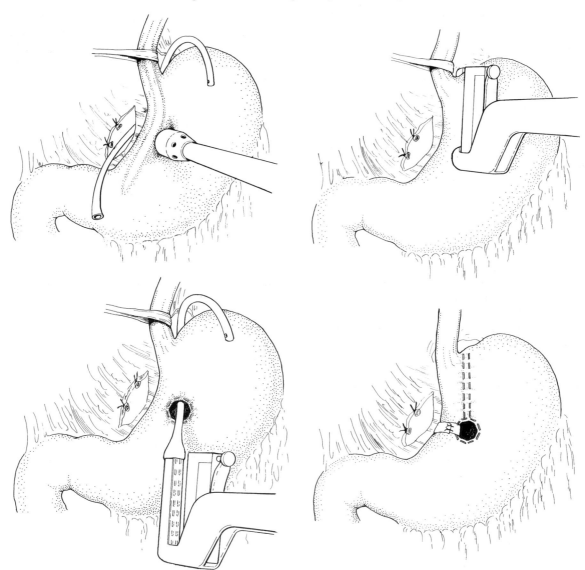

Fig. 17.33   Creating the stoma using the EEA

Fig. 17.34   Creating the pouch using the TA90

MINOR GASTRIC OPERATIONS

Gastrostomy

While the indications for open gastrostomy have decreased in recent years, percutaneous endoscopic gastrostomy has become more popular (Payne-James, 1992).

Open gastrostomy can be carried out under local or general anaesthesia. A small midline or left subcostal incision is used. If local anaesthesia is being used the parietal peritoneum should be infiltrated before the peritoneal cavity is entered. The anterior wall of the stomach is grasped with two pairs of Babcock's tissue forceps and the stomach is drawn onto the surface. The stomach is incised to allow insertion of a 12 or 14 French gauge Foley catheter whose balloon is then inflated. Leakage alongside the catheter is prevented in one of two ways. In Stamm's method two purse string sutures of a nonabsorbable material are inserted concentrically around the tube, the first 1 cm from the tube. This is then inverted by a second concentric suture some 2 cm from the tube. When drawn tight these sutures invaginate the catheter. To further reduce the risk of leakage, the anterior gastric wall is sutured to the parietal peritoneum. In Witzel's method a valve is created by burying the tube in a short tunnel in the stomach wall (Fig. 17.35). As with the Stamm's method the tube is brought out through a stab incision in the anterior abdominal wall, and the anterior stomach wall in the region of the tube is anchored to the parietal peritoneum of the anterior abdominal wall by interrupted sutures.

Percutaneous endoscopic gastrostomy is being used increasingly to deliver enteral nutrition particularly in patients with neurological swallowing disorders. It offers the advantage of greatly reduced morbidity and mortality compared to the open procedure. A fibreoptic endoscope is passed in the usual way into the stomach. The tip of the endoscope is directed towards the anterior abdominal wall where a second operator can identify it by transillumination and guide it to the ideal site for placement of the tube. A cannula is passed by the abdominal operator percutaneously into the stomach. He then passes a thread through this cannula. This thread is grasped under direct vision by the endoscopist using biopsy forceps and is drawn back through the mouth. The gastrostomy tube is securely anchored to the thread which is pulled by the abdominal operator, delivering the gastrostomy tube through the mouth and oesophagus into the stomach and out through the anterior abdominal wall. The tube is then secured in place by nonabsorbable sutures through the skin of the anterior abdominal wall.

Gastrostomy in children

Gastrostomy is now seldom used in neonatal surgery except for feeding purposes in delayed oesophageal procedures. Gastrostomy may, however, be necessary in children who are unable to swallow, for example spastic tetraplegia and in some children with cystic fibrosis so as to supplement nourishment. Where possible, endoscopic gastrostomy is preferred to an open operation.

Unless the abdomen has previously been opened a transverse incision 3 cm long is made in the left hypochondrium. Two concentric purse string sutures are placed high in the anterior wall of the stomach. The wall is then incised with a pointed scalpel, the margins of the opening are held apart with forceps so that a 10 Malecot catheter can be introduced with ease and the sutures are tied so as to invaginate the stomach wall around the catheter. The stem of the catheter is then brought out through a separate stab wound, the stomach wall sewn to parietal peritoneum around the catheter to prevent leakage and the incision is closed in layers. Finally the catheter should be withdrawn so that the bulbous expansion lies flush against the inner aspect of the stomach wall and the stem of the catheter fixed to abdominal skin with a silk suture. Unless adequately secured, the catheter may be passed down the stomach to obstruct the pylorus.

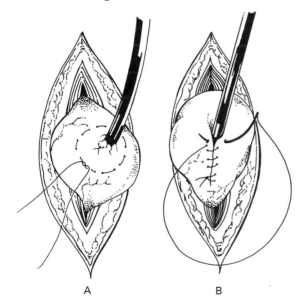

Fig. 17.35 (A) Gastrotomy by Stamm's method. The string suture closest to the tube has been tied and the purse string has been inserted and is about to be tied. (B) Gastrotomy by Witzel's method showing the tube being buried in a tunnel of stomach wall by continuous suture

CONGENITAL CONDITIONS

Congenital hypertrophic pyloric stenosis

This condition presents in babies within the first 5

weeks of life. Boys are four times more commonly affected than girls and the first born child is relatively at risk. The circular muscle of the pylorus is hypertrophied to produce a fusiform tumour between 1 and 2 cm in diameter causing partial or complete occlusion of the pyloric canal.

Diagnosis

The classical features of pyloric stenosis are forceful vomiting after feeds, visible gastric peristalsis and a palpable pyloric tumour. At the start of the illness the baby is otherwise healthy, but with time becomes progressively weaker from lack of nourishment and fluid loss. Both gastric peristalsis and the pyloric tumour become more obvious when the baby is fed. The tumour is most easily felt when the nurse feeding the baby sits with the infant cradled in the left arm, the surgeon sits on the left side of the nurse and palpates the baby's abdomen with the left hand. The middle finger of the left hand is placed over the right rectus muscle, half way between the xiphisternum and umbilicus and pressed both deep and medially. The tumour has a characteristic feel, likened to the tip of the nose.

Preoperative care. The baby's fitness for surgery is assessed and any dehydration or electrolyte imbalance corrected by intravenous infusion. A nasogastric tube is passed to allow gastric lavage and free drainage of stomach content.

Pyloromyotomy — Ramstedt's operation

The purpose of the operation is to split the hypertrophied muscle in the long axis of the pylorus leaving the underlying mucosa intact. The procedure is normally carried out under general anaesthetic but local anaesthesia is a practical alternative.

A 4 cm transverse incision (Fig. 17.36) is made in the right upper quadrant of the abdomen. The rectus abdominis muscle is divided in the line of the incision. The liver lies well below the costal margin in the new-born and must be retracted upwards. The stomach wall, which lies deep and medial to the incision, is lifted through the wound with blunt dissecting forceps and held with the aid of a wet gauze swab. The proximal part of the stomach is drawn down through the wound to provide extra mobility which allows the pylorus to be delivered with greater ease. The thickened pylorus is pinched between the finger and thumb so as to stretch the anterior wall and a 2 mm deep incision is made along the full length of the tumour in the avascular upper border (Fig. 17.37). The points of blunt curved artery forceps are introduced into the incision and spread from side to side to split the brittle muscle down to mucosa (Fig. 17.38). The remaining fibres can be broken with a blunt dissector. Care is taken not to damage the mucosa, particularly distally where

Figs 17.36–17.40 Pyloromyotomy for congenital pyloric stenosis

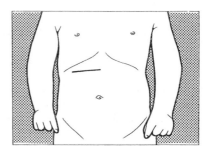

Fig. 17.36   Transverse incision high in right upper quadrant of abdomen

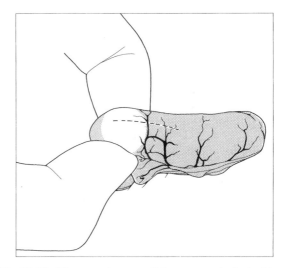

Fig. 17.37   The posterior part of the tumour pinched with finger and thumb to stretch the antimesenteric border. Dotted line indicates incision

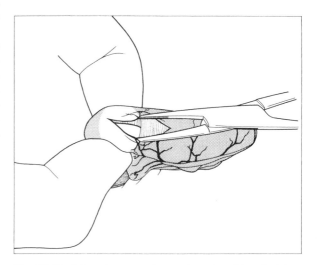

Fig. 17.38   Mosquito artery forceps introduced into incision and spread so as to split the hypertrophied muscle

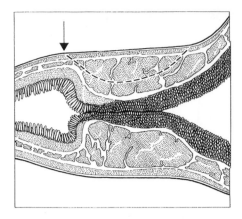

Fig. 17.39 Cross-section of hypertrophied pyloric muscle and line of incision. Arrow indicates the point where special care must be taken to avoid penetration of the mucosa

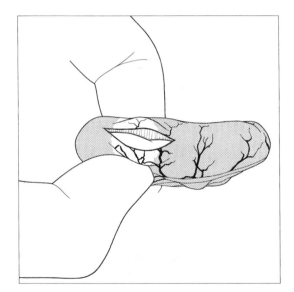

Fig. 17.40 Pyloromyotomy completed. Intact mucosa bulges into base of incision

the fornix of the duodenum lies close to the serosal surface (Fig. 17.39). When the dissection is complete the mucosa bulges freely into the base of the incision (Fig. 17.40). Bleeding points are easily coagulated with diathermy. The more general ooze from venous congestion will stop when the stomach is returned to the abdominal cavity. Finally the wound is closed in layers. If the mucosa is inadvertently opened during the procedure, it can be easily closed in a transverse manner with fine interrupted absorbable sutures and a nasogastric tube passed to decompress the stomach for 48 hours.

Postoperative care. A healthy breast fed baby can suckle 4 hours after operation and a bottle fed baby offered Dextrose Saline. In both it may be possible to establish a normal feeding pattern within 24 hours.

However, vomiting after pyloromyotomy is common and a more gradual approach may be needed. A debilitated baby should be maintained by intravenous infusion until oral feeding has been well established.

Duodenal atresia and stenosis

The incidence of duodenal atresia and stenosis is 1 per 6000 live births. The lumen of the duodenum develops in the embryo between 6 and 8 weeks after a period of mucosal proliferation and recanalization and the anomaly is probably established at this early stage. The duodenum is usually occluded at the level of the ampulla. The stomach and proximal duodenum are grossly hypertrophied and dilated and the duodenum distal to the obstruction is narrow. Although a wedge of pancreas may partly encircle the narrowed segment of duodenum, annular pancreas probably exists as a separate entity. If the obstructed duodenum has a normal outward appearance a mucosal diaphragm may be present.

Clinical presentation

There is a high incidence of associated abnormalities, 25% of babies having Down's Syndrome. Half of the babies with duodenal atresia are of low birth weight and maternal hydramnios is common. The presenting signs are copious vomiting which may be bile stained depending on the level of the lesion and either constipation or the passage of small, pale meconium plugs. In addition there may be a fullness in the epigastrium due to the dilated stomach and visible peristalsis. An erect abdominal X-ray will demonstrate the classical double bubble appearance of gas lying above one fluid level in

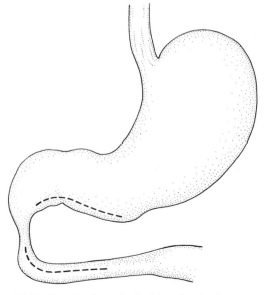

Fig. 17.41 Duodenal atresia. Incisions for duodeno-duodenostomy

the stomach and a second fluid level in the first part of the duodenum. For immediate management a nasogastric tube should be passed to prevent vomiting, an intravenous infusion established and the baby nursed in an incubator.

Treatment

At operation the obstructed segment is usually bypassed with a duodenostomy between dilated and narrowed duodenum immediately above and below the lesion (Fig. 17.41). However, when the atresic segment is more extensive a duodenojejunostomy may be necessary. Gastrojejunostomy should be avoided because of stasis and ulceration in the proximal duodenum. In the absence of an atretic segment a mucosal diaphragm should be considered and this may be demonstrated when an attempt is made to pass a tube through a gastrotomy and down through the duodenum. The duodenum can then be opened longitudinally, the mucosal diaphragm excised circumferentially and the duodenum closed transversely (Fig. 17.42).

As the baby is unlikely to feed normally for 2 or 3 weeks full nutritional needs should be provided early in the postoperative period by intravenous feeding.

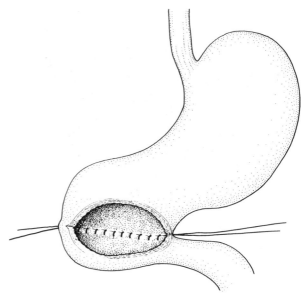

Fig. 17.42 Duodenal atresia. Partially completed anastomosis

REFERENCES

Alexander-Williams J 1981 Duodenogastric reflux after gastric operations. British Journal of Surgery 68: 685–687

Cuschieri A 1986 Surgical Management of severe intractable post vagotomy diarrhoea. British Journal of Surgery 73: 981–984

Hobsley M 1981 Dumping and diarrhoea. British Journal of Surgery 68: 681–684

Johnson A G, Baxter H K 1977 Where is your vagotomy incomplete? Observations on operative technique. British Journal of Surgery 64: 583–586

Kennedy T, Johnston G W, Love A H G, Connell A M. Spencer A M 1973 Pyloroplasty versus gastroenterostomy: Results of a double blind controlled trial. British Journal of Surgery 60: 949–953

Mason E E 1982 Vertical Banded gastroplasty for obesity. Archives of Surgery 117: 701–706

McGuigan J E, Wolfe M M 1980 Secretin injection test in the diagnosis of gastrinoma. Gastroenterology 79: 1324

Macintyre I M C, Millar A, Smith A N, Small W P 1990 Highly selective vagotomy 5–15 years on. British Journal of Surgery 77: 65–69

Payne-James J J, Kapadia S, Loft D E, Silk D B A 1992 Early experience with the Bower percutaneous endoscopic gastrostomy tube. Journal of the Royal College of Surgeons of Edinburgh 37: 34–36

Stabile B E, Passaro E 1976 Recurrent peptic ulcer. Gastroenterology 70: 124–132

FURTHER READING

Carter D C 1983 Peptic ulcer. In: Clinical surgery international, vol 7. Churchill Livingstone, Edinburgh

18

The spleen and portal hypertension

J. M. S. JOHNSTONE

Anatomy

The spleen lies between the fundus of the stomach and the diaphragm under cover of the left 9th, 10th and 11th ribs, its long axis being in the line of the 10th. Normally it lies entirely behind the midaxillary line, and does not project below the costal margin.

Its convex medial surface is related to the fundus of the stomach and the tail of the pancreas in front, and to the upper part of the left kidney behind. Its lower part is in contact with the left colic (splenic) flexure.

Peritoneal connections

The spleen is almost completely invested by peritoneum. At its hilum it is connected to the upper part of the greater curvature of the stomach by the *gastrosplenic (omentum)*, and to the posterior abdominal wall in front of the left kidney by the *lienorenal ligament.* These ligaments each consist of two layers, one layer being formed by peritoneum of the lesser sac (Fig. 18.1).

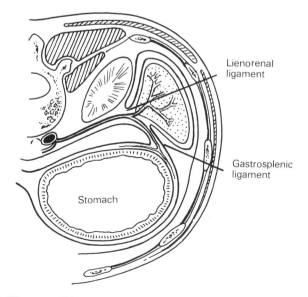

Lienorenal ligament

Gastrosplenic ligament

Stomach

Fig. 18.1 Diagram to illustrate the peritoneal folds attached to the spleen, and their contained blood vessels

Vessels

The splenic vessels are large in proportion to the size of the organ, and are very thin-walled. The *splenic artery* arises from the coeliac, and runs a tortuous course to the left along the upper border of the pancreas, crossing the front of the left kidney; it reaches the spleen between the layers of the lienorenal ligament, and divides into 5–8 branches which enter the hilum. Other branches, the *short gastric* and *left gastro-epiploic arteries*, pass onwards between the layers of the gastro-splenic ligament to reach the stomach. The *splenic vein* runs to the right behind the pancreas, and joins the superior mesenteric vein to form the portal vein; its tributaries correspond to the branches of the artery.

INDICATIONS FOR SPLENECTOMY

The conditions for which removal of the spleen may be required fall naturally into four main groups:

Rupture of the spleen

This is one of the commoner intraperitoneal injuries which may result from blows or crushes to the abdomen. In cases where the spleen is enlarged from disease, rupture may result from comparatively minor injuries. The spleen may be injured also in association with penetrating abdominal wounds. In a typical case signs of increasing intraperitoneal haemorrhage are present, and operation should be undertaken without delay, since it offers the only chance of recovery. Splenic suture has been recommended in order to conserve the spleen particularly in children, but is possible in less than 10% of cases (Tricarico, 1993). Splenectomy is usually required in order to control haemorrhage.

Delayed rupture

This equally dangerous condition may arise when the damage to the spleen is less severe. The laceration may then become temporarily sealed-off by omentum or by blood clot, or the bleeding may at first be confined within the capsule of the organ. In such cases the initial shock may be relieved by treatment and all symptoms subside. After a period of several days (or even of 2 or 3 weeks) symptoms suddenly recur; signs of serious intraperitoneal haemorrhage develop, and the case at once becomes of the gravest urgency.

Other conditions related to the spleen itself

Cysts, tuberculous infection, abscesses and tumours are rare in the spleen, but when they are confined to that organ, splenectomy should be carried out.

Aneurysm of the splenic artery

This is occasionally encountered, and may be a cause of sudden internal haemorrhage. The diagnosis is made usually at laparotomy in cases where rupture has already occurred. Treatment consists in splenectomy, combined with ligature of the artery on both sides of the aneurysm.

Total gastrectomy and upper partial gastrectomy

The spleen is usually removed as part of the resection, since this gives better access and allows more radical clearance of the glandular fields. Splenectomy may be included also in the operation of pancreatectomy.

Splenomegaly associated with blood dyscrasia

Enlargement of the spleen frequently co-exists in association with various altered conditions of the blood. The enlargement may occur because of congestion of the pulp cords, congestion of the venous sinuses, hyperplasia of the lymphatic tissue or hyperplasia of the red pulp. In some cases, more than one cause may be present. When red blood cells are abnormal, either congenitally as in *congenital spherocytosis*, or from acquired causes (*autoimmune haemolytic anaemia*), the passage of the red cell through the pulp cords is slowed, the cell becomes more fragile and its survival time is reduced. In these haemolytic anaemias the spleen is moderately enlarged because of pulp congestion. In portal hypertension, congestion of the venous sinuses occurs and is accompanied by proliferation of the cellular elements of the spleen. In the bulk of such an enlarged spleen sequestration of erythrocytes, granulocytes and platelets may occur, giving rise to considerable reduction in their numbers in the circulating blood (*hypersplenism*). Lymphatic hyperplasia occurs in the lymphoproliferative diseases and may give rise to a very large spleen with associated hypersplenism. Red pulp hyperplasia is found in infections, especially with parasites such as leishmaniasis and chronic malaria (*tropical splenomegaly*).

Haemolytic anaemia

In the condition of *congenital spherocytosis* there is an abnormal fragility of the red blood cells, which pass into the circulation in an immature form. In such cases splenectomy is, as a rule, most successful (Devlin, 1970). Although the red cell fragility is usually unaltered by the operation, the excessive blood destruction is arrested, and in most cases lasting cure, both of the anaemia and of the jaundice, is obtained. The optimum time to perform the operation is in late childhood or early adolescence, before liver changes have occurred. Performed in early childhood splenectomy is liable to be followed by acute and very serious infection (Cooper, 1984). The operation is uniformly and permanently successful in relieving the anaemia although the red blood cell abnormality persists (Macpherson, 1973). Patients undergoing splenectomy for haemolytic disease should have an ultrasound scan preoperatively since the detection of gall-stones is an indication for cholecystectomy at the same operation; the common bile duct should be examined by cholangiography and explored if necessary. In the acquired type of haemolytic anaemia, when the cause cannot be discovered and is, therefore, incapable of control, splenectomy is usually undertaken because of the failure of reasonable doses of corticosteroids to control the haemolysis. Experience shows however that the operation is less effective than in the congenital forms of the disease.

Idiopathic thrombocytopenic purpura

Splenectomy is followed by cessation of abnormal bleeding and restoration of the platelet count to normal in 60 to 80% of cases, the better results being obtained in cases with a short history. The initial treatment should be with corticosteroids up to a maximum of three weeks. Splenectomy is indicated in that time in short history cases and in all those with a long history of repeated relapses. At operation the discovery and removal of accessory spleens is of importance, since these may be responsible for a recurrence of the condition (Holme, 1984).

Other conditions

There are certain other diseases of the blood and reticulo-endothelial system where splenectomy is occasionally (but by no means consistently) successful. When anaemia is present, from whatever cause, splenectomy, by slowing down the rate of blood destruction, may have markedly beneficial effects. Even in conditions such as Hodgkin's disease, Gaucher's disease, and reticulosarcoma, in which splenomegaly with hypersplenism is often a feature, it may be justifiable to recommend splenectomy. Hypersplenism is in fact the main indication for splenectomy even where the primary disease is almost inevitably fatal. Although the operation cannot influence the final outcome of the disease, it may have considerable palliative value by slowing down the rate of blood destruction. Restoration of the blood count to normal often produces a worthwhile effect until such time as the marrow is overwhelmed by invading cells. Splenectomy as part of 'staging laparotomy' for Hodgkin's disease has been given up by most centres as the same information can be obtained from the more sensitive imaging techniques now available, for example CAT scanning.

Congestive splenomegaly (portal hypertension)
Splenectomy in this condition is considered on page 410.

TECHNIQUE OF SPLENECTOMY

Preparation
In nearly all patients requiring splenectomy, blood transfusion, both before and during operation, is valuable if not essential. In cases of ruptured spleen a delay of 1 to 2 hours, especially when used for resuscitation, is not associated with an increased mortality (Sargison, 1968). In the absence of transfusion facilities, the circulation may be temporarily sustained by infusion of dextran or plasma, to be followed by whole blood as soon as this is available. All patients undergoing elective splenectomy should be given *pneumovac* as protection against subsequent pneumococcal infection. Immediately preoperatively, Cefuroxime is administered and this is continued postoperatively until oral penicillin can be tolerated. Unless contra-indicated patients should receive prophylaxis against deep venous thrombosis with either heparin or alternative methods such as pneumatic cuffs to the legs during surgery. This is particularly important for this operation since splenectomy results in a rise in circulating platelets.

Incision
The best access to the spleen is obtained by a left rectus-splitting paramedian incision or by an oblique subcostal incision. The first incision may be extended laterally by a transverse cut which divides the outer fibres of the rectus muscle. In cases of ruptured spleen, the abdomen will often have been opened in the midline; this incision, extended laterally if necessary, should give adequate access. If a right paramedian incision has been employed, it may be best to close this and to make a left subcostal incision.

Mobilization of spleen
A hand is passed over the lateral surface of the spleen, between it and the diaphragm; the organ is lifted forwards and medially, and the posterior layer of the lienorenal ligament, which passes from it to the posterior abdominal wall and holds it in position, is divided

under vision. The underlying fascia is also divided but the scissors must not pass too deeply or the vessels may be damaged. Adequate exposure for this dissection is obtained by strong retraction of the left side of the wound while the spleen is drawn medially (Fig. 18.2). When the spleen is enlarged numerous vascular adhesions may be encountered. These are divided, if possible, under the guidance of the eye, and all haemorrhage arrested. A large pathological spleen may have dense adhesions to the under surface of the diaphragm which contain large veins. It is from these veins that hazardous bleeding can arise during the operation. Control is achieved by oversewing but can be more difficult than anticipated.

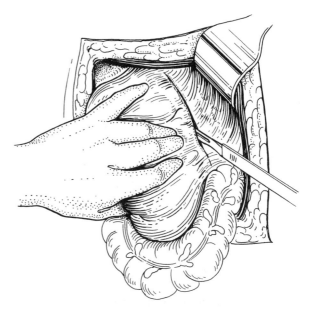

Fig. 18.2 Splenectomy. The spleen is lifted forwards and is mobilized by incision of the peritoneum passing from its lateral surface on to the posterior abdominal wall, i.e. the posterior layer of the lienorenal ligament

Once the spleen has been lifted from its posterior attachments, the gastrosplenic ligament (omentum), stretching between the spleen and the upper part of the greater curvature, is divided between clamps (Fig. 18.3). This fold contains the short gastric vessels which require to be ligatured. The spleen can then be delivered easily into the wound and the tail of the pancreas is carefully separated from the splenic hilum. Both the fundus of the stomach and the left colic flexure lie in contact with the spleen and must be safeguarded, all avascular fascial connections being divided. The splenic vessels are now exposed and may be approached from in front or behind. It is helpful at this stage to ligate the splenic artery in continuity 2 cm proximal to the spleen so as to allow the spleen to decongest and to reduce the

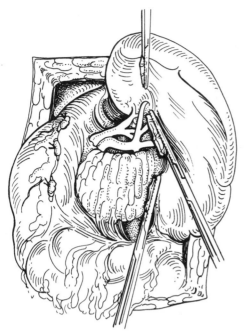

Fig. 18.3 Splenectomy. The gastrosplenic ligament is divided between clamps and ligatured. The thin anterior layer of the lienorenal ligament is then incised to expose the splenic vessels and the tail of the pancreas

risk of haemorrhage. Finally the artery and vein are ligatured individually.

Division of splenic vessels

The tail of the pancreas, which may partially obscure the vessels, is gently thrust aside by gauze stripping. A finger is passed behind the vascular pedicle, and the artery and vein are divided separately between clamps or ligatures. Gentle handling is most essential, since the vessels are exceptionally delicate and are easily torn.

Technique in cases of rupture

When splenectomy is being performed for rupture, a less deliberate exposure of the vascular pedicle is permissable. The spleen is delivered at the wound as rapidly as possible, and a hot moist pack is placed behind it. The combined pedicle — peritoneal and vascular — is then clamped and divided *in small sections at a time,* from below upwards. To obviate the risk of injury to neighbouring organs (particularly the tail of the pancreas), the clamps are applied as close as possible to the hilum.

Search for accessory spleniculi

This is essential when splenectomy is being performed for conditions of hypersplenism; otherwise the spleniculi may enlarge and give rise to recurrence. A single spleniculus may be more or less continuous with the

main spleen at either pole or at the hilum, being separated from it only by a constriction. Alternatively, one or more entirely separate spleniculi may be found within the layers of the gastrosplenic ligament.

Peritoneal toilet and closure

When the spleen has been removed, both the pedicle and the splenic bed are examined carefully, and bleeding points are dealt with, either by ligature or by underrunning suture. Drainage is necessary if there has been damage to the tail of the pancreas, or if haemorrhage has not been completely arrested. If the pancreas has been injured, sloughing of the wound may result from the escape of proteolytic enzymes.

Postoperative care

When severe anaemia is present blood transfusion may be required postoperatively. Thrombocytosis may develop during the first 10 days; it is important that blood specimens are taken to evaluate this so that the condition can be treated with Aspirin if it occurs. Any patient following splenectomy is in danger from major postoperative sepsis. Careful observation is therefore required and, if present, the condition must be treated vigorously. Penicillin should be continued indefinitely.

PORTAL HYPERTENSION

Increased pressure in the portal circulation, usually associated with enlargement of the spleen is due to an obstruction between the venous drainage of the gastro-intestinal tract and the heart. In practice the obstruction is usually situated in the portal system of veins. *Intrahepatic obstruction* is by far the most common and is due usually to cirrhosis of the liver in which the fibrotic changes have led to obliteration of the branches of the portal vein within that organ. *Prehepatic obstruction* occurs in the portal or splenic veins and is found most frequently in children although it may first manifest itself in adult life. It may be due to a congenital abnormality of the affected vein or, more commonly, to thrombosis occurring some years before the onset of symptoms. Umbilical vein sepsis in the new-born is the commonest cause of such thrombosis. Splenic enlargement and bleeding into the alimentary tract are the only features in the early stages; later atrophic changes develop in the liver. *Posthepatic obstruction* is rare except in tropical countries.

The main effect of portal hypertension is to cause gross engorgement of the anastomosing veins which connect the portal and systemic circulations. This is evidenced particularly by the development of oesophageal varices from which traumatic and devastating haemorrhage can occur. Some 40–50% of cirrhotic pa-

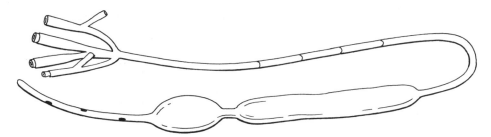

Fig. 18.4   Minnesota tube

tients die from their first haemorrhage. Other effects are splenomegaly; anaemia, leucopenia and thrombocytopenia, due mainly to pooling of blood in the spleen (hypersplenism); and ascites.

Conservative treatment of oesophageal haemorrhage
Bleeding can usually be controlled in the first instance by rest, transfusion, pitressin etc. or by passing a Minnesota tube (Fig. 18.4) which is designed to occlude the varices by direct pressure from a spherical balloon in the stomach and a cylindrical balloon in the lower oesophagus. There are separate channels for aspiration of the stomach beyond the gastric balloon and the oesophagus above the oesophageal balloon. The latter is especially important because of the ever present danger of aspiration. The balloons should not be left inflated for more than 24 hours; the tube is removed 24 hours later if bleeding has not occurred. Should these measures fail to control the bleeding, or should it recur soon after removal of the tube alternative nonoperative measures are available. The first of these is endoscopic sclerotherapy which is now standard practice in most centres but requires a skilled endoscopist and fibroptic endoscopic instruments (McKee, 1991).

An alternative nonoperative method is transhepatic embolization of the left gastric and short gastric veins. This is a highly specialized radiological technique in which a selective catheter is inserted percutaneously through the liver into an intrahepatic branch of the portal vein. The catheter having been guided into the appropriate vein small portions of gelatin sponge soaked in sclerosing material are injected. This has proved to be an excellent method of arresting haemorrhage although it cannot be regarded as a long-term solution (Henderson, 1979).

The development of these techniques means that emergency operative intervention for oesophageal haemorrhage in portal hypertension is less often required than hitherto. Such operations take the form of oesophageal transection rather than portal decompression which nowadays is seldom performed on an emergency basis.

Oesophageal transection
Earlier transthoracic operations, such as the Boerema-Crile and the Milnes Walker procedures have given way to oesophageal stapling (Spence, 1985) as the standard surgical method for the emergency control of oesophageal bleeding (Fig. 18.5). The great advantage of this technique is its avoidance of the need for a thoracic approach in a group of very ill patients. The abdomen is opened through an upper midline incision. The use of a manubriosternal elevator as employed in highly selective vagotomy greatly assists exposure. The overlying peritoneum is incised transversely at the point at which it is reflected from the anterior surface of the oesophagus onto the under surface of the diaphragm. The lower oesophagus is mobilized by blunt dissection preserving at least one vagus nerve. A longitudinal inci-

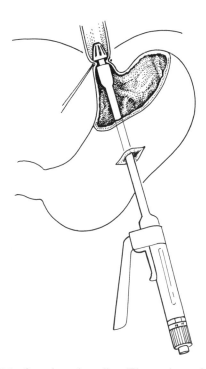

Fig. 18.5   Oesophageal stapling. The staple gun is inserted through a gastrotomy

sion is made on the anterior surface of the body of the stomach to allow insertion of the stapler. A No. 1 silk ligature is applied round the lower oesophagus approximately 2 cm above the oesophagogastric junction. It is tied to invaginate a cuff of the oesophageal wall between the two halves of the stapling capsule. The stapler is then closed to excise the core of the oesophageal wall and at the same time effect anastomosis with two rows of staples. The staple gun is carefully and gently withdrawn through the anastomosis and the gastrotomy. The latter is closed in routine fashion. The core of oesophageal wall is inspected for completeness. This simple procedure is highly successful in the majority of patients. Occasionally oesophageal stricture develops which may require dilatation at a later date.

Decompression operations

Survival in portal hypertension is determined mainly by the quality of liver function. The operative mortality in Child's (1957) groups A and B is in the region of 5%, whereas in group C it is around 40%. These facts together with the improvements in conservative measures (patients may be very successfully maintained with regular sclerotherapy see Clark, 1980) means that surgeons now tend to be selective in offering decompression operations. Such operations cannot reverse pathological changes in the liver but they may effectively prevent further haemorrhages, which in themselves are a serious menace to life.

There are two types of operations available: total and selective portalsystemic shunts.

Mesenteric arteriography is a valuable investigation if portal decompression is contemplated. It displays the arterial anatomy which may influence the choice of operation (an aberrant hepatic artery may contraindicate portocaval shunt) and, in its venous phase, outlines the portal venous system. If more information is required this may be obtained by either *transhepatic or transplenic venography*. Portal pressures can be measured at the same examination.

Total shunts

Those in which the whole of the portal system is decompressed by anastomosis of a systemic vein. This includes portacaval, mesocaval and proximal splenorenal shunts. Portacaval and mesocaval shunts result in diversion of the blood from the liver through a wide channel. It is associated with a low incidence of recurrent bleeding (10–20%) but a relatively high rate of encephalopathy (approximately 30% in Child's groups A and B). Splenorenal shunt is mainly indicated when there is hypersplenism necessitating removal of the spleen. The anastomosis being of smaller bore it is more liable to thrombosis and therefore to recurrence of oesophageal haemorrhage which occurs in 20–30%

but the incidence of encephalopathy is slightly lower than after portacaval anastomosis.

Selective shunt

This concept introduced by Warren (1967) involves decompression of the veins draining the oesophagus without deviation of portal flow from the liver (Shields, 1991). The main objective is to reduce the incidence of postoperative encephalopathy while decompressing the source of haemorrhage. The spleen is not removed. The splenic end of the divided splenic vein is anastomosed to the left renal vein. By division of left gastric, gastro-epiploic and umbilical veins, the splenic part is further separated from the remainder of the portal system. This is a technically more demanding operation than any variety of total shunt and should not be attempted by an inexperienced surgeon.

Portacaval anastomosis

An extended transverse right subcostal or, provided the patient is not obese or the liver greatly enlarged, a right paramedian incision give satisfactory access. The advantage of the latter is that it is also suitable for a mesocaval shunt should technical difficulty arise. The second part of the duodenum is reflected and the inferior vena cava exposed by incision of the overlying peritoneum. Its anterior surface is exposed from the caudate lobe to the level of the renal veins. The portal vein is exposed in the posterior part of the free border of the lesser omentum and is mobilized as far as possible. It is divided close to the liver and the upper stump is ligated. The lower end is implanted end-to-side into the inferior vena cava which has been partially occluded by an atraumatic clamp (Fig. 18.6).

Proximal (standard) splenorenal anastomosis

The operation comprises an anastomosis between the splenic and left renal veins, splenectomy having been performed. It is best carried out through a left thoraco-

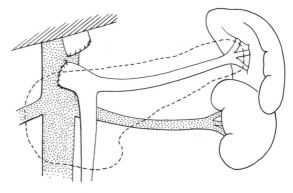

Fig. 18.6   Total shunt: end-to-side portacaval anastomosis

abdominal incision but a long subcostal incision has proved to be equally satisfactory. After the spleen has been removed the splenic vein is dissected out of its bed in the pancreas, its tributaries being divided between ligatures. The peritoneum over the left kidney is incised so that the renal artery and a segment of the vein may be controlled. An end-to-side anastomosis between the splenic vein and the left renal vein is carried out (Fig. 18.7).

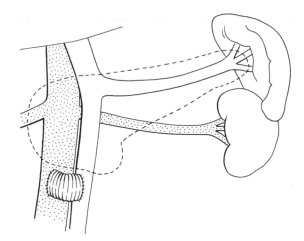

Fig. 18.8   Total shunt: mesocaval dacron 'H' graft

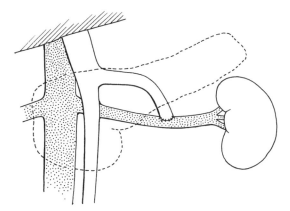

Fig. 18.7   Total shunt: proximal lienorenal anastomosis

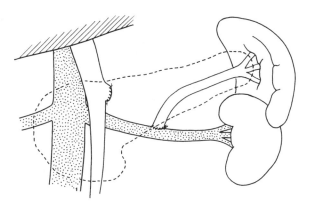

Fig. 18.9   Selective shunt: distal (Warren) lienorenal anastomosis

Mesocaval anastomosis
This is probably the easiest procedure for the inexperienced surgeon and the results are not significantly different from those of portacaval shunt. Through a midline incision the superior mesenteric vein is exposed at the lower border of the third part of the duodenum and by direct dissection through the posterior peritoneum the adjacent inferior vena cava exposed. A 20 mm woven or knitted Dacron graft is anastomosed as a bridge between the two vessels (Fig. 18.8).

Selective distal splenorenal shunt
Through a midline incision the small intestine is displaced to the right. The third and fourth parts of the duodenum are mobilized from the aorta to expose the left renal vein. The splenic vein is located by following up the inferior mesenteric vein to its junction. Separation of the distal splenic vein from the posterior surface of the pancreas, by division and ligation of the numerous fine tributary veins, is difficult and time consuming. At its junction with the portal vein the splenic vein is divided. The portal end is ligated and the splenic end anastomosed to the left renal vein (Fig. 18.9).

Complications
The most significant complication in patients who survive one of these shunting operations is *hepatic failure* of which a major manifestation is hepatic encephalopathy.

The latter occurs more commonly after a portacaval shunt (where the portal flow is totally diverted) than after a selective splenorenal anastomosis and this knowledge may influence the choice of operation. *Encephalopathy* is due to the toxic effects of breakdown products of protein digestion, which would normally be rendered harmless by deamination processes in the liver, but which, as the result of the shunt, are now poured directly into the systemic circulation. The risks of oesophageal bleeding, however, far outweigh those of encephalopathy. *Thrombosis at the site of anastomosis* occurs in a proportion of cases, particularly in small bore shunts such as the total splenorenal.

Other operations

Transthoracic oesophageal transection (the Milnes Walker operation)
The oesophagus is approached through the left chest. It is opened through a longitudinal incision in the muscular layers through which the mucosal layer is separated,

divided transversely and rejoined with a continuous catgut suture. This operation has largely been replaced by oesophageal stapling.

Splenectomy alone

This has been employed when the spleen is much enlarged, when the obstruction seems to be confined to the splenic vein, and when the liver is apparently healthy but this combination is rare. It is now seldom advised, since it precludes the possibility of a spleno-renal anastomosis at a later date, and, by encouraging portal vein thrombosis, it may also preclude a subsequent portacaval anastomosis.

Sub-cardiac gastric transection

This operation, as devised by Tanner (1958), is de-signed to arrest oesophageal haemorrhage by interrupting the venous communications between the portal and azygos (systemic) systems. The stomach is transected 5 cm below the cardia, and, all its vessels having been divided and ligatured, is immediately resutured. This operation carries a high mortality and is seldom performed today.

Oesophagogastrectomy

This may require to be undertaken as an emergency procedure, to arrest bleeding which is derived mainly from gastric varices. It is then a difficult and hazardous operation, but, in the presence of severe bleeding which cannot be controlled by simpler methods, there may be no other alternative. In rare cases, it may be the only elective procedure which is possible.

REFERENCES

Child C G, Donavan A J 1957 Current problems in management of patients with portal hypertension. Journal of the American Medical Association 163: 1219–1229

Clark A W 1980 Prospective controlled trial of injection scelerotherapy in patients with cirrhosis and recent variceal haemorrhage. Lancet 2: 552

Cooper M J, Williamson R C N 1984 Splenectomy: Indications, hazards and alternatives. British Journal of Surgery 71: 173–180

Devlin H B, Evans D S, Birkhead J S 1970 Elective splenectomy for primary hematologic and splenic disease. Surgery Gynaecology and Obstetrics 131: 273–276

Henderson J M, Buist T A S, Macpherson A I S 1979 Percutaneous transhepatic occlusion for bleeding oesophageal varices. British Journal of Surgery 66: 569–571

Holme T C, Crosby D L 1984 Elective splenectomy. Indications and complications in 102 patients. Journal of the Royal College of Surgeons of Edinburgh 29: 229–231

McKee R F, Garden O J, Carter D C 1991 Injection sclerotherapy for bleeding varices: risk factors and complications. British Journal of Surgery 78: 1098–1101

Macpherson A I S 1973 The Spleen. Charles C Thomas, Springfield, Illinois

Sargison K D, Cole T P, Kyle J 1968 Traumatic rupture of the spleen. British Journal of Surgery 55: 506–508

Shields R 1991 Bleeding oesophageal varices and the surgeon. British Journal of Surgery 78: 513–515

Spence R A J, Johnston G W 1985 Results in 100 consecutive patients with stapled oesophageal transection for varices. Surgery Gynaecology and Obstetrics 160: 323–329

Tanner N C 1958 Operative management of haematemesis and melaena; with special reference to bleeding from oesophageal varices. Annals of the Royal College of Surgeons of England 22: 30–42

Tricarico A, Sicoli F, Calise F, Iavazzo E, Salvatore M, Mansi L, 1993 Conservative treatment for splenic trauma. Journal of the Royal College of Surgeons of Edinburgh 38: 145–148

Warren W D, Zeppa R, Fomon J T 1967 Selective trans-splenic decompression of gastroesophageal varices by distal splenorenal shunt. Annals of Surgery 166: 437–455

19

The liver and the subphrenic space

O. J. GARDEN

Anatomy

The liver lies immediately below the diaphragm, mainly on the right of the median plane, only its thin left lobe being on the left. It is divided anatomically into two lobes, separated anteriorly and above by the attachment of the falciform ligament. The right lobe is the larger, and is related to the greater part of the right side of the diaphragm. In the recumbent position it is entirely under cover of the ribs; the gall-bladder is attached to its inferior surface. The left lobe stretches across the epigastrium towards the left hypochondrium and within the costal angle it is related to the anterior abdominal wall. The *porta hepatis* is a transverse cleft placed far back on the inferior surface of the right lobe. It transmits the portal vein, the hepatic artery and the hepatic ducts, together with lymph vessels and nerves. There is often a bridge of liver tissue of variable thickness between the two lobes and which covers the obliterated umbilical vein as it runs inferiorly to the left branch of the portal vein.

It should be noted that the line of division between the true right and left hemilivers runs in the plane of the gall bladder fossa and behind and to the left of the inferior vena cava (Fig. 19.1). These hemilivers are supplied by the right and left branches of the portal vein and hepatic artery. This discrepancy between anatomical and surgical divisions of the liver has produced considerable confusion in the surgical literature but the consensus view is that the major classical resections be referred to as hepatectomy or extended hepatectomy rather than lobectomy (*vida infra*).

Segmental anatomy

The falling morbidity associated with liver resection for tumour and trauma has emphasized the importance of knowledge of the segmental anatomy of the liver (Bismuth, 1982). The segmental anatomy is illustrated in Figure 19.2. The 8 segments are separated by the hepatic veins as they drain backwards into the vena cava and are based on their own segmental hepatic arterial and portal venous supply. The *left* hemiliver comprises 4 segments comprising segment I (caudate

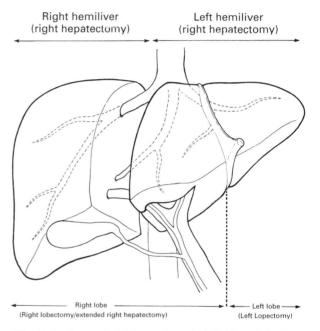

Fig. 19.1 Anatomical lobes and surgical division of the liver as seen on parietal surface

lobe) segments II + III (left lobe) and segment IV (quadrate lobe) which is often separated into an anterior (IV B) and posterior portion (IV A). The four segments of the *right* hemiliver are supplied by the segmental vessels arising from the anterior (segment V and VIII) and posterior (segment VI and VII) sectoral pedicles of the right branch of the portal vein and right hepatic artery.

The main venous drainage of the liver is via the hepatic veins to the inferior vena cava. The right hepatic vein drains the right hemiliver while the smaller left hepatic vein separates the two segments in the left lobe. This latter vessel has a common confluence with the middle hepatic vein which separates the right and left hemilivers as it runs in the plane between the gall bladder bed and the vena cava.

There are a variable number of small hepatic veins which drain direct from the caudate lobe (segment I)

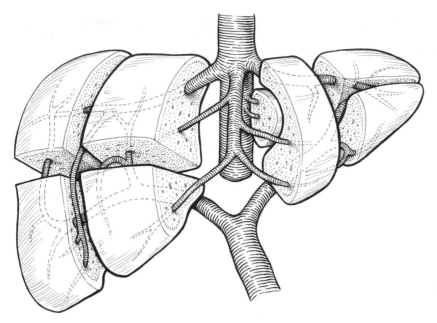

Fig. 19.2   Segments of liver as seen on the parietal surface with the main hepatic veins shown (after Couinaud)

into the inferior vena cava and in 20% of individuals there is an inferior right hepatic vein, the presence of which should be ascertained during right hepatectomy.

Peritoneal connections

The liver is clothed with peritoneum except at the 'bare area' on the back of the right lobe where it is in direct contact with the diaphragm. The peritoneum is reflected off the liver in four *double* folds — the coronary, left triangular and falciform ligaments, and the lesser omentum.

The coronary ligament is formed by the layers of peritoneum reflected on to the diaphragm from the upper and lower margins of the 'bare area'. Its two layers are separated by the vertical width of this area, but meet at its right-hand corner to form a free border to the ligament. The upper layer intercepts the hand which is passed backwards over the dome of the right lobe.

The left triangular ligament connects the upper surface of the left lobe to the diaphragm, and its two layers are in contact. The right triangular ligament is a redundant name given to the right free border of the coronary ligament.

The falciform ligament lies in the median plane. It is formed by peritoneum reflected from the upper and anterior surfaces of the liver to the diaphragm and linea alba down to the umbilicus. It provides the surface marking which separates the left lobe from the quadrate lobe.

The lesser omentum stretches from the porta hepatis to the lesser curvature of the stomach and the first 2.5 cm

of the duodenum. It separates the caudate lobe (segment I) from the left lobe (segments II + III). Its right free border forms the anterior boundary of the epiploic foramen; it contains the hepatic and common bile ducts, the hepatic artery and the portal vein. Temporary clamping of the structures by means of the Pringle manoeuvre can reduce blood loss during elective hepatic resection and during laparotomy for liver trauma.

The subphrenic space

This can be defined as that space which exists between the diaphragm above and the transverse colon and mesocolon below. Previously, considerable emphasis was laid on the division of the space into numerous compartments, but for practical purposes one may simply consider that there is a right and left subphrenic space, that on the right being divided into a supra and a sub-hepatic compartment.

SUBPHRENIC ABSCESS

A subphrenic abscess may follow perforation of an abdominal viscus or abdominal surgery (especially biliary or gastric surgery) and occasionally may result from direct extension of intrahepatic infection. Rupture of an abscess into the lung may result in a bronchobiliary fistula if there is associated biliary pathology. The right subphrenic space is involved in approximately 70% of patients, with subhepatic collections being more common than suprahepatic collections. Abscesses may be bilateral, a factor which may dictate the operative approach.

The incidence of subphrenic abscess is falling, possibly related to the greater use of prophylactic antibiotics in biliary surgery, improved techniques of bowel preparation, the use of antibiotic peritoneal lavage in combination with powerful systemic antibiotics in patients with a generalized peritonitis, and the recognition of the importance of anaerobic organisms in intraperitoneal infection.

Diagnosis

Clinical presentation of subphrenic abscess is often vague, and in patients on systemic antibiotics the classical features of infection are often suppressed. Bilioptysis (coughing up bile) will indicate the presence of associated biliary pathology. A persisting temperature and continued leucocytosis should raise suspicion of the condition. Occasionally patients complain of shoulder tip pain, or hiccoughs. Direct clinical signs are few, though some patients may be tender on percussion of the lower ribs. Associated chest pathology makes interpretation of chest signs difficult. Thoracic findings of atelectasis, pleural effusion and pneumonia are often present and may mislead the clinician.

Screening of the diaphragm may reveal an immobile diaphragm on the affected side, but fewer than 25% of patients demonstrate the classic radiological features of a raised hemidiaphragm with an effusion and some collapse above, and air/fluid level below. If present, the appearances are diagnostic.

The preferred method of investigation is by ultrasound scan, which is highly accurate in detecting fluid collections. Radioisotope scans using Gallium or Indium labelled leucocytes have been recommended to demonstrate intra-abdominal pus (Lucarotti, 1991) and may be of value in identifying other associated collections. Computerized tomography is more accurate than ultrasound and less operator dependent. Lesions as small as 2 cm may be identified and falsely negative examinations are uncommon.

If the diagnosis is established the usual approach is to avoid surgical intervention for localised collections which may be aspirated or drained percutaneously with ultrasound or CT scan guidance under systemic antibiotic therapy. If the diagnosis remains in doubt and the patient is receiving antibiotics, these should be discontinued and the situation allowed to clarify. Persisting uncertainty justifies exploration through an upper midline incision.

Surgical approaches

Previously, great emphasis was placed on the need to avoid encroaching on either the peritoneal or pleural cavity because of the risk of disseminating infection.

The availability of modern antibiotics has reduced considerably this risk and an *upper midline incision* is recommended to exclude bilateral suphrenic abscesses and collections elsewhere in the abdominal cavity and to enable inspection of any anastomosis for evidence of persisting leakage (Serrano, 1984).

The *posterior subpleural approach* has been described to drain abscesses in the subhepatic space, access to which is gained through the bed of the 12th rib. A lateral approach would be suitable for a right sided posterior subdiaphragmatic abscess. Access is gained through the bed of the 10th rib but contamination of the free pleura space can be avoided by securing pleura to diaphragm before entry to the abscess cavity.

A *limited anterior approach* may be considered when the abscess is thought to be situated in front of the liver but it is preferable to submit the patient to a formal laparotomy. Irrespective of which approach is used progressive diminution in the size of the abscess cavity may be checked by serial sinograms and/or ultrasound scan and the drain removed when the cavity has closed round it. Persisting discharge despite these measures may indicate inadequate drainage and repositioning of drains or re-exploration of the abscess may be required. Additional assessment by means of ultrasound or CT scanning may be useful.

Outcome

The overall mortality as a result of subphrenic abscess is extremely variable and is dependent on the underlying disease, the aetiology of the abscess and the patient population studied. The inability to diagnose and treat the primary cause of the subphrenic collection is associated with a poor outcome.

SURGICAL CONDITIONS OF THE LIVER

Trauma (see pp. 362 & 417)

Cystic disease of the liver

The most common form of cystic lesion of the liver is that of simple biliary cyst (Benhamou, 1988). With recent improvement in liver imaging it is apparent that the often reported incidence of 2% represents an under-estimate. The cysts which are found more commonly in the female are lined by biliary epithelium and contain serous fluid. In 50% of cases a solitary lesion is identified whereas in 10% of cases four or more cysts can be identified. Such cysts never communicate with the biliary tree and rarely give rise to symptoms. Abdominal distension, cholestasis, infection, haemorrhage, rupture and compression of the inferior vena cava and portal vein have been described (Fig. 19.3). Such cysts tend to recur following aspiration, and sclerosis by injection with alcohol is unlikely to be of value

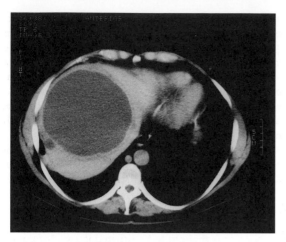

Fig. 19.3 CT scan showing a large biliary cyst in the right lobe of the liver and which became symptomatic as a result of haemorrhage into the cyst

for large symptomatic cysts. Surgical management is by deroofing which may be undertaken by laparoscopic means.

The cysts of polycystic liver disease have the same characteristics as simple biliary cysts and are associated with renal cysts. In this autosomal dominant condition, the complications are usually related to advancing renal disease which may require treatment by renal transplantation. These cysts often become symptomatic and may be a source of recurrent sepsis following transplantation. Deroofing of symptomatic hepatic cysts often meets with disappointing results.

Biliary cystadenoma of the liver is a rare condition being a thousand times less common than simple biliary cyst. There is a marked female predominance and one in four of such lesions will undergo malignant transformation. Biliary cystadenoma are lined by cuboidal or columner epithelium and contain mucous fluid. No communications are visible with the biliary tree but on ultrasound scanning papillary projections or septae may be visible. In the rare Caroli's disease, cysts are lined with biliary epithelium and contain bile. Cysts are multiple and communicate with the biliary tree. When found in association with congenital hepatic fibrosis, portal hypertension is often present. Caroli's disease may be complicated by cholangitis, jaundice, pancreatitis, liver abscess, amyloidosis and cholangiocarcinoma. Endoscopic percutaneous and surgical manipulation are best avoided in this condition and the role of liver transplantation in its management has yet to be established.

Pyogenic liver abscess

Liver abscess has become a more common condition with increasing radiological and endoscopic intervention of the biliary tree. Abscess may arise as a result of infection via the portal system (from appendicitis, diverticulitis), the hepatic arterial system (e.g. acute bacterial endocarditis), or by direct spread from a contiguous organ (e.g. gall-bladder). Abscess formation may follow blunt or penetrating injury and in up to a quarter of patients the source of infection is indeterminate (cryptogenic). Anaerobic organisms are common in cryptogenic infections and those arising from the portal system (e.g. *Strep. milleri*); coliforms and streptococci are present in most cases and are particularly frequent in infections arising from the biliary tree, while bacteraemia is probably responsible for abscesses with staphylococcus aureus or streptococcus (Lancefield A). The diagnosis is made from the history and might be confirmed by the presence of a raised white cell count and by positive blood culture. Radiological diagnosis is by means of ultrasound scan, and CT scanning may be useful to evaluate patients thought to have multiple hepatic collections.

The principles of treatment involve percutaneous drainage of accessible abscesses under ultrasound guidance, and antibiotic therapy selected on the basis of culture of blood and/or pus. Multiple small abscesses may require prolonged treatment with antibiotics for up to 8 weeks. Where the abscess is associated with other pathology such as in the biliary tree, it may be necessary to improve biliary drainage by surgical means or by placing endoscopically inserted stents. It is unusual to have to resort to open surgical drainage but where an abscess is suspected at laparotomy it may be located by needle aspiration or preferably by intraoperative ultrasonography. Once located, loculi are broken down, a large bore (28–32 French Gauge) tube drain is inserted and brought out through the abdominal wall at the nearest covenient point. In some cases chronic infection may give rise to a 'pseudotumour' which may require surgical excision before all sepsis can be eradicated.

Amoebic abscess

Amoebic abscess is a complication of amoebic dysentery caused by the parasite *Entamoeba histolytica*. Formerly confined to tropical countries, amoebiasis is occurring with increasing frequency in temperate zones as a result of immigration and intercontinental air travel. Approximately 10% of the world's population are asymptomatic carriers but only 1% of these develop invasive amoebiasis (Grewal, 1984). Hepatic infection results from migration of trophozoites from the intestine into the portal venous system. Up to 50% of patients with amoebiasis will show some evidence of amoebic 'hepatitis', but the incidence of true abscess formation is approximately 3%. It is likely that patients with 'hepatitis' would progress to true abscess formation in the absence of treatment.

The abscess is characteristically single and occupies the right lobe of liver. The histological features suggest that the principal pathology is a coalescence of multiple small areas of necrosis. Unlike pyogenic liver abscess, there is little surrounding tissue reaction, the 'abscess cavity' being lined by only a fine layer of granulation tissue separating it from normal liver. The contents of the abscess are usually bacteriologically sterile, and while the colour is variable the classic description is of 'anchovy sauce'. Trophozoites are identifiable in about 30% of cases.

The onset of symptoms may be sudden or insidious. Right upper quadrant pain and tenderness over the right lower ribs is almost invariable. Fever is present in over three quarters of the patients and may exceed 40°C. Hepatomegaly is detectable in 50%, but surprisingly, clinical jaundice is uncommon. Abnormal physical signs at the right lung base are common.

In patients suspected of the disease, fresh stool samples should be examined for cysts or trophozoites. Radiological investigations are similar to those for pyogenic liver abscess while serological studies are useful in distinguishing amoebic from pyogenic abscess. Diagnostic aspiration may be necessary in some patients but should always be preceded by drug therapy (vide infra).

Earlier diagnosis and prompt institution of treatment has reduced the incidence of the highly lethal complication of rupture and metastatic abscess.

Most amoebic abscesses respond to drug treatment, the size of the cavity being monitored by ultrasound. Metronidazole is the drug of choice at present, 800 mg t.d.s. for 10 days. Failure to respond within 24–48 hours usually indicates the presence of secondary infection in the abscess, colon necrosis or an incorrect diagnosis. Emetine hydrochloride or dehydroemetine are also very effective though potentially more toxic. Large abscesses may require closed needle aspiration in addition if there is no clear clinical response within 48 to 72 hours, or rupture appears imminent (Dietrick, 1984). A large bore spinal needle is introduced, after local anaesthetic infiltration, either over an obvious mass or through the right 9th intercostal space in the mid-axillary line. Ultrasonic guidance is essential in gaining access to the collection. Left lobe abscesses, though uncommon, may rupture into the pericardium (a lethal complication) but there is still considerable debate as to whether these should be aspirated to prevent this.

Open surgical drainage is rarely required, and even for the few cases who have secondary bacterial infection not responding to therapy, percutaneous aspiration is valuable. The overall mortality of amoebic abscess approximates to 4%.

Hydatid cyst of the liver
Hydatid disease, due to infestation with the *Echinococ-*

cus granulosus is uncommon in Great Britain but is endemic in the great sheep-rearing countries. The cyst commonly develops in the right lobe of the liver, where it may be mistaken for malignant disease or, if it extends upwards, for a subphrenic abscess. If it becomes secondarily infected an abscess will result; this may rupture into the pleural space and give rise to empyema or may rupture into the lung and result in a bronchobiliary fistula.

A diagnosis is made on the basis of the history, calcification on abdominal X-ray and the ultrasound finding of a cystic collection surrounded by a dense thick wall which may show areas of high echogenicity from calcification. Small cystic structures representing daughter cysts may be identified in the periphery of the main cyst or within the wall (Fig. 19.4). It is not usually necessary to undertake more sophisticated radiological investigations and percutaneous puncture should never be undertaken to establish the diagnosis. ERCP may be of value in patients with a hydatid cyst but who present with biliary colic suggestive of the passage of cyst and cyst debris into the main biliary tree. Organ imaging has to a large extent replaced the immunological diagnosis of hydatid disease in many parts of the world.

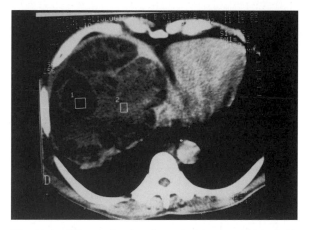

Fig. 19.4 CT scan showing the typical features of a hydatid cyst. The daughter nodules can be clearly seen lying beneath the thick cyst wall of the cyst which occupies the entire right lobe of liver

Chemotherapy with Mebendazole is of limited value; the most satisfactory treatment is complete excision of the cyst together with its contained parasites. The optimal approach is by means of an extended right subcostal incision. After the liver has been exposed and isolated by carefully positioned packs soaked in hypertonic saline, the cyst is aspirated following puncture with a cannula. Scolicidal agents should on no account be injected into the cyst since there is invariably a communication with the biliary tree which is at risk of

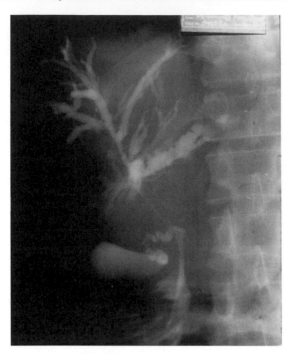

Fig. 19.5 Percutaneous transhepatic cholangiogram showing severe changes of secondary sclerosing cholangitis. A scolicidal agent had been injected into a hydatid cyst at the time of removal 3 years previously

secondary sclerosing cholangitis from the use of such agents (Fig. 19.5). The liver tissue is incised to expose the *ectocyst* or adventitious capsule, composed of condensed liver tissue. This is opened and the rubbery *endocyst* is brought into view. The endocyst is separated by blunt dissection from the ectocyst, to which it is usually only loosely adherent. Every effort should be made to remove the endocyst intact. If it ruptures during removal, the surgeon should satisfy himself, by careful inspection of the cavity, that the entire lining membrane together with any loose daughter cysts has been removed. In chronic long standing cysts it may be preferable to remove the fibrous ectocyst since this may minimise the risk of subsequent bile leakage, subphrenic collection and recurrence from contained daughter cysts (Belli, 1983). Such radical approach should only be undertaken by an experienced hepatobiliary surgeon. Some surgeons advocate packing the residual cavity with the greater omentum (Papadimitriou, 1970) but there is little evidence to support the routine use of this technique.

Other approaches have been advocated including the local freezing of the cyst's outer layer which allows its contents to be evacuated cleanly into a cone-shaped instrument which has become adherent to the cyst by the freezing process. There is much debate as to the most effective scolicidal agent but hypertonic saline is

considerably less toxic than formalin, alcohol and 0.5% silver nitrate solution.

Benign tumours

Non-cystic benign lesions of the liver are not uncommon. The lesion most often observed at ultrasound is the densely hyperechoic *haemangioma* which can in some patients reach a considerable size. Symptoms from such lesions are not common and intervention is only required if there is diagnostic doubt since rupture of these vascular lesions is extremely rare. Another not uncommon lesion which is encountered on palpation of the liver is that of *biliary hamartoma*. This subcapsular lesion has the appearance of a micrometastasis but its benign nature can be confirmed by biopsy and histology.

Fibronodular hyperplasia and *adenoma* cause considerable problems to the clinician because of the difficulties in differentiating between the two conditions on history and radiological evaluation. It is important to distinguish between the two lesions since fibronodular hyperplasia rarely causes symptoms and is not known to undergo malignant transformation (Foster, 1986). It tends to regress on observation and/or withdrawal of the contraceptive pill. Adenoma, like fibronodular hyperplasia, is an extremely vascular lesion which usually produces symptoms of pain as a result of haemorrhage within the tumour. Spontaneous bleeding is common. Because of the difficulties of distinguishing adenoma from hepatoma and the small risk that this benign lesion may undergo malignant transformation, resection should be undertaken. The two pathologies are differentiated classically on the basis of radiological imaging. Fibronodular hyperplasia often has a central fibrous scar visible on ultrasound scanning. This is one of the few situations where isotope scanning is of value since an adenoma usually appears as a filling defect whereas the Kupffer cells, in the fibronodular hyperplastic lesion, will generally take up isotope.

Malignant disease

Hepatoma is one of the commonest forms of malignancy in the world and may not often be resectable because of its association with cirrhosis. It is common in parts of the world where hepatitis B is prevalent. In the cirrhotic patient hepatoma often declares itself as a sudden deterioration in liver function often associated with extension of tumour into the portal venous system. Spontaneous haemorrhage from these highly vascular tumours is often fatal and dissemination to lymph nodes, peritoneum, lung and bone is extremely common. The best prospect of resecting such lesions is to pursue a policy of early detection by serial alpha-foetoprotein measurement and ultrasound scanning in susceptible individuals. Even patients with well-preserved liver function may tolerate only limited segmental or subsegmental resection (Garden, 1989).

In the non-cirrhotic patient the hepatoma may grow to a considerable size and only declare itself as a mass lesion or with pain. Despite their size such tumours may be amenable to resection by extended hepatectomy since the unaffected lobe of the liver may have undergone considerable hypertrophy to compensate for the presence of this space occupying lesion.

Alpha-foeto-protein levels are usually low or normal particularly in the fibrolamellar variant which tends to have the best prognosis. Diagnosis is made on the history and the radiological features of a solid mass lesion in the absence of any other primary tumour. CT scanning of the abdomen is essential in planning resection and excluding nodal or peritoneal involvement. Dissemination of disease is excluded by means of CT scan of the thorax and by isotope bone scan. Arteriography shows an extremely vascular lesion and infiltration of the portal vein and branches should be carefully assessed by means of ultrasound and the portal venous phase of mesenteric angiography. Percutaneous biopsy and fine needle aspiration should only be undertaken if resection is not contemplated because of the risk of haemorrhage and dissemination of tumour from the liver.

Other less common primary malignant tumours include *cholangiocarcinoma, haemangiosarcoma* and *haemangioendothelioma. Carcinoma of the gall-bladder* may present as an isolated mass involving the gallbladder but is rarely resectable at presentation. In a patient presenting with obstructive jaundice efforts should be focussed on relieving the obstruction of the biliary tree. If resection is possible this is usually undertaken by means of an extended right hepatectomy or segmental resections involving segments 4, 5 and 6.

With the lowering of morbidity and mortality rates for hepatic resection in patients with primary malignant disease it has become apparent that there is a group of patients with hepatic metastases from other organs who may be candidates for resection. Tumour spread may be direct as for adrenal carcinoma or more often bloodborne from the colon or kidney. Five year survival rates of up to 40% are reported for resection of isolated colorectal hepatic metastases and it may be justifiable to consider palliative resection of patients with symptomatic metastases such as those with carcinoid syndrome.

RESECTION OF THE LIVER

Provided there is no evidence of preoperative liver dysfunction extensive resection may be carried out with only temporary biochemical upset as normal liver tissue has considerable powers of regeneration. There is no one single reliable test of preoperative liver function. The surgeon therefore has to be guided by his own experience. Up to six segments can be resected but the extent of the resection is dictated by the degree of compensatory hypertrophy of the unaffected liver.

Indications and management

This may be indicated for benign and both primary and secondary malignant tumours of the liver. Hepatic resection may be required for tumours where there has been contiguous spread such as for adrenal, gall-bladder or primary bile duct tumours. Resection may be required for blunt abdominal trauma to the abdomen where there has been extensive disruption of hepatic parenchyma particularly in the right lobe of the liver.

Major resections of the liver should now carry an operative *mortality* of less than 5% and in the hands of experienced surgeons may be insignificant. Planned resection for tumour should be preceded by extensive investigations to exclude metastatic disease within the liver and elsewhere, and to determine the anatomy of the hepatic vasculature. *Arteriography* is useful in this regard since anomalies such as an aberrant right hepatic artery arising from the superior mesenteric artery may occur in up to 25% of cases. Operations must be covered by broad spectrum antibiotics, and careful attention must be paid to maintenance of acid base balance. Overzealous replacement of fluid losses may cause a rise in central venous pressure thereby increasing hepatic venous bleeding but central venous pressure should be carefully monitored. Cardiac output should be monitored when temporary clamping of the portal pedicle and/or infra- and suprahepatic vena cava is required to facilitate resection.

Evaluation of the tumour should continue in the operating theatre and the surgeon should take care to exclude dissemination of tumour into the peritoneal cavity or to lymph nodes. An experienced pathologist is required to undertake histological evaluation of the biopsies from the lesion or other nodules.

More use is being made of intraoperative ultrasonography to better localise the tumour mass with respect to the intrahepatic vasculature. This helps to plan the resection and ensures the absence of other lesions which may have not been detected on preoperation investigation. Intraoperative ultrasonography can be used to place a balloon catheter in the appropriate segmental branch of the portal vein before segmental resection is undertaken thereby minimising blood loss. *Complications* such as intra-abdominal sepsis and bile leakage will be kept to a minimum by sound surgical technique.

Such patients are best managed postoperatively in a high dependency or intensive care unit. Hypovolaemia should be avoided in the postoperative period to prevent acute tubular necrosis and to reduce portal venous flow which in turn may compromise hepatic function. These patients require regular assessment of blood glucose, electrolytes, prothrombin time and platelets during and after surgery. Using modern surgical techniques it is unlikely that patients will require large transfusions of blood or blood products.

Operative technique

Irrespective of the type of resection to be undertaken, the principles include preliminary dissection of the vessels in the porta hepatis with securing of the structures to allow a line of demarcation in the liver (Fig. 19.6). Attempts at control of the hepatic veins before dissection of the liver is inadvisable because of the risk of damage to the vena cava. The imprecise technique of finger fracture dissection has largely been replaced by use of ultrasonic surgical aspirators or dissection using a small straight arterial clamp (Kelly). Both techniques work on the principle of identifying the intrahepatic structures at an early stage and before they retract into the liver tissue. Vessels can therefore be diathermised or suture ligated before division. The transected surface of liver will usually remain dry if an anatomical resection is undertaken but haemostasis may be further secured by the use of tissue or fibrin glue.

The key to safe and succesful hepatic resection is to provide adequate exposure and to mobilise adequately the liver.

Right hepatectomy

A large right subcostal incision extended across the

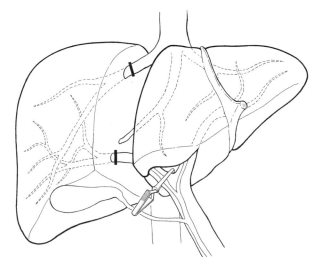

Fig. 19.6 Diagrammatic representation of the technique of right hepatectomy. The vessels are controlled at the porta hepatis (Step 1) prior to the transection of the liver along the line of demarcation (Step 2). The portal pedicles are secured within the liver (Step 3) and the hepatic veins suture ligated before delivery of the specimen (Step 4)

midline is more than adequate and access to the thorax should be avoided to minimise the risk of respiratory complication in the postoperative period. The incision can be extended upwards in the midline if required. The ligamentum teres is divided between ligatures and the falciform ligament incised back to the vena cava. The liver is mobilized from its bed by careful incision of the coronary ligament posteriorly to the vena cava taking care to avoid damage to the short right adrenal vein which may require suture ligation. It is preferable at this stage to identify and suture ligate any small hepatic veins draining from the back of the liver directly into the vena cava. No attempt is made to secure the right hepatic vein although it should be borne in mind that up to 25% of patients will have an accessory right hepatic vein which can be suture ligated during the mobilization of the liver. The structures at the porta hepatis are identified and it is preferable to undertake cholecystectomy at this stage. This facilitates exposure of the portal vein behind the common bile duct and hepatic artery. The right hepatic artery and right branch of the portal vein may be clamped and suture ligated at this point but it may be preferable merely to apply a vascular clamp to these structures. This will avoid inadvertent damage to the left hepatic duct as it sweeps across the midline to its confluence with the right hepatic duct. This manoeuvre will produce a clear line of demarcation between the devascularised right hemiliver and the left hemiliver running in the line of the gall-bladder bed, to the left of the inferior vena cava. Transection of the right hemi-liver should be undertaken approximately 5 mm from this line of demarcation to minimise blood loss and to avoid damage to the middle hepatic vein as it runs through this plane. Glisson's capsule is incised by diathermy at the proposed site of resection and the liver substance transected using the ultrasonic surgical aspirator or dissecting forceps. Small vessels and ducts crossing the plane of dissection are either diathermized or suture ligated with 3/0 silk or prolene before division. As the dissection proceeds backwards to the vena cava, the right portal pedicle can be secured if this has not already been done. The confluence of the right hepatic vein with the vena cava is identified and clamped before being oversewn with 3/0 or 4/0 prolene. The specimen can be removed taking care to avoid tearing any small hepatic veins which may have been missed as they pass directly from the liver into the vena cava.

If right hepatectomy is been undertaken for trauma, occlusion of the free border of the lesser omentum by a vascular clamp (Pringle's manoeuvre) will reduce blood loss from the liver before the vessels in the porta hepatis have been ligated. Such occlusion may be maintained for up to 20 minutes and in the elective situation can be well tolerated by the patient for up to 90 minutes.

It is usually unnecessary to pack the transected surface of the liver with omentum and two large tube drains are best passed through separate stab incisions to the right subphrenic space in the event of leakage of blood and bile.

Extended right hepatectomy

This operation has been incorrectly named as trisegmentectomy by Starzl (1982) since the procedure usually involves the sacrifice of at least five segments of the liver. The technique is similar to that of right hepatectomy but the dissection commences on the quadrate lobe side of the falciform ligament dividing between ligatures the small segmental vessels running to segment 4 (quadrate lobe). This dissection is continued backwards to the under surface of the quadrate lobe to facilitate division of the right branch of the portal vein and hepatic artery between clamps. A line of demarcation is produced to the right of the falciform ligament and this provides landmarks for incision of the capsule and transection of the hepatic parenchyma back to the vena cava. Care must be taken to avoid damage to the left hepatic vein which invariably has a common confluence with the middle hepatic vein as it joins the vena cava. The dissection usually proceeds quickly through an avascular plane before the right and middle hepatic veins are clamped and divided. Care must be taken to avoid damage to short hepatic veins which may be secured by careful mobilisation of the caudate lobe at the outset of the dissection.

Left lobectomy

The left lobe is mobilized by division of the ligamentum teres and falciform ligament. The lesser omentum (and left triangular ligament) are divided securing any small vessels between ligatures and taking care to avoid damaging the left hepatic vein which pursues a superficial course as it enters the vena cava at its confluence with the middle hepatic vein. The segmental branches of the left branch of the portal vein and the left hepatic artery are isolated and divided between ligatures as they pass in the fissure between the right and left lobe. It may be necessary to divide the small bridge of liver which often passes between the two lobes. Dissection can continue to the left of the falciform ligament securing vessels within the depth of the liver. This is a relatively avascular resection with the left hepatic vein being identified and divided over a vascular clamp before the specimen is delivered.

Left hepatectomy

The left hemiliver is mobilized in the same way as for left lobectomy and a cholecystectomy is performed.

The left branch of the portal vein and left hepatic artery are carefully indentified along with the left hepatic duct. The artery can be safely divided between ties although care must be taken in dissecting out the left branch of the portal vein since there are often one or two short branches passing posteriorly into the caudate lobe. The portal vein should be clamped and divided distal to these caudate branches if this lobe of the liver is to be preserved. Once a line of demarcation has been obtained the liver capsule is again incised using diathermy and dissection continues backwards and posteriorly, on this occasion to the left of the middle hepatic vein.

Wedge resection of liver

This technique may be employed for liver biopsy at laparotomy and for small peripherally located tumours. Since the operation transgresses anatomical boundaries there is often profuse haemorrhage which is difficult to control. If such a resection is warranted haemostasis is best controlled by individual suture ligation of vessels using 3/0 silk or prolene.

Segmental liver resection

Anatomical segmental resection of liver has largely replaced wedge resection of the liver. Such resections are preferable to classical hepatectomy if the location of the tumour or associated parenchymal liver disease leave insufficient liver to sustain normal hepatic function. The most common segmental resections are those to the anterior portion of the quadrate lobe (Segment 4) resection of the caudate lobe (Segment 5) (Bismuth, 1988), and I segmentectomy IV, V, VI for carcinoma of the gall-bladder. Such resections should only be done where the surgeon has an adequate knowledge of the segmental liver anatomy and where intraoperative ultrasonography is available to assist in the localisation of the tumour and adjacent hepatic vasculature. The use of an ultrasonic surgical aspirator ensures precise dissection between adjacent segments and isolation of supplying portal venous and arterial pedicles which can be controlled by suture ligation with silk or prolene. If the supplying segmental vessels cannot be identified before the hepatic parechyma is incised, temporary clamping of the porta hepatis (Pringle manoeuvre) may minimise blood loss during the procedure.

Needle biopsy of liver

Needle biopsy, in which a small core of liver is removed, is a useful technique in the investigation of liver disease but should be avoided if at all possible in the assessment of hepatic lesions being considered for resection. Three types of needle are commonly used, the Trucut needle, the Menghini needle, and the Vim-Silvermann needle, of which the first two are the most important. If diffuse liver disease is suggested the procedure is undertaken 'blind' by percutaneous puncture under local anaesthesia in the right 9th or 10th intercostal space in the mid-axillary line, or, if the liver is palpable, over the most superficial part. The patient must be able to co-operate by holding his breath in expiration while the needle is inserted into liver tissue.

If focal liver disease is anticipated, the procedure is best undertaken under ultrasound guidance or under vision at laparoscopy or at laparotomy so that the needle may be directed accurately to the area under suspicion (*target biopsy*). Care should be taken when biopsying a narrow left lobe of liver lest the needle pass through and damage the structures posteriorly.

The procedure is relatively safe, the principal risk being of haemorrhage, and it is essential that any coagulation defects are corrected beforehand. Rarely, haemobilia or the development of an intrahepatic arteriovenous fistula may follow.

REFERENCES

Belli L, Del Favero E, Marni A and Romani F 1983 Resection versus pericystectomy in the treatment of hydatidosis of the liver. American Journal of Surgery 145: 234–242

Benhamou J P and Mesu Y 1988 Non parasitic cystic diseases of the liver and ultrahepatic biliary tree. In: Blumgart L H (ed.) Surgery of the liver and biliary tract. Churchill Livingstone, Edinburgh, pp. 1013–1024

Bismuth H 1982 Anatomical surgery and surgical anatomy of the liver. World Journal of Surgery 6: 3–9

Bismuth H, Castaing D, Garden O J 1988 Segmental surgery of the liver. In: Nyhus L M (ed.) Surgery Annual 1988. Appleton and Lange, Norwalk, pp. 291–310

Dietrick R B 1984 Experience with liver abscess. American Journal of Surgery 147: 288

Foster J H 1986 Focal nodular hyperplasia, benign tumours and cysts. In: Bengmark S, Blumgart LH (eds) Liver surgery. Churchill Livingstone, Edinburgh

Garden O J, Bismuth H 1989 Cancer of the liver. In: Veronesi V, Arnesjo B, Burn I, Denis L, Mazzeo F (eds) European Handbook of Surgical Oncology. Springer-Verlag, pp. 622–635

Grewal R S 1984 Amoebic liver abscess. International Surgery 69: 137–139

Lucarotti M E, Virjee J, Thomas W E G, Leaper D J 1991 Intra-abdominal abscesses. Surgery 98: 2335–2341

Papadimitriou J, Mandrekas A 1970 The Surgical treatment of hydatid disease of the liver. British Journal of Surgery 57: 431–433

Serrano A, Dahl E P, Rubin R H et al 1984 Elective drainage of subphrenic abscesses. Archives of Surgery 119: 942–945

Starzl T E, Iwatsuki S, Shaw B W 1982 Left hepatic trisegmentectomy. Surgery Gynaecology and Obstetrics 155: 21–27

FURTHER READING

Bismuth H, Garden O J 1992 Regular and extended right and left hepatectomy for cancer. In: Nyhus L M, Baker R J (eds) Mastery of surgery. Little Brown and Co Boston

20

The gall-bladder, the bile ducts and the pancreas

D. C. CARTER, J. M. S. JOHNSTONE & I. B. MACLEOD

Anatomy

The gall-bladder is pear-shaped and about 10 cm long. It is attached to the inferior surface of the right lobe of the liver, and is enclosed within its peritoneal sheath. Its lower end or *fundus* is completely covered with peritoneum, and projects slightly beyond the free margin of the liver opposite the upper end of the linea semilunaris. The *body* and *neck* are covered only on three sides with peritoneum. They are attached anteriorly to the liver by loose connective tissue and are easily separated from it. The neck shows a dilatation, the *infundibulum* (Hartmann's pouch), which hangs downwards and is often connected to the duodenum by folds which may be either congenital or inflammatory in origin. The upper end of the neck narrows down to form the *cystic duct* which runs backwards and medially, and joins the common hepatic duct to form the common bile duct.

The gall-bladder is supplied by the cystic artery, which is usually a branch of the right hepatic artery (Fig. 20.1).

The bile ducts

The *right* and *left hepatic ducts* emerge from the liver through the porta hepatis, and unite to form the *common hepatic duct*, which is in turn joined by the cystic duct to form the *common bile duct*. This last duct is about 10 cm long; it runs downwards behind the first part of the duodenum, then through the head of pancreas and ends by passing obliquely through the

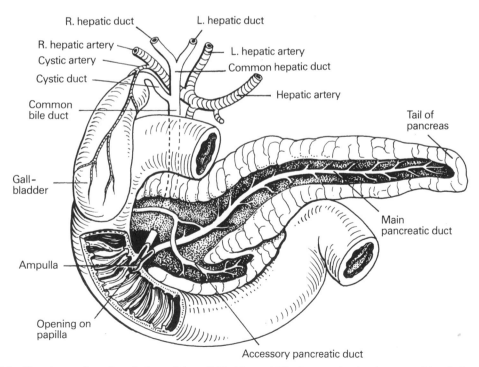

Fig. 20.1 Drawing to show the relations of the gall-bladder and bile ducts to the duodenum and head of pancreas

postero-medial wall of the second part. The extreme lower end of the duct is dilated to form the *ampulla of Vater* which lies partly within the duodenal wall.

Relations. The hepatic ducts and the supraduodenal part of the common bile duct lie in the right free border of the lesser omentum. The *hepatic artery* lies on the left side of the common bile duct, and the *portal vein* is behind it, these structures being all contained within the omentum. The *right hepatic artery* crosses behind the common hepatic duct, before it gives off its cystic branch. The lower part of the common bile duct descends behind the first part of the duodenum, and then lies in a groove on the back of the head of the pancreas or may tunnel the gland substance.

Anomalies. The above description of the relationship of the bile ducts and associated blood vessels is that given in the standard textbooks of anatomy. It should be noted, however, that considerable variations may exist; those which occur most commonly are shown in Figure 20.2. A knowledge of such 'anomalies' is of the greatest importance to the surgeon, for failure to recognize them at operation may lead to disaster. Thus, severance of an anomalous or accessory hepatic duct, without ligature of its cut-end, would result in biliary peritonitis, while inadvertent ligature of an abnormally placed right hepatic artery might produce a fatal hepatic infarction. Other anomalies render the right hepatic duct or the common bile duct very liable to injury.

The pancreas

This lies obliquely across the upper part of the posterior wall of the abdomen. Its *head* lies within the concavity of the duodenum, and is closely related to the lower part of the common bile duct. Its *body* lies behind

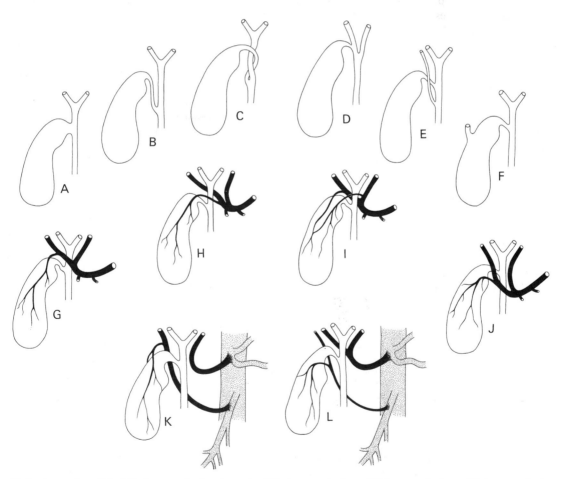

Fig. 20.2 Anomalies of the bile ducts and related arteries (A) short cystic duct; (B) long cystic duct; (C) long cystic duct winding round common hepatic duct; (D) cystic duct joining right hepatic duct; (E) Accessory hepatic duct joining common bile duct; (F) Accessory (*hepato-cholecystic*) duct passing directly into gall-bladder; (G) right hepatic artery crossing in front of common hepatic duct; (H) cystic artery arising low and crossing in front of common hepatic duct; (I) accessory cystic artery from left hepatic; (J) low division of hepatic artery; (K) right hepatic artery arising from superior mesenteric; (L) accessory right hepatic artery from superior mesenteric

the stomach, separated from it by the lesser sac of the peritoneum; the splenic artery runs along its upper border and the splenic vein is behind it. Its *tail* lies in contact with the spleen.

The pancreatic duct traverses the whole length of the gland, and ends by joining the common bile duct, either at the ampulla or at a slightly higher level. An *accessory pancreatic duct* may enter the duodenum about 2.5 cm higher up.

INDICATIONS FOR SURGERY AND CHOICE OF OPERATION

Cholecystitis and gall-stone formation are the most common disorders affecting the biliary tract. The great majority of stones develop within the gall-bladder, and those giving rise to symptoms are usually associated with inflammatory changes in the wall of the viscus.

Removal of the gall-bladder (*cholecystectomy*) is the standard procedure when the gall-bladder is diseased or contains calculi. Simple drainage of the gall-bladder (*cholecystostomy*) combined with removal of any stones present is occasionally indicated if severe inflammatory changes render the anatomy obscure, in very poor risk patients, or for preliminary drainage of the biliary tree obstructed by tumour in patients in whom later resection is contemplated.

Cholecystectomy has definite advantages over cholecystostomy:

1. it removes the site in which most gall-stones form, and thus reduces the risk of recurrence
2. it removes a focus of infection which may persist
3. it obviates the risk of persistent biliary fistula which may follow cholecystostomy
4. it eliminates the risk of carcinoma developing in a gallbladder which has been the seat of stone formation.

Increasingly, cholecystectomy is being carried out using the laparoscopic technique (page 354), but 'open' cholecystectomy may still be necessary if access to the region proves impossible laparoscopically, if a complication occurs during laparoscopy which requires conversion to an open procedure, or if laparoscopic equipment is not available.

Acute cholecystitis
In the majority of patients acute cholecystitis develops as a complication of gall-stones. *Acalculous* cholecystitis may occur, however, and has been reported in patients with severe multiple trauma, in septicaemia, and rarely as a result of embolization into the cystic artery in patients with atrial fibrillation. The acalculous variety tends to be more rapidly progressive than the calculous

type, frequently leading to gangrene of the gall-bladder wall, and early surgery is indicated.

The traditional management of calculous-acute cholecystitis is initially conservative, in the anticipation that in approximately 70% of patients the condition will settle (probably the result of an obstructing calculus disimpacting) allowing later elective cholecystectomy. Pain is relieved, pethidine by i.m. injection being suitable. Oral intake is stopped and adequate fluids given by i.v. infusion. If vomiting is a feature, a nasogastric tube is passed and aspirated hourly. Blood samples are taken for routine haematology, urea and electrolyte, standard liver function tests and blood culture, and antibiotic therapy started. Gentamicin, Cefuroxime, or Co-trimoxazole are suitable. Pulse and temperature are carefully monitored, and the patient re-examined at 4–6 hour intervals. Early confirmation of the diagnosis by ultrasound scan, or by intravenous cholangiography (provided liver function is satisfactory) should be undertaken in the first 24 hours. Improvement in the patient's condition will normally allow reintroduction of oral intake at 48 hours, discontinuation of antibiotics at 7 days, discharge from hospital at 7–10 days, and an appointment for readmission for elective cholecystectomy in 8–12 weeks' time. Indications to abandon this conservative regime and proceed to *early surgery* include:

1. failure to improve after 48 hours therapy
2. development of a tender enlarging mass in the right hypochondrium
3. development of rigors
4. features of general peritonitis (uncommon).

In recent years, increasing numbers of surgeons have favoured a policy of early surgery. Treatment is initiated as above, fluid and electrolyte deficiencies corrected, the diagnosis confirmed and, provided there are no specific contraindications to surgery, the patient is prepared for surgery on an elective operating list within 48–72 hours of admission to hospital. Antibiotics are continued for 3 days postoperatively unless it is necessary to explore the common bile duct, when they should be continued for 5 days. Advantages of this policy include:

1. shorter total period of hospitalization
2. prevention of the development of serious complications such as empyema (which carries a mortality of 10%)
3. operation is often technically relatively simple during the first week of the illness, oedema making dissection of tissue planes easier. The operative mortality of *planned* early cholecystectomy is similar to that of elective cholecystectomy
4. approximately 20% of patients leaving hospital

after initial conservative therapy require emergency readmission with a recurrent acute episode prior to their planned elective procedure.

Choice of operation

The writer recommends the policy of early surgery in acute cholecystitis, with the proviso that it is undertaken by a surgeon with considerable experience in surgery of the biliary tract. Cholecystectomy with peroperative cholangiography is the procedure of choice. This is usually possible using the standard technique (see p. 430), but any difficulty in visualizing the anatomy of the cystic duct and Calot's Triangle should dictate that dissection begins at the fundus and works towards the cystic duct. Haemorrhage is a little greater than with the standard technique, but risk of inadvertent damage to the common bile duct or right hepatic artery is minimized. Espiner has recently described a technique which avoids the necessity of ligation of the cystic artery. Using diathermy, dissection is carried out in the submucosal plane of the gall-bladder working from the fundus towards the cystic duct, which is amputated as soon as tissues in the free border of the lesser omentum are reached. Cholecystostomy is now infrequently practised, but may be indicated in some difficult patients as may be met if an initial conservative policy has failed, and is indicated if the surgeon is inexperienced.

Chronic cholecystitis and gall-stones

The incidence of gall-stones has increased markedly in recent years, this increase being most evident in men and in young women (in whom use of the contraceptive pill may be implicated). Surgical treatment is usually advised once the diagnosis is made, even in those patients in whom the stones are 'symptomless'. Some 50% of such asymptomatic patents will develop symptoms of biliary colic within 5 years, and the possible development of carcinoma of the gall-bladder following squamous metaplasia of the mucosa should always be borne in mind. Patients who have had one or more attacks of biliary colic usually accept readily the advice to undergo surgery, but patients with milder symptoms such as flatulent dyspepsia may not. Such patients, and those who are considered poor operative risks, should be advised about a fat reduced diet and considered for treatment with gall-stone dissolving agents such as chenodeoxycholic acid (*Chendol*) or ursodeoxycholic acid (*Destolit*).

Dissolution therapy is not suitable in the following situations:

1. calcified stones (10–15% of all stones)
2. nonfunctioning gall-bladder, or obstructed cystic duct
3. stones larger than 1 cm diameter
4. liver disease or jaundice
5. inflammatory bowel disease present
6. women of child bearing age.

Diarrhoea is a common side-effect, although reported to be less frequent with *Destolit* than with *Chendol*. Treatment should be continued for 3 months following disappearance of the stones, which may take up to 2 years. Stones may reform after discontinuing therapy, as the underlying lithogenicity of the bile is not permanently altered.

Ultrasonic shock wave lithotripsy, to shatter the gall-bladder stones, is an alternative non-operative treatment which has found favour particularly in Germany. It requires expensive equipment, and it has really been superseded as a consequence of the rapid rise in popularity of laparoscopic cholecystectomy.

Obstructive jaundice

If an attack of biliary colic is followed by jaundice it is very likely that a stone has entered the common duct. Many such stones pass spontaneously into the duodenum, and initial treatment is medical, anticipating improvement in liver function. Endoscopic retrograde cholangiopancreatography (E.R.C.P.) is then carried out to demonstrate the anatomy and check on the presence or absence of residual duct stones. If present, a papillotomy is performed and the stones removed using a balloon catheter or a stone 'basket' This procedure should be carried out under antibiotic cover. Later, elective cholecystectomy, using either the open or laparoscopic technique, is undertaken. In young patients with residual stones, many surgeons would prefer open cholecystectomy with supraduodenal exploration of the bile duct and extraction of the stones, as the long-term effects of endoscopic papillotomy in young patients have not yet been adequately documented.

Persistent jaundice following biliary colic indicates that a stone has become impacted in the common bile duct. Early ERCP and papillotomy after careful preparation is indicated to prevent further liver damage from back pressure and from the almost invariable cholangitis. Rigors indicate bacteraemic episodes from *cholangitis*. After obtaining blood cultures, broad spectrum antibiotic therapy is started, the patient is adequately hydrated, and after correction of any coagulation defects (usually an extended prothrombin time ratio) ERCP is undertaken. Cholecystectomy and surgical exploration of the common bile duct is undertaken if ERCP is unsuccessful — for example, this is frequently the case after a previous Polya partial gastrectomy.

Steadily deepening jaundice, without preceding biliary colic suggests obstruction of the common bile duct by malignant disease or chronic pancreatitis. Malignant disease may be primary in the head of the pancreas, in the bile ducts or in the peri-ampullary region, or may be secondary from a more distant primary. Ultrasound and CT liver scan will demonstrate the presence of hepatic metastases and show the diameter of the common bile duct.

If these investigations suggest metastatic disease and the common bile duct is of normal calibre it is wise in most patients to obtain a tissue diagnosis by Fine Needle Aspirate (FNA) under ultrasound guidance, or alternatively by liver biopsy using a Trucut needle under vision provided by a laparoscope.

If extrahepatic obstruction is indicated by a dilated common bile duct the site and nature of the obstruction should be delineated by ERCP, supplemented when necessary by *percutaneous transhepatic cholangiography* (PTC) (Fig. 20.3).

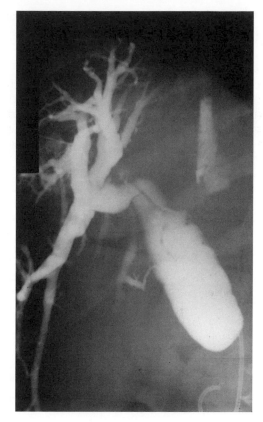

Fig. 20.4 Contrast X-ray showing biliary obstruction, relieved by a 'pig-tail'. catheter which has been inserted in retrograde fashion using an endoscope

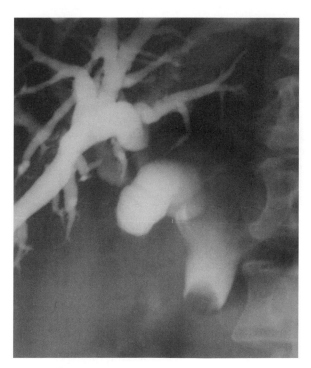

Fig. 20.3 Percutaneous transhepatic cholangiogram showing obstructing calculus at the lower end of bile duct

lieve the jaundice should be undertaken. Increasingly, endoscopists contribute significantly to the palliation of malignant obstructive jaundice by the insertion of a biliary endoprosthesis (Fig. 20.4). In some patients with small peri-ampullary tumours who are considered unfit for surgery, an endoscopic papillotomy may be undertaken to relieve the jaundice. If endoscopic intubation fails, pigtail catheters (Fig. 20.5) or endoprostheses (Fig. 20.6) may be inserted percutaneously. In some cases, a combined approach is used. In general terms, low obstruction is best palliated endoscopically, while obstructions near the porta hepatis usually need percutaneous intubation.

Peri-ampullary carcinomas and carcinomas at the lower end of the common bile duct may be suitable for resection (Whipple's operation q.v.). Many surgeons consider that resection for carcinoma of the head of the pancreas does not yield results sufficiently superior to simple bypass to justify such a major procedure even in those patients in whom it is technically possible. In this condition, in patients with metastatic disease and in patients with benign stricture from chronic pancreatitis, some form of drainage or bypass procedure to re-

GENERAL CONSIDERATIONS IN TECHNIQUE

Preparation for operation

All diseases of the biliary tract are likely to be associated with some disturbance of liver function. As operation is not usually a matter of urgency, some time should be spent in preoperative preparation. A high carbohydrate diet should be prescribed to ensure adequate stores of liver glycogen, and in the iller patient

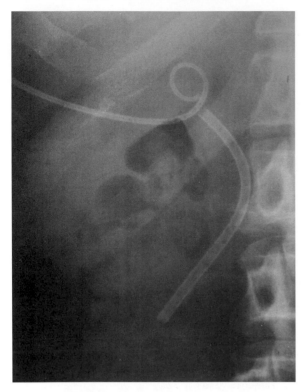

Fig. 20.5 Plain X-ray showing 'pig-tail' drainage catheter and biliary endoprosthesis inserted percutaneously

high carbohydrate intravenous infusions employed. Adequate preoperative intravenous hydration is important and is particularly so in the jaundiced patient (q.v.). Broad spectrum antibiotic therapy is used in the acute case, and where exploration of the common bile duct is anticipated. Gross obesity, common in patients with gall-stones, is a relative contraindication to elective surgery, and every encouragement should be given to the patient to lose weight before operation. Regrettably, such advice often 'falls on deaf ears', and continuing symptoms necessitate operation in less than ideal circumstances.

Any operation on the biliary tract should be approached with the maximum possible information and adequate time for investigation should be provided. In elective surgery most of the investigations will have been performed on an outpatient basis. Ultrasound scanning is now the usual 'screening' procedure (Muir, 1983), while oral cholecystography or intravenous cholangiography are less frequently used than formerly. Suspicion that the common bile duct may require to be opened demands accurate delineation of its anatomy by ERCP or PTC or both.

Preparation in jaundiced patients
Both morbidity and mortality are higher following sur-

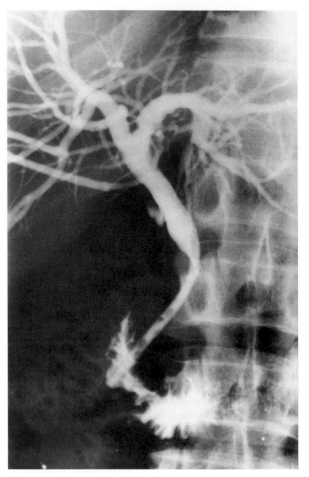

Fig. 20.6 Contrast X-ray confirming the position of the endoprosthesis within a malignant stricture

gery in jaundiced patients than in non-icteric subjects. The increased risks are:

1. *Haemorrhage.* In obstructive jaundice there is impaired absorption of the fat soluble vitamin K due to failure of bile salts to reach the intestine. This leads to failure to synthesize prothrombin, and an extended prothrombin time ratio (PTR)*. If the PTR is increased, it should be corrected before operation by the parenteral administration of vitamin K; 10 mg per day by i.m. or i.v. injection is normally adequate. In patients with severe intrinsic liver disease there may be a more general failure in synthesis of clotting factors. A full coagulation screen should be ordered and fresh frozen plasma made available for the perioperative period (p. 26).

---

*Now often referred to as I.N.R. (International Normalised Ratio of prothrombin time).

2. *Infection.* The majority of patients with obstructive jaundice, and virtually all of those in whom the cause is gall-stones, have infected bile. Antibiotic therapy in the elective case should be administered parenterally, beginning with the premedication and continued for 3–5 days. Gentamicin, Cefuroxime, or Co-trimoxazole are suitable.

3. *Acute renal failure.* Renal tubular function is compromised to a greater or lesser degree in jaundiced patients due to a direct action of bilirubin on the tubules and to a degree of vascular shunting in the kidney leading to relative cortical ischaemia. Episodes of hypotension due to haemorrhage or infection are more likely if the patients, as many of them are, are hypovolaemic prior to surgery. Adequate *preoperative* hydration is essential to minimize the risk of acute renal failure, and frequently obviates the need for preoperative mannitol infusion so favoured by anaesthetists. An intravenous infusion is set up to aim for a minimum urinary output of 2000 ml/day. The patient will frequently require bladder catheterization a day or two preoperatively to ensure accurate recording. All patients should be catheterized once anaesthesia has been induced, in order to monitor urine output during the operation, and hourly in the postoperative period.

4. *Liver failure.* When combined with acute renal failure, the patient has the hepato-renal syndrome. Adequate preoperative carbohydrate intake and hydration, combined with measures to control infection and minimize haemorrhage should reduce considerably the risk of this severe complication.

Position of the patient
The patient should lie supine on an operating table which can accept X-ray cassettes for preoperative chol-angiography (Fig. 20.7). A careful check should be made that the biliary area lies over the aperture in the cassette carrier allowing X-rays to reach the films. The patient should be tilted 15° down to his or her right, either by placing a rubber wedge under the patient's left side or by tilting the table itself. This manoeuvre carries the common bile duct away from the line of the vertebrae and allows easier interpretation of cholangiogram films.

Incision
Open biliary surgery may be undertaken through one of a variety of incisions.

Right paramedian
Either rectus displacing or rectus splitting. This is most suitable for patients with a narrow costal angle, and most easily allows a full laparotomy.

Kocher's subcostal
In stout patients with a wide costal angle this incision allows easier access to deeper structures than the paramedian incision.

Mayo-Robson (Hockey stick)
This is a combination of a paramedian and a medial subcostal incision.

Right upper quadrant transverse
This is the author's preferred incision and provides the most cosmetic scar, a significant consideration when many patients are young women. The incision can be carried across the midline if required to improve access.

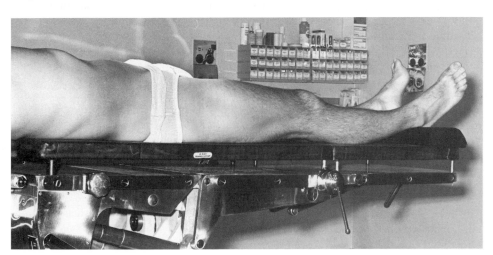

Fig. 20.7   Patient in position for operation on the biliary system. The X-ray translucent operating table top, to allow insertion of X-ray plates for cholangiography, is shown. Note that the ankles are supported by a rubber pad to prevent pressure on the calves (see p. 32)

Upper midline

Some surgeons prefer to operate on the biliary tree through a midline incision while standing to the *left* side of the patient.

Preliminary exploration

In the absence of acute inflammation, a careful examination of the entire biliary system should be carried out before any decision is made as to operative procedure. The stomach and duodenum are examined first, and are then packed-off out of the way. The gall-bladder is palpated for calculi, particular attention being paid to the infundibulum in which a calculus may be overlooked, and the condition of its wall is noted. The cystic duct is now brought into view by drawing the gall-bladder upwards and to the right. Any adhesions or peritoneal folds connecting the gall-bladder to the duodenum or colon are divided, and bleeding points are ligatured. The cystic duct is examined by palpation down to the point where it joins the common hepatic duct to form the common bile duct. The condition of these ducts also should be investigated as routine. The supraduodenal part of the common duct lying in the right free border of the lesser omentum is palpated between the index finger in the epiploic foramen and the thumb in front. If the foramen is not patent the duct can be palpated by pressing it backwards against the vertebral column. The retroduodenal part of the common duct may be palpated by placing the finger tips of the left hand along the lateral border of the second part of the duodenum, and by pressing them medially against the thumb, which is placed firmly against the groove between pancreas and duodenum. By this method the consistency of the pancreas can be determined at the same time, and any abnormality noted. If the appendix is accessible it is examined and, if necessary, removed — either immediately or towards the end of the operation.

In the presence of jaundice special precautions must be observed. In view of the risk of haemorrhage, exploration is reduced to a minimum; gentleness is more than usually essential, and even the smallest vessels should be caught and ligatured. Attention is directed mainly to the common duct and to the pancreas, for it is in these situations that the cause of the obstruction is most likely to be found. The appearance of the gall-bladder is a useful guide to diagnosis. If the gall-bladder is contracted and fibrotic the obstruction is most likely to be caused by a stone impacted in the common duct. If the gall-bladder is dilated the obstruction is often due to some cause other than stone (*Courvoisier's law*). In this latter case particular attention should be paid to the head of the pancreas. If the whole pancreas is enlarged and of rubbery consistency the condition is probably one of chronic pancreatitis. If stony hardness or nodularity is present and affects mainly the head of the pancreas, it is more likely to be due to carcinoma. A palpable nodule at the ampulla suggests a carcinoma of this region.

Choice of procedure as determined by operative findings

Following the preliminary exploration, the next step is to obtain *operative cholangiogram* films, preferably after direct cannulation of the cystic duct. The cystic duct is isolated and its junction with common hepatic duct and common bile duct noted. The cystic duct is clamped or ligated at its junction with Hartmann's pouch. A second ligature of absorbable material is passed around the duct close to its junction with common hepatic duct. The cystic duct is now incised between the ligatures, a metal or plastic catheter introduced, and held in place by tightening the second ligature with one throw. Three films (Fig. 20.8) are usually taken following injection of 2 ml, 3 ml and 5 ml of 25% *Biligram*. Features to note on the films are:

1. evidence of duct dilation (normal diameter < 7 mm)
2. presence of filling defects (stone, tumour, occasionally blood clot)
3. evidence of flow of dye into duodenum
4. particular attention should be paid to the anatomy of the lower end of the common bile duct — more detail may be obtained if necessary by placing a small piece of dental film directly behind the second part of duodenum
5. the configuration of the biliary tree as a whole.

On occasion, because of the tilt of the patient to the right, the left hepatic duct system is underfilled. If doubt exists, further films should be taken after removing the tilt.

Prior isolation of the cystic duct may be difficult or dangerous in a patient with severe acute cholecystitis, or the cystic duct may prove in some patients to be too narrow to cannulate. In such cases, cholangiogram films may be obtained after direct needle puncture of the common bile duct. The puncture wound should then be occluded by a fine suture (e.g. 3/0 Dexon), but even so, postoperative leakage of bile from the puncture site is not uncommon.

Routine operative cholangiography is no longer recommended. A selective policy of cholangiography is advised, obtaining films on those patients with a history of jaundice, patients with a dilated common bile duct, and patients with multiple small stones. It may be omitted in patients with carcinoma of the head of pancreas with a clear preoperative diagnosis and confirmatory findings at laparotomy in whom the intention

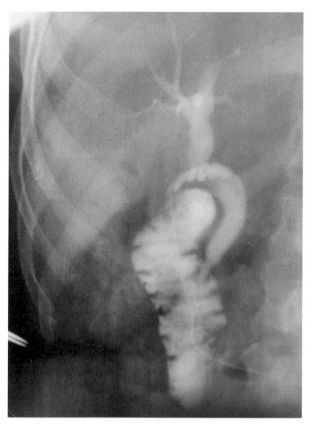

Fig. 20.8   X-ray film of normal operative cholangiogram

is to carry out palliative bypass surgery. Operative ultrasound, using a small probe, is used by some as an alternative to or as complementary to operative cholangiography.

For patients with calculous disease, cholecystectomy should be the aim, with the decision to explore the common bile duct being largely determined by the cholangiogram films, provided these are of reasonable quality. Occasionally, in patients with severe acute cholecystitis, a determined attempt to carry out cholecystectomy will be dangerous, and cholecystostomy with extraction of the intravesical stones is the more prudent course, particularly if the surgeon is inexperienced.

Transduodenal sphincteroplasty, or choledochoduodenostomy may be indicated for an impacted stone at the lower end of the common bile duct, stricture at the ampulla, or multiple stones in the common bile duct. The alternative of a later endoscopic papillotomy should be considered in such patients particularly if the patient is frail.

Obstruction due to chronic pancreatitis will normally be dealt with by a bypass procedure (cholecysto- or choledochojejunostomy). Obstruction due to small

ampullary carcinoma without evidence of spread should be treated by pancreaticoduodenectomy if the patient's overall condition permits.

CHOLECYSTOSTOMY

The indications for this operation have already been discussed. In cases of acute cholecystitis, a provisional decision to perform cholecystostomy may be made before the abdomen is opened. The operation may then be planned accordingly; local anaesthesia can be employed if desired, and a small incision (vertical or oblique) made directly over the fundus of the gall-bladder. If the diagnosis of acute cholecystitis is confirmed, adhesions are separated only sufficiently to expose the gall-bladder, and no further exploration is attempted.

The gall-bladder is carefully surrounded with moist packs, and an Oschner aspirator attached to suction inserted into the fundus of the gall-bladder to aspirate the liquid contents. When no more bile can be aspirated, light tissue forceps are applied to the gall-bladder wall on each side of the aspirator, which is then withdrawn. The opening is enlarged with scissors to a length of 2 to 3 cm, and the remaining contents (usually gall-stones and biliary 'mud') are evacuated with a scoop or with fenestrated forceps, a large spoon or special receiver being held against the opening in order to catch any escaping bile or debris. Two fingers are then passed deeply along the outside of the gall-bladder, and the neck of the viscus and the cystic duct are carefully palpated. Any further calculi detected are milked upwards until they are within reach of the scoop or forceps (Fig. 20.9). Care must be taken not to overlook a stone impacted in the cystic duct. The interior of the gall-bladder is then explored with the finger, and is dried with a swab held on forceps; this is rotated in order to entangle and remove any small stones which remain.

A 24 FG Latex Rubber Winsbury White or Foley catheter is introduced into the gall-bladder as far as its middle and sutured with 2/0 chromic catgut to the edge of the opening. Closure of the opening around the tube is effected by a purse-string suture of 2/0 chromic catgut or (if the gall-bladder wall is thickened or friable) by one or two interrupted sutures (Fig. 20.10). The tube drain should be brought to the surface through a stab incision separate from the main wound using the shortest route. If the gall-bladder fundus lies close to the parietal peritoneum, it should be attached to it using chromic catgut sutures — alternatively omentum may be brought up and sutured to the fundus. Lavage of the area with an antibiotic solution is advisable prior to closure of the wound, and use of a small suction

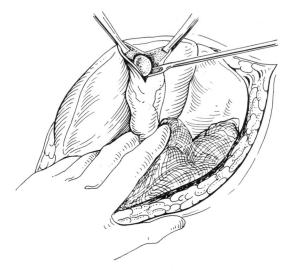

Fig. 20.9 Cholecystostomy. The technique of removing stones from the gall-bladder is depicted

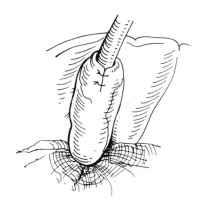

Fig. 20.10 Cholecystostomy. The gall-bladder has been repaired around a drainage tube

drain (e.g. *Redivac*) from the subhepatic space is recommended.

After-treatment
The tube is attached to a closed system bile drainage bag and allowed to drain freely for 7–10 days, when a tube cholecystogram should be undertaken to check for the presence of residual stones in the gall-bladder or common bile duct. If the X-rays show no residual calculi and a normal common bile duct, the tube drain may be removed at this stage. In this situation a decision to undertake elective cholecystectomy will be determined by whether or not the patient develops symptoms. More than 50% will be asymptomatic during the next 5 years, so that an expectant policy is justified.

If the cholecystogram demonstrates the clear presence of stones, or blockage of the cystic duct (most

likely from a stone) the tube should be left in situ for a further 3 to 4 weeks and consideration given to planned cholecystectomy (which is likely to be difficult and therefore should be undertaken only by an experienced surgeon) or to instrumental removal of the stones through the tube track. Removal of the cholecystostomy tube in the presence of obstruction is likely to lead either to a persisting mucous fistula or to recurrent infection in the gall-bladder.

Should the X-rays reveal a gall-bladder clear of stones or obstruction, but a stone or stones in the common bile duct, the ideal treatment is endoscopic papillotomy and removal of the stones in view of the difficulties of surgery following cholecystostomy.

OPEN CHOLECYSTECTOMY

All steps of the operation must be carried out under direct vision. The patients are often obese and access is difficult, so that an adequate exposure is essential. Suitable incisions are described on p. 427.

The first step consists in careful packing-off. The first pack is placed in the lower part of the wound, displacing duodenum, transverse colon and small intestine downwards; a second pack is placed medially to cover and retract the stomach. A third pack may be inserted laterally to fill the right kidney pouch. Deep retractors are then placed in position, and are held by the assistant so as to give the best exposure.

There are two principal methods of removing the gall-bladder. In the generally advocated *retrograde* method, the cystic duct and cystic artery are divided first, and the gall-bladder is then stripped off towards the fundus. In the alternative method the separation of the gall-bladder is commenced at the fundus.

The retrograde method
This has the great advantage that the cystic duct and cystic artery are clearly identified before division, this part of the operation being carried out at an early stage before the deeper parts of the operation field can become obscured by haemorrhage. The risk of injury to the common duct or to the right hepatic artery is therefore greatly reduced.

When distension of the gall-bladder prevents ready access to the ducts, or if there is thought to be any danger of rupture, the contents should be aspirated, the puncture opening being afterwards closed with a stitch or clamp. A forceps is then applied to the infundibulum of the gall-bladder, and is used to draw the viscus gently forwards and to the right (Fig. 20.11). The junction of the cystic and common ducts is now displayed by snipping the overlying peritoneum and by gauze

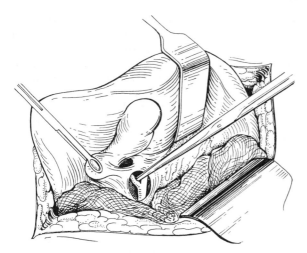

Fig. 20.11 Cholecystectomy by the retrograde method — exposure of the cystic duct at its junction with the common hepatic duct, in the right free border of the lesser omentum

stripping. This dissection may take some time since the ducts are often obscured by fat or by oedematous connective tissue.

Occasionally the cystic artery runs anterior to the cystic duct, obscuring access. It should then be divided between nonabsorbable sutures, a procedure usually left until later in the operation. An absorbable ligature (Dexon, Vicryl or catgut) is now placed loosely around the cystic duct close to its junction with the common bile duct. Any stones in the cystic duct should be milked towards the gall-bladder and the cystic duct clamped or ligated (Fig. 20.12) close to Hartmann's pouch. The cystic duct is now opened between the

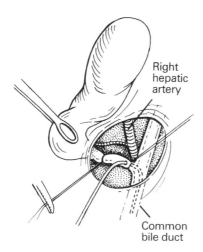

Right hepatic artery

Common bile duct

Fig. 20.12 Cholecystectomy. The cystic duct has been ligated and a cannula has been inserted into the common bile duct for cholangiography. The cystic artery has been identified

ligatures, any stones remaining in the duct removed, a bacteriology swab taken for culture, and the cannula introduced for operative cholangiography (see p. 428). The cannula is left in place until the films have been viewed, lest further films are required. When satisfactory films are obtained, the cannula is removed, the ligature close to the common bile duct fully tightened and the cystic duct divided.

Gentle traction on the cystic duct and careful sharp and gauze dissection keeping close to the upper part of the gall-bladder neck will now reveal the cystic artery (if not previously divided) in its usual position crossing the triangle of Calot. It should be doubly ligated with silk or linen and divided between the ligatures.

The gall-bladder is now attached by little more than the peritoneal sheath which binds it to the inferior surface of the liver. Its neck is drawn forwards away from the liver and a finger is insinuated between the two. The finger is made to work its way gently upwards separating the gall-bladder from its bed. As the separation progresses the peritoneal reflection on each side is divided with scissors. An attempt is made to retain a fringe of peritoneum on each side, with which the gall-bladder bed can be covered. To enable this to be done, the peritoneum should if possible be stripped for a short distance from the sides of the gall-bladder before being divided. Some haemorrhage occurs from minute vessels which pass directly to the gall-bladder from the substance of the liver, but if the separation is carried out in the correct plane the bleeding is relatively slight and can be arrested by pressure with a hot moist pack or by light coagulation with the diathermy electrode. If an aberrant duct (*hepato-cholecystic duct*) is encountered entering the gall-bladder directly from its bed (see Fig. 20.2) it should be secured and ligatured. It is a good plan to delay the final separation of the gall-bladder until its bed has been dealt with, for the partially separated viscus can be used as a convenient retractor (Fig. 20.13).

If it has been possible to conserve peritoneal fringes at each side of the raw area, these are brought together by continuous or interrupted sutures, if necessary to control haemorrhage, since the raw area seldom if ever produces any harmful effects.

Drainage should be provided as there may be leakage of bile from the cystic duct if the ligature slips, from the gall-bladder bed, or from the common bile duct if it has been punctured for cholangiography. Some postoperative oozing of blood may also occur, particularly if the gall-bladder was badly inflamed, with the potential for development of an infected collection in what is usually a contaminated area. Two *Redivac* suction drains are recommended, one leading from the subhepatic space and one from the right suprahepatic space,

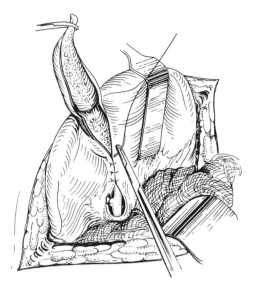

Fig. 20.13 Completion of cholecystectomy by the retrograde method. The partially separated gall-bladder is used as a retractor to allow exposure for haemostasis. Sutures are rarely necessary

brought out separately from the wound. These drains would normally be removed at 48 hours unless there is continuing drainage of bile (Hoffman, 1985).

Depending on the incision and the surgeon's preference, the wound is closed in layers or by the mass suture technique.

'Fundus first' method

This method is advised only when difficulties (particularly severe inflammatory changes) prevent the ducts being displayed in the first steps of the operation, so exposing them to great danger if dissection near the cystic duct and common bile duct is continued. Paradoxically, however, the fundus first method also carries risks of injury particularly to the common bile duct and right hepatic artery. Excessive traction on the mobilized gall-bladder may pull these structures out of their normal alignment, rendering them liable to be clamped or included in a ligature (Fig. 20.14).

Separation of the gall-bladder is commenced at the fundus, the peritoneal sheath being divided with scissors at each side where it is reflected on to the liver. It is most desirable that the cystic duct and cystic artery should be clearly defined before the gall-bladder is removed. If, however, owing to adhesions, isolation of these structures is thought to endanger the right hepatic artery or the common duct, it is far better to leave part of the neck of the gall-bladder in situ. More bleeding is encountered using this technique than using the retrograde method, where the cystic artery is controlled at an earlier stage.

Espiner (1982) has described a modification of the

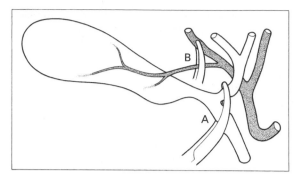

Fig. 20.14 Accidents liable to occur at cholecystectomy — inclusion of the common bile duct (A) or the right hepatic artery (B) in clamp or ligature

fundus first method which he considers particularly suitable for the very thickened and inflamed gall-bladder, in which the separation of the gall-bladder bed is carried out in the submucosal plane using diathermy. This obviates the requirement to control the cystic artery and minimizes the risk of danger to the common bile duct.

Risks of the operation

The chief danger lies in the possibility of injury to one of the main bile ducts or to the right hepatic artery. Unless the junction between the cystic and common ducts is clearly demonstrated, a segment of the common duct may be inadvertently clamped or included in a ligature (Fig. 20.14), so that biliary obstruction may result. Undetected section of a duct — possibly an abnormally placed or accessory one — may lead to biliary peritonitis or to an external fistula. The right hepatic artery may be ligatured in mistake for the cystic artery, or may be included in the ligature applied to it (Fig. 20.14); this accident may cause a fatal issue owing to massive liver necrosis. To obviate these dangers two simple rules should be observed at any operation for cholecystectomy:

1. The junction of the cystic and common ducts should be displayed beyond the slightest possibility of doubt, before any clamp or ligature is applied.

2. The cystic artery should be ligatured separately, and only after it has been clearly identified by its course to the gall-bladder.

Haemorrhage

Haemorrhage from a torn cystic artery or from a slipped ligature is likely to be profuse, and injudicious attempts to arrest it may damage important structures in the vicinity. A large pack should be placed against the bleeding area, *and left in situ for 2 or 3 minutes*; when it is removed the bleeding vessel can usually be secured without difficulty. If necessary, the hepatic artery may be temporarily occluded by a light bowel clamp placed on the free border of the lesser omentum.

Accumulation of bile
This may occur in the right subphrenic or subhepatic region, even when provision for drainage appears to have been adequate. Upper abdominal or chest pain associated with tachycardia and a persistently low blood pressure (the Waltman-Walters syndrome), are cardinal signs, and the condition is often mistaken for coronary thrombosis. If there is any suspicion that such an accumulation is present, an ultrasound scan should be performed, and if positive no time should be lost in re-exploring the abdomen, since immediate and dramatic relief is obtained from evacuation of the bile. Unless this is done the patient's condition rapidly deteriorates.

Cholecystectomy for carcinoma
A very early carcinoma may be detected only after the gall-bladder has been removed and opened up; in such cases the prognosis is reasonably good. More often, however, the gall-bladder is hard and nodular from an infiltrating growth. A segment of the adjacent liver tissue should then be removed along with the gall-bladder (p. 417). When there is naked-eye evidence of extension of the disease to the liver it is probably too late to hope for a cure, but partial hepatectomy may be considered.

CHOLEDOCHOTOMY

Choledochotomy (opening and exploration of the common bile duct) is indicated when the operative cholangiogram reveals filling defects or stricture. If facilities for operative cholangiography have been omitted or are not available, the palpation of a stone is a clear indication for exploration of the duct. Reliance on the classical indications for exploration, for example, a dilated or thickened duct, recent jaundice, multiple small stones in the gall-bladder with a wide cystic duct results in a negative exploration rate of approximately 50%. Negative exploration of the common bile duct increases mortality, morbidity and duration of hospital stay in comparison with simple cholecystectomy.

Supraduodenal choledochotomy
This approach is the method of choice since the supraduodenal portion of the duct, lying in the free border of the lesser omentum, is relatively accessible. Exploration of the duct is, in the majority of cases, for suspected calculi, and the gall-bladder will have been removed earlier in the operation.

The second part of duodenum should be fully mobi-lized ('Kocherized') after incision of the peritoneum lying lateral to it. This is usually avascular, though some vessels may require ligation close to the region where the common bile duct passes behind the duodenum. Mobilization of the duodenum and head of the pancreas should be carried as far as the left side of the inferior length of the common bile duct, to allow the second part of duodenum to be brought forward into the wound. A pack is now placed posterior to the duodenum in Morison's pouch.

The peritoneum over the supraduodenal portion of the common duct is incised and the anterior surface cleared of peritoneum and fatty tissue over a distance of 1.5 cm. One or two small vessels in the immediate supraduodenal region may require to be controlled either by fine ligatures or by haemoclips. If, due to gross inflammatory changes, there is some doubt as to the actual location of the common bile duct it may be identified by aspirating bile through a fine bore needle.

Exploration of the duct
Stay sutures of 2/0 chromic catgut are now inserted near the borders of the duct and a 1 cm longitudinal incision made between them into the duct (Fig. 20.15). A bacteriological swab is taken of the bile escaping through the incision, and the bile is aspirated through a fine bore sucker. Some small floating stones may emerge with the first rush of bile, and these should be

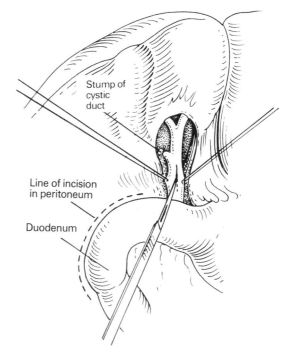

Fig. 20.15 Method of opening the supraduodenal part of the common bile duct by incision between stay sutures

retrieved. An attempt should now be made *gently* to milk any palpable stones towards the choledochotomy incision, whence they may easily be removed using gall-stone forceps.

Removal of calculi

The duct is now formally explored for residual stones, palpable or otherwise. A wide variety of instruments is available for this purpose. Rigid bougies or forceps (e.g. Maingot's, Desjardins's) are most frequently used, but unless great care is exercised damage to the duct, particularly at its lower end, may result, with subsequent stricture formation. It is therefore recommended that the initial exploration be made with a Fogarty biliary catheter (Fig. 20.16).

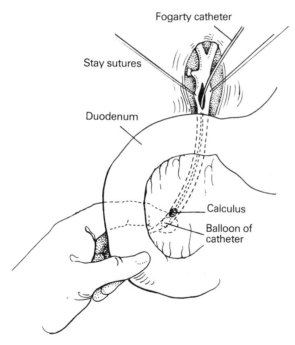

Fig. 20.16   Removal of a calculus in the lower part of the common bile duct using a Fogarty biliary catheter

Retrograde exploration is undertaken first. The common bile duct is lightly compressed between finger and thumb below the choledochotomy incision. The catheter is passed upwards and guided into the right hepatic duct and advanced as far as it will go. The balloon is now inflated until slight resistance to downward traction is felt, and the catheter is pulled downwards, maintaining inflation to provide slight resistance. Any calculi appearing at the choledochotomy incision are removed by forceps. The procedure is repeated for the left hepatic duct and then for both ducts in turn until the surgeon is satisfied that the upper biliary tree is clear.

Prograde exploration is now undertaken. The duct above the choledochotomy is occluded between finger and thumb, or using light occlusion forceps, and the Fogarty catheter passed into the duodenum (judged by the distance it has passed) and the balloon inflated. Confirmation of its position in the duodenum is made by palpation of the inflated balloon. The balloon is now partially deflated while maintaining upward traction until the balloon is felt to come through the sphincter. It is then re-inflated to maintain slight resistance to traction and the catheter pulled upwards until calculi, or the balloon, appear at the choledochotomy incision. Calculi are removed. The procedure is repeated until the surgeon is content that no calculi remain.

Should the Fogarty catheter fail to enter the duodenum (usually due to an impacted and palpable stone) further gentle exploration with a metal biliary scoop or Maingot's forceps, using the left hand to guide the instrument into position, will usually result in a successful extraction. Management of the impacted and apparently immoveable stone will be considered later.

Given that at this stage in the operation the surgeon feels that he has cleared the ducts, the common bile duct and hepatic ducts are irrigated with saline to wash out any calculous debris or blood clots and postexploratory cholangiogram films are taken. Dissatisfaction with films obtained by injecting dye through the T-tube (usually due to failure to outline the lower end of the common bile duct because dye does not pass through as a result of spasm of the sphincter of Oddi) led Gunn (Fox, 1984) to describe a technique using a fine (8 FG) Foley catheter. The catheter is first inserted upwards through the choledochotomy incision, and the balloon inflated to occlude the common hepatic duct. Dye is now injected to display the upper biliary tree and a film is taken. The balloon is deflated, the catheter inserted downwards, the balloon inflated to occlude the common bile duct and dye injected to display the lower biliary tree. Provided the ampulla is not occluded by a stone, the extra pressure obtained using this technique will allow dye to pass into the duodenum and fully display the lowest part of the common bile duct. Usually, two films are taken. Exploration of the duct system under vision using a *choledochoscope* is of added benefit if the necessary equipment and skills are available (Berci, 1988).

Drainage

Following demonstration of a satisfactory duct system T-tube drainage of the common bile duct should, in the author's view, be routine. Some surgeons omit this step, especially if the exploration has been negative, but the opportunity subsequently to obtain high quality films of the duct system in the X-ray department is lost. A relatively fine Latex rubber T-tube (10 or 12 FG)

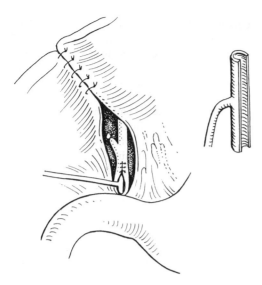

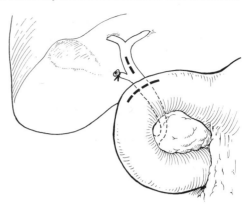

Fig. 20.18 Incisions in bile duct and duodenum for choledochoduodenostomy

Fig. 20.17 T-tube drainage of the common bile duct. The incision in the duct is sutured *above* the emerging limb of the tube in order to avoid any drag on the suture line when the tube is withdrawn

should be used. The long limb of the T-tube is brought out through the *lower* end of the choledochotomy incision (Fig. 20.17), which is closed in one layer of continuous fine absorbable suture (e.g. 3/0 Dexon), and brought to the surface through a stab incision, taking the most direct route.

Antibiotic lavage of the operation area prior to closure of the main wound is recommended, and small bore *Redivac* drains are led both from the subhepatic and suprahepatic spaces.

Postoperative check films are taken on the 7th–10th day usually following 2 to 3 days of intermittent clamping of the T-tube and, if satisfactory, the tube is removed. There may be a small bile leak following removal which rarely persists for more than 48 hours.

The impacted stone

If a stone remains impacted at the lower end of the common bile duct despite routine measures to remove it, the surgeon has essentially 3 choices, determined by the fitness of the patient, or availability of endoscopic skills:

1. To leave the stone where it is, drain the common bile duct by T-tube for 2 to 3 weeks to allow inflammation to settle, and invite an expert endoscopist to carry out endoscopic papillotomy. This has attractions for the very sick patient, but the truly impacted stone does provide the endoscopist with some difficulties, and stones over 15 mm in diameter are not suitable for the technique.

2. Leave the stone where it is and carry out *choledochoduodenostomy*. A transverse incision is made in

the duodenum close to the lower end of the previously made vertical choledochotomy incision (Fig. 20.18). The anastomosis is performed in one layer of interrupted inverting sutures of 3/0 absorbable material — knotted on the inside (Figs 20.19–20.21).

3. Remove the stone via a *transduodenal sphincteroplasty*. An oblique anterolateral incision is made in the second part of duodenum in a position determined by the palpable stone. Stay sutures are now inserted in

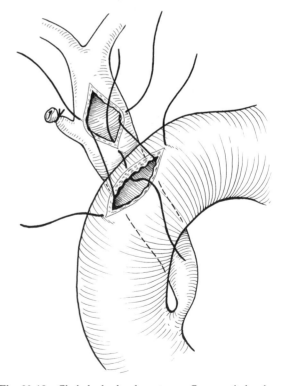

Fig. 20.19 Choledochoduodenostomy. Corner stitches have been placed for anastomosis between the common bile duct and the first part of duodenum

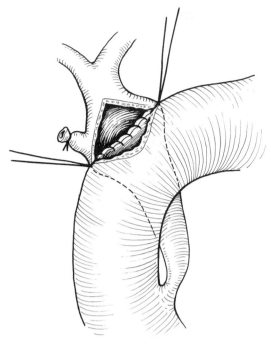

Fig. 20.20 Choledochoduodenostomy. Posterior layer has been completed

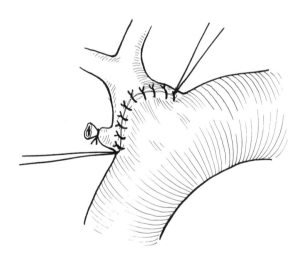

Fig. 20.21 Choledochoduodenostomy completed

the medial wall of the duodenum on either side of the ampulla (Fig. 20.22). Using a knife, an incision is made directly over the stone which is then extracted. The incision in the wall of duodenum and lower end of bile duct is now enlarged, using sphincteroplasty scissors, to a minimum length of 1.5 cm and converted to a formal sphincteroplasty by approximating duodenal and bile duct mucosa using interrupted 3/0 absorbable sutures. Care must be taken to ensure apposition of mucosae at the apex of the incision. The duodenotomy incision is now closed in its own line in two layers.

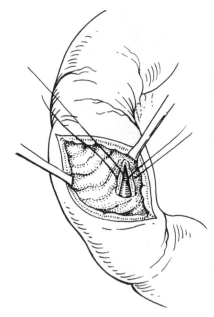

Fig. 20.22 Transduodenal sphincteroplasty

Supraduodenal T-tube drainage is not normally necessary following this procedure (Carter, 1983) and the choledochotomy incision is closed in one layer using a continuous 3/0 absorbable suture.

The retained stone

Despite apparently satisfactory postexploratory films obtained at operation, the T-tube cholangiogram obtained 7–10 days after operation may demonstrate one or more stones that had been missed at operation (Fig. 20.23). Again, several management options are available:

1. Leave the T-tube to drain for a further 7–10 days and then repeat the cholangiogram. Up to 40% of filling defects will have disappeared, either because they were not stones (e.g. blood clot, air bubble), or, if they were, have passed spontaneously.

2. Institute *irrigation* of the common bile duct through the T-tube. Intermittent irrigation through the T-tube using bile acids has been favoured, and heparin suggested, but there is little hard evidence that they provide better results than irrigation with saline. The method may be continued for up to 3 weeks, but is unlikely to be successful if the retained stone lies in the biliary tree above the level of the T-tube, and is contraindicated if a stone is impacted at the lower end of the bile duct preventing flow of dye into the duodenum. Check cholangiograms are taken through the T-tube every few days to assess progress.

3. *Endoscopic papillotomy* may be undertaken 2 weeks after surgery. The stone may be left to pass spontane-

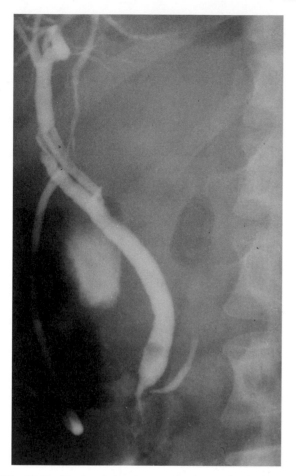

Fig. 20.23   T-tube cholangiogram showing retained calculus

ously after papillotomy, or it may be extracted at the time of papillotomy using a Dormia basket, or Fogarty type catheter. This technique is not suitable for stones retained high in the biliary tree, and may be unsuccessful if the stone is very firmly impacted at its lower end.

4. *Instrumental removal via the T-tube tract* (Burhenne, 1988). This technique, which should be delayed for 4 weeks after operation to allow maturation of the T-tube track, may be used for retained stones anywhere in the biliary tree, but is particularly suitable for stones in its upper part. The original injunction to use a large bore T-tube (> 14 FG) so as to permit this technique, no longer prevails, as the T-tube track may be dilated using graduated dilators before introducing the cannula down the track. Under fluoroscopic control, a Dormia basket or Fogarty type catheter is manipulated into position around or beyond the stone, which is then drawn out along the T-tube track.

5. *Reoperation* will be required in the event of failure or non-availability of the preceding techniques. Such reoperations are difficult and supraduodenal re-exploration particularly so, so that preference is given to a

transduodenal approach with sphincteroplasty for stones in the lower parts of the duct.

OTHER OPERATIONS ON THE BILE DUCTS

Immediate repair of injuries
Most injuries to the bile ducts follow operative misadventures. They are due usually to failure to isolate and to ligature separately the cystic duct and cystic artery at the operation of cholecystectomy or to lack of care in freeing the duodenum at gastrectomy. The common bile duct is the one most frequently damaged. Such injuries are potentially serious and should be dealt with at once provided that the situation is not aggravated by unskilled attempts at repair.

End-to-end suture
This is the ideal method of repair of a divided duct, but as a rule it is practicable only when the condition is discovered at or very soon after the injury, for at a later date considerable retraction together with periductal fibrosis will have occurred. The cut ends are identified; the upper is usually traced without difficulty from the escape of bile; the lower may have retracted behind the duodenum, which must then be mobilized by division of the peritoneum along its lateral border. This allows the duodenum to be brought up towards the porta hepatis, so that the cut ends of the duct may be approximated without tension. It is advisable that the anastomosis should be effected over a latex rubber tube: this not only forms an effective splint, but also serves to maintain the lumen of the duct. If a T-tube is used, it should be brought out through a separate opening in the lower segment of the duct at least 1 cm below the suture line (Fig. 20.24), and the anastomosis made over its upper limb. The cut ends of the duct are united by interrupted sutures of fine catgut, and the suture line is reinforced by repair of the surrounding fascial layers.

Late repair or reconstruction of ducts
Secondary repair of a severed or stenosed duct is one of the most difficult of operations. The duct is likely to be buried in dense scar tissue, and the ends may be widely retracted. The most successful method of reconstruction is to effect an anastomosis between the upper stump of the duct and a defunctioned (Roux) loop of jejunum, as shown in Figure 20.25 (Bismith, 1978). This is done by transecting the bowel 25 to 30 cm below the duodenojejunal flexure, and by bringing the lower cut end upwards in front of or behind the transverse colon, to be joined to the upper stump of the biliary duct. Direct suture may be possible to a stump of bile duct or to the left hepatic duct if this can be

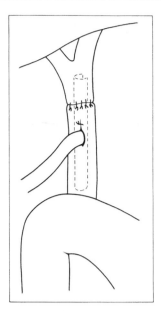

Fig. 20.24 Repair of bile duct over T-tube brought out through opening at lower level

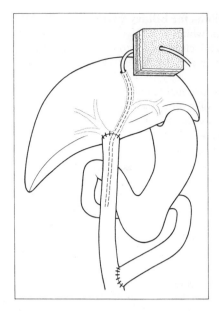

Fig. 20.26 Alternative method of splinting the anastomosis, the tube being led upwards through the liver substance before reaching the exterior

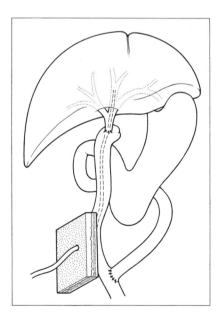

Fig. 20.25 Reconstruction of bile duct by the use of a *Roux* loop of jejunum. A latex tube splints the anastomosis, and is led down through the jejunal loop for about 10 cm before being brought out through the abdominal wall

exposed (Blumgart, 1988). The 'mucosal graft' technique described by Rodney Smith (1980) is applicable where no duct stump remains; by bringing into contact mucosa of bile duct and jejunum, it reduces the risk of re-stenosis. A soft latex tube within the anastomosis and brought out through the abdominal wall (Fig. 20.25) may be extruded by peristalsis and it is preferable to

bring the tube to the surface through the liver substance (Fig. 20.26). By this latter method the tube can remain in situ for 6 to 12 months; it can be clamped so that no external leakage of bile occurs; it will stay in place until removed by the surgeon, and until then can be used for irrigation of the reconstructed duct. This method greatly reduces the risk of progressive stenosis, which is always liable to occur after operative repair.

Strictures of the common bile duct

These may result from injury or from fibrosis following some inflammatory lesion. A common type of stricture occurs at the lower end of the duct, the most likely cause being a stone which has been impacted sufficiently long to set up a fibrotic reaction.

When stenosis involves only the orifice of the duct, it may be dealt with either by transduodenal surgical sphincteroplasty (see Fig. 20.22) or by endoscopic papillotomy. For sphincteroplasty, a probe is passed into the duct orifice which is then slit upwards for 1 to 2 cm. The mucosal layers of duct and duodenum are then united by interrupted absorbable sutures on each side.

When the stricture is thought to be too high or too long to be treated by simple incision of the duct orifice, short-circuiting operations offer the best prospect of success. The upper part of the duct, which is likely to be much dilated, can usually be anastomosed without undue difficulty to the duodenum — *choledochoduodenostomy* (see Fig. 20.20). Alternatively, a Roux loop of jejunum may be employed for the anastomosis (Figs 20.25 & 20.26).

Operations for biliary fistula

A fistula which follows the operations of cholecysto-stomy and choledochostomy usually closes spontane-ously within a week or 10 days after withdrawal of the tube.

A *persistent* fistula may close spontaneously even after a period of several months, so that surgical interference should not be too hastily considered. However, the anatomy should be defined by ERCP, and, if serious loss of bile is occurring, early treatment is indicated. The operative procedure will depend upon the conditions present.

A fistula following cholecystostomy is likely to be due to stricture of the cystic duct or to an impacted calculus, in which case the discharge will consist mainly of mucus. Cholecystectomy is usually curative.

Biliary fistula following cholecystectomy may be due to accidental wounding of a duct during the operation. Often the accident becomes evident only after several days, from profuse discharge of bile from the wound, or from signs of a subhepatic collection. When the injury to the duct has been relatively slight, or if it is only a small accessory duct that has been severed, a large proportion of the total bile may pass normally to the intestine, and spontaneous healing may then be expected. If, however, the common duct or one of the main hepatic ducts has been completely severed, spontaneous cure is impossible, and immediate operation is required.

If a fistula persists after choledochostomy, it is likely that the lower part of the common duct is obstructed — possibly by a residual stone, or by fibrosis associated with chronic pancreatitis. A residual stone may be removed endoscopically at or after ERCP; a *short* stricture of the lower end of the common bile duct may be treated by endoscopic papillotomy. If a stone cannot be removed endoscopically, surgical removal via the supraduodenal or transduodenal route is indicated. If the equipment is available ESWL (extracorporeal shock wave lithotripsy) may be considered. Strictures not amenable to endoscopic treatment should be treated by one of the reconstructive or short-circuiting operations already described.

ANASTOMOSIS OF GALL-BLADDER TO GASTROINTESTINAL TRACT

The operations described under this heading are designed to short-circuit irremediable obstruction of the common bile duct, such as may be caused by carcinoma or by chronic pancreatitis. They are seldom applicable to cases of common duct obstruction due to the effects of gall-stones, for the gall-bladder is then likely to be shrivelled and fibrotic, or otherwise unsuit-able for anastomosis; in many cases it will have been removed at a previous operation.

Cholecystogastrostomy

This is technically the easiest operation since the distended gall-bladder usually lies in contact with the pyloric part of the stomach. It is now seldom employed, however, since it has certain serious disadvantages: bilious vomiting due to the large quantities of bile which may be passed directly into the stomach, and an irritative cholangitis due to regurgitation of gastric contents into the biliary passages.

Technique

The gall-bladder is emptied by a trocar and cannula inserted on the inferior aspect of the fundus. Light occlusion clamps are applied to the fundus, and to the nearest portion of stomach. The clamps are laid side by side, and lateral anastomosis is carried out by the standard technique, the first line of sutures being placed so that the opening made by the cannula can be enlarged to form the anastomosis. An opening 2 cm in length is adequate.

Cholecystoduodenostomy

This is technically very difficult, and has no special advantages. It is therefore seldom performed.

Cholecystojejunostomy

Bypass using a loop of jejunum is the operation most commonly performed. A loop of jejunum some 45 cm below the duodenojejunal flexure is selected and brought up in front of the colon for the purpose of the anastomosis. The operation is completed by making an entero-anastomosis between the afferent and efferent loops of jejunum (Fig. 20.27). This not only prevents obstruction of the bowel by kinking, but diverts much of the bowel contents from the site of the anastomosis. More complete diversion is obtained by utilizing a defunctioned (Roux) jejunal loop of jejunum. Though technically more demanding to surgeon and patient than the standard cholecystojejunostomy it is preferred in the fitter patient and in those whose obstruction is of benign aetiology and consequently have a longer life expectancy.

Tumours of the bile ducts

Carcinomas of the common bile duct are rarely amenable to excision. Occasionally a carcinoma of the lower end of the common bile duct may be resected by *pancreaticoduodenectomy*. Rarely it may be possible to resect a tumour of the common hepatic duct, restoring biliary drainage through a Roux loop of jejunum.

Usually only palliative treatment is possible. In the case of tumours involving the lower common bile duct, cholecyst- or hepaticojejunostomy may be employed,

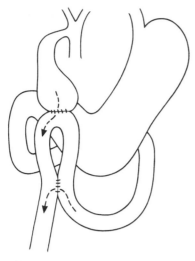

Fig. 20.27   Cholecystojejunostomy with entero-anastomosis

or drainage provided by endoscopic insertion of a biliary endoprosthesis through the tumour from the duodenum. In tumours involving the duct system at the level of the common hepatic duct or above, percutaneous intubation is the simplest palliative procedure. Anastomosis between a Segment III bile duct and a Roux loop of jejunum is favoured in fitter patients or if the obstruction is of benign aetiology (see page 437). Some of these tumours may be very slow growing and occasionally prolonged survival follows palliation.

BILIARY ATRESIA

In this text the term biliary atresia is used to include classical extrahepatic biliary atresia, biliary hypoplasia and choledochal cyst. In 10% of babies with biliary atresia a dilated bile duct proximal to an atretic segment is found below the level of the porta hepatis in the free margin of the lesser omentum. In the remainder, hypoplastic or atretic ducts extend proximally within the substance of the liver. In clinical practice it is important to differentiate between obstructive jaundice of biliary atresia and cholestatic jaundice of neonatal hepatitis. This must be done with some urgency as the treatment of biliary atresia is by operation within 6 to 8 weeks of birth so as to prevent irreversible damage to the liver. The distinction, however, is not always clear as there appears to be an area of overlap between the two conditions. The classical view of biliary atresia and neonatal hepatitis as separate entities is now in doubt and it is more probable that both are part of a spectrum of change in the biliary system from damage either viral or by foetal bile salts.

A diagnosis of obstructive jaundice should be considered in a baby with conjugated hyperbilirubinaemia and acholic stools who becomes icteric within a few days of birth or in whom 'physiological' jaundice fails to clear. Other causes of hepatitis, for example infection, galactosaemia and alpha 1 antitrypsin deficiency must first be excluded. The distinction between biliary atresia and neonatal hepatitis is then made on the basis of a technetium[99m] iminodiacetic acid (IDA), ultrasound and percutaneous liver biopsy. The histological changes of bile ductule proliferation, fibrosis and bile stasis are seen in biliary atresia whereas giant cell transformation is typical of neonatal hepatocytes.

The management of a baby with a diagnosis of biliary atresia is by operation. An operative cholangiogram is first performed through the fundus of the gall-bladder (Howard, 1983). The free margin of the lesser omentum is then dissected. When the obstruction is extrahepatic, a dilated duct is found and bile drainage can be achieved by means of a choledochoenterostomy fashioned with a Roux loop. Alternatively the dilated duct can be dissected proximally, divided at the level of the porta hepatis and porto-enterostomy performed. More often, however, only a hypoplastic or atretic duct is present; the fine stricture is then dissected proximally with great care to an area of fibrous tissue at the porta hepatis. The fibrous tissue at this level may contain fine ductules; the tissue is therefore divided and, once again, a porto-enterostomy performed using a *Roux* loop (Kasai, 1959). The role of liver transplantation is at present undecided but is normally reserved for infants in whom drainage is unsuccessful.

Although there has been some success with Kasai's operation, the earlier results were disappointing. Babies died of liver failure or, in later years, children died of haemorrhage from portal hypertension secondary to cirrhosis. The failure of surgery may have been, in part, related to delay in operation, failure to establish satisfactory bile drainage and ascending cholangitis. Recognition of the importance of early operation within 6 weeks of life has improved results significantly (Tagge, 1991).

OPERATIONS ON THE PANCREAS

Operations on the pancreas are performed relatively infrequently and are often difficult so that pancreatic surgery is best concentrated in specialist hands.

Surgery may be indicated for:

1. *inflammatory disease*
   a. acute pancreatitis
   b. chronic pancreatitis
2. *tumours*
   a. benign
   b. malignant
3. *trauma*

Surgical approach to the pancreas

In most patients excellent access is provided by a bilateral Kocher ('rooftop') or transverse epigastric incision extending from costal margin to costal margin. In patients with a narrow costal angle, a long midline incision may be preferred. The head of the pancreas is exposed by full Kocherization of the duodenum (page 433) and by downward displacement of the hepatic flexure after incising the lateral and superior peritoneal attachments. This allows inspection and palpation of the anterior and posterior aspects of the entire head of the pancreas and its uncinate process. The anterior aspect of the body and tail of the pancreas is exposed by serial ligation and division of the gastrocolic omentum along most of its length, allowing full access to the lesser sac. Access to the posterior aspect of the body and tail may be needed when palpating the pancreas to detect a small apudoma or when the splenic vein is required for a porto-systemic shunt. It can be provided by incising the peritoneum along the inferior border of the pancreas (taking care to preserve or formally ligate the inferior mesenteric vein as it passes to the splenic vein), or by forward mobilization of the spleen and distal pancreas after division of the lieno-renal ligament.

INFLAMMATORY CONDITIONS OF THE PANCREAS

Acute pancreatitis

Acute pancreatitis remains a difficult and dangerous condition which still has a mortality rate of up to 10%. The outcome is difficult to predict when the patient is first seen. In most cases the signs and symptoms abate within 48–72 hours on conservative management, but about one in four patients will prove to have severe disease with progression to complications, and of these, about one in four will die. Objective prognostic factor grading systems (Ranson, 1974; Blamey, 1984) are of great value in the early identification of patients with severe disease who will require more vigorous management.

In the United Kingdom, acute pancreatitis is commonly associated with gall-stones (50% of cases) or alcohol abuse (up to one-third of cases). In 10–15% of cases, no causal factor can be implicated, but there is increasing evidence that many of these idiopathic cases are associated with small gall-stones or the presence of biliary sludge (defined as bile which contains cholesterol crystals and calcium bilirubinate granules). Miscellaneous causes of acute pancreatitis include abdominal trauma, hyperparathyroidism, hyperlipidaemia, hypothermia, cardio-pulmonary bypass, certain drugs (e.g. corticosteroids) and iatrogenic causes (e.g.

ERCP and endoscopic papillotomy, gastric surgery, biliary surgery).

The overall plan of management is as follows:

1. establish the diagnosis
2. institute conservative management with adequate control of pain and vigorous resuscitation
3. identify and treat aetiological factor such as gall-stones, alcoholism or hyperparathyroidism
4. monitor to detect and treat complications (e.g. pancreatic and peripancreatic necrosis, pseudocyst, abscess or bleeding).

Establish the diagnosis

The diagnosis is based on consideration of the history and clinical findings, presence of hyperamylasaemia (80–90% of cases), and the demonstration of a swollen pancreas on ultrasonography or CT scanning. It is now unusual to find acute pancreatitis unexpectedly at laparotomy. Although unnecessary surgery should be avoided whenever possible, there are some patients in whom hyperamylasaemia is absent or unimpressive (less than 1000 units/1) and in whom abdominal conditions requiring urgent surgical treatment cannot be excluded without laparotomy (see below).

Conservative management

Pethidine is usually recommended for analgesia in the belief (mistaken) that it causes less spasm of the sphincter of Oddi than morphine. A nasogastric tube is passed to keep the stomach empty and avoid further vomiting, although there is little objective evidence that this is beneficial. An intravenous infusion is established and adequate amounts of fluid and electrolyte (and, if necessary, colloid) are administered as assessed by the patient's circulatory state and urine output. In severe pancreatitis, a CVP line is helpful and hourly urine output is monitored after inserting a urethral catheter. Many patients are hypoxic so that oxygen should be administered and arterial blood gases monitored. In some cases, assisted ventilation will be required. Broad spectrum antibiotics are reserved for specific indications although some surgeons prescribe them in patients with gall-stone pancreatitis because of the high risk of associated infection in the biliary tree. Anticholinergic drugs and glucagon were once used to 'rest' the pancreas while aprotinin (Trasylol) was used as a proteinase inhibitor; none of these agents was effective and they are no longer prescribed. Peritoneal lavage was also advocated in patients with severe disease but failed to reduce the incidence of complications and mortality (Mayer, 1985).

Identification and treatment of aetiological factors

Detection and eradication of gall-stones are the key

issues (Carter, 1989). Ultrasonography is normally a reliable means of detecting gall-stones within the gall-bladder and defining dilatation of the biliary tree. It is not so reliable in the detection of small stones at the lower end of the common bile duct, and with the ileus of acute pancreatitis, gas within the gastrointestinal tract often obscures the gall-bladder. If gall-stones are demonstrated unequivocally by ultrasonography and the patient settles on conservative management, cholecystectomy can be undertaken safely later in the same hospital admission (Osborne, 1981). Operative cholangiography should be undertaken at the time; in the majority of cases there is no indication to explore the bile duct in that the stone(s), which impacted transiently at the ampulla of Vater to give rise to the acute pancreatitis, will have passed spontaneously into the duodenum.

If the initial ultrasonography is equivocal, the investigation should be repeated after about a week has elapsed and the ileus has resolved. If gall-stones are still suspected, but cannot be excluded, ERCP is undertaken subsequently.

In some patients, gall-stones are demonstrated or suspected but the patient has *severe* acute pancreatitis which does not settle promptly on conservative management. Under these circumstances, urgent ERC can be used to define whether gall-stones are indeed present and the bile duct can then be cleared by endoscopic papillotomy. It was feared that this approach might exacerbate the attack of pancreatitis, but provided that contrast is not injected into the pancreatic duct, controlled study has shown that the incidence of complications (and perhaps mortality) are reduced (Neoptolemos, 1988). This endoscopic approach now enables urgent biliary surgery to be avoided in critically ill patients, but once the attack has settled, cholecystectomy is still advocated to reduce the risk of recurrent pancreatitis.

Detection and management of complications

Necrotising pancreatitis

In most patients, acute pancreatitis is a mild oedematous inflammation which settles within a few days. In contrast, some patients develop a severe, life threatening, necrotizing form of the disease with both pancreatic and peripancreatic necrosis (Beger, 1989). Necrotizing pancreatitis should be suspected in patients who have severe disease on admission and who fail to settle promptly on conservative management. Persisting pain, tachycardia, leucocytosis and organ failure (e.g. adult respiratory distress syndrome, renal failure, liver failure) all point to the development of necrosis and in many cases, to the fact that infection has supervened. Early detection of necrosis is aided by serial measurement of circulating levels of the acute phase protein, C-reactive protein (CRP) and by the use of the APACHE-II scoring system. If a rising CRP level and/or APACHE-II score strengthens the clinical suspicion of necrosis, a CT scan should be performed urgently. Contrast is instilled to outline the stomach and the duodenum, and contrast is also injected intravenously to obtain a dynamic or 'angio'-CT scan in which areas of necrosis are identified by their failure to 'light up' with contrast. Necrosis can be classified as focal, extensive or subtotal and some surgeons routinely aspirate material from necrotic areas to determine whether infection is present. Limited necrosis may not require surgical intervention, and the importance of clinical assessment cannot be overemphasized. However the presence of extensive necrosis, particularly when infected, is almost always an indication for surgical intervention.

If intervention is needed, an epigastric transverse or bilateral subcostal incision is needed to provide generous access to the entire pancreas and lesser sac. All necrotic material is removed by blunt necrosectomy using the index finger, and thorough débridement rather than formal pancreatic resection is now advocated. Bleeding can be problematic but is usually controllable by suture ligation. Some surgeons rely on simple drainage of the lesser sac following débridement, whereas many now reconstitute the lesser sac (by repairing the gastrocolic omentum) and insert multiple drains to allow lesser sac lavage in the post-operative period. Lavage may have to continue for days or even weeks depending on the nature of the effluent. Before closing the abdomen a gastrostomy is advisable to avoid prolonged nasogastric aspiration in patients with persisting duodenal ileus, and a feeding jejunostomy enables the gut 'downstream' of the duodenum to be used to provide luminal nutrition and avoid the need for TPN. It may be possible to remove the gall-bladder without undue risk in patients with gall-stone pancreatitis, but in general, the bile duct should be left alone in patients with necrotizing pancreatitis unless there is frank obstructive jaundice and insertion of a T-tube is required. Clinical judgement is needed to determine whether all layers of the wound should be closed primarily or whether the superficial layers of the wound should be left open. Some surgeons practice 'laparostomy' under these circumstances, leaving the wound open beneath sterile drapes or film, so that the lesser sac can be checked periodically to ensure that further necrosis has not developed. Patients with necrotizing pancreatitis usually require a period of intensive care followed by high dependency nursing. Surgical re-intervention is often needed to deal with further development of necrosis and infection, and many weeks of hospitalization may be necessary.

Abscess formation

Abscess formation following an attack of acute pancreatitis is usually the consequence of infection of a localised area of necrosis. The abscess often becomes manifest during the second or third week of the illness in a patient who has failed to settle completely on conservative management. Recurrent pain, pyrexia and leucocytosis suggest the diagnosis, and this may be confirmed by ultrasonography or CT scan. External drainage is indicated and can often be achieved by percutaneous insertion of a catheter without recourse to laparotomy.

Pseudocyst formation

Pseudocysts are common after pancreatitis but most will disappear spontaneously unless larger than 5 cm in diameter. Persisting pain, grumbling hyperamylasaemia, and in some cases, development of a palpable or visible mass, may reflect development of pancreatic pseudocyst. In some patients the pseudocyst compresses the stomach and duodenum causing vomiting or compresses the common bile duct to produce jaundice. As with abscess formation, 2 or 3 weeks may elapse before the pseudo-cyst becomes manifest. Ultrasonography is an excellent method of confirming the diagnosis.

If possible, drainage should be delayed to allow the pseudocyst wall to thicken and mature, but undue delay should be avoided in case further complications (notably infection, bleeding and rupture) ensue. The conventional method of draining a pseudocyst is formal surgical drainage into the stomach, duodenum or jejunum. At the time of drainage a biopsy from the cyst wall is obtained to exclude a cystic pancreatic neoplasm. *Pseudocyst-gastrostomy* was the operation most frequently performed. The anterior wall of the stomach is incised longitudinally to expose the bulging back wall of the stomach overlying the pseudocyst. A needle is then inserted into the collection and a sample obtained to check that there has been no bleeding into the collection and to allow bacteriological culture. The posterior wall of the stomach is then incised longitudinally over a distance of 3–4 cm and the cyst contents aspirated. Any loculi within the collection are broken down and necrotic material is removed. Bleeding from the posterior gastrotomy is controlled by full thickness mattress sutures of non-absorbable material placed around the margin. The pseudocyst cavity normally closes rapidly following effective drainage. *Pseudocyst-jejunostomy* using a Roux loop of jejunum is a little more time consuming but allows more effective dependent drainage and is now often preferred, particularly when the collection is found to be bulging through the transverse mesocolon. On occasions, pseudocysts compressing the duodenum may be more effectively dealt with by *pseudocyst-duodenostomy*.

Percutaneous aspiration under ultrasound control offers an alternative to surgical drainage, particularly in sick patients. A drainage catheter can be inserted but external drainage is frequently followed by the development of a fistula, a complication which has no significance after internal surgical drainage. In general, internal drainage of pseudocysts is preferred to external drainage, although using a combination of endoscopy and percutaneous radiology it is now possible to insert a stent between the lumen of the stomach and pseudocyst, thus avoiding operative intervention.

Bleeding

Acute pancreatitis may be complicated by bleeding into the retroperitoneum, lesser sac, pseudocyst or pancreatic duct (and from there to the gastro-intestinal tract). Haemorrhage under these circumstances may be life threatening and results from tissue necrosis with erosion into major blood vessels such as the splenic artery. Urgent operation may be mandatory but, if time permits, angiography may be an invaluable means of locating the source of haemorrhage and arresting it at least temporarily, by embolization of the bleeding vessel.

Indications for surgery in acute pancreatitis

The indications for surgery in acute pancreatitis can be summarised:

1. *When there is doubt as to the diagnosis.* This is now a rare indication for surgery given the improvements in diagnostic methods. Peritoneal lavage or laparoscopy may avoid unnecessary laparotomy in some cases but on occasions laparotomy may still be needed when an intra-abdominal catastrophe such as intestinal ischaemia cannot be excluded. If the diagnosis of acute pancreatitis is made for the first time at laparotomy, the abdomen is normally closed without drainage. If the patient has severe disease with extensive necrosis, necrosectomy may be indicated with institution of lesser sac lavage, gastrostomy and jejunostomy as described above. If gall-stones are found in association with acute pancreatitis at emergency laparotomy, clinical judgement is needed to decide whether it is safe to remove the gall-bladder. Regardless of whether cholecystectomy is undertaken, exploration of the common bile duct is usually inadvisable under these circumstances, and at most a T-tube should be inserted into the duct if it is obviously distended and the patient has obstructive jaundice.

2. *Deterioration in the patients condition.* The development of necrosis, particularly when associated with infection, may require urgent laparotomy.

3. *Treatment of complications.* Surgery may be needed to deal with complications such as abscess, pseudocyst, bleeding and obstructive jaundice.

4. *Treatment of gall-stones.* Gall-stones should be eradicated during the same hospital admission once the acute attack of pancreatitis has settled.

Chronic pancreatitis

Indications for surgery

The diagnosis of chronic pancreatitis is not in itself an indication for surgery and many patients can be managed conservatively. Intractable pain is the cardinal indication for operation. Less common indications include formation of a pseudocyst or abscess, obstructive jaundice, bleeding, duodenal obstruction, splenic vein thrombosis (with left sided portal hypertension, hypersplenism, and bleeding gastric/oesophageal varices), and pancreatic ascites or fistula formation. The pain of chronic pancreatitis can be devastating and often persists despite dietary manipulation (avoidance of fatty foods), and prescription of pancreatic exocrine supplements (e.g. Creon) and analgesics, including in many cases, opiate analgesics. Splanchnic nerve block provides transient relief at best and is usually a waste of time. Abstinence from alcohol is encouraged in patients with alcoholic pancreatitis but is notoriously difficult to achieve.

Ultrasonography and CT scanning detect calcification, pancreatic swelling, and dilatation of the pancreatic duct and biliary system, and may reveal complications such as pseudocysts and splenic vein thrombosis with splenomegaly.

Pancreatography provides an invaluable 'road map' which may influence the choice of operation; it can usually be obtained by ERCP but if this fails, antegrade pancreatography under ultrasound control or operative pancreatography may be needed. Pancreatic function tests are of limited value in diagnosis and management. The essential questions regarding pancreatic function are (1) does the patient have diabetes mellitus, (2) if diabetes is present, does it require dietary manipulation, oral hyperglycaemic agents or insulin for its control, and (3) does the patient have clinical evidence of steatorrhoea (pale bulky greasy stools which have a particularly offensive smell, float and are difficult to flush away).

Surgical options in chronic pancreatitis

Sphincteroplasty. Very few patients develop chronic pancreatitis because of a stricture in the terminal portion of the pancreatic duct. It follows that very few patients will benefit from the operation of transduodenal sphincteroplasty in which the openings of the bile duct and pancreatic duct into the duodenum are widened. It is now possible to carry out endoscopic sphincterotomy followed by removal of ductal calculi and/or insertion of stents into an obstructed pancreatic duct system.

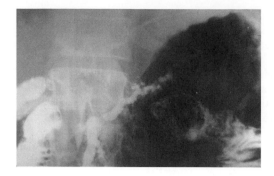

Fig. 20.28   Pancreatogram showing dilated duct

Although the definitive place of such endoscopic procedures is as yet unknown, their use might occasionally be considered if ductal narrowing is confined to the termination of the pancreatic duct.

Longitudinal pancreatico-jejunostomy. When the pancreatic duct is dilated, a pancreatic drainage procedure may be considered. Approximately 30–40% of patients requiring surgery for chronic pancreatitis have a duct system which is sufficiently dilated (diameter of more than 0.8–1.0 cm) for this procedure (Fig. 20.28). The operation has a lower operative morbidity and mortality than pancreatic resection, and conserves pancreatic exocrine and endocrine function. The gastrocolic omentum is divided widely to give full access to the lesser sac. The anterior surface of the pancreas is exposed fully and the duct is then incised and opened. The object is to create a long anastomosis between the opened pancreatic duct and the side of a Roux loop of jejunum brought up through a window in the transverse mesocolon. Ideally, the pancreatic duct is opened throughout the body and tail, the incision extending as far as possible into the head of the gland. All calculi are removed from the open duct, bleeding is controlled by suture ligation, and a one layer anastomosis is fashioned using interrupted sutures of a delayed absorption material such as polydioxanone (PDS). As shown in Figure 20.29, the blind end of the Roux loop should be laid on the tail of the pancreas, so that the same loop can be used to drain the biliary system if indicated at this or subsequent operation. Triple drainage has also been described in which the same loop of jejunum is used to drain the pancreatic duct, bile duct and stomach (if there is duodenal obstruction as well), although many surgeons would opt for pancreaticoduodenectomy (Whipple operation) under such circumstances. On completion of pancreaticojejunostomy, intestinal continuity is restored by an end-to-side jejunostomy some 40 cm below the mesocolon.

Distal pancreatectomy. If chronic pancreatitis is confined to the body and tail of the gland, distal pancreatectomy can be used to relieve symptoms. Such patients

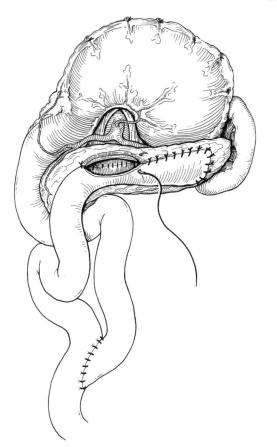

Fig. 20.29 Pancreatic duct drainage using *Roux-en-Y* pancreaticojejunostomy

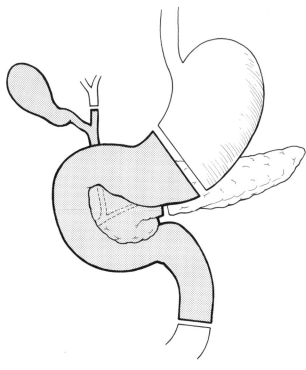

Fig. 20.30 Extent of resection in pancreaticoduodenectomy

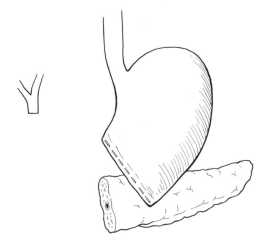

Fig. 20.31 Structures remaining after pancreaticoduodenectomy

frequently have a stricture which has given rise to distal obstruction and inflammation. The spleen is preserved if at all possible, but the degree of inflammation may make mobilization of the pancreas so difficult that splenectomy is unavoidable. The gland is transected to the right of the inflamed area and the duct is oversewn to minimize the risk of leakage postoperatively.

Near-total (80–95%) distal pancreatectomy was once a popular operation for chronic pancreatitis. However, pain was not always relieved in patients with extensive inflammation, and insulin-dependent diabetes and troublesome steatorrhoea were often precipitated. In modern practice, distal pancreatectomy usually means loss of about 40% of the pancreas so that endocrine and exocrine insufficiency may be avoided.

Pancreatico-duodenectomy. The Whipple operation (Whipple, 1946) is indicated when disease is maximal in the head of the gland, when the pancreatic duct is not sufficiently distended for pancreaticojejunostomy, when there is significant biliary obstruction, or when cancer of the head of the pancreas cannot be excluded (Fig. 20.30). Fibrosis usually makes the operation more difficult because of obliteration of tissue planes

but also makes for a more secure anastomosis between pancreatic remnant and the jejunum. Intestinal and biliary continuity is usually restored as shown in Figure 20.32. Some surgeons do not remove the gastric antrum and prefer pylorus-preserving pancreatico-duodenectomy on the grounds that this may cause less disturbance to gastrointestinal function.

Total pancreatectomy. This is very much a last resort procedure given that insulin dependent diabetes is inevitable and that major nutritional problems may

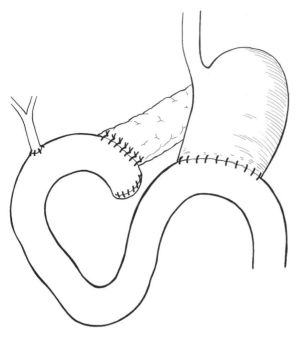

Fig. 20.32 Reconstruction following pancreaticoduodenectomy

follow the total loss of pancreatic exocrine function. The operation has an appreciable morbidity and mortality (5% in some series) and long-term survival is often compromised by complications due to the brittle diabetes, continuing alcohol abuse and addiction to narcotics. Total pancreatectomy and the Whipple operation can be achieved without resection of the duodenum, but it is arguable whether the increased difficulty of the surgery is justified by the results.

Overall, the results of surgery in chronic pancreatitis are disappointing but with careful selection and skilled surgery, some 70% of patients are pain free or substantially improved when assessed 5 years later. Results are particularly poor in patients who cannot abstain from alcohol, continue to have problems with drug dependence, and have difficulty managing their diabetes.

TUMOURS OF THE PANCREAS

Benign tumours of the pancreas
Benign tumours of the pancreas are rare. They may be functioning or non-functioning. Of the non-functioning tumours, cystadenomas can grow so large that they cause pressure effects on neighbouring structures and produce a palpable abdominal mass. The lesion is usually a multilocular serous cystadenoma (mucinous cystadenomas are more often malignant) and resection of the affected part of the pancreas (Whipple operation or distal pancreatectomy) is usually curative.

Insulinomas are the commonest benign functioning tumours of the pancreas but even their incidence is only 1 per million of the population per year. The lesion is usually less than 1 cm in diameter and can be dealt with by enucleation once found. Preoperative aids to localization include endoscopic ultrasonography, angiography and percutaneous transhepatic sampling of insulin levels in the splenic, portal and superior mesenteric veins. Useful as these aids may be, full mobilization of the entire pancreas and thorough bimanual palpation by a skilled surgeon are the keys to success. It was once taught that insulinomas were more common in the distal pancreas, and that failure to identify the lesion at operation was an indication for 'blind' distal pancreatectomy. It is now apparent that insulinomas are evenly distributed throughout the pancreas, and that failure to find the lesion is an indication to close the abdomen, control hypoglycaemia with diazeoxide, and revaluate the patient after an interval of months. In about 5% of cases the insulinoma proves to be multifocal and the patient is likely to have multiple endocrine neoplasia (MEN 1). In a further 5% of cases the insulinoma is malignant. Malignancy should be suspected when the diameter of the lesion exceeds 1 cm and pancreatic resection rather than enucleation should then be considered unless it is obvious that the patient has widespread metastatic disease.

Other functioning tumours such as gastrinomas, VIPoma (VIP = vasoactive intestinal peptide) and glucagonomas can be benign but are more often malignant. In some cases the tumour appears histologically to be of neuroendocrine origin but immunohistochemistry and search for circulating peptide products prove negative. In general, such non-functioning neuroendocrine tumours have a better prognosis than adenocarcinomas of the pancreas even when malignant, and resection should be undertaken if possible, even if it is clear that this is a palliative procedure.

Malignant tumours of the pancreas
Carcinoma of the pancreas now has an annual incidence of around 10 new cases per million of the population. The great majority of cases are ductal adenocarcinomas; carcinomas of acinar origin are relatively rare and cystadenocarcinomas are extremely rare. The cancer arises most frequently in the head of the pancreas and the patient presents with obstructive jaundice, often in association with weight loss and abdominal pain or discomfort. Only 10–20% of patients are potential candidates for resection in that local invasion and/or metastatic spread are often revealed by investigation, or the patient is too elderly or infirm to be considered for radical surgery. Cancers arising in the body and tail of the pancreas present even later than cancers of the pancreatic head, are often associated with extensive local

spread as evidenced by abdominal and back pain, and are rarely resectable.

Periampullary cancers (i.e. cancers arising at or within 1 cm of the papilla of Vater) and cancers of the common bile duct are less common than pancreatic cancer, but may present earlier with obstructive jaundice, are more often resectable and thus have a better prognosis. Whereas 5-year survival rates in pancreatic cancer are close to zero, rates of about 40% are reported for patients with biliary and periampullary tumours following radical resection.

Assessment of pancreatic cancer
Ultrasonography is an invaluable means of demonstrating extrahepatic biliary obstruction and may also show the mass lesion in the pancreas and any hepatic metastases. Endoscopic retrograde cholangiopancreatography (ERCP) may reveal obstruction of the common bile duct and pancreatic duct (the so-called double duct sign of pancreatic cancer). Percutaneous transhepatic cholangiography (PTC) is now seldom performed as ERCP is usually preferred by the patient, provides information about both biliary and pancreatic ducts, and can be used for therapeutic as well as diagnostic purposes in that a biliary stent can be inserted to relieve jaundice. The radiological diagnosis of cancer should be confirmed histologically or cytologically whenever possible by percutaneous sampling of lesions under radiological guidance. CT scanning is no more accurate than ultrasonography in revealing the local extent of pancreatic cancer, but is a more accurate means of detecting hepatic metastases. Selective angiography was used until recently to detect vascular anomalies (e.g. right hepatic or common hepatic artery arising from the superior mesenteric artery), and detect invasion of major vascular structures (e.g. superior mesenteric vessels or portal vein) that precluded resection. In some centres laparoscopy including laparoscopic ultrasonography, has now displaced angiography in the evaluation of resectability.

Resection of pancreatic cancer
If a patient has potentially resectable cancer of the head of pancreas (or periampullary area or common bile duct), careful pre-operative preparation is imperative. Deeply jaundiced patients will benefit from endoscopic insertion of a stent to allow liver function to return to normal over a period of 4–6 weeks. Anaemia is corrected and abnormal coagulation (e.g. extended prothrombin time) is rectified. In the immediate pre-operative period, renal function is assessed and adequate hydration is ensured by establishing an intravenous infusion on the day before surgery. A urinary catheter is inserted once the patient has been anaesthetised, and hourly urine output is monitored thereafter.

Prevention rather than belated recognition of the hepatorenal syndrome is the key to success when undertaking such major operations in jaundiced patients. Antibiotics are given prophylactically to cover the operation (e.g. piperacillin 4 g i.v. at induction, repeated at 4 hours if needed). If the patient has frank cholangitis, a combination of cefotaxime, ampicillin and metronidazole may be appropriate although with endoscopic or percutaneous stenting it is now unusual to have to undertake major pancreaticobiliary surgery in the face of such sepsis. If resection is to be undertaken, 4 units of blood should be crossmatched and available.

Upon opening the abdomen, the liver is carefully inspected and palpated to detect any metastatic disease. Intraoperative ultrasonography is very useful in this context, but the increasing use of laparoscopy and laparoscopic ultrasonography should mean that very few patients are found at this late stage to have metastatic disease that precludes resection. The pancreatic tumour is then palpated and its mobility assessed. Resection is contraindicated if inspection of the inferior aspect of the transverse mesocolon reveals tumour invasion. The duodenum and head of pancreas are then mobilized as on page 441, and the tumour is palpated bimanually. Careful inspection will reveal whether the superior mesenteric vein is involved by unresectable cancer. Any suspiciously enlarged or hard lymph nodes may be sent for frozen section examination and transduodenal Trucut biopsy can be used to establish the nature of the pancreatic mass if this is still uncertain.

If the tumour is still considered to be resectable, mobilization of the second and third parts of the duodenum continues until the superior mesenteric vein comes into view as it crosses the duodenum. The greater curvature of the stomach is then mobilized, commencing at the junction of the body and antrum and moving distally, ligating and dividing vessels in the gastrocolic omentum. The right gastro-epiploic vein is dissected meticulously and divided between ligatures just before its termination in the superior mesenteric vein below the neck of the pancreas. This last step should give access to the tunnel which runs between the front of the portal vein and the back of the neck of the pancreas. At this stage, all tributaries passing from the head of pancreas and uncinate process to the superior mesenteric vein are divided between ligatures; even the tiniest veins may give rise to massive bleeding if torn from the portal vein by careless handling.

The right gastric artery is next divided between ligatures as it runs on to the lesser curve of the stomach and the descending branches of the left gastric vessels are divided between ligatures at the gastric incisura. A linear stapling device is used to transect the stomach at the junction of body and antrum. The distal stomach is now swung over to the right, giving access to the gastroduodenal artery which is divided between ligatures as it leaves the genu of the common hepatic artery to pass down to the front of the pancreas.

Attention is now turned to the biliary tree. The gallbladder is dissected from its bed and the cystic artery is divided between ligatures. The cystic duct may also be divided at this stage or left attached. The common bile duct and lower common hepatic duct are mobilized and the duct is divided just above the entry of the cystic duct. Continued spillage of bile is prevented by applying a Bulldog clamp. The portal vein is now exposed and the continuity of the dissection plane behind the neck of the pancreas is established by gently passing a pair of forceps into the tunnel previously entered below the neck of the pancreas. Undue emphasis is often placed on this manoeuvre as an 'early' step in establishing resectability. This is not an 'early' step in the operation, and even if there is no fixation between the portal vein and back of the neck of the pancreas, fixation may yet become apparent more posteriorly in the last stages of the resection.

The proximal jejunum is now mobilized by division of its feeding blood vessels between ligatures. The ligament of Treitz is incised to free the duodenojejunal flexure and the proximal jejunum is divided using a linear stapler. This allows the fourth part of the duodenum to be brought behind the superior mesenteric vessels and into the main dissection field on the right side of the abdomen. The neck of the pancreas is now divided with a knife taking care to protect the portal vein behind. This step is made easier by inserting stay sutures into the upper and lower aspects of the neck of the pancreas. Bleeding from the cut pancreas may still be troublesome. Individual bleeding points in the distal pancreas are oversewn but bleeding from the resection specimen is best controlled by prior application of a vascular clamp such as a Satinsky clamp if this is feasible.

The pancreas is now left attached by remaining venous tributaries, the inferior pancreatico-duodenal vessels, and the surprisingly thick band of fibroareolar tissue which is still present posteriorly. Remaining venous tributaries are carefully displayed, ligated and divided, and the remaining fibrous attachments are best dealt with by clamping small bridges of tissue within sets of artery forceps in much the same way that a thyroidectomy is performed. The portal and superior mesenteric veins are obvious throughout these last stages and should not be in jeopardy. What is less often appreciated is that excessive retraction of the specimen to the right may bring the superior mesenteric artery into danger by pulling it into the operating field behind the superior mesenteric vein. Once the specimen has been removed, meticulous haemostasis is obtained.

Reconstruction commences with pancreaticojejunostomy. The cut end of the pancreas is freed for a few centimetres from the portal and splenic veins so that sutures can be inserted into the back of the pancreas under direct vision. Many variants are possible but this author uses one layer of interrupted delayed absorbable suture (PDS) to create an unstented end-to-side anastomosis between the cut end of the pancreas and the full thickness of the side of the upper jejunum. The pancreas is often friable and it is essential to take good bites of tissue. If the friability is such that there are major anxieties about anastomotic disruption, total pancreatectomy should be considered. However, total pancreatectomy leads inevitably to brittle diabetes and total loss of exocrine function and is not performed lightly. Some surgeons never attempt to create a pancreaticojejunostomy, preferring to oversew or staple the cut end of pancreas. There is little evidence that this manoeuvre reduces the incidence of leakage and pancreatic fistula formation, and it is not recommended.

The operation is completed by creating an end-to-side anastomosis (one layer of interrupted PDS) between the common hepatic duct and the jejunum just distal to the pancreaticojejunostomy, and by constructing a gastrojejunostomy to the more distal jejunum. Some surgeons stent the biliary-enteric anastomosis using a T-tube, a procedure which allows use of contrast radiology in the postoperative period to assess anastomotic integrity. Most surgeons place one or two suction tube drains in the operating field prior to closure of the abdomen.

It must be emphasised that a multitude of technical variations on the Whipple operation have been described. One of the more important variants is the pylorus-preserving operation in which the stomach remains intact and the upper resection margin passes through the first part of the duodenum.

Palliation of pancreatic cancer
Jaundice and pruritis can usually be relieved by nonsurgical means in patients who because of age, infirmity or extent of disease are not candidates for resection. In most cases, a stent can be inserted endoscopically. If this fails a guide wire placed through the stricture using a percutaneous transhepatic route can be used by the endoscopist to get a stent up into the biliary tree, the so called 'rendezvous' technique. Alternatively, the endoprosthesis can be inserted from above using a percutaneous transhepatic approach. Insertion of such stents is not without complications (pancreatitis, bleeding, perforation) and reinsertion may be needed if the stent silts up and blocks as they tend to do after about 3 months. Duodenal obstruction also proves troublesome in 10–15% of patients. Despite these drawbacks, mean survival after stenting is no different from that following surgical palliation (about 4 months), and the patient is spared the discomfort and risks of operation.

Surgical by-pass may be indicated when resection

proves not to be feasible at operation, when there is duodenal obstruction, and when the patient is relatively young and fit. Cholecystojejunostomy and gastrojejunostomy was once the standard operation under these circumstances but removal of the gall-bladder and construction of a Roux-en-Y hepaticojejunostomy provides more effective long term relief of jaundice. Cholecystojejunostomy must certainly be avoided when there is low entry of the cystic duct into the common bile duct, a situation which predisposes to early blockage by tumour and the return of jaundice. Opinions vary as to whether gastrojejunostomy should be performed prophylactically in patients who do not have frank duodenal obstruction at the time of operation. This author recommends gastrojejunostomy, while at the same time recognising the cruel paradox that those patients who need gastrojejunostomy most, often appear to benefit from it least.

PANCREATIC TRAUMA

Pancreatic trauma may result from penetrating or non-penetrating injury, and may occasionally result from surgery (e.g. splenectomy, difficult gastrectomy).

In patients with abdominal injury, hyperamylasaemia should alert the surgeon to the possibility of pancreatic damage and provide an indication for laparotomy in its own right. Similarly, the presence of a high amylase concentration in the return fluid following lavage is an indication for surgical exploration. At laparotomy, the presence of a retroperitoneal haematoma or significant bruising in the root of the transverse mesocolon, means that full exposure of the pancreas and duodenum is mandatory (p. 441). Much depends on whether the gland is simply contused or whether there has been disruption of major elements of the pancreatic duct system. Mild contusion is dealt with by drainage alone. Severe contusion of the body and tail of the gland with injury to the main pancreatic duct is best dealt with by distal pancreatectomy, oversewing the cut end of the pancreas. Similarly, transection of the pancreas by blunt compression against the lumbar spine is treated by distal resection. Trauma to the head of pancreas is much more difficult to deal with; if there has been major injury to both pancreas and duodenum, a Whipple resection may be advisable. Regardless of the nature of pancreatic surgery following trauma, adequate post-operative drainage must be provided and broad spectrum antibiotics are prescribed.

REFERENCES

Beger H G 1989 In: Carter D C, Warshaw A L (eds) Pancreatitis. Churchill Livingstone, Edinburgh pp 107–119

Berci G 1988 Choledochoscopy. In: Blumgart L H (ed) Surgery of the liver and biliary tract. Churchill Livingstone, Edinburgh, ch. 29

Bismith H, Franco D, Coriette M B, Hepp J 1978 Long term results of Roux-en-Y hepaticojejunostomy. Surgery Gynaecology and Obstetrics 146: 161

Blamey S L, Imrie C W, O'Neill J, Gilmour W H, Carter D C 1984 Prognostic factors in acute pancreatitis. Gut 25: 1340–1346

Blumgart L H 1988 In: Surgery of the liver and biliary tract. Churchill Livingstone, Edinburgh, pp 905–909

Burhenne H J 1988 In: Blumgart L H (ed) Surgery of the liver and biliary tract. Churchill Livingstone, Edinburgh, pp 605–610

Carter A E 1983 The transduodenal peri-ampullary approach to common bile duct calculi. Annals of the Royal College of Surgeons of England 65: 183–184

Carter D C 1989 In: Carter D C, Warshaw A L (eds) Pancreatitis. Churchill Livingstone, Edinburgh, pp 58–70

Espiner 1982 Emergency cholecystectomy: towards guaranteed safety. In: Wilson E H, Marsden A K (eds) Care of the acutely ill and injured. John Wiley, New York, p 385

Fox J N, Gunn A 1984 Common bile duct exploration by a balloon catheter technique. Journal of the Royal College of Surgeons of Edinburgh 29: 81–84

Hoffman J, Lorentzen M 1985 Drainage after cholecystectomy. British Journal of Surgery 72: 423–427

Howard E R 1983 Extrahepatic biliary atresia: a review of current management. British Journal of Surgery 70: 193–197

Kasai I M, Susuki S 1959 A new operation for 'noncorrectable' biliary atresia; hepatic porto-enterostomy. Shujutsu 13: 733

Mayer A D, McMahon M D, Corfield et al 1985 A randomised trial of peritoneal lavage for the treatment of severe acute pancreatitis. New England Journal of Medicine 312: 369–372

Muir B, Rimmer S, Redhead D N, Buist T A S, Best J K 1983 The radiological assessment of the obstructed biliary tree. Journal of the Royal College of Surgeons of Edinburgh 28: 233–239

Neoptolemos J P, Carr-Locke D L, London N J et al 1988 Controlled trial of urgent endoscopic retrograde cholangiopancreatography and endoscopic sphincterotomy versus conservative treatment for acute pancreatitis due to gallstones. Lancet 2: 979–983

Osborne D H, Imrie C W, Carter D C 1981 Biliary surgery in the same admission for acute pancreatitis. British Journal of Surgery 68: 758–761

Ranson J H C, Rifkind K M, Roses D F, Fink S D, Eng K, Spencer F C 1974 Prognostic signs and the role of operative management in acute pancreatitis. Surgery Gynaecology and Obstetrics 139: 69–81

Smith R 1980 In: Maingot R (ed) Abdominal operations, 7th edn. Appleton-Century-Crofts, New York, p 1251

Tagge D U, Tagge E P, Drongowski R A, Oldham K T, Coran A G 1991 A long-term experience with biliary atresia: reassessment of prognostic factors. Annals of Surgery 214: 590–598

Whipple A O 1946 Observations on radical surgery for lesions of the pancreas. Surgery Gynaecology and Obstetrics 32: 623

21

Operations on the appendix

R. F. RINTOUL

Anatomy (Fig. 21.1)
The appendix is normally 8–10 cm long and 6–8 mm in diameter, but great variations occur. Its wall has the same coats as the large gut, but contains numerous aggregations of lymphoid tissue. It is attached at its base to the posteromedial aspect of the caecum just below the ileocaecal junction. The three taeniae coli of the caecum converge to end at this point and are used as a guide to the appendix. The surface marking of the base of the appendix is usually said to be at *McBurney's point* — at the junction of the lateral and middle thirds of the line joining the anterior superior spine and the umbilicus — but it is commonly more inferiorly and medially.

In most cases the appendix has a complete peritoneal covering, with a well-formed mesentery, the *meso-appendix,* derived from the posterior layer of the mesentery of the lower end of the ileum. The artery of the appendix, a terminal branch of the ileocolic, runs along the free edge of the mesentery, giving off two or three branches during its course. The mesentery may extend to the tip of the appendix or may terminate about its middle. An additional fold of peritoneum, usually avascular (the inferior ileocaecal or 'bloodless' fold of

Treves), may be present, extending from the proximal part of the appendix to the front of the terminal inch of the ileum.

Different positions of the appendix (Fig. 21.2)
The base of the appendix is variable in position, since the caecum enjoys a certain amount of mobility. The rest of the appendix is freely movable, and may occupy one of several positions: (1) it may curl round the lower pole of the caecum and pass upwards on its lateral side — *paracolic position* (3%); (2) it may pass upwards behind the caecum — *retrocaecal position* (70%); (3) it may extend more or less transversely to the left, passing either in front of or behind the terminal part of the ileum (2%); (4) it may hang downwards into the pelvis — *pelvic position* (25%). The retrocaecal and pelvic positions are the commonest. In the former the greater part of the appendix may be embedded within the serous coat of the posterior caecal wall, or, if this part is not covered with peritoneum, it may lie in the retro-peritoneal tissues. In acute appendicitis with local peritoneal irritation, the site of maximal tenderness gives some indication of the position of the appendix. In rare cases the caecum (through developmental arrest of its descent) is absent from the right iliac fossa, and

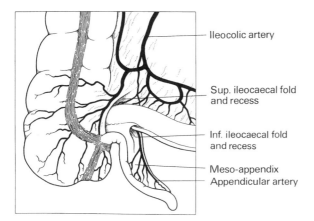

Fig. 21.1 Anatomy of the appendix and ileocaecal region (After Grant)

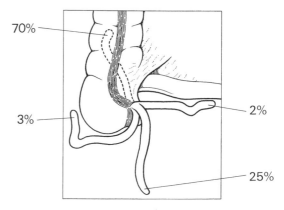

Fig. 21.2 The more common positions for the appendix and the relative frequency with which they are found

together with the appendix it must then be sought high up below the right lobe of the liver.

INDICATIONS FOR APPENDICECTOMY

Acute appendicitis

In most cases of acute appendicitis which are seen in the early stages of the attack, operation should be carried out without delay. The pathological process may be either catarrhal appendicitis or obstructive appendicitis but the history and clinical examination are little more than pointers to the diagnosis of either type. It is possible for catarrhal appendicitis to settle but operation should as a rule be advised in all cases since there is an invariable tendency towards recurrence. An exception may be made in those cases where the attack is obviously passing off, and where, for various reasons, it may be desirable to postpone operation until a more convenient time. Appendicitis during pregnancy should be treated on its own merits since the risk of appendicectomy during pregnancy is less than the risk of peritonitis — both to the pregnancy and to the patient herself — should the appendicitis fail to settle with conservative treatment.

The availability of suitable antibiotics has made a major impact on the management of acute appendicitis and, in particular, in the treatment of peritonitis and of late cases. Provided that antibiotics *are available,* all stages of appendicitis can be treated in the same manner, even including an appendix mass.

However, in hospitals where the supply of antibiotics *is limited,* some degree of caution must be exercised where the patient is not seen until 48–72 hours after the onset of symptoms. *Provided that there are no signs suggestive of general peritonitis,* it is probable either that the attack is passing off or that the infection is being successfully localized. The second alternative requires special consideration, for it constitutes a contraindication to immediate operation. Definite evidence of localization is obtained from the palpation of a tender mass in the right iliac fossa — a mass formed by the matting together of omentum and bowel around the inflamed appendix. As long as the infection remains localized there is little danger, whereas any attempt to remove the appendix entails the breaking down of protective adhesions, with the risk of spreading the infection to the general peritoneal cavity. The initial treatment of such a *localizing* appendicitis is conservative, and is described on page 457.

In children and in the elderly early operation should be advised since there are special dangers of delay. In children the appendix is thin-walled, and what appears to be a mild catarrhal inflammation may proceed rapidly to gangrene and perforation. Both in childhood and in old age there is less tendency to localisation, and the risks of general peritonitis are considerable. Unless, therefore, a definite mass is palpable, operation should not be delayed.

Recurrent or chronic appendicitis

In the absence of any acute attack, chronic appendicitis may be diagnosed from the existence of a 'grumbling' pain in the right iliac fossa. In addition there may be general malaise or various digestive symptoms — the so-called *appendix dyspepsia* (Kerr, 1962). Once the appendix has become inflamed, further attacks at gradually shortening intervals are to be expected although, in the elderly, the appendix may be replaced by fibrosis. Appendicectomy during the quiescent stage is attended by the minimum of risk and discomfort to the patient, and should not be delayed until a subsequent attack develops. It is usually curative.

Carcinoma of appendix

In a very small proportion of cases a tumour of the appendix is found. Appendicectomy is satisfactory in the treatment of an adenocarcinoma which is confined to the mucosa but its diagnosis depends on routine histology of all appendices. Right hemicolectomy may be advisable if the base of the appendix is involved but is not necessarily curative (Evans, 1990).

Carcinoid tumour of the appendix

The appendix is the most common site for gastrointestinal carcinoid tumour. A small tumour of the distal appendix is adequately removed by appendicectomy but, if histological examination shows involvement of the base of the appendix, right hemicolectomy is advisable (Parkes, 1993).

EMERGENCY APPENDICECTOMY

Incision

A right gridiron or *Lanz* incision is commonly employed, centred over the site of maximal tenderness. Some surgeons prefer a midline incision to provide wider access for exploration and peritoneal lavage if there is doubt about the diagnosis. However, the majority, preferring to act upon a preoperative diagnosis of appendicitis, make an incision in the right iliac fossa and examine only the organs that lie in the vicinity of the appendix. In most cases, access through the smaller incision is adequate and allows the patient to make a rapid recovery.

In a small proportion of cases, however, difficulty is encountered and the incision is then enlarged. An alternative approach is the muscle-cutting iliac incision (Rutherford Morison). This is, in fact, the incision which results when a gridiron is enlarged, the internal oblique and transversus muscles being divided in line with the fibres of the external oblique. The advantages of this incision are those of wide access, and the fact that a more direct approach is obtained in cases where the appendix is retrocaecal in position.

Technique

As soon as the peritoneum has been opened there may be an escape of exudate. Unless this is frankly purulent or malodorous it does not indicate that general peritonitis is present. More often the fluid is the result of peritoneal reaction to the local inflammation; it is then odourless, clear or slightly turbid, and is usually sterile. A sample is collected for bacteriological examination and all exudate in the neighbourhood of the wound is removed by gentle swabbing or by the use of suction.

The caecum is identified and is very gently withdrawn towards the wound. It is easily distinguished from small bowel by the presence of taeniae coli. Occasionally in visceroptotic cases the transverse colon is withdrawn in mistake for the caecum, but it should be recognized at once from the fact that it has omentum attached to it. The caecum is grasped in a moist pack by the left hand and is gently withdrawn towards the lower end of the wound, when the appendix should follow it into the wound. If the appendix does *not* come into view, it is located by a finger passed along one of the taeniae coli towards the point where the taeniae meet at the appendix base. The appendix is then felt as a tense resistant cord, lying in most cases lateral to or behind the caecum. The appendix is delivered partly by traction on the caecum, and partly by gentle pressure exerted by a finger below it. If the appendix is adherent, no force must be used to 'hook' it out of the wound but the right index finger may be passed along it towards its tip, any filmy adhesions being gently disrupted. If dense adhesions are present these should be separated or divided under the guidance of the eye, and with the assistance of suitable retractor. Sometimes, as the result of previous inflammation, the appendix is sharply kinked and is bound in the right iliac fossa or to the brim of the pelvis. Such bands can be divided with safety and without risk of causing haemorrhage if the knife is kept to the lateral side of the appendix.

Wherever difficulty is encountered, especially when the appendix occupies the retrocaecal position, it may be necessary to enlarge the wound, to pack off the rest of the peritoneal cavity, and to free the appendix under direct vision. Omentum which is firmly wrapped round the appendix may be separated or ligatured and divided a short distance away, the adherent part being removed along with the appendix. A retrocaecal appendix may lie free behind the caecum or it may be bound down to the posterior wall of the gut. Often the distal part is extraperitoneal, in which case it may be completely buried behind the caecum. The incision should then be enlarged upwards and laterally so that the caecum can be turned over and the appendix dissected out under direct vision.

The part of the caecum to which the appendix is attached is retained outside the wound, while the remainder is returned to the peritoneal cavity. The appendix is raised up and is held taut by a pair of Babcock's forceps applied near its tip (Fig. 21.3). The mesentery is clamped with one or more pairs of artery forceps, and is divided and ligatured. If the meso-appendix is short and oedematous it may be necessary to clamp and divide it within the peritoneal cavity. In such cases care must be taken that the stump of the mesoappendix does not slip out of the forceps while it is being tied-off, and it is an advantage to employ a transfixing ligature. When the inflammatory process has extended into the meso-appendix, this structure should be clamped and divided as far away as possible from the appendix.

A forceps is momentarily applied to the base of the appendix exactly at the point of its junction with the caecum, and a ligature is tied around the crushed area. It assists in the subsequent control of the stump if the ends of this ligature are kept long and are retained in forceps. A purse-string Lembert suture is inserted in the caecal wall around the base of the appendix (Fig. 21.4). Forceps are then applied to the appendix 5 or 6 mm distal to the ligature, the intervening lumen having been emptied by pressure of the blades. A swab is placed underneath to absorb any escaping contents, and the appendix is divided close to the forceps (Fig. 21.5). The stump ligature is cut short and the stump is invaginated with slender forceps while the purse-string suture is tightened (Fig. 21.6). The appendix, together with the knife, swab and forceps, which have been contaminated by contact with the mucosa, are placed in a bowl and are removed from the field of operation. Sometimes the proximal end of the appendix is buried by inflammatory swelling of the caecal wall, and care should then be taken that the entire organ is removed. When the caecal wall is friable or oedematous it is wiser not to attempt to bury the appendix. In fact, many surgeons leave the appendix stump unburied in all cases (Engstrom, 1985), but this must be accompanied by the appropriate antibiotic lavage.

Before the abdomen is closed the ligatured meso-appendix is re-examined for bleeding. In all cases where there has been peritonitis, the involved areas are thoroughly irrigated with tetracycline 0.1% solution (pagee 365). The wound is also cleaned with the solution. When the returned fluid looks clear, it is unnecessary to leave a drain either in the peritoneal cavity or

Figs 21.3–21.6 *Technique of appendicectomy*

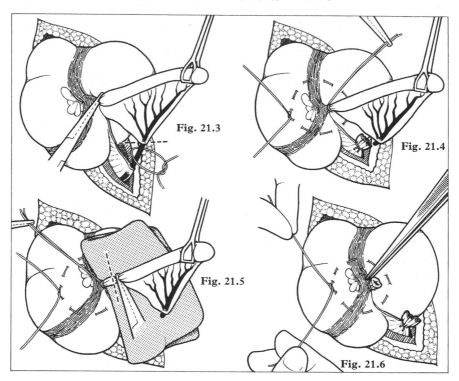

Fig. 21.3

Fig. 21.4

Fig. 21.5

Fig. 21.6

Fig. 21.3 Meso-appendix clamped and divided; base of appendix crushed with forceps

Fig. 21.4 Meso-appendix tied off; appendix ligatured at base; purse-string suture inserted

Fig. 21.5 Appendix clamped distal to ligature and about to be divided against swab

Fig. 21.6 Appendix stump about to be invaginated before tightening of purse-string suture

wound (Krukowski, 1988, 1990). The operation is completed by suture of the wound in layers.

Retrograde removal of the appendix

Frequently the base of the appendix is more accessible than the tip. This is especially likely to occur when the appendix occupies the retrocaecal position — when its inflamed distal end may be adherent to the posterior wall of the caecum, or may even be buried within the serous coat. In such cases the retrograde method of removal may often simplify the operation. Two pairs of artery forceps are insinuated through the meso-appendix and are applied to the base of the appendix 5-6 mm apart. The proximal forceps is removed and the appendix is ligatured in the groove that has been crushed. It is then divided close to the distal forceps and the proximal stump is either invaginated or not, depending on the circumstances (see above). The appendix, with its cut end still occluded by the forceps, is now freed by careful dissection, and by successive clamping and cutting of its mesentery from base to tip it is removed (Fig. 21.7). The mesentery is then ligated.

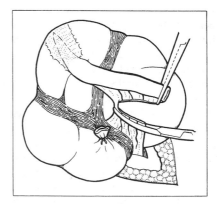

Fig. 21.7 Retrograde appendicectomy — a method to be considered when the base of the appendix is more accessible than the tip

ANTIBIOTICS IN APPENDICITIS

Bacterial contamination of the peritoneal cavity from a perforated appendix or from an acutely inflamed appendix is due to the synergistic effect of *E. coli* and

Bacteroides. The removal of an apparently normal appendix frequently results in wound infection with these organisms, hence the need for antibiotics in all patients undergoing appendicectomy. These should include a broad spectrum antibiotic such as Gentamicin or a Cephalosporin to deal with the gram negative organisms *and* Metronidazole which is particularly active against the Gram positive Bacteroides. Dosage depends on the anticipated contamination, varying from a single preoperative dose of metronidazole to therapeutic dosage of two antibiotics for several days. The routine use of peritoneal lavage with 0.1% tetracycline solution, where there has been peritonitis, plays an important part in the control of infection — see page 365 (Stewart, 1980).

General peritonitis

This is most likely to occur when the perforation is near the base of the appendix, for this part is not so readily shut-off by adhesions. It may appear also as a later complication, when a collection of pus, which is at first localized, overflows into the general peritoneal cavity.

When peritonitis due to appendicitis is diagnosed clinically it is advisable that operation should be delayed for an hour or two, in order to give treatment which will improve the patient's general condition. Such preoperative treatment consists in the institution of continuous intravenous infusion, nasogastric suction and antibiotic therapy. Delay in diagnosis without deterioration in the patient's general condition may persuade the surgeon to continue with conservative treatment but it is wiser to explore the abdomen for drainage, antibiotic lavage and appendicectomy.

At operation the diagnosis is apparent as soon as the abdomen has been opened, from the presence of frankly purulent or dark-coloured fluid — usually with the putrid smell of bowel organisms. The existence of general peritonitis — unlike that of localized peritonitis or abscess — demands that every effort should be made to remove the appendix. Simple drainage alone will not suffice, for, since the perforation is not effectively sealed-off, further contamination is usually inevitable. Appendicectomy should be carried out as expeditiously as possible, care being taken to ensure removal of the faecalith which has caused the perforation. All pus is evacuated and the peritoneum is thoroughly washed out with tetracycline solution.

POSTOPERATIVE COMPLICATIONS

Such complications as may occur after any abdominal operation have already been discussed (pp.349–352). Those which are associated more specifically with appendicectomy may be mentioned briefly here.

Pelvic abscess

This should be suspected if fever or tachycardia persist, and cannot be ascribed to wound infection, or to a pulmonary condition. The diagnosis may be confirmed by rectal examination, when a boggy and tender mass can be detected anteriorly. Where facilities exist for ultrasound scanning, a pelvic abscess may be confirmed by this examination and aspiration carried out under ultrasound guidance. Most pelvic abscesses, however, resolve under conservative treatment, the pus being absorbed, or they burst spontaneously into the rectum. Deliberate evacuation per rectum is very seldom required, and should be reserved for cases where the abscess is soft and bulging into the rectal wall (Fig. 21.8). This is done by penetrating the rectal wall with a long haemostat — if possible under direct vision, as can be obtained by the use of a vaginal speculum placed within the anal canal.

Subphrenic abscess and paralytic ileus

The treatment of these conditions is discussed on pages 412 and 462.

ACUTE APPENDICITIS WITH PERFORATION (LIMITED ANTIBIOTICS)

The management of the more complicated cases of appendicitis depend on the availability of antibiotics and alternative procedures are required in circumstances *where the supply of antibiotics is limited.*

Localized peritonitis or abscess

When abscess formation is diagnosed clinically, operation may be contra-indicated (p. 457). Frequently, however, an abscess is discovered only at operation from the presence of a mass of inflammatory adhesions around the appendix. It is probable in such cases that the appendix has perforated, and that pus is enclosed within the mass. The most essential aim of the operation is now to avoid spreading the infection to the general peritoneal cavity. The incision is enlarged if necessary, its medial side is lifted forwards with a retractor, and the mass is carefully surrounded with hot moist packs. Retractors are inserted, and under direct vision the mass is gently explored with the finger in an attempt to identify the appendix. If pus is encountered, it is immediately swabbed away. In the majority of cases the appendix is isolated without great difficulty and is removed in the usual way, but all manipulation should be reduced to a minimum. When the caecum is fixed by inflammatory adhesions the appendicectomy may require to be carried out in the depths of the wound and invagination of the stump should then be omitted. Before the packs are removed the appendix

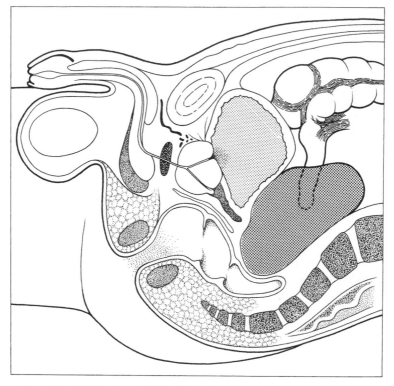

Fig. 21.8   Pelvic abscess bulging into the rectum (After Hamilton Bailey)

area and wound may be irrigated with 0.1% Tetracycline or alternative antibiotic solution. Sometimes the appendix is found to have become divided into two parts at the site of perforation; care must then be taken that the entire organ is removed. A faecalith which has escaped through the perforation may be found lying loose in the abscess cavity. It is essential that it is removed.

Drainage

The wound is closed around a drain which extends down to the infected area and into the pelvis. Either a tube or a corrugated plastic drain may be employed. When the appendix has been retrocaecal in position, it reduces the risk of peritoneal contamination if the drain is brought out as far laterally as possible, through the upper angle of the wound. Whatever type of drain is used, the wound should never be closed tightly around it, for it is essential that there should be free egress for infected exudate. This is particularly important when a tube drain is used; there must be room for exudate to escape, not only through its lumen, but also alongside it.

When a large abscess is present or when the appendix is found to be surrounded by friable inflammatory tissues which bleed readily to the touch, appendicectomy entails the risk of inflicting serious trauma or of spreading the infection. In such cases *it is wiser to be content with simple drainage alone.* Appendicectomy can

be carried out with comparative safety at a later date (p. 458).

Drainage following general peritonitis

Whenever possible the appendix is removed, as already described, since further contamination will otherwise continue. If limited antibiotics are available, thorough peritoneal irrigation is carried out with saline until the returning fluid is clear. It is best to drain the pelvis by means of a tube brought out through a stab wound above the symphysis pubis — and here *suction drainage* (p. 345) has special advantages. Additional drainage of the appendix area through the main wound is usually advisable; if this is omitted, the wound at least should be drained or loosely sutured, so that there is ample space for inflammatory products to escape to the surface. Even in a grossly infected wound delayed primary wound closure is contraindicated (Pettigrew, 1981).

The suprapubic drain is usually removed after 48 hours, by which time it will have ceased to function; a local drain is shortened gradually as the discharge diminishes.

APPENDIX ABSCESS OR MASS (LIMITED ANTIBIOTICS)

The term 'appendix abscess' is applied in a wide sense

to include any type of localizing appendicitis where a definite mass has formed in the region of the appendix. This finding is most likely to be present in patients who come to examination 48 hours or longer after the onset of symptoms. The mass is formed by the matting together of omentum and bowel round the inflamed appendix. Unless the mass is situated in the pelvis it can usually be detected on abdominal palpation.

In most cases the appendix has perforated, and a collection of pus is enclosed within the mass of adhesions. If perforation has not occurred the term 'abscess' is strictly incorrect — the condition is rather one of localized plastic peritonitis. In either case the presence of a mass is an indication that the infection is adequately circumscribed and walled-off from the general peritoneal cavity. The initial treatment in such cases should always be conservative, since removal of the appendix entails the risk of damaging the inflamed and friable bowel in the vicinity, and of spreading infection to the general peritoneal cavity. The mortality of cases treated conservatively — with limited antibiotics — is much lower than that of cases subjected to immediate operation.

Conservative treatment

This, as first described by Ochsner and Sherren, is advised for all cases of acute appendicitis where operation, for one reason or another, is withheld. It may be employed, therefore, both in the early case when conditions are unfavourable for operation, and in the late case where it is believed that the infection is being successfully localized.

The details of the method may be summarised as follows:

1. The patient is nursed propped-up, in order to encourage any peritoneal exudate to gravitate towards the pelvis.

2. Available antibiotic therapy is given if there are signs of toxicity.

3. For the first 24–48 hours nothing is administered by mouth, except sips of water or ice. An adequate fluid intake is maintained by intravenous infusion, and nasogastric suction is installed. After 24–48 hours, provided that all symptoms are subsiding and bowel sounds are present, fluid diet is commenced and is gradually supplemented. Solid food is withheld until pulse rate and temperature have returned to normal.

4. A careful record is kept of the pulse rate and temperature. The pulse rate is much the more important; at the commencement of treatment it should be recorded at hourly intervals.

5. Strong analgesics should be avoided if possible, since they may mask symptoms which demand operation.

6. Too frequent examination of the abdomen is avoided, but it is helpful to outline the mass on the patient's abdominal wall so as to compare one examination with the next.

7. Suppositories are administered after the third day.

The majority of cases react favourably to this treatment. The pulse rate and temperature fall and pain is relieved. The lump becomes less tender, shrinks steadily in size and ultimately disappears. Any pus which is present is absorbed. It is essential, however, that the treatment should be carried out under the care of the surgeon who has accepted responsibility for the case, for at any moment it may require to be abandoned in favour of operation. When the method is employed in children or in the elderly, particularly careful supervision is essential.

Indications for operation

Unless all symptoms subside, and there is a steady improvement in the patient's general condition, operation should be considered. *The most dangerous sign is a rising pulse rate* — hence the necessity for frequent recording in the early stages of treatment. If this sign is present, operation should be carried out without delay. A pulse rate which remains high (e.g. above 95 or 100) is also an indication for operation, but is not a matter of such urgency. A raised temperature is of less importance in the early stages, provided that the pulse rate is steady or falling, but a persistently high or swinging temperature indicates that operation will be required. Continued pain, vomiting or diarrhoea usually demands that conservative treatment should be abandoned. If there is spreading tenderness or resistance — signs which suggest an incipient general peritonitis — immediate operation should be undertaken.

In a proportion of cases the abscess, although remaining successfully localized, shows no sign of shrinking. Operation will then be required, but it may with advantage be deferred until the abscess, as shown by a dull note on percussion, has come into contact with the abdominal wall (Fig. 21.9) for it can then be approached extraperitoneally. The operation should consist of simple drainage alone, no attempt being made to remove the appendix.

Technique of simple drainage

The best approach is by a small muscle-cutting iliac incision, made just to the lateral side of the summit of the mass. All muscle layers are divided in the line of the skin incision (p. 341). The peritoneum, which is usually thickened and oedematous, is incised with care since it may be adherent to the underlying mass. Its medial leaf is held forwards with a retractor, and a gauze pack is inserted below it. The mass is then gently explored with a finger directed laterally and backwards.

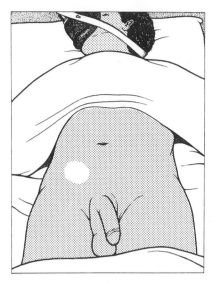

Fig. 21.9   Appendix abscess in contact with the abdominal wall

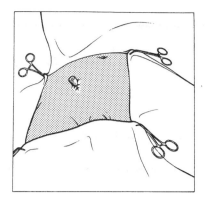

Fig. 21.10   Abscess drained through small incision; drainage tube in situ

The abscess cavity is usually located without difficulty, and a varying quantity of malodorous pus escapes. Adhesions which form loculi within the cavity are very gently broken down with the finger. A soft tube or corrugated drain is inserted into the cavity and the wound is loosely closed around it. *When the abscess is in contact with the abdominal wall,* drainage is a very simple procedure and can be carried out under local anaesthesia. A 3–4 cm incision is made directly over the mass; pus is located with sinus forceps or with the finger, and while it is still flowing, a tube is introduced into the abscess cavity (Fig. 21.10).

Subsequent appendicectomy

The patient must be impressed with the necessity of having his appendix removed at a future date. The operation should be postponed, however, until all inflammatory reaction has subsided unless symptoms recur.

When the abscess has resolved under conservative treatment alone, appendicectomy is performed about 2–3 months later. Where simple drainage has been carried out a period of 3–6 months should be allowed to elapse. There is then usually a remarkable absence of adhesions. The appendix may be reduced to an attenuated cord; sometimes it looks surprisingly normal. In the elderly it may have been destroyed by the inflammatory process so that it is not always essential to persuade such a patient to undergo elective appendicectomy.

REFERENCES

Engstrom L, Fenyo G 1985 Appendicectomy: assessment of stump invagination versus simple ligation: a prospective, randomised trial. British Journal of Surgery 72: 971–972

Evans D A, Hamid B N A, Hoare E M 1990 Primary adenocarcinoma of the appendix. Journal of the Royal College of Surgeons of Edinburgh 35: 33–35

Kerr J A 1962 Appendix dyspepsia. British Journal of Surgery 49: 437–442

Krukowski Z H, Irwin S T, Denholm S D, Matheson N A 1988 Preventing infection after appendicectomy: a review. British Journal of Surgery 75: 1023–1033

Krukowski Z H 1990 Appendicitis. Surgery 86: 2044–2048

Parkes S E, Muir K R, Al Sheyyab M, Cameron A H, Pincott J R, Raafat F, Mann J R 1993 Carcinoid tumours of the appendix in children 1957–1986: incidence, treatment and outcome. British Journal of Surgery 80: 502–504

Pettigrew R A 1981 Delayed primary wound closure in gangrenous and perforated appendicitis. British Journal of Surgery 68: 635–638

Stewart D J 1980 Generalised peritonitis. Journal of the Royal College of Surgeons of Edinburgh 25: 80–90

22

Operations on the intestines

D. C. C. BARTOLO, J. M. S. JOHNSTONE, I. B. MACLEOD & R. F. RINTOUL

Anatomy

The small intestine

This lies in coils which are found in all parts of the abdominal cavity below the liver and stomach, and which bear no fixed relationship to each other. The coils are covered to a varying extent by the greater omentum which hangs down in front of them. The *jejunum* begins at the duodenojejunal flexure at the left side of the body of the 2nd lumbar vertebra, and is about 2 m in length The *ileum*, which is 3 m to 4 m long, is continuous with the jejunum and ends in the right iliac fossa by joining the medial side of the caecum. The jejunum, which has a thicker and more vascular wall than the ileum, lies mainly to the left and above, but there is no definite line of demarcation between the two. The small intestine has a complete peritoneal covering, and, being attached by a long mesentery to the posterior abdominal wall, it is freely movable except at its two ends.

The *mesentery* contains between its two layers the blood vessels (*jejunal and ileal branches of the superior mesenteric*), the lymphatics and the nerves of the small intestine. Its roots or line of attachment to the posterior wall is no more than 15 cm long; it extends obliquely downwards and to the right from the duodenojejunal flexure. Distally the mesentery fans out to its attachment along the length of small gut.

The colon

This can be distinguished from small bowel by its sacculated structure, and by the presence of taeniae coli and appendices epiploicae. The *caecum* normally occupies the right iliac fossa; it is completely clothed with peritoneum, but has no mesentery so that it is relatively fixed in position. The *ascending colon* is bound down to the posterior wall, and is covered with peritoneum only on its front and sides. The *right colic (hepatic) flexure* lies on the right kidney immediately below the liver. The *transverse colon* is freely movable since it has a complete peritoneal investment with a mesentery — the *transverse meso-colon*. It is very variable in position, and may hang down nearly to the pelvis. It is easily recognized from the attachment of the greater omentum to its lower border. The *left colic (splenic) flexure* lies behind the stomach on the lateral border of the kidney and on the diaphragm to which it is attached by the phrenico colic ligament. The *descending colon*, like the ascending colon, is covered by peritoneum only on its front and sides, and is fixed in position. Both flexures have a partial peritoneal covering similar to that of the ascending and descending colons; they are the most fixed parts of the large bowel. The *pelvic colon* hangs down as a loop in the pelvis, and forms a reservoir where solid faeces accumulate. Its extremities lie fairly close together — hence its liability to volvulus. It begins at the brim of the pelvis, and ends opposite the middle of the sacrum by becoming the rectum. It is relatively mobile having a complete peritoneal investment and a mesentery — the *pelvic meso-colon*.

Arteries of the colon

The caecum and ascending colon together with the terminal few centimetres of the ileum, are supplied by the *ileocolic* and *right colic* arteries, the transverse colon by the *middle colic* — all branches of the superior mesenteric. The descending and pelvic colons are supplied by the *upper* and *lower left colic (sigmoid)* arteries, from the inferior mesenteric. Between these arteries there is a free anastomosis by marginal vessels lying close to the bowel.

Lymphatic drainage of the colon (Fig. 22.1)

This is of great importance in regard to the spread of carcinoma (see also p. 477). Glands draining the colon fall into four main groups — *epicolic* glands lying on the surface of the bowel wall; *paracolic* glands between the layers of the meso-colon close alongside the bowel; *intermediate* glands along the branches of the mesenteric arteries; and *central* or *principal* glands around the main trunks of these vessels.

The lymphatic drainage from the different parts of the colon bears a direct relationship to the arterial blood supply. Thus, drainage from the right side of the

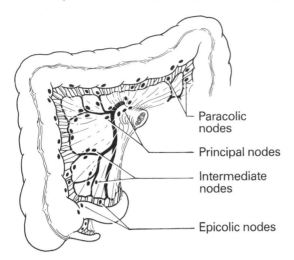

Fig. 22.1   Anatomy of the colonic lymphatic drainage

colon takes place to glands related to the entire course of the ileocolic and right colic arteries, and extending right up to the origin of these arteries from the superior mesenteric. The middle three-fifths of the transverse colon drains to glands around the middle colic artery. The splenic flexure, the descending colon and the pelvic colon, drain to glands around the branches and main trunk of the inferior mesentric artery.

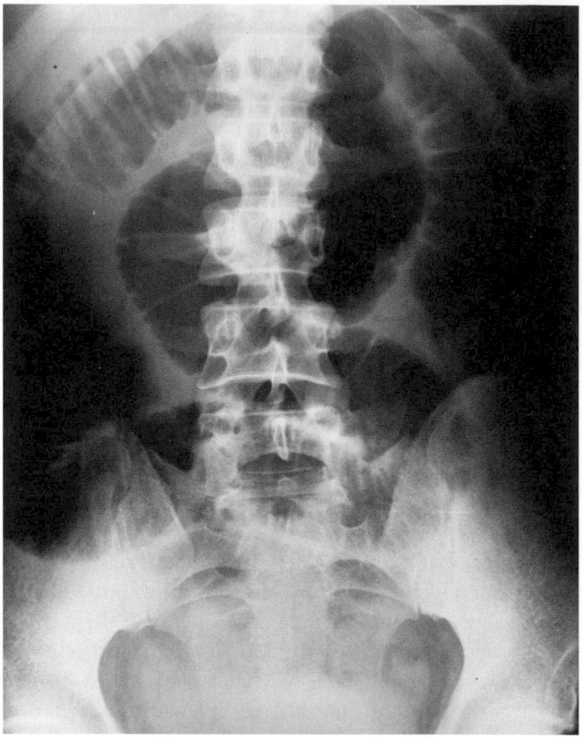

INTESTINAL OBSTRUCTION: GENERAL CONSIDERATIONS

Most cases of intestinal obstruction are mechanical in origin, and are due to occlusion of the lumen of the bowel, caused by changes in its wall or by compression or constriction from without. Strangulation of the bowel may complicate this type of obstruction, and adds greatly to the seriousness of the condition. Occasionally, usually in postoperative cases, there is no mechanical obstruction, and the stoppage is due entirely to paralysis of the bowel wall. The effects, however, are very similar.

Before any treatment, conservative or operative, can be planned, it is essential to assess (1) whether the obstruction is mechanical or paralytic; (2) its probable level, and (3) whether any element of strangulation is present. A decision on such points is reached by the taking of a detailed history and by careful examination of the patient, including inspection of the vomitus and material voided after an enema. Erect and supine plain abdominal X-rays are mandatory (Figs 22.2–22.5). In the healthy state the small and scattered collections of gas in the small bowel cast no definite radiological shadow; a variable quantity of gas is seen in the colon, but this is evacuated completely after an enema. When

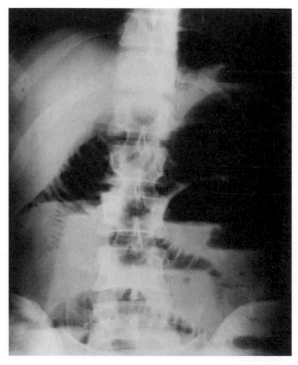

Fig. 22.2   Lower small bowel obstruction; supine X-ray film showing distended loops

Fig. 22.3   Erect film in the same case showing fluid levels

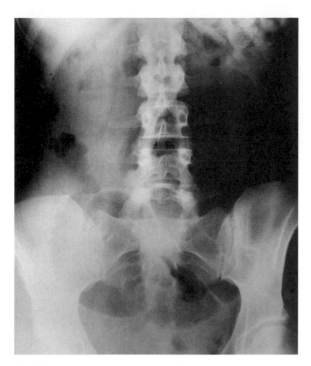

Fig. 22.4   An erect film showing distended caecum due to volvulus

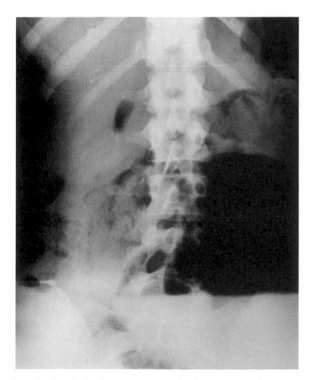

Fig. 22.5   Supine film of caecal volvulus with fluid levels

small bowel obstruction is present (unless at an unusually high level) gas-distended loops of bowel above the obstruction are shown lying transversely across the abdomen, and may contain fluid levels. In obstruction large collections of gas may be shown in the colon, both proximal and distal to the obstruction; the larger collection is usually proximal, and is not evacuated after an enema. If gas remains in any part of the colon after an enema colonic obstruction probably exists. In suspected large bowel obstruction, sigmoidoscopy should be undertaken. It may allow confirmation of the presence of carcinoma, and it may prove therapeutic, e.g. in some patients with volvulus of the sigmoid colon.

Mechanical obstruction

This includes simple occlusion and occlusion combined with strangulation. Except when the obstruction is at an unusually high level, it is characterized invariably by colicky pain as the bowel above the obstruction contracts in an attempt to overcome it. In some cases the nature of the obstruction can be determined or conjectured before operation. In others the diagnosis must await laparotomy. The obstructive lesions which give rise to typical diagnostic features are listed on Table 22.1.

Strangulation

This may complicate most of the common types of mechanical obstruction except carcinoma of the colon. Its existence should be suspected in the following conditions:

1. when an irreducible external hernia is tense and tender
2. when the pain is severe and comes in frequent spasms, or becomes constant and localized
3. when there is elevation of temperature and pulse rate
4. when tenderness or rigidity or *rebound tenderness* is present
5. when the white cell count is elevated
6. when a state of shock exists; this suggests that a large segment of bowel is involved, as in mesenteric occlusion. The effects of this last condition are in every way similar to those of strangulation, and it can be considered under the same heading
7. if pain persists for more than 2 hours after effective gastroduodenal suction has been installed.

Level of obstruction

This has considerable bearing on the indications for operation, and on the necessary preparation should operation be considered. The distinguishing features of obstruction at different levels are set out in Table 22.2.

Table 22.1   Differential diagnosis in intestinal obstruction

Intussusception in infancy	Occurs usually in a healthy child during the first year. Sudden onset of severe colicky pain, followed by passage of blood-stained stool. Elongated mass palpable in umbilical region; RIF 'empty'. Blood on finger after rectal examination
External hernia*	An irreducible swelling at any of the hernial orifices furnishes an obvious cause for obstruction. Examination for such should never be omitted
Adhesive obstruction**	This is at once suspected if there has been any previous abdominal operation — especially if for peritonitis
Gall-stone ileus	Usually in elderly women. Insidious colicky pain. Previous history may suggest gall-stones. X-ray shows distended small bowel and may show gas in the biliary tree. Diagnosis seldom make before laparotomy
Mesenteric vascular occlusion	Should be suspected if the obstruction is accompanied by a shock-like state of collapse — especially if patient suffers from degenerative vascular disease. Blood-stained stool may be passed
Carcinoma of the colon	By far the commonest cause of obstruction in older patients. Insidious in onset. Progressive constipation and distension. Growth may be palpable, or its site determined by radiography
Volvulus of the colon	Usually pelvic colon. Tense tympanitic swelling placed centrally in abdomen. A blood-stained stool may have been passed or an enema may be returned blood-stained. Radiograph shows extreme distension confined to a single loop of bowel, which is often ∩-shaped

* The commonest cause of small bowel obstruction in the Third World
** The commonest cause of small bowel obstruction in the Western World

Paralytic ileus

This condition results from paralysis of the intestinal musculature leading to cessation of peristalsis, progressive abdominal distension and profuse vomiting. Colicky abdominal pain is absent, though the patient may be uncomfortable from the distension, and on auscultation no bowel sounds are heard.

A short period of ileus, usually only a few hours, follows most intra-abdominal procedures. If the ileus persists for more than 48–72 hours it is regarded as 'refractory', and may be due to intra-abdominal sepsis,

to hypoxia or to electrolyte imbalance, particularly deficiencies of potassium, calcium or magnesium. Retroperitoneal trauma, either deliberate (as in renal or spinal surgery) or accidental, is frequently followed by ileus, and the mechanism may be reflex through the autonomic nervous system. A similar mechanism may account for the ileus seen in patients immobilized in a spinal plaster cast (The Cast Syndrome). Ileus is a frequent finding in circulatory shock of whatever cause and may be due to a combination of hypoxia and catecholamine overactivity.

Peritonitis, resulting from perforation of an intra-abdominal viscus or abscess produces an ileus due to paralysis of the plexus of Auerbach. A localized ileus is frequently seen in the vicinity of localized intra-abdominal inflammation (e.g. a dilated loop or loops of small bowel in the right iliac fossa in the abdominal X-ray of a patient with appendicitis) and this may occasionally be of sufficient degree to produce the clinical features of mechanical small bowel obstruction.

Intestinal pseudo-obstruction

The condition of acute colonic pseudo-obstruction was described by Ogilvie in 1948. It presents with clinical and radiological features of mechanical large bowel obstruction although no obstructing lesion exists. Radiologically, gas may be seen extending down to and including the rectum, but frequently there is a sharp 'cut off' of gas in the transverse or descending colon, making distinction from mechanical obstruction difficult. Inco-ordinated autonomic activity on the colon is thought to be responsible. Gross dilatation of the colon is common with risk of caecal perforation, so that a high index of suspicion is required. Some 90% of patients have serious extra-intestinal metabolic or systemic dysfunction. The condition may be chronic or recurrent in some cases and a familial form has been described.

Conservative or preoperative treatment

Certain forms of therapy now used as routine in the preoperative treatment of intestinal obstruction may so relieve the patient's symptoms and improve his general condition that operation can be deferred indefinitely. In cases of paralytic ileus they have almost entirely replaced operation. Their routine adoption in all cases of intestinal obstruction, combined with the correct timing of operative intervention, has led to a significant reduction in mortality.

The essentials of conservative or preoperative treatment are suction drainage of the gastrointestinal tract, and intravenous infusion (Fig. 22.6) to restore fluid and electrolyte balance.

Suction drainage

This has, as its object, the removal of fluid and gas

Table 22.2   Diagnosis of level of obstruction

Level of obstruction	Onset	Pain	Dehydration	Distension	Radiographs
High small bowel	Sudden	Upper abdominal. Variable severity: may be continuous	Extreme	Absent	May show 'gasless' abdomen or may show distension of duodenum or first jejunal loop
Low small bowel	More gradual	Central abdominal, severe, colicky	Less marked	Moderate: central in position	Gasless small loop of small bowel on supine film, usually lying transversely. Fluid levels on erect films
Large bowel	Usually insidious	Central or lower abdominal. May be colicky or generalized; discomfort due to distension	Slight except in late stage	Progressive: extreme in late stage: peripheral except in volvulus	Gas shown in the colon mainly proximal to obstruction: this is not evacuated after an enema

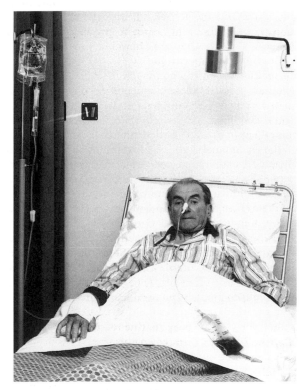

Fig. 22.6 Intravenous 'drip' infusion and nasogastric drainage into a polythene bag to allow for siphonage

from the stomach and upper intestine. By so doing it usually abolishes vomiting and brings about progressive relief of pain and distension. It greatly facilitates operation, should this be required, and obviates the risk of vomitus being inhaled during anaesthesia. *Gastric or gastro-duodenal* suction is established by means of simple plastic tube which can be passed without difficulty through a nostril. This is usually effective in re-

lieving distension not only of the stomach, but also of the greater part of the small bowel — due probably to the reversed peristalsis which commonly exists in the obstructed state, and to the fact that intestinal peristalsis is inhibited by gastric distension, and is restored when this is relieved. Frequent, usually hourly, aspiration may be carried out by syringe, or continuous suction applied using a low-pressure suction pump. If continuous suction is used a double lumen tube, with one lumen to allow air to be drawn into the tube is advised (e.g. the Salem Sump Tube made by Argyle). This will prevent mucosa being sucked into the tube and effectively blocking it.

Intravenous infusion
The patient with acute small bowel obstruction has usually suffered a serious loss of fluid and electrolytes from the out-pouring of intestinal secretions into the distended bowel above the obstruction — whether the fluid stagnates in the bowel, or whether it is lost by vomiting. If he has been sick for several days, the total deficit of water and sodium may run to several litres of water and several hundred millimoles of sodium. Such deficits may have been partly restored by the transfer of intracellular water and by the mobilization of bone sodium. Restoration of the estimated *total* of fluid should not therefore be attempted too rapidly, since overloading of the circulation may result. In the average case of obstruction it will usually suffice to give 1 litre of normal saline and 1 litre of glucose solution before operation is undertaken. Administered at the rate of a fast 'drip', this total of 2 litres can be given in the space of 2 to 3 hours, which is usually both an adequate and justifiable time to spend in preoperative preparation. Hourly urine output should be monitored after urethral catheterization; fluid should be given to maintain an output of more than 50 ml per hour. In the severely ill patient, the CVP should also be monitored.

High small bowel obstruction
Characterized by profuse vomiting, the patient's greatest need is for fluid and electrolytes. These needs are effectively met by intravenous infusion, while the vomiting is abolished by suction drainage. Alkalosis is likely to be present, since the vomiting of acid gastric juice predominates, but this is satisfactorily corrected by normal saline given intravenously (p. 22). If the obstruction is due to simple kinking of the bowel it may be completely relieved by this treatment. In any case, there is seldom any great urgency for operation since strangulation is rare. If the patient's general condition is improved, and if such improvement is maintained, conservative treatment may be continued for several days if necessary.

Low small bowel obstruction
The need for fluid therapy (except in the late case) is less urgent, but such therapy, together with suction drainage, should always be installed before the patient is submitted to operation. In obstruction due to bands or adhesions, complete (even if only temporary) relief may be obtained by such treatment. Operation can then be undertaken later — and with much greater safety, when the acute symptoms of obstruction have been relieved, and fluid and electrolyte balance has been restored.

Late cases of small bowel obstruction
The fluid loss is too great for the deficit to be made up by the transfer of intracellular fluid. In consequence the blood volume is reduced and the patient exhibits all the signs of shock. The *first priority* in treatment is restoration of the circulatory volume, and, with this object in view, whole blood, plasma or dextran should be administered (Wilkinson, 1973). Electrolyte solutions, given in the stage of shock, will serve only to increase the hypoproteinaemia, and may lead to pulmonary oedema. As soon as the blood volume has been restored, the patient can, if necessary, be submitted to operation. Electrolyte solutions are then infused during the operation, and are continued into the postoperative period as required. A fluid balance chart must, of course, be kept throughout the period of intravenous therapy (p. 23).

Colonic obstruction
These methods of preoperative treatment have a more limited application here. They should always be employed, however, in cases where vomiting or dehydration have occurred, or where gross distension is present.

In cases of suspected *strangulation* there is no justification for any undue delay, but suction drainage and intravenous infusion should be installed before the patient is taken to the operating theatre. When shock is present, operation should be delayed until the blood volume has been restored by whole blood, plasma or dextran solution.

Paralytic ileus
Suction drainage and intravenous infusion form the basis of modern therapy, and in most cases the condition resolves completely under this treatment. All purgatives and other drugs which stimulate peristalsis are avoided, and the bowel is left completely at rest to recover in its own time. This treatment can be continued for 2 weeks or longer if necessary, until bowel sounds return or flatus is passed. The suction may then be discontinued for a trial period of a few hours; if vomiting occurs it is at once reinstalled. In the reflex type of paralytic ileus the effect of guanethidine and prostigmine may be tried (Neely, 1971): by abolishing sympathetic inhibition this may bring about the return of peristalsis.

Indications for operation
In small bowel obstruction without suspicion of strangulation, the indications for operation depend largely on the response to conservative treatment. The patient's condition is assessed at 2-hourly intervals by clinical examination, which includes measurement of the abdominal girth, estimation of the fluid loss obtained by aspiration and the urinary output. If the response to treatment is satisfactory, operation may be delayed until conditions are considered to be most favourable. Failure to respond to conservative treatment may well indicate strangulation (p. 461), particularly if the patient's pulse rate continues to rise. Persistence with such treatment can then lead to disaster and the patient's only hope of survival lies in prompt operative treatment.

In acute colonic obstruction, especially when distension is marked, operation should be carried out without undue delay. Ischaemic rupture of the caecum may occur and is a real risk when the transverse diameter of the caecum on the abdominal film is greater than 12 cm.

Paralytic ileus
Operation is indicated if there is suspicion of intra-abdominal infection or that a mechanical element may exist. In long persisting paralytic ileus (12–14 days) a mechanical element may have resulted from matting together of intestines by fibrinous exudate.

In paralytic ileus, or in intestinal pseudo-obstruction, colonic distension may be so great that rupture of the large bowel becomes a risk. Decompression of the colon by tube caecostomy may be required. Alternatively, in skilled hands, decompression by colonoscopy may be undertaken.

LAPAROTOMY FOR INTESTINAL OBSTRUCTION

Operation for intestinal obstruction — except when this is due to an external hernia — will usually take the form of an exploratory laparotomy. Its primary object is to save life by relieving the state of obstruction which exists. In certain cases this can be accomplished effectively by some simple procedure such as the division of a constricting band or adhesion. Otherwise it may be necessary to deal with the obstruction by short-circuiting or (in the case of the colon) by drainage of the bowel to the exterior. Resection of a segment of small bowel may be rendered necessary by the presence of strangulation, infarction or tumour. Strictures due to Crohn's disease present a special case, and may be dealt with by resection or, if the stricture is short, by stricturoplasty.

In carcinoma of the colon (the commonest cause of obstruction in elderly patients), a second object of laparotomy is to assess the possibility of radical removal of the tumour. In obstructing carcinomas of the right colon and transverse colon, right hemicolectomy or extended right hemicolectomy is preferred. In obstructing carcinomas in the left colon there is an increasing tendency to resection and primary anastomosis, but this requires an experienced surgeon and a fit patient. If distension is great, it is best to carry out a staged procedure — for example preliminary decompression by loop transverse colostomy followed by later resection and anastomosis, or preferably a Hartmann type of resection (see page 509) followed by later anastomosis.

Anaesthesia

A good anaesthetic with complete relaxation is essential in order to reduce the surgeon's difficulties in dealing with distended and unruly coils of bowel. The skilled anaesthetist will probably choose some form of inhalation anaesthetic, with tracheal intubation, and combined with a relaxant drug. Gastroduodenal suction carried out during anaesthesia prevents vomiting or inspiration of stomach contents. When such expert assistance is not available the advantages of spinal anaesthesia should be considered.

Incision

A midline incision centred on the umbilicus is preferred to a paramedian incision and is suitable for most patients with obstruction. A transverse subumbilical incision is satisfactory for patients with small bowel obstruction or obstructing lesions of the right colon, and is advised particularly in patients with chronic respiratory problems. Transverse incisions are preferred also in neonates and young infants (see p. 342). Hae-

mostasis should be meticulous and diathermy or staples may be used in division of the rectus.

If the patient already has a suitable previous incision the same site should be used. The new incision should start above or below a previous vertical incision, or lateral to a transverse one, so that the peritoneal cavity may be entered without risk of damaging adherent bowel. Bowel or omentum adherent to the inner aspect of the scar may then be dissected free under direct vision.

A clear peritoneal exudate is usually present when intestinal distension is marked. A bloodstained exudate suggests either some form of strangulation or of mesenteric occlusion, while a seropurulent exudate indicates an inflammatory cause for the obstruction.

Following any operative procedure necessary, it is advised that the incision is closed using a continuous mass suture of No. 1 Prolene or nylon incorporating peritoneum and muscle layers. Continuous No. 1 PDS (slowly absorbable) is becoming increasingly popular, as suture sinus formation is not a problem. Continued abdominal distension is common for a few days after operation for intestinal obstruction and chest complications are frequent, so that the strain on the wound is great.

Location of the obstruction

Sometimes the cause of the obstruction is at once apparent — as when the loop of a colonic volvulus presents in the wound. More often, however, nothing can be seen except distended coils of small bowel. In such cases the first step in the operation is to inspect the caecum. This can be done by retracting the right margin of the wound and by packing distended coils of small bowel away to the left.

If the caecum is distended the obstruction must be in the colon. By far the commonest cause of such obstruction is carcinoma. Growths which give rise to colonic obstruction are usually in the left side of the colon; these growths are of the constricting or 'string' type, and may easily be missed if the surgeon is expecting to find a large tumour mass. The colon should, therefore, be methodically examined, and this should always be done *from below upwards.*

If the caecum is collapsed the obstruction is in the small bowel. A search is then made in the right iliac fossa or in the pelvis for a collapsed loop of small bowel and this is traced proximally until the obstruction is reached. The actual direction in which the bowel must be traced is determined in the following manner. The loop is held in the long axis of the body, and a finger is passed deeply along the left side of its mesentery. If the finger finds itself guided inevitably to the left iliac fossa or to the left side of the vertebrae, the proximal end of the loop lies towards the thorax. If the finger is guided into

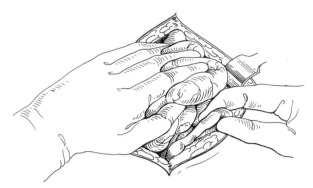

Fig. 22.7 Laparotomy for intestinal obstruction of uncertain origin. Distended coils of small bowel are kept as far as possible within the abdomen, while a search is made for a collapsed loop

the right iliac fossa or to the right side of the vertebrae, the loop is inverted, i.e. its proximal end lies towards the feet. During the search for the cause of the obstruction, distended coils of bowel should if possible be kept within the abdomen (Fig. 22.7); any coils which cannot be retained are covered by warm moist packs.

When, as frequently occurs, the operation is impeded by gaseous distension of the small bowel the bowel should be deflated. This is best done by 'milking' back small bowel content from proximal jejunum into the duodenum and thence stomach, from where it may be aspirated through the nasogastric tube by the anaesthetist (Fig. 22.8). It is seldom necessary to carry out needle aspiration of the small bowel.

Gross gaseous distension of the colon should be dealt with by inserting a fine bore needle obliquely through a taenia coli in the transverse colon and attaching it to

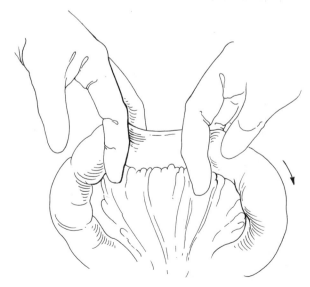

Fig. 22.8 Method of 'milking' back small bowel content

a low pressure suction apparatus — if a transverse colostomy is contemplated the proposed site of the colostomy should be used. Occasionally a further needle may need to be inserted in sigmoid colon. It is advisable to oversew the puncture sites with a Z suture of 2/0 chromic catgut to minimize the risk of leakage from the site during further manipulations.

Bands and adhesions
These are likely to have resulted from a previous operation — especially if performed for some condition complicated by peritonitis. In other cases they are congenital — as in the case of the band which is sometimes found stretching from the umbilicus to the ileum about 60 cm from its lower end, and which is the remains of the vitello-intestinal duct. The ileal end of the duct may remain open to form a Meckel's diverticulum. A loop of small bowel may become wound round the band or may be ensnared by it.

Bands and small adhesions are divided under direct vision. The remnants of any band should be removed in order to prevent a possible recurrence. The constricted area or the site of adhesion on the gut is examined carefully; if it is damaged it is infolded by *Lembert* suture. If there has been gross distension the bowel may be deflated by aspiration; alternatively a temporary enterostomy may be performed (p. 474).

Where a complicated mass of adhesions is present, separation of the loops of bowel may be difficult and carry an attendant risk of damage to the bowel. When such a situation exists it is better to short-circuit the obstruction by making a lateral anastomosis above and below the involved bowel. Sometimes more than one anastomosis is necessary (p. 473). If the length of bowel to be bypassed is such that there is a risk of producing a short-bowel syndrome, adequate bowel must with great care be dissected free to reduce this risk.

Recurrent adhesive small bowel obstruction
Some unfortunate patients are subject to repeated episodes of adhesive small bowel obstruction. Glove powder has been incriminated in the past, and the modern starch powders are not above considerable suspicion. Starch free gloves should always be used in intraabdominal surgery.

In patients with multiple adhesions, where recurrent obstruction is considered to be likely, or in those where it has already occurred, a number of authors consider that some form of plication procedure, allowing the intestine to take regular folds, will reduce the risk of further obstruction. Noble (1937) described his intestinal plication procedure, whereby the small intestinal loops, after lysis of adhesions, are sutured to one another in ordered fashion (Fig. 22.9). The procedure is laborious and carries a risk of intestinal fistula forma-

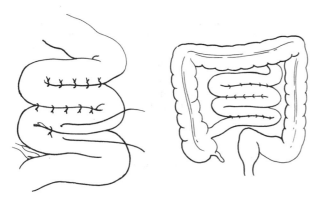

Fig. 22.9 Noble's plication procedure

tion. A simpler technique is transmesenteric plication, as described by Childs, 1960 (Fig. 22.10).

Baker (1959), and more recently Munro & Jones (1978), have advocated the use of a jejunal tube brought out through a jejunostomy to act as an internal splint holding the bowel in gentle curves and preventing kinking while adhesions form. The polyvinyl tube, 300 cm long, and with a double lumen, one leading to an inflatable balloon and one for drainage, is inserted into the jejunum approximately 20 cm distal to the

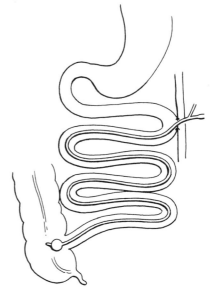

Fig. 22.11 Operative intubation in the treatment of complicated small bowel obstruction

duodenojejunal flexure. It is then guided along the small bowel into the caecum, when the balloon is inflated (Fig. 22.11). The tube is removed 12 days postoperatively.

Internal strangulation

This term is applicable when the blood supply of a loop of bowel has been endangered by an obstructing constriction. If the bowel is considered to be non-viable (p. 543), resection and anastomosis must be carried out.

Intussusception

Intussusception occurs with invagination of bowel so that the apex is carried distally by peristalsis. Depending on the segment involved, the lesion is described as ileoileal, ileocolic or colocolic. The condition is most common in babies between 3 and 9 months who develop an ileocolic intussusception, probably from hyperplasia of Peyer's patches secondary to a virus infection. In older children and adults, a Meckel's diverticulum, Henoch Schonlein purpura, or a bowel neoplasm may be the underlying cause.

Intussusception presents initially with bouts of colicky abdominal pain which may continue for a variable interval before the signs of bowel strangulation and obstruction develop. During such bouts of pain a baby will scream, go red in the face and draw its knees up to the chest; as the pain subsides the baby lies pale and lethargic. Vomiting may be a feature and constipation follows after bowel content distal to the intussusception has been passed. At a later stage the typical red current jelly stool may be seen. When the abdomen is relaxed

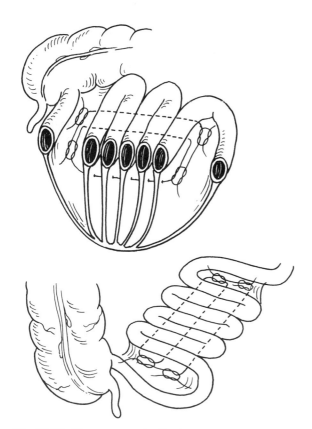

Fig. 22.10 Transmesenteric plication

between bouts of pain it may be possible to feel a sausage-shaped mass above the umbilicus in the line of the transverse colon. Occasionally the intussusception will progress further along the bowel and the apex can be felt on rectal examination. However, the clinical picture is often inconclusive and the diagnosis can then be confirmed on a barium enema examination which will outline the apex of the intussusception within the lumen of the colon.

Management

Depending on the severity of the presentation it may first be necessary to correct fluid loss and electrolyte imbalance. In babies, hydrostatic reduction of an intussusception by barium enema or by air can often be successful when performed by an experienced radiologist. The procedure is, however, potentially dangerous and should not be attempted when strangulation of bowel or obstruction are suspected. Ideally the procedure should be performed with the baby anaesthetized and a theatre and surgeon available in case of failure or complication. In the adult, nonoperative treatment is not an option since the cause in ileocolic and colocolic intussusception is usually a malignant one.

At operation a transverse right sided lower abdominal incision will usually provide adequate access and can, if necessary, be extended towards the left. The thickened mass of the intussusception can be easily felt but, to obtain a better view, it may be helpful to deliver dilated proximal ileum through the wound. The intussusception is reduced by applying firm pressure over the apex, so as to push the intussuscipiens back along the line of the bowel; traction should never by applied to bowel proximal to the lesion. If this manoeuvre proves difficult, the intussusception should be wrapped in warm gauze and squeezed gently along its length so as to reduce oedema. Providing the wall of the caecum is undamaged, an appendicectomy may be performed so as to prevent confusion in the future. When reduction of the intussusception is incomplete or when the ileum is traumatized or ischaemic, the abnormal segment of bowel should be excised and an end to end ileocolostomy performed in two layers. In late cases where resection would result in almost complete excision of the colon, the method of colotomy described by Shah (1991), offers a less drastic alternative, excising only the gangrenous apex of the intussusception.

Small bowel volvulus

This may be primary in infants and young children. In older children and adults the condition is usually secondary to adhesions. Adhesions, if present, are divided, then the loop of bowel derotated. Non-viable intestine must be resected and intestinal continuity restored in end-to-end fashion.

Malrotation of bowel in infancy

Embryology

This condition may present as an isolated anomaly but may also be found in association with a diaphragmatic hernia or exomphalos. Between the fourth and twelfth weeks of pregnancy, the mid-gut is first displaced into the umbilical sac and then withdrawn back into the abdominal cavity. During this period the proximal and distal limbs of the mid-gut rotate in an anti-clockwise direction through 270° about the long axis of the superior mesenteric artery. As a result, the distal part of the duodenum passes behind the artery from right to left and the caecum passes in front of the artery from left to right so that it comes to lie in the right hypochondrium. Thereafter the caecum slowly descends to the right iliac fossa and the ascending colon and duodenum are fixed to the parietal peritoneum of the posterior abdominal wall.

The term 'malrotation' embraces both incomplete and abnormal rotation. The most common situation is that the gut rotates only 180° so that the duodenum lies partly behind or to the right of the superior mesenteric artery. Adhesions (Ladd's bands) pass from the caecum across the duodenum to the under surface of the liver (Fig. 22.12). Less commonly there may be nonrotation or, after initial rotation, the gut twists in a clockwise direction. Ladd's bands may partly or completely obstruct the duodenum and the narrow root of mesentery of the mid-gut predisposes to volvulus.

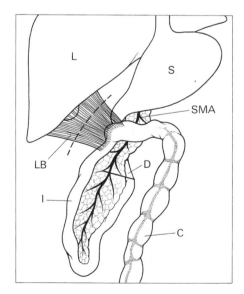

Fig. 22.12 Illustration of the most common type of malrotation. C-colon; D-duodenum; I-ileum; L-liver; LB-Ladd's bands; S-stomach; SMA-superior mesenteric artery

Clinical presentation

Symptoms may develop at any age but are more common in the neonate (Welch, 1983). Partial obstruction of the duodenum and intermittent volvulus may present with bile stained vomiting only; there may be little or no abdominal distension and meconium and changed stools are passed normally. Volvulus may, however, cause complete obstruction and strangulation. A plain abdominal X-ray may show either the 'double bubble' appearance of duodenal obstruction or the more generalized changes of small bowel obstruction. In incomplete obstruction a contrast follow through study will show the characteristic corkscrew appearance of the duodenum to the right of the midline and a contrast enema shows an abnormally high position for the caecum.

Treatment

In a baby with malrotation the immediate treatment is that of obstruction by nasogastric aspiration, intravenous infusion and correction of fluid and electrolyte imbalance. The underlying anomaly should then by corrected by operation.

The abdomen of the baby is opened through a transverse upper abdominal incision and the bowel delivered through the wound. A volvulus, if present, is usually twisted in a clockwise direction and can easily be corrected. It is important that Ladd's bands are completely divided so that the terminal ileum and caecum can be placed in the left hypochondrium (Fig. 22.13). This will expose the full length of the duodenum which can then be mobilized so that it lies freely to the right of the vertebral column. Finally, remaining adhesions between loops of bowel are separated. To ensure patency of the duodenum, the nasogastric tube can be manipulated from the stomach to the duodenum and on into the jejunum. An appendicectomy should be performed because of the abnormal position of the caecum. The abdominal wound is then closed in layers.

The postoperative management of malrotation is usually uncomplicated and oral feeding can be started after a few days.

Small bowel atresia

This condition is probably the result of ischaemic damage rather than a primary developmental anomaly (Louw & Barnard, 1955). It is one of the more common major congenital gastrointestinal abnormalities, the incidence being approximately one in 2500 live births. Bland Sutton (1889) described three types. In type I continuity of the lumen of the bowel is obstructed by a membrane; in type II the proximal and distal segments of the bowel are connected by a fibrous cord; and in type III the two segments are separated and there may be a 'V' shaped deficiency in the mesentery. Less commonly, multiple atresias are found or the distal bowel may be vascularized by a branch of the middle colic artery and arranged in a spiral form around a central vessel giving the appearance of 'apple peel'. The proximal bowel in atresia is normally grossly dilated and hypertrophied and the distal part may be partly ischaemic.

The baby born with jejunal or ileal atresia may be of low birth weight and there may be a maternal history of hydramnios. Associated congenital abnormalities may be present but they are less common than in duodenal atresia. The presenting sign is that of bile stained vomiting. Abdominal distension may be a feature particularly when the obstruction is distal. Although normal meconium or pale inspissated plugs may be passed initially, the baby thereafter becomes constipated. A plain erect and supine abdominal X-ray will show features of small bowel obstruction. When the atretic segment is distal the condition must be distinguished from meconium ileus, malrotation and Hirschsprung's disease and a barium enema may be of value.

The immediate management is that of obstruction; a nasogastric tube is passed, an intravenous infusion established and any fluid and electrolyte imbalance corrected. As part of the supportive care the baby should be nursed in an incubator. When the baby's condition is satisfactory a laparotomy is performed using a transverse upper abdominal incision. It is important to exclude further areas of atresia in the distal bowel and this is done by introducing a catheter and injecting saline into the lumen. The dilated part of the proximal

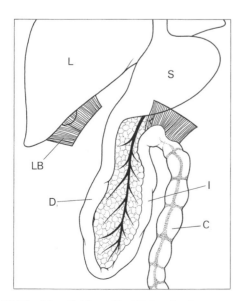

Fig. 22.13 After division of Ladd's bands, the caecum is place in the left hypochondrium and the duodenum is freed to lie to the right of the vertebral column. C-colon; D-duodenum; I-ileum; L-liver; LB-Ladd's bands; S-stomach

bowel is then generously resected as it may fail to develop effective peristalsis (Nixon, 1955). Because of the discrepancy between the dilated proximal and narrowed distal bowel an end-to-end anastomosis is impractical and an end-to-side anastomosis should be performed with a single inverting layer of fine sutures. In most babies a delay in normal feeding should be anticipated and intravenous nutrition started early in the postoperative period.

Impacted gall-stone or faecalith

On occasion, a gall-stone may pass into the lumen of the gut through a cholecystoduodenal fistula which has resulted from unsuspected cholecystitis. The calculus becomes impacted at any narrowing of the gut and causes intestinal obstruction. The diagnosis is suspected when air is noted in the biliary tree in addition to the X-ray features of small bowel obstruction.

Operation

The segment of bowel (usually the lower ileum) in which the concretion has become impacted is withdrawn from the wound; contents are milked away in both directions and clamps are applied. After careful packing-off the bowel is opened, if possible by a transverse incision, and the concretion is removed, either by expression or by the use of stone-holding forceps. The opening is repaired by two layers of suture. If the concretion is not too firmly impacted it may with advantage be moved proximally to a healthier part of the bowel which can be incised with greater safety.

Internal hernia

A coil of small bowel is occasionally imprisoned in a hole in the mesentery or omentum, or in a retroperitoneal fossa. The constricting ring should be gently stretched and the bowel withdrawn, after which the opening is closed by suture. If difficulty is encountered, the distended bowel should be emptied by aspiration (p. 466). Great care must be taken if the constricting ring requires to be divided, for severe haemorrhage may be induced. Strangulation is common in internal hernias, and if present, resection of the involved loop is mandatory.

Mesenteric vascular occlusion

This is a relatively uncommon and frequently fatal cause of intestinal obstruction. The occlusion may be the result of embolism to or thrombosis in the superior mesenteric artery, or thrombosis in the superior mesenteric or portal vein. In many patients the large vessels are not involved, the occlusion occurring widely in small arteries or veins.

Presenting symptoms and signs are vague in the early stages of the occlusion, so that the diagnosis remains unsuspected until a greater or lesser length of intestine has infarcted, providing the clinical features of peritonitis. Inferior mesenteric artery occlusion presents with severe lower abdominal pain and there may be little to find at laparotomy until bowel necrosis occurs.

On suspicion of the diagnosis, providing time and facilities permit, mesenteric angiography may be very helpful preoperatively, since any major arterial occlusion may be relieved surgically although small vessel or venous thrombosis is not amenable to this.

At laparotomy, if extensive established gangrene is present, attempts to restore arterial flow are not indicated. Resection of the involved intestine is required. In patients with potential for restoration of arterial flow, and intestine which is still viable (or of questionable viability) attention should be directed first to restoration of flow. An embolus is extracted using a Fogarty catheter via an arteriotomy in the main trunk of the superior mesenteric artery. If the block in the artery is due to thrombosis over an atheromatous plaque, an H-graft between aorta and superior mesenteric artery may be carried out. Following successful restoration of flow, areas of dubious viability may become clearly viable and intestinal resection can be lessened in extent, or even avoided. A 'second look' laparotomy after 24 hours has been recommended by some authors.

Operations on patients with mesenteric vascular occlusion should be covered by broad spectrum antibiotics (including an anti-anaerobe agent) and followed by anticoagulation. Adequate fluid replacement is essential, and requirements are particularly high in the patient who has successful restoration of flow.

Volvulus of colon

Rotation of a loop of bowel on its vascular pedicle occurs most commonly in the *pelvic colon* in the adult. It represents a good example of closed loop obstruction, allowing entry of some intestinal content from more proximal bowel, so that rapidly increasing distension of the loop occurs, while more proximal bowel may not be impressively distended. Compression of the blood vessels in the rotated pedicle compromises the blood supply to the loop, and this, added to the effect of distension, leads to a high risk of strangulation.

In volvulus of the sigmoid colon where there is no suspicion of strangulation, the condition may be treated conservatively by the careful insertion of a flatus tube via a sigmoidoscope into the distal limb of the volvulus. If done successfully, decompression of the loop occurs, allowing time for assessment of the patient and consideration of definitive elective treatment, for the condition, once it occurs, tends to be recurrent.

If the method is unsuccessful, or strangulation is suspected, laparotomy is undertaken through a lower midline or left paramedian incision. As soon as the abdomen is opened, the distended and congested pelvic colon presents. When the loop is only moderately distended it should be gently withdrawn from the abdomen and unwound by rotation between the two hands. When the pedicle can be inspected the direction for rotation is obvious — otherwise it must be discovered by trial and error; usually the twist has been in an anticlockwise direction. When the loop is too distended to be delivered through the wound there should be no hesitation in decompressing it by aspiration.

If the loop is non-viable, it *must* be resected. If the loop is viable it is still best resected, as recurrent volvulus is common, and various means of colopexy are relatively unsuccessful. If the patient's condition does not permit emergency resection, the sigmoid loop may be drained via a flatus tube inserted per rectum, or by performing a sigmoid colostomy. Later elective resection of the sigmoid loop is undertaken when the patient is fit.

Following emergency resection, the surgeon has 3 choices, determined by local conditions and by the general condition of the patient:

1. To perform an end-to-end reconstitution of colonic continuity. This is the preferred choice. The anastomosis should be in one layer, using interrupted inverting sutures of 2/0 or 3/0 gauge.

2. To bring both cut ends of bowel to the surface — the proximal end as an end colostomy, and the distal end separately as a mucous fistula (Mikulicz operation). Intestinal continuity is restored at a later date.

3. The length of distal bowel available may not permit its cut end being brought to the surface. In this event the distal cut end is oversewn in two layers and returned to the pelvis (leaving long non-absorbable sutures to mark its position), while the proximal cut end is brought out as an end colostomy (Hartmann's procedure). Intestinal continuity is again restored at a later date, but the procedure is usually technically more difficult than if a mucous fistula had been formed.

Volvulus of the caecum
This is less common. Right hemicolectomy is the preferred procedure and is mandatory if the bowel has been devitalized. If resection is not undertaken the caecum may be fixed in the right iliac fossa (caecopexy) by direct suture to parietal peritoneum, by using polyvinyl alcohol sponge (El-Katib, 1973), or by performing a tube caecostomy.

Postoperative obstruction
This is most liable to occur in cases of peritonitis. It may be either paralytic or mechanical in origin.

Paralytic ileus
The clinical features of this condition, the conservative

treatment and the rare indications for operation have been discussed (p. 462). An obvious source of infection should be sought, abscesses should be drained, and a leaking anastomosis repaired or resected. Simple repair of a leaking anastomosis may be unsatisfactory, and if resection is inadvisable for technical reasons a large bore tube drain should be led from the vicinity of the anastomosis to the exterior; this, in the further breakdown of the anastomosis, will lead to a controlled fistula rather than recurrent peritonitis. Prior to closure of the abdomen peritoneal lavage using 3 litres of a wide-spectrum antibiotic solution is advised. The wound should be closed using a mass suture technique.

Mechanical obstruction
This may be due to oedema of the bowel at the site of an anastomosis, or to kinking or compression by adhesions. Unlike paralytic ileus it occurs fairly late in the postoperative period — usually 5 to 10 days after operation, by which time the bowels may have moved normally. Colicky pains are present, and bowel sounds are heard on auscultation. The guiding principles in treatment are the same as in other types of mechanical obstruction — i.e. early laparotomy if there is no response to conservative treatment.

RESECTION AND ANASTOMOSIS OF SMALL BOWEL

Resection is always attended by some risk and should be avoided wherever possible. The most absolute indication arises when the blood supply of a segment of bowel has been so seriously interfered with that gangrene, if not already present, is considered to be inevitable. Resection may be required also in extensive injuries of a segment of gut, as may occur in penetrating abdominal wounds. The risks of resection are greatly increased in the presence of obstruction, which usually co-exists with strangulation, but when the bowel is considered to be non-viable (p. 543) such risks must be accepted.

Resection with end-to-end anastomosis
This is the standard procedure for re-establishing continuity of small bowel. Disparity in the sizes of ends to be joined is corrected by division of the narrower bowel obliquely, the greater length of bowel being, of course, retained on the mesenteric border.

Technique of resection (Fig. 22.14)
In order to ensure a satisfactory anastomosis the level of resection must be well to each side of the devitalized area. The affected loop is withdrawn from the wound until a sufficiency of healthy bowel has been delivered,

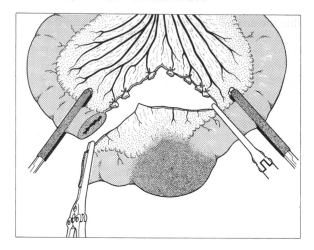

Fig. 22.14 Technique of resection in small bowel

and the wound and peritoneal cavity are protected with moist packs. At the levels selected for the section a hole is made in an avascular area in the mesentery close to the gut. The mesentery is now divided between these two points, in the line of a shallow V, the apex of which points towards the mesenteric root, the division being carried out by clamping with a succession of artery forceps, and by cutting with scissors. This is most satisfactorily achieved by displaying the vascular pattern of the mesentery by means of a bright light behind it. The forceps are then tied off; they should each contain a relatively small bite of mesentery owing to the danger of a ligature slipping. The segment of bowel to be resected is emptied by milking away its contents, and a crushing clamp is applied at each end. *The tip of this clamp should lie exactly opposite the line of division of the mesentery.* In order to ensure a good blood supply to the anti-mesenteric border it may be placed slightly obliquely, so that more of this border is removed. Light occlusion clamps are now applied to the healthy bowel 2.5 cm away from the crushing clamps. A swab having been placed underneath to absorb leakage, the bowel is divided close to the crushing clamps. The loop is now removed along with the crushing clamps still attached. The open ends of the healthy bowel protruding beyond the occlusion clamps are mopped out with small gauze pledgets held on forceps.

Technique of anastomosis
The occlusion clamps are approximated so that the open ends of bowel lie in apposition. The junction is effected by two complete layers of suture — a layer of through-and-through sutures, and a layer of *Lembert* sutures which do not penetrate the lumen. It is usually easier to insert the through-and-through suture first. This is commenced at the anti-mesenteric border, and is continued round the circumference of the bowel

until the starting point is reached, when it is tied to its own short end. A lock-stitch should be inserted at intervals to prevent a purse-string effect being produced. When the superficial cut edges are being approximated, the Connell type of suture (Fig. 22.15), which prevents eversion of the mucous membrane, may be employed as an alternative to the method shown on page 344. When this suture has been completed the clamps may be removed. The suture line is carefully inspected for oozing or haemorrhage, and additional stitches are inserted if necessary. The line of junction is now invaginated by *Lembert* suture (Fig. 22.16). Special attention should be paid to the point where the leaves of the mesentery separate to enclose the bowel (the 'mesenteric angle'), for here there is a small area of gut wall which is uncovered by serosa, and from which leakage may occur. It is an advantage to commence the suture at this point, and to pass the needle through both leaves of the mesentery close to the bowel, so that they are included in the first stitch. The suture is then continued round the circumference of the bowel until the starting point is reached, when it is passed through the mesentery and tied to its own short end. Finally, the gap in the mesentery is closed by interrupted sutures taking only small bites so as to avoid damage to vessels supplying the gut. The bowel is washed with saline or antibiotic solution before being returned to the peritoneal cavity. Drainage is not required unless there was perforation of the gut before operation.

SHORT-CIRCUITING OPERATIONS ON THE INTESTINES

These operations are carried out, as a rule, by lateral anastomosis, the technique of which has already been

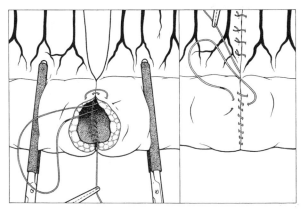

Fig. 22.15   **Fig. 22.16**

Fig. 22.15 & Fig. 22.16   End-to-end anastomosis of small bowel by two layer of continuous suture. The Connell suture shown in the first drawing prevents eversion of the mucosa

described (p. 347). In the case of such an operation on the colon the incision into the lumen should be made along one of the taenia, since the greater thickness of the muscular coat in this line ensures a more satisfactory anastomosis.

Short-circuiting of small bowel

This is the operation of choice when obstruction has been caused by a complicated mass of adhesions as may result from caseating mesenteric glands. Unless the length of bowel to be short-circuited is considered likely to result in 'short-bowel' problems no attempt should be made to free the adherent loops as damage to the bowel, or haemorrhage from mesenteric vessels may result. The anastomosis should be performed as close to the obstruction as possible. Most surgeons prefer a two-layer anastomosis in small bowel, using continuous sutures of 2/0 or 3/0 chromic catgut or Dexon. In some cases more than one anastomosis may be necessary.

Ileo-transverse anastomosis (Fig. 22.17)

This is employed most commonly in the treatment of tumours of the caecum and ascending colon. If the growth is removable the anastomosis forms part of the operation of right-sided *hemicolectomy*. If the growth is irremovable, ileotransverse anastomosis is valuable as a palliative procedure. It may also be used as an effective diverting procedure in ileocaecal tuberculosis with obstructive features, allowing chemotherapy to be used and obviating the necessity of resection.

When the operation is being carried out by itself (not as part of a one-stage hemicolectomy), it is usually best that the anastomosis should be effected with the ileum in continuity (i.e. not divided), in view of the possibility that the colonic lesion might give rise to obstruction — in which case, if the ileum were divided, a 'closed loop' would result. A segment of ileum, as near to the caecum as is found convenient, is brought up to lie without tension alongside the transverse colon at the junction of its proximal and middle thirds, so that a lateral anastomosis may be made. The stoma of the anastomosis should be about 4 cm in length.

In Crohn's disease affecting the terminal ileum and caecum and causing obstruction, right hemicolectomy is the preferred surgical treatment. This may not in some patients be technically feasible at the time of laparotomy. In this circumstance ileotransverse anastomosis with exclusion is preferred to in continuity anastomosis as it is associated with a lower incidence of continued or recurrent activity in the affected area of bowel. For this method, the ileum is divided in its terminal part, the distal cut-end is closed, and the proximal cut-end is joined to the transverse colon by end-to-side anastomosis.

Transverse-pelvic anastomosis (Fig. 22.18)

This is the procedure of choice in irremovable tumours of the splenic flexure, and has obvious advantages over a permanent transverse colostomy. Except in cases where the transverse colon is pendulous, the lower part of the descending colon may require to be mobilized by incision of the peritoneum along its lateral border, in order that the anastomosis can be effected without tension.

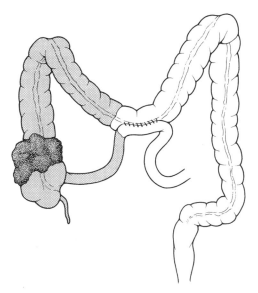

Fig. 22.17 Ileotransverse anastomosis (antiperistaltic) with the ileum in continuity. Stippling shows segment of bowel which is 'defunctioned'

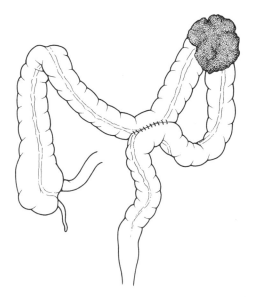

Fig. 22.18 Transverse-pelvic anastomosis, short-circuiting an irremovable tumour of the splenic flexure

OPERATIONS FOR EXTERNAL DRAINAGE OF THE INTESTINES (STOMA)

Drainage of the colon (*colostomy*) may be either temporary or permanent. Temporary drainage is performed for the immediate relief of obstruction or for the protection of a colonic anastomosis following resection of a distally placed tumour: it may be employed also in inflammatory conditions such as Crohn's disease, diverticulitis and intractable fistula-in-ano in order to 'defunction' the distal colon. Permanent drainage (i.e. the making of an 'artificial anus') is inevitable in the case of tumours which are irremovable and cannot be shortcircuited, or in which continuity of the bowel cannot be restored after excision. A colostomy may be formed in any mobile part of the colon but is usually either transverse or pelvic.

Ileostomy

Ileostomy following colectomy for inflammatory disease such as ulcerative colitis, is usually permanent (see p. 492) but a temporary loop ileostomy may be used as part of a 'pouch' operation (page 492) until healing is satisfactory.

Ileostomy in children

A temporary ileostomy may be necessary in a baby to relieve obstruction or to defunction ischaemic bowel in necrotising enterocolitis. Normally the decision to perform an ileostomy will be taken during an exploratory laparotomy. A separate stab wound is then made in the right iliac fossa of sufficient size so that a loop of ileum can be drawn through with ease (Fig. 22.19A). Within the abdomen the bowel should be fixed by a stitch placed between serosa and parietal peritoneum. On the outside, the loop of ileum is opened longitudinally and sewn to the skin margin with an everting suture so as to raise the stoma 3–4 mm (Fig. 22.19B).

The procedure for a permanent spout ileostomy in an older child with ulcerative colitis is the same as that used in the adult.

Management of an ileostomy

The ileostomy does not usually act for 12 to 24 hours after operation. It may then act profusely, however, and the sudden and unaccustomed loss of small bowel contents may lead to dehydration and salt depletion. For this reason, intravenous infusion should be maintained for at least the first 2 postoperative days and longer if oral intake does not replace fluids lost by the ileostomy. It is most important, if at all possible, to prevent excoriation of the skin by the ileostomy efflux, and for this purpose a collecting appliance (*ileostomy bag*) should be fitted immediately after the operation. The ileostomy

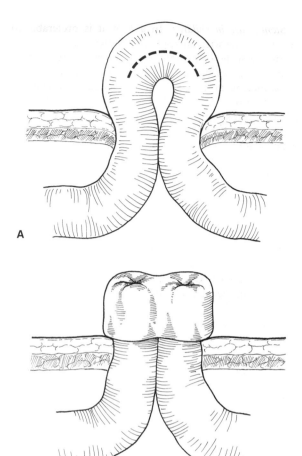

Fig. 22.19 Loop ileostomy. **A** – Loop pulled through incision. Dashes mark incision to bowel. **B** — Everted stoma 3–4 mm above skin

bags at present in use are designed to fit closely and firmly to the skin around the stoma. In some types there is a flange which can be made to adhere for as long as 3 or 4 days by means of special cement containing either a latex mixture, karaya gum or stomahesive, and to the rim of this flange a detachable or disposable bag is fitted. There are also one-piece disposable bags incorporating a small adhesive area. Other types of bag are not adherent, but depend upon a belt to hold the flange in position around the stoma.

After a week or two, the discharge becomes more solid, but it never develops the solidity of normal stools passed per rectum; it is, however, relatively odourless. In the early days there will be frequent difficulties because of looseness of the efflux, but the patient will soon learn to prevent such troubles by discovering which foodstuffs to avoid. When stability has been reached, the bowel acts shortly after meals, and usually remains quiescent at other times, except at night when it may move freely.

Stoma care in children. In a *baby* it is preferable to cover a stoma with an appliance rather than a dressing or nappy so as to prevent excoriation of surrounding skin and loss of blood from bowel mucosa which may be sufficient to cause anaemia. Suitable appliances, consisting of a flange and clip-on bag, are available in all age groups. The flange is made up of a stomahesive square carrying a 38 mm ring. The flange can be left in position for 2 or 3 days providing the seal is watertight and the bag is changed as necessary. The baby can be bathed in the normal manner and the stoma is cleaned with cotton wool soaked in warm water. The parents must be fully conversant with stoma care before the baby leaves hospital and the support which they received in hospital must be continued at home by a Health Visitor or District Nurse. The important role of the Stoma Therapist in co-ordinating this care cannot be overemphasized.

In an *older child*, in addition to the physical problems of the stoma, there may be profound psychological disturbance which may become accentuated with puberty. The disturbance may be such as to cause behavioural problems and this should be recognized. The management of both child and family requires particular skills and understanding. Under favourable circumstances, a child will learn to manage the stoma independently at about the age of 8; he or she should be able to attend a normal school and take part in a full range of outdoor activities including swimming. In many cases of ulcerative colitis and familial polyposis, however, permanent ileostomy can now usually be avoided by using the operation of restorative proctocolectomy using a J-ileal pouch anastomosed to the rectal stump.

Caecostomy

Drainage by caecostomy is now rarely required and is indicated for devitalization of the caecum resulting either from pseudo obstruction (p. 462) or caecal gangrene (p. 487).

Transverse colostomy

The technique for making a loop colostomy is described in the section on colonic carcinoma (p. 488).

Opening the colostomy

In the presence of obstruction, it is usual to open the colostomy at the initial operation. This is carried out with diathermy or by simple incision; if possible, the opened mucosa is sutured to the edge of the skin incision so as to minimize formation of fibrous tissue. In non-obstructed cases, wound infection can be avoided if the opening is delayed for 2 or 3 days after the operation. To achieve simple and speedy opening, a single blade of a Cope's clamp is applied to the bowel at operation. On removal of the clamp, crushed tissue is trimmed without pain or bleeding.

Defunctioning transverse colostomy

Any colostomy may be regarded as 'defunctioning' if it is so constructed that faeces are prevented from entering the bowel distal to it. This is a most desirable aim if a resection is to be carried out later, for the distal part of the colon bearing the tumour or the inflammatory mass is placed completely at rest; it regains its normal size and tone, and, if faeces from the proximal colon is prevented from entering it, its bacterial content becomes greatly reduced. The operation for resection and primary anastomosis can then be carried out under the best possible conditions — in a defunctioned segment of colon (which is empty, inactive and relatively sterile) although total defunctioning may only be obtained by dividing the colon and bringing each end out through a separate opening in the abdominal wall.

Pelvic colostomy

This is most commonly performed as part of the operation of abdominoperineal excision of the rectum for carcinoma. In such cases it is usually an *end-colostomy* (single stoma), and will, of course, be permanent. The technique is described on page 508.

A pelvic colostomy of *loop* type (with eventually a double stoma) may be indicated as a palliative measure in the case of obstructing and irremovable growths of the rectum. It may be employed also in nonmalignant strictures and gunshot wounds of the rectum, and in intractable cases of fistula-in-ano, when it may be only temporary.

For the simple loop colostomy a small left gridiron incision is used. It should not lie too near the anterior superior spine, lest this interfere with the accurate fitting of a colostomy appliance. The pelvic colon is identified and withdrawn. If it is fixed by a short mesentery it is mobilized by dividing the peritoneum on the lateral side as it is reflected on to the left iliac fossa. The site for the stoma should be in the upper part of the mobile loop of pelvic colon, in order that prolapse of the bowel may be avoided. The loop is retained on the skin surface by sutures to peritoneum and layers of abdominal wall in order to avoid the need for a supporting rod. The colostomy is normally opened after 2 or 3 days (p. 475).

Pelvic colostomy has no place in the treatment of acute obstruction, since, owing to the solid nature of the faeces in this part of the colon, immediate drainage is unsatisfactory.

Care of colostomy

This, like the management of an ileostomy (p. 474), has been made very much easier by the development of disposable plastic bags which can be made to fit very accurately around the stoma, either by an adhesive flange or by the use of a belt. Since, however, the efflux from a colostomy, unlike that from an ileostomy, is solid or semisolid, a watertight junction between skin and collecting appliance is by no means so necessary. Most patients will prefer a close fitting appliance, since it will make the stoma almost odourless and interfere very little with daily activities. It is possible, should appliances not be available, to manage the colostomy with a pad of wool held in position by a belt or by an elastic girdle of the 'roll on' type.

Colostomy in children

A colostomy is most often used in a baby or infant in the management of anorectal agenesis and Hirschsprung's disease both to relieve obstruction and as a preliminary to a definitive operation. It is important to prevent spill-over of bowel content; this can be ensured by separating the proximal and distal limbs of bowel so as to form a split colostomy. The construction must be such that the flange of an appliance fits comfortably round the proximal stoma and forms a watertight seal with the surrounding abdominal wall. Normally the colostomy is placed either in the right hypochondrium using right transverse colon or in the left iliac fossa using descending or sigmoid colon.

A transverse incision 3 or 4 cm long is made through the abdominal wall. The underlying colon is mobilized and a loop drawn through the incision (Fig. 22.20A). The bowel is divided transversely at the apex of the loop and the mesentery divided sufficiently so that proximal and distal limb lie without tension at either end of the incision. It is important that both limbs are fixed on the inside of the abdominal wall with stitches placed between serosa and parietal peritoneum to prevent prolapse. The incision between the two limbs is then closed in layers. The proximal limb is sewn to the

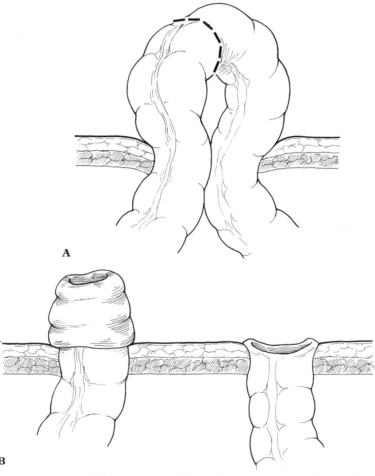

A

B

Fig. 22.20 Split colostomy. **A** – Loop of colon exteriorised. Dashes show line of transection of colon. **B** – Two stoma separated 1.0 cm; proximal stoma everted 3 mm above skin and distal stoma flush with skin

skin margin with an everting suture to raise the stoma 3 or 4 mm and the distal limb is sutured flush with the skin (Fig. 22.20B).

Stoma care in children
(See p. 475).

Closure of colostomy

This procedure is only applicable where a temporary colostomy has been formed for the relief of obstruction, the protection of an anastomosis or in order to rest or 'defunction' the colon. The safety of the distal bowel to resume its normal function must be ascertained by appropriate examination, possibly including contrast X-ray and endoscopy. The operation may involve intra-peritoneal dissection if the colostomy is other than of the loop type and full bowel preparation is then required. The restoration of bowel continuity in such cases is identical to the methods applicable to primary anastomosis following resection of colonic carcinoma. Limited preparation is appropriate to closure of a loop colostomy.

Operation
An elliptical incision is made around the colostomy opening about 0.5 cm from the mucocutaneous junction (Fig. 22.21). Bowel is separated, by sharp dissection, from the layers of the abdominal wall as far as the peritoneum which is gently separated from the deep layers of the muscles. The edges of the opening in the colon, which still have a narrow margin of skin attached, are excised. The defect in the anterior wall of the colon is repaired by sutures placed in the transverse axis of the bowel, inverting the mucosa. The bowel is now allowed to fall back (Fig. 22.22) or is gently pushed into the depths of the wound. If it has been possible to separate the peritoneum in the manner described, the bowel should lie well below the level of the muscles. The wound is repaired in layers, a small drain being left extending down to the suture line in the bowel (Fig. 22.23). Sometimes leakage of faecal matter occurs, but it usually ceases spontaneously within a few days.

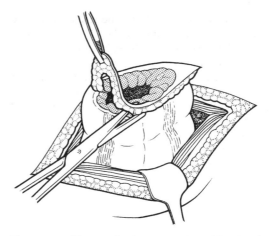

Fig. 22.22 Closure of colostomy — bowel freed and mucocutaneous junction trimmed

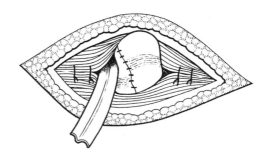

Fig. 22.23 Closure of colostomy — suture in transverse axis and drain inserted

CARCINOMA OF THE COLON

Surgery for colon cancer is based upon three premises: an understanding of principles and strategy — of what is right and proper for each situation; an appreciation of the appropriate techniques for colonic mobilization and resection; and the needs of effective reconstruction.

Strategy

It is reasonable to divide the large bowel into right half of colon, left half of colon, sigmoid and colorectum. These areas correspond approximately to vascular-lymphatic supply and drainage. A cancer operation is one which, in addition to the primary and adjacent bowel, removes the lymph node field which is illustrated in Figure 22.1. This involves a wide mesenteric resection and dissection carried up to the feeding artery, irrespective of whether this compromises bowel to a greater extent than would appear necessary. Cancer operations can then be rationally based upon these vascular patterns. For a right sided lesion in caecum or ascending colon a formal right hemicolectomy (Fig. 22.24) will remove the ileocolic vascular territory

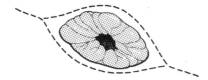

Fig. 22.21 Closure of colostomy — skin incision

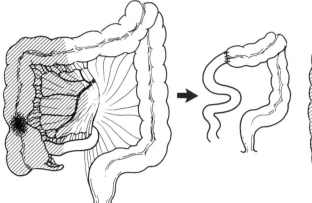

Fig. 22.24   The operative resection for a right sided tumour

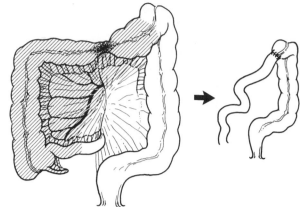

Fig. 22.26   The extent of resection for a transverse colon tumour

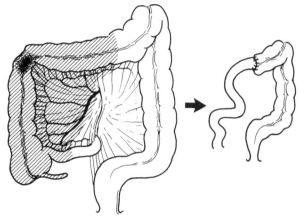

Fig. 22.25   Extended colectomy for a hepatic lesion

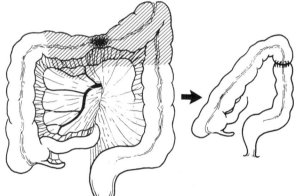

Fig. 22.27   Alternative resection for a transverse colon tumour

but permit preservation of the distal ileum and thus of the enterohepatic bile salt circulation. Even in the presence of an obstructing lesion such a resection can usually be followed by a primary reconstruction (see *Obstruction* below). Right hemicolectomy can be extended to embrace the hepatic flexure (Fig. 22.25) and transverse colon (Fig. 22.26) lesion, and the same principles apply. The further this concept is extended, the more water absorbing surface is inevitably removed and thus the greater the likelihood of troublesome diarrhoea for the patient. In consequence, though occasionally a hemicolectomy which embraces splenic flexure, descending colon or even sigmoid carcinoma is expedient (obstruction; synchronous multiple tumours; an unprepared bowel; palliative resection in the presence of metastases), it is more usual to carry out an adequate local procedure (Fig. 22.27–22.29) with reconstruction by colocolostomy. In all instances the resection is based upon the main feeding and draining vessels which are accompanied by lymphatics and lymph nodes.

The more distal the lesion the more difficult it be-

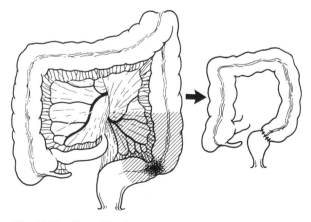

Fig. 22.28   Sigmoid colectomy

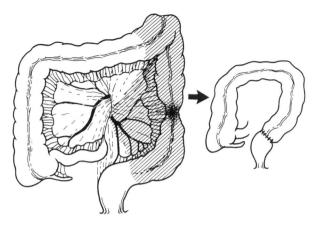

Fig. 22.29 Left hemicolectomy

comes to effect reconstruction, while at the same time undertaking an adequate cancer operation. Until recently it has been accepted that a cancer of the large bowel spreads almost equally distally as proximally and that in the rectum a large distal margin is required so necessitating in low tumours an abdominoperineal excision and a permanent colostomy (see Fig. 23.7). The pathological support for this view is not well defined and increasingly a distal rectal stump, perhaps no more than 2–3 cm beyond visible tumour, is being preserved for reconstruction (Williams 1984, Williams et al 1983, Heald and Ryall, 1986). When the whole rectum must be excised for a very low tumour, reconstruction can be carried out so long as the anal canal can be preserved with an adequate cancer resection. If the distal resection leaves 6 cm which, together with the anal canal, can be preserved, function is better than when the anastomosis is to the anal canal (Karanjia et al 1992). Colo-anal anastomoses can be constructed either using an endo-anal approach or by stapling the mobilized left colon onto the top of the anus. Unfortunately function after colo-anal anastomosis is less than satisfactory, because of loss of the rectal reservoir. This leads to urgency because defaecation cannot be deferred. Thus in elderly patients, and those with weak sphincters, it is preferable to construct a rectal reservoir, using a J pouch constructed from two 8 cm limbs of distal colon. The apex of the reservoir can then be anastomosed to the anus using one of the techniques described above (Nicholls et al 1988).

Tactics

Bowel preparation
Surgery on the colon is, while faeces are present, like stepping into a cesspool. Every effort should be made to have a completely empty colon before surgery. Indeed it is a criterion of excellence that this should be so. An empty bowel can be achieved by:

1. Oral cathartics.
2. Antegrade lavage by the use of either:
   a. constant infusion by a nasogastric tube of up to 12 l of saline over 3 hours, or
   b. one of the ethylene glycol solutions.

These methods cannot work in obstructed patients which include not only those admitted as emergencies, but also patients with slowly progressive but high grade stenosis. In such circumstances it is traditional to say that resection is contraindicated, or resection may be undertaken but primary reconstruction is not to be done. Such a view may no longer prevail in that the bowel can be prepared on the operating table (see The *management of obstruction* below).

Perioperative antibiosis
Though oral antibiotics as a method of 'sterilizing' the bowel have been shown to be effective in reducing septic wound complications, they carry the risk of intestinal superinfection and are not now recommended. There is by contrast ample evidence to support the safety and efficacy of perioperative antibiosis, either systemically or by local application. Some form of such prophylaxis should be routine. My present preference is:

Cefuroxime 1.5 Gm and
Metronidazole 500 mg

both given i.v. at induction of anaesthesia followed by two further doses at 8-hourly intervals. The postoperative doses can be omitted following straight forward resections. In addition, at the conclusion of the operation the operative site and general peritoneal cavity is washed out with at least a litre of saline containing 1 g/l of tetracycline. Some 200 ml of the same solution are used to irrigate the superficial layers of the wound. There are many alternative techniques for chemoprophylaxis.

Other tactical measures
In large bowel surgery these include: correction of preoperative anaemia; reversal of starvation (though not prolonged preoperative nutritional support) and avoidance of low blood pressure states which adversely affect colonic blood flow.

Operative techniques
Rather than describe each operation, the general surgical techniques appropriate to all colonic surgery will be given. From these the operations can easily be assembled to deal with any individual lesion.

Position on the operating table
For surgery of the right colon the patient lies supine and the surgeon stands to the patient's right (Fig. 22.30). In all other circumstances it is strongly recommended

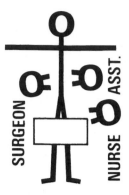

Fig. 22.30   Position of operating team for right hemicolectomy (Reproduced with permission from Dudley, 1977)

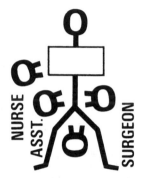

Fig. 22.31   Position of operating team for left colon procedures (Reproduced with permission from Dudley, 1977)

that the lithotomy-Trendelenberg (Lloyd Davies) position is used and that the surgeon is on the patient's left (Fig. 22.31). This not only facilitates assistance — a second assistant if available can be between the legs — but allows the surgeon freedom to change his position or move from, say, a handsewn to a peranal stapled procedure, or even to resort to an abdomino-perineal excision (p. 505) as necessary. The disposition of the operating team is shown in Figure 22.31 and though unfamiliar to many at first, has proven most satisfactory in use over the last 20 years. Mobilization of the splenic flexure is facilitated if the operator stands between the legs.

Incision

Planned right sided surgery can be carried out through a transverse incision at the level of the umbilicus and which must cross both rectus sheaths. Such an approach may even facilitate the dissection of a bulky lesion in the proximal transverse colon from the lower border of the third part of the duodenum. Indeed, my current preference is to use transverse incisions for all colo-rectal resections, as they afford excellent access, and have a low incidence of postoperative herniation.

If a stoma is required, the incision can be made a little lower. Many surgeons use generous vertical midline incisions because they provide access to all parts of the abdomen.

Midline incisions are closed with a single layer of loop No 1 Polydioxonone with 1 cm deep bites. It is my preference to close transverse incisions using a layered technique with the same suture material, since this leads to a less bulky scar.

Exploration

A full laparotomy is undertaken in a systematic manner, ascertaining in particular the nodal status and the presence or absence of hepatic metastases. Synchronous or other neoplasms in the large bowel have been largely eliminated by preoperative barium enema and/or endoscopy but the colon should be carefully palpated. In circumstances where neither of the preoperative investigations has been done the flexible fibreoptic sigmoidoscope can be inserted into the empty residual bowel to ascertain its normality.

Principles of mobilization

The colon is, at the final stage of gastrointestinal rotation, firmly tucked back against the posterior abdominal wall in the lumbar groove and anchored by the parietal peritoneum of the lateral paracolic gutters. It follows that the only intrinsically free parts are the

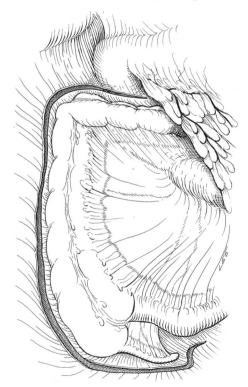

Fig. 22.32   Mobilization of the right colon

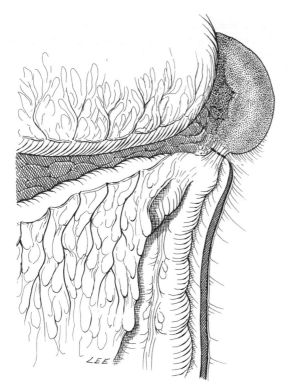

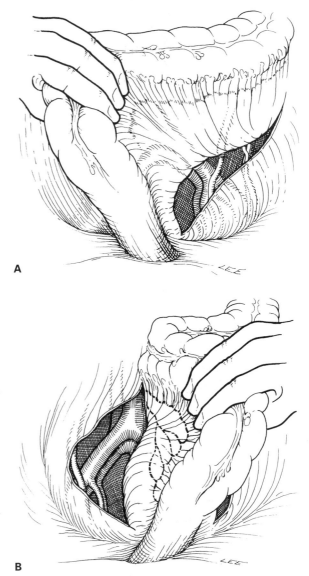

Fig. 22.33 Mobilization of the left colon and splenic flexure. Note the 'adhesion' to the lower pole of the spleen

Fig. 22.34 **A** Division of the left side of the sigmoid mesentery. **B** Mobilization of the sigmoid colon from the right

transverse and sigmoid colons and these are held at the hepatic and splenic flexures and at the junction of distal sigmoid and rectum. Mobilization of the colon requires division of these parietal peritoneal attachments: in the right paracolic gutter in order to free the caecum, ascending and proximal transverse colon (Fig. 22.32); in the left paracolic gutter to mobilize the left half of the transverse and descending colon (Fig. 22.33) where, in addition, a very constant band connecting the left edge of the omentum and the lower pole of the spleen should be divided early in order to avoid tearing the splenic capsule. In the transverse colon the omentum may be detached from the colon along its bloodless union by turning it up and slitting with the scissors along Pauchet's bloodless line; or the omentum may be taken down from the epiploic vessels and incorporated in the resection as shown in Figure 22.33. In either event, it is important to lift the omentum forwards and medially from the splenic flexure so as to divide the highest part of the peritoneum lateral to and above the colon — the so-called left phrenocolic 'ligament'. Turning the dissection medially at this point allows the operator access to the left end of the transverse mesocolon below the splenic hilum and pancreatic tail. The sigmoid colon and hence the upper rectum are mobilized by incision of the two leaves of the sigmoid mesentery (Fig. 22.34A & B). On the left (A) the common

iliac vessels and ureter are found with the gonadal vessels laterally; on the right the dissection begins over the front of the bifurcation (B) and may have been preceded by flush ligation of the inferior mesenteric artery (see below). The distal sigmoid and upper rectum are freed by extending the two sigmoid mesenteric cuts downward and anteriorly across the floor of pelvis behind the bladder in the male and uterus in the female (Fig. 22.35). The late Mr T McW Miller, a colleague of Eric Farquharson's, pointed out that this U shaped incision is best made early in the procedure before the anatomy is distorted.

Once any or all of these incisions in the parietal

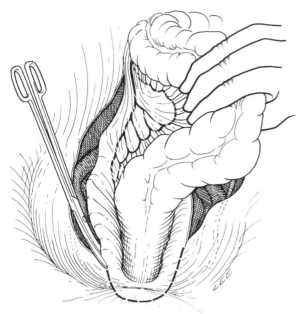

Fig. 22.35 The peritoneal mobilization required to free the rectosigmoid

peritoneum are made — and this should be done by insinuating the blades of the scissors under the peritoneum and raising the layer so that the cut is made under direct vision — the dissection takes place in the *fascia propria*. This is a dense meshwork of connective tissue in which the retroperitoneal structures are embedded; it must be formally entered and opened up. In particular, sweeping the fascia propria away from the posterior aspect of the mesentery of ascending and descending colons makes sure the gonadal vessels and, more medially, the ureter are displaced on to the posterior abdominal wall. In the case of the ureter such dissection should proceed as required downwards over the iliac vessels and brim of the pelvis so that the ureter is displaced laterally and the mesocolon medially.

Vascular mobilization

The cancer operations of right hemicolectomy, transverse colectomy, left hemicolectomy and sigmoid resection are based upon the above peritoneal mobilizations and the division of the vascular supply of the segment at its root so that a fan shaped area of mesentery and its contained lymph nodes can be removed in one piece. Wide mesenteric resection is regarded by most as essential. In the classical approach to resection the peritoneal mobilization is done first, traction is applied to the colon so freed, in order that the vascular pedicle can be drawn into view and divided. Some years ago Turnbull, at the Cleveland Clinic, suggested that such a way of proceeding by handling the tumour, invited the detachment and embolization of tumour cells to the liver. He recommended a 'no touch' tech-

nique in which vascular and mesenteric division was undertaken first, so isolating the tumour. Though the figures he adduced to support this approach do not stand up to rigorous analysis, the technique is rational, elegant and the present writer's preference. It has the additional advantage that it permits clear delineation of a line of good vascularity in the rare circumstances where the marginal artery and vein are incomplete. In addition, in tumours where it is possible to get beyond the growth before mobilization is begun, the possibility of intraluminal spread by detachment can be guarded against by tying a tape tightly around the bowel 4 cm proximal and distal to the lesion.

Whether the mobilization is done lateromedially or mediolaterally the vessels should be divided as close to their root as is possible. Though the anatomy is moderately constant, no assumption can be made and each vessel is dissected and formally displayed.

For *right hemicolectomy* the middle colic/ileocolic trunk is identified to the right of the fourth part of the duodenum (Fig. 22.36), a procedure that can be made easier by dividing the peritoneum below the terminal ileum (lower arrow Fig. 22.34) and insinuating the finger upwards behind the ileocolic mesentery. For transverse colectomy the middle colic trunk alone is ligated in the same position. For any tumour at or beyond the splenic flexure it is best, if an adequate node

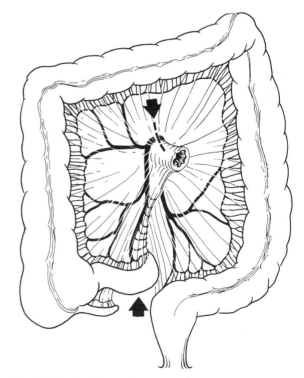

Fig. 22.36 Arteries supplying the colon – branches of superior and inferior mesenteric. Arrows show initiation of right mediolateral colonic mobilization

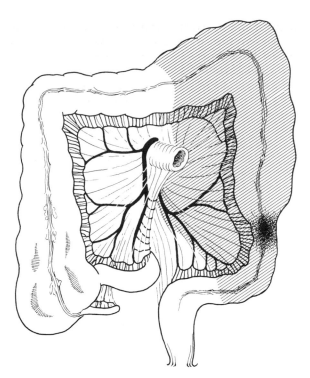

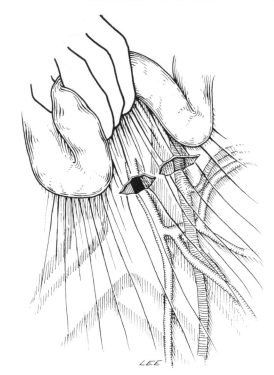

Fig. 22.37 Early ligation of the inferior mesenteric trunk delineates the bowel which must be resected in left colectomy

Fig. 22.38 The division of the inferior mesenteric artery and vein

dissection is to be achieved, to make a flush ligation of the inferior mesenteric trunk and to remove bowel as indicated in the shaded area of Figure 22.37. As long as the marginal supply is satisfactory the splenic flexure is mobilized (see above) for more distal tumours rather than resected. To dissect the inferior mesenteric vessels the fourth part of the duodenum is mobilized by dividing the peritoneum which flows from its lower border on to the anterior face of the infrarenal aorta (Fig. 22.38). This exposes the artery on the left antero-lateral face of the aorta with the vein more in the mesenteric substance laterally. When both have been ligated and divided the distal ligatures may be left uncut to provide traction against which the division of the mesenteric leaves laterally is undertaken and the peritoneal mobilization on the right side of the sigmoid mesentery (see Fig. 22.34B) carried down the front of the aorta and over the pelvic brim and sacral promontory in front of the *left* common iliac vein.

We have now completely described colonic mobilization with the exception of the two ends. Proximally, the medially-turning branch of the ileocolic artery runs along the upper border of the terminal ileum as a marginal vessel and is simply divided, usually preserving as much terminal ileum as possible so as to maintain the enterohepatic bile salt circulation and so prevent diarrhoea. At the distal end the situation is more complex. When restorative resection of a distal sigmoid tumour

is undertaken the bowel will have been mobilized as already described. The rectosigmoid junction is next lifted out of the pelvis by: first mobilizing the whole mass of the bowel and bulky perirectal fat from behind by blunt dissection in the hollow of the sacrum; and second, by entering the plane anterior to the rectum. By these two moves the proximal rectum is brought up but remains enveloped in a fatty/vascular sheath, laterally (lateral rectal 'ligaments') and behind (the superior rectal artery and vein). The former can usually be divided freely but the latter is dissected piecemeal and sectioned between ligatures until only a relatively narrow muscular-mucosal tube of rectum remains. For sigmoid and upper to mid-rectal tumours where a restorative resection is to be done, it is strongly recommended that the splenic flexure is fully mobilized and swung down on to the pelvic brim so, when most if not all the rectum has been removed, to lie in a floppy and redundant manner in the hollow of the sacrum. Failure to do this may result in a stretched and potentially ischaemic bowel.

Restoration of continuity

Sutures. In the last decade or so it has become apparent, particularly thanks to the work of John Goligher (1984), that imperfections in colonic anastomoses are relatively common. Both clinical leaks with either general peritonitis or a faecal fistula occur in upwards of 8–10% of most series and subclinical leaks — detected by radiological contrast examination — in anything from an extra 10 to 50% depending on the site of anastomosis and the skills of the operator. Though many factors — blood supply, the quality of bowel preparation, prolonged operating time and age, for example — have been implicated, it remains fundamental that a technically satisfactory anastomosis without tension is the key to success. Individual series with low radiological leak rates (3–5%) have been published which bear out the importance of technique.

The conventional two layer anastomosis with an inner 'all coats' continuous suture of absorbable material to make the junction haemostatic and watertight with an outer layer of interrupted nonabsorbable material to ensure serosal apposition (when contiguous serosal surfaces are present) has become established as the norm (p. 346). Yet from the days of Halsted there have existed several theoretical, experimental and practical arguments against it. The theoretical and experimental is that healing takes place chiefly on the serosal aspect and that all-coats apposition does not contribute to this. Both experimental and practical observations show that continuous full thickness sutures produce linear necrosis by strangulation and that the best clinical results with handsewn anastomoses have been those which did not use a two layer technique but relied simply on an outer interrupted coaptation. An additional factor is that two layer anastomosis may be associated with snagging between the two sutures — inner and outer — (Fig. 22.39) which makes necrosis between the sutures wellnigh inevitable.

These problems suggest that a one layer reconstruction is the ideal. Absorbable, relatively non irritant materials such as 4/0 polydioxone are the sutures of choice and an extramucosal but otherwise full thickness suture

exploits the strength of the submucosa but allows mucosa to regenerate across the suture line.

The bowel is carefully prepared so that there is a good blood supply. It is important not to clear the bowel excessively, since this may compromise the

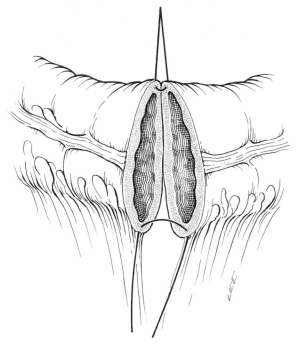

Fig. 22.40 Stay sutures placed for single layer anastomosis

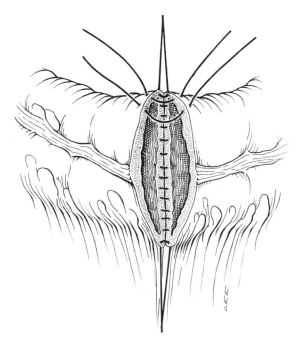

Fig. 22.41 Principles of single layer extramucosal anastomosis

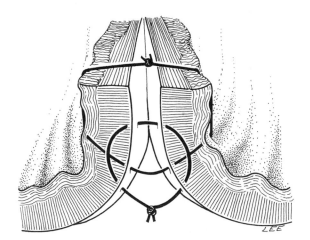

Fig. 22.39 Snagging of the two layers – a danger of conventional anastomosis

blood supply. Every stitch is precisely inserted through bowel wall. Stay sutures are next placed (Fig. 22.40) so that gentle tension permits unequal lumens to be brought into opposition. If the terminal ileum is the proximal opening then an oblique division is often required to avoid a major discrepancy between ileum and colon. Next, sutures are placed precisely with 1–1.5 mm bites through all layers except the mucosa. With a fully serosa-covered mobile bowel the knots are placed externally (Fig. 22.41) but there need be little hesitation in tying towards the lumen if this is more convenient. All sutures are best placed on each aspect before any is tied. The end result is a 'butt-ended' extramucosal apposition (Fig. 22.42). The stay sutures are finally tied and although mesenteric defects are frequently closed, the author does not consider this is necessary (Fig. 22.43).

For those who still feel more comfortable — albeit without any evidence — with a 2-layer anastomosis, an inner layer of continuous 4/0 polydioxone (PDS or maxon) is gently inserted either after the posterior all coats row or, if the anastomosis can be turned round to expose either face, before the outer layer is done.

Stapling. Since the dawn of modern surgical time, surgeons have sought alternative, more precise techniques of co-apting tissues, particularly hollow tubes. The initial devices everted tissue edges but more recently inverting techniques which closely approach tried and established hand sutured methods have been introduced. Numerous rechargeable or disposable devices are available, all working on the principle of bringing the two ends of bowel together over an 'anvil' and then inserting staples through the full thickness of the bowel wall, while at the same time cutting a central core with a circular knife (Fig. 22.44A, B). The result is a full thickness but single layer interrupted anastomosis either with a row or a staggered double row of staples. The anastomosis heals as does a single layer suture procedure but there may be delay in mucosal apposition.

Stapling devices do not provide an easy alternative to hand suturing for the beginner. They are precision instruments which exact the same need for care in the preparation of the bowel and precise insertion of the purse string (Fig. 22.45). A fine sense of tissue apposition is needed before the device is fired, though aids are now available to assess tissue thickness (Fig. 22.46). There is no doubt that stapling can achieve a sound anastomosis. Many surgeons currently regard it as the appropriate technique for a low sigmoid tumour which after adequate distal resection requires anastomosis of the descending colon or splenic flexure below the peritoneal reflexion. The device is inserted from below and purse string applied to proximal and distal bowel, tightened and the instrument fired. It can then be with-

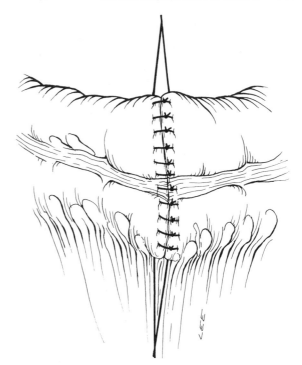

Fig. 22.42

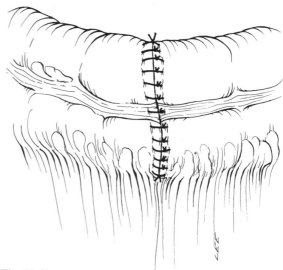

Fig. 22.43

Figs 22.42 & 22.43   The anastomosis completed

drawn per anum. For details of technical problems and practical advice the reader is referred to the recent publications (see p. 498).

The obstructed case

Left sided tumours in particular tend to narrow the bowel lumen; the patient presents as an emergency

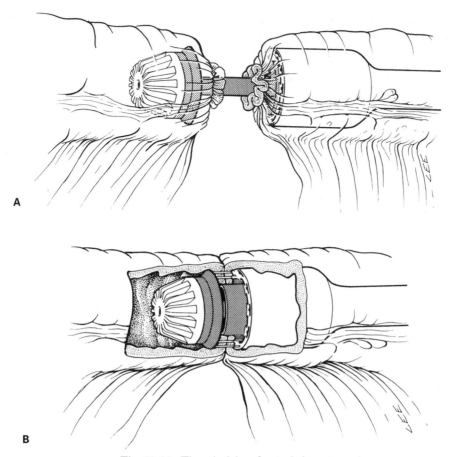

Fig. 22.44   The principles of a stapled anastomosis

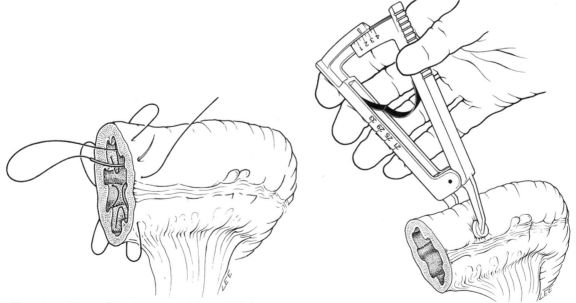

Fig. 22.45   The preferred purse string for a stapled anastomosis. Very small bites should be taken

Fig. 22.46   Method of assessment of tissue thickness

with acute colonic obstruction or with subacute obstruction so that there is banked up faeces and gas behind a narrow lumen. The one situation merges into the other.

In acute or acute-on-chronic obstruction the danger lies in progressive caecal dilatation with the development of a gangrenous patch and ultimate rupture. A profound degree of gaseous distension of the colon and/or right iliac fossa tenderness are the only indications for really urgent surgery. Otherwise most patients can be tided over a day or two for more leisurely assessment and an operation at a more convenient time. Nevertheless, it is unusual before operation to be able to empty the colon proximal to the lesion to the high standard now deemed mandatory for definitive colonic surgery.

The conventional answer to this situation has been to establish a proximal defunctioning colostomy (Fig. 22.47A) and then after a variable interval to resect the tumour, either eliminating the colostomy (Fig. 22.47B) or leaving it for closure at a later stage. The disadvantages of this safe approach are logistic and humanitarian: the long expenditure of hospital time and resources; and the inconvenience of a temporary colostomy. Some patients do not reach the second or third stage because of complications or progression of their disease.

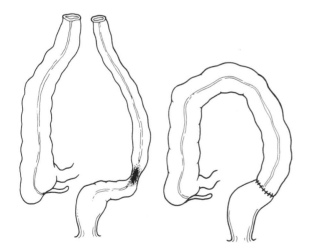

Fig. 22.47 Conventional management of the obstructed case

The alternatives are three. Immediate resection with an end colostomy followed by second stage reconstruction (Fig. 22.48); as a variant on this immediate resection, end colostomy and closure of the distal stump (Hartmann's procedure) again followed by later reconstruction (Fig. 22.49); an immediate resection and primary anastomosis. The first two are safe procedures when the bowel is unprepared. The last has great attraction in terms of short hospital stay, particularly

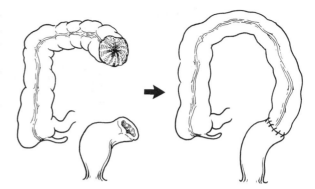

Fig. 22.48 Immediate resection and mucous fistula followed by reconstruction

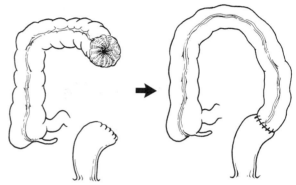

Fig. 22.49 Hartmann's resection followed by reconstruction

if there are circumstances which make the patient's life expectancy short (e.g. a locally advanced tumour or hepatic metastases).

Laparotomy in obstruction

The major cause of colonic distension is gas which contrasts with the usually liquid content of small bowel. It follows that fine needle aspiration of the colon will deflate the bowel and permit safer and easier exploration. This is achieved by attaching a 21 SWG needle to a suitable adapter and so to the suction line. The moment the abdomen is opened and distended transverse colon presents, the needle is inserted obliquely through a taenia (Fig. 22.50). Firm pressure is exerted in the flanks to drive the air up into the transverse colon. Within a few moments a tense, friable and awkward colon is collapsed and exploration and subsequent action much facilitated. The following situations are encountered:

Caecal gangrene

The presence of this potentially lethal complication rests on the competence of the ileocaecal valve. Thus the ileum is of normal diameter. Consequently, if the

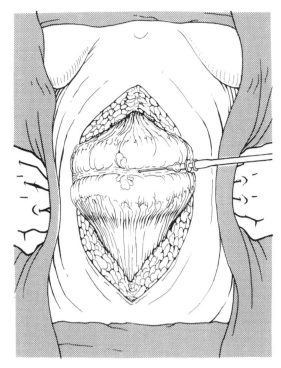

Fig. 22.50 Technique for colonic decompression in obstruction

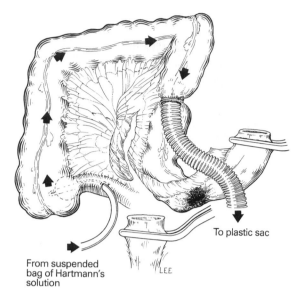

Fig. 22.51 Technique for antegrade on table irrigation in obstruction

tumour is right sided, right hemicolectomy and primary anastomosis can be done. In a left sided tumour there are three options: an extended right hemicolectomy and primary anastomosis; the same with a terminal ileostomy and mucous fistula; or exteriorization of the gangrenous patch as a caecostomy. Circumstance and experience dictate the most appropriate choice, but it cannot be too strongly emphasized that the only appropriate caecostomy is one which brings the caecal wall to the surface. After laparotomy, decompression and assessment, a small muscle cutting incision is made in the right iliac fossa, the caecum brought to the surface and healthy bowel wall beyond the gangrenous patch stitched with carefully placed absorbable seromuscular sutures to the parietal peritoneum. The patch is next excised and a submucosa to subcutaneous tissue junction fashioned (see below). Though the result may appear somewhat untidy, it is usually possible to apply a stoma bag and control the effluent quite satisfactorily. Tube caecostomies do not work and should not be done.

Caecal devitalization not present
In the absence of caecal gangrene but the presence of obstruction and a loaded bowel, a right or proximal left sided tumour may still be subjected to primary resection. The alternatives already discussed are appropriate to more distal lesions.

It remains only to consider in more detail the possibility of primary anastomosis. The contraindications have always been the loaded, unprepared bowel. Some years ago Muir proposed that this might be emptied by retrograde lavage. The technique has been modified to combine it with the desirable features of preoperative whole gut irrigation. The procedure is illustrated in Figure 22.51. The tumour is mobilized in the usual manner. The bowel is intubated proximal to the tumour but distal to the proposed site of resection with semirigid corrugated tubing and a wide bore Foley catheter is inserted into the caecum via a small ileotomy. Antegrade irrigation is now undertaken with warm Hartmann's solution, breaking up faecal masses by gentle finger pressure. Irrigation is continued until the effluent is clear. The bowel is then amputated at the site of election. Experience has shown that though distended before on table irrigation, it will now have come down to normal size and is suitable for primary anastomosis either by suture or staples. The ileal catheter can be removed or preferably left to permit an antegrade radiological study of the colocolonic suture line on the 6th to 8th day.

Temporary stomata
Indications for these in colonic surgery have already been discussed and the technique of caecostomy described.

Transverse colostomy is made on the right side and if possible the hepatic flexure is mobilized so that there is not a redundant proximal loop which can subsequently prolapse. The usual circumstance is when a laparotomy incision has already been made. Then the temptation

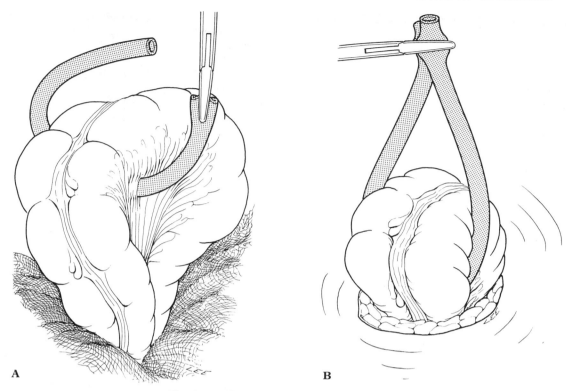

A

B

Fig. 22.52   The technique of transverse colostomy

to make a large hole for the colostomy should be resisted, as should the urge to bring it out through the same incision. A 2-finger vertical or transverse opening suffices and avoids the problems of prolapse, paracolostomy hernia and infection. The cut is taken directly through all layers in the abdominal wall, haemostasis attained and the size of the opening tested by passing the fingers through it. A convenient 6 cm length of transverse colon is stripped of greater omentum and drawn out through the wound either with a Babcock's forceps or by passing a loop of soft rubber tubing around it (Fig. 22.52). The bowel is best attached to the parietal peritoneum internally by four sutures of synthetic absorbable material (Vicryl: Dexon) and to the anterior rectus sheath or external oblique aponeurosis similarly. A rod may now be inserted beneath the loop but is rarely necessary and the old fashioned glass rod and looped rubber tubing is obsolete. More complex devices with subcutaneous plastic inserts are described but, in the writer's opinion, are quite unnecessary. A soft clamp is applied across the loop so as to prevent any inflammable gasses from being ignited by the diathermy, and the colostomy opened forthwith by a longitudinal incision made with that device. Its margins are stitched to the parieties. In all instances this is best done with an absorbable suture passing extramucosally in the bowel and subcuticularly

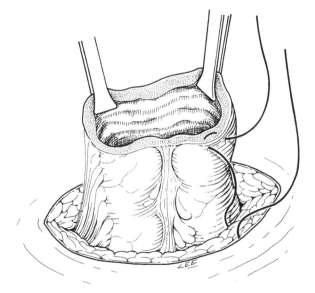

Fig. 22.53   Suturing the colon to the skin

in the skin (Fig. 22.53) (the illustration demonstrates the suture on an end colostomy as might be required after resection without anastomosis).

A useful alternative which the author prefers is to use a loop ileostomy. A trephine is made through the rectus muscle. A transverse incision 5 cm long is made in the rectus sheath, and the muscle fibres are split vertically. A loop of terminal ileum is delivered through the wound. An incision is then made through about three quarters of the distal margin, and the proximal ileum is everted to form a spout. The everted bowel is carefully sutured to the skin over a plastic rod, which prevents retraction of the bowel. Although sero-serosal sutures prevent retraction and the formation of a flush stoma, they should be kept to a minimum to facilitate closure at a later date.

OPERATIONS FOR OTHER INTESTINAL CONDITIONS

Meckel's diverticulum

In 2% of the population the segment of vitello intestinal duct joining the ileum persists on the anti-mesenteric border as a diverticulum within 80 cm of the caecum. The diverticulum may contain ectopic gastric and pancreatic tissue and gastric secretion may cause peptic ulceration in adjacent ileal mucosa. The clinical problems associated with a diverticulum are gastrointestinal haemorrhage, obstruction, acute abdominal pain and intussusception. Rarely the entire vitello intestinal duct may persist, establishing a fistula between the ileum and the umbilicus. Preoperative diagnosis of Meckel's diverticulum is difficult but in some patients labelled technetium pertechnate will demonstrate ectopic gastric mucosa. When discovered incidentally at laparotomy, it should probably be removed because of the high risk of associated pathology (Hutchinson, 1981).

Haemorrhage is most common in children under 3 years of age and it is usually accompanied by abdominal pain. Blood loss is variable; it may be insidious, resulting in iron deficiency anaemia, or sufficiently severe to cause melaena or the loss of fresh blood from the rectum.

Intestinal obstruction may result from volvulus of ileum round a persistent band that runs from the apex of the diverticulum to the umbilicus or internal herniation of small bowel caught under an adhesion between the diverticulum and adjacent mesentery. Obstruction may occur in any age group including the neonate.

Acute inflammation of the diverticulum may resemble appendicitis. For this reason the distal ileum must be carefully inspected when a normal appendix is found at laparotomy. On rare occasions the diverticulum will be found at the apex of an *intussusception* and is presumed to have been the cause.

Operation

A choice must be made between either diverticulectomy or excision of that segment of ileum carrying the diverticulum followed by end-to-end anastomosis.

The latter is favoured when the bowel adjacent to the diverticulum is oedematous or the site of a peptic ulcer, or when the ileum is of small calibre so as to ensure complete excision of ectopic tissue.

A *diverticulectomy* is performed by applying light occlusion clamps to the ileum after ligation of any supplying vessels. The diverticulum is then excised at its base and the bowel wall closed transversely in two layers (Fig. 22.54).

Crohn's disease

Regional ileitis
The acute form of this disease is indistinguishable clinically from acute appendicitis, and as a rule it is diagnosed only when the abdomen has been opened for the purpose of appendicectomy. The terminal segment of the ileum is found to be deeply congested, thickened and oedematous. Its mesentery is also much thickened, and contains enlarged glands. Usually the inflammatory process ceases abruptly at the ileocaecal junction, but the caecum also may be involved (*ileocolitis*).

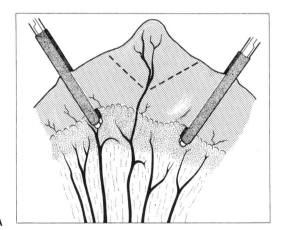

A

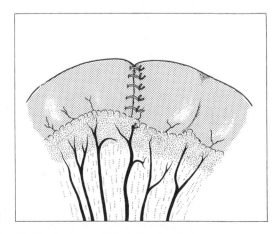

B

Fig. 22.54 Excision of Meckel's diverticulum

Abscess formation may result from perforation of the gut, but owing to adhesions general peritonitis is rare.

When the disease in its acute phase is encountered at operation for appendicectomy, no definitive procedure should be undertaken, but the appendix may be removed unless the caecum is heavily involved. About 80% of cases resolve spontaneously.

The chronic form of regional ileitis may be a legacy of one or more acute attacks, but not infrequently it appears to develop insidiously. It is characterized by mucosal ulceration, accompanied by great thickening of the submucous and muscular layers owing to granulomatous and fibro-fatty infiltration. Similar changes are found in the mesentery, and the caecum may frequently be involved in continuity with the ileum. The clinical features are those of sub-acute or intermittent obstruction, resulting from reduction in the lumen of the gut, and also diarrhoea of intermittent type. An abdominal mass may be present or the patient is noted to have suffered weight loss, malabsorption and anaemia. Fistula formation may occur — either to the exterior, or to adjacent organs such as the bladder.

Operation. Since Crohn's disease affects the whole gastrointestinal tract, surgical excision can not effect a cure (Williams, 1991). Surgery is largely confined to the management of complications such as perforation, obstruction, abscess or fistula formation. Short fibrous strictures can be opened by multiple *stricturoplasties,* incising in the line of the bowel and suturing transversely. *Resection* must be limited to macroscopically involved bowel, disease-free anastomotic margins no longer being considered essential. There is always a tendency, whatever operation is employed, for the disease to recur at a higher level and further bowel may need to be resected at a later date. Bypass procedures, such as *ileotransverse anastomosis*, are less satisfactory than resection but may be required if the bowel mass is fixed.

Segmental inflammatory bowel disease (Crohn's colitis)
Long or short segments of colon become involved by a *granulomatous* process, the changes of which are very similar to those of Crohn's disease as it affects the ileum. There is gross thickening and rigidity of all coats of the bowel, leading to a 'hosepipe' appearance, with uniform constriction of the lumen although obstructive symptoms develop less frequently than in the small bowel. It tends to involve the right side of the colon in the first instance, and to spread distally towards the rectum, so that the whole colon may eventually become affected. It is frequently associated with peri-anal suppuration (Marks, 1990) or the disease may be confined to the rectum and anal canal (Morson, 1990).

The characteristic of Crohn's colitis as seen at colonoscopy is the 'cobblestone' appearance of the mucosa. This examination also defines the extent of the condition, its segmental distribution giving rise to 'skip lesions'. Unfortunately, in many patients, a clear distinction cannot be made between Crohn's colitis and ulcerative colitis since the prognosis following surgery for Crohn's colitis is less predictable than for ulcerative colitis.

The treatment is by excisional surgery, limited to the diseased bowel. When the greater part of the colon is involved, either a threequarter colectomy with ileorectal anastomosis, or a total proctocolectomy with permanent ileostomy, will be required. In the case of localized lesions, early surgical intervention is advisable if it is difficult or impossible to exclude carcinoma.

Ileocaecal tuberculosis
Intraabdominal tuberculosis is still relatively common, is diagnosed with difficulty (Underwood, 1992) and may only be confirmed following resection of an inflammatory bowel mass for suspected Crohn's disease. Resection requires a 5 cm margin of healthy tissue rather than a formal right hemicolectomy, specific chemotherapy being given postoperatively. If tuberculosis is suspected before operation, the patient should be prepared with the appropriate antibiotics; drug sensitivity can be checked by submitting operative tissue for bacteriological studies.

Ulcerative colitis
Medical treatment of this disabling condition is of value when the disease is mild or is localized to the rectum but it is now generally accepted that in a severe or established case the changes in the colon are irreversible. Thus there is little prospect of cure unless the diseased bowel is removed. Apart from the general ill-health caused by loss of blood, mucus and fluid from the ulcerated bowel, operation may be required for life-threatening toxic dilatation, for stricture or fistula formation, or because of the risk of carcinoma (Lennard-Jones, 1990). This is a very real risk in patients with a history of 10 years or more and in those with extensive colitis, particularly if it developed during childhood. Such patients, who do not otherwise agree to surgical treatment, should have colonoscopy and multiple random biopsies every 2 years (O'Kelly, 1991).

Steroid therapy, while it has not proved to be curative, is of undoubted value in tiding the patient over an acute phase of the disease, and in improving his general condition to an extent where radical surgery becomes a relatively safe procedure. Such treatment should be combined with replacement of protein, which may have been lost in large quantities from the ulcerated bowel. It should be noted that some surgeons have blamed steroid therapy for causing extreme friability and even perforation of bowel, and advise against its use for longer than 2 weeks if no remission occurs. This suspicion is not confirmed by Goligher (1984).

The present aim of surgery in ulcerative colitis is to remove all the affected bowel. The choice lies between complete excision of both colon and rectum (*total proctocolectomy*), and excision of the colon alone, continuity of the alimentary tract being re-established by *ileorectal anastomosis*. The standard proctocolectomy is completed by fashioning a *permanent ileostomy*. However, the alternative procedure of *ileo-anal pouch anastomosis* is becoming increasingly popular for ulcerative colitis, the operation being known as *restorative proctocolectomy*. Its use requires specialised training, particularly in view of the importance of patient selection and the experience necessary to deal with complications. The principal advantage is the absence of a permanent ileostomy but the patient has to accept the associated frequency of bowel action. Depending on the patient's circumstances, a permanent ileostomy may be preferable.

Total proctocolectomy with permanent ileostomy
This procedure is still regarded by many surgeons as the best choice (Kumar, 1990), since a single operation eradicates the disease and eliminates the risk of malignancy. The rectum is usually involved by the disease to a greater or lesser extent, and, if the changes are irreversible, its normal function (including that of reservoir action) cannot be restored. If the colon alone is removed, and the rectum retained, the patient may continue to suffer from intractable diarrhoea, and may therefore be little benefited by the operation; furthermore, there is the risk of cancer. With total proctocolectomy, the patient must accept either an ileo-anal pouch or a permanent ileostomy, but the latter may be regarded as the price which he has to pay for health, if not for life itself. An ileostomy is not as grievous an affliction as might be supposed. With modern appliances to collect the ileostomy efflux, the majority of patients adapt themselves well to their disability and lead a normal life, the ileostomy interfering little with business, social or sporting activities.

The operation of total proctocolectomy may be carried out, after suitable preparation, as a single procedure or in two stages in a seriously ill patient. The latter leaves the rectum to be excised at a later date, either as an abdomino-perineal resection or as a restorative resection with formation of an ileo-anal pouch.

The technique of total proctocolectomy starts with excision of the rectum, usually by the synchronous combined method, but, because of the nonmalignant nature of the condition, a more restricted dissection is permissible; there is therefore less risk of interference with sexual function. The entire colon is then mobilized and its mesentery divided. The site of the ileal division is selected by careful attention to its blood supply, usually about 15 cm from the ileocaecal junction. The proximal cut-end, occluded by a clamp, is laid aside

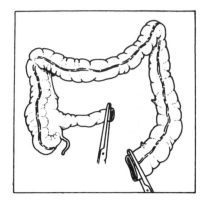

Fig. 22.55 Subtotal colectomy as performed for ulcerative colitis or for diffuse polyposis of the colon

while the ileostomy site is prepared. The ileostomy is then fashioned.

Technique of ileostomy. Ileostomy is most commonly performed as part of a one-stage proctocolectomy. It may be performed also in combination with a 'three-quarter colectomy' (Fig. 22.55), as the first stage of a total proctocolectomy. Great care should be taken with the siting and fashioning of the ileostomy stoma, since it is largely upon the accurate fitting of a collecting appliance that the success of the operation will depend. Following excision of the colon, the proximal end of ileum is brought to the surface in the right iliac fossa, through a small incision separate from the main wound, and at such a distance from it that the skin for 3–4 cm around will be free from scarring. The ideal position for the stoma is equidistant from the umbilicus, the anterior superior spine and the fold of the groin but it is advisable to confirm this in each patient by applying an ileostomy bag prior to operation, adjusting the site if necessary. A *circular* incision, 2 cm in diameter, is recommended, since it reduces the likelihood of subsequent stenosis from contraction of the scar. For the same reason, the external oblique aponeurosis, or the anterior rectus sheath, is incised in cruciate manner. The ileum, held by a clamp, is brought out so that at least 5 cm projects above the skin surface (Fig. 22.56), and is anchored by a stitch between its mesentery and the external oblique aponeurosis. The peritoneal space to the right of the emerging ileum (*the para-ileal gutter*) is closed by a running suture, which unites the cut edge of the mesentery to the peritoneum of the floor and lateral side of the right iliac fossa. Alternatively, the terminal ileum is passed along an *extraperitoneal tunnel* fashioned by the surgeon's fingers, starting within the abdomen (Goligher, 1984). Finally, the terminal half of the projecting ileum is turned back as a cuff, and the cut edge of mucosa is joined to the skin margin with 6 to 8 interrupted sutures (Fig. 22.56). As a result the ileostomy stoma takes the form of a

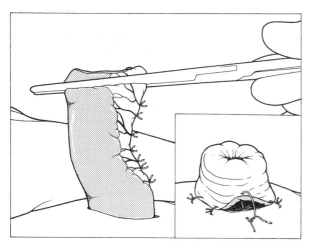

Fig. 22.56 Technique of ileostomy

completely epithelialised nipple or 'bud'; this fits accurately into the aperture of an ileostomy bag, so that the risk of leakage is diminished and skin damage is avoided.

The ideal of a reservoir or continent ileostomy devised by Kock (1976) has been largely superseded by the restorative procedure, anastomosis being achieved between a similarly constructed ileal pouch and the anal canal (Rombeau, 1992). The availability of stapling instruments has simplified the procedure but it should only be done by suitably trained surgeons.

Ileostomy in children. The indications for emergency ileostomy and the method of construction in infants is described on p. 474. The procedure for a permanent spout ileostomy in an older child with ulcerative colitis is the same as that used in the adult.

Complications of ileostomy. Difficulties of control are common, especially in less intelligent patients who cannot manage to fit their appliances correctly. They may well result, however, from an unsatisfactory ileostomy. Ideally, the efflux should drop directly into the bag, without contaminating the flange or disturbing its adherence to the skin — hence the necessity for an ileostomy which projects outwards from the skin surface. An ileostomy which is flush with the skin is very difficult to control. Excoriation of the skin around the stoma should not occur unless the ileostomy or the appliance are unsatisfactory. Relief may be obtained by changing to an alternative bag or one which is retained in position by a belt. Intestinal obstruction may occur from failure to close the para-ileal gutter, in which a loop of small bowel may become entrapped. Stenosis of the stoma, which may develop insidiously, is a frequent cause of ileostomy dysfunction. Because of the degree of obstruction produced, normal evacuation ceases, and is replaced by the continual passage of wind and watery fluid; associated with this there may be vomiting, colicky pains and abdominal distension.

Refashioning of the ileostomy should at once be undertaken in cases where, because of stenosis or difficulties of control, the existing stoma is in any way unsatisfactory. It is usually best to perform laparotomy, and to bring out the ileum anew, through a new circular incision in a part of the abdominal wall where the surrounding skin is smooth and healthy.

Colectomy with ileorectal anastomosis
This operation is designed to preserve normal sphincter control and retain the rectum as a natural reservoir but its use is restricted to cases where the rectum is either healthy or shows minimal involvement by the disease. With the development of pelvic pouch procedures, ileorectal anastomosis is now seldom indicated but may be suitable for an older patient with minimal rectal disease. Because of the risk of developing carcinoma in the rectal stump, patients must be kept under careful supervision including regular sigmoidoscopy.

The technique of ileorectal anastomosis is very similar to that described for restorative resection of the rectum except that it is often possible to preserve the whole or the greater part of the rectum, and that it is the ileum, instead of the left colon, that is brought down for the anastomosis.

Diverticulitis
This degenerative and inflammatory condition affects mainly the left side of the colon, the changes being maximal in the pelvic loop. It can give rise to symptoms and signs closely resembling those of carcinoma, and both radiological and sigmoidoscopic examination may fail to establish the diagnosis. On this account surgical intervention may be required.

At operation, often the first sign to be noted is an obvious increase in the mesenteric and pericolic fat of the pelvic colon. The bowel wall itself is thickened from muscle hypertrophy, and the changes vary from slight induration to an enormous mass involving the greater part of the pelvic colon (*peridiverticulitis*). Even at operation the condition may be difficult to distinguish from carcinoma. Owing to surrounding reaction, a peridiverticular mass is usually more fixed than a carcinoma, except when this is very far advanced. It involves a longer segment of gut, tapering-off gradually; it tends therefore to be sausage-like or spindle-shaped, and its limits are less clearly defined.

Treatment
With increasing experience of bowel resection for carcinoma, treatment of diverticulitis has become much more radical, and resection can often be considered especially if, as is frequently the case, malignancy cannot be excluded. A one-stage operation is usually possible unless inadequate bowel preparation or sepsis indicate

the dangers of proceeding with a primary anastomosis. Resection is carried out on lines very similar to those described for carcinoma of the colon, except that, when malignancy can be excluded, clearance of the glandular fields need not be so extensive.

Not infrequently certain *complications* of diverticulitis, such as intestinal obstruction, paracolic abscess, perforation or fistula formation, bring the patient to urgent surgery.

Intestinal obstruction is dealt with as described on pages 462 & 475 by a defunctioning transverse colostomy or resection.

Paracolic abscess. This usually comes to lie in contact with the abdominal wall, and may present as a visible swelling, confirmed by ultrascanning as being due to an abscess. In such cases, it can be evacuated safely through a small stab incision placed over its most prominent part.

Perforation is a most serious complication, since its very occurrence indicates that the infection is not walled-off by adhesions, and a degree of generalized peritonitis therefore results. The condition is likely to be diagnosed preoperatively as an appendix peritonitis. At operation, this diagnosis seems at first to be confirmed by the putrid smell of bowel organisms in the peritoneal cavity, but the appendix is found to be normal; further search may then disclose either a peridiverticular mass in relation to the pelvic colon, or merely some congestion and thickening of its wall, together with an increase in pericolic fat. The perforation itself may be difficult to find, but if identified should be closed by a plug of omentum or any other available tissue. Frequently, however, the changes in the colon may be comparatively slight, and the diagnosis of perforated diverticulitis may be reached only because no other cause can be found to account for the presence of malodorous pus in the pelvis. Such cases may be treated by peritoneal lavage (with 0.1% tetracycline solution) and drainage alone, for the perforation will often heal spontaneously, and there may be no recurrence. This applies particularly in the case of the aged, in whom perforated diverticulitis is comparatively common. Such patients who will not withstand immediate resection or are unlikely to come to resection later should not be burdened with a colostomy, unless this is necessary as a life-saving measure, or because a faecal fistula develops and persists after the drainage operation.

When the bowel shows gross disease, the initial treatment may be by a defunctioning transverse colostomy and later resection or by primary resection. Depending on the surgeon's experience, bowel continuity may be re-established at the same operation or later although the incidence of complications is greater when surgery is undertaken in stages (Underwood, 1984). Exteriorization of bowel ends following resection is described on page 509 (Hartmann's operation).

Colovesical fistula is a not uncommon complication of diverticulitis of the colon. Its treatment is discussed on page 636.

Haemorrhage occurs more often from diverticulosis than from diverticulitis and does not usually require operation — mainly because of the difficulty in locating the site of bleeding and hence the segment of colon which should be removed.

Polypoid disease of the colon

Two main types of polypoid tumours are recognized — *adenomata* (90%) and *villous papillomata* (10%). An adenoma may produce bleeding, prolapse or discharge. A villous papilloma more commonly results in profuse mucus discharge which may sometimes result in electrolyte depletion — particularly of potassium. Although essentially benign, each type has a risk of developing invasive cancer. This risk is much greater in the villous group whereas, the larger the adenoma, the greater the risk. All polypi should therefore be treated energetically, with the possible exception of an adenoma less than 1 cm in diameter. If they occur singly or in small numbers they are likely to be of the acquired type rather than inherited.

Single or isolated polypi

These are found most commonly in the pelvic colon or rectum (80%), but any part of the large bowel may be involved. If they can be viewed through a sigmoidoscope they may be destroyed by fulguration or removed by diathermy snare. In clinics where a colonoscope is available, endoscopic removal of polypi can be extended to all parts of the colon should the necessary expertise be available. Sessile polyps *above the peritoneal reflection* should not be treated in this way for fear of perforating the gut. Should such polypi be identified or suspected they should be subjected to colonoscopic inspection before a decision is made on treatment. A much less satisfactory alternative is laparotomy with systematic examination of the whole colon by palpation. If a polyp (detected as a mass, which does not appear to be faecal, within the bowel lumen) is milked by the fingers in either direction, the serous surface may show a dimple at the site of attachment (unless this lies on the mesenteric border), and a local excision of the tumour-bearing area can then be carried out. Larger polypi, or multiple ones confined to one segment of bowel, are treated by partial colectomy. After the removal of polypi whether locally or by partial colectomy, review of the patient should include yearly colonoscopy (Williams, 1992) or double contrast barium enema. This is necessary for several years after operation — if not for the rest of the patient's life.

Familial adenomatous polyposis (FAP)

In this rare condition (which, although inherited, does not appear usually until late childhood or early adult life) the development of carcinoma is practically certain, unless surgical treatment is carried out in the early and benign stage. Since the greater part of the colon is likely to be involved with many hundreds of polyps, a very radical excision is required, and is justified by the otherwise hopeless prognosis. Where the rectum is not seriously involved, *colectomy with ileo-rectal anastomosis* (Fig. 22.57) is a safe operation with a good functional result. Following this operation it is now recognised that polyps in the retained rectum regress in size and number but reassessment at least every 6 months is essential (Thomson, 1990). Polyps of more than 5 mm diameter may be controlled by diathermy fulguration. *Restorative proctocolectomy*, using an ileo-anal pouch anastomosis, is now used in only a minority of patients with FAP who have large sessile adenomas in the upper or mid-rectum. Patients who develop a carcinoma in the rectum require *total proctocolectomy with permanent ileostomy*.

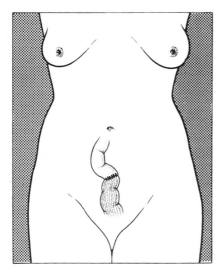

Fig. 22.57 Ileorectal anastomosis following subtotal colectomy

Hirschsprung's disease

Pathology

In this condition the autonomic innervation of the distal bowel is abnormal and causes partial or complete obstruction to the normal passage of faeces. It is thought that the normal craniocaudal migration of neuroblasts in the bowel wall is incomplete; hence the abnormal segment always includes the distal rectum and extends proximally for a variable distance. The classical histological feature of the condition is the absence of ganglion cells from Auerbach's and Meissner's plexus but, in addition, the nerve fibres in the myenteric plexus are increased both in number and size. The normal bowel proximal to the aganglionic segment is secondarily hypertrophied and dilated whilst the abnormal segment is relatively narrowed (Fig. 22.58). Hirschsprung's disease is arbitrarily divided into short or long segment according to whether the aganglionic segment is confined to the rectum and sigmoid colon or extends proximal to the junction between the descending and sigmoid colon.

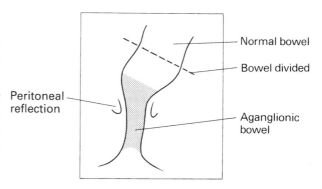

Fig. 22.58 Hirschsprung's disease longitudinal section of rectum showing the abnormality and level of bowel division

Clinical presentation

The incidence of the condition is one in 5000 births and the male to female ratio is 4 to 1. Babies with the condition are of normal birth weight and, with the possible exception of Down's syndrome, associated anomalies are rare. The clinical presentation varies from complete or partial obstruction in the new born to chronic constipation in the older child. Necrotising enterocolitis is a dangerous complication of the condition, presenting paradoxically with diarrhoea and, unless recognized and treated appropriately, it may be fatal. The diagnosis of Hirschsprung's disease is confirmed by demonstrating the histological features on a punch rectal biopsy of mucosa and sub-mucosa taken 2 cm above the dentate line. A barium enema may outline a 'coned' segment between the dilated nominal segment of bowel and the relatively narrowed distal aganglionic segment. Rectal manometry can be used to demonstrate the absence of normal relaxation of the internal sphincter in response to rectal dilatation.

Operation

The surgical management of the condition depends on the clinical presentation. In a baby with obstruction it may be possible to clear the bowel content by gentle rectal irrigation with warm saline; alternatively an emergency colostomy should be performed. In the absence of acute obstruction the diagnosis can first be established by investigation and a colostomy then fashioned prior to the definitive operation. According to preference, either a right transverse colostomy is made or a left iliac colostomy using the distal part of normal bowel. The definitive operation follows after an interval of 3 to 6 months. When the condition presents in the newborn, it is customary to delay the procedure until the baby is 9 months or reaches 10 kg in weight.

Excision of the aganglionic segment in Hirschsprung's disease presents two problems; first the technical difficulties of a low anastomosis close to the anorectal junction, and second the risk of damage to the pelvic splanchnic nerves. The different techniques designed to overcome these problems are important and have relevance to sphincter conserving operations in adult surgery. In Swenson's operation (1948), the bowel is divided above the aganglionic segment and the two ends oversewn (Fig. 22.59). The aganglionic bowel is then drawn inside-out through to the perineum by forceps introduced through the anal canal. Normal bowel is drawn down through the invaginated abnormal seg-

ment and anastomosed 2 cm from the mucocutaneous junction. The anastomosis is then pushed back through the anal opening to its normal position. In Duhamel's operation (1960) normal bowel is once again divided (Fig. 22.60). A tunnel is made from the pelvic floor posterior and lateral to the rectum and opened into the posterior wall of the anal canal at the level of the dentate line. Normal bowel is drawn down through the tunnel so that it lies alongside the rectum. The adjacent walls of rectum and small bowel are stapled and divided longitudinally so as to form a common cavity. Rectal sensation is thus preserved within the cavity, the normal bowel provides peristalsis and division of the internal sphincter reduces outlet resistance. In Soave's ano-rectal-pull through (1960), the muscle wall of the rectum is left in situ. This is achieved by circular myotomy of the pelvic floor so that the distal dissection to the anal canal can be performed in a sub-mucosal plane. Normal bowel is drawn down through the muscle cuff and left with a stump projecting beyond the

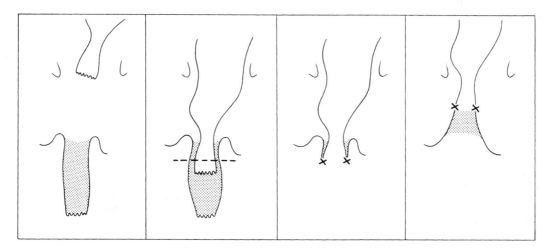

Fig. 22.59   Swenson's pull-through operation

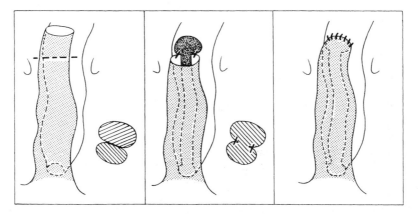

Fig. 22.60   Duhamel's operation

anal opening. After an interval, during which the normal bowel becomes fixed in position by adhesions, the stump can be excised. In a modification of this procedure, which eliminates the need for a second operation, normal bowel is anastomosed to anal mucosa. This can be achieved using a technique similar to that used by Swenson but only the rectal mucosa is pulled inside-out.

An alternative to rectosigmoidectomy is to reduce the outlet resistance of the aganglionic segment by anorectal myectomy. This was first used for older children with ultra short segment Hirschsprung's disease. More recently myectomy has been used in combination with anterior resection in children with more extensive aganglionosis (Orr & Scobie, 1979). Anorectal myectomy is performed with the child in the lithotomy position. An incision is made at the mucocutaneous junction on the posterior wall of the anal canal and a plane dissected between mucosa and underlying muscle. The strip of muscle, 0.5 to 1.0 cm in width, including the internal sphincter, is excised along the length of the aganglionic segment.

REFERENCES

Baker J W 1959 A long jejunostomy tube for decompressing intestinal obstruction. Surgery Gynaecology and Obstetrics 109: 519

Bland Sutton J 1889 Imperforate ileum. American Journal of Medical Science 98: 457

Childs W A, Phillips R B 1960 Experience with intestinal plication and a proposed modification. Annals of Surgery 152: 258

Dudley H A F 1977 Operative dispositions and ergonomics. In: Rob C, Smith R (eds) Operative surgery: general principles, breast and hernia. Butterworths, Sevenoaks, p 17

Duhamel B 1960 A new operation for the treatment of Hirschsprung's disease. Archives of Diseases of Childhood 35: 38

El-Katib Y 1973 Volvulus of the caecum: caecopexy by polyvinyl alcohol sponge. British Journal of Surgery 60: 475

Goligher J C 1984 Surgery of the anus, rectum and colon, 5th edn. Baillière Tindall, London, p 497, 828

Heald R J, Ryall P E 1981 Meckel's diverticulum. Journal of the Royal College of Surgeons of Edinburgh 26: 86–88

Hutchison G H, Randall P E 1981 Meckel's diverticulum. Journal of the Royal College of Surgeons of Edinburgh 26: 86–88

Karanjia N D, Schache D J, Heald R J 1992 Function of the distal rectum after low anterior resection for rectal carcinoma. British Journal of Surgery 79: 114–116

Kock N G 1976 Present status of the continent ileostomy; surgical revision of the malfunctioning ileostomy. Diseases of the Colon and Rectum 19: 200

Kumar D, Williams N S 1990 Surgical Management of Ulcerative Colitis. Hospital Update 16: 113–120

Lennard-Jones J E, Melville D M, Morson B C et al 1990 Precancer and cancer in extensive ulcerative colitis: findings about 401 patients over 22 years. Gut 31: 800–806

Louw J H, Barnard C N 1955 Congenital intestinal atresia. Observations on its origin. Lancet 2: 1065

Marks C G 1990 Anal lesions in Crohn's disease. Annals of the Royal College of Surgeons of England 72: 158–159

Morson B C 1990 Pathology of Crohn's disease. Annals of the Royal College of Surgeons of England 72: 150–151

Munro A, Jones P F 1978 Operative intubation in the treatment of complicated small bowel obstruction. British Journal of Surgery 65: 123–127

Neely J, Catchpole B 1971 Ileus: the restoration of alimentary-tract motility by pharmacological means. British Journal of Surgery 58: 21

Nicholls R J, Lubowski D Z, Donaldson D R 1988 Comparison of colonic reservoir and straight colo-anal reconstruction after rectal excision. British Journal of Surgery 75: 318–320

Nixon H H 1955 Intestinal obstruction in the new born. Archives of Diseases of Childhood 30: 13

Noble T B 1937 Plication of small intestine as prophylaxis against adhesions. American Journal of Surgery 35: 41

Ogilvie H 1948 Large intestine colic due to sympathetic deprivation: a new clinical syndrome. British Medical Journal 2: 671

O'Kelly T J, Mortensen N J McC 1992 Surgical management of ulcerative colitis. In: Johnson C D, Taylor I (eds) Recent advances in surgery No 15. Churchill Livingstone, Edinburgh

Orr J D, Scobie W G 1979 Anterior resection continued with anorectal myectomy in the treatment of Hirschsprung's disease. Journal of Paediatric Surgery 14: 58

Rombeau J L 1992 Operative and perioperative treatment of inflammatory bowel disease. Current Opinion in Gastroenterology 8: 694–702

Shah A J 1991 Colotomy with minimum resection for advanced irreducible intussusception. Journal of Paediatric Surgery 26: 42–43

Soave F 1966 Hirschsprung's disease: Clinical evaluation and details of a personal technique. Zeitschrift fur Kinderchirurgie Suppl. 66

Swenson O, Bill A H 1948 Resection of rectum and rectosigmoid with preservation of the sphincter for benign spastic lesions producing megacolon. Surgery 24: 212

Thomson J P S 1990 Familial adenomatous polyposis: the large bowel. Annals of the Royal College of Surgeons of England 72: 177–180

Underwood J W, Marks C G 1984 The septic complications of sigmoid diverticular disease. British Journal of Surgery 71: 209–211

Underwood M J, Thompson M M, Sayers R D, Hall A W 1992 Presentation of abdominal tuberculosis to general surgeons. British Journal of Surgery 79: 1077–1079

Welch G H, Azmy A F, Ziervogel M A 1983 The surgery of malrotation and mid gut volvulus: a nine year experience in neonates. Annals of the Royal College of Surgeons of England 65: 244–247

Williams C B, Fairclough P D 1992 Colonoscopy. Current Opinion in Gastroenterology 8: 37–49

Williams J G, Wong W D, Rothenberger D A, Goldberg S M 1991 Recurrence of Crohn's disease after resection. British Journal of Surgery 78: 10–19

Williams N S, Dixon M F, Johnston D 1983 Re-appraisal of the 5 cm rule of distal excision for carcinoma of the rectum: a study of distal intramural spread and of patients' survival. British Journal of Surgery 70: 150

Williams N S 1984 The rationale for preservation of the anal sphincter in patients with low rectal cancer. British Journal of Surgery 71: 575–581

FURTHER READING

Keighley M R B, Grobler S P 1993 Results of restorative proctocolectomy in ulcerative colitis. In: Taylor I, Johnson C D (eds) Recent advances in surgery 16. Churchill Livingstone, Edinburgh

Mortensen N 1990 New thoughts and methods in colorectal cancer. In: Hadfield J, Hobsley M, Treasure T (eds) Current surgical practice, vol 5, Edward Arnold, London

Nicholls J, Bartolo D, Mortensen N 1993 Restorative proctocolectomy. Blackwell, Oxford

Thomas P E, Taylor T V 1991 Pelvic pouch procedures. Butterworth–Heinemann, Oxford

23

Operations on the rectum and anal canal

D. C. C. BARTOLO, J. M. S. JOHNSTONE & R. F. RINTOUL

Anatomy

The rectum

This is the direct continuation of the pelvic colon, and, when straightened out, is about 12 cm in length. It begins opposite the third piece of the sacrum, and follows the curvature of the sacrum and coccyx; it ends 2.5 cm beyond the tip of the coccyx by making an acute angle concave backwards with the anal canal.

The rectum has three lateral curvatures or *flexures* — the upper and lower being convex to the right, and the middle convex to the left. Corresponding to the flexures, *horizontal folds*, consisting of mucous and circular muscle coats, project into the lumen of the gut (Fig. 23.1). The lower third of the rectum is somewhat dilated, and is termed the *ampulla*.

Relations. The upper third of the rectum is clothed with peritoneum anteriorly and on each side; the middle third is covered only in front, while the lower third is entirely devoid of peritoneal covering because it lies below the peritoneum of the pelvic floor. The upper two-thirds is related anteriorly to the recto-vesical (or recto-uterine) pouch and to its contents (a coil of ileum or pelvic colon and the retroverted uterus that is normal in 20% of females). The lower third is related in the male to the base of the bladder, with the seminal vesicles and vasa deferentia intervening, and, below this, to the prostate; in the female it is related to the posterior vaginal wall. Posteriorly, the rectum lies first in front of the sacrum and coccyx, and then the raphe of the levatores ani, which converge on it from the side walls of the pelvis.

Blood supply (Fig. 23.2). Arteries supplying the rectum are the *superior, middle and inferior rectal,* and the *middle sacral.* The superior rectal, a single vessel formed as the continuation of the inferior mesenteric, divides into two branches, which run down the posterior wall of the rectum. The middle and inferior rectal arteries are bilateral; the middle arises from the internal iliac artery in the pelvis and the inferior is a branch of the pudendal artery in the perineum. The middle sacral is a single twig branching directly from the aorta. The veins

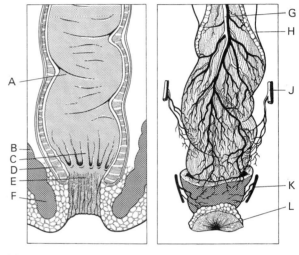

Fig. 23.1   **Fig. 23.2**

Fig. 23.1   Musculature and internal structure of rectum and anal canal (coronal section)

Fig. 23.2   Blood supply of rectum and anal canal (posterior view)

Annotations for Figures 23.1 and 23.2 (A) Horizontal fold; (B) Levator ani; (C) Anal columns; (D) Internal sphincter; (E) Pectinate line; (F) External sphincter; (G) Superior rectal vessels; (H) Peritoneum; (J) Middle rectal vessels; (K) Inferior rectal vessels; (L) Anus

drain partly into the portal system by the superior rectal vein and partly into the systemic veins through the middle and inferior rectal and middle sacral veins. Thickened bands in the investing fascia accompany the middle rectal vessels, stretching between the rectum and the side walls of the pelvis and are termed *lateral ligaments.*

Lymph drainage. Lymph vessels of the rectum drain first to glands lying alongside the viscus and within its fascial sheath (*pararectal glands*). From the pararectal glands related to the upper two-thirds of the rectum further drainage occurs mainly to glands in the pelvic mesocolon, along the course of the superior rectal and inferior mesenteric vessels. From the lowermost pararectal glands efferents pass laterally across both surfaces of levator ani to glands alongside the internal iliac and common iliac vessels.

The anal canal

This is 4 cm in length, and passes downwards and backwards from the lower end of the rectum to the anal orifice which is defined arbitrally as the point where the anal canal begins to increase in diameter. The upper two-thirds of the canal is surrounded by the internal sphincter, a condensation of the lowermost circular fibres of the rectum. The physiological external sphincter, composed of striated muscle, is in effect the levator ani fibres as they encircle the anal canal. The important feature is the puborectalis sling — those fibres of levator which, arising from the pubis, pass backwards and around the canal just distal to the internal sphincter but fused with it. The levatores ani are inserted into the sides of the canal between the overlapping internal and external sphincters.

The mucous membrane of the anal canal is loosely attached, and in the upper part presents a number of longitudinal folds, called *anal columns*; these are joined at their lower ends by crescentic folds termed *anal valves*. The level of the valves is marked by a white wavy line the line of Hilton or *pectinate line*. The part of the canal above this line is lined by columnar epithelium, the part below by modified stratified epithelium, which at the anal orifice takes on the character of true skin. The skin around the anal orifice contains numerous sebaceous and sweat glands.

Relations. Anteriorly the anal canal is related in the male to the apex of the prostate and to the membranous and bulbous parts of the urethra; in the female it is related to the lower third of the vagina. On each side the levator ani separates the canal from the ischiorectal fossa. Posteriorly the canal is related to the tip of the coccyx and to the anococcygeal raphe.

Blood supply is derived from descending branches of all three rectal arteries. Corresponding veins communicate with each other in a plexus (*haemorrhoidal plexus*) lying in the anal cushions which are analagous to erectile tissue and complete the closure of the anal canal.

Lymph drainage. Lymphatics from the upper part of the anal canal accompany the inferior rectal vessels across the ischiorectal fossa, and pass to internal iliac (*hypogastric*) glands. Lymphatics from the lower part of the canal and from the anal margin drain to the superficial inguinal glands on both sides.

The ischiorectal fossa is a wedge-shaped space filled with fat, lying on each side of the anal canal. Its base lies downwards at the skin surface, and its thin edge, which is directed upwards, lies along the attachment of levator ani to the fascia covering obturator internus. It is bounded medially by the levator and anal canal, and laterally by the ischium covered by obturator internus. The *internal pudendal vessels* run forward in the substance of its lateral wall; they give off the *inferior rectal vessel*, which cross the fossa to reach the bowel.

PROCTOSCOPY AND SIGMOIDOSCOPY

For proctoscopy in the average patient, whose bowels have already moved on the day of examination, no special preparation is required. This may apply equally well to sigmoidoscopy, since small masses of solid faeces do not materially interfere with the examination. In preparation for flexible sigmoidoscopy, a phosphate enema in conveniently given about an hour before the examination.

A male patient may be examined in the knee-elbow position, but the left lateral position, with the buttocks over the edge of the table (see Fig. 23.3) is preferred by most patients. Unless the patient is excessively nervous, an anaesthetic is unnecessary and should be avoided, since, in the unconscious patient, there is an inescapably greater risk of damage to the bowel. Both proctoscope and sigmoidoscope should be well lubricated before use.

Proctoscopy

The proctoscope (or anal speculum) enables a visual examination to be made of the lower part of the rectum and the anal canal. With the obturator in situ, the instrument is introduced gently and with due regard to the direction of the anal canal, i.e. in a line pointing forwards towards the umbilicus. When its point is felt to have passed the resistance offered by the sphincters and to have entered the rectum, its direction is altered so that it points posteriorly towards the hollow of the sacrum, and in this line it is inserted to its fullest extent. The obturator is removed and a light is directed into the speculum. The mucous membrane of the rectum is examined, and any abnormalities such as inflammation, ulceration or tumour are noted. The speculum is now slowly withdrawn, when the internal end of the anal canal will be seen to close over it. If internal haemorrhoids are present they will project into the speculum at this stage, and their number, size and position should be noted.

If the proctoscope requires to be reinserted, it should be completely withdrawn and the obturator refitted.

Sigmoidoscopy

By the use of the rigid sigmoidoscope, which is about 30 cm in length, the whole of the rectum and the lower part of the pelvic colon can be examined. The instrument is passed through the anal canal in a direction towards the umbilicus (Fig. 23.3). *As soon as its point is*

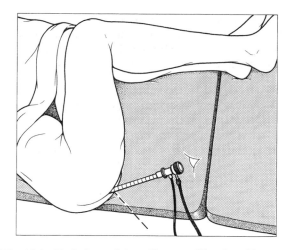

Fig. 23.3 Technique of sigmoidoscopy. The sigmoidoscope is introduced through the anal canal in the direction shown by the broken line. It is then advanced, under direct vision, around the hollow of the sacrum

felt to have entered the rectum all further introduction must be carried out under direct vision. The obturator is therefore withdrawn; the glass eye-piece and light-carrier are fitted, and the bellows is attached. The sigmoidoscope is now directed posteriorly (Fig. 23.3), so that it lies in the line of the rectum, and by circumduction of the instrument the rectal wall is thoroughly examined. The horizontal folds are encountered and are easily circumvented as the sigmoidoscope is passed upwards. As it follows the sacral curve its point must gradually be directed more anteriorly towards the pelvirectal junction, which often lies a little to one side, usually the left. As the bowel is sharply kinked at this level, the introduction of the instrument into the pelvic colon is the most difficult part of the operation, but, by careful manipulation always under direct vision, and by gentle inflation of the bowel, the lumen can usually be made to open out in advance of the instrument. By continuing in the same manner the sigmoidoscope can, in favourable cases, be passed up to its full extent, so that the greater part of the pelvic colon can be examined.

During the introduction of the sigmoidoscope, and again during its withdrawal, the condition of the bowel wall and the presence of any tumour formation are noted. The colour of a tumour is almost invariably a brighter red than that of the surrounding mucosa. The proliferative type of carcinoma has an irregular nodular surface which is friable and bleeds easily; in a growth of the ulcerative type the appearance of the raised everted margin is characteristic. A simple tumour is usually pedunculated; if it is smooth and lobulated it is probably a tubular adenoma. Simple growths of sessile type may be difficult to distinguish from carcinoma and in such cases a portion should be removed for biopsy, by

means of special long forceps introduced through the sigmoidoscope. Various inflammatory conditions have their own characteristic appearance which usually involve the entire bowel under inspection whereas a tumour tends to be localized. Thus, if no normal mucosa can be seen, the condition is probably inflammatory.

When a tumour is encountered, and if it does not obstruct the passage of the instrument, it is an advantage to examine the bowel above, in order to ascertain the extent of the growth, and to ensure that a second tumour at a higher level is not missed.

Flexible fibreoptic sigmoidoscope
Flexible sigmoidoscopy is now the initial investigation for a patient with rectal bleeding for which a cause cannot be established with the proctoscope. It is commonly carried out on an out-patient basis, the only necessary preparation being a phosphate enema given immediately prior to the examination. Since over 70% of colon cancers arise in the distal colon, inspection of the bowel up to the full length of the instrument — 60 cm — will detect a worthwhile proportion of malignant lesions with greater certainty than a barium enema. Biopsy of any abnormal lesion is submitted for histological examination and the distance between the abnormality and the anal margin is noted. Inflammatory bowel disease may also be diagnosed and its extent assessed, including the presence of 'skip lesions'. Flexible sigmoidoscopy is ideal for detecting polyps and for obtaining appropriate biopsies. If necessary, the examination is complemented by barium enema or colonoscopy.

WOUNDS AND INJURIES

Injuries of the anal canal and rectum are commonly caused by the patient sitting or falling astride on some sharp object such as a spiked railing. Injury less commonly results from a severely fractured pelvis with mobile bony fragments and may be overlooked because of damage to other organs. Penetration of the rectal wall, or even of the mucosa alone, is liable to give rise to a severe pelvic cellulitis, to which both streptococci and anaerobic organisms contribute. Where the peritoneum has been entered peritonitis may result.

It is important to note that such injuries may occur in the absence of any external damage, particularly with a fractured pelvis. A slender object may pass into the anal canal or rectum before penetrating its wall, and rupture of the rectum may occur simply as the result of a blow on the anal region. In such cases of suspected internal damage the bowel should be carefully examined under an anaesthetic. The sphincter is stretched, and the examination is carried out both by the finger and by the aid of a proctoscope.

Lacerations of the anal canal are best left open and packed with gauze. If a penetrating wound of the rectum is found, it is rarely possible or desirable to repair it by primary suture. It is wiser to be content with providing free drainage through the anal canal. This is done by leaving a corrugated drain or a loosely inserted gauze pack in contact with the damaged area, and by bringing it out through the anus. Drainage may be further improved by division of the sphincter in the midline posteriorly. If the damage to the rectum is severe it may be advisable to provide complete rest to the part by means of a temporary colostomy. Broad spectrum antibiotics are given in full dosage.

In all cases a careful watch must be kept for the development of pelvic cellulitis, and a secondary operation for drainage of the perirectal tissues may be required.

In wounds of the buttocks and perineal region the wound should be enlarged if necessary to permit of careful exploration, in order that penetration to the rectum does not pass undetected. If the rectal wall is seen to be torn no attempt should be made to suture it, but free drainage of the perirectal tissues is provided, by enlarging the wound as necessary and by the insertion of a gauze pack. If the tear is a large one the advisability of a colostomy should be considered. At the same time an opportunity is taken to examine for, and to exclude, any intraperitoneal injury.

Intraperitoneal injuries. Penetration to the peritoneal cavity may be suspected, either at the initial clinical examination, or after the condition of the rectum has been more fully investigated in the operating theatre. In either case an immediate laparotomy should be carried out *as the first step in operative treatment.* If an intraperitoneal rupture is found it is repaired in two layers, and a drain is left in the pelvis. Unless the rupture is a comparatively small one a pelvic colostomy should be performed. Lavage with 0.1% tetracycline solution is carried out in all cases.

Gunshot wounds of the rectum are particularly serious, owing to their inaccessibility, the frequency of damage to other structures, and especially because of the risks of a virulent infection of the retroperitoneal tissues. Early exploration of the wound is therefore essential; devitalized tissues are excised, and free posterior drainage of the perirectal space is provided through a curved incision in front of the coccyx. In nearly all cases a colostomy should be performed.

BENIGN TUMOURS AND STRICTURES OF THE RECTUM

Benign tumours of the rectum and of the colon

These have the same pathology and frequently co-exist.

Their great importance lies in the tendency which they show towards malignant change. The classification of such tumours (polypoid disease) of the colon has already been described (p. 494).

Tumours of the lower half of the rectum can be detected easily by the examining finger, and, if pedunculated, may be delivered through the anus. Tumours at a higher level in the rectum are diagnosed by sigmoidoscopy. If the tumour is sessile and of large size, or shows any evidence of induration, biopsy should be performed in view of the serious suspicion of malignancy. When an apparently benign tumour is found in the rectum, careful search by flexible sigmoidoscopy and double-contrast barium enema, or by colonoscopy, should be made for another lesion, especially a carcinoma, at a higher level, for the association of such lesions is a very common one.

Benign tumours in the lower rectum

If the tumour is pedunculated and can be delivered at the anus, its removal presents no difficulty (Fig. 23.4). Sessile (papillomatous) tumours, when small, may be excised also per anum. When the rectal wall is lax, the part bearing the tumour may be drawn through the anus; the affected area of mucosa is then excised with the diathermy knife, and the defect is closed by suture. Otherwise the sphincter must be stretched and subsequently held open by retractors to allow access. Sometimes, when the tumour is small, an artificial pedicle may be created by traction, and this can be dealt with by a transfixing ligature, prior to division.

Benign tumours in the upper rectum

These may be dealt with, through a short operating sigmoidoscope, by fulguration with a diathermy electrode, or by removal with the diathermy snare. Such methods should not be used when the tumour is above the peritoneal reflection (unless it is pedunculated), because of the risk of perforating the bowel; in such cases it is safer to approach it by laparotomy.

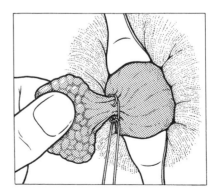

Fig. 23.4 Method of removing a pedunculated rectal polyp which can be delivered at the anus

In view of the inescapable risks of malignant change — either in further tumours developing or in undetected tumours already present, systematic re-examination of the patient is essential for many years after operation — if not for the duration of his life. For the first two years after operation sigmoidoscopy and double contrast barium enema or colonoscopy are advised every 6 to 12 months; in the absence of recurrence the interval between examinations may be progressively lengthened, but the patient is told to report at once if bleeding recurs.

Large tumours and those suspected of malignancy
If the tumour is too large for local excision, or if there is evidence that it has undergone malignant change, one of the operations described for carcinoma of the rectum must be undertaken. If the tumour is situated in the mid or upper part of the rectum, and *if tumours elsewhere in the bowel have been excluded,* a sphincter-conserving resection is ideal.

Benign strictures of the rectum
These result most commonly from injuries, from chronic inflammatory conditions such as proctitis or Crohn's disease, or from infections such as lymphogranuloma inguinale. Occasionally they may be due to excessive fibrosis following irradiation treatment of carcinoma of the cervix uteri or following a low rectal anastomosis. When the stricture is not too far advanced, and is sufficiently low for the finger to reach above it, regular dilatation with bougies may suffice in treatment. Low-level ring strictures, such as may result from postoperative scarring, may be treated first by *internal proctotomy,* i.e. division of the constriction from within with a probe-pointed knife. A finger passed upwards through the stricture is used as a guide, and several shallow incisions are made in the posterior half of the circumference of the constricting ring. Dilatation with bougies is immediately carried out; this is repeated daily for several days, and thereafter at longer intervals.

Localized strictures which cannot be dilated satisfactorily may, provided no active inflammation is present, be treated by one of the methods of sphincter-conserving resection described for carcinoma or by the circular stapling device alone (Ross, 1980).

Tubular strictures and those associated with severe inflammatory reaction can be treated only by colostomy. When the inflammation has subsided it may be possible to restore evacuation through normal channels, or to perform a sphincter-conserving resection. More often, however, the colostomy will be permanent. In some cases the inflammatory condition is progressive and causes chronic invalidism from continued pain, fever and rectal discharge; radical excision of the rectum should then be advocated.

PROLAPSE OF THE RECTUM

In the less severe varieties of this condition — *partial prolapse,* the everted tissue consists of mucosa alone which is both lax and redundant. A mild degree of partial prolapse occurs in association with prolapsing haemorrhoids and effective treatment of the haemorrhoids is usually curative. *Complete prolapse,* in which the entire thickness of the rectal wall is extruded, is essentially a sliding hernia of the anterior rectal wall through the anal canal. If the protrusion is longer that 5 cm, it is probable that a peritoneal sac prolonged downwards from the rectovesical or recto-uterine pouch lies between the two layers of rectal wall forming the anterior part of the protrusion (Fig. 23.5).

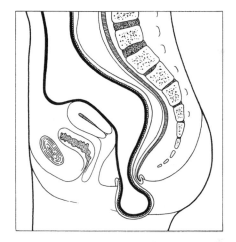

Fig. 23.5 Drawing to show the relation of the peritoneum to a complete prolapse of the rectum

Minor degrees of partial prolapse, especially when they occur in children or in old people, are treated by conservative measures including the avoidance of constipation and straining at stool.

Injection therapy
Suitable for cases of partial prolapse. Its objective is to secure fixation of the lax mucosa to the underlying muscular coat. This may be achieved by the injection of 5% phenol in almond oil into the submucous layer, as in the 'high injection' treatment of haemorrhoids (p. 511). Through a proctoscope, five or six injections, each of 2 ml are given at the first treatment; these are spaced around the circumference of the bowel at as high a level as possible. The results are at best uncertain.

Radical operations
The main difficulty in attempting cure of complete pro-

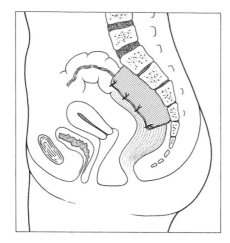

Fig. 23.6 Wells's operation for rectal prolapse

lapse is control of the patient's associated incontinence. Abdominal rectopexy should achieve this in approximately 75% of cases although not all patients are suitable for an abdominal procedure.

Implantation of plastic sponge material (Fig. 23.6)
This operation, devised by Wells in 1959, is simpler than any hitherto described, and is successful in a high proportion of cases (McCue, 1991). The technique is relatively straightforward, and the operation is well tolerated by elderly patients. The rectum is mobilized as for anterior resection, and, with its vascular pedicle intact, is lifted forwards from the hollow of the sacrum. A sheet of polyvinyl alcohol sponge, 3 mm thick and 8 to 10 cm square, is attached to the fascia in front of the sacrum, from the promontory down to the 3rd or 4th segment inserting all sutures into the presacral fascia before passing them through the sponge. The rectum is then drawn firmly upwards; the sheet of sponge is folded around it, to cover all except the anterior one-quarter or one-fifth of its circumference, and is secured by three or four stitches uniting its lateral margins to the bowel wall. Finally the peritoneal flaps are sutured in front of the bowel or against its sides, so that the sponge is completely buried. The effect of the plastic sponge is to provoke a vigorous fibrotic response, so that the rectum becomes anchored against the sacral hollow by firm adhesions. In most cases, this effectively cures the prolapse, and although incontinence cannot always be abolished it is usually much improved. Marlex mesh is an alternative material which may be used, a combined anterior and posterior rectopexy being advocated in patients with a deep recto-uterine or rectovesical pouch.

Anterior resection of the rectum
As performed for carcinoma, this has been advocated

as an effective method of treating rectal prolapse, since the bowel usually becomes firmly adherent to the sacrum at the level of the anastomosis. The splenic flexure is mobilized and proximal descending colon is divided to ensure healthy colon for the anastomosis. The lower rectum is fixed to the presacral fascia with non-absorbable sutures (Duthie, 1992).

Repair of the defect from above, without resection of bowel
This method has been superseded by rectopexy. It was designed to deal directly with the factors causing the prolapse — the abnormally deep rectovesical or recto-uterine pouch and the lax or atonic condition of the pelvic floor. Following mobilization of the bowel, the puborectales muscles were drawn together by three or four sutures of unabsorbable material in front of the rectum, or occasionally behind the rectum if tension prevented anterior suture. However, deficient tissues often led to poor results and a varying degree of incontinence.

Amputation of the prolapse from below
Full thickness resection (*rectosigmoidectomy*) is no longer practised in UK. The similar but lesser procedure of mucosal resection, devised by Delorme in 1900, is occasionally advocated for patients unfit for an abdominal procedure. It involves excision of lax mucosa from the fully everted prolapse and plication of the underlying muscle layers followed by reanastomosis of the mucosa over the plicated rectal wall. The results are inferior to abdominal procedures (Duthie, 1991).

The Thiersch operation
Of limited use in the palliation of rectal prolapse. A ring of silver wire or nylon suture, or a band of silicone rubber (Jackaman, 1980) is inserted within the fibres of the weakened external sphincter to deter the prolapse of rectum through the anus. It may be inserted under local anaesthesia and is tied sufficiently tightly to admit one finger.

CARCINOMA OF THE RECTUM

The principles of surgery for rectal carcinoma are similar to those for colonic carcinoma, as described on page 477. The approach to operation will, to some extent, be influenced by the findings at sigmoidoscopy and the degree of fixity of the growth as assessed by rectal examination.

Biopsy
It is essential that histological confirmation of tumour is obtained since the finding of an anaplastic carcinoma, with poor prognosis, will influence the choice

of operation. Although it may be technically possible to restore bowel continuity, this is not usually advisable for a tumour of Dukes' Stage C (often anaplastic) where local massive recurrence of tumour would lead to recurrence of bowel symptoms. The presence of liver metastases, detected by ultrasound or CAT scan and confirmed at laparotomy, is an indication for conservative surgery and the avoidance of a colostomy in a patient whose life expectancy is limited.

Choice of operation

In 60 to 70% of patients suffering from carcinoma of the rectum, radical removal of the tumour can be carried out with a reasonable prospect of cure. In such cases the operation is designed to remove the growth in its entirety, along with any regional extensions or metastases. If continuity cannot be re-established, a permanent colostomy must be performed.

Three main types of operation are carried out at the present time for carcinoma of the rectum:

1. Abdominoperineal excision is the operation of choice for all tumours in the lower half of the rectum. Classically it implies the removal of the entire anorectum together with the lower pelvic colon, and the establishment of a permanent colostomy. Where facilities exist, it is usually carried out by the *synchronous combined method* (Fig. 23.7).

2. Conservative resection with preservation of the anal sphincters is the operation of choice for all early growths involving the upper rectum or pelvirectal junction (*rectosigmoid*). The advent of the EEA (end-to-end anastomosis) stapling gun allows for restoration of bowel continuity after excision of virtually the whole rectum, although it may not always be advisable that this is attempted.

3. Abdominal excision alone (*Hartmann's operation*) is a valuable procedure in old or debilitated patients, in

whom abdominoperineal dissection is too formidable, or in whom, because of general or local conditions, restorative resection is impracticable. It does not obviate a permanent colostomy, but, the anal canal being left in situ, the patient is spared the additional strain and recovery entailed by a perineal dissection.

It is generally agreed that no final choice of operation can be made until the situation and extent of the growth have been investigated by laparotomy. This is necessary in order to confirm that the growth itself is removable, and that there are no metastases in other organs or inaccessible lymph glands, such as might invalidate the operation. Furthermore, it is seldom possible before laparotomy to determine the type of operation best suited to the individual case.

Preoperative treatment

Preparation along the lines described for bowel preparation is essential (p. 479), and the policy of perioperative antibiosis (p. 479) also applies.

Abdominoperineal excision

Restorative resection or complete removal of the rectum?
Until relatively recently and with a few notable exceptions, tumours of the extraperitioneal rectum have been managed by total removal of that organ and permanent colostomy. As indicated on page 477, the pathological and physiological basis for this irreversible ablative procedure is not now regarded as well found and, provided the rectum and its enveloping fascia are carefully dissected en bloc, and provided also the operator is confident about reconstruction, tumours as low as 2–3 cm from the dentate line can be treated by restorative resection. The exception must be those in which there is a high risk of early recurrence because of extensive pararectal infiltration and clinically involved nodes. Here palliation is better achieved by abdominoperineal resection. In addition, there will always remain some tumours in which adequate surgical clearance cannot be achieved without removal of the tissues and associated lymph nodes as shown in Figure 23.8.

Abdominal dissection
The standard operation in the United Kingdom is done synchronously by two teams with the patient in the Lloyd Davis position and a urethral catheter in situ (Fig. 23.9). The colostomy position is determined the day before, preferably with the co-operation of a stoma therapist. The abdominal mobilization proceeds as described (p. 480) to separate the rectum, down to the levator ani and puborectalis, from its surrounding structures — behind in the hollow of the sacrum, laterally in relation to the rectal ligaments and in front. Anteriorly in the male this involves careful dissection in

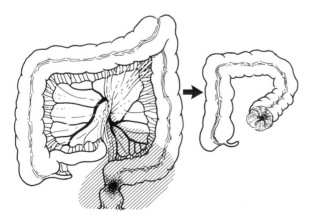

Fig. 23.7 The extent of resection in abdominoperineal excision of the rectum

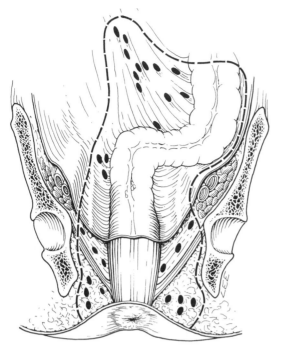

Fig. 23.8 Drawing to show the tissues removed with a tumour in the distal rectum. Wide removal of the pelvic mesocolon with its contained glands can be carried out

the retrovesical and retroprostatic space, displacing the seminal vesicles forward. The whole fibrofatty mass encircling the rectum is thus freed and the rest of the dissection must be completed from below, though the abdominal operator can and should assist the perineal worker by identifying the planes. At all times, care should be taken to preserve the sympathetic and parasympathetic nerves. Once the inferior mesenteric artery has been ligated, a plane is developed between the mesentery of the sigmoid colon and the pre-aortic tissues. The nerves lie in a fascial envelope surrounding the aorta. This should be preserved without dissection onto the aorta. Mobilisation is continued towards the promontary of the sacrum. Here, the two branches of the autonomic nerves can be seen. Laterally, branches enter the rectum. These need to be carefully severed, thereby preserving the main nerves which then lie on the side walls of the pelvis. Traditionally, this manoeuvre was carried out bluntly with the hand. This is inadvisable since the nerves can easily be avulsed. Once the correct plane has been entered, the nerves can be easily identified. The next important aspect is to ensure that the whole mesorectum is removed in its entirety. There is a tendancy to cone medially towards the rectum. With advanced tumours, this may actually go across the lateral margins, making the resection inadequate. A

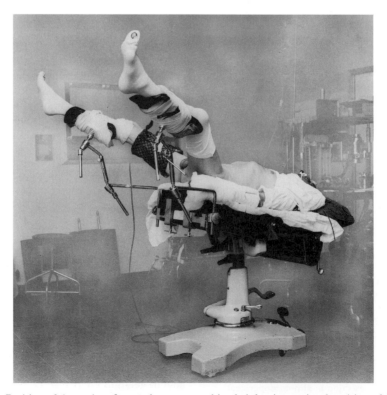

Fig. 23.9 Position of the patient for synchronous combined abdomino perineal excision of the rectum

Lloyd Davies retractor with a lip enables a clear view of the side walls of the pelvis to be seen. The lateral ligaments are a condensation of parietal pelvic fascia which are normally avascular. Distally, the middle rectal artery can be ligated if necessary, but frequently diathermy coagulation suffices. The posterior dissection now proceeds in an anterio-inferior direction beneath the mesorectum. Loose areolar tissue is separated to reveal the levator ani muscles below. Anteriorly, the plane deep to Denonvilliers' fascia should be entered at the level of the seminal vesicles. On the antero-lateral aspects, lie the nervi erigentes which should be preserved if possible. Once the fascia which is relatively thick, has been divided, the rectal muscle tube is seen, and dissection proceeds along the rectal wall anteriorly behind the prostate which is separated anteriorly.

Perineal dissection

The anus is closed with a subcutaneous purse string — 1 silk on a half circle needle is suitable (Fig. 23.10). A transverse incision is made in the perineum half way between vaginal orifice and anus in the female or just posterior to the perineal raphe in the male. From the centre of this, encircling incisions are carried back around the anus at a distance from it of about 2 cm to meet at the tip of the coccyx. The transverse incision is deepened to expose the transverse perinei muscle and its posterior fibres split, allowing access to the retroprostatic space in the male (Fig. 23.11). The urethral catheter is a useful guide at this point and should be felt only distantly through the soft tissues surrounding the

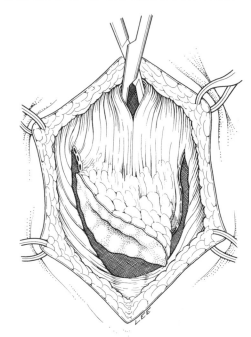

Fig. 23.11 Dissecting the perineum

urethral bulb. As this dissection is carried upwards the fibres of puborectalis are encountered to either side as they pass anteroposteriorly. At this point the encircling incisions are deepened through the fat of the ischiorectal fossa. Posteriorly the coccyx is encountered with, on either side, the firm fibrous origin of the levator ani. Either the coccyx is detached from the sacrum by cutting through the sacrococcygeal joint with a knife or, as the writer prefers, the levator insertion is cut in the midline at the coccygeal tip. Either manoeuvre permits the blades of a scissors to be inserted into the gap in the midline which is so produced and the levators to be divided forwards close to the pelvic wall (Fig. 23.12). Entry is thus made into the retrorectal space where the abdominal operator is encountered.

Division of the levators is next carried forward to meet the point where the puborectalis fibres have been identified anteriorly. By a combination of sharp and blunt dissection the musculofibrous tissue here is divided off the back of the prostate and dissection then carried up behind the bladder to meet the abdominal operator. The latter then divides the colon at an appropriate place to permit it to be passed through the abdominal wall at the colostomy site and the specimen is delivered per anum. In the female it is permissible, but not desirable, to remove the posterior vaginal wall, in which case the perineal and abdominal dissections join in the posterior vaginal fornix. Healing of the vagina is said to be satisfactory but there is little objective evidence on this point.

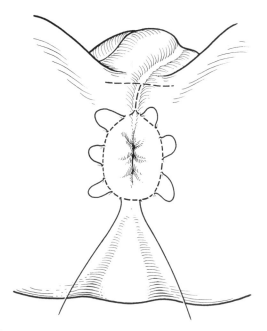

Fig. 23.10 The anal purse string

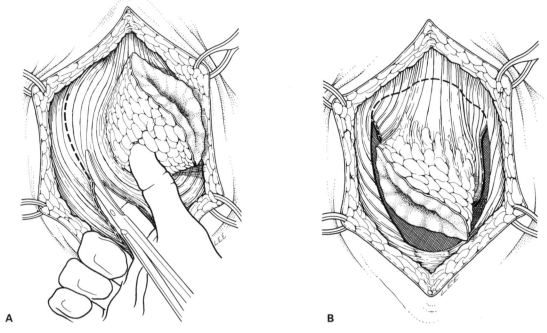

Fig. 23.12   Dividing the levators

Establishing the colostomy

Either an extraperitoneal or intraperitoneal method can be used. If the former, the edge of parietal peritoneum, formed when the sigmoid is mobilized, is raised and a blunt dissection made outside it round the lateral aspect of the abdominal wall to the colostomy site. A disc of skin is excised and the abdominal wall cut through in all layers in two directions at right angles; the resulting gap must easily take two fingers without any feeling of grip. The colon is then drawn through behind the peritoneum and stitched to the skin (Fig. 22.52 p. 489).

If the colostomy is established intraperitoneally, there is a danger of herniation lateral to the colon in the old paracolic gutter. This gap must be obliterated by either a running or a close series of interrupted sutures of silk or braided nylon passed from the lateral aspect of the colon wall to the parietal peritoneum (Fig. 23.13).

Closure of the pelvic floor and perineum

No attempt should be made to close the pelvic peritoneal cavity. A few absorbable sutures (catgut, dexon, vicryl or polydioxanone) are inserted to draw the fatty margins of the ischiorectal fossa together and the skin closed with soft absorbables, with a suction drain led out through a stab incision. If there has been contamination or if there is tension, it is better to leave the wound open and lightly packed with dry gauze. At 4–5 days, the pack is removed under general anaesthesia

and the wound will usually rapidly contract to heal by second intention in 2–3 weeks.

It has been suggested that there is less likelihood of adhesion of small bowel to the pelvic floor if the omentum is pedicled on one gastro-epiploic vessel and brought down into the pelvis. This manoeuvre is recommended if the perineal wound is to be left open.

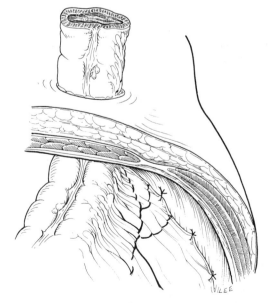

Fig. 23.13   Closure of the lateral paracolic gutter (exposure through transverse abdominal incision)

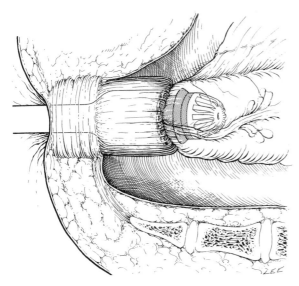

Fig. 23.14 The final stage of transanal stapled anastomosis

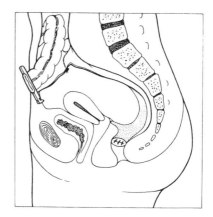

Fig. 23.15 Anterior (transabdominal) resection of the rectum with permanent colostomy — Hartmann's operation

Anterior resection of the rectum

The technique for mobilization of the upper rectum has already been described in the section on colonic carcinoma (p. 481). Dissection within the pelvis proceeds on the lines of the abdominal dissection in the synchronous combined operation. Continuity of bowel is most safely established by the stapling gun (Fig. 23.14) although suturing is preferred by many surgeons. The rectum should be irrigated with a tumouricidal agent such as povidone iodine prior to transection of the rectum. This may prevent seeding of exfoliated tumour cells into the pelvic parietes. This is particularly important when stapling, since the device is passed up into the pelvis and will contaminate the tissues with faecal residue containing tumour cells.

For a sutured anastomosis deep in the pelvis, the posterior row of sutures must be inserted *prior* to approximation of the gut ends if accuracy of apposition is to be achieved. In skilled hands, sutured colo-anal anastomosis can be achieved by the perineal approach (Parks, 1982), although as outlined in chapter 22, a colonic reservoir may be constructed in selected cases to improve bowel function.

Abdominal excision alone with permanent colostomy

This method may be preferred in selected patients (p. 505) or as a first stage procedure in the presence of obstruction (p. 487). *Abdominal dissection* is carried out as already described and a terminal colostomy is made. The distal stump of rectum is closed by sutures (Fig. 23.15) and the peritoneum of the pelvic floor is repaired above it.

Palliative procedures

Removal of the primary growth, where this is practicable, is the best method of palliation. The presence of metastases in the liver or elsewhere should not therefore preclude an excision, provided, of course, that the growth is not fixed by malignant infiltration to surrounding tissues. It is obvious that, when the excision is considered to be purely palliative, extensive clearance of the glandular fields is unnecessary, and that sphincter-conserving resections have a special application.

Fulguration of the tumour

When the patient is too enfeebled to stand an excision, and when the main symptom is bleeding, this may sometimes be arrested by fulguration with the diathermy electrode, or with the laser, carried out if necessary at several sessions. Considerable shrinkage of the growth may result, and symptomatic relief may be obtained for many months (Gingold, 1983).

Colostomy alone

This should be considered when the growth appears to be irremovable, but it should not be advised as routine in all such cases. When obstruction exists or threatens to develop at an early date, or when the patient's life is made miserable by tenesmus or continual discharge, colostomy may provide a considerable measure of relief during the time that is left to the patient. Occasionally after colostomy there is an astounding improvement in both general and local conditions. Fixation of the growth may be due mainly to inflammatory reaction; it may diminish or even disappear with free drainage of the bowel above, so that radical removal may become practicable after a course of radiotherapy. Even in apparently fixed growths, therefore, the possibility of radical cure at a later date should not be entirely discounted. Colostomy is contraindicated in advanced malignancy with widespread metastases or carcinomatosis peritonei. Unless obstruction is present the patient will be made more miserable by a colostomy, and is unlikely to live long enough to derive any benefit from it. In such cases *there is no evidence to show that colostomy prolongs life.*

ANAL FISSURE

The fissure is most commonly situated in the midline posteriorly. It varies in appearance from a superficial crack in the mucosa to a long oval-shaped ulcer, with indurated or undermined edges, and in the base of which plain muscle fibres may be exposed. At its external end there is usually a hypertrophied and oedematous tag of skin, the *sentinel pile.* The fissure is invariably associated with sphincteric spasm, which is not only the main cause of pain, but which also keeps up the irritation and delays healing.

Treatment directed towards correction of constipation will, in many cases, lead to healing of a recent fissure. The application of analgesic ointments will result in pain relief and relaxation of sphincteric spasm. In some cases, daily use of an anal dilator will be found helpful but its use may be required over a prolonged period.

Sphincter injection
This method of treatment is infrequently employed but may be of value where urgent relief of pain is required. With the patient in the *right* lateral position, a wheal of local anaesthetic is raised 2.5 cm posterior to the anus in the mid line. The needle is then advanced into the sphincteric muscle for injection of lignocaine 1ml of 2% plus sodium tetradecyl sulphate 0.05 ml (Antebi, 1985), the site of injection being guided by the surgeon's left index finger which has been inserted through the anal canal.

Operation
General anaesthesia is usually necessary to achieve adequate anal dilatation.

Simple stretching of the sphincter
In many cases this is successful in effecting a cure. It should be noted that it is the *internal,* rather than the external sphincter which requires to be stretched, since it is this muscle which underlies the fissure. Stretching is carried out slowly and gently until the orifice admits three or four fingers without difficulty.

Sphincterotomy consists in division of the fibres of the internal sphincter, this muscle being identified by palpation after the anal canal has been stretched and everted. Relief of pain is usually quite dramatic and is almost certainly due to the abolition of spasm. A bivalve speculum is introduced into the anal canal, and is gradually opened to expose the fissure and to put the

fibres of the internal sphincter on the stretch. These fibres are then completely divided to just above the dentate line, to expose the smooth conjoined longitudinal muscle lying underneath. The wound is prolonged outwards on to the peri-anal skin, so that a 'sentinel' pile, if present, can be excised. Any well developed commissural fibres of the subcutaneous external sphincter are divided also, in order to avoid a ridge. Many surgeons prefer a lateral sphincterotomy although greater skill is required in identifying the internal sphincter (McDonald, 1992).

Excision
When the fissure is a chronic one, or shows much induration, it is probable that complete excision is the operation of choice. After the sphincter has been stretched two pairs of light tissue forceps are placed on the mucocutaneous junction well to each side of the fissure, and are drawn downwards until the entire fissure comes into view. With a sharp knife, the fissure and its fibrous tissue covering is then cleanly excised by an elliptical incision which is deepened down to the fibres of the internal sphincter. To ensure free drainage the ellipse, which includes the sentinel pile, should be carried well out on to the peri-anal skin, where it should be at least 1 cm in breadth (Fig. 23.16). The sphincteric fibres immediately deep to the fissure may be divided at the same time. Thereafter the floor of the wound should be completely smooth and free from ridges or hollows (Fig. 23.17).

After-treatment
After either sphincterotomy or excision, bleeding is arrested by the application of a gauze swab, a corner of which may be tucked into the anal canal. If necessary for haemostasis, a small pack may be held firmly in place by a suture which is retained for 24 hours. The wound is covered with wool and secured with a T-bandage. The dressings are changed daily, but subse-

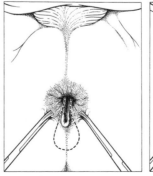
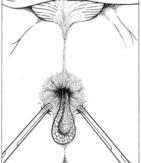

Fig. 23.16   **Fig. 23.17**

Figs 23.16 & 23.17   Excision of an anal fissure

quent repacking of the wound should not be required. Hot sitz-baths are instituted as early as possible, and gentle cleansing with soap and water is carried out after each evacuation. There is usually almost complete relief of pain immediately after operation, and healing may be expected to be complete in from 10 days to 3 weeks. The bowel motions should be kept soft for several months after operation, since, if constipation is allowed to exist, there is a considerable risk that the fissure may recur.

HAEMORRHOIDS

External haemorrhoids

True external haemorrhoids (i.e. covered with skin alone) are not very common. Usually they are no more than small skin tags, which require no treatment unless they become irritated or inflamed. In such cases they may, when quiescent, be snipped off with scissors or treated with the Cryoprobe, so that a flat surface results. Frequently they co-exist with internal haemorrhoids or fissure, and their removal should then be included in the operation for the more troublesome condition.

Peri-anal haematoma. This is often incorrectly referred to as a 'thrombosed external pile', but it is in reality a small haematoma due to the rupture of an anal venule. It is usually 4 or 5 days before the patient seeks advice; by this time the period of maximum discomfort has passed, and, unless the haematoma is a large one, no treatment is required, as the clot will shrink and disappear in a further few days. When the condition is seen soon after its onset, a small incision may be made under local anaesthesia, and the clot evacuated.

Internal haemorrhoids

Internal haemorrhoids, or intero-external haemorrhoids (which lie at the mucocutaneous junction, and have a covering partly of mucosa and partly of skin) are much more common. In those cases which are not relieved by adjustment of the dietary fibre, aperients or suppositories, the choices of treatment are injection, rubber banding, cryosurgery, infrared coagulation, anal dilatation or excision.

Conservative treatment

Injection therapy

This gives satisfactory results in selected cases of internal haemorrhoids. It has the advantage over operation that the patient can be treated as an outpatient but a course of several injections is frequently required. Injection treatment is most satisfactory when the piles are small and cause no symptoms other than bleeding at defaecation. Prolapse of the haemorrhoids during defaecation is not necessarily a contraindication to injection, provided that they can be replaced.

Injection treatment must not be employed in cases of external piles, or of internal piles which tend to remain prolapsed outside the anal sphincter, in view of the danger that sloughing may result. It is contraindicated also in the presence of infection.

The patient is placed in the knee/elbow or in the lateral position. A well lubricated anal speculum is introduced, and the number, size and arrangement of the haemorrhoids are carefully noted. They present in three distinct groups, with one or more in each group — left lateral, right anterior and right posterior. This is due to the anatomical arrangement of the blood vessels supplying the anal cushions (Thomson, 1975).

The method of *high injection* is generally employed. The term denotes an injection made into the submucous coat of the bowel above a group of piles (Fig. 23.18). Its object is to cause thrombosis of the vessels draining the piles and to promote a localized fibrosis which will lead to retraction of the lax mucosa. Where possible a special syringe and needle should be used; the latter is long enough to use through a proctoscope, and is bent at an obtuse angle; it has a shoulder about 1 cm from its point, so that too deep penetration is avoided. The solution advocated is 5% phenol in almond oil, and up to 5 ml may be injected in each situation. It is best to make the first injection in the quadrant which presents the largest pile mass. The injection should be carried out slowly, and the fluid should be seen to raise a pale swelling which spreads immediately deep to the mucosa. A white wheal appearing at the site of puncture indicates that the solution is being injected into the mucosa with consequent risk of local necrosis; the needle should be withdrawn immediately and another site selected. Similar injections may be made above other pile masses in the remaining quadrants, or this may be postponed until

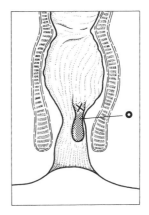

Fig. 23.18   Internal haemorrhoids — site for high and low injections

another session. It is not advisable that more than three injections should be made at any one treatment.

After treatment

The patient is instructed to avoid prolonged standing or strenuous exercise for a few days, and to keep the bowel motions soft by a regular aperient. If a pile prolapses during defaecation it should be replaced immediately. Further injections are carried out if required at fortnightly intervals. They are given normally in those quadrants which have not already been injected, and in which piles are present.

Rubber band ligature of the pedicle of each haemorrhoid may be carried out without anaesthesia in the manner of injection described above but using a special applicator. The pile may be drawn into the instrument with forceps or using a specially designed suction tube. The results of out-patient treatment are superior to those following injection (McDonald, 1992).

Cryosurgery of haemorrhoids is an alternative procedure but has been superseded by rubber band ligature. The cryoprobe is applied to the haemorrhoidal mass and liquefaction of frozen tissue occurs over the ensuing 2 or 3 weeks.

Infrared coagulation is obtained using an appropriate probe and a one second exposure at each site. Its use is limited by the expense of the equipment.

Manual dilatation of the anus, as advocated by Lord (1969), aims to dilate the sphincter to accept 4 fingers of each hand and to maintain sphincter laxity by regular use of a specially designed dilator. General anaesthesia is required but the patient need not be detained in hospital. Incontinence is a common complication of this method.

Operation

Operative removal of haemorrhoids is indicated when they are of significant size, and especially if they tend to remain prolapsed outside the anal sphincter.

Preparation

The bowel should be thoroughly cleared out before operation, in order to minimize faecal contamination, and to promote quiescence of the colon for the first few days of the postoperative period. An aperient is given 24 hours before operation, and thereafter the patient is kept on a fluid or nonresidue diet. An enema is not usually required but a low washout (of the rectum alone) may be given early on the morning of operation. It is customary to employ general or low spinal anaesthesia, and to operate with the patient in the lithotomy position.

Dissection–ligature operation

This is the most widely practised operation at the

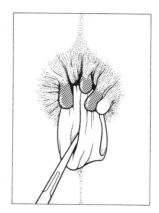

Fig. 23.19   Method of withdrawing internal haemorrhoids by the use of a dry gauze swab

present time (McDonald, 1992). The anal sphincter is gently stretched between the two index fingers. A dry swab is pushed into the rectum, and is then partially withdrawn, when the haemorrhoids will appear alongside it (Fig. 23.19). They are picked up individually with artery forceps, and each is then dealt with in turn. In the case of intero-external piles two forceps are applied; one to the mucous part and one to the cutaneous part. The pile is drawn downwards, and with a pair of scissors, a V-shaped cut is made through the overlying mucosa at its junction with the skin. If the pile is intero-external in type, the cut is commenced in the skin just at its external border (Fig. 23.20). By blunt dissection with the scissor points the submucous space is opened up until the pile is entirely stripped from its bed, and is attached only by its vascular pedicle, and by a narrow

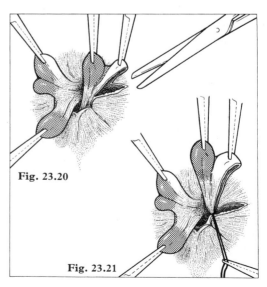

Fig. 23.20

Fig. 23.21

Figs 23.20 & 23.21   Haemorrhoidectomy by the dissection-ligature technique.

strip of mucous membrane. Care is taken not to elevate any of the fibres of the external sphincter in the dissection. A ligature of strong thread or catgut is used to transfix and tie the pedicle as high up as possible (Fig. 23.21), and the distal part is cut off. After all the piles have been dealt with, two fingers are introduced into the anal canal, to ensure that no stenosis has been caused. A large pad of gauze liberally smeared with sterile vaseline is applied to the anus. This is secured with a T-bandage, which is firmly tied, so that the pressure exerted will tend to prevent oedema. Some surgeons leave a small soft rubber tube within the anal canal; this gives warning of haemorrhage but, although it allows the passage of flatus, it may increase the patient's discomfort.

Submucosal haemorrhoidectomy is a modification of the ligature operation which avoids suture of anal mucosa with the pedicle and does not result in any raw areas to cause fibrosis. It is, however, technically difficult and may result in some blood loss.

Clamp and cautery operation

This method is now frequently described as obsolete, but it has certain advantages over the dissection-ligature operation, in that it involves no opening up of the tissue planes by dissection — a factor of some importance in view of the potentially septic character of the operative field. A special clamp is employed; its blades are guarded with ivory or plastic plates which protect the skin from burning. Additional protection is provided by pads of moist wool or gauze placed around the clamp, between it and the skin. The clamp must always be applied radially to the anal orifice, and both an external and an internal pile may therefore be clamped together (Fig. 23.22). The greater part of the pile mass is then cut away with scissors, only a little of its substance being left projecting beyond the clamp. The copper cautery specially designed for the operation is heated over a gas ring; it is applied at a black heat, so that the pile stump projecting beyond the clamp is slowly burned away. The surface area of the cautery is sufficiently large to heat up the blades of the clamp; in this way the tissue grasped by the clamp is thoroughly seared, so that the haemorrhage is effectively arrested. The only objection to this old-fashioned cautery is that a gas ring is seldom readily available in a modern operating theatre. The electric cautery or the diathermy knife are unsatisfactory substitutes, since they are ineffective in arresting haemorrhage, while the coagulating current penetrates too deeply into the tissues (Chamberlain, 1970).

After-treatment

The foot of the bed is elevated for 24 to 48 hours after operation, in order to reduce congestion. Retention of

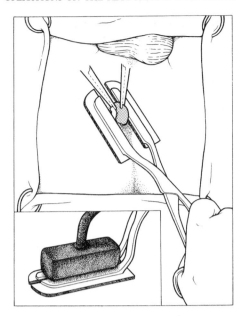

Fig. 23.22 Haemorrhoidectomy by the 'clamp-and-cautery' method. Inset shows copper cautery block applied to the Smith's pile clamp

urine is a fairly common complication, especially in older men, and may require attention. The bowels are kept confined if possible for several days, and to assist in this a fluid diet only is allowed. Small doses of liquid paraffin or of magnesia emulsion may be given daily after the first day. Pain from defaecation can be relieved by the introduction of local anaesthetic ointment into the anal canal. Twice-daily sitz baths are very comforting and promote rapid healing. Recurrence of the piles is rare, except in the chronically constipated.

Thrombosed or strangulated piles

It is generally taught that removal of haemorrhoids in the 'acute' stage is contraindicated, in view of the risk of spreading infection, especially to the portal tract (*pylephlebitis*); also, because the haemorrhoids are very friable, they bleed readily, and ligatures tend to cut through.

Conservative treatment, therefore, is commonly employed until the acute condition has subsided. The patient is confined to bed with its foot raised on blocks. Pain is relieved by moist compresses containing ice and by sedatives as required. In cases seen early, it may be possible, under an anaesthetic, to reduce the prolapsed piles after stretching the sphincter. Surgery is then undertaken later in the quiescent stage.

The results of such treatment are not impressive. Ten days or more may elapse before the protruding mass shrinks within the anus and this is a painful and distressing time for the patient. When he has recovered from the attack, he still has to face operation at a later date. Even when the prolapse can be successfully reduced, it frequently recurs within a few hours.

It now appears that the dangers of operation in the acute stage have been exaggerated (Smith, 1967). Dissection should obviously be reduced to the minimum, but crushing clamps can safely be applied to the pile pedicles which are relatively normal, and the protruding masses cut off. The stumps are then ligatured or over-sewn. The 'clamp-and-cautery' method is particularly suitable for use in such conditions.

ANORECTAL ABSCESSES

Peri-anal abscess

A subcutaneous abscess
This lies under the skin at the anal margin (Fig. 23.23A). It results usually from inflammation of a sebaceous follicle, or from infection through some superficial abrasion. It should be opened by a cruciate incision, and any undermined edges are cut away. The injection of a small quantity of local anaesthetic into the skin renders the operation quite painless.

A submucous abscess is less common. It is located under the mucosa of the anal canal (Fig. 23.23B), and is due frequently to infection which has entered an anal gland through an anal crypt. The patient experiences severe pain and the diagnosis may be missed if digital examination of the anal canal is omitted. The abscess usually bursts spontaneously, but if necessary it should be opened by incision, access having been obtained by stretching of the anal sphincter.

Ischio-rectal abscess

The presence of brawny induration to one or other side of the anus, accompanied by throbbing pain, justifies the diagnosis of ischiorectal abscess (Fig. 23.23C). Drainage should always be provided without delay. If redness of the overlying skin or signs of fluctuation are awaited, the abscess is very liable to rupture into the bowel, in which case a fistula is almost certain to result. If early incision is carried out this sequel can usually be prevented. Spread to the ischiorectal fossa of the opposite side is not uncommon; this complication also is avoided by early incision.

Operation
It is most essential that the incision should be a large one. Not only must it provide free drainage, but it should also be sufficiently large to ensure that the wound will heal from its deepest part outwards. It is no kindness to the patient to employ a small incision, for satisfactory healing is then unlikely to be obtained unless the surface wound is kept open by continual repacking which is always an uncomfortable and tedious procedure. A large cruciate incision is recommended, one limb of which radiates towards the anus; it is deepened through skin and fascia, and the corners are then cut away, so that the final opening represents the entire floor of the abscess cavity (Figs 23.24 & 23.25). Fibrous septa are broken down with the finger or by further incisions, and the whole cavity is then carefully packed with gauze. In some series, satisfactory healing has followed suture of the abscess cavity after curettage (Ellis, 1960; Lindhus, 1989).

After-treatment
The packing is normally removed after about 48 hours. When the external opening has been made sufficiently large repacking can be dispensed with, but sitz baths should be commenced as early as possible. Healing

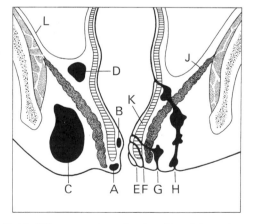

Fig. 23.23 Diagram to show the situation of the various anorectal abscesses and fistulae.
Abscesses: (A) subcutaneous; (B) submucous; (C) ischiorectal; (D) pelvirectal
Fistulae (E) superficial or extra-sphincteric; (F) intersphincteric; (G) trans-sphincteric; (H) extrasphincteric
Normal anatomy (J) levator ani; (K) internal sphincter; (L) peritoneum

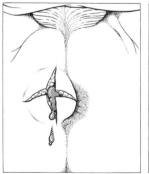
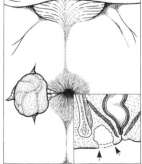

Fig. 23.24   **Fig. 23.25**

Figs 23.24 & 23.25   Method of opening an ischiorectal abscess by cruciate incision. Inset shows how the entire floor of the abscess cavity is removed

should occur steadily from the depths outwards, the time taken depending, of course, upon the size of the cavity. The wound must be inspected regularly, and, if there is any sign that surface healing is progressing too rapidly, gauze packing should at once be reinstituted, the pack being renewed each day.

A chronic ischiorectal abscess may be tuberculous. The fat normally occupying the ischiorectal fossa is replaced by tuberculous granulation tissue and caseous material. Local treatment is on similar lines to that described for an acute abscess. All caseous material should be removed, and the wall of the fossa gently curetted with a sharp spoon and sent for histological examination, bacteriological culture and sensitivities. Antituberculous chemotherapy is instituted on confirmation of the disease.

Pelvi-rectal abscess

This type of abscess is situated above the levator ani muscle, between it and the rectum (see Fig. 23.23D). It originates from some septic process in the pelvis, e.g. pelvic cellulitis. It may track downwards through the levator ani to become ischiorectal in location, or it may burst directly into the rectum. The treatment consists in providing drainage by the most accessible route — usually through the ischiorectal fossa. At operation it will be evident that pus is tracking downwards through an opening in the levator ani muscle; this opening should be enlarged to provide adequate drainage.

FISTULA-IN-ANO

The condition is usually a sequel to some variety of anorectal abscess, the infection arising within an anal gland and most frequently involving the intersphincteric plane. It is most likely to occur in cases where incision has been too long delayed, or where the drainage has been inadequate. The external opening of the fistula lies at the skin surface, usually to one or other side of the anus, and at a varying distance away. From this the fistulous track passes towards the mucous membrane of the bowel. The majority of fistulae are comparatively superficial, in that the track lies immediately deep to the skin and mucous membrane (*superficial or extrasphincteric*, 16%) or traverses the fibres of the internal sphincter to involve the intersphincteric plane to a variable extent (*intersphincteric*, 54%). Fistulae passing through both sphincters (*trans-sphincteric*, 21%) are less common (Marks, 1977). If the external opening is in front of the transverse line bisecting the anus the track may be more or less straight, and open into the corresponding quadrant of the anal canal. Most fistulae, however, pursue a curved course and enter the anal canal in the midline posteriorly, even when the opening is found anteriorly.

A high level fistula (*extrasphincteric*, 3%), which is a sequel usually to pelvirectal abscess, passes deep to both sphincters and traverses the levator ani, to enter the rectum at a high level.

The different types of fistula are shown diagrammatically in Figure 23.23.

Operation

The essential aim in treatment is to lay the fistulous track widely open or to excise it completely, and to ensure that the wound heals from the depths outwards.

The preoperative treatment is similar to that described for haemorrhoidectomy. A general or low spinal anaesthetic is employed, and the patient is placed in the lithotomy position. After gentle stretching of the sphincter the fistulous track is explored with a probe, which should be either curved or easily bendable. Frequently the probe passes without difficulty by way of the fistula into the anal canal. By the aid of a finger introduced into the bowel, it is then bent round or manipulated in such a way that its tip can be brought out at the anus. When the probe cannot be made to locate the internal opening, careful search must be made under vision for an abnormality in the anal canal — usually in the midline posteriorly. The probe is gently passed through the internal opening and its tip is brought out at the anus.

The fistula may now be laid widely open by division of all tissue between it and the skin surface, i.e. by cutting down on the probe. If the fistula has been present for many months, epithelium will have grown into it and it is then better to excise the track completely with the probe in situ (Fig. 23.26). The wound should be piriform or triangular in shape with its wider part externally. In the case of trans-sphincteric fistulae, the superficial fibres of the external and internal sphincters are included in the excision. Any ramifications of the main track are dealt with in the same way. Irregularities on the floor of the wound and any overhanging skin edges are cut away, so that there can be no interference with free drainage (Fig. 23.27) and the wound is packed with gauze. Even if the fistulous track is believed to have been cleanly and completely excised, it is seldom advisable to attempt to close it by suture.

For a trans-sphincteric fistula, in which the greater part of both sphincters must be divided, a two-stage operation is usually required in order to reduce the risk of anal incontinence.

A two-stage operation may be advisable when the track pursues a curved course ('horse-shoe fistula'). In such cases, a ligature of stout silk is passed on a probe or aneurysm needle through the deep part of the track and is loosely tied. At the first operation the external and lateral part of the track, which is usually subcutaneous, is excised (Figs 23.28 & 23.29). The silk ligature serves to identify the residual track so that, when

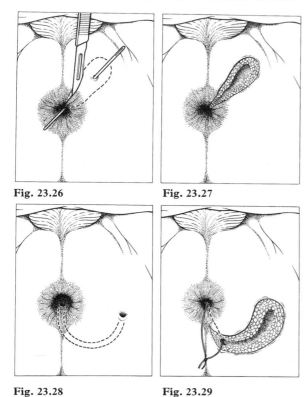

Fig. 23.26   **Fig. 23.27**

Fig. 23.28   **Fig. 23.29**

Figs 23.26 & 23.27   Excision of a superficial anal fistula passing directly into the anal canal

Figs 23.28 & 23.29   First part of a two-stage operation for a deep fistula pursuing a curved course into the bowel, excision of the superficial and lateral part of the track. A silk ligature identifies the residual fistula to be excised at the second stage

the first wound has healed (except for the new external opening of the fistula at its medial end) the remainder of the track entering the bowel is dealt with by a further excision (Williams, 1991).

Multiple fistulae

In longstanding fistulae it is common to find several external openings scattered around the anus particularly in the suprasphincteric or extrasphincteric type. They are likely to be connected to each other by subcutaneous tracks, but to share a common track by which they communicate with the bowel. Operative treatment should be carried out in two or more stages, the subcutaneous or communicating tracks being excised in the first instance. It is not advisable to divide sphincteric fibres in more than one place at the same operation. Excised tissue is examined for Crohn's disease if this has not already been suspected.

High level fistula

The track in this type of fistula cannot be laid open into the bowel, nor can it be completely excised, since it extends to too high a level in the rectum. A circular incision is made round the external opening, and the fistulous track is cored out along with a generous margin of surrounding tissue, including the levator ani muscle, to as high a level as possible. If it is possible to define the rectal defect and to close it with a mucosal advancement flap (Seow-Choen, 1992), healing will proceed rapidly. Otherwise, the large wound is carefully packed with gauze and allowed to granulate outwards. The internal opening in the rectal wall may then close spontaneously. If not, a temporary pelvic colostomy, preferably of defunctioning type (p. 474), should be advised. As the result of complete rest to the bowel, healing may occur.

Tuberculous fistulae are characterized by multiple tracks with widespread undermining of skin. In general, treatment is carried out on the lines described. All tracks are laid open as far as possible, and undermined skin is excised; unhealthy wound surfaces are cauterized with the diathermy electrode. Complete division of the external sphincter is contraindicated, since, owing to impaired healing power, incontinence may result. Antituberculous chemotherapy should be instituted.

After-treatment is very similar to that described for abscesses. The necessity for repacking the wound depends upon the type of fistula. In superficial fistulae the excision wound is comparatively shallow, so that packing is both unnecessary and difficult to retain. When, however, the track has been deeply situated, a narrow and relatively deep cleft is inevitable, and in such cases careful cleansing and repacking should be carried out after each bowel movement. Otherwise, superficial healing is liable to occur, with stagnation of pus in the depths of the wound; in such cases recurrence of the fistula is a probable result.

OTHER CONDITIONS AFFECTING THE ANUS

Carcinoma of the anus or anal canal

Some 3% of rectal carcinomata are of squamous type arising either at the anal margin or at a higher level within the canal, the latter being three times commoner than the former (Morson, 1979). There are two varieties, those involving the peri-anal skin or anal margin, and those arising within the anal canal above the dentate line, each carrying a very different prognosis. In the first type, the upper margin of the growth is often visible on everting the anus, and a finger detects no abnormality within the canal; this type is of relatively low malignancy, and can be treated by local excision (Madden, 1981). In the second variety, the growth may not be visible at all on inspection, but is at once detected within the canal by the examining finger;

such growths are much more malignant, and should be treated by radical excision of the anorectum.

Columnar epitheliomata are sometimes encountered; they arise immediately above the dentate line or represent the downward extension of a rectal tumour. Basal celled carcinomata are occasionally reported; they may be superficial, locally aggressive or metastasising (Nielsen, 1981).

Local excision by diathermy is suitable for early marginal growths confined to one quadrant of the anus and arising below the dentate line. The growth is excised with the diathermy knife, together with a generous margin of surrounding skin and with the underlying fibres of the external sphincter aiming for a clearance of 2.5 cm; the wound is left open to granulate. Provided that the puborectalis sling remains intact, incontinence does not normally result.

Radical excision of the rectum

More advanced growths and those involving the anal canal rather than the perianal skin should be treated by radical excision of the rectum by the abdominoperineal method. An extra wide excision of the perianal tissues must be undertaken.

Irradiation therapy

Some encouraging successes have been obtained by this method of treatment alone, but in general the results are less satisfactory than those of excisional surgery. Certain cases may be dealt with by a combination of radiotherapy (which causes the growth to shrink) and subsequent excision.

Treatment of the inguinal glands

It should be noted that glandular swellings may be due simply to infection, and may subside rapidly after effective treatment of the primary growth. If, however, the swellings persist for more than 2 or 3 weeks, or if their hardness suggests that they are metastatic in nature, assessment of their malignant potential is made by fine needle aspiration (FNA) cytology and a block dissection of the glands is carried out if necessary (p. 669).

In inoperable cases the severe pain and anal incontinence of the terminal stages may be relieved by a palliative colostomy.

Anal incontinence

Most cases of incontinence of the anal sphincter are due to accidental or obstetrical injuries, or are the result of operations in the anorectal region. Some may result from congenital abnormalities or their treatment.

Many types of repair have been described, but no one has proved entirely satisfactory, for by any method failures are common, owing to the high incidence of infection with dehiscence of the wound. It is, therefore, often advisable to establish a defunctioning colostomy prior to repair.

Direct repair of the sphincter

If the sphincter has not been too extensively damaged, an attempt should be made to reconstitute it by suturing together its divided ends. Probably the most promising methods are those which depend on the use of stainless steel wire as suture material. This does not predispose to infection, and engenders a minimal tissue reaction. A crescentic incision is made just lateral to and centred over the defect, excising all underlying scar tissue. A fringe of mucosa is mobilized and sutured to restore the mucosal tube. The cut or torn ends of the sphincter muscle are identified and brought together with some overlap using mattress sutures of No. 40 SWG stainless steel wire (Browning, 1984). The residual wound is allowed to heal by granulation.

Plastic methods of repair

These may be undertaken as a preferable alternative to a colostomy, in cases where the sphincter is considered to be irreparable. In Thiersch's operation a ring of silver wire, silicone rubber tubing or nylon is passed round the anus, and is tied sufficiently tightly to admit one finger. It will allow motions to be passed, but at the same time will give considerable support to the anus. The alternative procedure of gracilis muscle transposition is still advocated in specialized centres (Christiansen, 1990).

Pruritus ani

In cases where no treatable cause can be discovered, or where local applications have failed to bring relief, recourse may be had to injection treatment.

Injection of alcohol

Under general or low spinal anaesthesia, the affected area may be 'stippled' by multiple subcutaneous injections of 95% alcohol. The needle punctures are made about 1 cm apart; the needle is thrust vertically through the skin, and usually not more than 0.25 ml is injected at each site. There is some danger of the skin sloughing if these quantities are exceeded. If successful this treatment may give complete relief of symptoms for several months or even years (Stone, 1926).

Cryosurgery

Of value in the elimination of unhealthy skin tags which aggravate pruritis ani. Several applications may be required before a smooth moisture-free anal margin is obtained.

Anorectal malformations

The incidence of this relatively common and important condition is 1 in 3000 births. The malformation devel-

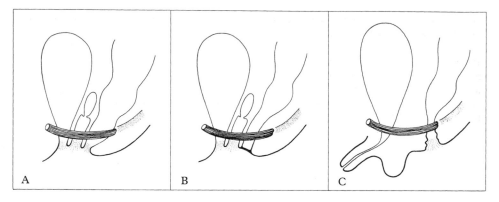

Fig. 23.30 High anorectal anomalies
A. Rectal atresia with recto-vaginal fistula
B. Rectal atresia with recto-urethral fistula
C. Rectal atresia with rectovestibular fistula

ops in the foetus between 4 and 10 weeks. During this period, the cloaca is divided into a urogenital chamber anteriorly and rectum posteriorly by a septum that grows caudally to the cloacal membrane. On the surface, the ectodermal pit overlying the rectum becomes the lower part of the anal canal. The more severe malformations form at an earlier stage of development. 33 different types were described at an international conference in Melbourne in 1970 which illustrates the complex nature of the problem. However, the important practical distinction is between the high and low types. In a high anomaly, the bowel ends above the levator ani but in the low anomaly the bowel passes down through the limbs of the puborectalis sling.

Classification

The more common malformations are best understood in relation to development. High anomalies (Fig. 23.30), which include rectal atresia with or with-

out fistula, develop at a relatively early stage as a result of incomplete division of the cloaca. In rectal atresia the normal bowel ends above the levator ani, occasionally blind, but more commonly connected by a fistula to the prostatic urethra in the male and to the posterior wall of the vagina or vestibule in the female. In contrast the low anomalies (Fig. 23.31), which include ectopic anus, covered anus and anal stenosis, develop at a later stage. It is suggested that an ectopic anus results from incomplete migration of the anus back across the perineum. The opening may be perineal in the male or perineal, vulval or vestibular in the female. The covered anus probably results from overgrowth of the anal folds and as a result the underlying rectum and anal canal are normal. The covered anus appears either as a membrane which may be crossed by a median bar or as a fine superficial fistulous tract running forward in the midline of the perineum. Anorectal fibrosis may be caused by incomplete involution of the cloacal mem-

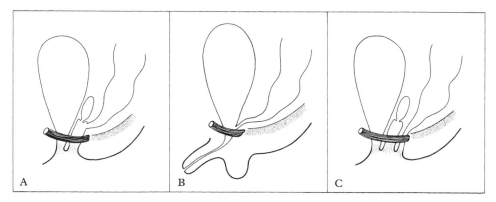

Fig. 23.31 Low anorectal anomalies
A. Vulva ectopic anus
B. Covered anus
C. Anorectal stenosis

brane. Normally a narrow rigid fibrous ring can be felt but occasionally fibrosis may extend along the length of the canal.

The uncommon high anomaly of atresia of the middle third of the rectum in which the proximal rectum and anal canal are normally formed but are joined by a fibrous band is difficult to explain by the sequence of events described above.

Clinical presentation

The clinical diagnosis is normally made during examination of the newborn baby. However, anorectal fibrosis and marginal displacement of an ectopic anus may be missed and present later in life with chronic constipation. In a baby with a high anomaly, no bowel opening is immediately seen but meconium may stain the urine of a male or may be passed from the vagina in a female. In a baby with a low anomaly the opening is visible when the perineum is examined. Care must be taken to differentiate between rectal atresia with a rectovestibular fistula and a vestibular ectopic anus. The former runs deep in close relation to the vagina and is supported by the puborectalis whereas the latter runs backwards in a superficial plane (Figs 23.30C and 23.31A).

The distinction between high and low anomalies is not always clear. The value of radiology in this respect is debatable; the position of gas in the distal bowel in relation to the puborectalis can be demonstrated on a lateral X-ray taken at the level of the greater trochanter with the baby inverted and the hips flexed (Stephens & Smith, 1971) but the result must be interpreted with caution. An X-ray of the sacrum, however, is important as sacral agenesis may be associated with abnormal pelvic innervation. An intravenous pyelogram should also be performed in the first month of life to exclude an associated urinary tract abnormality.

Operation

A *high type* of malformation is treated by a transverse or left iliac colostomy according to preference and a definitive operation performed when the baby is 9 months or 10 kg. The operation is approached through a transverse lower abdominal incision. The distal bowel is mobilized by careful dissection to preserve the pelvic splanchnic nerves and the fistula is divided. The puborectalis sling can be felt with the tip of a finger pushed down into the pelvis in the midline immediately behind the posterior wall of the urethra or vagina. A perineal incision is then made over the anal dimple which can be recognized by stimulating the underlying fibres of the superficial external sphincter. Forceps are passed through the perineal opening to the abdominal cavity and are directed through the limbs of the puborectalis by a finger placed deep in the pelvis. The bowel is then

drawn down through the tunnel and anastomosed to perineal skin. An initial sacral approach to safeguard the puborectalis sling may be preferred (Stephens & Smith, 1971). The tip of the coccyx is separated from the sacrum to provide access to the front of the levator ani. The sling can then be identified under direct vision and marked. An endorectal dissection may be used to preserve the pelvic splanchnic nerves which are closely related to the fistula (Rehbein, 1959). The distal dissection of the rectum from the peritoneal reflection is continued at a submucosal plane. The muscle wall of the rectum is thus left in position and an opening made in the distal part so that the bowel can be pulled down through the muscle cuff toward the perineum.

The *low type* of malformation should be treated within 48 hours of birth if the bowel is obstructed. An ectopic anus is treated by a cutback operation. The anal mucosa and overlying skin are divided with scissors in a posterior direction. The cut edges of mucosa and skin are then sewn together. If the blade is allowed to pass too deeply, the puborectalis may be damaged. Although a cutback operation is described for treatment of a vestibular ectopic anus, some surgeons consider it undesirable in view of the proximity of the vagina. Instead, the vestibular opening can be circumcised, the distal bowel freed by dissection and then transposed to the normal position. A covered anus may be treated either by excision of the membranous covering or by tracing proximally the fine fistulous tract; the mucosa of the anal canal is then stitched to skin. In anorectal stenosis the rigid band should be divided using a longitudinal incision and mucosa and skin stitched together in a transverse plane. It is essential that, after the initial treatment of a low anomaly, anal dilatation is continued daily for three months to ensure an adequate and supple opening. Failure to do this may result in constipation and secondary rectal inertia which can be extremely difficult to manage.

Results

Continence can be described as excellent, meaning no accidents; good, meaning occasional accidents; and unsatisfactory. In children with low type malformations continence should be excellent in the majority and good in the rest; in those with high malformations approximately one third have an excellent result, one third are good and the remainder are unsatisfactory. In expert hands, however, the unsatisfactory group can be as low as 10% (Nixon, 1978).

PILONIDAL SINUS

Pilonidal sinuses are found in the midline of the natal cleft overlying the coccyx or lower part of the sacrum.

They were formerly ascribed to a defect in development, leading to subcutaneous inclusion of epidermal structures, but it now seems more likely that they are acquired lesions, resulting from penetration of the skin by hairs or infection within a hair follicle. There are often two or more sinus openings, leading to tracks of varying depth; these are lined by squamous epithelium and not infrequently contain hairs (hence the name, *pilonidal sinus*).

Most patients come first to treatment on account of suppuration related to the sinuses, and abscesses commonly form either in the natal cleft or to one or other side; such abscesses may discharge spontaneously through an existing sinus, or may require to be opened. Thereafter, the infection may clear up completely, and no further trouble is experienced. More often, however, the discharge persists; either continuously, or after periodic abscess formation.

Surgical treatment should usually be advised when there have been two or more infective episodes, or when the discharge shows no sign of clearing up. Although several conservative procedures have been described (Mansoory 1982), the usual treatment — and probably the most effective one — is complete excision of the sinus tracks, together with all their ramifications.

Technique of excision

The operation is carried out with the patient in the left lateral or in the inverted-V position. An elliptical incision is made to include all sinus openings, and is deepened vertically until all diseased tissue has been detected. Coloured dye injected into the sinus track for identification during operation does not always reach the smaller sinuses and it is preferable to look carefully for granulation tissue during the dissection. If it is apparent that one of the ramifications of the sinus has been opened, a wider line of excision must be followed. Wide clearance down to sacrococcygeal fascia is not necessary, provided all the sinus tracks have been excised (Allen-Mersh, 1990).

Primary wound suture

When there has been no recent infection, it may be justifiable to suture the wound in an attempt to obtain healing by first intention. This offers the prospect of rapid cure, but the slightest infection may lead to a discharging sinus and a recurrence of the disease. If primary suture is carried out, every effort must be made to avoid leaving dead space in the wound, for such will undoubtedly predispose to infection. Various methods of closure may be employed. The tissues on each side of the wound may be mobilized by undercutting, so that they can be approximated without undue tension. Alternatively, the wound may be closed in layers, with a large number of buried sutures. Midline suturing fails,

however, to flatten the natal cleft and may lead to recurrence. To obviate this, numerous plastic procedures have been described (Toubanakis, 1986) but require special skills to avoid flap tip necrosis.

Gauze packing without suture

This entails a somewhat tedious convalescence, but has the advantage of effecting a permanent cure in nearly every case. No sutures whatever are inserted for closure; the wound is left widely open, and is packed either with dry gauze or with a non-adherent dressing which is held in place by sutures (Figs 23.32 & 23.33). The pack is removed in 2 or 3 days. The large cavity which is present at this stage may occasion some misgivings but it is virtually painless and heals with amazing rapidity by granulation from the depths outwards. After the initial pack has been removed only a flat dressing is required. For cleansing and irrigation of the wound sitz baths are taken twice daily. Dressings are simplified and wound healing encouraged by the use of silicone foam sponge dressing (Wood, 1975). The sponge is renewed weekly, and is changed daily by the patient himself.

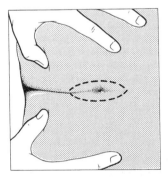

Fig. 23.32 Pilonidal sinus before operation. The opening of the sinus is seen between the index fingers

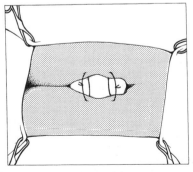

Fig. 23.33 Excision completed and wound packed with gauze. (The stitches serve only to retain the pack in position)

Healing is rarely complete before 4 or 5 weeks, but the patient can be discharged from hospital in 7 to 10 days or earlier if a silicone dressing is available. He is instructed to continue with daily baths and requires no treatment other than the simple dressings which he himself can apply.

COCCYGECTOMY

Removal of the coccyx is indicated occasionally when it is the seat of pain due to dislocation or malalignment of the bone in relation to the sacrum, or to arthritic changes at the intervening joint. Such conditions may result from childbirth or from other forms of local trauma. The lesion may be at the articulation between the 1st and 2nd coccygeal segments, and not at the sacrococcygeal articulation; in such case the distal segments alone are removed.

Before any operation is contemplated there should be *definite* evidence of deformity, or of arthritis (indicated by acute pain when the coccyx is moved on the sacrum by a finger in the rectum and a thumb externally). Pain in the coccygeal region, *coccydynia,* is common in young women, and frequently follows a fall on the buttocks. It may persist for months or even years, but definite evidence of deformity or arthritis is usually lacking, and there is likely to be a functional element in the complaints. In these cases coccygectomy is contraindicated, since the pain persists after operation. Relief can often be obtained by injection of local anaesthetic on both surfaces of the coccyx.

The operation of coccygectomy is a simple one. Through a longitudinal incision the coccyx is freed first at its tip and on each side, and disarticulation is carried out with a scalpel at the joint affected. The coccyx is then drawn backwards and is dissected off the underlying fascia. The knife is kept close to the bone in order to avoid injury to the fascia or to the middle sacral artery.

REFERENCES

Allen-Mersh T G 1990 Pilonidal sinus: finding the right track for treatment. British Journal of Surgery 77: 123–132

Antebi E, Schwartz P, Gilm E 1985 Sclerotherapy for the treatment of fissure-in-ano. Surgery, Gynaecology and Obstetrics 160: 204–206

Browning G G P, Motson R W 1984 Anal sphincter injury. Management and results of Parks' sphincter repair. Annals of Surgery 199: 351

Chamberlain J, Johnstone J M S 1970 The results of haemorrhoidectomy by clamp and cautery. Surgery, Gynaecology and Obstetrics 131: 745

Christiansen J, Sorensen M, Rasmussen O 1990 Gracilis muscle transposition for faecal incontinence. British Journal of Surgery 77: 1039–1040

Duthie G S, Bartolo D C C 1991. Pathophysiology and management of rectal prolapse. In: Taylor I, Johnson C D (eds) Recent advances in surgery No 14. Churchill Livingstone, Edinburgh, Ch 11

Duthie G S, Bartolo D C C 1992. Abdominal rectopexy for rectal prolapse: a comparison of techniques. British Journal of Surgery 79: 107–113

Ellis M 1960 Incision and primary suture of abscesses of the anal region. Proceedings Royal Society of Medicine 53: 652

Gingold B S, Mitty W F, Tadros M 1983 Importance of patient selection in local treatment of carcinoma of the rectum. American Journal of Surgery 145: 293

Jackaman F R, Francis J N, Hopkinson B R 1980 Silicone rubber band treatment of rectal prolapse. Annals of the Royal College of Surgeons of England 62: 386–387

Lindhus E, Gjode P, Gottrup F, Holm C N, Terpling S 1989 Bacteriocidal antimicrobial cover in primary suture of perianal or pilonidal abscess. Acta Chirurgica Scandinavica 155: 351–354

Lord P H 1969 A day case procedure for the cure of third degree haemorrhoids. British Journal of Surgery 56: 747

McCue J L, Thomson J P S 1991. Clinical and functional results of abdominal rectopexy for complete rectal prolapse. British Journal of Surgery 78: 921–923

McDonald P 1992 Haemorrhoids and anal fissure. In: Johnson C D, Taylor I (eds) Recent advances in surgery No. 15, Churchill Livingstone, Edinburgh, Ch 7

Madden M V, Elliot M S, Botha J B C, Louse J H 1981 The management of anal carcinoma. British Journal of Surgery 68: 287–289

Mansoory A, Dickson D 1982 Z-plasty for treatment of disease of the pilonidal sinus: Surgery, Gynaecology Obstetrics 155: 409

Marks C G, Ritchie J K 1977 Anal fistulas at St Mark's Hospital. British Journal of Surgery 64: 84–91

Morson B C, Dawson I M P 1979 Gastrointestinal pathology, 2nd edn. Blackwell, Oxford, p 741

Nielsen O V, Jensen S L 1981 Basal cell carcinoma of the anus — a clinical study of 34 cases. British Journal of Surgery 68: 856–857

Nixon H H 1978 Surgical conditions in paediatrics. Butterworth & London, p 93

Parks A G, Percy J P 1982 Resection and sutured colo-anal anastomosis for rectal carcinoma. British Journal of Surgery 69: 301–304

Rehbein F 1959 Operation for anal and rectal atresia with recto-urethral fistula. Chirurgia 30: 417 (Year Book Medical Publishers, Chicago)

Ross A H M 1980 Rectal stricture resection using the EEA auto stapler. British Journal of Surgery 67: 281–282

Seow-Choen F, Nicholls R J 1992 Anal fistula. British Journal of Surgery 79: 197–205

Smith M 1967 Early operation for acute haemorrhoids. British Journal of Surgery 54: 141

Stephens F D, Smith E D (eds) 1971 Anorectal malformations in children, Year Book Medical Publishers, Chicago

Stone H B 1926 Pruritus ani, treatment by alcohol injection. Surgery Gynaecology and Obstetrics 42: 565

Thomson W H F 1975 The nature of haemorrhoids. British Journal of Surgery 62: 542–552

Toubanakis G 1986 Treatment of pilonidal disease with the Z-plasty procedure (modified). American Surgery 52: 611–612

Wells C 1959 New operation for rectal prolapse. Proceedings Royal Society Medicine 52: 602

Williams J G, MacLeod C A, Rothenberger D A Goldberg S M 1991 Seton treatment of high anal fistulae. British Journal of Surgery 78: 1159–1161

Wood R A B, Hughes L E 1975 Silicone foam sponge for pilonidal sinus: A new technique for dressing open granulating wounds. British Medical Journal 3: 131

FURTHER READING

Goligher J C 1985 Surgery of the anus, rectum and colon, 5th edn. Baillière Tindall, London

Parks A G, Gordon P H, Hardcastle J D 1976 A classification of fistula in ano. British Journal of Surgery 63: 1

Parks A G, Stitz R W 1976 The treatment of high fistula in ano: Diseases of the colon and rectum 19: 487–525

24

Abdominal herniae

J. M. S. JOHNSTONE & R. F. RINTOUL

OBLIQUE INGUINAL HERNIA

Anatomy

The inguinal canal, which is about 4 cm in length, runs obliquely between the muscles, aponeuroses and fasciae of the abdominal wall above the medial part of the inguinal ligament. Its internal end is the *deep inguinal ring,* an opening in the transversalis fascia 1 cm above the midinguinal point, and immediately lateral to the inferior epigastric vessels. Its external end is the *superficial inguinal ring,* a triangular aperture in the aponeurosis of external oblique situated immediately above the pubic tubercle. The base of the ring is formed by the inguinal ligament; its margins (*crura*) are sewn together at the apex, which points laterally and upwards, by the *intercrural fibres.*

Boundaries. The *anterior wall* is formed in its whole length, by the aponeurosis of external oblique, and in its lateral third by the lowest fibres of internal oblique arising from the inguinal ligament. The *posterior wall* is formed in its whole length by the transversalis fascia, and in its medial half by the conjoined tendon. The *roof* is formed by the lower borders of internal oblique and transversus, which arch over the canal before fusing together to form the conjoined tendon. The *floor* is the grooved upper surface of the inguinal ligament, and of its reflection on to the superior ramus of the pubis.

Contents. In the male, the main contents of the canal are the *spermatic cord* and the vestigial remnant of the *processus vaginalis,* the fetal prolongation of peritoneum which accompanies the testes in its descent into the scrotum. In the female, the canal transmits the *ligamentum teres uteri (round ligament).* The *ilio-inguinal nerve* lies in the medial part of the canal and emerges through the superficial ring. The *iliohypogastric nerve,* which is not strictly a content of the canal, but which is displayed when the canal is opened, lies on the front of internal oblique a little above its lower border.

The spermatic cord consists of the vas deferens with its artery, the testicular artery, the pampiniform plexus of veins (its bulkiest constituent), lymph vessels and sympathetic nerves. The cord has 3 *coverings:* (1) the internal spermatic fascia derived from fascia transversalis at the deep ring, (2) the cremasteric muscle and fascia derived from internal oblique, and (3) the external spermatic fascia derived from external oblique aponeurosis at the superficial ring.

Oblique inguinal hernia

The *sac,* or peritoneal tube through which the abdominal contents protrude, accompanies the spermatic cord in its oblique course, and is enclosed within its coverings usually lying anterior to the structures of the cord proper. The neck of the sac, which is often constricted, lies at the deep inguinal ring, lateral to the inferior epigastric vessels. The *coverings* of the sac, from within outwards are those of the cord *plus* deep fascia, superficial fascia and skin.

Aetiology and types of sac. It has long been taught that, even in the adult, most oblique inguinal herniae are of congenital origin, the sac being formed by the processus vaginalis, which either wholly or in part has failed to become obliterated, and that, although the sac is present from birth, the hernia may not appear until adult life. The sac is usually of the *funicular* type, terminating below in a blind end or *fundus:* this is attributed to the fact that only the upper part of the processus has remained open, while the rest has become obliterated. The evidence in favour of such a congenital origin for adult herniae is not, however, convincing, and many surgeons now believe that most of these herniae are acquired, the sac being formed as a true protrusion of the parietal peritoneum through the inguinal canal. In support of this belief, there is the important finding that when operation for oblique inguinal hernia is followed by a recurrence, the sac is noted in almost 50% of cases to be again an oblique one; this proves that an oblique hernia can be acquired. In infants and young children there is no doubt that the hernia is congenital: in males the entire processus vaginalis may have remained patent, in which case the sac is of the *vaginal* type, extending down to the testis to become continuous

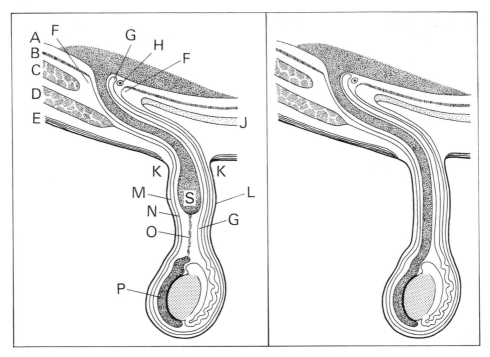

Fig. 24.1   **Fig. 24.2**

Figs 24.1 & 24.2   Schematic drawing to show the relations and coverings of an oblique inguinal hernia; also the two common types of sac — *funicular* in Figure 24.1, *vaginal* in Figure 24.2. A — peritoneum; B — transversalis fascia; C — transversus; D — internal oblique; E — external oblique; F — margins of deep ring; G — vas deferens; H — inf. epigastric art.; J — conjoined tendon; K — margins of superf. ring; L — ext. spermatic fascia; M — cremasteric fascia; N — int. spermatic fascia; O — processus vaginalis; P — tunica vaginalis; S — sac

with the tunica vaginalis; in females the sac is necessarily funicular, being developed from a blind process of peritoneum accompanying the round ligament.

Selection of patients
Oblique inguinal hernia should as a rule be treated by operation. This advice is given in spite of the fact that, in many surgeon's hands, the end-results of surgical treatment are disappointing, in that the recurrence rate is in the region of 10%. This is to a large extent avoidable if a careful technique is followed, despite the fact that the inguinal canal has to be left open in order to transmit the spermatic cord. The aim should be to have a recurrent rate of around 1% (Devlin, 1986). The smaller the hernia, and the shorter its duration, the more certain are the prospects of operative cure. Surgical intervention should be advised therefore even although the hernia is small and is causing no symptoms, for there is an invariable tendency for it to increase in size and for symptoms to develop. With modern anaesthesia (local, regional or general) there are few contraindications to operation. In general, a truss should be prescribed only when the patient refuses surgery; it is at best an unpleasant encumbrance, and its use for any length of time causes pres-

sure atrophy of the muscles around the hernial orifice, thus reducing the chances of a successful operation, should this be desired at a later date. Whether a truss is worn or not (for there are few trusses which do not slip occasionally and allow the hernia to protrude), the danger of strangulation is always present, and is one of the most cogent arguments in favour of operation. This danger is greatest when the orifice is narrow, or when the hernia is partly irreducible. If there have been temporary attacks of incarceration, or of threatened strangulation, operation should not be delayed.

Preparation for operation
If the patient is to have an elective operation, the arrangement should allow this to be done when his general health is at its optimum. Any chest affliction should be treated, if necessary, by physiotherapy or operation postponed until the season of the year when his respiratory function is at its best. This will minimize postoperative problems and reduce the strain placed on the repair by an explosive cough.

Choice of operation
While there is almost universal agreement as to the

advisability of surgery, opinions differ regarding the best method of operative repair.

In the truly congenital herniae of infancy or childhood, where a preformed sac is undoubtedly present, removal of the sac alone — *simple herniotomy* — is all that is required. In adult cases of hernia the same operation may be considered adequate by those surgeons who believe that the aetiological concept of a congenitally preformed sac applies. Its use should be restricted, however, to younger patients, in whom the deep ring is unstretched and the musculature of the canal appears to be sound. It is probable that the majority of surgeons at the present time prefer to carry out some form of reconstructive operation in all adult cases. Thus, in patients over the age of 16 years, the operation has 2 parts: (1) removal of the sac, (2) repair of the defect.

Anaesthesia

Local, regional or general anaesthesia may be used, depending on the needs of the patient and availability of the necessary skills. *Marcain* 0.25% with adrenaline 1 in 400 000 solution is suitable for inguinal field block anaesthesia, up to a maximum of 2 mg/kg body weight. The same solution may be combined with general or spinal anaesthesia to provide up to 12 hours of post operative pain relief.

Inguinal herniotomy in children

Inguinal herniae in children are of congenital origin and associated with a patent processus vaginalis which extends partly or completely along the spermatic cord in boys and the round ligament in girls. Such herniae are common, the incidence being 10 per 1000 live births. Boys are affected 10 times more frequently than girls and, in approximately 1 in 5 of such children, the condition is bilateral.

The presenting sign is that of an intermittent or persistent swelling which appears over the pubic tubercle and may extend down towards the scrotum. The swelling, if present, can be reduced with a characteristic gurgling sensation. Alternatively, thickening of the spermatic cord can be felt when the cord is under light traction and rolled between finger and thumb. A hernia which appears in early infancy is at risk of becoming strangulated and operation should be carried out as soon as possible.

Operation

Inguinal herniotomy is a safe and effective operation which can, under normal circumstances, be performed as a day case procedure. In most children under 5 years of age the internal inguinal ring lies deep to the external ring and the foreshortened inguinal canal can be explored without opening the external oblique aponeurosis.

A skin crease incision 2–3 cm in length is made just above the pubic tubercle (Fig. 24.3) and the superficial and deep abdominal fascia divided. The external spermatic fascia is then split in the line of the cord, exposing the bluish coverings of the cord. Using blunt dissecting forceps, the spermatic cord is cleared of adherent tissue and delivered through the wound and held with a light vascular sling (Fig. 24.4). With the cord under light traction the coverings over the proximal half are divided longitudinally. In order to secure the correct plane, it is helpful to make a small incision in the coverings through which the contents stand proud. The incision can then be extended with ease (Fig. 24.5). The

Figs 24.3–24.6 *Inguinal herniotomy in children*

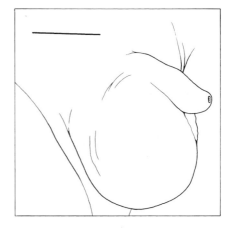

Fig. 24.3 Skin crease incision above pubic tubercle

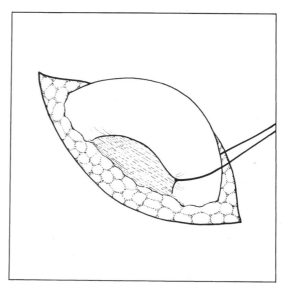

Fig. 24.4 Cord delivered through wound. A vascular sling is used for traction

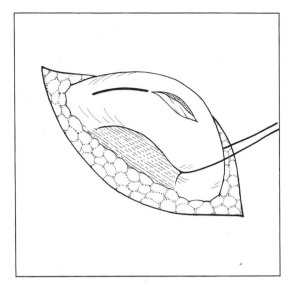

Fig. 24.5 Coverings incised allowing contents to bulge through

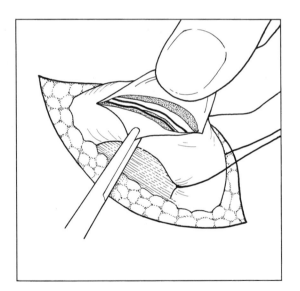

Fig. 24.6 Sac cleared circumferentially and vas and vessels lying underneath

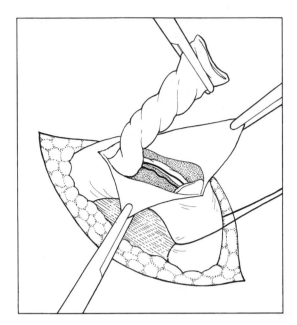

Fig. 24.7 Divided sac traced proximally and twisted

cut edges of the cord coverings are gripped with forceps and held aside so as to expose the content of the cord. The hernial sac, which may have an opaque appearance, will be found lying in front of the vas deferens and the testicular vessels (Fig. 24.6).

When the processus vaginalis is complete the hernial sac is lifted at a point in the proximal part of the cord and cleared circumferentially of adherent tissue, particular care being taken with the closely adherent vas and vessels. Artery forceps can then be placed across the hernial sac. The sac is divided distal to the forceps and the open fundus left in situ. With gentle traction on the forceps, the proximal part of the sac is traced towards the inguinal ring. The dissection is complete when the neck of the sac is reached as indicated by the presence of extraperitoneal fat. The sac is twisted to exclude intraperitoneal content (Fig. 24.7), the neck of the sac is ligated and the sac distal to the neck excised. When the processus vaginalis is incomplete the fundus of the sac will be seen and the dissection started from that point. It is important that the testis be replaced and manipulated well down into the scrotum and the alignment of the spermatic vessels checked to exclude torsion. The wound is then closed with a single absorbable suture in the deep fascia and a subcuticular absorbable skin suture.

Inguinal herniotomy prior to reconstruction

Technique
The classical incision is made 2.5 cm above and parallel to the medial three-fifths of the inguinal ligament but a more horizontally placed skin-crease incision will be found to produce a more acceptable scar. The superficial epigastric and superficial external pudendal vessels are secured. The incision is deepened until the aponeurosis of external oblique is exposed, and the superficial inguinal ring, through which the cord emerges, is identified. The external oblique aponeurosis is divided in the line of its fibres, the incision being placed so that it opens into the ring in its upper medial part if a satisfactory overlapping is to be achieved later in the operation. Forceps are applied to the two cut edges; the

upper leaf is retracted to expose the conjoined muscles arching over the cord, and the lower to expose the upper surface of the inguinal ligament. The ilioinguinal and iliohypogastric nerves are identified and safeguarded. The cord, with which is included the hernial sac, is lifted up from the medial part of the incision, and is spread out on the finger. Its coverings are incised longitudinally, and are further separated by blunt dissection, care being taken to avoid injuring the spermatic veins. If the hernia is recent and is completely reducible, recognition of the sac may be a matter of some difficulty. It appears as a pearly-white structure, lying as a rule anterior to the components of the cord proper. In adults it is almost invariably of the *funicular* type, and is more easily isolated if its fundus, the crescentic border of which lies transversely across the cord, is defined first and is held in artery forceps. Further separation of the sac is then effected by gauze stripping. Care must be taken that the vas deferens, which is palpable as a firm cord, is not detached along with the sac in the process of stripping. As the separation proceeds, traction is applied to the sac and the stripping is continued until the neck comes into view. This is identified from the presence of an adherent pad or collar of fat. The inferior epigastric vessels lie to its medial side, and care should be taken that they are not injured. When separation is complete the sac is opened at some distance from its neck, and a finger is intro-

duced into its interior to ensure that it is empty of contents. In general it is better that the sac should be completely separated before it is opened, for otherwise during the process of separation, the opening become extended as a split proximally beyond the neck of the sac — a complication to be avoided if possible. When, however, the sac is very adherent, it can often be more easily separated if it is opened and a finger introduced at an early stage. Glassow (1973, 1984), with an experience of over 50 000 such herniae, stresses the importance of freeing the sac right up to the deep ring. Adherent contents are freed from the sac and returned to the abdomen.

The sac is now drawn strongly downwards, and a transfixion ligature is applied immediately above its neck. When the neck is wide, care must be taken that underlying bowel is not transfixed or caught up in the ligature. In such cases it is an advantage to twist the sac at its neck, in order to occlude it before the ligature is applied. The sac is amputated 1 cm below the ligature *prior* to cutting the ligature so that there is adequate control of the stump in the event of bleeding. If the ligature has been applied at a sufficiently high level, the stump will immediately retract well above the deep inguinal ring to lie flush with the general peritoneum.

In the case of *scrotal* herniae, where the fundus of the sac may not come easily into view, there is no objection to leaving the distal part of the sac in situ. The sac is

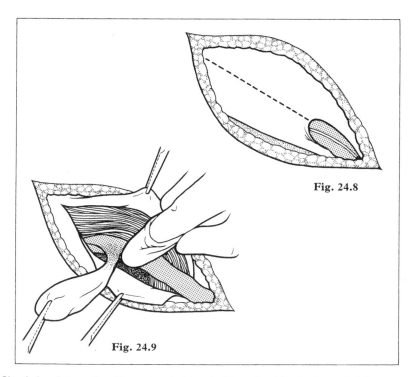

Fig. 24.8

Fig. 24.9

Figs 24.8 & 24.9   Simple herniotomy for oblique inguinal hernia. Line of incision in external oblique aponeurosis, and separation of the sac by gauze dissection

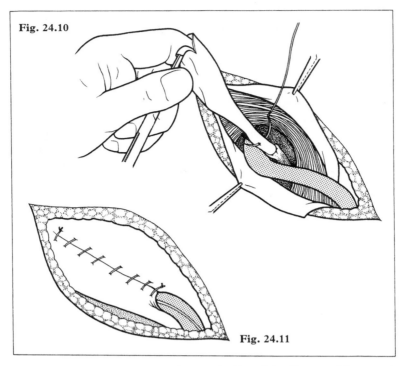

Fig. 24.10

Fig. 24.11

Figs 24.10 & 24.11   Simple herniotomy for oblique inguinal hernia. Transfixion-ligature of the sac as its neck, and repair of oblique aponeurosis

first separated for a short distance from the cord structures, and is then divided transversely. The distal part is dropped back, while the proximal part is cleared up to its neck and removed in the usual way. This method obviates the dissection required to deliver the sac from the depths of the scrotum, and greatly reduces the risk of subsequent haematoma formation.

Reconstructive procedures

The Bassini method of repair
This classical operation was first described by Bassini in 1888. It consists essentially in strengthening the posterior wall of the inguinal canal in its lateral part, by stitching the lower border of the conjoined muscles and tendon down to the inguinal ligament *behind the cord.*

After the sac has been removed, the cord together with the ilio-inguinal nerve, is held out of the way by drawing the lower leaf of the external oblique aponeurosis downwards superficial to it (Fig. 24.12). The lower border of the conjoined muscles and tendon and the upper surface of the inguinal ligament are carefully cleared of fat and areolar tissue. The muscles and tendons are lifted forwards with dissecting forceps and five or six stitches are inserted at about 1 cm intervals between them and the inguinal ligament. The most lateral suture is inserted first, picking up tissue at the margins of the deep ring and the ring around the emerging cord.

In placing these initial stitches, great care must be taken not to injure the external iliac vessels which lie immediately deep to the inguinal ligament. To avoid such an accident the actual ligament alone should be lifted forwards on the point of the needle, before the stitch is passed. The most medial suture is placed under the periosteum overlying the pubic tubercle. All stitches should be introduced at different depths into the inguinal ligament, in order that they may not cause splitting of the ligament along the line of sutures.

It is particularly important that the stitches should not be tied too tightly or they will cause strangulation of the muscular fibres, which then become replaced by weak scar tissue. Care must be taken that the ilio-hypogastric nerve is not included in any suture. The conjoined muscles should lie snugly around the cord in the lateral part of the wound, thus giving support to the deep inguinal ring. In the approximation of the muscles to the inguinal ligament, *it is essential that there should be no tension on the sutures,* for this may determine the failure of the operation. If the approximation cannot be made without tension, the case is unsuitable for simple Bassini repair, and some other method of reconstruction should be considered.

Finally, the cord is allowed to fall back on the strengthened posterior wall of the canal. The aponeurosis of external oblique is repaired, either by simple suture, or preferably by overlapping (Figs 24.14

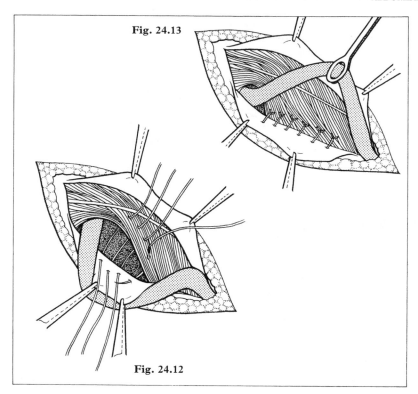

Fig. 24.13

Fig. 24.12

Figs 24.12 & 24.13   The Bassini method of repair in inguinal hernia — approximation of the conjoined muscles and tendon to the inguinal ligament, behind the spermatic cord; this is held out of the way, under cover of the lower flap of external oblique

& 24.15). The reconstituted superficial ring should fit snugly around the cord, but it must not be too tight or atrophy of the testis may result; it should admit the tip of the little finger without difficulty, in addition to the cord. After careful haemostasis the wound is closed by suture of the superficial fascia and skin.

Suture material. The type of suture material to be used is a matter of choice, and many conflicting views have been expressed. Dexon, nylon, linen and silk thread, and stainless steel and tantalum wire have all been advocated. Of these, monofilament nylon is the best since the multiple knots required for interrupted

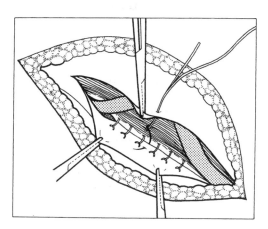

Fig. 24.14   Inguinal herniorrhaphy — third stage. The upper leaf of the external oblique aponeurosis is mobilized and drawn down *in front of the cord* to be stitched to the deep surface of the inguinal ligament

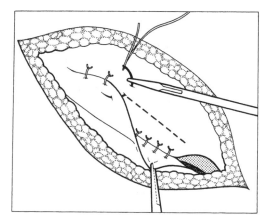

Fig. 24.15   Inguinal herniorrhaphy — fourth stage. The lower leaf of the external oblique is stitched against the upper leaf thus overlapping it, so that a strong anterior wall to the canal is constructed

thread may lead to troublesome sinus formation. Of greater importance, the continuous frictionless suture distributes tension evenly (Wantz, 1989).

Modification of the Bassini repair and alternative methods
Most other methods of inguinal herniorrhaphy are based essentially upon the Bassini operation, but are designed to avoid such tension as may be inseparable from this method. In general they serve to occlude the gap between the conjoined muscles and the inguinal ligament, by methods other than that of simply stitching these structures together.

The Shouldice operation. The essential steps in this method of repair of the posterior wall are (1) double breasting of fascia transversalis in order to tighten and narrow the deep ring, (2) approximation of conjoined tendon to inguinal ligament in two layers. The operation depends on removal of the cremaster muscle from that portion of spermatic cord which lies within the inguinal canal so that clear identification can be made of transversalis fascia as it is reflected on to the cord at the deep ring. This is the optimum method of repair, provided the surgeon has been given the necessary instruction.

Relaxation incisions, designed to relieve tension at a Bassini repair, may be made either before or after the repair has been carried out. In the 'muscle-slide' operation as described by Tanner (1942) the upper leaf of the external oblique aponeurosis is elevated and retracted upwards, so that a curved incision can be made in the aponeuroses of the internal oblique and transversus where they form the anterior rectus sheath. This incision begins over the pubic crest, passes vertically upwards about 4 cm from the midline, and then turns laterally to end 2 cm from the lateral border of the rectus muscle a hand's breadth above the pubis. The lateral leaf of this incision at once retracts downwards owing to the tone of the conjoined muscles, which are now found to lie without tension alongside the inguinal ligament (Fig. 24.17).

Repair by nylon darn. A monofilament nylon suture has inherent strength and produces no tissue reaction. The advantage of a nylon darn lies in the continuous suture which does not result in any localised areas of tension. However, the original description by Moloney (1948) stressed that the material used for the darn matters less than the care of the operator. The posterior wall is repaired in two layers with particular care to support the deep ring.

Implantation of foreign material. Gauzes or meshes made of tantalum wire or nylon, or materials such as polyvinyl alcohol sponge or marlex mesh, have been implanted with success in cases where there is a large defect as in a recurrent hernia.

Overlapping of the external oblique aponeurosis
In the author's opinion this is a most important part of any operation for inguinal hernia. The strength of the inguinal canal lies in its obliquity, and for this a strong external oblique is indispensable (Fig. 24.18). In nearly all inguinal herniae the external oblique aponeurosis is weak and bulging over the greater part of the canal, the degree of weakness being directly proportional to the size of the protrusion. It is not enough to narrow the deep ring and to strengthen the posterior wall of the canal, for the hernia will recur if the deep ring lacks the support which it can derive from a strong anterior wall to the canal. This can readily be provided by over-

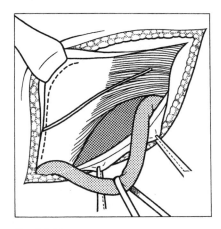

Fig. 24.16

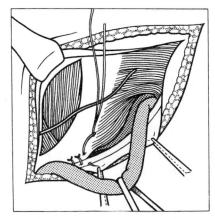

Fig. 24.17

Figs 24.16 & 24.17 The 'muscle-slide' operation in inguinal herniorrhaphy. An incision is made in the aponeuroses of internal oblique and transversus near the medial border of the rectus muscle, where they form its anterior sheath. This relaxes the lower border of these muscles, which now lie alongside the inguinal ligament without tension (After Tanner)

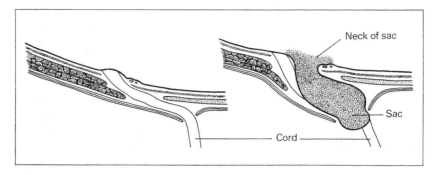

Fig. 24.18   Obliquity of the inguinal canal — one of the most important factors in its strength — requires a strong anterior wall as well as a strong posterior wall. Unless the external oblique is repaired strongly *in its normal relationship to the cord,* much of this obliquity is lost, and recurrent herniation is more liable to take place

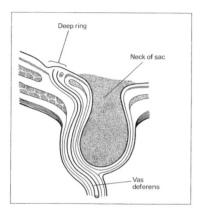

Fig. 24.19   Schematic drawing to show the relations and coverings of a *direct* inguinal hernia

lapping the external oblique aponeurosis *in front of the cord* (Figs 24.14 & 24.15). Since the aponeurosis is invariably lax, the overlapping can be effected with ease and without any undue tension.

Preperitoneal approach

This method of approach to inguinal herniae has been advocated by certain workers, notably in America. The incision is made through the muscles *above* the inguinal canal; it is deepened as far as the peritoneum, and it is in this plane that the hernia is approached. The sac is identified at its neck, i.e. where it enters the canal, and is withdrawn inwards before being removed. The posterior wall of the canal is then repaired by stitching the aponeurosis of transversus to the deep surface of the inguinal ligament.

The operation is more difficult and more time-consuming than the standard approach through the inguinal canal. It does not allow any reconstruction of the anterior wall of the canal, and this, in the author's opinion, is an important factor in preventing recurrence.

After-treatment

Surgeons who believe in the benefits of early ambulation (p. 349) may allow their patients to get up within a few hours of operation, or may even operate on them as outpatients (Farquharson, 1955; Ruckley, 1978). It seems certain that there is nothing to be gained in the average case of inguinal hernia by postoperative rest in bed. Unrestricted mobilization should be encouraged but the patient should refrain from heavy lifting for 2–3 months depending on his occupation.

Operation in the female

The inguinal canal is opened as in the male. The sac is separated from the round ligament and is amputated at its neck. Should the separation prove difficult the ligament may be removed along with the sac. If the inguinal canal is weak it is completely obliterated with sutures, the round ligament being disregarded.

DIRECT INGUINAL HERNIA

Anatomy

A direct inguinal hernia traverses only the medial part of the inguinal canal, and does not, therefore, pursue the oblique course taken by the spermatic cord. It protrudes from the abdominal cavity through the inguinal triangle (triangle of Hesselbach), which is bounded medially by the rectus muscle, laterally by the inferior epigastric vessels, and below by the inguinal ligament. It passes forwards, either below the arch of the conjoined muscles or through a weak area in the conjoined tendon, and finally emerges through the superficial inguinal ring. It seldom descends completely into the scrotum, but exceptions occur.

The sac, which is often wider at its neck than at its fundus, and which may be no more than a bulging of the peritoneum, is usually found lying posterior to the spermatic cord. Its coverings are the same as in oblique hernia, except that the covering it receives from transversalis fascia is not derived from the margins of the deep ring. If the sac passes through a weak area in the conjoined tendon, it receives a fascial covering from this structure instead of from internal oblique.

Selection of patients

Direct inguinal hernia occurs most commonly in patients of the obese or flabby type, or in those of asthenic build with poor muscular development or a chronic cough. It differs from oblique hernia in that it is never congenital, and in the fact that it invariably results from, or is associated with, weakness of the abdominal muscles particularly those which form the conjoined tendon. Operative cure is, therefore, a matter of greater difficulty than in the oblique hernia and the key to success lies in a careful reconstructive operation.

Direct inguinal herniae, as compared with oblique herniae, do not show the same tendency to increase in size, and, since the sac is wide-necked, there is seldom any risk of strangulation. It is unnecessary, therefore, to advise operation where the hernia is small, symptomless, and showing no increase in size. An unsuccessful operation with recurrence increases the risk of strangulation since the resultant defect is smaller, and has more rigid margins, than the initial hernia.

Operation

An incision is made as for oblique inguinal hernia and the external oblique is divided. The sac is sought for behind the cord, and is easily separated from it. It is freed up to its neck by blunt dissection and by gauze stripping. This must be done gently, or the inferior epigastric vessels which lie to the lateral side of the neck may be wounded (Fig. 24.20). Care must be taken also not to injure the bladder which lies in the extraperitoneal fat at the medial side of the sac, and may be adherent to it. If there is difficulty in separating the sac, or if bleeding is caused, close proximity of the bladder should at once be suspected.

The sac is opened and any contents are returned to the abdomen. If it is a wide-necked one, it is impracticable to deal with it by the method of transfixion-ligature; it is better to cut away the redundant part, and to repair the peritoneum at its base by continuous suture as in laparotomy. If the patient is obese and access is difficult, this suture may be inserted in mattress fashion *before* cutting away the excess tissue. Additional coverings of the sac are dealt with in the same manner. When the sac is no more than a slight bulging of the peritoneum, it should be ignored, and the treatment directed solely towards repair of the muscular defect. The cord should be carefully examined to exclude the presence of an oblique sac which sometimes coexists. If such a sac is found it is dealt with in the usual manner, and any lipoma of the cord is removed in order to reduce cord bulk.

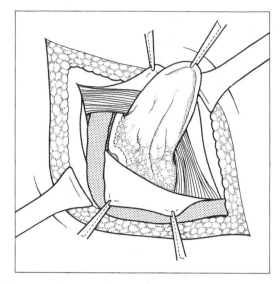

Fig. 24.20   Direct inguinal hernia — appearances at operation. Note the inferior epigastric artery lying lateral to the neck of the sac

Reconstructive measures

Owing to weakness of the conjoined muscles, and to the large gap which is usually present between these and the inguinal ligament, a simple Bassini repair is unlikely to be successful. The choice of operation is largely a matter of individual preference. Probably the majority of surgeons at the present time will choose to repair the defect by 'darning' with some material such as monofilament nylon; repair by the Shouldice method is preferable if the surgeon has received the necessary training. If the defect is particularly large, marlex mesh or a similar sheet of foreign material may be inserted.

When, as is frequently the case, the patient is an old or elderly man, with very poor muscles, no hesitation should be felt in removing the testis, since this allows complete obliteration of the inguinal canal to be carried out, and almost entirely obviates the risk of recurrence. In all cases where the advisability of orchidectomy might be considered, permission should if possible be obtained before operation.

SLIDING HERNIA

This condition may present both in indirect and in direct inguinal herniae. The term 'sliding' hernia denotes that some or all of the hernial contents lie *outside* the peritoneal sac. A part of the colon which is devoid of mesentery (the caecum on the right side and the pelvic colon on the left side), or a portion of the bladder, is found to be incorporated in the posterior wall of the sac, and is therefore not reducible in the ordinary way, owing to the fact that the sac forms part of its peritoneal coverings. It the condition is not recognized, and an attempt is made to clear the sac in the customary manner, the vessels of the colon or bladder are very liable to be torn. When the neck of the sac is unusually bulky, when it does not separate easily, or when bleeding is induced, a sliding hernia should at once be suspected.

Ordinary ligature and removal of the sac at its neck are impossible and the following method of repair has been recommended. A U-shaped incision is made in the peritoneum at a distance of about 2 cm from the bowel, so that a fringe of peritoneum remains on each side (Fig. 24.21), and is carried upwards beyond the neck of the sac. The bowel is then elevated; its retroperitoneal surface is covered by stitching together the peritoneal fringes on each side, and the gap in the posterior wall of the sac is closed by suture (Fig. 24.22). The bowel which has been freed from the sac and reperitonized is replaced within the abdominal cavity. The neck of the sac is closed securely by a purse-string suture and the rest of the sac cut away.

Many surgeons believe, however, that such elaborate methods are unnecessary, and are content with removing the free portion of the sac below the attached viscus. The peritoneum is then repaired and the whole is returned to the abdomen. Whatever method is adopted, special attention must be paid to a sound reconstruction of the canal, since this is always weak, and the chances of recurrence are considerable.

FEMORAL HERNIA

Anatomy

The femoral canal is the medial of the three compartments of the femoral sheath; this is formed by a prolongation into the thigh of the fascia transversalis and of the fascia iliaca, which line respectively the anterior and posterior abdominal walls. The lateral compartment of the sheath contains the femoral artery, and the intermediate one, the femoral vein. The femoral canal is about 2 cm in length, and is funnel-shaped. It lies on pectineus under cover of the cribriform fascia and the upper margin of the saphenous opening.

The femoral ring, which is the name given to the internal orifice of the canal, is relatively rigid. It is bounded

Figs 24.21 & 24.22   *Method of repair in a sliding hernia containing the caecum*

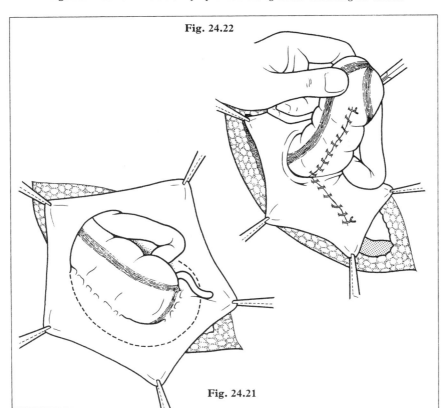

Fig. 24.22

Fig. 24.21

Fig. 24.21   Line of incision in peritoneum forming posterior wall of sac
Fig. 24.22   Caecum peritonised posteriorly and defect in sac sutured

anteriorly by the inguinal ligament and posteriorly by the pectineal line of the pubis. Laterally, it is related to the femoral vein, and medially to the free edge of the *lacunar ligament*. *The pectineal ligament* (of *Cooper*), a thickened band running along the pectineal line of the pubis, incorporated in its periosteum, forms an additional posterior boundary to the femoral ring. The ring is normally occluded by a pad of fatty tissue containing a lymph gland, and known as the femoral septum. The inferior epigastric artery crosses the upper lateral margin of the ring; a branch of this, constituting an *abnormal obturator artery*, may descend along the lateral (or less commonly medial) margin of the ring (McMinn, 1990) and is in danger of being wounded in an operation for strangulated femoral hernia.

Femoral hernia

The sac descends through the femoral canal, and turns forwards through the saphenous opening, the cribriform fascia, which covers the opening, being thinned-out in front of it. It may then turn upwards and laterally for a short distance in front of the inguinal ligament.

The *coverings* of the sac are (1) fat and lymphoid tissue derived from the femoral septum (2) transversalis fascia derived from the anterior wall of the canal, (3) cribriform fascia and (4) superficial fascia and skin.

Indication for operation

Femoral hernia occurs most commonly in women, especially those who have borne children. There are few contraindications to surgical intervention, and operative treatment should almost invariably be advised since, owing to the narrowness of the orifice, there is an ever-present danger of strangulation. The hernia may be approached either from below or from above the inguinal ligament.

The 'low' operation

This was for many years the standard operation, and in the writer's opinion, should still be regarded as the procedure of choice, unless strangulation is present.

Removal of the sac

The incision is made 1 cm below and parallel to the inguinal ligament. If the hernia is irreducible, it will present as a swelling which emerges through the saphenous opening. The actual sac is often surprisingly small. It is covered by the thinned-out cribriform fascia, and is deeply embedded in condensed fatty tissue; these structures must therefore be incised and separated before it can be isolated. It is freed by gauze dissection up to its neck, which is seen to emerge through the femoral canal, and is then opened at its fundus. Any contents are returned to the abdominal cavity; omentum is often adherent and requires to be separated, but if it is free at the neck the adherent part may be removed. When the neck of the sac is constricted by a tight femoral ring, so that the return of contents is difficult, the ring may be gently dilated by a finger passed upwards outside the sac. The neck of the sac is

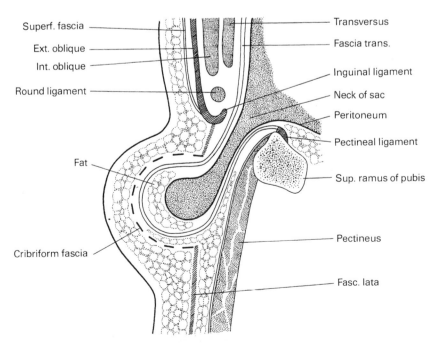

Fig. 24.23 Schematic drawing to show the relations and coverings of a femoral hernia

freed from the margins of the canal, if necessary by a few touches of the knife. It is drawn down so that it can be ligatured by transfixion at the highest possible point, and is cut off. The stump should then retract, or should be pushed upwards, well above the canal. Suture of the coverings over the stump helps to achieve this objective.

Closure of the canal?

It is held by some that this is an important part of the operation, and that it can be done effectively only at the level of the femoral ring. The fact that the ring is inaccessible from the 'low' approach has been used as an argument against this operation. In cases where the canal is narrow, it will be effectively blocked by the remnants of the sac coverings sutured over the stump of the sac. When the femoral canal is wide and the inguinal ligament lax, it may be possible to place sutures between the pectineal ligament and inguinal ligament from below.

Alternatively, sutures may be inserted between the inguinal ligament and fascia over pectineus muscle, inserting *all* sutures before tying any (Fig. 24.26). Many surgeons are content with a still lesser procedure merely to obliterate the space formerly occupied by the hernial protrusion, by two or three stitches which pick up the fasciae forming the floor and the lateral margin of the saphenous opening. Care must be taken not to injure the femoral vein, which lies immediately postero-

lateral to the saphenous opening; the vein should, therefore, be protected by a finger placed upon it while the stitches are being introduced.

The 'high' operation

This operation was first performed by Annandale in 1876, but is usually associated with the name of Lotheisen. It gives more generous access than does the 'low' approach, and is considered to be the better procedure when strangulation has occurred. It allows the sac to be dealt with more easily at its highest point, and provides direct access to the femoral ring, should it be desired to attempt closure of this. Its main disadvantage is that it involves very wide opening (and therefore weakening) of the inguinal canal. An effective repair of the posterior wall of the inguinal canal is therefore necessary with this approach (Nicholson, 1990). It is an operation of greater magnitude than that required by the low approach, and in an elderly patient this is a point worthy of consideration.

Method of approach

The incision is similar to that used for inguinal hernia, but it may be placed a little nearer to the inguinal ligament. The inguinal canal is opened by division of the external oblique aponeurosis; the cord or round ligament is displaced, and the conjoined muscles are drawn upwards. The transversalis fascia is divided in

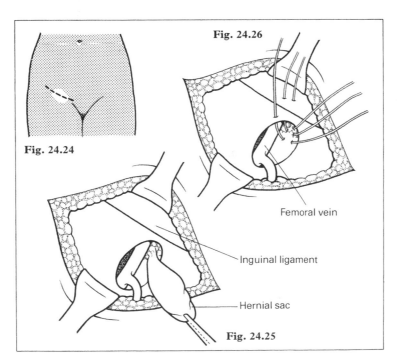

Fig. 24.26

Femoral vein

Inguinal ligament

Hernial sac

Fig. 24.24

Fig. 24.25

Figs 24.24–24.26   The 'low' approach to a femoral hernia. Drawings to show the incision employed, the relationship of the sac to the inguinal ligament and saphenous opening, and the method of obliterating the femoral canal

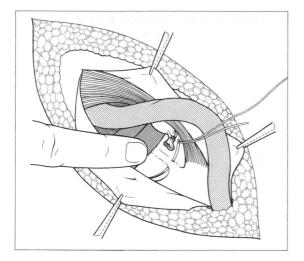

Fig. 24.27   The 'high' operation for femoral hernia. The sac is exposed at its neck through an approach made above the inguinal ligament. It is drawn upwards through the canal and removed at its neck. The femoral ring is then obliterated by stitches which draw down either the inguinal ligament (as shown here), or the conjoined tendon, to the pectineal ligament, the femoral vein being protected by the finger

the line of the incision, care being taken to avoid injury to the inferior epigastric vessels which ascend from the midinguinal point. Extraperitoneal fat is wiped aside by gauze stripping until the sac can be seen entering the femoral canal. The bladder is sometimes adherent on the medial side, and must be carefully safeguarded. If the sac is empty and if it is not too adherent to its surroundings, it can often be withdrawn without difficulty from above, by gentle traction on a pair of forceps applied to its neck. If not, the lower margin of the wound is retracted, and the sac is isolated from below as in the 'low' operation; it is then opened at its fundus and any contents dealt with, after which it is manoeuvred upwards through the canal and is delivered above the inguinal ligament. Finally, the sac is removed flush with the general peritoneum.

Closure of the canal

The lower leaf of the external oblique aponeurosis is drawn downwards, and the deep surface of the inguinal ligament is cleared of fatty and areolar tissue. The femoral ring is now obliterated by stitching either the conjoined tendon or the inguinal ligament down to the pectineal ligament. Two or at the most three sutures of unabsorbable material should be used. While the sutures are being placed the external iliac vein must be protected by the finger, and care should be taken that it is not compressed when they are tightened.

The inguinal canal is repaired in the usual way, care being taken to reconstruct the posterior wall where this has been weakened by the exposure.

McEvedy's approach

This approach, which was first described in 1950, has all the advantages of the transinguinal approach, and gives better access — but without weakening the inguinal canal.

In the original description of the operation (McEvedy, 1950), a vertical incision was employed, but an oblique incision, placed in a skin crease above the medial part of the inguinal ligament, gives equally good access and is now preferred. The anterior rectus sheath in its lower part is incised 2 cm medial to the *linea semilunaris,* and the rectus muscle is displaced towards the midline. The transversalis fascia is divided to expose the peritoneum, on which the inferior epigastric vessels are displayed as they run upwards on its surface (Fig. 24.28). The hernial sac is identified where it enters the femoral canal, and in most cases which are reducible can be drawn up without difficulty; it is then ligatured and removed. In irreducible or strangulated herniae, it is necessary first to clear the sac below the inguinal ligament, and, to enable this to be done, the lower margin of the wound is retracted strongly downwards; the sac is then opened at the fundus and its contents dealt with, after which it is withdrawn upwards through the canal. The femoral ring may now be obliterated by one of the methods already described, after which the wound is repaired by allowing the rectus muscle to fall back into place, and by suture of its anterior sheath.

UMBILICAL HERNIA

Umbilical hernia in children

This is discussed with anomalies of the umbilicus on page 539.

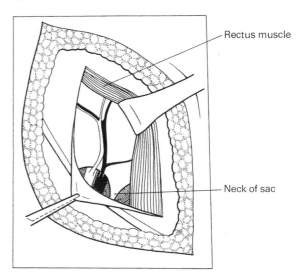

Rectus muscle

Neck of sac

Fig. 24.28   McEvedy's approach to a femoral hernia (for description, see text)

Umbilical hernia in adults

This occurs most commonly in middle-aged or elderly women. The contributory causes are obesity and repeated child-bearing, which result in stretching and thinning-out of the linea alba, together with wide separation of the recti. The hernia normally occurs through a weak area in the linea alba either above or below the actual umbilicus, so that it is strictly *para-umbilical* in type. The deeper layers of the aponeurosis form a well defined margin to the aperture, which is as a rule roughly circular in outline. The superficial layer becomes stretched out over the protruding peritoneal sac; since it stretches unevenly, it becomes split and forms fibrous septa, which cause the sac to be divided up into loculi. The fundus of the sac is often adherent to the skin of the umbilical cicatrix. The most frequent contents are portions of large and small intestine, together with omentum; these contents tend to become adherent both to the fundus of the sac and to each other.

Owing to the loculation of the sac and to the presence of adhesions the hernia is usually irreducible, and there is a very real danger of intestinal obstruction, with or without strangulation of the bowel — a complication in which the mortality may be high.

Even in reducible cases any form of belt or appliance is unlikely to be effective in controlling the hernia or in preventing its enlargement. Operation therefore should almost invariably be advised.

Preoperative treatment

Since many of the patients are in poor condition, careful preparation is essential. Gross obesity should be treated by dietetic measures. Cardiac and renal functions are investigated, and regular action of the bowels is secured. Careful skin preparation is especially important, for the crease below the protuberance is frequently ulcerated or infected.

Mayo's operation

In this operation, after the hernial sac and contents have been dealt with, the defective linea alba is repaired by overlapping across a transverse axis. This has definite advantages over any repair in a vertical line, since a satisfactory degree of overlapping can be obtained without tension, and the sutures are subject to less strain in the postoperative period.

Treatment of the hernial sac and contents. A transverse elliptical incision is made enclosing the umbilicus and the skin covering the hernia. It should extend laterally on each side for at least 5 cm beyond the protuberance. It is deepened through the subcutaneous fat until the glistening surface of the aponeurosis is exposed. *The neck of the sac is generally free from adhesions, and should always be opened first.* To enable this to be done the

aponeurosis is cleared centrally from all directions, until the neck of the hernia is exposed at the level where it emerges through the linea alba. A small incision is made in the fibrous coverings of the neck at any convenient point on its circumference, and is carefully deepened until the sac itself has been opened. A finger is now introduced and is passed round the inside of the sac to determine the presence of any adhesions. The remaining circumference of the neck of the sac is then divided with scissors, the finger being used to protect the contents from injury. The central 'island' comprising the sac together with the attached ellipse of skin and fat is now joined to the abdomen only by the contents passing into the sac. These contents are carefully examined. If they consist of omentum alone, this may at once be clamped and divided in small sections at a time, after which each segment of tissue is transfixed and ligatured. If, as is frequently the case, bowel is seen entering the sac, a finger is introduced alongside, and is passed towards the fundus; a segment of the sac wall free from adhesions is sought for, and is opened up as far as possible. The sac is now gradually turned inside-out, so that the contents come freely into view, and can be gently peeled off its interior. Dense adhesions within the loculi of the sac are frequently present; their separation rarely presents much difficulty, but it must be carried out carefully and without undue haste. Adherent omentum may be removed along with the sac. Adhesions between adjacent coils of bowel — such as might give rise to subsequent obstruction — are separated as far as is practicable, and the hernial contents are returned to the abdominal cavity.

Repair of the abdominal wall. No attempt is made to separate the peritoneum from the margins of the defect in the linea alba, or to suture it as a separate layer unless this can be achieved with ease. The opening is enlarged laterally on each side by a transverse incision so that comfortable overlapping of the aponeurosis can be obtained. The recti are usually so widely separated that their sheaths are not normally opened. The two leaves of the aponeurosis together with the peritoneum are then sutured in the overlapping position, it being a matter of convenience which flap is placed anteriorly. The suture material used (nylon, silk, wire, etc.) will depend upon the surgeon's preference. For the first stage of the overlap a series of four or five mattress sutures is employed. These are introduced so that they will draw the free edge of one flap for a distance of 4 cm under cover of the other flap. In order to promote more ready adhesion between the two flaps, the aponeurosis of the deeper flap is carefully cleared of all fatty tissue. The overlapping is then completed by suturing the free edge of the superficial flap against the deep flap. Details of the technique are shown in Figures 24.29–24.32. All dead space in the wound is

Figs 24.29 & 24.30 *Mayo's operation for umbilical hernia — treatment of the sac*

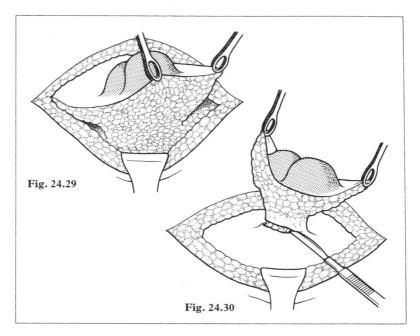

Fig. 24.29

Fig. 24.30

Fig. 24.29   Clearance of the aponeurosis centrally towards the neck of the sac
Fig. 24.30   Circular division of the neck of the sac and its fibrous covering

Figs 24.31 & 24.32 *Mayo's operation for umbilical hernia — repair by overlapping*

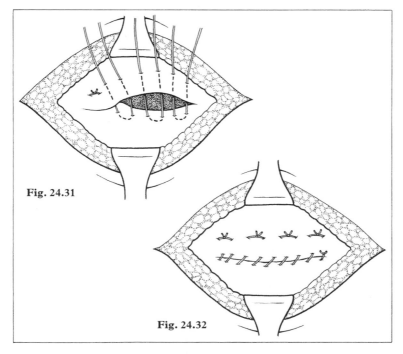

Fig. 24.31

Fig. 24.32

Fig. 24.31   Mattress sutures inserted to draw one flap under cover of the other
Fig. 24.32   Overlapping completed by suturing down free edge of superficial flap

obliterated by suture if possible. Open drainage should be avoided since it may predispose to infection, but the use of a vacuum drain (p. 345) for a large wound can be recommended. The vacuum drain should be retained for several days since too early removal often results in infection.

After treatment. The method of transverse repair has the great advantage that it allows the patient to be nursed from the outset in the fully propped-up position. This not only brings about relaxation of the sutured aponeurosis but is also much more comfortable for the patient, who is often prone to cardiac or respiratory embarrassment.

ANOMALIES OF THE UMBILICUS IN CHILDREN

Umbilical hernia

This condition is relatively common and is due to incomplete closure of the umbilical ring. Since this process may continue during the first three or four years of life, it is possible that the condition will resolve spontaneously. The hernia is seen as a forward protrusion of the umbilicus which becomes tense with straining and is easily reduced when the child is relaxed. A hernia that persists after three or four years should be treated by operation.

Operation

The operation is performed through a curved skin incision below and parallel to the inferior margin of the umbilicus (Fig. 24.33). The subcutaneous fat is divided to expose the linea alba and the medial margin of the rectus sheath on either side. The hernial sac protrudes through a circular opening in the midline,

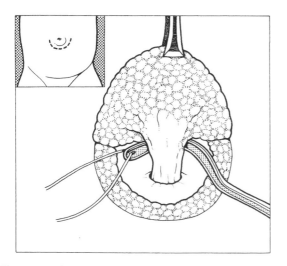

Fig. 24.33 Repair of umbilical hernia in an infant and child

towards the apex of the umbilicus and is covered by a condensation of fascia that is continuous with the linea alba. The junction of fascia and linea alba is defined and forceps pressed round above the umbilicus to provide traction. The hernial sac rarely contains viscera but should nevertheless be opened with care. To achieve this, the fascia over the inferior half of the neck of the sac is first divided to expose the underlying peritoneum which, in turn, is opened and the interior of the sac inspected. The neck of the sac is then transected leaving a circular deficit in the linea alba and peritoneum, which can be closed in one layer in a transverse manner with interrupted Vicryl sutures. During closure, the apex of the umbilicus should be fixed to the linea alba with a subcutaneous stitch and the skin edges are then sewn together. When there is excessive redundant skin, this can be excised, leaving an oval deficit so as to give the appearance of an umbilicus.

Exomphalos

This is a congenital abnormality in which viscera protrude through a defect in the abdominal wall into the base of the umbilical cord. The viscera are contained by a semi-transparent covering made up of amniotic membrane and peritoneum separated by Wharton's jelly. The umbilical cord is attached either to the apex or to the side of the lesion near the base. The condition is arbitrarily divided into minor and major depending on whether the defect is smaller or larger than 5 cm. The content of an exomphalos varies from a few coils of ileum to most of the abdominal viscera including liver, spleen, stomach, small bowel and colon. Malrotation is common (p. 468), remnants of the vitello-intestinal duct may persist (p. 540) and a diaphragmatic hernia may be present (p. 110). In two-thirds of babies there is an associated congenital abnormality. Of particular interest is the relationship between exomphalos, macroglossia and gigantism (EMG), the Beckwith Wiedman Syndrome.

The diagnosis of exomphalos may be made on antenatal ultrasound and is obvious at birth. There may be a history of maternal hydramnios and amniotic alpha fetoprotein may be raised (Brock, 1976). Surprisingly, the membranous covering is rarely ruptured during delivery. A baby with exomphalos should be carefully examined to exclude associated congenital anomalies. In the immediate management, a nasogastric tube is passed to empty the stomach and an intravenous infusion is started. The blood sugar should be monitored as hypoglycaemia is a feature of EMG.

Treatment

In the past, exomphalos has been successfully treated by painting the membranous sac with mercurochrome. An eschar forms which is later sloughed and the underlying granulation tissue is gradually epithelialised. The disadvantages of this method are that underlying visceral anomalies remain undetected and, because the process of epithelialisation is slow, the baby may remain in hospital for several months. However, the technique remains suitable for babies unfit for operation although antiseptics other than mercurochrome are used to avoid the danger of mercury poisoning.

Operation

Where possible an exomphalos should be treated by operation. The sac is excised with a circumferential incision at the junction of membrane and skin. The umbilical vessels and urachus are identified and ligated. After the bowel has been carefully inspected an attempt is made to return the viscera to the abdominal cavity. If successful, the defect in the abdominal wall is closed in two layers. However, a large lesion is not easily reduced and forcing prolapsed viscera back into a relatively small abdominal cavity may restrict respiration by splinting the diaphragm and impair venous return by pressure on the inferior vena cava. In this situation an attempt can be made to increase the capacity of the abdominal cavity by stretching the abdominal wall from within. Failing this a choice can be made between closing the defect in a single layer with the skin or a staged repair using a temporary prosthesis. After skin closure alone an incisional hernia is inevitable and can be repaired if necessary at a later date. In the latter, a pouch of Dacron reinforced silastic sheet is sutured to the margin of the defect and after an interval of seven to ten days a further attempt is made at a formal two layer closure of the abdominal wall (Allen, 1969).

The postoperative care includes nasogastric suction and intravenous infusion until the baby feeds normally. When the defect has been closed with difficulty, ventilatory support may be needed for the first 24–48 hours. If delay in normal feeding is anticipated, feeding by the intravenous route should be started.

Gastroschisis

In many respects gastroschisis is similar to exomphalos and only the important differences need to be considered below.

In gastroschisis the gut is eviscerated through a defect in the abdominal wall immediately adjacent and usually to the right of the umbilicus but the bowel lies free as there is no covering membrane. The embryogenesis is uncertain; it may be similar to that of exomphalos but an alternative view is that the lateral ectodermal fold of the abdominal wall is unsupported by underlying mesoderm and breaks down. The prolapse is normally limited to midgut which is oedematous, apparently short and covered with a fibrinous exudate. A degree of malrotation is inevitable. Curiously the incidence of associated congenital anomalies is small. The diagnosis, as with exomphalos, may be made antenatally on ultrasound and is obvious at birth.

Treatment

The immediate management is to place the lower half of the baby, including the lesion, in a polythene bag — the intestinal bag used in abdominal surgery is suitable. The bag serves to protect the bowel, limits fluid and heat loss and allows inspection of the abdominal wall. It may be necessary to support the viscera with moist packs to avoid drag on the mesenteric vessels. In the early management a nasogastric tube is passed and plasma should be given intravenously to replace the loss of protein rich fluid from the exposed serosal surface. There is no alternative but to treat gastroschisis by operation as there is no membranous covering, and it is an advantage if primary closure can be achieved (Filston, 1983).

Operation

The viscera are carefully examined before being returned to the abdominal cavity and loose matter is removed. The abdominal defect is relatively small and is normally extended by a longitudinal midline incision. The technique of closure of the abdominal wall is the same as for exomphalos.

In the *postoperative management,* early oral feeding is often unsuccessful because of the oedematous condition of the bowel and intravenous feeding should be started.

Patent vitello-intestinal duct

Incomplete involution of the vitello-intestinal duct may result in a persistent fistulous communication between the distal ileum and umbilicus. The patent duct is seen as a mucosal lined opening at the umbilicus which may discharge small amounts of meconium and flatus. The duct itself is of little consequence but there is a danger of prolapse and of volvulus, and early operation is therefore advisable. The prolapse of ileum through the duct may give the lesion a curious T-shaped or horned appearance (Fig. 24.34).

Operation

The abdomen is opened through a 2 cm transverse incision lateral to the umbilicus. The umbilicus is excised in continuity with the duct, care being taken to identify and ligate the umbilical vessels and the urachus. A short segment of ileum bearing the proximal end of the duct is then excised (Fig. 24.35).

Urachus

A patent urachus may be suspected when there is a clear discharge from the umbilicus. A fleshy swelling

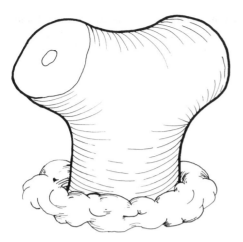

Fig. 24.34 'T' shape of ileal prolapse through vitello-intestinal duct

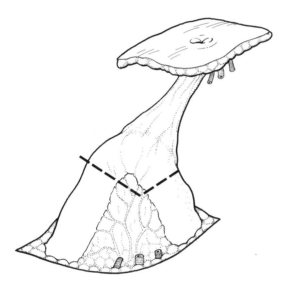

Fig. 24.35 Patent vitello-intestinal duct between umbilicus (excised with ellipse of skin) and distal ileum. Dashes show line of bowel resection

may be present or the umbilicus may appear normal. Outlet obstruction of the bladder can coexist and a cystogram is therefore performed, the contrast being introduced through a catheter inserted at the umbilicus.

Operation

A patent urachus should be closed by operation. The approach is similar to that used for a patent vitello-intestinal duct. The umbilicus is first mobilized with the urachus in continuity and the umbilical vessels ligated and divided. The urachus is traced to the fundus of the bladder where it is divided and the bladder repaired in two layers.

EPIGASTRIC HERNIA

This term is applied to herniae occurring in or near the midline between the umbilicus and the xiphisternum. There is usually no more than a small protrusion of extraperitoneal fat through a defect in the linea alba, but a slender peritoneal sac may also be present.

Operation is indicated for the relief of local discomfort or of the 'dyspepsia' which is commonly present as a result of increased pressure within the hernia following a large meal.

A vertical or transverse incision is employed. The fatty protrusion, and sac if present, are ligatured and removed; the defect in the linea alba is then closed by simple suture or by overlapping.

INCISIONAL HERNIA

A hernia developing in the site of a previous operation occurs most commonly as the result of wound infection which has led to healing by weak scar tissue. Inadequate wound repair following abdominal surgery may also be responsible (Ellis, 1983). Other causes are injury at operation to the nerves supplying the abdominal wall and severe bouts of coughing in the postoperative period. Part of the abdominal wall, with the exception of skin, becomes unable to support the intraperitoneal structures and this results in an abnormal protrusion or hernia. The peritoneal sac is often covered by little more than a thin layer of unhealthy skin.

Clinical types

Two distinct types of incisional hernia require to be considered for they present rather different problems in treatment.

In the first type, there is a wide defect in the aponeurotic or muscular layer of the abdominal wall with smooth and regular margins which are easily defined. The hernia takes the form of a diffuse bulge through the defect; it reduces spontaneously as soon as the patient lies down, and there appears to be no risk of strangulation. There is no urgency about operation except for the patient's comfort since an abdominal support may prove equally helpful. One of the considerations in advising operation is that there is adequate space within the reconstructed abdomen to accept the hernial contents and that the patient's breathing will not thereby be compromised.

In the second type of incisional hernia, conditions are different. The defect is often relatively small and irregular, and two or more such defects may be present in the same scar. The contents, which are normally both bowel and omentum, are matted together and are often adherent to a loculated peritoneal sac, so that the hernia is partially or wholly irreducible. The hazard lies in the narrow neck of the defect. No form of support is likely to be effective, and may increase the risk of strangulation, which is a particularly serious complication. Every effort should be made, therefore, to persuade such patients to accept surgery. The patient can assist in the success of the operation by achieving a weight/height ratio which is near normal for his/her age.

Operation

An elliptical incision is made enclosing the area of unhealthy skin, and is prolonged sufficiently to give adequate access. The outer edges are undercut, and are reflected beyond the limits of the hernial protuberance; since they are often adherent to the sac, the reflection must be carried out with great care. The incision is then deepened to the aponeurosis, and the dissection is continued inwards towards the margins of the defect. If the sac is no more than a redundancy of peritoneum, and if it is not too adherent to the skin, it may be possible to free it and to replace it unopened within the abdominal wall. More often, however, it is loculated and very adherent. It is then better to open it around its neck, and to free the contents by turning it inside out, in the manner described for umbilical hernia. Adherent omentum may be ligatured and removed along with the sac. Any adhesions involving bowel should be separated as far as practicable, before the hernial contents are returned to the abdomen.

The type of repair to be adopted depends on the size and situation of the hernia, and on the amount of scar tissue present. The following methods may be considered.

Anatomical restoration. This is the ideal method of repair, and is suited to small herniae where scarring is minimal. The edges of the defect are excised, and by careful dissection the surrounding abdominal wall is separated into its constituent layers — usually peritoneum, fleshy muscle and aponeurosis. Each layer is freed sufficiently to allow it to be sutured individually and without tension.

Closure of the defect using nylon. This method is applicable to any hernia where there are rigid margins capable of holding suture. It is important to use a continuous suture with bites in the abdominal wall up to 2.5 cm from the edges to be sutured so that a generous suture length to wound-length ratio results. The suture must allow for the increase in wound length which results from abdominal distension and a suture length four times greater than the wound is advised (Jenkins, 1980).

Other materials. An incisional hernia repaired with a continuous non-absorbable suture has a risk of developing 'button hole' defects at the puncture sites of each 'bite' of suture. This problem may be overcome, in selected cases, by the use of an absorbable monofilament material such as polydioxanone (Krukowski, 1987).

Onlay graft of foreign material, such as tantalum gauze or polypropylene mesh (Molloy, 1991) may be used where the defect is large.

OBTURATOR HERNIA

Obturator hernia is very uncommon. It is encountered most frequently in elderly women who have lost weight. The herniation occurs through the obturator foramen usually along the narrow canal traversed by the obturator vessels and nerve. Strangulation is therefore liable to ensue.

The abdominal approach

The condition is usually discovered only after laparotomy has been performed for intestinal obstruction, a coil of small bowel being found passing into the obturator foramen. In such circumstances the patient is tilted into the Trendelenburg position, and the general peritoneal cavity is carefully packed off in order to avoid contamination by toxic exudate escaping from the sac. It may be possible to extricate the imprisoned bowel by drawing it back into the general peritoneal cavity, but no more than the gentlest traction must be employed. If necessary the fibres of the obturator membrane which constrict the neck of the sac are carefully incised. The obturator vessels have no constant relationship to the sac, and are therefore liable to be injured in whatever direction the incision is made. After the bowel has been released the sac may be withdrawn into the abdomen and removed; if this presents any difficulty, it is sufficient to close its neck by suture.

The femoral approach must be employed if the bowel cannot be freed from the abdominal aspect, and it is the method of choice when the condition is diagnosed before operation. A vertical incision is made extending downwards from the inguinal ligament 2 cm medial to the femoral vessels. The adductor longus is retracted medially, and the fibres of the pectineus are separated or divided, so that the obturator externus is exposed. The sac is usually found lying on the surface of this muscle, having emerged at its upper border or between its fibres. The sac and contents are dealt with in the usual manner, and the space which was occupied by them is obliterated by suture.

STRANGULATED HERNIA

A hernia is said to be strangulated when the contents are constricted in such a way that interference with

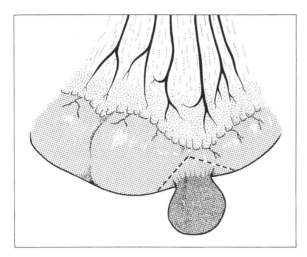

Fig. 24.36 Richter's hernia — suitable for *partial* resection, by the method indicated

their blood supply results. When a loop of bowel is involved in the constriction, intestinal obstruction is also present — except possibly in the case of *Richter's hernia* (Fig. 24.36), where only part of the circumference of the gut is affected.

Preparation

Operations for strangulated hernia are among the most urgent in surgery. Not only is acute obstruction usually present, but the patient suffers from additional toxaemia due to absorption of toxic products arising from devitalisation of the imprisoned bowel. The high mortality in this condition results from failure to appreciate its potential seriousness and is clearly linked with the duration of symptoms (Andrews, 1981). Nevertheless, despite the urgency for operation, preoperative treatment should not be neglected (p. 462). This should include prophylactic antibiotics against bowel organisms.

When there has been much vomiting, or when the patient is in poor condition, local anaesthesia may with advantage be employed. This occupies more time, but it causes less shock and reduces the risk of postoperative complications.

Operation

In general the operation is very similar to that described for non-strangulated cases, but certain important differences should be noted:

1. The hernial sac contains a varying quantity of dark-coloured fluid derived from devitalised bowel or omentum. When the vitality of bowel is seriously unpaired this fluid is highly toxic and is swarming with organisms. If possible the sac should always be opened at its fundus and the fluid evacuated before the con-

striction is relieved, as otherwise there is a serious risk of contaminating the peritoneal cavity.

2. After the constriction has been divided, the hernial contents must be carefully examined before they are returned to the abdominal cavity. They should be drawn down well out of the wound, so that the constricted areas, which often sustain the greatest damage, can be inspected and healthy tissue identified beyond. Sometimes the contents slip back before the constriction has been divided, or even before the sac has been opened. In such cases it is essential that the affected parts should be sought from within the peritoneal cavity and brought out for examination; fortunately they usually remain in the vicinity of the sac.

3. It should be remembered that the operation has been undertaken not to cure the hernia but to save life, and that its essential part has been completed as soon as the hernial contents have been returned to the abdomen. The defect in the abdominal wall is dealt with as effectively as possible, but the simpler methods only should be employed.

Viability of the bowel

When a loop of bowel has been damaged by the strangulation, the question of its viability must at once be decided. The damage may affect only localised area of the bowel wall, either at the convexity of the loop or at the *constriction rings,* or it may involve the entire loop which has been imprisoned within the hernia.

The decision is one of supreme importance, especially if the circumference of the bowel is affected. The inexperienced surgeon is probably apt to decide too hastily that the damage is irreparable, and to proceed at once to resection and anastomosis. Even though the bowel is deeply congested and oedematous, with haemorrhages into its wall, and possibly with some loss of its normal lustre, it may still be capable of recovery. The affected loop should be covered with a hot moist towel, in order to stimulate any possible circulation within it, and the anaesthetist is asked to flood the lungs with oxygen. After an interval the bowel is carefully re-examined. Frequently the discoloration will be found to have become noticeably less, and there may be a return of the normal lustre. The stimulus of the heat applied may induce a peristaltic wave of contraction, and, if this can be seen to pass uninterruptedly along the damaged segment, it is irrefutable evidence of its viability. Such a contraction may be induced also by gentle flicking with the finger of the healthy bowel on the proximal side. If doubt still exists as to the viability of the loop, it is justifiable to wait for 4 to 5 minutes, applying fresh towels at intervals.

When the vitality of the bowel is more seriously impaired, the fluid within the sac is likely to be turbid and foul-smelling. The bowel is ashen-grey or even black in colour, and is completely lustreless; its wall is flaccid and sodden to the touch — its consistence being compared to that of wet blotting paper. In addition there is likely to be thrombosis of the associated mesenteric vessels. In such cases the bowel is almost certain to be non-viable, but if the slightest doubt exists it should be treated in the manner described, in order that any possibility of its recovery should not be overlooked.

Treatment of devitalized bowel

In the great majority of cases it is the small bowel which is affected. The choice of procedure then varies according to the severity and extent of the damage. *Localised* areas of impaired vitality (or even of frank gangrene), not involving the entire circumference of the gut, can be treated satisfactorily by the relatively simple procedures of infolding or partial resection. If, however, the damage extends over a wider area, the only practicable treatment is by resection and anastomosis.

Infolding is obtained by Lambert sutures which take up the seromuscular coat on each side of the damaged area. The line of sutures should lie in the transverse axis of the gut, so that narrowing of the lumen will not be produced.

Partial resection is preferable when localized gangrene is present such as occurs in cases of Richter's hernia

(Fig. 24.36). Light occlusion clamps are applied to the healthy bowel on each side, and after careful packing-off the gangrenous area is cleanly excised. Repair is effected in the transverse axis by two layers of suture.

Resection and anastomosis. Under modern conditions of anaesthesia and of pre- and postoperative care, the dangers of this operation have been considerably reduced. Even in very old or seriously ill patients the operation is often surprisingly well tolerated. The technique of resection prior to end-to-end anastomosis is shown in Figure 24.37. This is the procedure of choice when there is no great disparity in the size of the bowel above and below the segment to be resected (see also p. 471). When such disparity exists, the narrow segment of bowel is divided obliquely, opening up the anti-mesenteric border or incising along it.

In the rare cases where a segment of colon has been devitalised by inclusion in a strangulated hernia, it should be excised between clamps and the ends left on the surface, as in the Mikulicz operation (p. 471). Only when obstruction is minimal, and the operating conditions ideal, should a primary anastomosis be attempted.

Treatment of strangulated omentum

Even if viable, strangulated omentum should always be excised, since if returned to the peritoneal cavity it may

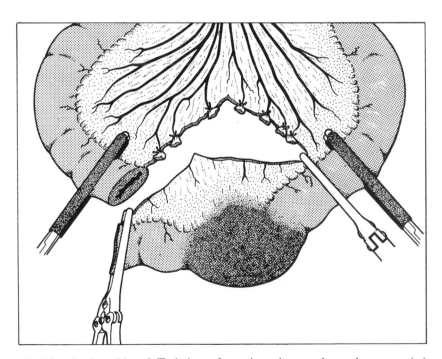

Fig. 24.37   Strangulated hernia of small bowel. Technique of resection prior to end-to-end anastomosis (see also Figs 22.15 & 22.16, p. 472)

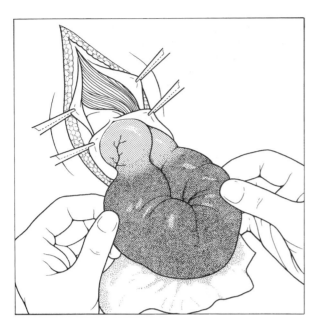

Fig. 24.38 Strangulated inguinal hernia. The sac has been opened to expose the site of constriction (After Hamilton Bailey)

set up adhesions. The pedicle is clamped and divided in small sections at a time, after which each segment is transfixed and ligatured.

Strangulated inguinal hernia

The constriction is usually caused by the narrow neck of the sac, and is situated therefore at the level of the deep ring. When skin and fascia have been divided the tense sac is at once seen emerging through the superficial ring; this ring is divided and the inguinal canal is opened up in the usual manner. The sac is gently separated from surrounding structures, and is delivered at the wound. A small fold of it is picked up with forceps, and is opened so that the contained fluid is evacuated externally. The sac is now drawn downwards, and is slit up beyond the level of any constriction, a grooved director being used if necessary to protect the contents from injury. Should the constriction appear to be at the level of the superficial ring, it is better that the sac should be opened and the fluid evacuated before this ring is divided. When the sac is a large one it may be left in situ, its neck being cut across and the opening into the general peritoneal cavity is closed by suture.

Strangulated femoral hernia

One of the 'high' approaches (Lotheisen or McEvedy) is generally advised since it allows the constriction at the level of the femoral ring to be divided under the guidance of the eye; furthermore, it provides better

access for the investigation and treatment of damaged bowel. As soon as the skin and fascia have been divided, the lower part of the wound is retracted, and the sac is cleared and opened at its fundus. The femoral ring is now exposed above the inguinal ligament, and the constriction is investigated. This may be due to narrowness of the neck of the sac itself, or to pressure from the pectineal part of the inguinal ligament (*lacunar ligament*). In the latter case the ligament is incised sufficiently to allow the sac to be freed. If an abnormal obturator artery is present it can, from the 'high' approach, be seen and avoided, or at least secured without difficulty. The neck of the sac is now divided against a grooved director, which has been slipped upwards from the fundus. The contents are then drawn out above the inguinal ligament, and are dealt with as their condition demands. If the hernia is of the Richter's type, the imprisoned bowel is very apt to slip back into the abdomen as soon as the constriction has been relieved, but in every case it must be sought for and its condition carefully investigated.

If difficulty is experienced in freeing the hernial contents, as may occur in obese subjects, it may be justifiable, in a very ill patient, to divide the inguinal ligament or to detach its medial end from the pubic tubercle. When the hernial contents and sac have been dealt with, the free end of the ligament is sutured against the pectineal ligament, thus obliterating the femoral ring. Such a drastic step, however, should seldom be required. If, for any reason such as that of infection in the wound, the repair gives way, a most unpleasant type of inguinofemoral herniation results. This is extremely difficult to repair, since the integrity of the inguinal ligament — a structure which is vital to the whole anatomy of the groin — has been destroyed. An attempt may be made to reattach it to the pubis by means of wire or nylon sutures passed through drill holes in the bone.

Strangulated umbilical hernia

As a rule the strangulation occurs not at the neck of the sac, but in one of the loculi. Operation is carried out on the same lines as described for non-strangulation cases. When the patient is in poor condition, the defect is repaired by simple suture.

Strangulated incisional hernia

This is most likely to occur when the hernia has developed in a lower abdominal scar when multiple small defects may be present. It is a particularly serious condition, since the early symptoms of strangulation may be masked, and gangrene of the bowel will often be found to have occurred. Operation is carried out as described on page 541.

REFERENCES

Allen R G, Wrenn E L 1969 Silan as a sac in the treatment of omphalocoele and gastroschisis. Journal of Paediatric Surgery 4: 3–8

Andrews N J 1981 Presentation and outcome of strangulated external hernia in a District General Hospital. British Journal of Surgery 68: 329–332

Brock D J H 1976 Mechanisms by which amniotic-fluid alpha-fetoprotein may be increased in fetal abnormalities. Lancet 2: 345–346

Devlin H B, Gillen P H A, Waxman B P, MacNay R A 1986 Short stay surgery for inguinal hernia: experience of the Shouldice operation, 1970–1982. British Journal of Surgery 73: 123–124

Ellis H, Gajraj H, George C D 1983 Incisional hernias: when do they occur? British Journal of Surgery 70: 290–291

Farquharson E L 1955 Early ambulation with special reference to herniorrhaphy as an out-patient procedure. Lancet 2: 517–519

Farquharson E L 1955 Some problems in the treatment of hernia. Annals of the Royal College of Surgeons of England 17: 386–399

Filston H C 1983 Gastroschisis — primary fascial closure. Annals of Surgery 197: 260–264

Glassow F 1973 The surgical repair of inguinal and femoral hernias. Canadian Medical Association Journal 108: 308–313

Glassow F 1984 Inguinal hernia repair using local anaesthesia. Annals of the Royal College of Surgeons of England 66: 382–387

Jenkins T P N 1980 Incisional hernia repair: A mechanical approach. British Journal of Surgery 67: 335–336

Krukowski Z H, Matheson N A 1987 'Button hole' incisional hernia: a late complication of abdominal wound closure with continuous non-absorbable sutures. British Journal of Surgery 74: 824–825

McEvedy P G 1950 Femoral hernia. Annals of the Royal College of Surgeons of England 7: 484–496

McMinn R M H 1990 Last's anatomy, 8th edn. Churchill Livingstone, Edinburgh, p 397

Molloy R G, Moran K T, Waldron R P et al 1991 Massive incisional hernia: abdominal wall replacement with Marlex mesh. British Journal of Surgery 78: 242–244

Moloney G E, Gill W G, Barclay R C 1948 Operations for hernia. Technique of nylon darn. Lancet 2: 45–48

Nicholson S, Keane T E, Devlin H B 1990 Femoral hernia: an avoidable source of surgical mortality. British Journal of Surgery 77: 307–308

Ruckley C V 1978 Day care and short stay surgery for hernia. British Journal of Surgery, 65: 1–4

Tanner N C 1942 A 'slide' operation for inguinal and femoral hernia. British Journal of Surgery 29: 285–289

Wantz G E 1989 Ambulatory hernia surgery. British Journal of Surgery 76: 1228–1229

FURTHER READING

Clinical Guidelines on the Management of Groin Hernia in Adults. Report of a Working Party convened by The Royal College of Surgeons of England 1993

25

General urology

T. B. HARGREAVE

INVESTIGATIONS

Urological surgery is concerned with diseases and injuries of the kidneys, ureters, bladder, urethra and the male genital tract. The morphology and function of these structures, the site, nature and extent of disease involving them, and the effects these diseases have on other parts of the urinary tract and on the patient's general health, can be so accurately assessed, that in most cases the appropriate operation can be predetermined, the patient properly prepared, and difficulties (during and after operation) anticipated. Nevertheless, the surgeon must always be prepared to modify the operation if unexpected anatomical or pathological features are encountered. Operation is now much more a means of treating disease, and much less a method of investigation.

Advances in other branches of medicine, such as radiation and medical oncology, nutrition, antibiotics, blood transfusion and anaesthesia enable us to operate more safely and more effectively, to operate on patients who would previously have been regarded as unfit for surgery, and to do operations which would otherwise be impossible.

In investigating patients with diseases of the urological or male genital tract, I need not remind you of the importance of taking a full history of the patient's present problems, previous health, family, occupation, social life, and of the medicines he or she takes or has taken; to carry out a thorough physical examination, and to do routine examinations of the urine and blood. In some patients enough information can be derived from these investigations alone to determine the appropriate treatment, but usually more detailed tests are required.

Straight X-ray (Fig. 25.1)
In the straight X-ray, which must extend from the 9th rib above and include both ischial tuberosities and the whole of the pubic symphysis below, the renal outlines, the psoas shadows, abnormal opacities and bony

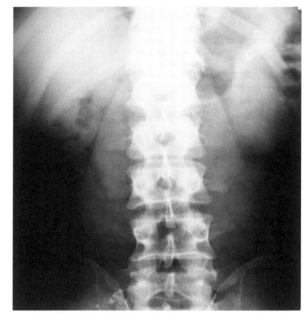

Fig. 25.1 Straight X-ray of the renal tract

lesions are looked for. Its value can be enhanced in some cases by taking oblique films, which should distinguish opacities in the gall bladder, costal cartilages or lymph nodes from those in the urinary tract.

Intravenous excretory urography
Intravenous or excretory urography has replaced the term intravenous pyelography because the procedure reveals the morphology, not only of the pelvis and calices of the kidney, but also of the renal parenchyma, ureters and bladder, and, furthermore, gives much information about the excretory functions of the kidney.

The *contrast media* presently used for intravenous urography are sodium or meglumine diatrizoate, iothalamate or metrizoate which are water soluble salts derived from triiodinated benzoic acid. In the kidneys they are all treated like Inulin which is excreted by glomerular filtration and neither absorbed nor excreted by the tubules. As side effects, which are rare and usually mild, seem unrelated to the dose, large volumes of the contrast media can be given and repeated if desired. Usually about 60 ml of a 50% solution (equivalent to 20 g of iodine) is given and repeated once or even twice if the early films are unsatisfactory. Some radiologists give a much larger initial dose, especially if renal function is subnormal.

Three phases can be recognised:

1. *The nephrographic phase* (Fig. 25.2) is seen in films made immediately the injection finishes while the contrast medium is in the glomeruli and tubules and rapidly being concentrated, as 80% of the water is reabsorbed in the proximal tubule. It shows the size, position and contours of the kidneys, and the ability of the glomeruli to filter plasma, and of the proximal tubules to reabsorb water. The quality of the nephrograms can be enhanced by taking tomograms (nephrotomography) although a second injection of contrast medium will be required.

2. *The pyelographic phase* (Fig. 25.3). The pelvicaliceal systems are seen in films made 5, 10, 15 and 20 minutes after injection. The clarity of the pictures depends on the amount of water reabsorbed in the distal tubule (under the influence of antidiuretic hormone) and is enhanced if the patient is dehydrated for some hours before the examination is started. It can be further enhanced if we prevent the dye escaping too quickly from the pelvis into the ureter and bladder, by tilting the patient into the Trendelenberg position or applying pressure to the anterior abdominal wall with a pneumatic cushion.

The ureters are seen best in films made after the compression is released. However, peristalsis interferes with the visualization of some parts of the ureters and their whole lengths can usually be seen only in retrograde ureterogram (p. 550). In patients with nephroptosis, stone or obstruction, erect, oblique or late films or tomograms, or films taken after the intravenous injection of Frusemide, are useful.

3. *Cystogram* (Fig. 25.4). The quality of the cystogram can be improved if the patient empties his bladder before the examination, and its value enhanced with oblique films. A post micturition cystogram should always be taken (Fig. 25.5). Although it is not a reliable means of measuring the amount of residual urine, it may reveal filling defects, the true size of acquired diverticula which fill as the bladder empties or early ureteric obstruction.

Ultrasound

Ultrasound waves cannot be appreciated by the human ear because they have frequencies above 20 000 cycles (20 000 hertz) per second. For ultrasonography, waves with frequencies of 1 to 5×10^6 cycles (1–5 megahertz) per second produced by ultrasound transducers are used. They are directed onto the object being studied and are reflected back by the interfaces separating tissues of different densities and different sound velocities. The echoes are analysed, displayed and stored.

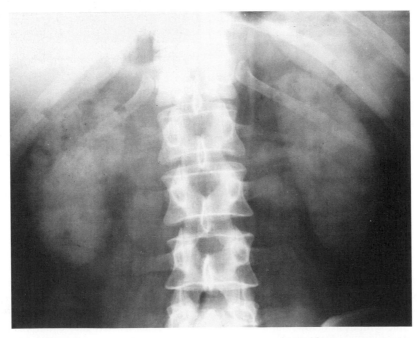

Fig. 25.2   Intravenous urogram taken 3 minutes after injection, showing the nephrographic phase

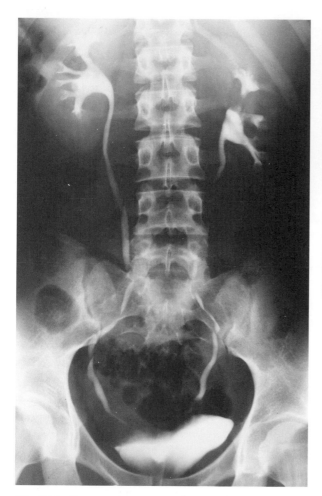

Fig. 25.3 Intravenous urogram taken 10 minutes after the injection, showing the pelvicaliceal system of the kidney and the ureters

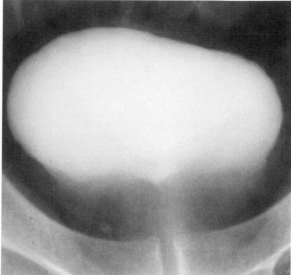

Fig. 25.4 Cystogram. Premicturition film showing the normal bladder

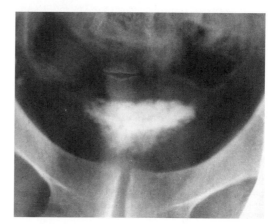

Fig. 25.5 Cystogram. Post micturition film

The delay between the transmission of the wave and the return of the echo reveals the depth of the object from the surface and the amplitude of the wave, its nature. The kidneys (Fig. 25.6) are easily recognizable by ultrasound, even if they are not functioning and their size, position, contours and the nature of any space occupying lesions can be appreciated. Furthermore, under ultrasound control, a needle can be inserted into the kidney to obtain a biopsy, into the pelvis to provide a percutaneous nephrostomy or an ante-grade pyelo-ureterogram or into a cyst. Ultrasound is also of value in some diseases of the bladder and prostate. A special probe is available for transrectal ultrasound and this can be used in conjuction with a percutaneous needle to take accurately located biopsies of any abnormal areas. This is particularly useful in the diagnosis and staging for men with prostate cancer.

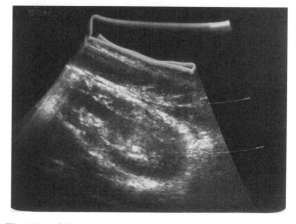

Fig. 25.6 Ultrasound scan of the kidney demonstrating kidney with a normal collecting system

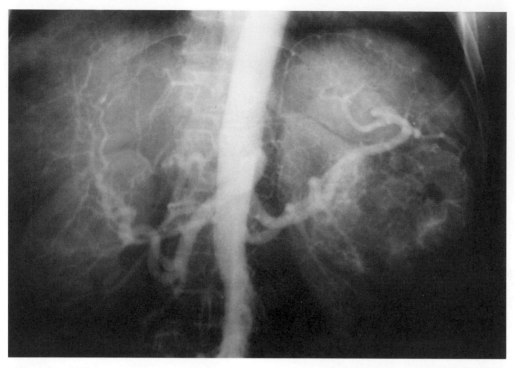

Fig. 25.7 Main stream aortogram showing a large tumour in the left kidney and a normal right kidney

Angiography

Main stream aortography and selective renal angiography are carried out by the Seldinger technique in which the catheter is passed directly, using a needle and guide wire, into a femoral artery. Main stream aortography (Fig. 25.7) shows the number, position and distribution of the renal arteries. Selective renal angiography has three phases: the arterial (Fig. 25.8); the nephrographic and the venous. Angiography is valuable for the investigation of patients with hypertension, or with injuries, or arteriovenous anomalies. It used to be the standard investigation for renal tumour but, in most cases, the information required for management can be obtained from ultrasound scans. The value of arteriography can be enhanced by the injection of adrenaline which constricts normal vessels, but not tumour ones. In patients with tumour or vascular abnormalities, the 'feeding' or main artery can be embolized by the injection through the catheter of absorbable gelatin foam or occluding springs, or by the distension of a ballooned catheter (Fig. 25.9).

Retrograde pyelography

Retrograde pyelography began in 1906 using, at first, aqueous solutions of colloidal silver and later sodium iodide, and was the only means of examining the upper urinary tract until the early 1930s when the synthesis of the water soluble organic iodine compounds made

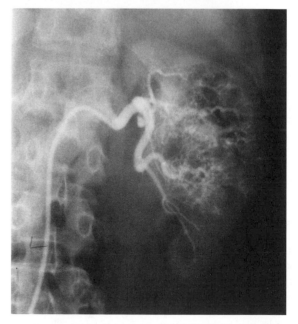

Fig. 25.8 Selective left renal angiogram showing a large tumour in the left kidney

intravenous urography a safe and efficient procedure. The author now uses the same contrast media for retrograde pyelography as for intravenous urography, but in a lower concentration of 20 to 30%.

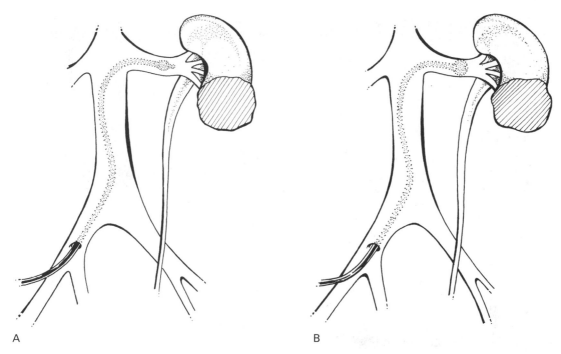

A   B

Fig. 25.9   Renal artery embolisation

Nowadays, we carry out retrograde pyelography much less often than we used to, partly because it involves cystoscopy and ureteric catheterization (p. 567) (which can so easily induce or exacerbate infection, particularly in obstructed kidneys) but predominantly because intravenous urography, ultrasonography and radionuclide and CAT scanning provide, with less trouble and danger, good pictures of the anatomy of the kidneys. Furthermore, they tell us much about function. However, retrograde pyelograms may still be required to show the pelvicaliceal systems of obstructed or otherwise poorly or nonfunctioning kidneys; to clarify the exact relationship of opacities to the urinary tract, or the size and nature of filling defects in the ureters or pelvicaliceal system and to reveal the whole length of a ureter. (The whole length of a ureter is rarely seen in an intravenous urogram (IVU)) (Fig. 25.10). The normal renal pelvis has a capacity of about 5 or 6 ml. If too much contrast medium is injected into the ureteric catheter, backflow or extravasation (Fig. 25.11) can easily be produced and not only makes interpretation of the films difficult or even impossible, but may cause septicaemia.

Ureteric catherization, though not necessarily pyelography, is also necessary if we want to collect separate specimens from each kidney, for biochemical or cytological examination. Retrograde pyelo-ureterograms are best made under a screen and image intensifier, but, if carried out using Braasch or Chevasseur cath-

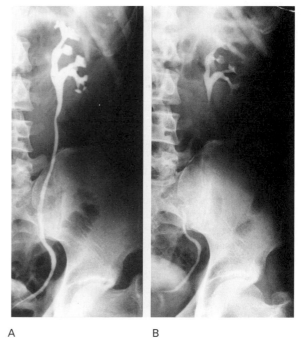

A   B

Fig. 25.10   (A) Retrograde pyelo-ureterogram, using a Braasch catheter, revealing the whole length of the ureter. (B) IVU, in same patient, for comparison

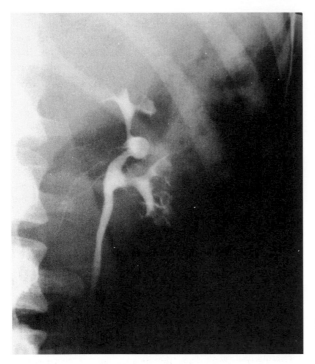

Fig. 25.11   Pyelovenous and pyelotubular backflow

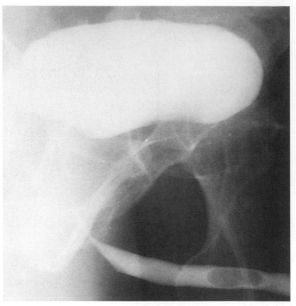

Fig. 25.12   Ascending urethrogram

eters (p. 570), have to be made on the endoscopic table.

It is vital to fill the ureteric catheter with the contrast medium before it is introduced so that air bubbles are not injected, because they may be confused with tumours or stones.

Antegrade pyelo-ureterography

Dye can be injected through a needle inserted into the renal pelvis under X-ray or ultrasonic control, if pictures of the ureter or pelvicaliceal system are needed and cannot be obtained by other means.

Ascending or retrograde urethrocystography
(Fig. 25.12)

This procedure is carried out by inserting a 14F catheter into the external meatus and inflating the balloon with 2–3 ml of water.

A 10–25% solution of one of the water soluble contrast media is injected slowly and carefully so that the dye does not extravasate into the corpora or cause oedema. Anteroposterior and oblique films are taken and show the urethra clearly as far as the external sphincter. Considerable pressure is usually required to force the dye through the external sphincter into the bladder, and the membranous and prostatic parts appear narrow because they only open when the bladder contracts.

It is important to fill the catheter with the contrast medium otherwise air bubbles will be introduced and spoil the films.

Cystogram

Adequate cystograms are often obtained during intravenous urography, especially if the patient empties his bladder just before the examination commences. Nevertheless, to demonstrate diverticula, vesico-ureteric reflux and bladder injuries, or to obtain micturating (voiding) cystograms with pictures of the bladder neck, the prostate, and membranous parts of the urethra, cystograms (Fig. 25.13) are best done by injecting a 10% or 20% solution of one of the water soluble contrast media directly into a catheter passed through the urethra into the bladder.

Pedal lymphangiography (Fig. 25.14)

This is best carried out by injecting indigocarmine mixed with 1% lignocaine hydrochloride into the skin and subcutaneous tissues of a webbed space on the dorsum of the foot. A 27 g needle can be inserted into one of the lymphatic channels when they become visible some 5 to 10 minutes later and 5–6 ml of ethiodized oil containing 37% of iodine is then injected. X-rays show lymph vessels 1 hour and lymph nodes 12–24 hours after the injection. The lymph nodes seen are the inguinal ones and those along the common and external iliac vessels and the aorta. The lymph nodes alongside the internal iliac vessels are not shown, so the procedure is of limited use in patients with prostatic or bladder tumours.

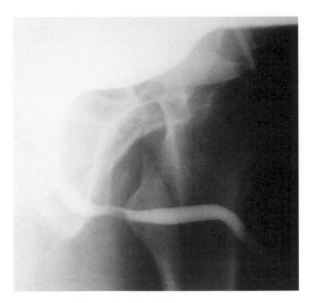

Fig. 25.13   Micturating cystogram

Some of the fat soluble contrast leaks into veins, especially if the lymphatics are obstructed and can cause pulmonary embolism. The procedure is particularly dangerous in patients with lung disease and must always be preceded by a chest X-ray.

Venography (Fig. 25.15)
Radiographs of the inferior vena cava and the renal veins can be obtained by applying the Seldinger technique through the femoral vein and are of value in patients with renal cell carcinoma or renal vein thrombosis. The technique can be used to collect venous blood from the vena cava and each renal vein for the estimation of rennin production in patients with hypertension.

Nuclear medicine
The procedures used in nuclear medicine are non-invasive, require little if any preparation, cause few side effects and are unaffected by bowel or gas shadows.

Renography (Fig. 25.16)
A renogram can be made using either ^{131}iodine — or ^{123}iodine-labelled iodohippurate, or ^{99m}technetium labelled diethylene tetramine pentacetic acid (DTPA).

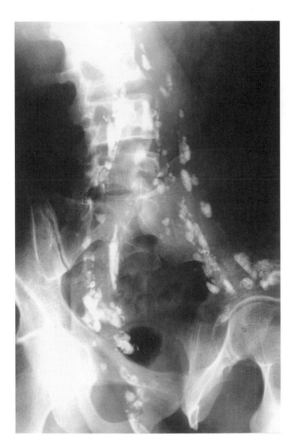

Fig. 25.14   Lymphangiogram showing normal lymph nodes along the common and external iliac vessels and aorta

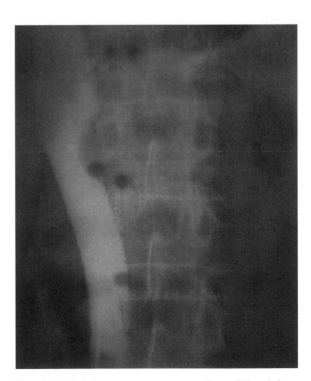

Fig. 24.15   Inferior vena cavogram revealing a filling defect in the left side of the vena cava at the level of the renal vein. The defect is caused by an extension of the renal cell carcinoma seen in the intravenous urogram (which is a feature of all inferior vena cavograms) of the left kidney

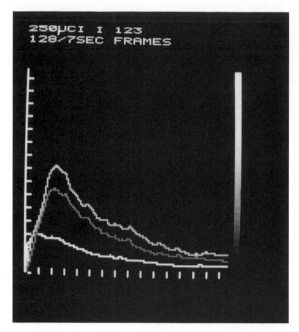

Fig. 25.16   Renogram showing normal curves from both left and right kidney (the lower curve represents the blood level of the isotope)

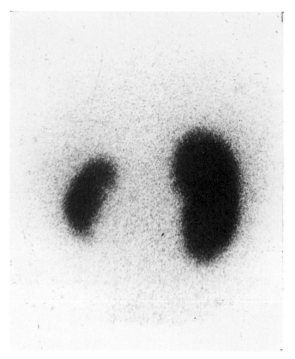

Fig. 25.17   Radionuclide renal scan showing a normal right kidney and a small left one. (The detector camera is applied posteriorly)

The curves obtained have three components: a vascular phase, which lasts about 20 seconds, is a steep rise and depends on the arterial supply to the kidneys; a secretory phase, which lasts up to 5 minutes, depends on the amount of dye filtered at the glomerulus and excreted by the tubules; and an excretory phase which falls rapidly as the dye drains out of the kidney into the pelvis and ureter. Obstruction hinders the third phase and can be shown more easily if the patient is given Frusemide.

Renal scan (Fig. 25.17)
The ^{99m}technetium-labelled chelates diethylene tetramine pentacetic acid (DTPA) and dimercapto succinic acid (DMSA) are used and the images recorded by gamma cameras. For dynamic imaging DTPA is used; it is excreted by glomerular filtration and the scan provides in picture form the same information that the renogram does in graphic form. For static imaging DMSA is used; it is taken up by normally functioning parenchyma and tells us more about morphology than function.

Bone scan (Fig. 25.18)
This is carried out using ^{99m}technetium-labelled phosphate or diphosphonate compounds. Scans can show metastases at an earlier stage than X-rays, particularly in patients with prostatic carcinoma; however, the changes are non-specific and must be compared with

the appropriate conventional X-rays. If the scan is positive and the X-ray negative, metastases are the likeliest cause.

Urodynamics (Fig. 25.19)
For many years cysto-urethroscopy and cysto-urethrography have proved to be satisfactory means of studying the structure of the bladder and the urethra. Now urodynamics provides a means of studying their function, and helps to elucidate the causes of incontinence, frequency, urgency and the severity of obstruction. The most useful measurements are the residual urine, the bladder capacity, the bladder pressures and the urine flow rates, but much else can be measured with the sophisticated apparatus now available.

A 2-way catheter is passed into the bladder. The bladder is emptied and the amount of urine recovered is the residual. One limb of the catheter is connected to a fluid reservoir and the other to a pressure recorder. The pressure recorded from the bladder is a combination of the detrusor pressure and the general intra-abdominal pressure. The latter can be measured with a rectal catheter, and when subtracted from the bladder pressure, gives us the intrinsic bladder or detrusor pressure. The flow rate is measured with a flow meter; and if apparatus is available, a micturating cystogram (p. 552) can be done at the same time. The bladder

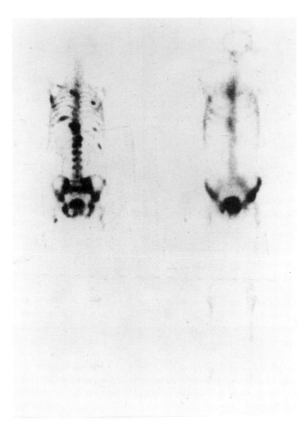

Fig. 25.18 Bone scan revealing multiple hot spots in the pelvis, lumbar and thoracic spine. As X-rays of these areas were normal, hot spots were considered to be caused by metastic disease

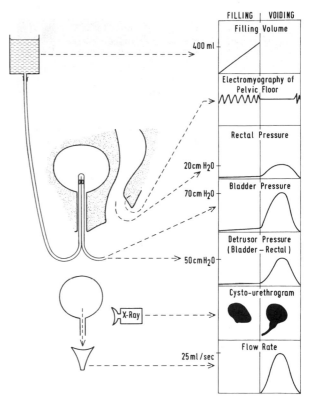

Fig. 25.19 Urodynamics

only contracts properly when it is full (300 ml +) and flow rates and residual urine should only be measured when the patient passes urine because he wants to, not because he's told to.

Computerized axial tomography (CAT scanning)
In CAT scans many X-rays are taken, from all angles, of one thin section of the body by rotating the tube through 360°. The X-rays are received by a scintillator detector which integrates and transforms the images into one picture. As each picture shows only one thin section of the body a large number of pictures are needed to show the whole of the abdomen or chest. The size, shape and position of the kidneys, and the size and nature of space occupying lesions is revealed (Fig. 25.20). CAT scans also show calcification or stones too small to be revealed in conventional X-rays. Retroperitoneal swellings like para-aortic glands are also clearly demonstrated, so that the procedure is particularly valuable in a patient with a testicular tumour.

Magnetic resonance imaging (MRI scanning)
At first sight the scans look similar to CT but in fact the technology is completely different and MRI scans are better at showing pelvic organs than CT. The patient is placed in a magnetic field and this field is rotated. The changing field alters the spin of water atoms and causes emission of radio waves. These can be measured and compiled into images.

URETHRAL CATHETERIZATION

Although the complications of urethral catheterization occur less often now than they used to, and can be better treated, they can still be serious or long lasting when they do occur, and catheterization should only be used as an investigative procedure, if the information required cannot be obtained by noninvasive and safer methods.

Indications
Urethral catheterization is employed:

1. to empty the bladder in most patients with acute and clot retention and in many with chronic retention
2. to empty the bladder before operating on pelvic viscera like the rectum or uterus and to fill the bladder before some operations on the bladder and prostate

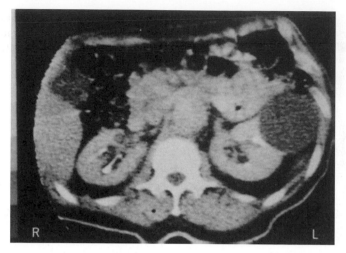

Fig. 25.20   CAT scan. This reveals that the right kidney, or at least the thin section revealed in this picture, is normal. The left kidney contains a large cyst (Reproduced from Sutton D 1980 A textbook of radiology, 3rd edn, Churchill Livingstone, Edinburgh, by kind permission of the author)

3. to instil antiseptics like Noxythiolin (Noxyflex) or Chlorhexidine 1/5000 into the infected bladder, or tumour inhibitors like Ethoglucid (Epodyl) into the neoplastic bladder
4. to measure residual urine, bladder capacity and other urodynamic parameters
5. to carry out cysto-urethrography in the investigation of bladder, vesico-ureteric, vesico-urethral and urethral disease
6. in patients with, or liable to develop, acute renal failure so that the urinary output can be measured hourly
7. in the treatment of neuropathic bladder disorders following diseases or injuries of the nervous system and other causes of urinary incontinence
8. as a means of draining, and keeping empty, the bladder after operations on the bladder, prostate and urethra and after some gynaecological and rectal operations
9. to determine the nature and extent of urethral and bladder injuries.

Catheter type

If the catheter is to be removed as soon as the bladder is emptied or filled or fluid is injected, a non-ballooned catheter of the Nelaton, Harris or Jacques type made of polyvinyl chloride (PVC)(Fig. 25.21) can be used; on the other hand, if the catheter is to be left in, a ballooned (Foley) or Gibbon catheter (Fig. 25.22) should be used.

Ballooned catheter

Two way Foley (Fig. 25.23). This is called two-way because it has two channels, one for urine drainage, the

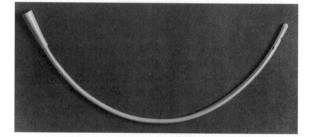

Fig. 25.21   Jacques catheter (Courtesy of Eschmann)

other, which is much smaller, for inflating the balloon which retains the catheter in the bladder. Sterile water or saline should be used to distend the balloon. If air is used, the balloon floats on the surface of the urine and the bladder does not drain properly.

Three way Foley (irrigating catheter (Fig. 25.24). This has three channels: one for urine drainage, one for inflating the balloon, and one, which opens just below the tip of the catheter, for continuous irrigation. The three-way Foley is predominantly used after endoscopic and open operations on the bladder or prostate (with a closed drainage system) to prevent clot retention. It can also be used for the continuous irrigation of a very infected bladder.

Foley catheters are made of latex, which is elastic and strong, and has a low toxicity. However, after 9 or 10 days, encrustations form around the drainage holes which progressively restrict urinary flow. Some latex catheters are coated on the inside or the outside (or both inside and outside) with silicone or teflon. Such coated catheters are smoother and less likely to encrust, but they are expensive.

catheters are constructed entirely of silicone. They are less irritant than latex or coated latex, but expensive, and generally only for people who require longterm catheterization.

'Haematuria' Foley catheters (Fig. 25.25). These are latex catheters whose walls are reinforced with nylon thread. They can withstand, without collapsing, the strong suction necessary for the removal of blood clots, and the three way ones are often used after prostatic surgery.

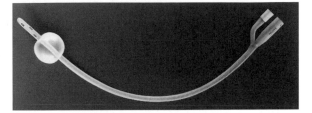

Fig. 25.25   Foley catheter — haematuric type(Courtesy of Eschmann)

Catheter size

If the catheter is too small, urine leaks around its sides; if too large, it can irritate the urethra. The French (F) — often called Charriere (CH) — gauge is used for sizing catheters, endoscopes, and many other tubes used in medicine. Dividing the French gauge by 3 gives the outside diameter of the tube in mm, i.e. an 18F catheter has an outside diameter of 6 mm. In adults, a 12–16F or CH catheter is adequate if the urine is clear, but a 20 or 22F should be used if the urine is turbid or blood stained. The balloon sizes of the Foley catheter range from 3–5 ml; 5–10 ml; 30 ml. and 75–100 ml; the smallest is used with 8 or 10F catheters; in adults a 30 ml is used although often no more than 10 ml is introduced. The full 30 ml should be used after prostatectomy otherwise the balloon may be displaced into the prostatic cavity, especially if traction is applied to the catheter to control venous bleeding (p. 647).

The inflated balloon of a Foley catheter provides a large surface area for the deposition of calcium phosphate and the formation of stones. As little fluid as necessary should be inserted into the balloon and it is good practice, although not always possible, to deflate the balloon for a few minutes each day or week in patients requiring prolonged catheterization. Some catheters are made for females only. The commonest are two way catheters with a shorter shaft length than the male ones. A double ballooned catheter (Fig. 25.26) is also available; the distal balloon (below the eyes) retains the catheter in the bladder; the other balloon is inflated outside the external meatus and prevents the shaft moving within the urethra, reducing, some believe, the risk of infection.

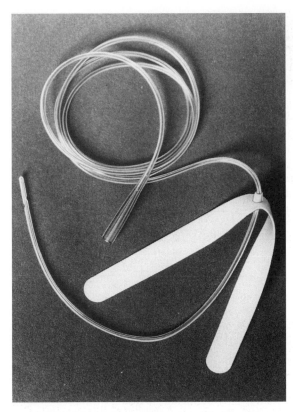

Fig. 25.22   Gibbon catheter (Courtesy of Eschmann)

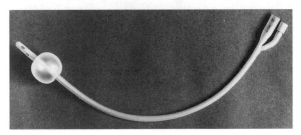

Fig. 25.23   Foley catheter two way (Courtesy of Eschmann)

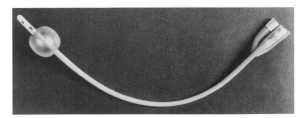

Fig. 25.24   Foley catheter three way (Courtesy of Eschmann)

Early ones were liable to delaminate, when the outer coating broke away from the latex and remained in the bladder after the catheter was removed, but this is not likely to happen with the present day ones. Some Foley

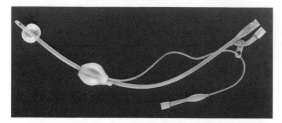

Fig. 25.26 Catheter with two balloons (Courtesy of Eschmann)

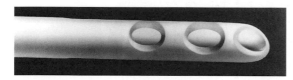

Fig. 25.27 Whistle tip catheter (Courtesy of Eschmann)

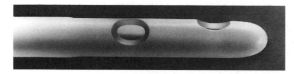

Fig. 25.28 Catheter with solid end and side eyes (Courtesy of Eschmann)

Various tips are available with two and three way Foley catheters; some have a terminal eye as well as side ones (Whistle tip) (Fig. 25.27), others only side eyes and a solid end (Fig. 25.28) which can be used with an inducer (Fig. 25.30).

Procedure

The procedure of urethral catheterization must be carried out with the most rigorous aseptic precautions and gentleness, otherwise infection can easily be introduced or exacerbated, or the urethra damaged, and the patient discomforted. If the patient is excessively apprehensive he can be given pethidine or diazepam intravenously before the procedure starts. The procedure, often done in the patient's bed in the ward, is best done in a dressing room or theatre, and the operator should wear sterile gloves. The patient is placed supine; in males, the legs are separated; in females, the knees are bent then separated with the feet together. The genitalia are cleaned with an aqueous antiseptic solution (spirit irritates the skin). In males, the penis is held in a sterile swab, the prepuce retracted and all smegma removed; in females, the labia should be separated with one hand while the meatus is cleaned (from before backwards) and only released after the catheter has been inserted. Sterile towels are used to prevent the catheter or operator's hands touching the skin or bedclothes. The urethra is filled with an antiseptic

anaesthetic gel (Lignocaine hydrochloride 1 or 2% with chlorhexidine 0.25%) using the nozzle supplied with the tube (both nozzle and tube are supplied sterile). Two minutes are allowed for the local anaesthetic to become effective while the catheter is prepared.

Most catheters are now supplied sterile and are often double-wrapped. When the outer pack is carefully removed by an assistant, the operator can handle the sterile inner pack. This is opened to expose the distal end of the catheter which is then well lubricated. (Petroleum products like liquid paraffin dissolve latex, and must not be used). The catheter is then slowly fed into the urethra out of the inner tube, elevating the penis in the male, and keeping the labia separated in the female. When the catheter reaches the bladder, urine drains through it. If a balloon catheter is being used the catheter is advanced a little further into the bladder before the balloon is inflated. The catheter is then connected to a drainage bag providing a closed drainage system. The bag should have a one way valve which will prevent urine returning to the bladder if the bag is lifted or sat upon.

Difficulties

In women catheterization is usually easy because the urethra is short, wide and straight, although sometimes the external meatus is hidden within the vaginal introitus.

In males catheterization may obviously be difficult if the patient has a urethral stricture or enlarged prostate, but may also be difficult if the external meatus is narrow (attempts to force a catheter through the meatus can cause a fissure and later a stricture). The patient may be apprehensive and his muscles in spasm, but, gentleness, patience and appreciation of the sensitivity of the urethra and the value of using plenty of lubricating gel and rotating movements, usually succeed in guiding the catheter safely into the bladder.

The catheter should be anchored securely to the thigh with elastoplast (Fig. 25.29).

A catheter introducer can be inserted into a Foley catheter to facilitate introduction, but great care must be taken because false passages can easily be made. The *Maryfield* introducer is of value to those experienced in the use of urethral dilators. If a catheter cannot be passed, the procedure should be abandoned until the urethra can be further investigated, and, if the patient has retention, the bladder can be drained by a suprapubic cystostomy (p. 622). Sometimes the balloon of a Foley catheter cannot be deflated when we wish to remove it. The first thing to do is to cut the valve off the balloon channel and try to deflate the balloon by applying a syringe directly to the channel. If this is unsuccessful, wait 12 hours, because the balloon may gradually and spontaneously deflate. If still un-

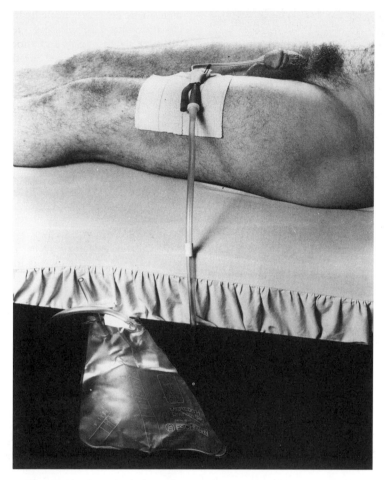

Fig. 25.29   A method of securing a catheter at the thigh with strapping

successful, injecting liquid paraffin down the main drainage channel may dissolve part of the balloon. Over inflation is not recommended because it often leaves pieces of latex in the bladder. A stylet from a ureteric catheter can be placed down the balloon channel and used to puncture the balloon. If all else fails, or if inability to deflate the balloon is associated with retention and instant relief required, the balloon can be punctured with a 19 g spinal needle passed suprapubically, transvaginally or transrectally, after first ensuring that the bladder is partially distended.

ENDOSCOPY (CYSTO-URETHROSCOPY)

Mainly due to the work of Professor H H Hopkins, endoscopy has improved enormously over the past two decades, for the following reasons:

1. Fibre illumination (which has replaced the small delicate, unreliable terminal incandescent bulb previously used in urology) provides a powerful safe and reliable lighting system, suitable not only for endoscopic procedures, but also for still and cine photography, and the use of teaching attachments. The light is produced by a large quartz iodine lamp housed in the light source box. It is transmitted to the fibre light pillar of the telescope by a flexible cable made up of glass fibre bundles wrapped in a protective sheath of coiled metal wadding and coated with rubber or plastic. The light is then transmitted down the telescope by another set of glass fibre bundles which are incorporated in the wall of the telescope.

Glass tubes can transmit not only light, but also images (fibre optics) and are widely used for this purpose by gastro-enterologists. Although we use rigid telescopes for cysto-urethroscopy, flexible ones, using fibre optics, have been developed for the inspection of the ureter and pelvicaliceal systems with a larger one for the bladder.

2. The invention of the rod lens telescope. In the conventional telescope, the lenses were made of glass and the spaces between them filled with air; in the rod

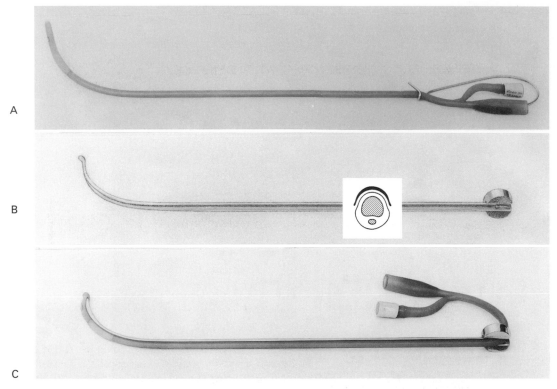

Fig. 25.30   A. Foley catheter mounted on a wire stretcher. B. The *Maryfield* introducer for Foley catheters. C. The catheter is stretched along a groove on the convex surface of the instrument as shown on the inset in B

lens telescope the lenses are narrow spaces of air and the spaces between them are filled with glass rods. This change augments the amount of light transmitted from object to viewer, the optical resolution and the field of view.

3. The improved methods of coating the fibre optics reduces the amount of light lost by reflection.

The basic endoscopic examination system (Fig. 25.31) consists of a sheath which is a straight hollow metal tube from 17F to 24F for adults, but as small as 8F for infants. The end of the sheath may be straight or slightly bent, but is always made with little if any beak or curvature, so that it can be used for examining the urethra with a fore-oblique telescope, as well as the bladder. The proximal end of the sheath has one, or usually two side channels, each controlled by a small tap, for the supply of fluid. Sometimes these channels are on a rotating collar and sometimes they are fixed. Although sheaths of 17F–18F upwards accept the standard telescopes, and can be used for inspection, the sheath size determines the size of ureteric catheters, electrodes, or biopsy forceps that can be used, and for adults a 21F sheath is probably best. The latter will accept the pinch biopsy forceps and one 9F electrode or two 6F catheters, but a larger sheath is needed for stone crushing forceps.

An obturator inserted into the sheath prevents the open end of the sheath damaging the urethra as it is passed into the bladder.

Nowadays the obturator is often not used and the sheath is passed with the fore-oblique or direct view telescope so that the urethra can be visualized from the external meatus to bladder neck as the instrument is slowly passed. (Some manufacturers supply a special hollow obturator for this purpose, but it is not necessary). Urethroscopy can be done after the bladder has been examined, but it is better done first. To examine the urethra requires a steady flow of irrigating fluid, otherwise the urethral walls collapse onto the end of the telescope and only a red haze will be seen.

When the tip of the sheath is in the bladder, the obturator or telescope is removed and the bladder emptied. The bladder is then filled with sterile water or saline, and fully examined.

Telescopes (Fig. 25.32)
The rigid telescopes used in cysto-urethroscopy are classified by the angle of view they provide into fore-oblique, lateral, direct and retrograde. The fore-oblique telescope usually provides a 30° angle, but with some manufacturers, it is 12° or 20°. This telescope can be used with the inspecting sheath to examine the

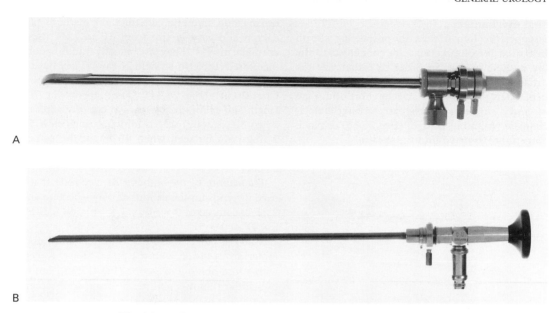

A

B

Fig. 25.31 Cystoscope — the sheath, a telescope and the short bridge

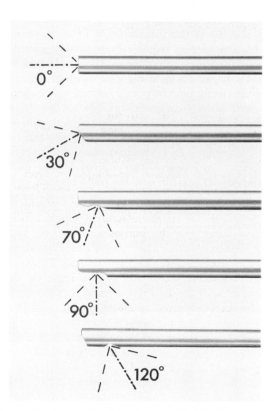

Fig. 25.32 The angle of the view provided by different telescopes

urethra, prostate, bladder neck and the trigone and posterior wall of the bladder; and with biopsy forceps, stone crushing forceps, catheter deflecting mechanisms and most resectoscopes. Telescopes are the most ex-pensive items of urological endoscopes and if the surgeon can afford only one telescope, the fore-oblique is the one to buy. To examine the bladder properly, however, a lateral 70° telescope is needed. It can also be used with the catheter deflecting mechanism (Albarran lever) but not with biopsy or stone crushing forceps or resectoscopes. The anterior wall of the bladder, and in patients with prostatic hypertrophy, the base can be best seen with the retrograde (120°) telescope; however, in most patients, the fundus can be seen well enough with the 70° telescope if the abdomen is compressed, the patient tilted or the bladder only partly filled, so that the purchase of a retrograde telescope, which is rarely used, may be unnecessary.

The direct viewing telescope (0°) is used with some models of resectoscopes and is perhaps the best for ure-throscopy or visual urethrotomy; but most surgeons use a resectoscope with a fore-oblique (30°) telescope which can also be used for urethroscopy and visual urethrotomy.

The fibre light sources and fibre light cables of one manufacturer can be used with the endoscopes of another, using adapters that are freely available. Unfortunately, interchangeability finishes there, and so far as the rest of the endoscopy set is concerned, it is advisable to buy a matched set from one maker, because the telescopes, sheaths, forceps etc., of one maker, are, sadly, not interchangeable with those of another.

Urethroscopy should be done in all male patients, but is essential when carrying out endoscopy on patients with benign or malignant prostatic disease, bladder tumours, and urethral diverticula or strictures.

Deflecting mechanism

The telescopes are longer than the inspection sheath and, when used for observation, are connected to the sheath by a short bridge. In order to catheterize the ureters, diathermize a bladder tumour or take biopsies from the bladder, the telescope and the short bridge are removed, and a single or double catheterizing deflecting mechanism (Albarran Bridge) (Fig. 25.33) or pinch biopsy forceps are inserted into the sheath.

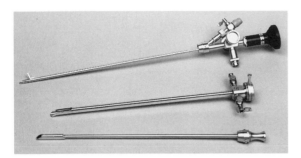

Fig. 25.33 Catheter deflecting mechanism (Albarran bridge) with sheath and obturator (Courtesy of Key Med.)

The catheter deflecting mechanism has, at its distal end, a platform on which the ureteric catheter or electrode rests. This platform can be raised or lowered by rotating a wheel at the proximal end of the instrument (Albarran lever) and the catheter thus guided visually into the ureter or the electrode onto the tumour. The one or two openings at the proximal end of the catheter deflecting mechanism can be kept closed by taps. However, if catheters or electrodes are being passed, these taps have to be left open.

In these circumstances the openings are occluded with perforated rubber nipples which grip the catheter or electrode and prevent the irrigating fluid from leaking out. Ureteric catheters are made of plastic or dacron and vary in size from 3F to 12F. (Size 5F is normally used.) They are usually radio-opaque and, therefore, visible in straight X-rays. They have various tips, plain, whistle tip or with bulbs (Braasch or Chevasseur) (Fig. 25.34). They are about 70 cm in length and calibrated by rings in cm (the adult ureter is 25 to 30 cm long) with additional rings each 5 cm, so 2 rings can be seen when 10 cm of the catheter has passed into the ureter, 3 at 15 cm, 4 at 20 cm and 5 at 25 cm.

The calibre of the catheter or electrode that can be used depends on the calibre of the inspection sheath. A 21 F sheath takes 2 × 6F or 1 × 8F; and a 17F sheath 2 × 4F or 1 × 5F.

Mucosal biopsies can be accurately and safely taken under direct vision with the pinch biopsy forceps used with a fore-oblique telescope (Fig. 25.35), but biopsies of bladder tumours and the prostate are best and most easily taken with a resectoscope.

Resectoscope

Many feel that only a urologist should use a resectoscope, and use of this instrument in urethral, prostatic and bladder surgery requires some general comment. Transurethral resection of the prostate or a bladder tumour by untrained, inexperienced surgeons, especially if they are using poor or poorly maintained equipment can cause serious complications, but so can the performance of any open or endoscopic procedure in similar circumstances. The general surgeon who can easily refer his patients to a urologist, may well decide to do no resections or any other urology for that matter; but the general surgeon who has to do his own urology must learn to use a resectoscope, at least, for patients with bladder tumours and fibrous, malignant, and the smaller hypertrophied prostates, because it is the best way to treat these conditions.

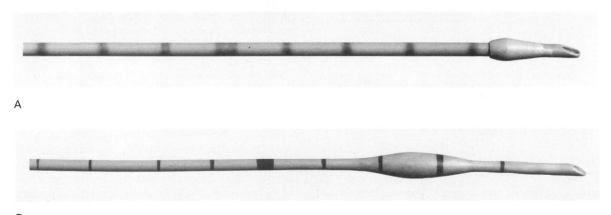

A

B

Fig. 25.34 Ureteric catheters. (A) Braasch; (B) Chevasseur

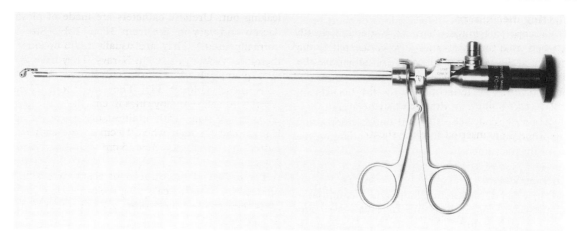

Fig. 25.35 Pinch biopsy forceps. These are used with a fore-oblique telescope through a cystoscope or resectoscope sheath (Courtesy of A C M I Ltd)

There are many types of resectoscopes, but they all consist of an outer sheath, a working element which moves the diathermy loop backwards and forwards; a telescope which is usually a fore-oblique but sometimes a direct viewing one (Fig. 25.36).

The sheath is made of fibre glass or stainless steel with a fibre glass tip so that the diathermy current is not transmitted down the sheath as the loop is with-drawn into the sheath at the conclusion of a cut. How-ever, fears that emission of the current down the sheath in this way would burn the urethra, and even the opera-tor, seem exaggerated, and some surgeons use an all metal noninsulated sheath.

The sheath sizes vary from 24F to 28F, but, since the larger sheaths are much more likely to damage the ure-thra and leave strictures, most surgeons use a 26F sheath.

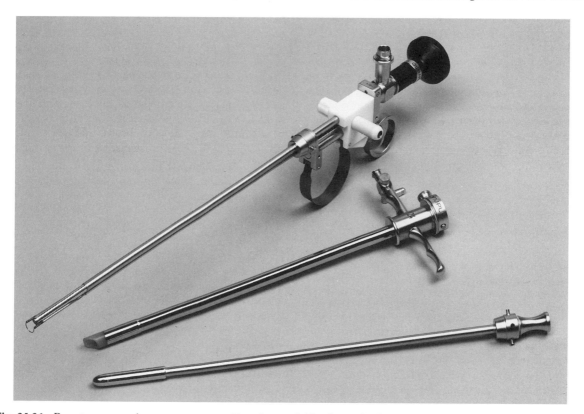

Fig. 25.36 Resectoscope — the resectoscope working element (with telescope), sheath and obturator (Courtesy of Key Med.)

The end of the sheath can have a long or short beak, and those used with direct vision telescopes have no beak at all. The long beak covers the whole journey of the loop and is perhaps safer, but most urologists prefer the short beak. The fluid inlet tap on the sheath is usually fixed, but on some sheaths rotates. The sheath can be passed blindly into the bladder with an appropriate obturator, but is best passed under vision using the appropriate telescope, 30° or 0° depending on the make of the instrument.

The working element

This carries and moves the loop and fits into the sheath, the telescope fitting into it. There are many different types of working elements, but each can be used with any adult sized sheath and with each the loop moves about 2.5 cm. They fall into 3 groups including two spring loaded groups. (1) The Baumrucker type in which the spring aids the return of the loop to the extended position, and in the resting state, the loop projects out of the sheath; (2) the Iglesias type in which the spring aids the cutting action of the loop and in the resting state the loop is inside the tip of the sheath; and (3) a group without spring assistance at all. Of these, the Iglesias type is the safest because the patient will not be burnt if someone accidentally treads on the diathermy pedal.

The resection is carried out while fluid flows into the bladder, and the working element and telescope have to be removed from the sheath at regular intervals to empty the bladder. A continuous flow resectoscope was introduced in 1975 by Iglesias, but balancing the inflow and outflow is not easy, and most urologists still prefer the conventional resectoscope.

Various loops can be fitted. The loop electrode is used for cutting and vessel coagulation; but roller and ball electrodes are available for vessel coagulation and a knife electrode for incising a bladder neck or ureteric orifice.

Technique of endoscopy

Position (Fig. 25.37)

The patient's legs should be separated and the thighs flexed to 45°. This is a half lithotomy position; the full one makes endoscopy difficult.

Anaesthesia

General anaesthesia is preferred because it facilitates the examination and allows for painfree biopsies, electro coagulation or resection and a satisfactory bimanual examination. An adequate endoscopic examination, however, can be done using intravenous diazepam and injecting lignocaine gel 1% antiseptic (which contains

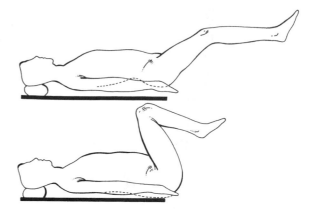

Fig. 25.37 Position of the patient for urological endoscopic procedures is shown in the upper figure. The lower figure shows the lithotomy position which is unsuitable for endoscopy

lignocaine hydrochloride 1% and chlorhexidine gluconate solution 0.25%) into the urethra.

Procedure (Fig. 25.38)

The instrument sheath and obturator are well lubricated (liquid paraffin, K.Y. jelly or lignocaine gel) and allowed to fall down the urethra and into the bladder under its own weight, depressing the instrument in the male to allow the beak to traverse the membranous and prostatic parts of the urethra. Once the instrument is in the bladder the obturator is removed and the bladder emptied. However, most urologists now prefer to pass the instrument under direct vision, so that they can view the entire length of the urethra before it is affected by instrumentation. For this purpose the fore-oblique or direct telescope is inserted into the sheath using the short bridge; the instrument is then passed slowly down the urethra continuously irrigating in order to prevent the urethra collapsing on to the end of the telescope and obscuring the view. In this way, the spongy, membranous and prostatic parts of the urethra are seen in turn. Once in the bladder, the bladder neck, trigone and posterior wall of the bladder are examined before removing the telescope and emptying the bladder. The bladder is then filled with 250 to 300 ml of sterile water or saline and carefully examined with the 70° telescope. Vision may be obscured by a number of factors and can often be improved if the bladder is washed out a few times (Fig. 25.39).

The bladder

All parts of the bladder are carefully examined by moving the cystoscope in and out and gradually rotating it. It is probably easier to start at the bladder neck at 6 o'clock viewing the bladder as the cystoscope is moved

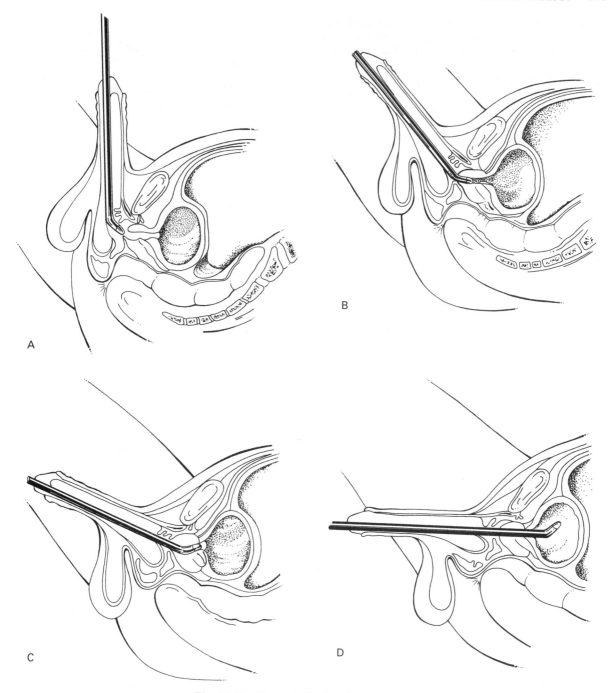

Fig. 25.38   The method of passing cystoscope

in as far as it will go and then out again, rotating it a few times and repeating the movement (Fig. 25.40) and continuing this way until the instrument has rotated 360° and all the bladder has been inspected. If the cystoscope is moved closer to any suspicious areas, they will be magnified and seen more clearly. The ante-rior wall of the bladder or the bladder pouch that forms behind an enlarged middle prostatic lobe may not be seen even with the 70° telescope, but can be seen with the retrograde telescope (120°). If a retrograde telescope is not available, these parts may still be visualized with the 70° telescope if pressure is applied to the anterior abdominal wall or the anterior rectal wall or if the patient is tilted into a Trendelenberg position. The trigone of the bladder is always redder than the rest of the bladder and failure to appreciate this accounts for the apparent epidemics of trigonitis that occur whenever a new surgeon starts doing cystoscopies.

Both ureteric orifices should next be examined (see Fig. 25.53); they are situated some 2 or 3 cm above the posterior bladder neck at 4 and 8 o'clock at the lateral angles of the interureteric bar. The easiest way to find the ureteric orifices (which may be difficult or even impossible to locate if the bladder is inflamed or trabeculated, or the middle prostatic lobe much enlarged) is to find the interureteric bar in the midline posteriorly then follow it to the left and right. Sometimes the intravenous injection of indigocarmine (with frusemide, if the examination is done under general anaesthesia, and the patient is dehydrated) may help to locate an orifice if one can see the dye emerging from the ureter, although the dye rapidly diffuses and mixes with the fluid in the bladder, and obscures the view (Fig. 25.39). The air bubble is seen in the highest part of the bladder (the fundus) and obscures the mucosa underlying it. This mucosa can be examined if the air bubble is moved by tilting the patient. (If a large air bubble enters the bladder as it is being filled, the patient may complain of pneumaturia, the first or second time he passes urine after the examination).

Although the bladder neck and posterior urethra were examined with the 30° fore-oblique telescope, they should be examined a second time with the 70° telescope. The bladder neck cannot all be seen in one view, but suc-

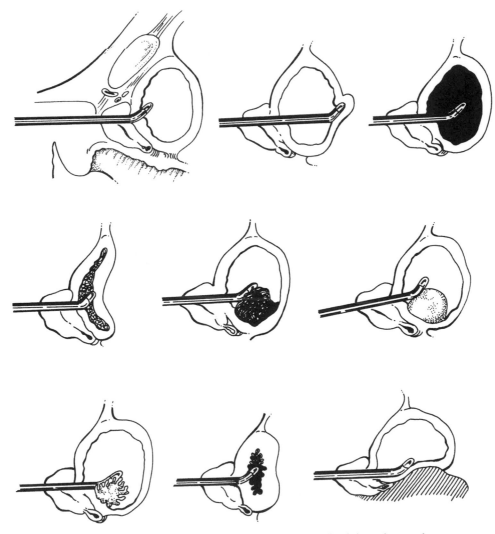

Fig. 25.39   The factors which may obscure the view obtained through an endoscope

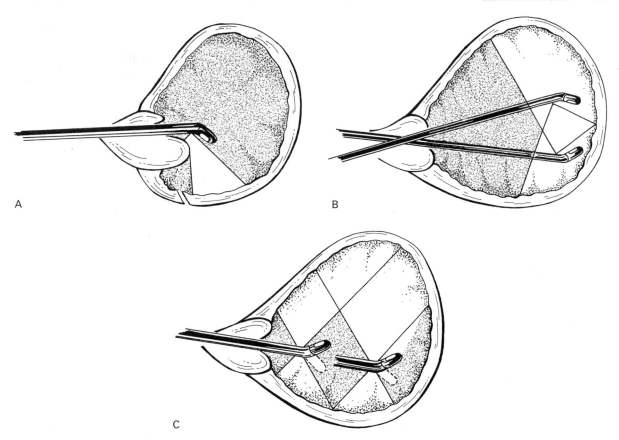

Fig. 25.40 The fields of view obtained with various positions of the telescope and the means by which the whole bladder can be examined by moving the cystoscope

cessive views seen as the instrument is rotated through 360° reveal its shape. Common conditions seen at GU endoscopy are shown in Figs 25.41–25.52.

Retrograde catheterization

The indications for this procedure (p. 550) and apparatus required (p. 562) have been discussed. At one time retrograde pyelograms were made often instead of intravenous ones as a means of determining whether or not the upper urinary tract was normal. Nowadays they are done, if at all, to elucidate an abnormality seen in IVU, ultrasound or other investigation, and it is safest to do one side at a time.

With the inspection sheath catheter deflecting mechanism (Albarran lever) and telescope (either 70° or fore-oblique can be used), the catheter is threaded through until its tip can be seen emerging into the bladder from the end of the instrument. By moving the endoscope the ureteric orifice can be located and the catheter tip approximated to it (Fig. 25.54). The tip of the catheter can then be pushed into the orifice by

moving the whole endoscope or only the Albarran lever; once the catheter is in the ureter the stylet should be removed, either completely, or 1 cm or 2 cm at a time, as the catheter is pushed 25 to 30 cm up the ureter.

At this stage some 10 cm of catheter still projects out of the cystoscope; this is pushed down the cystoscope and into the bladder until the end of the catheter is flush with the rubber nipple. The cystoscope is then carefully removed, making sure the platform is first lowered, leaving the 10 cm of ureteric catheter sticking out of the external meatus. Its end is inserted into some collection appliance like a small bottle with a rubber cap. Once X-rays have been made or collections completed, the catheter is removed. In many units the patient is transferred from the theatre to an X-ray department before the retrograde films are taken. It is important to do this expeditiously, especially if the catheter could not be passed up the whole length of the ureter; otherwise, the catheter may be found coiled up in the bladder and no longer in the ureter because of

Figs 25.41–25.52   *Cystoscopic photographs*

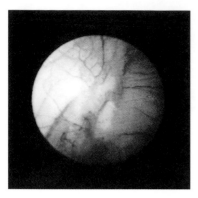

Fig. 25.41   Normal ureteric orifice

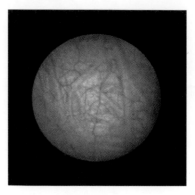

Fig. 25.42   Bladder trabeculation

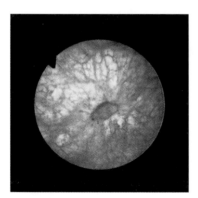

Fig. 25.43   Bladder diverticulum

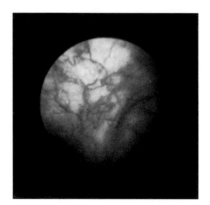

Fig. 25.44   Simple patchy cystitis

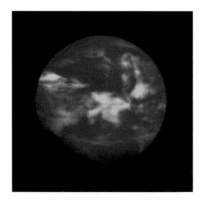

Fig. 25.45   Tuberculous ulcer

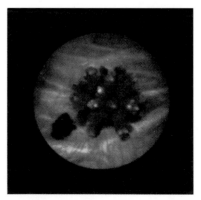

Fig. 25.46   Bladder calculi

Figs 25.41–25.52 *Cystoscopic photographs*

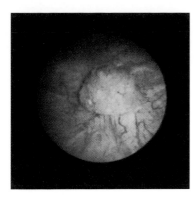

Fig. 25.47   Papillary bladder tumour

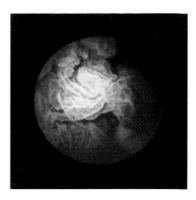

Fig. 25.48   Bladder carcinoma

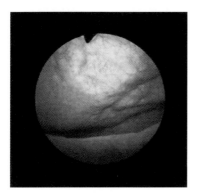

Fig. 25.49   Bladder neck and beyond

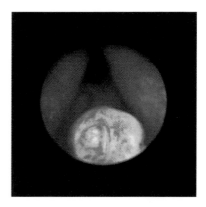

Fig. 25.50   Normal verumontanum and lateral lobes

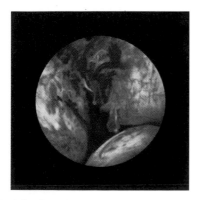

Fig. 25.51   The three lobes of prostate

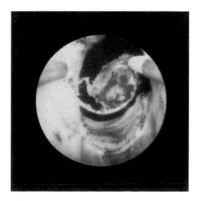

Fig. 25.52   Resection of the prostate

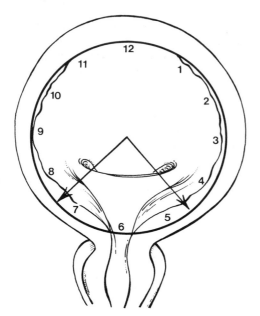

Fig. 25.53   The ureteric orifices

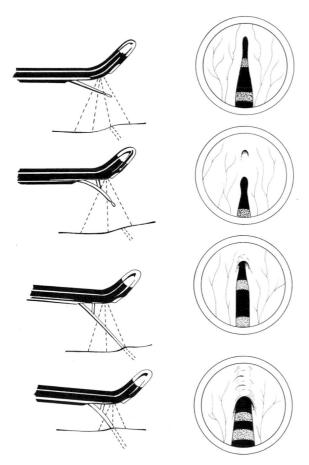

Fig. 25.54   The method by which a ureteric catheter is introduced into the ureter

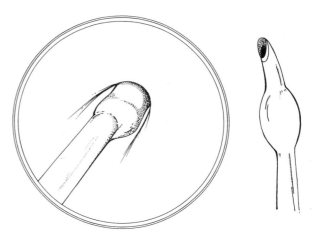

Fig. 25.55   Method of using Braasch or Chevasseur ureteric catheters

extrusion by ureteric peristalsis. Failure to pass a catheter does not mean the ureter is obstructed, nor does success mean it is not.

Ureteric catheterisation may introduce or aggravate infection, it may also aggravate obstruction by causing oedema. For this reason, retrograde pyelograms and ureterograms are often made using a bulb catheter of Braasch or Chevasseur (Fig. 25.55) type. The tip of the catheter is inserted into the ureter and the bulb impacted in or against the orifice to prevent dye effluxing into the bladder when it is injected into the catheter. Contrast medium 25% is slowly injected into the catheter, and ascends to fill the ureter and pelvicaliceal system, and X-rays can be taken. As only 1 or 2 cm of the catheter are inserted, the procedure is done with the cystoscope tip in the bladder, and with the operator viewing the ureteric orifice to ensure that the catheter does not dislodge during the examination.

Ureteroscopy

Four recent developments have changed our management of ureteric disease and upper tract obstruction:

1. the ability to do antegrade imaging studies
2. the ureteric stent
3. percutaneous drainage of the obstructed tract
4. the rigid ureteroscope.

A note of warning. The calibre of the rigid ureteroscope is relatively large in relation to the size of the normal ureter and complications may occur, including ureteric stricture, ureteric rupture and urine extravasation. The inexperienced surgeon would be wise to use one of the well-tried standard techniques. Most of these standard techniques are not under direct vision but, despite the advent of the rigid ureteroscope, they still have a role. It may be better to subject a patient to an open operation than to risk stricture of the ureter and a lifelong problem.

The ureteroscope

The design of the ureteroscope is still evolving. The choice lies between a rigid instrument and flexible one, between long and short or between larger and smaller calibre instruments. Rigid ureteroscopes either have an inbuilt telescope (the operating ureteroscope) or a straight changeable telescope (the diagnostic ureteroscope). The original instruments were long (40 cm) but it is now realised that for stones in the upper one third of the ureter the push-pull technique or transrenal ureteroscopy is safer and a new range of 'short' ureteroscopes (33 cm), designed for these purposes has been introduced. Flexible ureteroscopes have not become widely accepted because of expense, limited life of the instrument and small size of the operating channel.

Optics of the rigid ureteroscope

Because of the length and narrow sheath, ureteroscopes are liable to bend and this may distort the optics. This is particularly true for the longer rigid scopes when crescent-shaped black areas may seriously interfere with vision. A technique that is sometimes useful when using the older 40 cm ureteroscopes is to introduce it through a 26 or 27 F urethral sheath to minimise cross-axis stress in the urethra.

The short ureteroscope

The instrument is essentially the same as the cystoscope but of narrower calibre (9F) and longer (33 cm). Either direct or offset 0° telescopes are available. The *direct* telescope allows the passage of flexible instruments — such as a fine lithotron probe, stone basket or ureteric catheter — through the offset operating port. When the *offset* telescope is used rigid instruments such as a fine ultra sound probe can be used. The design varies between different manufacturers and the following features should be taken into account. The beak should be oblique and not square ended or else the instrument is very difficult to pass. The telescope should be stabilised and not free in the sheath, otherwise it moves around under stress and the view becomes obscured by the side or beak of the sheath. A certain amount of bending is inevitable and this should be allowed for in the telescope construction.

Accessories

The following accessories are available

- fine flexible and rigid biopsy forceps
- ureteric stone baskets of various designs
- flexible probe for the electrohydraulic lithotripter
- rigid probes for the ultrasound lithotripter

Indications for ureteroscopy

1. Stone extraction from the lower one third of the ureter. Stone extraction from the middle one third provided the stone size is 8 mm or less
2. Diagnosis of ureteric filling defects where other means such as urine cytology have failed
3. Diagnosis of ureteric colic where repeated imaging fails to show a calculus
4. Diathermy or resection of ureteric tumours.

Contra-indications

1. Previous ureteric surgery or known ureteric stricture. This probably includes most, if not all, tuberculous and bilharzial strictures
2. If the instrument will not easily proceed despite adequate dilatation of the ureteric orifice and intramural part of the ureter
3. Patient unfit for general anaesthesia.

Technique of ureteroscopy

1. The procedure should be undertaken with the patient under general anaesthetic. If stone extraction is to be attempted it must be remembered that, should the procedure fail, open operation could be necessary and, unless this can be done in the same operating theatre, a second anaesthetic may be needed. The anaesthetist should be warned of this to allow for the possibility of an early second anaesthetic. It must also be remembered that if the instrumentation is successful then up to 33 cms (40 cms if only an older instrument is available) of narrow probe will be within the patient. It is therefore important that the patient is well relaxed and does not cough in the middle of the procedure and snap the ureteroscope.

2. The ureter is straightened by having the legs in the lithotomy position but in men this may accentuate angulation of the urethra. Thus in women a full lithotomy position may be used but in men the legs may have to be lowered.

3. The procedure should be covered by prophylactic antibiotics.

4. A preliminary cystoscopy is undertaken to exclude any urethral stricture or any other bladder abnormality. The site of the ureter is noted.

5. It is often necessary to dilate the ureteric orifice. This can be achieved by using graduated metal bougies or ureteric dilators passed through the cystoscope. Possibly the easiest way, although more expensive, is to use a 4 or 5 F Fogarty arterial embolism catheter. The balloon takes approximately 1 cc and dilates about 14 F. Dilation of the intramural ureter is easy with the Fogarty but because the balloon is round it is necessary to balance it at the ureteric orifice to achieve dilation of the meatus.

6. The cystoscope is withdrawn and the uretero-scope is passed into the bladder under direct vision.

7. The ureteric orifice is visualised and the uretero-scope angled so that the ureteric lumen can be seen leading away from the orifice. The ureteroscope is maintained at this angle and passed along the lumen. If the instrument does not easily pass the orifice it helps to pass a fine catheter or the stone basket or a guide wire a few centimetres up the ureter to act as a guide for the instrument. The ureteroscope should be rotated so that the longer lip of its beak is posterior and enters the orifice in contact with posterior wall.

8. Once the ureteroscope is in the ureter it is advanced one or two centimetres and then rotated through 180°. It is then further advanced gently and the angle of entry is constantly adjusted to keep the ureteric lumen in view. If the ureter is excessively angled or of narrow calibre further passage becomes increasingly difficult and the procedure should aban-doned. Previous ureteric operation leaves a ring of contraction and it is usually not possible to proceed beyond this point. If a ring of scar tissue is seen this can be dilated with the 9 F balloon catheter.

Although it is possible to reach the level of the renal pelvis it is now recognized that stones in the upper one third of the ureter are best managed from above. It helps if the patient is on a screening table as the level achieved can then be checked.

Complications of ureteroscopy

In most series there is about an 80% success rate with stone extraction and a 10% complication rate. The main complications are sepsis, perforation and stric-ture. About 1% of patients may require open operation; ureteric reimplantation is sometimes necessary. Com-plications are most likely to occur during the learning period of both the technique and the indications and undoubtedly they will diminish with experience. The complications of open surgery must also be borne in mind.

Bimanual examination

Once the endoscopy is completed, the bladder emptied and the instruments removed, a bimanual examination should always be done. Under general anaesthesia with an empty bladder, bimanual examination can deter-mine the local extent of bladder and prostatic tumours, or detect lesions of vagina, cervix, uterus, rectum, colon or pelvis that are associated with or indeed the cause of urinary problems.

FURTHER READING

Gow J G, Hopkins H H 1978 Handbook of urological endoscopy. Churchill Livingstone, Edinburgh
Hargreave T B 1990 Practical urological endoscopy. Blackwell Scientific, Oxford
Lees W R 1984 Abdominal ultrasonography. Blackwell, Oxford
Lloyd-Davies R W, Gow J G, Davies D R 1983 A colour atlas of urology. Wolfe Medical, London
Mitchell J P 1981 Endoscopic operative urology. John Wright & Son, Bristol
Sherwood T 1990 Imaging radiology. In: Chisholm G D, Fair W (eds) Scientific foundations of urology. Heinemann Medical, Oxford, p 17

Turner-Warwick R, Whiteside C G 1982 Urodynamic studies. In: Chisholm G D, Williams D I (eds) Scientific foundations of urology, 2nd edn Heinemann, London, p 442
Uszler J M, Holmes J H, Boswell W D 1983 Radionuclear and Radiographic Techniques. In: Massry S G, Glassock R J (eds) Textbook of urology. Williams & Wilkins, Baltimore, p 12.3
Whitfield H N, Hendry W F (eds) 1985 Textbook of genito-urinary surgery, vol. 1. Churchill Livingstone, Edinburgh

Anatomy of the kidney

The kidneys have a characteristic shape and measure about 11 by 6 by 4 cm. They lie on the posterior abdominal wall opposite the 12th thoracic and first three lumbar vertebrae (Fig. 26.1). Their long axes are slightly oblique, so that the upper poles are nearer one another than the lower. The right kidney is pushed down by the liver and lies at a lower level than the left one. *The hilum* is a vertical slit on the medial border of the kidney. It opens into a space called the renal sinus, lies about the level of the 1st lumbar vertebra some 4 cm from the midline and transmits the ureter, blood vessels, sympathetic nerves and lymphatics (Smith, 1983).

Structure of the kidney
The kidney is enveloped by a *fibrous capsule* and consists of the parenchyma and the collecting system. The *parenchyma* has an outer cortex which is pale and

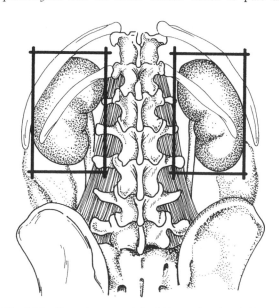

Fig. 26.1 Posterior view of the kidneys showing their relationships with the thoracic and lumbar vertebrae and the ribs

granular and composed of glomeruli and proximal and distal tubules, and an inner medulla which is striated and composed of the loops of Henle and the collecting tubules. The medulla is divided into a number of pyramids, the apices of which are called papillae and invaginate the minor calices. The *collecting system* comprises the 8 to 10 major calices which embrace the papillae and which unite to form 2 to 4 major calices. These in turn unite to form the pelvis which is funnel shaped and tapers to become the ureter.

The *renal fascia* encloses the kidney, the adrenal gland and the perinephric fat. It consists of anterior and posterior layers which blend laterally with the retroperitoneal tissues, superiorly with the diaphragmatic fascia and medially invest the blood vessels and renal pelvis. The extraperitoneal fat lies outside the renal fascia and is sometimes called *pararenal fat*.

Relations
Posteriorly the upper part of the kidney lies on the diaphragm which separates it from the 11th intercostal space, the 12th rib and the pleura (Fig. 26.2); the lower part on the psoas major, quadratus and transversus muscles, the subcostal vessels and the subcostal, iliohypogastric and ilio-inguinal nerves (Fig. 26.3). *Anteriorly* the right kidney is related to the 2nd part of the duodenum and the right colic flexure; the left, to the pancreas and splenic vessels. *Laterally* the right kidney is related to the hepatic flexure and the ascending colon; the left, to the left colic flexure and the descending colon (Fig. 26.4).

The pedicle of the kidney
This consists of the vein, artery and ureter or renal pelvis (from before backwards) the sympathetic nerves and the lymph vessels. The right renal vein is short and, therefore, more difficult to deal with at operation than the left one and more likely to be invaded by a renal cell carcinoma. The renal artery often has two main branches. Sometimes accessory or aberrant arteries enter the kidney above or below the hilum and may pass behind or in front of the ureter.

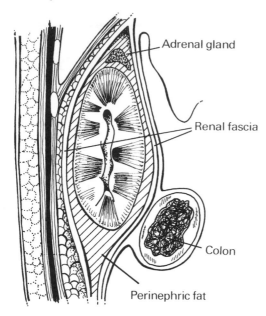

Fig. 26.2 A sagittal section of the kidney showing its relationships to the pleura, adrenal gland and colon

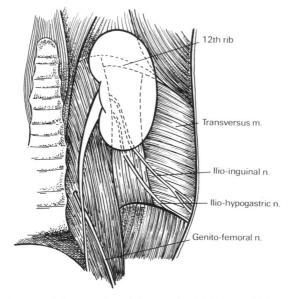

Fig. 26.3 The posterior relations of the left kidney which are the diaphragm above and the psoas, quadratus lumborum and transversus muscles, separated by the iliohypogastric and ilioinguinal nerves, below

The adrenal glands
These are small yellow bodies which lie on the superomedial aspect of the kidneys. They are enclosed within the renal fascia, but separated from the kidney by a fascial septum (see also p. 602).

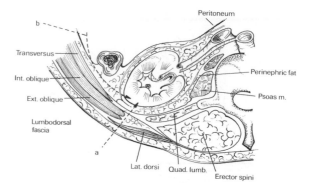

Fig. 26.4 A transverse section of the body at the level of the first lumbar vertebra showing the relationship of the left kidney and the renal pedicle. The lumbar approach (a) and the transperitoneal anterior approach (b) are indicated

SURGICAL APPROACHES TO THE KIDNEY

Position of the patient for posterolateral incisions
The patient is placed on his sound side, with his back, at which the surgeons stands, brought over towards the edge of the table. The leg next to the table is fully flexed at the hip and knee; the upper leg is extended (Fig. 26.5). The patient is maintained in this position by a back support or strapping. To increase access, the trunk should be flexed laterally by raising the 'kidney bridge' if the table has one, or 'breaking' the table to lower the feet and the head. A support for the upper arm prevents the shoulder from sagging forwards and makes the arm and hand easily accessible to the anaesthetist.

Lumbar subcostal approach
This approach can be used for some operations on the kidney and the renal pelvis and for most operations on the upper ureter. In fat patients, and for operations on high kidneys for large tumours and for reoperations, it provides a poor exposure and cannot easily be extended and most surgeons prefer the lateral approaches made through or above the 12th or 11th rib. The subcostal incision can be extended anteriorly, but it is not easy to extend it posteriorly and superiorly by excising or mobilizing the 12th rib if access is restricted. Investigations can image the kidney and assess disease so accurately that the surgeon should know what incision is best before starting the operation.

Incision (Fig. 26.6)
This begins below the angle between the 12th rib and the lateral border of sacrospinalis and is carried downwards and forwards in a curved line between the 12th rib and the iliac crest.

It usually stops 4 to 5 cm above the anterior superior spine, but can be extended forwards to the lateral bor-

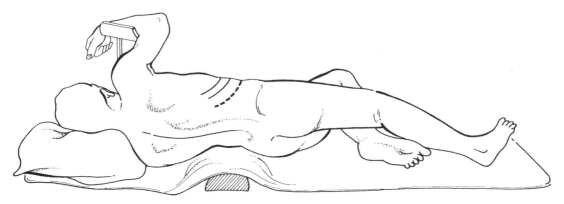

Fig. 26.5   Position of patient on the operating table for posterolateral approaches to the kidney. Note the flexed lower limb and the extended upper one

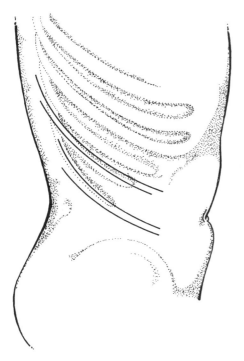

Fig. 26.6   The skin incisions for the various posterolateral exposures of the kidney. From below upwards, the subcostal approach, the twelfth rib approach, the eleventh rib approach and the thoraco-abdominal incision through the tenth intercostal space

Figs 26.7–26.9   *The lumbar exposure of the left kidney*

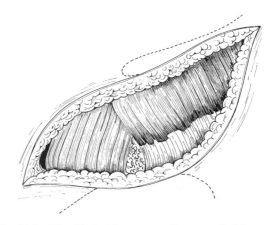

Fig. 26.7   The skin incision exposes the external oblique muscle anteriorly and the latissimus dorsi posteriorly. Between them is the lumbar triangle

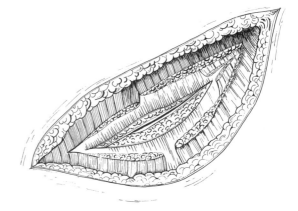

Fig. 26.8   Once the posterior fibres of the external oblique and the anterior fibres of the latissimus dorsi are divided in the line of the skin incision, the serratus posterior inferior posteriorly, and the internal oblique muscle anteriorly, are exposed. They are divided to expose the renal fascia. A self-retaining retractor can now be inserted

der of the rectus muscle or beyond. The skin incision exposes the muscle fibres of latissimus dorsi and serratus posterior inferior posteriorly, and of the external oblique anteriorly. They are incised in the same line as the skin incision to expose the quadratus lumborum posteriorly, the internal oblique anteriorly and the three fused layers of lumbodorsal fascia, which form a strip of fibrous tissue about 3 cm wide between them. The lumbodorsal fascia is incised or split transversely in

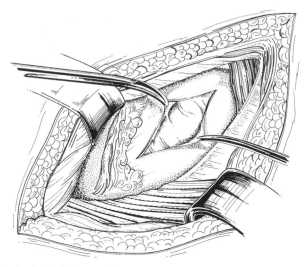

Fig. 26.9 The renal fascia is picked up well posteriorly so that it is not confused with the peritoneum. It is incised exposing perinephric fat and the kidney which can then be mobilized

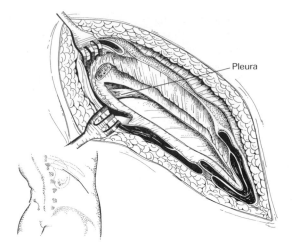

Fig. 26.10 Twelfth rib approach. The skin incision is made along the line of the twelfth rib starting at the angle posteriorly and continued into the abdomen as far as necessary. The rib is resected subperiosteally taking care to avoid, if possible, the pleura which descends below the level of the twelfth rib

front of the lateral border of the quadratus lumborum exposing extraperitoneal fat (Figs 26.7–26.9). Two fingers or a swab on forceps can be inserted into this space and used to separate the peritoneum from the deep surface of transversus and to protect it as the transversus and internal oblique are divided in the line of the incision. The subcostal nerve and vessels passing downwards and forwards within the deep layers of internal oblique can often be retracted. If they are in the way the vein and artery can be divided between ligatures, but every effort should be made to preserve the nerve.

Closure of the incision
The patient is straightened by lowering the kidney bridge or straightening the table so that the wound margins fall together. The retroperitoneal space should be drained with a tube, a strip of corrugated plastic, or a Redivac drain. The muscles are repaired in three layers; the author uses number 1 chromic catgut for each layer.

12th rib approach
This approach provides better access to the kidney and is little, if any, more difficult than the subcostal incision (Fig. 26.10).

The incision starts a little medial to the lateral border of sacrospinalis, directly over the angle of 12th rib and is continued forwards along the rib and carried beyond its tip as far as required, depending on the build of the patient and how complex the operation is expected to be. The latissimus dorsi and the serratus posterior inferior muscles are divided. The periosteum over the 12th

rib is incised in the line of the incision and the rib freed subperiosteally using a periosteal elevator. If the lower border is freed first, a finger can be introduced behind the rib to protect the pleura (which extends below the 12th rib) while the rest of the rib is freed; the rib is divided near its angle and the anterior part removed. The bed of the rib, consisting of the periosteum on the inner surface of the rib and some fibres of the diaphragm, is incised and the extraperitoneal fat exposed. Two fingers or a swab on forceps can now be inserted anteriorly to push the peritoneum forwards off the deep aspect of the transversus muscle and kept there to protect the peritoneum as the incision is extended forwards by cutting the external and internal oblique and the transversus muscles. The incision can be extended anteriorly if necessary by dividing the rectus sheath and muscle. The pleura can be identified in the medial part of the rib bed and safeguarded as the incision is extended medially. If the 12th rib is absent or very short, the incision can be made along the 11th rib. In other words, it is the last palpable rib that is excised, usually the 12th but maybe the 11th. The renal fascia is then incised and the kidney exposed.

Supracostal incision (see Turner-Warwick, 1980)
This incision is usually made above the 12th rib, but if the 12th rib is short or absent it can be made above the 11th rib. It provides as good an exposure as resecting the rib but has advantages, as the rib provides a sound foundation for retracting the lower part of the incision and adds strength to the final wound. The skin incision, like that used for rib resection, is made over the rib but for the supracostal approach it starts some 4 or

5 cm further back over the rib. The upper and medial aspects of the rib are mobilized extraperiostally if possible, (subperiosteally if not) aiming to avoid the pleura because this is meant to be an extrapleural approach. Once fully mobilized, the rib can be easily rotated downwards on its single articulation with the 12th thoracic vertebra. Mobilization must extend back as far as this joint and include division of the costovertebral ligament, otherwise the rib may be fractured as it is retracted. If the rib is fractured it should be removed because it may sequestrate. The incision is extended forwards through the muscles of the anterior abdominal wall as described for the incision resecting the 12th rib.

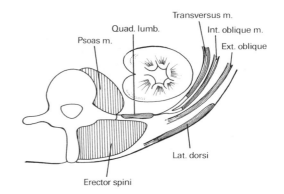

Fig. 26.11

Lumbotomy

This exposure is used by many surgeons for simple operations on the renal pelvis or upper ureter. It gives less access than the lumbar incision, especially in fat people, but can be extended upwards by resecting a small segment of the 12th or even 11th rib.

The patient is placed in a lateral position, but as this is a posterior incision the upper shoulder and buttock are allowed to roll forward, exposing more of the back than for the posterolateral incision (Fig. 26.11).

A vertical skin incision is made downwards from the 12th or 11th rib to the iliac crest along the lateral border of the sacrospinalis, and the latissimus dorsi is incised or split in the same line. Retracting forwards the free posterior border of the external oblique exposes the 3 cm wide strip of fused lumbodorsal fascia at the lateral edge of the quadratus lumborum. This fascia is incised vertically and the retroperitoneal space entered (Fig. 26.12).

Thoraco-abdominal approach

This approach is made through the bed of the 10th rib or through the 10th intercostal space, and affords an excellent exposure of the renal pedicle and kidney. A long incision is made over the 10th intercostal space and continued across the costal margin downwards and forwards to the midline or even across the midline to the lateral edge of the opposite rectus. The thoracic component of the incision is deepened through the muscles of the space and the pleura is opened. The abdominal component is deepened through the oblique abdominal muscles and one or both recti and the peritoneum opened. The diaphragm is incised in the line of the incision. On the left the colon and on the right the colon and duodenum are reflected medially and the kidney and its pedicle exposed.

Nagamatsu incision

This is an extrapleural extension of the incision excising the 12th rib. It is used by some surgeons for

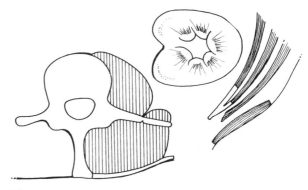

Fig. 26.12

Figs 26.11 & 26.12 Lumbotomy incision. The skin incision is a vertical one along the lateral edge of the sacrospinalis exposing the latissimus dorsi. Incising the latissimus dorsi in the same line the free posterior edge of the external oblique is seen and retracted forwards exposing the fused layers of lumbar dorsal fascia and the external and transversus muscles taking origin from them. The fused layers of lumbar dorsal fascia are incised vertically exposing the renal fascia which is then opened

the exposure of large renal tumours and certainly provides a wide exposure. The incision is the same as the one used for 12th rib resection. The 12th rib is resected and the incision extended anteriorly as described, but the posterior end is extended vertically upwards across the angles of the 11th and 10th ribs, incising the latissimus doris and serratus posterior inferior and excising a 2.5 cm segment from the angles of the 11th and 12th ribs. It provides a large antero-superior flap of skin, muscles and ribs which when retracted gives an extensive exposure.

Exploratory technique for posterior approach

Pleura

No matter how much care is taken, it is inevitable that the pleura will occasionally be opened when the kidney is exposed by resecting the 12th or 11th rib, or by a supracostal incision. Little disturbance results at the time because most patients are on some form of positive pressure anaesthesia; but if air remains in or can be sucked into the pleural cavity postoperatively, the patient may develop respiratory difficulties.

Some surgeons suture the pleura (more easily done with the supracostal than the rib resection exposures) while the anaesthetist hyperinflates the lungs; some leave in a tube, one end in the pleura and the other in a basin of water, removing it when the wound is sutured and the anaesthetist hyperinflates the lungs; it is preferable to close the pleura, but leave in a water seal drain which is removed 24 or 48 hours after operation when a chest X-ray shows that the lung is reinflated.

Exposure and delivery of the kidney

The muscles are retracted and the loose retroperitoneal fatty tissue exposed. The renal fascia is identified in the posterior part of the wound behind the peritoneum. It is opened between forceps and the opening is enlarged by cutting with scissors or scalpel or stretching with the fingers. The smooth glistening surface of the renal capsule may be seen, but is usually hidden amid perinephric fat. With fingers, forceps or scissors the kidney in its capsule is carefully separated from the perinephric fat and from the peritoneum which may be adherent anteriorly. The upper pole of the kidney is anchored to the diaphragm by strong fibrofatty bands which should be divided and ligated. The adrenal gland is separated from the kidney by fascia and unlikely to be disturbed if the dissection is kept close to the kidney. Equally easily separated are the colon and duodenum on the right side and the colon and pancreas on the left side. The kidney can be mobilized and brought out of the wound without difficulty when there are no surrounding adhesions. In many patients, however, because of infection, stones or previous operations, the kidney is densely adherent to surrounding structures and the posterior abdominal wall and can be mobilized only with great difficulty. In some circumstances the dissection must be patiently pursued with great care to avoid damaging pleura, diaphragm, renal pedicle, duodenum and even the liver, the spleen, the pancreas and the vena cava.

Anterior approach

This approach is often preferred for the removal of a large renal cell carcinoma, for the exploration of an injured kidney and the treatment of hydronephrosis, but it is not very suitable for the removal of stones or for operations on an infected kidney. It is, however, ideal for most operations on the pelves of horseshoe or ectopic kidneys or of other kidneys which have failed to rotate because in such kidneys the pelvis and pelviureteric junctions lie anteriorly, not medially.

A subcostal or a paramedian incision, depending on the build of the patient, can be used for benign disease but for renal cell carcinoma a larger incision is essential (Fig. 26.13). A useful one starts at the tip of the 12th rib on the affected side and extends transversely and slightly upwards across the midline to the opposite costal margin, dividing both recti (Fig. 26.14). It can be extended backwards along or above the 12th rib if

Figs 26.13 & 26.14 *Anterior approach to the kidney*

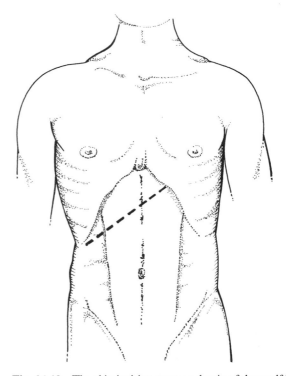

Fig. 26.13 The skin incision starts at the tip of the twelfth rib and is carried below and more or less parallel to the costal margin across the midline to the opposite costal margin

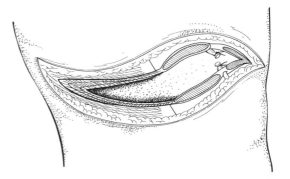

Fig. 26.14 The incision is deepened through the oblique muscles of the abdomen laterally and the rectus medially to expose the peritoneum, and can be extended anteriorly by dividing the opposite rectus muscle or posteriorly through or above the twelfth rib

necessary. The peritoneum is opened and the falciform ligament is divided between forceps and ligated. Small bowel is packed into the opposite side of the abdomen. The peritoneum of the posterior wall is incised along the lateral aspect of the ascending colon, hepatic flexure and second part of the duodenum on the right side, or descending colon and splenic flexure on the left side and the colon is mobilized and displaced medially to expose the anterior surface of the kidney and its pedicle.

NEPHRECTOMY

The surgery of the kidney has become increasingly conservative and far fewer nephrectomies are done for hydronephrosis, stones, infection, trauma or vascular disease than used to be the case. Even for malignant disease some surgeons now favour more conservative operations than nephrectomy, particularly in patients with impaired renal function or low grade tumours.

Indications

Nephrectomy is indicated in:

1. Patients having renal transplants or chronic dialysis if their own kidneys are infected or considered the cause of uncontrollable hypertension.

2. Patients with a nonfunctioning or very poorly functioning hydronephrotic, infected, ischaemic or stone containing kidney on one side and a normal kidney on the other.

3. Patients with unilateral renal hypertension, when it is thought better to remove the kidney rather than reconstruct the artery.

4. Patients with renal tuberculosis in whom the organisms are resistant to chemotherapy, or chemotherapy is otherwise considered inappropriate.

5. Some patients with a severely traumatized kidney or renal pedicle on one side and a normal kidney on the other.

6. Patients with malignant disease of the kidney. For renal cell carcinoma a radical nephrectomy is considered better than a simple nephrectomy and for transitional cell tumours, a nephro-ureterectomy better than a nephrectomy.

Nephrectomy

The kidney is exposed and mobilized. By gentle dissection with scissors or gauze the pedicle is cleared on both aspects and the major vessels separately identified. The main renal artery lies behind the vein in front of the renal pelvis, but there may be other blood vessels passing to or from the upper or lower poles of the kidney, arteries that arise from the renal artery or aorta or veins which join the renal vein or vena cava.

All vessels should be dealt with separately if at all possible to reduce the risks of a ligature slipping and of an arteriovenous anomaly forming.

Whether the vessels should be ligatured in continuity before being divided, or clamped and divided before ligation, is a matter for personal preference and expediency although the first method is safer. The artery is separated from investing fat, which is often firm and fibrous, and nerve fibres. Two ligatures are placed on the aortic side and one on the kidney side using a right angled forceps like an O'Shaughnessy and the artery divided between them (Figs 26.15 & 26.16). The renal vein is similarly dealt with. Be careful not to pull too hard on the kidney while placing the ligatures around the vein, otherwise you may tear the vein off the inferior vena cava, and have some anxious minutes wondering why you ever took up surgery!

The right renal vein is short and may be difficult to ligate in the way described; if so, apply a Satinsky clamp laterally on the vena cava where the vein enters. Divide the vein distal to the clamp and suture the cava with a 5/0 arterial suture before the clamp is removed.

If the kidney has been operated on before or is infected and there are dense adhesions, it may be impossible to identify, isolate and ligate the vessels in the way described. In such cases the pedicle can be clamped en masse and the kidney removed, leaving sufficient tissue beyond the clamp that can be picked up with forceps, separately ligating the stumps of the main vessels before removing the clamp. If even this procedure is impossible, the pedicle may be ligated en masse. To do this the pedicle is divided on the distal side of two heavy kidney clamps. The deeper clamp is slowly removed as a ligature is tied on the proximal side; a second ligature is then applied and tightened as the superficial clamp is removed. It is tempting to use No. 1 silk or nylon to ligate the vessels of the renal pedicle. To use nonabsorbable materials, however, when removing an infected kidney often causes a persistent sinus or recurrent infection, which only heals when the suture material is extruded or removed, and removing it by operation is not easy. The author uses No. 1 chromic catgut whether the kidney is infected or not. The kidney, attached now only by the ureter, is drawn forwards; the ureter is freed downwards to a convenient level and divided between ligatures (Figs 26.17 & 26.18). Dense adhesions, likely to be found if the kidney is infected, or has been previously operated on, add greatly to the difficulties of the operation. Some can be anticipated by making an incision that provides a generous exposure and by cross matching the patient for several more units of blood than is usual for a simple nephrectomy. It is often useful to open deliberately the peritoneum at an early stage of the operation to free the liver and duodenum on the right side or the spleen

Figs 26.15–26.18 *Left nephrectomy*

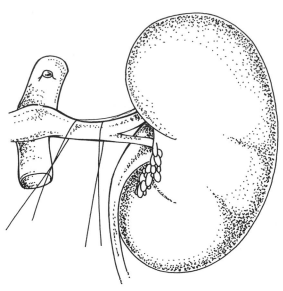

Fig. 26.15 The renal vein is exposed and gently separated from the artery. Two ligatures are placed around the vein

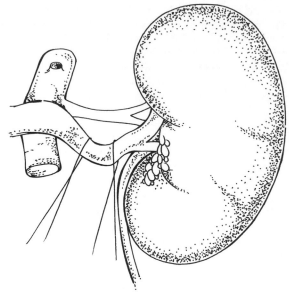

Fig. 26.16 The artery is displayed by gentle downwards traction on the ligatures around the vein. (Because the vein lies anterior to the artery it may seem easier to ligate it first. This is a mistake because it congests the kidney)

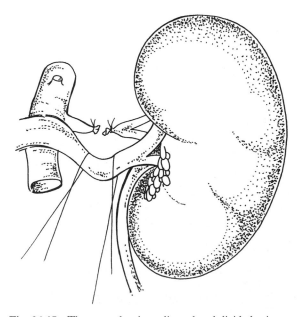

Fig. 26.17 The artery has been ligated and divided prior to ligation of the vein. Two ligatures can be placed on the aortic side and one on the renal side for safety. (It is important at this stage to look carefully for aberrant or accessory vessels)

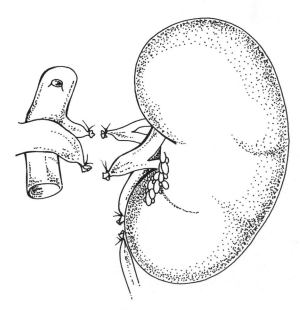

Fig. 26.18 The ureter is divided between ligatures at a convenient level and the kidney is then removed

and colon on the left side, as these structures may not be seen easily if an extraperitoneal exposure alone is attempted. If it proves impossible to mobilize the kidney in the plane between capsule and fat, a subcapsular nephrectomy can be done. An incision is made through the renal capsule on the lateral aspect of the kidney and by finger and gauze dissection, the plane of cleavage between it and the kidney is opened up. The separation is continued on all surfaces as far as the pedicle, where the everted capsule must be incised (Fig. 26.19) so that the vessels of the pedicle can be dissected out. This can be very difficult and the procedure should only be done when a careful and patient effort to mobilize the kidney in its capsule proves impossible.

Nephrectomy for renal cell carcinoma

Nephrectomy for renal cell carcinoma (sometimes known as hypernephroma or adenocarcinoma) differs in several ways from nephrectomy for nonmalignant disease. Firstly it is more radical and involves the removal of all the perinephric fat and the adrenal gland; secondly it involves ligation of the veins at an early stage in the procedure so that malignant cells are not

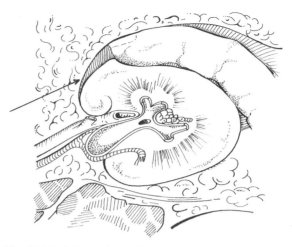

Fig. 26.19 Subcapsular nephrectomy. The finger is mobilizing the kidney in the plane between parenchyma and renal capsule. Once the front and back and lateral aspects of the kidney have been mobilized in this way it is essential to divide by sharp dissection the capsule of the kidney anteriorly (arrowed) to expose the renal pedicle

Figs 26.20 & 26.21   *Renal artery embolization*

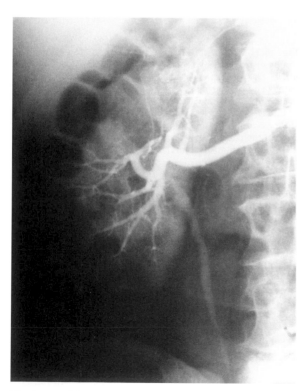

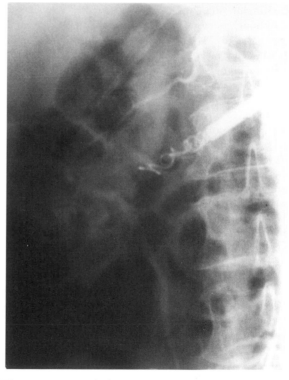

Fig. 26.20 Right renal arteries outlined by selective renal angiography.

Fig. 26.21 Several occluding springs have been inserted into the renal artery. The springs carry thrombogenic tails of Dacron strands which cannot be seen on the X-ray

disseminated to other parts of the body as the kidney is handled and manipulated and thirdly the tumour, especially when it involves the right kidney, often grows along the renal vein and into the inferior vena cava and in these circumstances it is essential to open the vena cava and remove the tumour within, but considerable care has to be exercised otherwise a tumour embolus can be caused. Fourthly many surgeons now embolize the renal artery with a balloon catheter, occluding spring or gelatin foam, some days before operation. This procedure obviously facilitates the operation by reducing the amount of bleeding, and it may also have some beneficial immunological effects. Embolization is done by selective renal angiography (Fig. 26.20) and the main renal artery is occluded with a balloon catheter (see Fig. 25.9) which has to be left in place until operation, or by the insertion of a spring with thrombogenic tails of dacron strands or pieces of soluble gelatin foam (Fig. 26.21). The second of these is best. The procedure usually causes pain and fever, which resolves within a day or two. It is by no means certain how long to wait after embolization before carrying out nephrectomy, but 2 or 3 days is usual. At that time oedema around the kidney aids mobilization; later oedematous tissue becomes fibrous and operation more difficult. Angiography and inferior caval venography carried out before operation suggest the size, position and extent of the tumour (Fig. 26.22).

Although a large posterolateral incision through or above the rib, a Nagamatsu or a thoraco-abdominal incision can and often are used, an anterior incision is preferred. This can be a long paramedian or transverse incision, or a subcostal one (see p. 578). The patient is placed supine and elevated on the affected side with sandbags to an angle of 45°, i.e. halfway to a lateral position and an anterior incision is made.

First the renal vein is gently mobilized using a right-angled clamp. A ligature is passed round the vein, but it is not tied at this stage unless the artery has been embolized preoperatively, otherwise the kidney swells, congests and bleeds. Next the artery is located behind the vein in fibrofatty tissue. It is mobilized, ligated and divided. If the right renal vein or the inferior vena cava contain tumour, special care must be exercised to avoid dislodging a tumour embolus, and an attempt must be made to remove tumour from the vein.

In these circumstances the right renal artery is best ligated at its origin from the aorta medial to the vena cava. Occlusion clamps should be applied to the inferior vena cava above and below the renal veins, and to the left renal vein, and any lumbar veins entering the vena cava between them ligated. The inferior vena cava is opened and the tumour removed by suction. The incision in the vena cava is closed with a 5/0 arterial suture and the renal vein ligated.

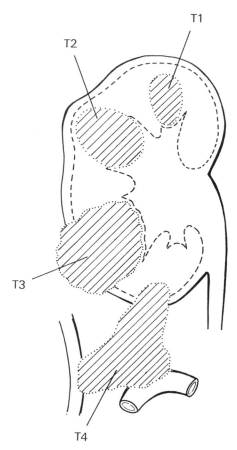

Fig. 26.22   The local extent of renal cell carcinoma. This can be expressed as its T stage.

T1. The tumour is confined to the parenchyma of the kidney and neither disturbs the outline of the cortex nor invades the collecting system

T2. The tumour is confined to the parenchyma of the kidney but distorts the outline of the kidney and invades or distorts the collecting system

T3. The tumour extends through the capsule into perinephric fat

T4. The tumour extends through the perinephric fat and involves adjacent viscera or muscles

Once the pedicle has been dealt with the kidney can be mobilized and removed with its perinephric fat, the adrenal gland and as much renal fascia as possible. Haemostasis is secured and the wound is closed with drainage.

Renal cell carcinomas are relatively radioresistant and much controversy surrounds the place of radiotherapy. Few regard routine preoperative or postoperative radiotherapy of much value, but postoperative radiotherapy is worth considering if tumour is found in the regional lymph nodes at the time of operation. These nodes are involved in as many as 20% of patients with renal cell carcinoma. Some patients have abnormal blood findings such as an elevated ESR and less often polycythemia, hypercalcaemia or other abnormalities. Such changes can be used as tumour markers to assess the progress of the disease after treatment.

How should we treat patients who have metastases when first seen? If a metastasis seems solitary and is in a site amenable to surgery, both it and the primary can be treated. If the metastases are multiple the problem is much more difficult and filled with unanswerable questions; should we do a nephrectomy? should we just embolize the kidney? should we do neither? Well, no one knows, but it is obviously sensible to remove the kidney if the patient has pain or bleeding, and probably sensible to remove it if the patient has bony or pulmonary metastasis because there is evidence that such metastases may regress when the primary tumour is removed.

Hormone therapy using either medroxyprogesterone acetate (Provera) 100 mg t.d.s. or androgens may be useful and without side effects. No other chemotherapeutic agent or combination of agents offers much at the present time although several are on trial.

Haemorrhage from the renal pedicle

This may occur if a mass ligature has been applied and slips, if the pedicle is inadvertently divided while mobilizing an adherent kidney, or if the clamps slip or are pulled off the pedicle before the ligatures are applied. Profuse haemorrhage obscures all structures.

On the right side profuse bleeding often comes from a hole in the inferior vena cava. No attempt should be made to secure the bleeding vessels by plunging forceps into a pool of blood in the hope that the vessels and nothing else will be picked up. Instead two or more gauze packs are pressed into the wound for at least 10 minutes. When the gauze packing is slowly removed the haemorrhage should have slowed enough for the severed vessels to be seen and secured. A tear in the inferior vena cava may be controlled by a Satinsky clamp and repaired with a continuous suture of 5/0 arterial silk.

Large hydronephrotic kidney

The removal of a large hydronephrotic kidney is facilitated if the fluid is first aspirated through a large bore needle inserted into the posterior surface of the hydronephrotic sac. The collapsed sac is then easily mobilized and removed.

NEPHRO-URETERECTOMY

In nephrectomy for nonmalignant disease or renal cell carcinoma the ureter is divided at a convenient level, only a small part being removed. If the ureter is dilated, tuberculous or one in which reflux has been demon-

strated, it should all be removed with the kidney. Similarly, in patients with transitional cell tumours of the calices or pelvis of the kidney or the ureter, the whole length of the ureter, including the intramural part should be removed with the kidney, unless a conservative approach is needed because the kidney is solitary, the disease bilateral, renal function poor or the tumour small and of low grade. The operation can sometimes be done through one incision, but it is best and most easily done through two. Firstly the kidney is mobilized through an appropriate posterolateral or anterior incision removing perinephric fat and renal fascia if the operation is being done for malignant disease. The vessels of the pedicle are separately ligated. The ureter, which is all that now holds the kidney, is mobilized as far down as possible, but not divided. The kidney is then dropped back into the retroperitoneal space and the incision closed over it. The patient is transferred to the supine position and a transverse suprapubic incision is made through skin and rectus sheath with retraction of the recti or a low oblique muscle cutting incision through the oblique muscles and transversus is made (Fig. 26.23). The transversalis fascia is incised and the peritoneum retracted medially. The mobilized kidney is located in the retroperitoneal space and lifted out of the wound. The ureter can then be easily traced down to the bladder. In nonmalignant cases to open the bladder is unnecessary and the lower ureter can be pulled up and ligated flush with the bladder wall. In malignant cases the whole ureter, including the intramural part and the ureteric orifice must be removed together with a cuff of bladder, and to do this means opening the bladder. The bladder, thereafter, is closed in two layers with plain catgut and kept empty with a catheter for a week. The wound is drained through the lower incision.

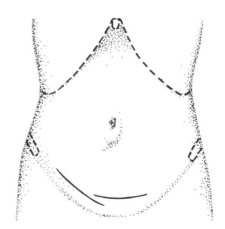

Fig. 26.23 The position on the anterior abdominal wall of the suprapubic or oblique incision used to mobilize and remove the lower end of the ureter in the operation of nephro-ureterectomy

PARTIAL NEPHRECTOMY

This operation, once popular for the treatment of patients with calculus or tuberculosis of the kidney, was particularly recommended for patients who had a stone or stones in one calix, in the belief that removing the calix would prevent recurrence of stone. However, it is no longer considered justifiable to remove a large piece of normally functioning kidney because the cause of stone formation is hardly confined to one calix and there is now much evidence to show that stones recur no more frequently after nephrolithotomy than they do after partial nephrectomy. In stone disease, therefore, a partial nephrectomy would now be considered appropriate treatment only if the pole containing the stone was seriously fibrosed or infected and has been shown to contribute little, if anything, to overall renal function.

In tuberculosis, too, partial nephrectomy is rarely, if ever done now, because if the disease is localized enough to be curable by partial nephrectomy, it should respond to chemotherapy alone. Partial nephrectomy nowadays, therefore, is mostly carried out for renal cell or transitional cell tumours of the kidney when the more radical procedures are inappropriate because the kidney is solitary, the disease bilateral, renal function poor, or the tumour small and of low grade; or for some renal injuries.

Operation

The kidney is exposed by the appropriate posterolateral incision and fully mobilized. The vessels of the pedicle are cleared of all fat and displayed. If a branch of the renal artery appears to be supplying the area or part of the area of the kidney to be removed it can be ligated but only after temporary occlusion confirms that it does not also supply some part of the kidney that is to be left; the capsule is incised in the coronal plane over the pole to be removed and reflected back as two flaps, one anterior and one posterior (Fig. 26.24).

Next the pedicle needs to be occluded while the kidney is resected. At normal temperature the kidney can withstand complete ischaemia without permanent damage for only about 15 minutes. This time can be extended by using inosine or by cooling. Inosine is a purine nucleotide and 30 to 60 mg/kilo is injected into a peripheral vein 10 minutes before operation or into the renal artery just before the occlusion clamp is applied. It protects the kidney from the effects of total ischaemia for 1 hour (provided preoperative renal function was satisfactory). Cooling the kidney to 15°C or 20°C can provide up to 2 to 3 hours protection against complete ischaemia and can be achieved by packing 2 to 3 kg of crushed ice around the mobilized kidney

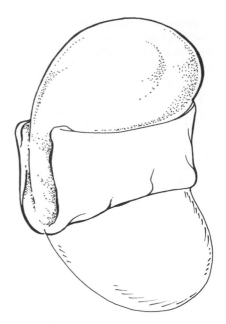

Fig. 26.24 Partial nephrectomy. The capsule is incised in the coronal plane and reflected upwards

for about 10 minutes, by irrigating the outside and the inside of the kidney and the pelvis caliceal system with ice cold water, or by circulating cold water through two heat exchange coils applied to the surface of the kidney. With all methods of cooling the temperature inside the kidney must be measured with a telethermometer probe and not allowed to fall below 15°C. A vascular occlusion clamp is applied across the pedicle. The kidney is divided transversely at the level of raised capsular flaps or with short anterior and posterior flaps at the appropriate plane, taking great care to avoid the main vessels and the renal pelvis (Fig. 26.25). Further slices can be removed if the initial resection was inadequate. The opened vessels and calix are closed with fine catgut sutures and the occlusion clamp then removed, and any other bleeding vessels are controlled with sutures; the capsule is folded back over the raw surface of the kidney and loosely sutured with catgut (Fig. 26.26). Occasionally, it can be helpful to use a staple gun. This is applicable where the lower pole is to be removed and the renal substance is not too thick. It is not necessary to mobilize the capsule or to identify vessels as these are taken care of by the line of staples. The wound should be drained. Some renal cell carcinomas are so well encapsulated that they can almost be enucleated if it is thought best to treat them conservatively.

Transitional cell tumours of the pelvicaliceal system present special problems if they are unsuitable for the radical treatment described; some in the renal pelvis can be removed locally if they are pedunculated or by resecting part of the pelvis (like a pyeloplasty); tumours

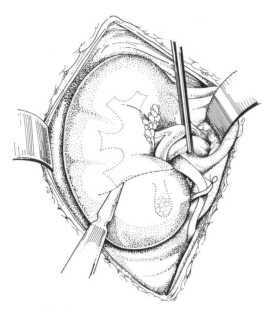

Fig. 26.25 Partial nephrectomy. The renal vein and artery have been temporarily occluded with a vascular occlusion clamp. A small vessel to the lower pole of the kidney has been ligated. The incision made to remove the lower pole of the kidney passes through the neck of the lower calyx which contains stones

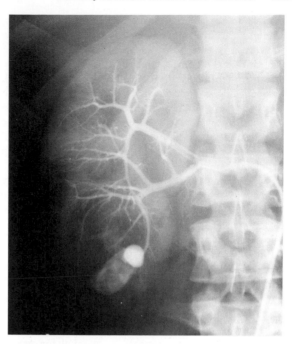

Fig. 26.27 Secondary haemorrhage after partial nephrectomy. Selective angiogram of a patient with severe secondary haemorrhage 10 days after a right nephrolithotomy. It demonstrates that the haemorrhage was due to the formation of an aneurysm which was cured by embolizing its feeding artery with gelatin foam

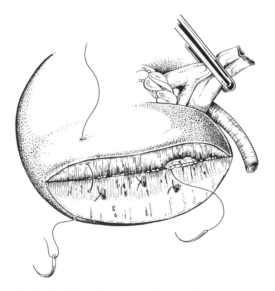

Fig. 26.26 Partial nephrectomy. The excision exposes the neck of the calix and opens a number of blood vessels. The neck of the calix can be closed with 4/0 catgut sutures although this is not absolutely necessary. The opened vessels are stitched or ligated and this can be difficult because renal parenchyma is friable. Once haemostasis has been secured the flaps of renal capsule are folded back over the divided lower pole of the kidney and loosely secured with sutures. It is probably unwise and unnecessary to suture the parenchyma of the kidney with mattress sutures as some advise, provided haemostasis has been satisfactorily secured by ligating or suturing the open vessels themselves

in the calix can be treated by partial nephrectomy. However, transitional cell tumours are often much more extensive than the X-rays suggest and it is necessary to examine the whole pelvicaliceal system before proceeding with a conservative operation thought suitable after inspecting the X-rays. This can be done with a nephroscope passed through a small incision in the renal pelvis, but if one is not available, a cystoscope can be used.

The major complication of partial nephrectomy is secondary haemorrhage which may be due to vascular abnormality rather than infection and can often be stopped by embolizing the feeding artery at selective renal angiography (Fig. 26.27).

STONES

The condition of stones in the bladder has been known since 4800 B.C. Lithotomy is one of the earliest operations and was practised by the ancient Greeks and Romans. Even in the 19th century it was still the most commonly performed of all operations. Primary bladder stones form almost exclusively in males, especially male children below 5 years of age, and are still endemic in such parts of the world as India, Turkey, Thailand, China, Egypt and Sudan but are now unknown in Western Europe and North America.

In affluent countries upper urinary tract stones, almost unmentioned in medical literature before 1900, are becoming commoner, and now affect about 2 to 4% of the population at some time during their lives. Not only do they occur in affluent societies, but in the most affluent parts of such societies; thus professional workers are 10 times more likely to develop them than unskilled workers.

The treatment of renal tract stones has completely changed in the last 10 years with the advent of the extracorporeal shock wave lithotripter and by the development of ureteroscopy. Hence, traditional stone operations are becoming historical procedures in many countries. It is sometimes argued that lithotripters are too expensive but there are now a variety of machines — manufactured in developing as well as developed countries — and strict cost benefit analysis should enable almost all countries to invest in this technology. It is cheaper to break stones up as an outpatient procedure rather than have patients in hospital for several days with all the discomfort of an open operation. There will be instances where traditional operations must be performed and for that reason the descriptions remain in this book. Also there may still be some countries where lithotripsy is not available.

Diagnosis

The signs and symptoms of stones in the upper urinary tract will not be discussed here; the diagnosis can only be confirmed if the stone is passed or demonstrated radiologically.

About 90% of upper urinary stones contain calcium usually as calcium oxalate or calcium phosphate and, with infection, magnesium ammonium phosphate. Calcium stones are more opaque than soft tissues like muscle and kidney and can be seen in straight X-rays if they overlie soft tissue, but if they overlie bone of the ribs, transverse processes or sacrum, they may not be visualized. Nor may they be seen, even though overlying soft tissue, if they are small. Calcium stones tend to be about the same density as the contrast media used for urography and, in urograms, are either not seen at all or appear as filling defects and may, like uric acid stones, be confused with tumours or air bubbles. Of the stones that do not contain calcium, about 5% are made of uric acid; 1 or 2% of cystine and the few remaining ones of Xanthine or matrix.

Uric acid stones are no more opaque than soft tissues and can only be seen in pyelo-ureterograms as filling defects; cystine stones contain sulphur, but although slightly more opaque than soft tissues appear in straight X-rays only if the patient is thin and the X-ray of high quality. It follows that many stones, even ones containing calcium, do not show up in a straight X-ray and if the patient's complaints suggest a renal or ureteric stone, further investigations are necessary.

Indications for operation

Once the diagnosis is made and confirmed radiologically treatment can be considered under various headings:

1. Urgent symptoms such as severe pain, severe infection or acute renal failure require urgent treatment.

2. Investigations to identify risk factors that predispose to stone are desirable in most stone patients and essential in those with recurrent or bilateral stones. For calcium stones, the major risk factors are metabolic and include the excretion of excessive quantities of calcium, phosphate or oxalate; low urinary volumes; a low urinary pH and a reduction in the urinary agents such as uric acid and the acid mucopolysaccharides which inhibit crystallization. Other risk factors include anatomical abnormalities which interfere with the free flow of urine by causing obstruction, reflux or stasis and infection. Cystine stones only occur in patients with cystinuria, who can be easily identified by estimating the amount of cystine in a 24 hour specimen of urine. Uric acid stones tend to occur in patients with gout, or with excessive amounts of uric acid in the blood or urine for other reasons (Robertson, 1982).

3. Treatment of the stones.

Management of stones with lithotripsy, ureteroscopy and percutaneous lithotomy

Small stones in the renal pelvis (less than 2 cm) can be managed by most lithotripters. The main complication is that the stone pieces may collect in the ureter to form a *steinstrasse* (stone street). This may necessitate ureteroscopy. In some centres a prophylactic ureteric stent is placed prior to lithotripsy in order to encourage stone fragments to pass down the ureter and into the bladder.

Larger stones in the renal pelvis are difficult to break up without the need for many treatment sessions and in these cases there is often combined management by preliminary percutaneous nephroscopy (see below) and lithotripsy for the remaining fragments. Stones in the *upper ureter* may be pushed back into the renal pelvis with a catheter and then broken up by lithotripsy ('push bang'). Stones in the *middle ureter* may either be treated by lithotripsy or by ureteroscopic laser lithotripsy. Stones in the *lower ureter* are generally dealt with by ureteroscopic extraction either with a stone basket or by laser lithotripsy.

The exact techniques of the above procedures will depend on the equipment available but a further description of percutaneous nephroscopy is given.

Percutaneous nephroscopy

Recently the scope of endoscopic urology has been increased by the realization that endoscopes introduced into the renal pelvis directly through a skin puncture obviate the need for much of open renal surgery. At first, normal cystoscopes were used but now special instruments have been developed. The major indication for percutaneous endoscopic surgery is the removal of renal calculi but the techniques have also been used for the treatment of transitional cell cancers in the renal pelvis and to relieve pelviureteric obstruction. The technique is clearly established for renal calculi and, despite the advent of the extracorporeal shock wave lithotripter, there will remain a number of situations where percutaneous surgery is the treatment of choice. The other indications, namely renal pelvic transitional cell tumours and pelviureteric junction obstruction are not so well established and we must wait for the longer term results before giving up well established open operative techniques.

Organization of a percutaneous service

There are two stages of the procedure to consider, access to the kidney to form a tract followed by procedures that can be performed through the tract. Whether these are performed by the surgeon or the interventional radiologist will depend on local arrangements. Close cooperation between the urologist and interventional radiologist is extremely helpful for many reasons. When starting percutaneous work it is better for the interventional radiologist to place the tract. This is mainly because the skill of placing a tract under X-ray or ultrasound control is not normally one that the surgeon has trained for and it takes time to learn, whereas the use of the new endoscopic instruments is quickly learned by the surgeon who is already competent at cystoscopy. Another reason for cooperation is that the position of the tract is critical if percutaneous procedures are to be successful. This is relevant in the emergency situation when the interventional radiologist may be asked to perform emergency decompression by placing a nephrostomy. If the radiologist is aware of the possible subsequent surgical requirements then the emergency tract can be appropriately placed to allow a later definitive percutaneous procedure through the same tract. The advantages for the urologist to learn the whole procedure including tract placement and dilatation are to do with logistics of performing one stage procedures and fitting percutaneous work into an existing urological operating schedule. In addition there are advantages when the whole procedure is performed in the sterile environment of the operating theatre rather than in the X-ray department.

Percutaneous renal work may be organized as a two stage or one stage procedure. If a two-stage procedure is planned, many favour the initial tract being made under local anaesthesia and the subsequent dilatation to full working diameter is done as a second stage under a general anaesthetic. The choice of the number of stages is up to individual centres and the facilities that are available with regard to X-ray, screening and operative intervention. Increasingly most units are now utilizing single stage procedures as it is possible to make a rapid, safe, nephrostomy tract without significant complications or bleeding.

Special instruments for renal endoscopy

New instruments have been developed for percutaneous renal surgery. In addition some instruments can be used both in the bladder and kidney e.g. the Mauermeyer stone punch and the optical urethrotome and indeed the nephroscope may be used to deal with urethral calculi. The nephroscope sheath has an inner tube to allow continuous irrigation. The outer sheath is usually supplied with a hollow obturator to allow the instrument to be passed over a guide wire into the renal pelvis. The telescope is offset at an angle to allow a straight instrument channel so as to accommodate stone forceps, ultrasound probes etc as with the ureteroscope (p. 571).

Technique

The normal position for the operation is prone or prone oblique depending on the operator's preference. It is important that the thorax and pelvis are well supported so that there is no obstruction to venous return during the operation. The arms must also be properly supported and the ulnar nerves and the feet protected from undue pressure. Sometimes it helps to place a cushion under the kidney to be operated on in order to immobilise it to some extent. Placing pillows under the thorax and pelvis will ensure that the rest of the abdomen can move, allowing the patient to breathe or be ventilated.

Any approach into the renal parenchyma will be associated with bleeding and the choice of route should be through the least vascular part of the renal parenchyma. With the patient in the prone oblique position, the approach is made through the lower pole of the kidney via an inferior calyx. The distance between the skin puncture and the calyx should be as short as possible as this makes subsequent dilatation easier and allows greater operative mobility. The optimal site is selected under X-ray screening. This may be below or just beyond the tip of the 12th rib. For a high kidney or for access to the middle or upper calyces the puncture may be through the 11th or 10th interspace. The chosen calyx is punctured using a 22G needle with a 0.018″ wire and a special thin catheter. The angle of approach into the calyx is approximately 30 degrees to the skin but this is quite variable. The procedure is monitored by ultrasound or fluoroscopy. If possible the guide wire is advanced down the ureter and then it is much less likely to become dislodged during the dilatation. Once the guide wire is in position a 2 cm stellate skin incision is made at the point of skin entry to allow the dilators to pass through the skin without resistance. There are 3 methods of making a tract into the kidney and it is wise to learn more than one method: (1) metal telescoping dilators, (2) the Amplatz dilating system and (3) balloon catheter dilatation. When the tract is dilated an operating sheath is placed in position and the nephroscope can be inserted.

Classical operations for stone

Renal calculi
Renal calculi less than 1 cm in diameter may pass themselves, and should be observed; larger ones should be removed if they are responsible for recurrent pain, obstruction, progressive hydronephrosis or hydrocalicosis, persistent infection or bleeding; if they are increasing in size or if the kidney is solitary. If they are larger than 1 cm, but causing no symptoms it is tempting to wait and see what happens. This is sensible if the stone is in a calix, but if it is in the pelvis further trouble is inevitable and it should be dealt with.

Pyelolithotomy
In this procedure the stone is removed through an incision in the renal pelvis and it is an ideal operation also for the removal of stones from the calices if they are accessible. For stones in an intrarenal pelvis and for staghorn stones an extended pyelolithotomy of Gil-Vernet type can be done (p. 588). Stone fragments can be removed by coagulation pyelolithotomy (p. 589).

Nephrolithotomy
The stone, usually one in a calix, is removed with an incision through the parenchyma of the kidney. A radial incision damages the kidney less than other incisions. Stones in two or more calices are best removed through separate small radial incisions rather than one big coronal incision. Nephrolithotomy can be combined with pyelolithotomy for the removal of multiple or staghorn calculi.

Partial nephrectomy (p. 584)
Formerly a popular method for treating stones in one calix (usually a lower calix) as a means not only of removing the stone but also of preventing others forming; it is no longer popular and nowadays such stones would be treated by pyelolithotomy or nephrolithotomy. The pole containing the stone would only be removed if it was very scarred or infected.

Nephrectomy
A nephrectomy may be the appropriate operation if one kidney contains multiple stones or a staghorn stone, and has little function or much infection and the other kidney is normal, especially if the patient is elderly.

Percutaneous pyelolithotomy
This procedure has developed because of the ease with which needles can now be inserted percutaneously into the collecting system of a kidney under radiological or ultrasound control. The track made by the needle is progressively dilated with special dilators until it will admit a cystoscope or nephroscope. (This takes some days.) The stone can then be removed from the pelvis or calix with biopsy forceps or a stone dislodger of the Dormia type (p. 607) or fragmented with an ultrasound lithotripter.

Pyelolithotomy
The kidney is exposed by a subcostal or lumbotomy incision if the pelvis is extrarenal, the stone solitary and not large, the patient thin and the kidney neither too high nor previously operated upon; otherwise it should be exposed through or above a rib.

Before mobilization is started the upper ureter should be found and secured with a tape or plastic or silicone tube. This serves two purposes, it prevents stone fragments falling into the ureter if the stone crumbles while it being removed, and secondly, it acts as a guide to find the pelvis. As the renal pelvis is covered anteriorly by the renal vein and artery, it is best approached posteriorly. The operation can often be done without fully mobilizing the kidney if the stone is medium sized and lies in an extrarenal pelvis not previously operated on.

The upper ureter and posterior aspect of the bluish coloured pelvis are exposed by dissecting off perinephric fat which is often very adherent to the pelvis and separated with difficulty. The pelvis is incised transversely or longitudinally between stay sutures of 3/0 silk and the stone is gently removed (Fig. 26.28).

Usually, however, it is easier, once the ureter is controlled by a tape, to mobilize fully the kidney which can then be supported by a netelast sling while the posterior aspect of the pelvis is freed of fat and opened between stay sutures.

Extended pyelolithotomy (see Gil-Vernet, 1983)
For stones in an intrarenal pelvis and for staghorns the procedure is extended to demonstrate the pelvis within the renal sinus. The kidney is fully mobilized after the ureter is secured, and the posterior aspect of the renal pelvis or upper ureter is exposed. The thin connective tissue which passes from the renal capsule to the pelvis and seals the entry into the renal sinus is opened by blunt dissection (Fig. 26.29). The dissection is continued into the sinus between muscle and the pelvis and

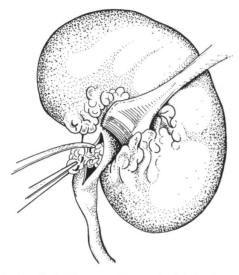

Fig. 26.28 Pyelolithotomy. The renal pelvis has been opened longitudinally and the stone is being removed. A transverse incision, if there is room, is favoured by many surgeons

its adventitial tissue using blunt dissection with scissors or wet pledgets aided by Gil-Vernet retractors which are specially designed for the purpose, when the whole pelvis and caliceal necks can be exposed without damaging any retropelvic arteries or veins. The pelvis is opened transversely and the incision can be extended into the necks of the calices if the stone is a staghorn one (Fig. 26.30).

Large stones are often partly adherent to the mucosa and best removed by gently easing them out using a Macdonald or Watson-Cheyne dissector rather than grasping them with forceps which may crush the stone and make the procedure more difficult than it need be (Fig. 26.31).

If the caliceal extensions of a staghorn calculus are bigger than the necks of the calices containing them, they can be cut from the pelvic part of the stone with heavy scissors or bone cutters, and removed through separate nephrolithotomy incisions as attempts to drag them into the pelvis will only damage the caliceal necks. Once the stone or stones have been removed the pelvis should be thoroughly washed out with sterile water or saline and a contact X-ray taken to ensure that the kidney has been cleared of all stones or stone fragments. The author sutures the pelvis incision loosely with 4/0 dexon or catgut suture, though this is not necessary for small incisions. The wound must be drained for 3 or 4 days because some urine leaks out after operation, no matter how well the pelvis is closed.

Coagulum pyelolithotomy (see Dees, 1981)

This procedure is complementary to one of the other forms of pyelolithotomy and is one method of removing tiny stones and gravel from the pelvicaliceal systems after the main stone has been removed. The pelvic incision is tightly sutured around a 14 or 16 F Malecot or De Pezzer catheter and the upper ureter is occluded by a tape. The pelvis is emptied by aspiration and its capacity determined by injecting sterile water or saline. Human or bovine albumin in liquid form, equal in volume to about 90% of the pelvic capacity is injected through the catheter; at the same time thrombin solution equal in volume to 10% of the pelvic capacity is injected through a needle inserted into the pelvis or catheter. The two substances mix and rapidly form a clot or coagulum. Five minutes later the pelvis is reopened and the coagulum, together with the gravel and small stones entrapped in its meshes is removed.

Nephrolithotomy

This is the appropriate procedure for removing caliceal

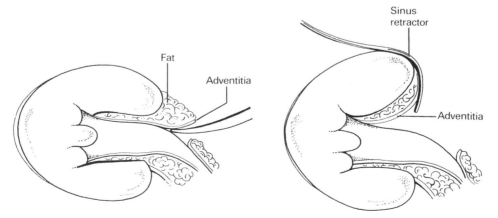

Fig. 26.29 Extended pyelolithotomy. The plane between the muscle of the renal pelvis and the adventitial tissue of the renal sinus must be developed to expose the intrarenal part of the renal pelvis without damaging arteries or veins

Figs 26.30 & 26.31   *Extended pyelolithotomy*

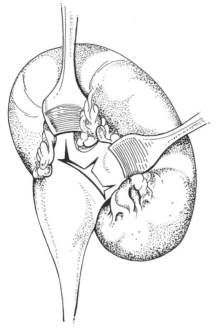

Fig. 26.30   Retractors of the Gil-Vernet type are used to retract the fat of the renal sinus and expose the intrarenal pelvis which has been incised transversely. The incision can be extended into the neck of one or more calices if necessary

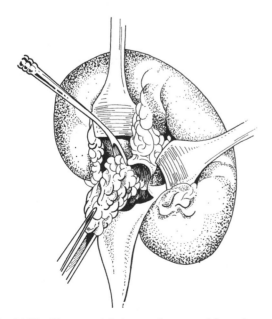

Fig. 26.31   The stone is being gently removed from the pelvis and the calices, often easier done using a dissector as illustrated rather than stone holding forceps

stones too large to be extracted through the caliceal neck by a pyelolithotomy; the expanded caliceal portions of staghorn calculi and other caliceal stones that cannot be removed by pyelolithotomy or extended pyelolithotomy because of adhesions from previous operations or an abnormal distribution of vessels in the renal sinus. If the stone is large, is lying in a middle or lower calix and is palpable on the external surface of the kidney, it may be tempting to proceed with nephrolithotomy without fully mobilizing the kidney or opening the renal pelvis, but this is not advisable. The kidney is exposed through or above the 12th rib, the ureter is secured, the kidney fully mobilized and the vessels of the pedicle fully displayed. The pelvis is opened, as in the operation of pyelolithotomy, and the pelvic stones or pelvic component of a staghorn stone, if any, removed. The caliceal stone can sometimes be palpated on the external surface of the kidney, but its exact position within the kidney can usually only be determined by palpating it through the open pelvis with forceps, probe or finger (if the calix is dilated) or by probing through the exterior of the kidney with a 19 g needle. The pedicle should always be clamped in order to reduce blood loss. This can be done without special precautions if the calyx can be cleared within 15 minutes; otherwise the patient should be given Inosine or the kidney should be cooled (p. 584) (Fig. 26.32).

The pelvicaliceal system is thoroughly irrigated with sterile water or saline before the incisions in the kidney and pelvis are closed with 4/0 catgut. When multiple stones or large soft stones have been removed, an X-ray should be made before completing the operation to ensure that stones or stone fragments have not been left in the kidney, because they will inevitably grow and cause trouble later. Small flexible X-ray films in equally flexible sterile plastic cassettes are available. They are applied directly to one surface of the mobilized kidney so that the kidney lies between film and the tube of a portable machine. A detachable cone, previously sterilized, can be attached to the X-ray tube and its wider distal end placed on or around the kidney. If metal clips are applied to the netelast sling supporting the kidney the position of stones can be accurately plotted from the X-ray. Many surgeons routinely make an X-ray before and after removal of stones and this should certainly be done if the stones are large or multiple.

Drainage

The site of operation should always be drained after pyelolithotomy and nephrolithotomy no matter how straightforward the operation and how well the pelvis was sutured, because urine almost invariably leaks out for a few days. The drain used must be one that leaves a track so that any urine that leaks after the drain is removed can escape and does not accumulate. For this

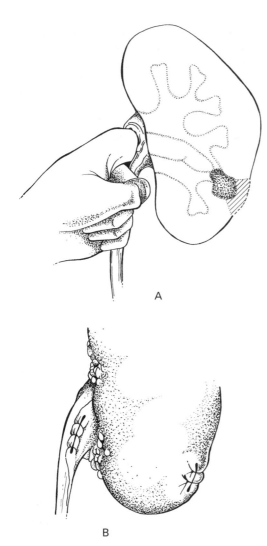

A

B

Fig. 26.32 Nephrolithotomy. The kidney has been mobilized and the renal pelvis opened. The stone is located in its calix using, in this case, finger. (If a finger is used in this way it must be used gently and carefully, and can be used safely only if the pelvis and necks of the calices have become dilated by obstruction. Otherwise it is much safer to use a probe or forceps, or to locate the stone by inserting a fine needle through the outer cortex. Once the stone is located it can be removed by a transverse incision made through the parenchyma of the kidney into the calix

reason a Redivac drain should not be used alone. A persistent fistula occurs if a stone is inadvertently left and obstructs the pelvis or ureter, but otherwise a urinary leak should stop, and may be assisted to do so by passing a ureteric catheter up the ureter and leaving it in place for a day or two.

Haemorrhage
Primary haemorrhage should be controlled at the time of the operation; secondary haemorrhage, which occurs

7 to 10 days after operation may still be a problem. It is as often due to some vascular abnormality at the site of the nephrolithotomy incision as to infection (p. 585). At one time a nephrectomy was often the only means of stopping the bleeding from secondary haemorrhage, but now the responsible vessel can usually be detected and occluded by selective renal angiography (p. 550).

Infection
Since many kidneys operated on for stone are already infected, wound infections are not uncommon and should be treated with the appropriate antibiotic. It is sensible to give patients with urinary tract infection an antibiotic before operation.

Renal function
Pyelolithotomy preserves or improves the function of the kidney. Nephrolithotomy, on the other hand, may reduce it because the incision or incisions are made through parenchyma, some at least of which is normal. Multiple radial nephrotomies, however, seem to do less damage than longitudinal incisions, especially the lateral longitudinal incision (through Brodel's line) that splits open the kidney. The removal of staghorn calculi, even from infected scarred kidneys, generally improves function.

ACUTE RENAL FAILURE

Acute renal failure is a sudden and severe reduction in renal function which causes serious defects in the regulation of the body's internal environment. It is usually associated with anuria or oliguria, but can occur when the urinary output is normal. The causes may be prerenal, renal or postrenal in origin (Newsam, 1981).

Prerenal acute renal failure
Prerenal acute renal failure is caused by impairment in renal perfusion. The reduced blood flow lowers the glomerular filtration rate and filtration stops altogether if the renal artery pressure falls below 35 mmHg. Impaired perfusion may result from (1) a low blood volume caused by the loss of blood, or plasma, or of fluid and electrolytes or (2) from conditions like myocardial infarction, pulmonary embolism, or septicaemic shock, when the blood pressure falls despite a normal blood volume.

In prerenal acute renal failure, renal function usually recovers if the blood pressure and blood volume are restored to normal. If impaired renal perfusion persists, however, acute tubular necrosis or (less often) renal cortical necrosis occurs.

Renal causes of acute renal failure

Any cause of prerenal acute renal failure or nephrotoxic agents can lead to acute tubular necrosis (which is reversible) or to renal cortical necrosis (which is not). Acute glomerulonephritis, malignant hypertension, poly-arteritis, leptospirosis, fat embolism, Goodpasture's syndrome and disseminated intravascular coagulation can all present as acute renal failure and such paren-chymal diseases of the kidney must be kept in mind, when there is no definite history of hypotension.

Chronic renal disease usually progresses insidiously, but an intercurrent infection, a gastro-intestinal upset, causing dehydration or even Tetracycline ingestion (which produces a hypercatabolic state) can precipitate patients into acute renal failure. Acute or chronic renal failure of this kind is suggested by a history of ill-health and the presence of a normocytic anaemia. Plain X-rays of the abdomen or high dose urography may reveal the outlines of scarred and contracted kidneys.

Postrenal acute renal failure

Obstruction in the urinary tract causes back pressure which reduces glomerular filtration and may stop it completely. If obstruction involves both kidneys or a solitary kidney, acute renal failure occurs. Relief of the obstruction restores renal function, unless back pressure and infection have destroyed a considerable amount of renal parenchyma. A postrenal cause should be suspected if the patient has complete anuria, periods of anuria alternating with periods of polyuria, renal colic with analgesic abuse or diabetes, necrosed papil-lae or cancer of the bladder, cervix or prostate, which can all spread to involve both ureters.

Early diagnosis and early treatment are important in postrenal failure, and it is essential to exclude obstruc-tion when the cause of impaired renal function is not obvious. In the early stages of obstruction before much structural damage has occurred, intravenous urography or renography provides the diagnosis but the only way to be certain whether or not obstruction is present is to carry out cystoscopy and attempt ureteric catheteriza-tion and ureteropyelography. An antegrade pyelogram, if the necessary skill is available, will provide diagnosis and treatment at a single procedure.

Treatment of postrenal acute renal failure

This consists of relieving obstruction by removing or bypassing the cause as soon as possible and only in the most exceptional circumstances is it advisable to dialyse the patient first.

Retrograde ureteric-catheterization

This is usually carried out to confirm that obstruction is the cause of the acute renal failure, and to relieve it if the catheters can be negotiated beyond the obstruction into the renal pelvis, where they are left. Although ureteric peristalsis pushes them down into the bladder within a few days, the procedure provides time to plan and carry out an elective procedure. However, ureteric catheterization often fails and may introduce or ex-acerbate infection in an obstructed kidney, and must be carried out with scrupulous attention to asepsis. If ureteric catheterization fails the cause of the obstruc-tion can be removed if the patient is reasonably fit and the operation appears straightforward, for instance a stone in a renal pelvis. Otherwise, temporary diversion by nephrostomy, pyelostomy or ureterostomy is required.

Nephrostomy (Figs 26.33–26.37)

This operation diverts urine from the ureter by drain-ing it to the exterior and is often done as part of some other procedure like pyeloplasty. On its own it is indi-cated in patients with pyelonephrosis or obstructive acute renal failure who are unrelieved by ureteric catheterization and considered unfit or unsuitable for a more extensive procedure. The operation is now usually carried out by inserting a needle into the kidney percutaneously under radiographic or ultrasonic con-trol, threading a guide wire through it and hence placing a stent in the pelvis of the kidney (Fig. 26.38). The tip of the stent curls up once it is in the pelvis in order to retain it in position. Most stents are small (5F) and liable to become blocked. However, instruments are now available to dilate the track to a size that will admit a large Malecot catheter (Fig. 26.39) or even a cystoscope. An open nephrostomy may still be needed for pyonephrosis or an infected hydronephrosis although it can make later conservative renal operations like pyeloplasty very difficult. A lumbotomy or postero-lateral incision is required. It is tempting, once the kidney is exposed, to stretch a Malecot or De Pezzer catheter tightly onto an introducer and push it blindly through a small incision on the lateral aspect of the kidney in the hope that it will go into a calix or the renal pelvis. It is better and safer to expose and open the renal pelvis, to pass a probe through the pelvis and lower calix and out through the lower pole of the kidney after tying a De Pezzer or Malecot catheter to the distal end (Cabot's method) (Fig. 26.40).

The wound is closed round the tube which can be brought out through a separate stab incision inferiorly. A loop nephrostomy can be used instead of a De Pezzer or Malecot catheter (Fig. 26.41).

Pyelostomy

The pelvis can be drained by a tube which is inserted into the pelvis at open operation. The procedure is less satisfactory than nephrostomy and not recommended.

Figs 26.33–26.38 *Percutaneous nephrostomy*

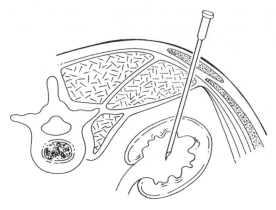

Fig. 26.33 A needle is inserted into the renal pelvis under ultrasound control

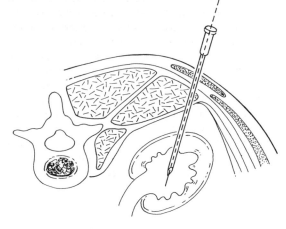

Fig. 26.34 A guide wire is passed through the needle

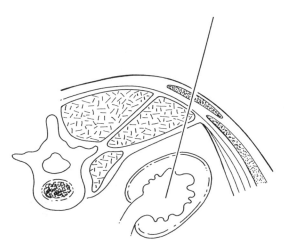

Fig. 26.35 The needle is removed

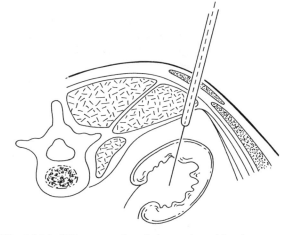

Fig. 26.36 Dilators are threaded over the guide wire to enlarge the tract

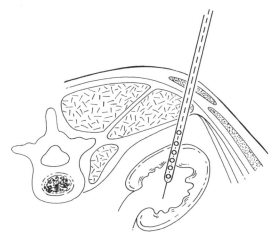

Fig. 26.37 The stent is passed over the guide wire

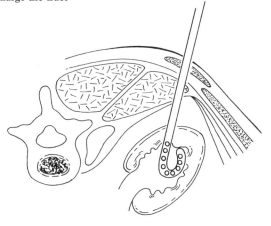

Fig. 26.38 The end of the stent curls in a pigtail fashion when the guide is removed

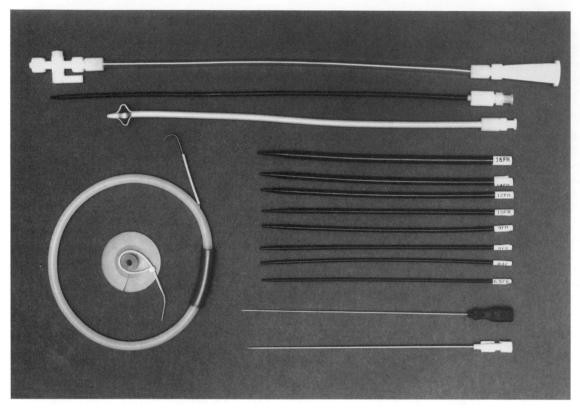

Fig. 26.39   Percutaneous Malecot nephrostomy set

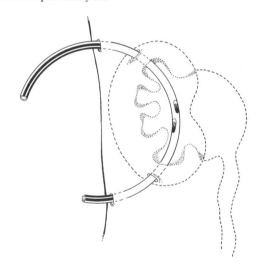

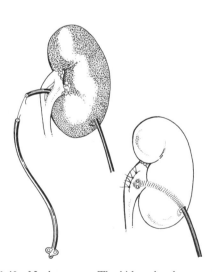

Fig. 26.40   Nephrostomy. The kidney has been mobilized and the pelvis opened. A probe is passed through the pelvis, lower calix and out through the lower pole of the kidney. A Malecot catheter is tied to the end of the probe and withdrawn through the lower pole of the kidney so that the bulb of the catheter lies in the renal pelvis. The tube can then be brought out through a separate stab incision below the wound

Fig. 26.41   Method of making a loop nephrostomy. The two open ends of the tube are connected to a single tube by a Y connection and thus drawn into one appliance. The probe has to be passed through the pelvis, calix and parenchyma of the kidney twice, once through the upper pole and once through the lower pole. Positioning the tube so that the holes lie in the calices or the renal pelvis is not easy. Many tubes, however, are radio-opaque and the position of the tube can be adjusted if it fails to drain properly. The advantage of the loop nephrostomy is the ease with which the tube can be changed

Ureterostomy

Temporary ureterostomy is sometimes an easier procedure than nephrostomy for the urgent relief of obstructions involving the lower end of a ureter. The upper third of the ureter is exposed by a muscle cutting incision. There is no advantage in using a T tube; it is preferable to pass a simple tube through a small incision in the ureter up to the renal pelvis and bring the other end out through a separate stab incision. A Gibbon catheter (see Fig. 25.22), with the solid tip removed, is useful because the flanges on this catheter can be secured to the skin with sutures or tape.

When the patient's renal function has recovered, the cause of the obstruction can be assessed and appropriate elective treatment decided. This may just involve removal of pelvic or ureteric stones, but calculus anuria is not common and most patients with obstructive acute renal failure have a disease like retroperitoneal fibrosis (p. 618) or malignant disease of cervix, prostate or bladder and pose much greater problems. The former will be explored in the appropriate way unless the kidney is solitary, but the latter can pose many problems, of which the surgical ones may be the least. In the presence of incurable or recurrent malignancy obstructing the ureters, it might be kinder to let the patient die of renal failure. If the disease causes acute renal failure before it has been treated, it is usually worth bypassing the obstruction by nephrostomy or ureterostomy.

PERINEPHRIC ABSCESS

A perinephric abscess forms in the perinephric fat, which lies between the renal capsule and renal fascia. The infection, usually staphylococcal, originates in a small abscess or carbuncle in the cortex of the kidney or spreads from a distant infection by the blood stream and the kidney itself is usually remarkably normal. Severe gram negative infections of the kidney, particularly those associated with staghorn calculi, do extend into perinephric fat, but tend to cause low grade inflammation with fibrous adhesions rather than an abscess. The problem with perinephric abscess is not the treatment, which is straightforward, but the diagnosis, which can be difficult because the lesion, like subphrenic abscess, is deeply situated and produces few, if any, local signs until it very advanced. In the early stages the features are those of a nonspecific febrile illness with malaise, anorexia, myalgia, intermittent fever and gradual loss of weight with leucocytosis and an elevated ESR. A swelling does not appear in the loin for some time, or may be undetected by an inadequate examination. The swelling renders the normally concave loin, first flat, later convex and can only be appreciated if we look down the back of the sitting patient.

In a straight X-ray the abscess often reveals itself because it obliterates the psoas shadow, displaces the colonic flexure and kidney, elevates the diaphragm and sometimes causes a small effusion on the base of the lung. Intravenous urography may reveal the displacement of the kidney most clearly, but is often of little more help than the straight X-ray unless the abscess is secondary to gross renal disease. Ultrasonography should reveal the mass around the kidney.

By the time a perinephric abscess is diagnosed it is usually beyond cure by chemotherapy alone and should be exposed and drained through a subcostal posterolateral incision. The incision is made below and parallel to the 12th rib dividing muscles in the same line. A finger can then be inserted into the retroperitoneal space and the abscess drained.

HYDRONEPHROSIS

Hydronephrosis means dilatation of the pelvis and calices of the kidney and implies, unless the word hydroureter is added, that the ureter is normal. When it is not secondary to stone, stricture, tumour or other obvious disease it is called idiopathic or congenital and it is the congenital type which is treated by pyeloplasty or, if little useful function remains, by nephrectomy.

The cause of *congenital* hydronephrosis is still not known. The kinks, adhesions and high insertion of the ureter are regarded as effects and not causes. Although all surgeons regard an aberrant artery to the lower pole of the kidney (found in 70% of patients with congenital hydronephrosis) an aggravating factor, few consider it the cause. The obstruction is probably functional rather than physical and caused by some defect of the musculature of the pelvi-ureteric junction that prevents contraction waves, and therefore urine from passing through, but no less amenable to pyeloplasty because of that. Although it has been recognised for many years that not all hydroureters are obstructed (some for instance are dilated because of vesico-ureteric reflux) only recently has it been widely appreciated that not all hydronephrotic kidneys are obstructed. The best example of this is seen in the kidney after pyeloplasty, which, no matter how successfully it relieves symptoms and obstruction, leaves the calices and sometimes the pelvis as dilated as before. Kidneys may also be hydronephrotic, but not obstructed after vesico-ureteric reflux is cured, or in the condition of hydrocalicosis.

Before pyeloplasty, therefore, it is essential to demonstrate not only hydronephrosis, but also obstruction. This can be done most easily by taking late films at the time of intravenous urography, by renography, radionuclide scanning, or in doubtful cases by Whitaker's test. In Whitaker's test, a needle is inserted into the renal pelvis percutaneously or at open operation and used to measure pressures in the renal pelvis while perfusing it at a flow rate of 10 ml/min. The renal pelvis pressure minus the bladder pressure (measured simultaneously) gives the relative pressure (RP). An elevated RP (15 cm water) indicates obstruction. The assessment of hydronephrosis is further complicated because the obstructed type (and it is the commonest) may be chronic or intermittent (Whitaker, 1977).

In the chronic type, the pelvis and calices are permanently dilated as seen on X-ray whether the patient is in pain or not. In the intermittent type, the dilatation comes and goes and can be detected only if the X-rays are taken when the patient has pain or is given intravenous Frusemide; at other times the kidney may appear normal or nearly normal. Hence there are kidneys that are obstructed, but not always dilated, and others which are dilated, but not obstructed. Pyeloplasty is an operation which relieves obstruction enabling the kidney to drain better; it should only be done if the hydronephrotic kidney is obstructed; on the other hand, it should not be denied to those patients whose symptoms suggest renal obstruction, but whose pyelogram is relatively normal, until the X-rays or renograms have been repeated during an episode of pain or diuresis. If, in cases of obstructive hydronephrosis, the *ureter* is also dilated the cause and treatment of the disease will be entirely different. If the upper ureter is seen in the intravenous urograms the distinction is easy; if not, its normality must not be assumed and it should be demonstrated by retrograde ureterogram. Doing this with a Braasch or Chevasseur catheter is less likely to cause oedema and infect the obstructed kidney, but even then is best done immediately before operation and under the same anaesthetic. If the findings are unexpected, operation is avoided. The *principles* of the

operation of pyeloplasty are to excise the pelviureteric junction and remake a new one that is wide, dependant and spouted; to excise the redundant part of the renal pelvis and to preserve the aberrant vessels especially those that cross anterior to the pelviureteric junction, by displacing them behind the new pelviureteric junction (Fig. 26.42).

Many methods of pyeloplasty fulfil these requirements, but none perhaps so well as the Anderson Hynes pyeloplasty (called the dismembered Foley pyeloplasty in America) which is suitable for all types of congenital hydronephrosis.

Pyeloplasty

The kidney is exposed through or above the 12th rib although some surgeons use an anterior subcostal or paramedian approach. The redundant pelvis is excised. The pelviureteric junction is reformed by suturing, with 4/0 catgut or dexon, the spatulated ureter to the lower part of the pelvis providing a new pelviureteric junction that is wide spouted and dependant. If an aberrant vessel is present the anastomosis is made in front of it. The upper part of the pelvis is closed with the same suture material. Many surgeons use a Cummings catheter (Fig. 26.43) which acts both as a splint across the anastomosis and a nephrostomy tube, and is removed some 7 days after operation; others use two separate tubes so that the splint can be removed a day or two before the nephrostomy tube.

CONGENITAL ANOMALIES OF THE KIDNEY

Congenital hydronephrosis is one congenital anomaly of the kidney that often requires surgical treatment, solitary cyst is another, but few of the many other ano-

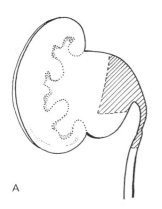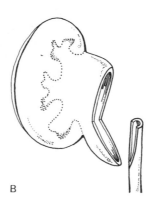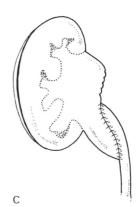

A   B   C

Fig. 26.42 Anderson–Hynes pyeloplasty for congenital hydronephrosis: (A) the amount of renal pelvis and upper ureter to be excised. (B) the means by which the upper end of the ureter is spatulated thus facilitating reconstruction of a wide pelviureteric junction. (C) the anastomosis completed, the ureter being sutured to the lower cut half of the pelvis forming a dependant, wide and spouted anastomosis. The upper part of the cut pelvis is sutured (the operation resembles and is derived from the Billroth 1 gastrectomy)

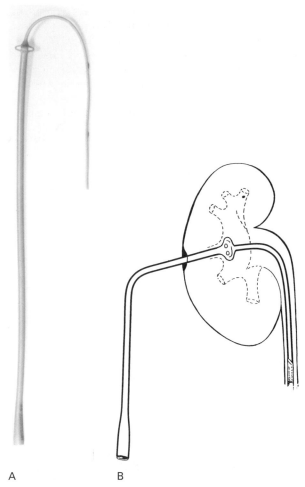

A   B

Fig. 26.43 Cummings catheter. The narrow part of the catheter passes through the anastomosis and down into the ureter. The expanded part of the catheter with the Malecot wings lies in the renal pelvis and the wider tube is brought out through the calix and parenchyma, and acts as a nephrostomy. Thus one tube is used as both splint and nephrostomy. (Courtesy of G U Manufacturing Co)

malies require operation unless affected by secondary disease processes such as stone, infection, obstruction (to all of which anomalous kidneys are more liable than normal) injury or tumour. Nevertheless, surgeons must be familiar with all common and many of the uncommon congenital anomalies, otherwise they may mistake the images they produce in X-rays, ultrasonic, radionuclide and CAT scans for disease, and be confused by their abnormal site, morphology and blood supply during operations for secondary disease processes.

Details of congenital abnormalities of the kidney need not be described here although the problems they may present before and during surgery should be anticipated.

Intrarenal pelvis
Most kidneys have an extrarenal pelvis which can be exposed easily because most of it lies outside the renal sinus. Some kidneys have an intrarenal pelvis. The latter is small, lies wholly within the renal sinus and appears as if the upper ureter enters the renal sinus and breaks up into major calices without first forming a pelvis. Operations, such as pyelolithotomy, are more difficult on intrarenal than extrarenal pelves. The presence of an intrarenal pelvis can usually be recognised in the preoperative X-rays.

Unrotated kidney (sometimes called malrotated)
(Fig. 26.44)
The metanephros, which becomes the adult kidney, develops in the caudal part of the embryo. At first the renal pelvis lies anterior to the kidney and some calices lie posteromedially and some posterolaterally. As the kidney ascends to its adult position in the loin it also rotates through 90%, the left one clockwise, the right one anticlockwise so that the pelvis comes to lie medial to the kidney and the calices all lie laterally. If the kidney fails to rotate the pelvis remains anterior to the kidney and some calices point medially. The kidney looks abnormal but usually functions normally.

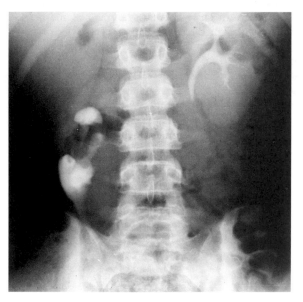

Fig. 26.44 i.v.u. showing an unrotated right kidney

Ectopic kidney (Fig. 26.45)
An ectopic kidney is one that has neither ascended nor rotated. It lies in the pelvis on or below the brim with an anterior pelvis and receives its blood from a number of small arteries; a renal artery develops only if and when the kidney ascends. Despite its appearance it usually functions satisfactorily unless secondarily diseased.

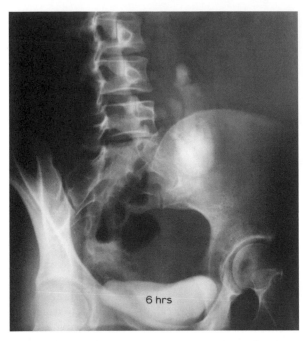

Fig. 26.45 i.v.u. showing an ectopic kidney which is also hydronephrotic

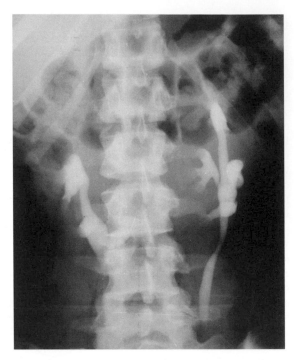

Fig. 26.46 i.v.u. showing a horseshoe kidney

If an i.v.u. fails to reveal a kidney the pelvic films must be inspected carefully for an ectopic kidney.

Fused kidneys
Of the several ways in which kidneys may be joined to each other, the commonest is the horseshoe anomaly in which the kidneys lie on their own side of the midline, but are joined together at their lower poles by a bridge made of renal fibrous tissue (Fig. 26.46). The horseshoe kidney like other fused kidneys is unrotated and usually lies at a lower level than normal. Each requires treatment only if it is secondarily involved by disease, and there is no point in dividing the bridge joining the kidneys in the hope that they will assume the positions they should have attained during the fourth month of intrauterine life. Operations on horseshoe, ectopic and unrotated kidneys are often easier than expected because they lie at a low level and have anterior pelves.

Duplication
Duplication of the renal pelvis with partial or complete duplication of the ureter is probably the commonest congenital anomaly of the urinary tract. Secondary disease processes often involve only one moiety or half of a duplex kidney and a heminephrectomy is often the appropriate treatment. Heminephrectomy is easier than the operation of partial nephrectomy on a normal kidney because each moiety has its own pedicle and is often clearly demarcated from the other.

The two pelves of a duplex kidney are unusual; the upper one rarely has more than 2 calices and in the lower the calices tend to be short and crowded together. If both moieties are functioning the condition can easily be recognized. If only one moiety is working, however, the abnormal appearance may be confused with gross disease of the pelvis of a normal kidney.

RENAL INJURIES

The kidneys are small, mobile and well protected by muscles, ribs, other viscera and the spine; nevertheless, they may be damaged by the perforating injuries of knives or gunshot wounds, by the blunt trauma or by the deceleration of road traffic accidents, sports injuries or falls. Perforating injuries, often complicated by infection or vascular problems like arteriovenous fistulae, are uncommon in the UK and most renal injuries are caused by blunt trauma or deceleration when the kidney is crushed between ribs and spine, impaled by a fractured rib or transverse process or torn from its pedicle. 80% of perforating injuries of the kidneys are associated with injuries to other viscera, whereas the injuries caused by blunt trauma or deceleration are either solitary or associated with skeletal injuries to the ribs, transverse processes or spine (Guerriero, 1982).

Classification

Injuries of the kidney can be classified into 4 groups: (1) Contusion (2) Laceration (3) Fragmentation or (4) Major vessel injury: (Fig. 26.47). Haematuria is the commonest finding but the amount of bleeding does not necessarily correlate with the severity of the injury; with severe injuries to major vessels haematuria may be slight and transient. Despite the large renal blood flow, severe shock is not a feature of renal injury and its presence suggests that other viscera are also damaged. Once the patient has been resuscitated and injuries to other structures assessed (and treated if they are lifethreatening) attention can be focused on the renal injury.

A straight X-ray may reveal injuries to ribs, transverse processes or spine, and a soft tissue mass obliterating the outline of the kidney and the psoas shadow. An intravenous urogram is essential; it reveals the presence and function of the uninjured kidney and gives some information about the injured kidney. Bruised kidneys often look surprisingly normal, lacerated ones can be recognized by their depressed function and by the extravasation of contrast medium into perirenal tissues. Nonfunction implies that the kidney is fragmented or the major vessels severely damaged and arteriography should be carried out. Ultrasonography and radionuclide scanning are useful in following the progress of the patient, but of limited help in establishing the extent of the injury when the patient is first seen. Patients with *contusions* (Group 1) and *lacerations* (Group 2) can be treated conservatively (unless there are associated injuries).

Many patients with a *fragmented kidney* can also be treated conservatively unless bleeding is persistent and severe, when the kidney should be explored and an attempt made to suture the lacerations or remove only part of the kidney. But nephrectomy is often the only solution, provided the other kidney is normal. *Injury of the renal vessels* usually involves intimal tears with secondary spasm and thrombosis, or partial or complete transection of the renal artery, and can only be distinguished from a fragmented kidney by angiography because the kidney is nonfunctioning on the intravenous urogram. Haematuria is often transient in patients with injuries of the renal artery, but retroperitoneal bleeding can be extensive with transection, particularly partial transection, when contraction of the vessel widens the hole.

As the kidneys can withstand ischaemia for only 15 minutes little is to be gained by exploring injuries of the pedicle, but careful follow up is essential as many develop hypertension.

A fragmented kidney or injured pedicle can be explored through a posterolateral incision, but is best explored through an anterior one, which allows examination of other viscera and an easier approach to the renal pedicle. Sometimes (especially in patients with perforating wounds) a renal injury is suspected only when a retroperitoneal haematoma is found during the course of a laparotomy for the exploration of other injuries. It is tempting just to explore and deal surgically with the kidney. However, an intravenous urogram should be done on the table as it is impossible to assess the functional state and integrity of the other kidney by palpating or even looking at it. All patients should be followed up for some time after injury, especially those who had lacerations, fragmentation or injuries of the renal artery because complications such as vascular abnormalities or hypertension can develop silently.

OTHER RENAL CONDITIONS AND OPERATIONS

Renal cysts

Solitary cysts are rare. They are usually situated in the cortex especially towards the lower pole, and communicate with neither the pelvis nor the calices. Their importance lies in the fact that they may be difficult to distinguish from neoplasms, but 95% are detectable by ultrasound scanning. Percutaneous puncture of the cyst under X-ray or ultrasonic control may be attempted; if clear or straw-coloured fluid is obtained, the cyst is outlined with radio-opaque medium. Simple aspiration is curative in 30 to 40% of cases. If operation is undertaken, it is wise to excise only the projecting part of the cyst (Fig. 26.48).

Polycystic disease is not amenable to surgery, since the cysts are scattered throughout the substance of both kidneys. Complications such as pain, bleeding or infection may be relieved (even if only temporarily) by Rovsing's operation, in which the kidney is exposed and all the larger cysts projecting on the surface are punctured or incised, but the correct treatment of polycystic disease is the treatment of the chronic renal failure it causes.

Nephropexy

Operative fixation of an abnormally mobile kidney is seldom performed since the undue mobility is often part of a generalized visceroptosis. Symptoms vary greatly and often bear little relationship to the degree of mobility and in many cases a considerable psychological element is present.

Nephropexy should, however, be considered (1) when symptoms appear to be related to the excessive mobility of the kidney, and are not relieved by an abdominal support (2) if intravenous urography or radionuclide scan demonstrate obstruction to the outflow of urine, (especially if there is also infection or hydro-

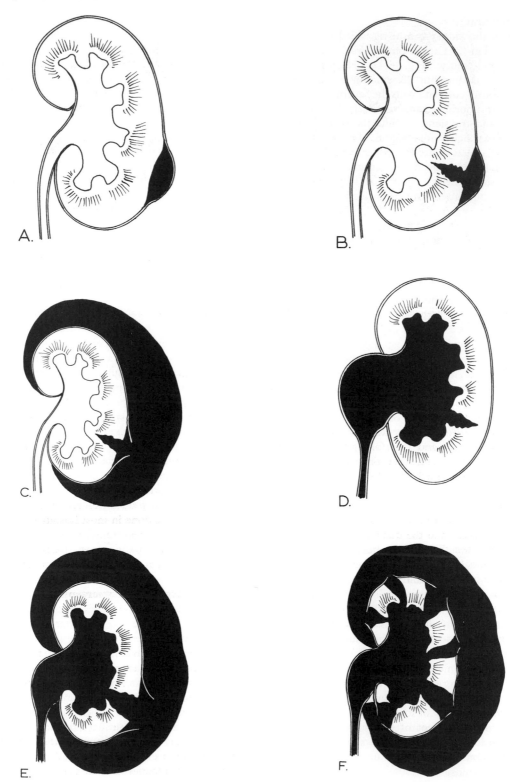

Fig. 26.47   Renal injuries. (A) Subcortical haematoma. (B) and (C) Lacerations involving the cortex but not the collecting system. (D) Laceration involving the collecting system but not the cortex. (E) Laceration involving both collecting system and cortex. (F) Fragmentation of the kidney

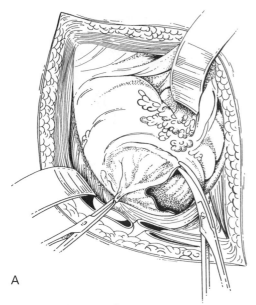

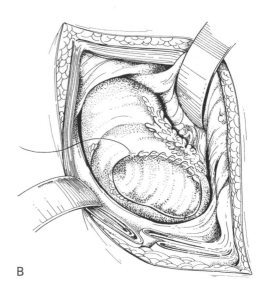

A   B

Fig. 26.48 Excision of solitary renal cyst. (A) The cyst has been deroofed and in (B) a running suture has been inserted around the cut edge of the cyst to control bleeding

nephrosis) or (3) if variations in urinary output occur because the renal artery is stretched and the kidney made ischaemic when the patient is erect.

When the patient is erect and the kidney ischaemic less sodium and therefore less water is excreted; when supine, the sodium and therefore water is excreted. Such patients complain that they pass little urine during the day, but much at night.

Technique
Probably the most effective method of anchoring the kidney is to stitch it to the quadratus lumborum. The kidney is exposed through a subcostal or lumbotomy approach and is delivered at the wound. The pelvis and ureter are carefully examined to exclude any organic obstruction to the urinary outflow. In order that the kidney may adhere to its muscular bed its posterior surface is cleared of all fatty tissue and is denuded of capsule except for a small strip near the convex border. The kidney is placed as high as possible with its upper pole under cover of the 12th rib and with the denuded area on its posterior surface in direct contact with quadratus lumborum. It is anchored to the lateral part of the muscle by three or four stitches. In order to promote adhesions, a sheet of polyvinyl alcohol sponge may be placed between kidney and the muscle, but is usually unnecessary.

Percutaneous operations on the kidney
Rapid progress is being made in the development of percutaneous renal operations, which now include

the long established needle biopsy, the insertion of nephrostomy tubes (Fig. 26.38), the aspiration of renal cysts and procedures such as removal or ultrasonic destruction of calyceal or pelvic calculi. Biopsy, electro-coagulation or resection of transitional cell tumours of the collecting system, and the dilatation and even incision of a narrowed pelviureteric junction are also being accomplished, all of which require special endoscopic instruments or other apparatus.

The first three procedures are relatively common-place and can be done in most hospitals with standard X-ray and ultrasonic facilities. The others are still experimental and are presently being done only on selected patients in a few specialized centres.

Renal ischaemia and hypertension
Renal ischaemia is now well recognized as a cause of hypertension. The two conditions most commonly encountered are atheroma of the renal artery, usually causing stenosis near its origin, and fibromuscular hypertrophy of the arterial wall, causing a more generalized constriction. The diagnosis is best made by *selective renal arteriography* (p. 550).

Surgery may be advised in otherwise fit patients who do not respond to medical treatment. The operations commonly employed are *thrombo-endarterectomy*, *splenic artery to renal artery anastomosis* and *bypass grafting*. If, however, the kidney is shrunken and atrophic, and frozen section examination of a biopsy section shows gross tubular atrophy and fibrosis, nephrectomy is indicated, provided that the other kidney is healthy.

Renal transplantation

The technique of renal transplantation is now well established although its use is confined to those centres with facilities for haemodialysis and with a surgeon experienced in the problems which may arise. In homotransplantation, with transfer of a kidney from a related donor or from a cadaver, graft survival at 1 year can be expected in well over 75% of cases. While the operative technique has been largely standardized, there remains the problem of rejection whereby the body's defence mechanisms attempt to discard the transplanted organ in much the same way as any foreign body or infective organism is rejected. Control of rejection has allowed transplantation of liver and heart to be carried out with increasing success. The complex mechanism of rejection can be controlled with immunosuppressive therapy but more major advances can be expected in the field of tissue-typing (a more detailed method of blood grouping) so that the cells of the donated kidney can be more accurately matched to the recipient patient.

The *main indication* for renal transplantation is in the treatment of chronic irreversible renal failure, as an alternative to chronic intermittent haemodialysis or in addition to it (Morris, 1979). The recipient must be fit enough to withstand a major surgical procedure, he should be free from systemic infection and should possess a normal lower urinary tract. The kidney itself must be free from disease and capable of good function. Its vessels should be of sufficient length to allow for a satisfactory anastomosis and it is preferable for it to have a single renal artery.

Technique

It is now standard practice to transplant a kidney to an extraperitoneal site in the contralateral iliac fossa. This makes it possible to re-establish the circulation in the kidney with the minimum of delay since the ureter lies anteriorly and can be dealt with after suture of the blood vessels. The renal vein is joined end-to-side to the external or common iliac vein and the artery is anastomosed end-to-end to the divided internal iliac artery. Finally, the ureter is implanted into the bladder.

OPERATIONS ON THE ADRENAL GLANDS

Partial or complete removal of the adrenal glands is a relatively safe procedure, linked to the availability of cortisone and its synthetic substitutes. The operation may be curative in cases of adrenal dysfunction (adrenogenital or Cushing's syndrome), and also of tumour formation, whether this involves the cortex or the medulla of the gland. It is no longer used in the treatment of metastatic carcinoma of the breast or prostate.

Except in the case of a tumour which has been clearly localised by CT scanning or arteriography (p. 555) to one or other side, both adrenal glands will require at least to be exposed and examined. In some cases, therefore, the operation will be a bilateral one.

Anatomy

The right adrenal gland

Triangular in shape, it lies partly on the diaphragm, and partly capping the upper pole of the kidney; anteromedially it is in contact with the vena cava, and anterolaterally, with the liver.

The left adrenal gland

Semilunar in shape, it also caps the kidney, but extends further down its medial border towards the hilum. Its anterior surface is closely applied to the pancreas and the splenic artery.

Each gland is embedded in fat and enclosed within the renal fascia, but is separated from the kidney by an incomplete fascial septum. It is attached lightly to the kidney below by loose connective tissue, and more firmly, to the diaphragm above by thickened fascial bands.

Arterial supply is derived from the aorta, the inferior phrenic and the renal arteries, but the individual branches from these vessels are seldom encountered at operation, for they divide before reaching the gland into a number of smaller vessels; these may be difficult to identify before division, but bleeding is seldom troublesome.

Venous drainage is usually by one large vein, which may however be duplicated; this is very easily torn, and the bleeding may be dangerous. On the right side the vein, which is very short, emerges on the anteromedial surface of the gland near the apex, and immediately enters the vena cava with which the gland is in contact. The left vein is longer; it emerges from the anterior surface of the gland near the lower pole, and joins either the inferior phrenic or the renal vein.

Surgical approach

The adrenal glands, like the kidneys, may be approached by the lumbar route, by the anterior (transperitoneal) route, or by the transthoracic route. The anterior route has the advantage that both adrenal glands can be exposed at the same time if preoperative investigations indicate bilateral disease. The conditions of the glands can then be compared, and a bilateral removal carried out if necessary. In suspected malignancy, para-aortic lymph glands can also be assessed. In ectopic ACTH syndrome, the anterior approach allows for exploration for a possible intra-abdominal primary tumour.

Adrenalectomy by the lumbar or transthoracic approach

This may be through the bed of the 10th, 11th or 12th rib (pp. 574–578), and may be either subpleural or transpleural. The upper pole of the kidney is delivered, and the adrenal gland is recognized from its orange colour which distinguishes it clearly from fat or pancreatic tissue. It is cleared first along its lateral border, and a finger is inserted behind it; it is then dissected free, all vessels — especially the large veins at its medial border — being secured as they are displayed. A search is made in the surrounding retroperitoneum for any islands of accessory adrenal tissue, and these, if present, are removed.

On the right side, the gland is gently rotated laterally by the use of a small rake retractor, so that the vessels related to its medial surface (Fig. 26.49), especially the large and dangerously short vein which joins the vena cava, can be cleared. Once this vessel has been safely secured, removal of the gland should present no serious difficulty. Ligaclips are particularly helpful for this procedure.

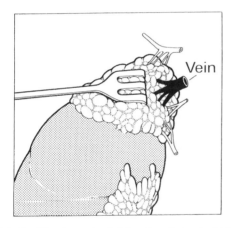

Fig. 26.49 Blood supply of right adrenal gland which is rotated laterally to expose medial surface. Note that there are considerable variations in the vascular pattern, but the veins are always much larger than the arteries which may divide into a large number of small branches before entering the glands

Technique of bilateral adrenalectomy by the anterior approach

The patient is placed in the dorsal position with the thoracolumbar region slightly arched over the raised bridge. A curved transverse incision, convex upwards and with its centre 5 cm above the umbilicus, may be employed. This provides much better access than a straight incision of the same length. Surgeons with experience in this field may use a midline incision.

The left adrenal gland is approached first, by incision of the posterior layer of the lienorenal ligament

(Fig. 18.2, p. 405). This incision should not be made too close to the spleen, since the peritoneum may then tear back on to the organ, with consequent bleeding. The spleen is turned forwards and to the patient's right, together with the tail and body of the pancreas and the splenic vessels, thus bringing the left kidney and adrenal gland into view. The adrenal gland is mobilized as described in the lumbar approach, its vessels are secured, and it is removed. The spleen and pancreas are then replaced in their original position.

The right adrenal gland is now sought for deeply in the subhepatic pouch, in the area bounded by the lower border of the liver, the right side of the vena cava and the renal vessels. A small gauze pack is laid deeply on the inferior surface of the liver, and by the use of a retractor placed against this the liver is gently drawn upwards. The kidney is then drawn downwards by pressure with the fingers and the posterior-wall peritoneum is incised around the upper pole and about 2.5 cm above it. Elevation of this curved peritoneal flap should now display the adrenal gland, which can be brought better into view by a finger inserted above it into the space between the two fascial layers enclosing it. The vein is identified and secured as described above and the gland is mobilized. The fascial connections between the gland and the kidney should be divided last, since otherwise the gland may become retracted upwards to a less accessible level.

Finally, the incision is repaired, suction drains being brought out at each end if there is doubt about haemostasis.

Adrenalectomy for cortical tumours

Cushing's syndrome results from excessive secretions of adreno-cortical hormones, due to hyperplasia of the adrenal cortex, an adenoma or an occasional carcinoma. The hyperplasia may result from excess ACTH production by the pituitary or inappropriate secretion of ACTH by a tumour, for example, of the bronchus. *Primary hyperaldosteronism* (Conn's syndrome) due to a solitary adenoma or bilateral hyperplasia causes hypertension and loss of potassium (Grondal, 1992).

In cases where the glands are *hyperplastic*, due to pituitary or ectopic ACTH stimulation, the usual policy in surgical treatment is to control the source of ACTH. If this is not possible, removal of the whole of each gland is required. When a unilateral *tumour* is present, the affected gland only is removed; if there are bilateral tumours, total adrenalectomy must necessarily be performed. If the tumour is still encapsulated on removal, the prognosis is reasonably good.

Adrenalectomy for medullary tumours

These tumours (*chromaffinomata* or *phaeochromocytomata*) are associated with paroxysmal or sustained hypertension. Since they are usually unilateral and larger than cortical tumours, averaging 5 cm in diameter, they can usually be localized by ultra sound scanning, selective venous sampling or by selective angiography (Fig. 25.8). Occasionally the tumour is malignant.

An anterior (transperitoneal) approach is preferred, since this enables the main veins to be ligated before any manipulation of the tumour can release adrenaline into the circulation, thereby causing a dangerous rise in blood pressure. Alpha adrenergic blocking agents should be administered preoperatively to control blood pressure and to minimize the effect of paroxysmal release of catecholamines. *Phenoxybenzamine* (10–20 mg twice daily) is usually given orally until several days before operation (Welbourne, 1980), when *phentolamine,* by intravenous infusion (5–60 mg in 5% dextrose, 0.2 to 2 mg per minute) should be substituted, the dose being carefully titrated against blood pressure. Arrhythmias during operation require intravenous lignocaine or a beta adrenergic blocker such as propranolol.

Substitution therapy. In order to combat possible hormone insufficiency, all operations on the adrenal glands should be carried out under cortisone control, and after total adrenalectomy administration of this hormone must be continued throughout life. After partial or unilateral adrenalectomy, the majority of patients eventually become independent of steroid therapy. The cortisone may therefore be withdrawn gradually, the length of time during which it is required varying from one patient to another. The dosage of steroids and the duration of such therapy are determined by the absence of signs of adrenal insufficiency when trial reductions are made. A suggested scheme of therapy is as follows:

1 to 2 hours before operation	100 mg of hydrocortisone (as sodium succinate) intravenously.
At the end of the operation	Repeat i.v. injection of hydrocortisone every 8 hours.
1st postoperative day	100 mg hydrocortisone i.v. every 8 hours.
2nd postoperative day	50 mg hydrocortisone i.v. every 8 hours.
3rd postoperative day	25 mg hydrocortisone i.v. every 8 hours.
4th postoperative day	25 mg hydrocortisone orally every 8 hours.
5th postoperative day	20 mg hydrocortisone in morning, 10 mg in evening, orally.

The maintenance dose of 30 mg hydrocortisone, or 37.5 mg of cortisone acetate daily, should at once be increased to 100 mg during any conditions of stress —

illness, accident or emotional disturbance, or if signs of adrenocortical deficiency appear — apathy, weakness, nausea, vomiting, etc.

Fludrocortisone in a daily dose of 0.1 mg has greater salt-retaining powers and may be employed to supplement cortisone during the first few days after operation.

Complications of adrenalectomy. Acute circulatory failure may be the first sign of adrenocortical insufficiency and may not be prevented by routine substitution therapy. It may occur with dramatic suddenness, usually within 48 hours of operation, and may terminate fatally. Treatment consists in the intravenous administration of 200 mg of hydrocortisone, every 2 hours if necessary. If profound shock is present, a simultaneous infusion of noradrenaline should be given.

Salt deficiency is likely to be mistaken for cortisone deficiency, for the clinical features are very similar. In the early postoperative period it may be prevented by fludrocortisone, or by daily estimations of serum electrolytes so that sodium chloride may be given intravenously. Symptoms which develop later may be treated by giving salt by mouth. Alternatively, a maintenance dose of fludrocortisone may be preferred.

Every patient who has undergone adrenalectomy should, on discharge from hospital, be issued with a printed card which he should carry with him at all times. This should contain advice on the indications for increasing the dosage of cortisone, and there should be an instruction that, if he is found in a state of collapse, hydrocortisone should be administered intravenously.

OPERATIONS ON THE URETER

Anatomy (see Gosling, 1982)
The ureter is a muscular tube 24 to 30 cm long and about 4 mm (12F) in diameter. Starting at the pelviureteric junction it passes down the posterior abdominal wall, crosses the pelvic brim and then runs medially and forward to the bladder. It is lined throughout by transitional cell epithelium and enclosed in a firm sheath of adventitial tissue derived from the retroperitoneal fascia.

Relations
The abdominal part of the ureter, accompanied by the testicular or ovarian vessels, is separated from the tips of the lumbar transverse processes by the psoas muscle. Anteriorly, peritoneum separates the right ureter from the third part of the duodenum, the right colic and the ileocolic vessels and the root of the mesentery; and the left ureter from the left colic vessels. However, as these structures are reflected medially with the peritoneum they are not usually seen in the extraperitoneal approaches to the ureter. The ureter is loosely attached

to, and lifted forwards with, the peritoneum and usually therefore found in the loose fat behind the peritoneum rather than on the psoas major muscle.

In the pelvis the ureter runs down the side wall, below the internal iliac artery to the level of the ischial spine, then forwards and medially in the fat above the levator ani muscle to the bladder, where it is surrounded by a plexus of veins. In males it is crossed anteriorly near the bladder by the vas deferens and overlapped by the upper end of the seminal vesicle. In females it is crossed by the uterine artery and vein in the broad ligament and runs immediately above the lateral fornix of the vagina at the side of the cervix uteri to reach the bladder.

The intramural portion of the ureter is about 1 cm long. It passes obliquely through the muscular wall of the bladder so that 5 cm separate the ureters as they enter the bladder but only 2.5 cm separate them as they open into the bladder at the upper angles of the trigone.

Blood supply

The ureters receive blood by transverse branches from various arteries in the abdomen and pelvis which feed a freely anastomosing plexus in the adventitial sheath. If this sheath is undisturbed a considerable length of the ureter can be mobilized without fear of ischaemic damage.

Exposure of the ureter

The upper third of the ureter, including the pelvi-ureteric junction, can be exposed through a posterolateral, subcostal or lumbotomy incision as described for exposure of the kidney (p. 574).

The middle third of the ureter lies in the iliac fossa and is usually exposed through a muscle cutting incision. The patient lies supine or has the shoulder and buttock of the affected side slightly elevated by a pillow or sandbag. The incision, centred on McBurney's point, extends from the midaxillary line posteriorly to the lateral edge of the rectus sheath anteriorly. The incision can be extended forwards or backwards depending on the extent of the operation and the build of the patient. The muscles of the anterior abdominal wall and transversalis fascia are divided in the same line as the incision and retracted. The unopened peritoneum is gently swept forwards and medially off the fascia covering the iliacus muscle with gauze or fingers. The ureter may be identified as it crosses the bifurcation of the common iliac vessels but more often is elevated along with the peritoneum and found in the loose fatty tissue alongside the spermatic or ovarian vessels. The ureter can be recognized by its white colour, by the blood vessels that run longitudinally in its adventitial coat, by its lack of branches and by its peristaltic contractions (which can

be stimulated if they are not obvious by pinching or tapping the ureter). However a dilated ureter may have a bluish colour or look too wide to be a ureter; furthermore peristalsis may not be obvious nor easily provoked.

If doubt exists, it is advisable to aspirate its contents with a fine needle and syringe before proceeding with mobilization. A normal ureter can usually be mobilized without great difficulty and secured with a sling of tape, a silicone tube or a piece of Paul's tubing. Difficulty may arise if it is bound down by firm adhesions from previous operations or infection. Mobilization is always facilitated by first securing the ureter above and below the lesion with slings before proceeding further.

The pelvic part of the ureter can be exposed through a low paramedian incision, a low oblique incision above and parallel to the inguinal ligament or a transverse suprapubic incision like that used for exposing the bladder or prostate (p. 622) (Fig. 26.50). The patient lies supine with the head of the table lowered. The incision is made through transversalis fascia but not through peritoneum (although some urologists consider that stones can be more easily removed from the pelvic part of the ureter if it is exposed transperitoneally). The peritoneum is reflected medially and the ureter found as it crosses the iliac vessels and enters the pelvis. The ureter is secured with tape or tube and the pelvic ureter can then be mobilized as far as the bladder. Apart from some vesical vessels, it is crossed anteriorly by the vas deferens in males; by the broad ligament and the uterine arteries and veins (which can be very large) in females.

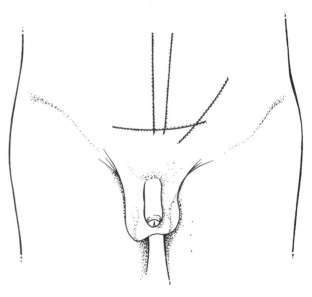

Fig. 26.50 Various skin incisions for the exposure of the lower third of the left ureter

The ureters are approached *transperitoneally* for such operations as ileal loop ureterostomy, or ureterocolic anastomosis and by some surgeons for the removal of stones from the ureter.

Transvaginal approach to the pelvic ureter through the lateral fornix of the vagina has been described for the removal of stones from the lower part of the ureter in women. It can only be done if the stone is easily palpable and even then is not very satisfactory because it is impossible to control the ureter with slings before incising it and the stone can easily be displaced upwards.

Ureteric stones

Stones do not form in the ureter, but pass from the kidney while they are still small. Some pass silently through the ureter and into the bladder; stones that pass through the ureter, which has a diameter of 10 F or less, can easily pass through the normal urethra which has a diameter of 26 F or more. Even small stones may arrest temporarily in the ureter, producing renal or ureteric colic and sometimes infection, haematuria or acute renal failure (p. 591). All stones with a diameter less than 5 mm, and many with a diameter between 5 and 7 mm, pass spontaneously into the bladder and it is wise to treat such patients conservatively unless there are good reasons for interfering. However, urgent relief is required for the patient with acute renal failure or severe infection. Less urgent operation is necessary if the patient has a ureterocele or stricture below the stone, persistent pain or progressive hydronephrosis. Stones tend to increase in size as they remain in the ureter and those more than 7 mm in diameter which are unlikely to pass without help should probably be given only about 3 months to do so. Smaller ones can be left much longer provided they are doing no harm. The patient should be followed up by straight X-rays and renography at 3 monthly intervals or earlier if symptoms or signs appear.

Stones that do not pass unaided have to be removed. In nearly all cases this can be done by ureteroscopy for stones in the middle and lower one third or by 'push bang' for stones in the upper one third. The classical operations of ureterolithotomy may occasionally be required, and are described on page 608.

Endoscopic methods

Stones in the intra-mural part of the ureter. Few stones that have travelled as far down the ureter as its intramural part have difficulty travelling the last few mm into the bladder; those that do can usually be removed endoscopically (Ford, 1983).

At cystoscopy, an oedematous ureteric orifice is usually seen, sometimes with the lower end of the stone visible within it. The ureteric orifice and the intramural part of the ureter over the stone can be incised with a Lane or Bee Sting meatome (Fig. 26.51). The stone then falls into the bladder or can be persuaded to do so by gently nudging it with the closed meatome (Fig. 26.52). The stone can be removed by irrigating the bladder through the cystoscope sheath with an Ellik evacuator (p. 646). Some surgeons prefer to incise the intramural part of the ureter over the stone leaving the ureteric orifice itself intact, believing that this procedure is less likely than the others to cause vesico-ureteric reflux. However this is a more difficult procedure because the incision can only be made with a diathermy knife passed through a resectoscope.

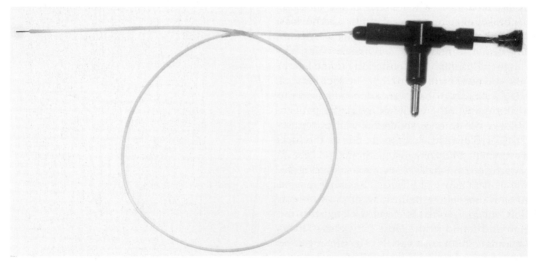

Fig. 26.51   Lane meatome. The handle of the instrument is connected to diathermy; the handle also contains a mechanism for extruding or retracting a small length of bare wire at the end of the instrument, which is insulated

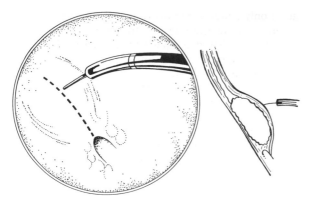

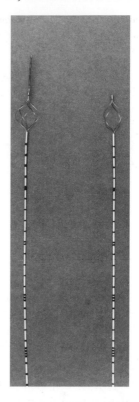

Fig. 26.52 Use of meatome. The bare wire is extruded and can be used for incision of the ureteric orifice. The incision can be made in the way illustrated from the outside but is often more easily accomplished if the wire is inserted into the ureteric orifice and pulled forward into the bladder as it cuts

Stones in the lower third of the ureter. Most stones that progress to the lower third of the ureter pass without interference into the bladder; those that do not can be removed by ureterolithotomy but, for stones smaller than 7 mm in diameter, it is worth attempting endoscopic methods, bearing in mind what damage can be inflicted on the ureter by some of the instruments available for the removal of stones from its lower third, especially when they are used in ways other than those recommended. Some surgeons pass one or two ureteric catheters up the ureter beyond the stone and leave them in for a few days. Others use stone dislodgers of one sort or another; the author favours the Dormia type (Fig. 26.53). The Dormia stone dislodger is a size 5 French ureteric catheter, the interior of which is occupied by four pliable stainless steel threads which project from the proximal end: when the threads are pushed forward a basket of spiral wires emerges from the distal end of the catheter; when the threads are pulled backwards the basket retracts into the catheter. The dislodger is passed through the catheterizing part of the cystoscope and into the ureter with the basket retracted. If it cannot be negotiated past the stone no more can be done although some surgeons dilate the ureter by opening the basket before it is withdrawn. If it passes beyond the stone the basket is opened and the dislodger slowly and gently withdrawn (Fig. 26.54) until its tip and the open basket are safely back in the bladder. No attempt must be made to close the basket while it is still in the ureter. If the stone is trapped in the basket it may be difficult to pull the dislodger and the trapped stone downwards into the bladder. In such circumstances, steady firm even traction should be applied for half an hour or more if necessary. If this still fails to dislodge the stone into the bladder the ureteric orifice can be split using the Lane meatome.

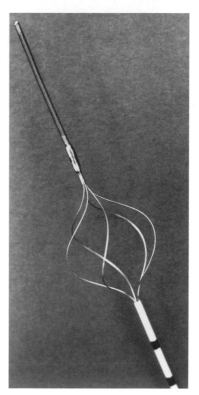

Fig. 26.53 Dormia stone dislodger (A) long and short tips (B) long tip

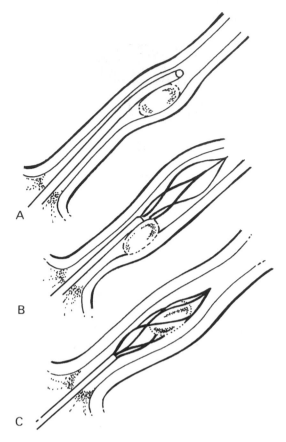

Fig. 26.54 Use of Dormia 'basket' (A) catheter tip passed beyond calculus (B) 'basket' opened (C) catheter and 'basket' withdrawn

If endoscopic measures fail it is worth waiting a few days before doing an open operation.

Ureterolithotomy (Figs 26.55–26.58)

It is essential to X-ray the patient on the operating table to confirm that the stone has not moved since the previous examination before making the incision. The ureter is exposed, and secured with a sling of tape, Paul's tubing or silastic tube above the level of the calculus. This facilitates mobilization of the ureter and prevents the stone slipping upwards to a level where it may be inaccessible from the approach employed — most likely if the ureter is dilated. After the ureter has been secured, the patient may be tilted into a Trendelenberg position which facilitates exposure, especially of the lower part of the ureter. The ureter is gently mobilized downwards as far as the stone which may be recognized by the fusiform swelling of the ureter it produces or by palpation. A second sling or a tissue forceps is applied across the ureter below the stone to prevent the stone or small fragments slipping downwards. The stone is steadied between the slings or

between a finger and thumb and a longitudinal incision is made through the ureter directly over it. This incision begins over the thickest part of the stone and extends upwards to a level just above its upper end. The stone can then be partly dislocated out of the ureter with a Watson-Cheyne or a Macdonald dissector and carefully removed with forceps, avoiding fragmentation. It is essential to mobilize the ureter as described, no matter how difficult this may be. Do not be tempted to open the ureter somewhere above the stone and hope to remove it by passing forceps down the ureter. It is not usually possible to dislodge the stone upwards and remove it through healthy ureter, although this is often described. However if you attempt to do this it is essential to have firm control of the ureter above the stone otherwise the stone might slip upwards to an inaccessible part of the ureter, even to the pelvis or calyces of the kidney. After removing the stone, insert a fine tube or ureteric catheter into the incision and wash out the ureter before and after removing the slings. Then pass a ureteric catheter upwards and downwards to make sure nothing has been missed. The incision in the ureter may be repaired with 3/0 or 4/0 absorbable sutures which do not penetrate the mucosa, although many urologists feel that it is unnecessary and leave the incision open (Fig. 26.58). Sometimes urine does not leak from an unsutured ureteric incision; more usually there is leakage for a few days whether or not the ureter is sutured and the area must be drained.

Transperitoneal ureterolithotomy

This is a safe procedure unlikely to be followed by intraperitoneal complications and is sometimes an easier way of removing stones in the lower third of the ureter than the more usual extraperitoneal approach. Some urologists favour this approach for all stones in the lower third of the ureter. An oblique or paramedian incision is made and deepened into the peritoneal cavity. The bowel is reflected and the ureter exposed by incising the peritoneum overlying it. The stone is removed in the way already described.

Transvaginal ureterolithotomy

In women some stones in the lower third of the ureter can be palpated vaginally and in such patients some surgeons recommend removing them through an incision in the lateral fornix of the vagina. With the patient in the lithotomy position an incision is made in the lateral fornix after appropriate retraction. The ureter is secured above the stone, which must be easily palpable for this procedure to be successful, and opened. The stone is removed, the ureter is sutured and the vaginal fornix loosely closed around a drain. There seems little risk of producing a ureterovaginal fistula but the procedure is not as easy as it sounds. The ureter can only be

Figs 26.55–26.58 *Ureterolithotomy*

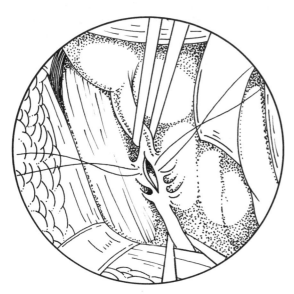

Fig. 26.55 The ureter is exposed and secured with a tape sling above the stone. The ureter has been opened between stay sutures over the stone

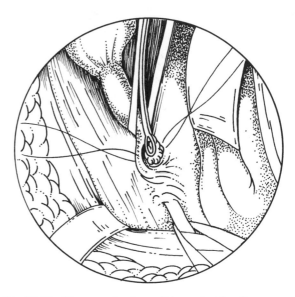

Fig. 26.56 The stone has been dislocated with a dissector and is now being removed with the stone-holding forceps

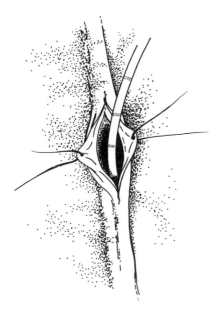

Fig. 26.57 The stone has been removed and a ureteric catheter is being passed down the ureter to ensure its patency

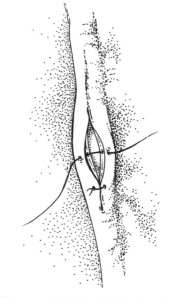

Fig. 26.58 The ureteric incision is being loosely sutured with stitches that do not pass through the mucosa

identified by palpating the stone within and it is usually impossible to secure and control the ureter above the stone before incising it. It is not difficult therefore to displace the stone upwards inadvertently and the patient must be advised before a transvaginal ureterolithotomy is attempted that it may be unsuccessful and an abdominal procedure may be required.

Injuries of the ureter and methods of repair (see Asmussen, 1983)

The ureter is more likely to be injured during pelvic operations, especially those on the uterus, than by road traffic accidents, falls or perforating wounds. It is important that the ureter should be identified and safeguarded at an early stage of such operations. When damaged, the ureter may be partially or completely divided, crushed by a clamp or occluded by a ligature or suture. If the accident is recognized at the time immediate steps should be taken to rectify matters. Removal of the constricting agent may be all that is required if the ureter has been clamped or occluded by ligature or suture but not divided, although there is some risk that a stricture or fistula may develop later.

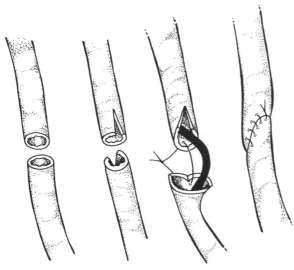

Fig. 26.59 End-to-end anastomosis of ureter. Each end of the ureter is spatulated. This results in a wide oblique anastomosis which is carried out with interrupted sutures over a ureteric splint

Incomplete tears may be loosely sutured with fine absorbable sutures that do not penetrate the mucosa and complete tears are treated if possible by an end-to-end anastomosis using absorbable sutures, diminishing the risk of stricture by spatulating the cut ends of the ureter before suturing (Fig. 26.59). Some surgeons make the anastomosis over a fine portex or silastic tube, leaving the lower end of the tube projecting into the bladder. The tube is removed some 7 or 10 days later with biopsy forceps through a cystoscope. If the injury involved the lower 5 or 6 cms of the ureter the most satisfactory procedure is to ligate the lower stump and reimplant the upper cut end into the bladder (p. 611). If the ureter can be neither repaired nor reimplanted into the bladder without tension even after hitching the bladder up to the psoas muscle (Fig. 26.60), a temporary cutaneous ureterostomy can be done by stitching a portex or silastic tube into the ureter and bringing the other end of the tube out of the skin through a separate stab incision, being careful to leave a reasonable length of tube within the patient so that the ureter is not dislodged too far from its anatomical position. The ureter can then be repaired by a second operation at a later date using a Boari pouch (p. 613) or by replacing the damaged segment of ureter with an isolated loop of ileum. Uretero-ureteric anastomosis i.e. anastomosing the cut end of one ureter into the side of the other ureter is not recommended because it then endangers the integrity of the opposite urinary tract.

In patients who are poor risks and whose opposite kidney is known to be healthy, the ureter may be ligated but renal atrophy by no means always ensues

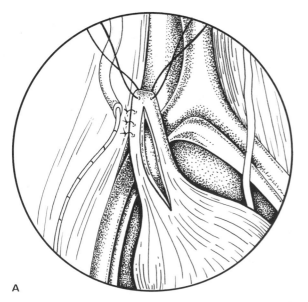

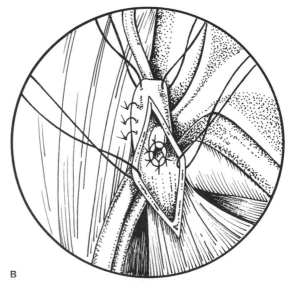

A   B

Fig. 26.60 The psoas hitch operation. (A) The right side of the bladder has been pulled up above the common iliac vessels and secured to the psoas muscle by three stitches. (B) These stitches are not tied until the reimplantation has been completed

and about 35% of patients so treated develop fistula or hydronephrosis and require nephrectomy. In many patients the ureteric injury remains unsuspected until some days after the operation when the patient develops renal pain, infection, or anuria (if the injury involves a solitary ureter or both ureters); or urine extravasates into the peritoneum or extra peritoneal tissues; or a fistula develops between ureter and vagina or skin. Sometimes the injury is never discovered because the obstructed kidney progresses silently to renal atrophy.

The elective repair of a damaged ureter (discovered some days after operation) should be delayed until the wound is fully healed and the patient fit. In the meantime an attempt can be made to introduce a ureteric catheter or stent endoscopically and if this fails a temporary ureterostomy or nephrostomy is necessary.

If the ureter has not been completely divided and a ureteric catheter can be passed, no more need be done and the ureter may heal. Otherwise the pelvis should be explored and the damaged ureter treated by reimplantation using a Boari pouch or end-to-end anastomosis.

Reimplantation of the ureter into the bladder (ureterocystostomy)

This procedure is used for *injuries* of the lower ureter and it is often the best means of treating lower ureteric *strictures*. It is the operation of choice for restoring continuity of the urinary tract following excision of the ureteric orifice and intramural ureter during removal of a bladder diverticulum or partial cystectomy, of preventing vesico-ureteric reflux and of treating megaureter. It is also part of the operation for renal transplantation. The method of approach and the technique of reimplantation vary according to the conditions present. *Transperitoneal approach* is likely to be employed if the ureter has been accidentally divided during an abdominal operation, otherwise an extraperitoneal approach is normally preferred since it obviates the risk of peritoneal complications. The ureter is exposed and divided as low down as conditions permit, ligating or excising the lower segment. The remaining part of the ureter is mobilized so that it pursues a fairly straight course to the bladder and lies without tension. Provided that its adventitial sheath remains intact there is little risk of ischaemic necrosis. Each side of the cut end of the ureter is split longitudinally for a distance of about 2 cm so that anterior and posterior flaps are formed for anchoring the ureter inside the bladder. A small incision is made in the posterior wall of the bladder above the normal ureteric orifice. The cut end of the ureter is then brought through this incision into the bladder and secured by suturing the ureteric flaps to the mucosa of the bladder with absorbable material. Fine sutures are then used to join the fibrous sheath of the ureter to the outside of the bladder. This method is

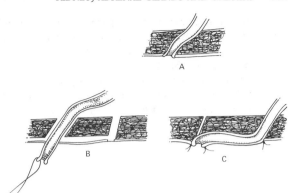

Fig. 26.61 The Politano–Leadbetter method of ureteric reimplantation. (A) shows the normal anatomy. (B) the intramural ureter has been mobilized and freed from the surrounding bladder and an incision has been made through the bladder above the ureteric orifice. (C) the ureter has been removed from the bladder, reinserted through the recently made incision, brought down through a subcutaneous tunnel and sutured to the margins of the old ureteric orifice

the simplest one of reimplanting the ureter but has to be modified or replaced by a different operation in most patients because it offers little if any protection against vesico-ureteric reflux, particularly if the ureter is dilated (Johnson, 1984).

If the operation is being carried out to cure vesico-ureteric reflux, the *Politano-Leadbetter operation* is appropriate (Fig. 26.61). The bladder is exposed through a transverse suprapubic incision and opened between stay sutures. The ureter is catheterized (Fig. 26.62) with a plastic or silastic tube (about 5 F in size) which is tied to the edge of the ureteric orifice with a fine catgut suture. A circular incision is made around the ureteric orifice and, by sharp dissection (Fig. 26.63) aided by traction on the tube, the intramural ureter is freed and drawn into the bladder. A right angled clamp of the O'Shaugnessy type is passed out of the bladder alongside the freed ureter and used to invaginate the posterior bladder wall some 5 or 6 cm above the ureteric orifice (Fig. 26.64). A small incision is made through the bladder wall onto the tip of the clamp which then appears inside the bladder. A suture is passed, by means of the clamp, between the two openings in the bladder and tied to the tube previously inserted into the ureter. Traction on the other end of the suture takes the ureter out of the bladder and in again through the newly made opening (Fig. 26.65). The ureter is drawn down through a submucosal tunnel (made by blunt dissection with scissors or forceps between this new opening and the old ureteric orifice) spatulated and sutured to the margins of the ureteric orifice using interrupted 4/0 absorbable material. The hole in the mucosa is closed with similar material (Fig. 26.66).

Figs 26.62–26.66   *Politano–Leadbetter method of ureteric reimplantation*

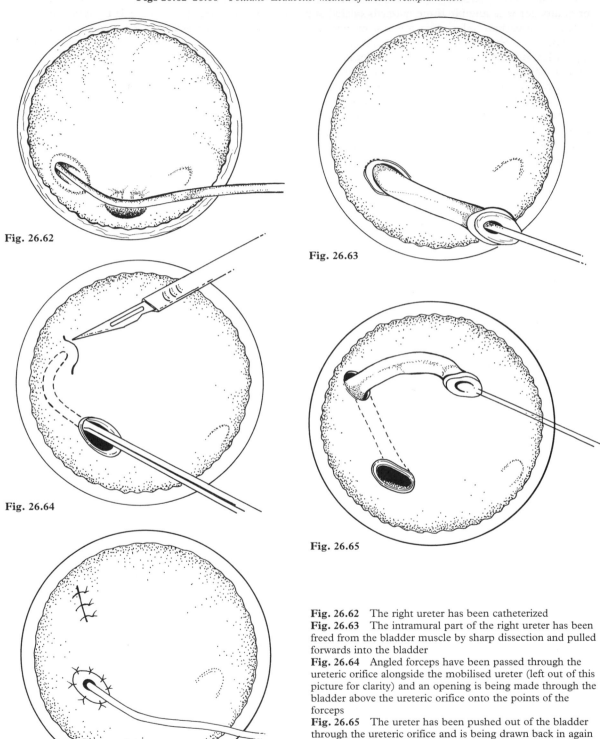

Fig. 26.62

Fig. 26.63

Fig. 26.64

Fig. 26.65

Fig. 26.66

Fig. 26.62   The right ureter has been catheterized

Fig. 26.63   The intramural part of the right ureter has been freed from the bladder muscle by sharp dissection and pulled forwards into the bladder

Fig. 26.64   Angled forceps have been passed through the ureteric orifice alongside the mobilised ureter (left out of this picture for clarity) and an opening is being made through the bladder above the ureteric orifice onto the points of the forceps

Fig. 26.65   The ureter has been pushed out of the bladder through the ureteric orifice and is being drawn back in again through the new incision

Fig. 26.66   The ureter has been brought down to the original ureteric orifice (to which it is now sutured) through the submucosal tunnel and the incision made into the bladder has been closed

The Politano-Leadbetter procedure is not suitable for adults nor is it suitable if the ureter is dilated and has to be tapered as well as reimplanted. In these circumstances the ureter is exposed by an extraperitoneal approach and freed down to the bladder. This is facilitated if the superior vesical vessels, and in women the uterine vessels also, are ligated and divided. The ureter is divided at the bladder and its lower end is ligated. The bladder is opened anteriorly and the proximal end of the ureter is brought into the bladder through a small stab incision in the posterolateral wall. A submucosal tunnel is fashioned downwards from this incision for some 5 cm and the mucosa (some distance above the ureteric orifice) is incised. The ureter is brought through the submucosal tunnel and sutured to the edges of the second incision.

If the ureter is very dilated (e.g. in patients with megaureter or reflux) the lower end should be tapered before it is brought through the submucosa tunnel. The ureter is tapered by excising a 'dart' from each side and suturing the defects with 4/0 catgut. The 'darts' must be longer than the length of the ureter incorporated into the submucosal tunnel. A splint can be left in if desired and removed later with cystoscopic biopsy forceps.

When the ureter is too short to be reimplanted into the bladder by these methods, a pedicled flap may be fashioned from the bladder wall (Boari), the intact bladder may be hitched up by stitching it to the psoas, an isolated segment of ileum may be used to bridge the gap, or (if the other kidney is normal) the kidney can be removed.

Boari flap (Figs 26.67–26.71)
This is used to bridge a long gap between ureter and bladder when treating strictures or injuries of the lower third of the ureter. The bladder has a good blood supply which is not compromised when the length of the flap is much longer than the base.

The ureter is mobilized and the superior vesical pedicle is divided. The flap is marked on the distended bladder with sutures or clips, cut with its base superolaterally, and folded upwards and backwards. A small incision is made through the posterior aspect of the flap about 2 cm from its cut edge and the ureter brought through it (Fig. 26.69). A submucosal tunnel is fashioned downwards for some 2 to 3 cm, opening the mucosa at its distal end. The cut end of the ureter is pulled through the submucosal tunnel into the lumen of the pouch with about 1 cm projecting. The projecting ureter can be spatulated and sutured to the margins of the opening or fliped and left projecting into the lumen like a nipple. It is best to splint the ureter with a 6–8 F portex tube leaving the distal end in the bladder so that it can be removed later. The flap and the bladder are closed with two layers of catgut and the site drained.

Urinary diversion operations (see Ashken, 1982)
Permanent diversion of urine is necessary in patients with malignant disease of the bladder either as part of the operation of total cystectomy or as a palliative measure when the growth is irremovable but causing severe symptoms; in patients with a contracted bladder due to tuberculosis, radiation or chronic interstitial cystitis (if conservative measures fail and bladder expanding operations are thought inappropriate); in some patients with vesicovaginal fistulae (particularly when caused by X-ray therapy or malignant disease and irreparable by operation); in patients with congenital extroversion of the bladder and in some patients with neurological disturbance of bladder function.

Transplantation of the ureters into the colon (ureterosigmoidostomy)
This operation, evolved from techniques originally described by Stiles and Coffey, is now considered an unsatisfactory means of urinary diversion. Its complications include (1) disruption and leakage from one or both anastomoses especially in patients who have had radiotherapy (2) renal infection caused by an obstruction at the anastomosis or reflux of colonic content into the ureter (3) hyperchloraemic acidosis (because colonic mucosa absorbs hydrogen and chloride from the urine) and (4) hypokalaemia from excessive loss of potassium-containing mucus.

Despite the external fistula and the need to wear an appliance permanently, diversion of urine to the skin using an ileal loop is the best and safest form of permanent diversion. A ureterosigmoidostomy may still be done however if a patient requires a diversion and refuses to have an external fistula. Before operation it is essential to determine the condition of the ureters and the function of the kidneys. Thickened or dilated ureters increase the hazards of the operation, but are not necessarily a contraindication.

The ultimate success of the operation depends on the ability of the anal sphincter to preserve continence when the colon is the receptacle, not only for faeces, but also for the entire urinary output. Assessment of the tone and contractility of the anal sphincter by rectal examination is not enough. If 250 or 300 ml of water can be retained in the colon for some hours during normal activities, the sphincters may be considered satisfactory.

The colon should be prepared as for colonic surgery (p. 479) and both ureters (if there are two) are transplanted at the same procedure, which can be done trans or extra peritoneally.

Trans-peritoneal approach. With the patient in the Trendelenberg position the lower abdomen is opened through a left paramedian or transverse incision and the small bowel is packed upwards. The right ureter is

Figs 26.67–26.71 *The Boari pouch*

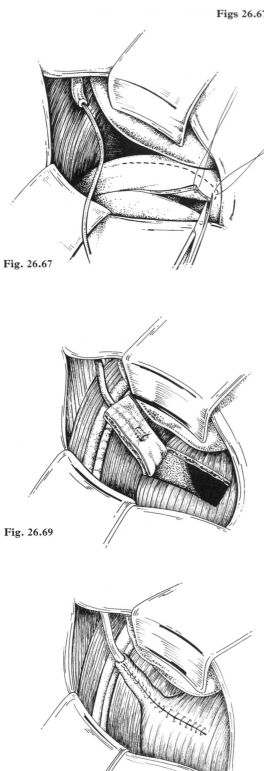

Fig. 26.67

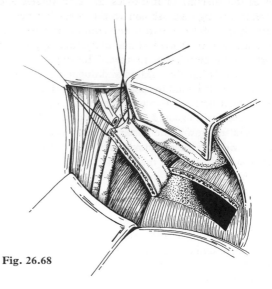

Fig. 26.68

Fig. 26.69

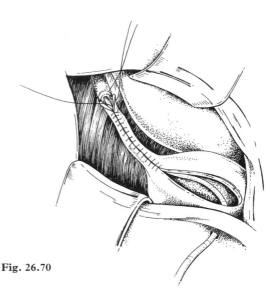

Fig. 26.70

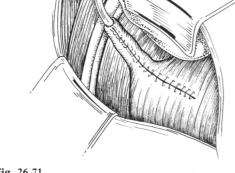

Fig. 26.71

Fig. 26.67 A long flap has been cut from the bladder with its base superolaterally and the ureter has been intubated
Fig. 26.68 The flap is raised
Fig. 26.69 The ureter has been anastomosed to the flap using a submucosal tunnel
Fig. 26.70 Alternatively, the ureter can be anastomosed to the edge of the flap
Fig. 26.71 The flap is closed

usually dealt with first. It is identified on the medial side of the caecum as it crosses the iliac vessels and delivered through an incision in the overlying peritoneum. It is mobilized with its adventitial coat down to the bladder and divided above a ligature applied as closely to the bladder as possible. The upper cut end is trimmed obliquely, and stay sutures are inserted (Fig. 26.72). It is laid alongside the lower part of the pelvic colon just above the pelvirectal junction, and a seromuscular incision 2 to 3 cm long is made in the bowel wall along the line in which the ureter lies comfortably without tension or kinking. The upper end of this incision is extended a little on either side, converting the linear into a T incision through serous and muscular coats only in the first instance. Flaps are carefully undermined with sharp and blunt dissection to separate them from the underlying mucosa at the lower end of the seromuscular incision, compatible in size with the obliquely cut end of the ureter. The mucous membrane of the colon is anastomosed to all coats of the ureter with interrupted 3/0 absorbable sutures (Fig. 26.73). When this has been completed, the edges of the seromuscular incision are sutured together over the ureter to provide protection and a valve, taking great care to avoid constriction of the lumen of the ureter especially at the upper end.

The peritoneum on the left side of the pelvic colon is incised along the 'white line' and the left ureter found. It is mobilized, like the right one, into the pelvis, divided above a ligature close to the bladder and transplanted into the colon in a similar manner to the right one, but usually at a slightly higher level (Fig. 26.74). Finally, the posterior peritoneal flaps are stitched to the bowel wall in front of the anastomosis which thus becomes extraperitoneal.

Extraperitoneal approach. This method has the advantage that the consequences of anastomotic leaks are less serious. It can be done through a single central incision or two oblique ones. The peritoneum is displaced medially, but unopened. The ureter is identified and freed downwards as far as possible to the bladder and divided above a ligature. An incision is made in the peritoneum, medial to the genital vessels and a loop of pelvic colon withdrawn. The edges of this peritoneal incision are stitched around the area of bowel selected for the anastomosis which is carried out by the technique already described. A similar operation is then undertaken on the opposite side. The site must be drained.

Many surgeons use splints of 5 F plastic or silastic tube; one end is inserted into the ureter for 10 cm and the other end is brought into the rectum and pulled out through the anus using a sigmoidoscope. Whether or not splints are used, the colon and the rectum should be kept empty for some days by inserting a rectal tube or a large (30F) Foley catheter.

Figs 26.72–26.74 *Ureterosigmoidostomy*

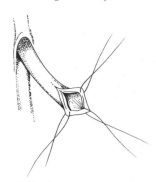

Fig. 26.72 The mobilized ureter spatulated and secured with stay sutures

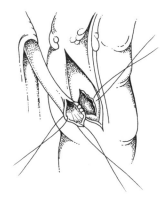

Fig. 26.73 Shows the colon illustrating the submucosal tunnel, intact mucosa above and an opening into the mucosa below. The full thickness of the ureteric wall is being sutured to the mucosa of the colon

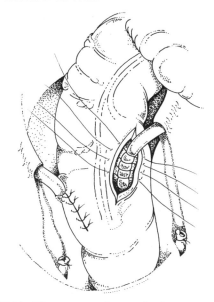

Fig. 26.74 The seromuscular coat has been sutured over the anastomosis of the right ureter. The left ureter has also been anastomosed and the sutures covering the anastomosis with seromuscular flaps have been inserted but not yet tied

Ileal conduit

The ileal conduit introduced by Bricker in 1958 has become the most popular method of permanent urinary diversion. The ultimate success of the operation depends upon the patients adjusting psychologically to the change in their way of life and of tolerating the appliance and managing it well enough to keep dry.

Before operation, time must be spent explaining the procedure to the patient and trying out the appliance (partly filled with water) on the intact skin. It is very helpful to introduce the patient to others who have had the same operation and who may answer questions the patient hesitates to ask of his medical advisers.

Operation. The bowel is prepared in the same way as for any small bowel resection. The best position for the stoma, predetermined by wearing the appliance on intact skin, is marked indelibly.

The abdomen is opened through a long left lower paramedian incision (Fig. 26.75). The appendix is removed, and the caecum is mobilized so that an isolated ileal loop will lie comfortably on the side wall of the abdomen, below or behind the caecum. Select a loop of terminal ileum which is not too near the ileocaecal junction (because of vitamin B_{12} absorbtion) which is healthy, which has not suffered radiation damage and which has a mesentery undistorted by calcified glands or adhesions. The loop must have a good blood supply; appropriate vessels are ligated after holding the bowel up and illuminating its mesentery with a powerful spot light while the loop is being prepared (Fig. 26.76). The loop most be long enough to extend without tension from the midline to some 5 cm beyond the site chosen on the skin for the stoma. The mesenteric incision can be much shorter on the left end of the loop, which will remain at or near the promontory of the sacrum, than on the right which has to emerge through the skin and form the stoma. The loop is then isolated, by cutting the bowel across at each end, and washed out with water or saline (Fig. 26.77). The continuity of the small bowel is restored in front of the isolated loop by an end-to-end anastomosis (p. 471). If the patient has previously had radiotherapy to the pelvis, the author does a one layered anastomosis using interrupted Nuralon sutures, inserted through all coats of the bowel except the mucosa. The ureters are then found (the right one by incising the posterior peritoneum on the medial aspect of the caecum, the left one by mobilizing the pelvic colon after dividing the peritoneum on its lateral aspect) mobilized and divided at a convenient level above the bladder. The left ureter is brought medially under the pelvic mesocolon to lie alongside the right one, both then emerging side by side through the incision in the posterior peritoneum, making sure that the left ureter does not form an acute angle, as it passes medially under the mesocolon, by mobilizing it well upwards. Various methods are available for implanting ureters into the loop, including the Wallace method or the Stiles method for patients who have previously had radiotherapy. In the *Wallace method* the ends of the ureter are spatulated by making a short slit anteriorly in each and their medial walls are sutured together to form one oval shaped stoma (Fig. 26.78). Each ureter is intubated for a distance of about 10 cm with 6 or 8 F (depending on the calibre of the ureters) polyvinyl or silastic tube, secured to the ureter with a stitch. A pair of forceps is passed down the ileal loop from the right to left and the tubes drawn through it. The oval stoma constructed from the lower ends of the ureters is stitched to the open left end of the loop with interrupted 3/0 catgut or dexon. The left end of the loop is then fixed by stitching it to the margins of the peritoneal opening. In the *Stiles* procedure (Fig. 26.80), the left end of the loop is closed with sutures or staples and the ureters are inserted separately into the loop. A splint is passed into each ureter and secured with a stitch. An Allis forceps is passed into the loop through the right end and a small incision made onto its opened jaws on the antimesenteric border some 2.5 cm from the left end of the loop. The ureteric splint is drawn through. A 2/0 catgut stitch is inserted into the loop about 2 cm to the right of the small incision made on the tips of the Allis forceps and brought out of the incision. It is then passed through one wall of the ureter (which can be spatulated) then passed back through the incision and out of the loop close to the entering thread. The ureter is pushed into the ileal loop and firmly secured by tying the suture. The right ureter is similarly inserted one cm or so to the right of the left one. The site for the stoma is prepared by excising a disc of skin and external oblique aponeurosis and incising the underlying muscles and peritoneum, making sure that the opening is wide enough to avoid narrowing the stoma. The stoma, with protruding ends of the splints, is slowly and very carefully withdrawn through the opening until about 5 cm projects. Any attempt to force it through may tear its mesentery and imperil its blood supply. The peritoneal aspect of the stoma is lightly scarified with a scalpel then everted or fliped so that some 2.5 cm projects beyond the skin (Fig. 26.79). The edge is sutured to the skin margin with dexon or catgut sutures. Finally the mesenteric defect is closed and the space lateral to the mesentery of the loop obliterated with a few sutures before the wound is closed with drainage. The splints are cut short so that 3 or 4 cm project from the stoma and an adhesive bag is applied.

Early complications include ileus, urinary leakage from

Figs 26.75–26.79   *Cutaneous ileoureterostomy*

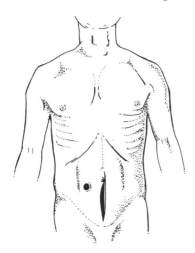

Fig. 26.75   Shows the incision, which can be a long midline or a left paramedian, and also the marking on the right side of the abdomen where the stoma will be

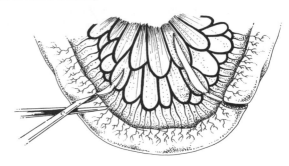

Fig. 26.76   The mesentery has been divided and vessels ligated on each side of the loop which is just being fashioned

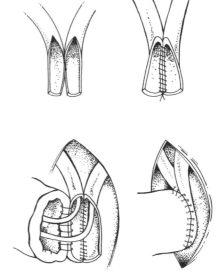

Fig. 26.78   The Wallace method of anastomosing the ureters to the open left end of the ileal loop. The lower ends of each ureter are approximated and spatulated. The medial aspects are sutured together to form one oval stoma. Each ureter has been separately intubated with a splint brought through the ileal loop from left to right and the oval stoma formed by the two ureters is being sutured to the left end of the ileum

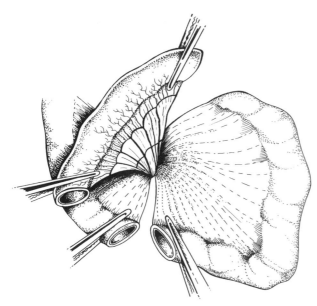

Fig. 26.77   The loop with its mesentery has been separated from the rest of the small bowel and ends of the ileum have been prepared for anastomosis (shown posterior to the loop for clarity)

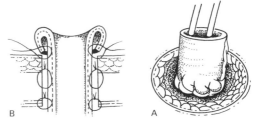

Fig. 26.79   The stoma has been constructed, evened or fliped and then sutured to the skin. Although many surgeons suture the stoma to deeper tissues as well, as illustrated here, the author tends not to do so

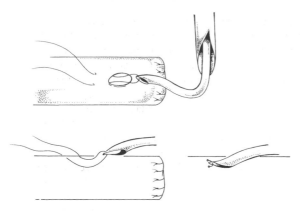

Fig. 26.80 Stiles method. The splint and forceps have been left out to improve clarity

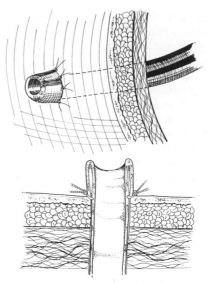

Fig. 26.81 Cutaneous ureterostomy. The ureter is brought through a separate stab incision away from the main wound used to exposed it and is everted or fliped, if that is possible, and sutured to the skin margin

the ureteric anastomosis or intestinal leakage from the small bowel anastomosis; later ones include stenosis of the stoma, parastomal hernia, ureteric obstruction, pyelonephritis, stone formation or intestinal obstruction. Reflux from loop to one or both ureters can often be demonstrated by X-rays made after the injection of radio-opaque media into the stoma (loopogram) but causes little problem because it is a low pressure system.

Transplantation of the ureter to the skin surface (cutaneous ureterostomy)
This operation, performed bilaterally as an elective procedure, was formally employed as an alternative to ureterocolic anastomosis but has been replaced by ureteroileostomy which has many advantages. The operation may still be useful however in patients who have only one ureter.

The middle third of the ureter is mobilized and divided as far down as possible, the lower end is ligated and the upper end is brought out through a small stab incision below the main incision (which should be much higher than usual so that it does not interfere with the positioning of the appliance). Its fascial sheath is sutured to the wound margin, so that it projects 2 to 3 cm beyond the surface. The protruding segment often sloughs away, leaving a meatus which tends to stenose. If the ureter is dilated it can sometimes be fliped or everted like the stoma of an ileal loop (Fig. 26.81). The procedure is obviously much simpler than an ileal loop, but much less satisfactory because the stoma stenoses and retracts, cannot easily be reconstructed and often has to be kept open with a small indwelling tube which has to be changed regularly. Nevertheless, it can be a useful operation if the aim is palliation and the patient's prognosis poor. Attempts to form a satisfactory stoma by incorporating the ureter

into a pedicle skin flap, enclosing it in the flaps of a Z incision or constructing a nipple ureterostomy by drawing the exteriorized part of the ureter into a cutaneous pedicle tube, are not always successful.

Ureterolysis

Retroperitoneal fibrosis
This reveals itself when it envelops and obstructs one or both ureters. It may also involve the aorta, the inferior vena cava or the common iliac vessels and it sometimes extends upwards to surround the heart and become one form of constrictive pericarditis (Ormond, 1981).

In some patients the fibrosis results from radiation therapy or the organization of a retroperitoneal haematoma from a leaking aortic aneurysm or other cause; in others it is the fibrous tissue of a scirrhous carcinoma containing so few malignant cells that they cannot easily be detected. The idiopathic form of the disease is the one requiring surgical correction and, as its name implies, the cause is unknown. Although it has been thought to be a neoplasm or autoimmune disease or a side effect of drugs like Methysergide (sometimes used in treatment of migraine), as little is known about the cause of idiopathic retroperitoneal fibrosis as about Peyronie's disease (p. 669) or Dupuytren's contracture (p. 201).

Patients with idiopathic retroperitoneal fibrosis present with renal failure, usually chronic but sometimes acute, or with other features of obstruction like pain or infection. The renal symptoms may be associated with, and sometimes overshadowed by, symptoms and signs of arterial or venous obstruction.

Treatment. If the disease is diagnosed early it is worth attempting treatment with glucocorticoids or drugs with glucocorticoid effects, but the patient must be carefully observed because, although retroperitoneal fibrosis is considered an insidious disease, it can advance very rapidly.

If the patient has acute or severe chronic renal failure, elective operation is deferred until renal function is improved by draining one or both kidneys by ureteric catheterization (and insertion of stents) or percutaneous nephrostomy although glucocorticoids can be given in the meantime. Both ureters are usually involved, although one side is worse than the other. If the disease is not too extensive, the patient fit and renal function satisfactory, it is tempting to deal with both ureters at one operation through an anterior incision; otherwise it is better to do one side at a time using a postero-lateral approach and freeing the ureter of what appears to be the best kidney.

Operation. After dissection enters the retroperitoneal space, the normal parts of the ureter, above and below the level of the fibrous plaque, are secured with tapes. The ureter is next separated and displaced from the fibrous tissue encasing and obstructing it. Fortunately this is often not difficult and the ureter can be lifted out intact after the fibrous tissue overlying it is cut or split. Sometimes however separation can be difficult and fraught with the risk of splitting open the ureter which is then very difficult to repair. Once the ureter is freed it is important to protect it from subsequent involvement in fibrous tissue, which may continue to increase. Some surgeons displace it laterally, securing it loosely to the quadratus lumborum muscle; others invaginate it into the peritoneum on the posterior abdominal wall with a few loose sutures.

If a small opening is inadvertently made into the ureter while it is being freed, it can be left or loosely sutured; if a large opening or split is made it is probably better to insert a stent rather than attempt repair. The stent can be a plastic or silicone tube, 6 or 7 F in diameter, 25 to 30 cm in length. One end is passed up the ureter so that its tip lies in the renal pelvis; the other end is passed down the ureter so that its terminal few centimetres lie in the bladder. The stent can be removed some time after the operation using a cystoscope and biopsy forceps. If the patient also has features of arterial or venous obstruction, an attempt should be made to free the affected vessels.

The operation does nothing for the cause, whatever that may be, of the disease. The fibrosis may later extend to involve blood vessels and even the ureters again no matter how well they are protected and patients must be followed up for a long time.

REFERENCES

Ashken M H 1982 Clinical practice in urology — urinary diversion. Springer Verlag, Heidelberg

Asmussen M, Miller A 1983 Clinical gynaecological urology. Blackwell, Oxford

Dees J E, Anderson E 1981 Coagulum pyelolithotomy. Urological Clinics of North America 8: 313

Ford T F, Watson G M, Wickham J E A 1983 Transurethral ureteroscopic retrieval of ureteric stones. British Journal of Urology 55: 626

Gil-Vernet J M 1983 Pyelolithotomy. In: Glenn J F (ed.) Urological surgery, 3rd edn. Lippincott, Philadelphia, p 159

Gosling J A, Dixon J S, Humpherson J R 1982 Functional anatomy of the urinary tract. Churchill Livingstone, Edinburgh

Grondal S, Hamberger B 1992 Primary aldosteronism. British Journal of Surgery 79: 484–485

Guerriero W G 1982 Trauma to the kidneys, ureters, bladder and urethra. Surgical Clinics of North America 62: 1047

Johnson J H 1984 Reimplantation of the ureter. Williams & Wilkins, London

Morris P J 1979 Renal Transplantation. In: Black D, Jones N F (eds) Renal disease, 4th edn, Blackwell Scientific Publications, Oxford, ch. 18

Newsam J E, Petrie J B 1981 Urology and renal medicine, 3rd edn. Churchill Livingstone, Edinburgh, p. 82

Ormond J K 1981 Idiopathic retroperitoneal fibrosis. In: Bergman H (ed.) The ureter, 2nd edn. Springer Verlag, Heidelberg

Robertson W G, Peacock M 1982 Risk factors in the formation of urinary stones. In: Chisholm G D, Williams D I (eds) Scientific foundations of urology, 2nd edn. Heinemann, London, p 267

Smith J W, Murphy T R, Blair J S G, Lowe K G 1983 Regional anatomy illustrated. Churchill Livingstone, Edinburgh

Turner-Warwick R 1980 Surgical access. In: Chisholm G D (ed.) Urology. Heinemann, London, p 402

Welbourne R B 1980 Some aspects of adrenal surgery. British Journal of Surgery 67: 723–727

Whitaker R H 1977 Hydronephrosis. Annals of the Royal College of Surgeons of England 59: 388–392

FURTHER READING

Blandy J P 1984 Operative urology, 2nd edn. Blackwell, Oxford

Farndon J R, Dunn J M 1992 Adrenal tumours. In: Johnson C D, Taylor I (eds) Recent advances in surgery. Churchill Livingstone, Edinburgh

Hargreave T B 1988 Practical urological endoscopy. Blackwell Scientific Publications, Oxford

McDougal W S (ed) 1984 Urology. In: Dudley H, Pories W J (eds) Rob and Smith's operative surgery, 4th edn. Butterworth, London

Sherwood T 1990 Imaging radiology. In: Chisholm G D, Fair W (eds) Scientific foundations of Urology, p 17

Whitfield H N, Hendry W F (eds) 1985 Textbook of genito-urinary surgery, vol. 2. Churchill Livingstone, Edinburgh

Wickham J E A, Miller R A 1983 Percutaneous renal surgery. Churchill Livingstone, Edinburgh

27

Bladder and prostate

T. B. HARGREAVE

Anatomy of bladder

The normal bladder has a capacity of 300 to 500 ml and lies in the pelvis. Its wall consists of smooth muscle separated from the internal lining of transitional cell epithelium by the lamina propria. When empty it is pyramidal in shape, with *an apex, a base, a superior surface, two inferolateral surfaces* and *a neck* which tapers to become continuous with the urethra. Only the superior surface and a small part of the base are covered with peritoneum (Fig. 27.1). As the bladder fills it becomes globular and the demarcation between its various surfaces is lost but its neck and base remain unaltered. When overdistended the bladder rises out of the pelvis into the abdomen pushing the peritoneum upwards. In infants, the bladder is an abdominal organ even when empty (Gosling, 1982).

The transitional cell epithelium is smooth and flat in the full bladder, but falls into transverse folds in the empty one. The *trigone* forms the base of the bladder. It is more vascular than the rest of the bladder, is firmly attached to the underlying muscle and smooth whether the bladder is full or empty. The *ureteric orifices* are found at the upper lateral angles of the trigone, and the bladder neck at its lower angle.

Relations

The *apex* of the bladder lies behind the symphysis pubis

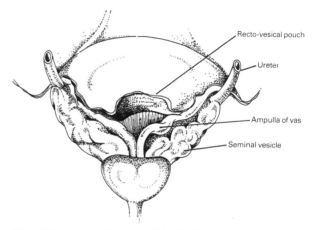

Fig. 27.2   A posterior view of the bladder

and is connected to the umbilicus by the median umbilical ligament (the fibrous remnant of the allantois). The *base* faces downwards and backwards and is separated from the rectum by the vasa deferentia and the seminal vesicles in the male (Fig. 27.2) and is closely related to the cervix uteri and the vagina in the female.

The *superior surface* is covered by peritoneum and related to ileum and pelvic colon and in the female to the body of the uterus. The *inferolateral surfaces* are separated from the pubis and from the floor and side walls of the pelvis by fat, and from each other by an ill defined border which disappears as the bladder fills. They lie below the peritoneum and are the parts of the bladder exposed by the suprapubic approach. The bladder is supported by thickenings of the pelvic fascia called the puboprostatic or pubovesical ligaments and by its attachments to the urethra and in the male to the prostate also.

The *retropubic space* (of Retzius) lies between the bladder and the pubis and contains fatty and areolar tissue. Below it is bounded by the puboprostatic or pubovesical ligaments, laterally by the side walls of the pelvis and superiorly it becomes continuous with the space between peritoneum and transversalis fascia.

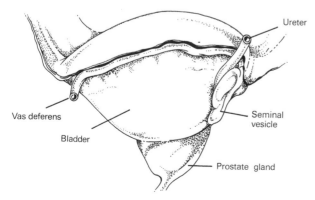

Fig. 27.1   A lateral view of the bladder

Blood supply

The bladder receives blood from the superior and inferior vesical, the middle rectal, the obturator and the pudendal arteries (all branches of the internal iliac artery). The vesical veins drain into the prevesical plexus or join the prostatic plexus which lies in the sulcus between bladder and prostate (plexus of Santorini). Both plexuses drain into the internal iliac veins.

Lymphatic drainage

Lymph from the bladder and the prostate goes first to nodes alongside the internal and common iliac and the obturator vessels, thence to the para-aortic nodes.

SURGICAL APPROACH TO THE BLADDER

The bladder can be approached endoscopically (p. 559), or openly by a suprapubic incision.

The suprapubic route is generally used for the treatment of bladder stones, diverticula, trauma and some tumours, for ureteric reimplantation or for access to the prostate gland. The operation is entirely extraperitoneal and usually through a transverse incision; for cystectomy the approach is intraperitoneal and usually through a vertical incision.

Technique

The operation is easier, particularly if the patient has had previous operations on the bladder or lower abdomen, if the bladder is filled with sterile water or saline through a catheter before operation. The table is tilted into a slight Trendelenberg position and illumination arranged so that light can be directed into the interior of the bladder. Although a vertical paramedian or midline incision can be used, the best approach is by a transverse one, because it heals better and is less liable to herniate. A transverse incision is made (see Fig. 27.47) in a skin fold about 2.5 cm above the pubis, opening the anterior rectus sheath with a transverse or U-shaped incision and freeing it from the underlying rectus and pyramidalis muscles by sharp dissection in the midline and by blunt dissection laterally. The lower flap of the rectus sheath can be split vertically in the midline down to the pubis to improve exposure of the retropubic space (see Fig. 27.48). (The U incision is useful because one or both limbs can be extended upwards to expose the lower ends of the ureters and even the lower pole of the kidney.) The recti and pyramidalis muscles are separated in the midline and retracted laterally although it is often better to divide the pyramidalis muscles transversely and reflect them with the rectus sheath.

The extraperitoneal fat and peritoneum are stripped upwards to expose the bladder wall which is easily recognized by its fasciculated appearance and by the many thin walled veins that course over its surface. The bladder wall is picked up at two points with tissue forceps or with stay sutures, opened vertically or transversely, and emptied by suction.

Difficulties and closure

The peritoneum may be inadvertently opened while exposing or opening the bladder especially if the two structures are adherent to each other after previous bladder or pelvic operations, but complications are unlikely if the peritoneum is repaired. The bladder is closed with continuous or interrupted absorbable stitches which should probably not penetrate the mucosa, although absorbable suture material rarely forms a nucleus for stone formation. A second layer of sutures can be inserted to invaginate the first layer, or to close the prevesical fascia over it. The rest of the wound is closed in layers and the retropubic or prevesical space is drained for 48 hours or sometimes longer.

SUPRAPUBIC CYSTOSTOMY

In this operation, a tube is placed in the bladder for drainage or as part of an operation on the bladder, prostate or urethra. As an operation on its own, when no more is done than drainage, it is much less frequently performed than formerly, and then only when urethral drainage is impracticable or is considered inadequate or unwise. When used in these circumstances, the operation can be performed openly or percutaneously under local anaesthesia.

Suprapubic cystostomy by open operation

This allows correct positioning of the tube, exploration of the bladder and the placement of the tube at a higher level on the abdominal wall than is possible by percutaneous methods; any future operations on the bladder are thus facilitated.

Technique

The bladder is exposed and a small incision is made into it as high as possible between two forceps or stay sutures. The bladder is emptied by suction and its interior explored with a finger to exclude calculi, diverticula and tumour. A self-retaining catheter of the De Pezzer, Malecot or Foley type (Fig. 27.3) is introduced

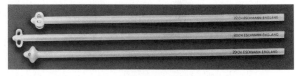

Fig. 27.3 Suprapubic catheters. Two Malecot above, and a De Pezzer below

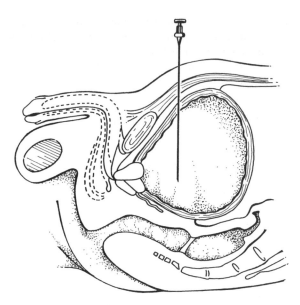

Fig. 27.4 Suprapubic cystostomy by the percutaneous method

and the bladder wall is sutured around it with one or two catgut stitches. The catheter is brought through a stab wound in the upper skin flap and anchored with a stitch prior to wound closure.

Suprapubic cystostomy by the percutaneous method (Fig. 27.4)

This method causes little discomfort to the patient and little scarring, but can only be done safely if the bladder is distended. It is the method of choice unless there are compelling reasons for exploring the bladder or for bringing the tube out at a high level.

Technique

Local anaesthetic (1 or 2% Lignocaine solution) is injected into the midline skin some 5 cm above the pubis. As the needle is advanced anaesthetic is injected into subcutaneous tissue, linea alba, extraperitoneal fat and bladder wall. The position and depth of the needle tip required to enter the bladder is recognized when urine can be aspirated. After a 5 minute interval for anaesthesia to develop, a 2 cm incision is made through skin and linea alba, and the suprapubic trocar and cannula are introduced into the bladder with a quick stabbing movement. It is best to introduce the needle — and later the trocar, cannula and catheter — directly backwards. To introduce them backwards and downwards is hazardous because they may pass below the bladder into the prostate.

The patient may experience momentary discomfort, but should have no pain if the anaesthetic has been correctly introduced. The trocar is withdrawn and the cannula is closed with a finger. A well lubricated Malecot or De Pezzer catheter stretched on an introducer is inserted and the cannula and introducer removed. The catheter is anchored to the skin margin with a stitch. Some 10 cm of catheter is left below skin level so that it is not forced out when the bladder contracts. One of the proprietary suprapubic cystostomy kits (Fig. 27.5) can be used, instead of a trocar and cannula with a Malecot or De Pezzer catheter.

INJURIES OF THE BLADDER

The bladder may be damaged by blows or crushing injuries to the lower abdomen or pelvis, by penetrating

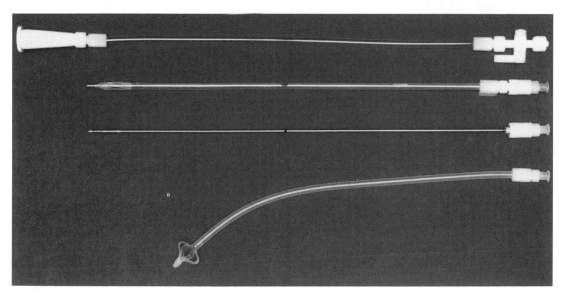

Fig. 27.5 Stamey suprapubic catheter set

wounds from sharp weapons or gunshot wounds (which are likely to be associated with damage to adjacent structures such as the rectum) or by fractures of the pelvis when the posterior urethra is also often injured. The bladder may be damaged during almost any major pelvic operation, especially hysterectomy, and during endoscopic resections of bladder tumours or the prostate. If recognized at the time, such injuries can be treated by simply keeping the bladder empty for some days after operation with a urethral catheter, although, if injured at an open operation, the bladder can be repaired with absorbable sutures as well. If not recognized at the time, urine or irrigating fluids extravasate into the extraperitoneal tissues and fistulae may develop between bladder and vagina or rectum. Intraperitoneal rupture, when urine extravasates into the peritoneal cavity, is uncommon and only occurs if the bladder is distended at the moment of injury.

The diagnosis should be made from the patient's history and inability to pass urine. The bladder distends if the urethra is injured, but a palpable suprapubic swelling may not be a distended bladder but a haematoma from a ruptured bladder, which will always be empty or contain only a small quantity of blood-stained urine.

If bladder rupture is suspected, a catheter should be passed and a cystogram made. If a catheter cannot be passed, the posterior urethra is probably injured and only operation will determine if the bladder is also injured. A ruptured bladder should be explored once adequate resuscitation has been achieved. If the tear is extraperitoneal, blood stained urine wells up from the retropubic space. An anterior tear is usually located without difficulty and can be closed. A posterior tear may not be seen until the bladder has been opened and even then may be difficult to repair. If the tear cannot be repaired satisfactorily, it is essential to drain the bladder by suprapubic cystostomy. In all cases the extravesical tissues must also be drained. If there is no evidence of extraperitoneal rupture, the peritoneum is opened, the intestines packed upwards and the upper surface of the bladder examined. If a tear is found it is repaired with two layers of stitches.

Both the peritoneal cavity and the bladder are carefully dried out and each is drained. After both extra and intraperitoneal ruptures the bladder may be kept empty with a urethral catheter, but it is wise to leave a suprapubic tube as well, if bladder repair was difficult.

DIVERTICULA OF THE BLADDER

Nearly all bladder diverticula are acquired as a result of increased intravesical pressure caused by obstruction to the urinary outflow. Congenital diverticula may occur at the vault (site of the urachus) or near the ureteric orifices where the part of the bladder derived from the cloaca joins the part derived from the mesonephric duct. The walls of congenital diverticula have the same structure as the bladder, whereas the walls of acquired diverticula have little if any muscle, and therefore little if any contractility. They fill and expand when the bladder contracts and empty when it relaxes. The urine within them stagnates predisposing to infection, stones, metaplasia and tumour. Most diverticula arise from the infero-lateral or posterior wall of the bladder close to a ureteric orifice. The opening of the diverticulum into the bladder (called the neck of the diverticulum) is smaller than the cavity of the diverticulum. Diverticula can be seen in the cystographic phase of an intravenous urogram, but their size, shape, position and relationship to the ureteric orifices can only be determined by cystoscopy and by cystography (Fig. 27.6), which must include micturating and postmicturition views (Fig. 27.7). Many diverticula cause little if any trouble after the associated obstruction has been dealt with, and excision is indicated only for those that are large or infected, that contain stone or tumour (Fig. 27.8), that obstruct a ureter or distort a ureteric orifice or cause vesico-ureteric reflux.

Methods of diverticulectomy

At operation, the diverticulum is completely excised leaving the bladder wall smooth. Small diverticula may be exposed through an intravesical approach. The bladder is opened by a suprapubic incision and the depth of the diverticulum is ascertained with finger or probe. The wall of the diverticulum is seized with tissue forceps (Fig. 27.9) and invaginated into the bladder (Fig. 27.10) to allow excision at its neck and closure of the defect in the bladder wall with catgut sutures. If this is considered unsafe, two or more pairs of tissue forceps are applied to the margin of the opening and a circular incision is made through the mucosa and muscular coats of the bladder wall around it. The severed neck of the diverticulum is drawn into the bladder and dissection is continued closely around the diverticulum with curved scissors until it can be removed. As the ureter lies close to the diverticulum, it is wise to insert a ureteric catheter into the ureter as soon as the bladder is opened and before any attempt is made to mobilize or remove the diverticulum. It is best to mobilize large diverticula extravesically (Figs 27.11–27.13), preserving the ureter which is often adherent to the wall of the diverticulum. The procedure is facilitated if the bladder is opened and a finger or pack placed in the diverticulum so as to combine intra- and extravesical dissection (Fig. 27.12).

Once the diverticulum is freed it is removed flush

Figs 27.6–27.8 *Bladder diverticulum on contrast X-rays*

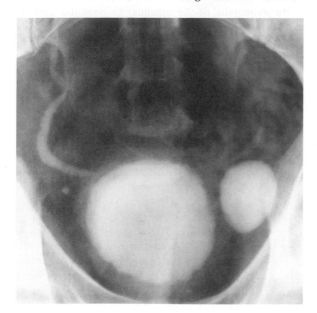

Fig. 27.6 Prevoiding phase

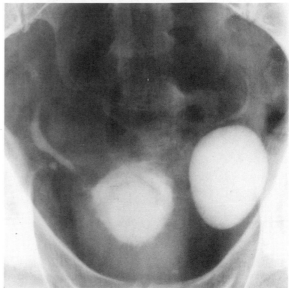

Fig. 27.7 Postvoiding phase. Note how the diverticulum expands as the bladder contracts

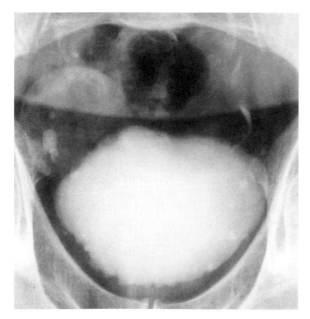

Fig. 27.8 A diverticulum arising from the right side of the bladder and filled with tumour

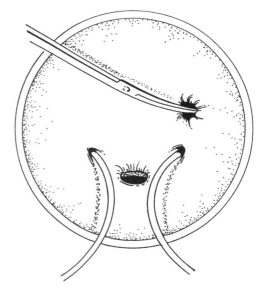

Fig. 27.9 Intravesical excision of bladder diverticulum. The ureters are 'protected' by ureteric catheters. The wall of the diverticulum is grasped with tissue forceps

with the bladder wall and the bladder is repaired. Both bladder and extravesical space must be drained. Sometimes a ureter opens into the diverticulum or is so close to the diverticulum that it has to be divided and reimplanted into the bladder after the diverticulum has been excised. When the fundus of the diverticulum lies posteriorly between bladder and rectum, and is densely adherent to rectum, it is best to leave some of the diverticulum rather than risk making a rectal fistula.

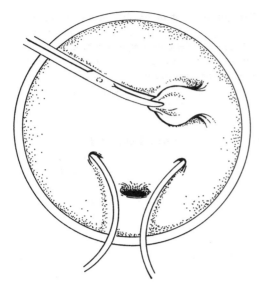

Fig. 27.10   Intravesical excision of bladder diverticulum. The diverticulum has been invaginated into the bladder

Figs 27.11–27.13   *Extravesical excision of bladder diverticulum*

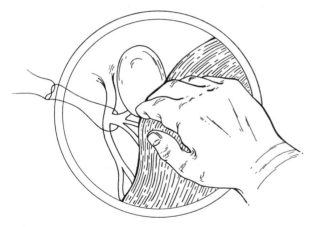

Fig. 27.11   The diverticulum is partially displayed and the superior vesical pedicle is ligated and divided

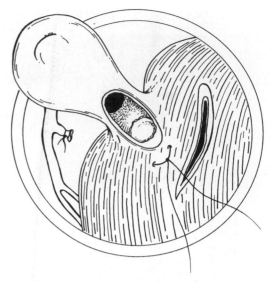

Fig. 27.12   The diverticulum is gradually and carefully mobilized and freed from colon, pelvis, ureter and bladder until only attached to the bladder by its neck. This procedure can be facilitated by inserting a finger or pack into the diverticulum through an incision in the anterior bladder wall

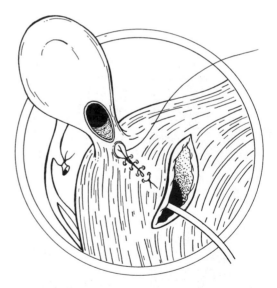

Fig. 27.13   The diverticulum is removed flush with the bladder wall, and the defect closed with absorbable sutures. Some of the fundus can be left behind to fibrose if densely adherent to rectum or colon

STONES IN THE BLADDER (See Husain, 1984)

Operations for the removal of stones from the bladder (lithotomy) were carried out before the time of Hippocrates, but only in the early part of this century were instruments constructed for treating bladder stones endoscopically. Primary bladder stones were very common in Britain until the end of the 19th century, but although still common in such developing parts of the world as Egypt, Thailand and Sudan, they are now all but unknown in Britain and other affluent parts of Western Europe and North America. Instead renal stones have become increasingly common and bladder stones (Figs 27.14 & 27.15) now only form in an infected or obstructed bladder or in one containing foreign material. The treatment of bladder stone depends as much on the primary disease as it does on the stone itself, and many stones eminently suitable for endoscopic removal are removed by open operation when the primary disease can be treated at the same time.

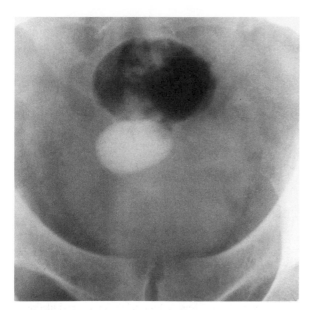

Fig. 27.14 Plain X- ray showing a large smooth bladder stone

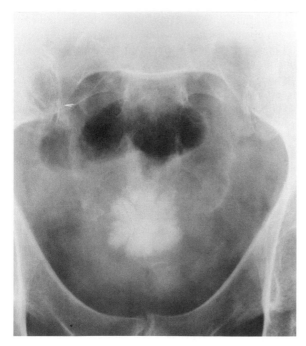

Fig. 27.15 Plain X-ray showing a bladder stone of Jackstone type

Stones smaller than 8 mm in diameter are usually passed spontaneously because the normal urethra measures 26F or more (i.e. 8.6 mm); if not, they can be washed out or gently removed intact with biopsy forceps through a resectoscope sheath.

Do not attempt to crush a stone, however small or soft it may appear, with biopsy forceps otherwise you can break the delicate hinge mechanism of the instrument and find the cups of the instrument fixed immobile in the open position.

Stones larger than 8 mm can be treated by litholapaxy or open operation.

Litholapaxy (see Mitchell, 1981)

In this procedure, a 'blind' or an optical lithotrite is passed through the urethra into the bladder and used to crush the stone into fragments small enough to be washed out of the bladder through a resectoscope sheath using an Ellik or similar syringe. Lithotrites are all large instruments (26F) which can easily damage the urethra, prostate or bladder while being passed, manipulated or rotated as the stone is grasped or crushed. There are several contraindications to their use:

1. Stones larger than 2 cm cannot be grasped between the jaws of a visualizing lithotrite and although stones up to 3 cm diameter can be crushed with a blind lithotrite by experienced hands, they are usually best removed by open operation.

2. Stones inside bladder diverticula, even ones smaller than 2 cm, cannot be safely grasped and crushed with a lithotrite and should be treated by open operation when the diverticula can also be removed.

3. Attempts to crush bladder stones in patients with large prostates are often unsuccessful and frequently followed by urinary retention or septicaemia or both. It is usually best to remove both stone and prostate by open operation, although if the prostate can be resected a lithotrite can be passed and the stone crushed when the resection is completed or at a second operation some weeks later.

4. Some bladder stones, particularly those with a high content of urate, are too hard to crush and best removed by open operation.

5. Attempts to crush stones in a very infected, congested bladder are frequently followed by severe bleeding or septicaemia and should only be made if the infection can be controlled by treatment with antibiotics.

6. In young boys the urethra is always too narrow to accommodate even a small lithotrite. In adults, a narrow, strictured urethra can be enlarged by dilatation or urethrotomy before litholapaxy but the procedure may well aggravate the stricture.

7. Stones that form around the balloon of a Foley catheter or the end of a suprapubic catheter can usually be crushed after the catheter has been removed; ones that form on fragments of catheters left behind in the bladder, or other foreign bodies inserted into the blad-

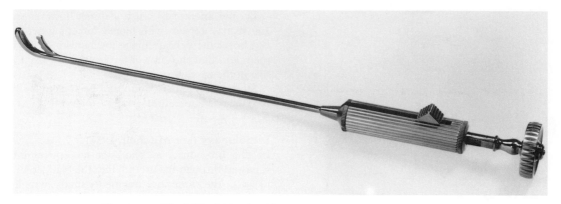

Fig. 27.16   The Miller Lithotrite (Courtesy of GU Manufacturing Co. Ltd)

der by the patient, are best removed by open operation when the foreign material can also be removed.

8. Phosphatic encrustations on the surface of bladder tumours may be mistaken for stones. They can usually be easily crushed and washed out even though attached to the bladder wall but the underlying mucosa must be carefully inspected and biopsied even if it looks reasonably normal.

Stones may form on nonabsorbable suture material — 'a hanging stone'. Such material is never used for suturing the bladder but may be inserted inadvertently through the bladder during operations on women for stress incontinence. Both stone and suture can usually be removed endoscopically.

Technique
The patient is prepared and placed in the same position as he would be for cystoscopy or transurethral resection and the X-rays should be reviewed. The urethra, prostate and bladder are examined endoscopically and a decision made about the appropriate procedure for removing the stones, remembering that strictures, infection and bleeding complicate litholapaxy more often than open operations.

'Blind' lithotrite
This instrument is safe if the operator knows what he is doing, unsafe otherwise (Fig. 27.16). After the preliminary endoscopic inspection, the whole cystoscope is removed leaving 100 to 150 ml of fluid in the bladder. With the jaws of the lithotrite closed and the instrument well lubricated, it is passed through the urethra into the bladder in the same way as a bougie or a cystoscope. Once its tip lies in the bladder the jaws are opened so that they face towards the centre of the bladder.

The instrument is gently moved, rotated from side to side and shaken as the jaws are gently opened and closed until the stone is felt between them. The stone is

gripped but not yet crushed, by partially tightening the jaws and the instrument is advanced into the bladder and rotated through 180° to make sure that mucosa is not also gripped. The stone is crushed by screwing the jaws of the instrument together. The procedure is repeated until all the stone appears crushed; the lithotrite is removed and replaced with a 24 or 26F resectoscope sheath, through which the fragments can be evacuated with an Ellik syringe. The bladder is then examined by inserting a telescope and short bridge into the resectoscope sheath. If any fragments remain they can be lifted out with biopsy forceps if they are small, or crushed by reinserting the lithotrite (after removing the resectoscope sheath and telescope) if they are large.

The greatest care and gentleness must be exercised when passing and repassing the resectoscope sheath and lithotrite.

The visualizing lithotrite
Visualizing or optical lithotrites tend to be smaller and less strong than 'blind' ones and should only be used for stones less than 2 cm in diameter.

Some visualizing lithotrites are inserted directly into the urethra (Fig. 27.17) while others are passed through a 26 or 27F resectoscope sheath (Fig. 27.18).

With each type, a direct view or fore-oblique telescope is passed through the centre of the instrument. The author prefers those that are passed through a sheath because the same sheath can be used for washing out the fragments and inspecting the bladder and the repassing of different instruments down the urethra is avoided. With modern lithotrites it is not usually difficult to see, grasp and crush the stone. Small fragments and dust may obscure vision, but can be removed by frequent irrigation. A urethral Foley catheter is retained for 2 or 3 days after litholapaxy.

The ultrasonic lithotripter
This instrument fragments stones by ultrasonic waves

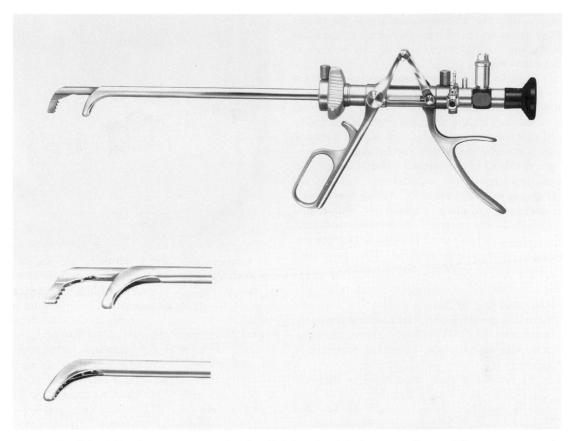

Fig. 27.17 Visualizing Lithotrite. The jaws are closed and lubricated and the instrument is passed like a cystoscope or bougie (Courtesy of Storz Ltd)

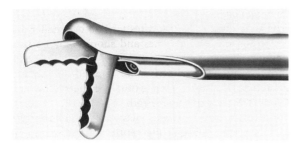

Fig. 27.18 Visualizing lithotrite. This instrument is passed through a resectoscope sheath. Detail shows the end of the instrument with the jaws opened (Courtesy of Storz Ltd)

applied directly to the stone with an ultrasonic transducer which is passed through a specially designed endoscope. The instrument incorporates a powerful suction system which prevents the stone moving out of contact with the vibrating transducer when it is being used. The instrument is no larger than an ordinary visual lithotrite and the ultrasonic waves do no damage to the bladder wall, thus distinguishing it from the electronic lithotripter which generates explosive discharges and which can damage the bladder wall. However, the ultrasonic lithotripter is very expensive and not yet in general use.

Vesicolithotomy

This is the name given to the open operation for the removal of bladder stone. The bladder is exposed and opened as already described and the stone is removed. The bladder is drained with a urethral Foley catheter for at least 3 days.

BLADDER TUMOURS

Most patients with a bladder tumour complain of painless haematuria; however, those with carcinoma in situ or squamous carcinoma often present with frequency, urgency and dysuria and may be thought to be suffering only from chronic cystitis and indeed they may have secondary infection. Many tumours reveal themselves as filling defects in the cystographic phase of the intravenous urogram (Fig. 27.19) and all can be seen at cystourethroscopy.

Only when the *stage of the tumour* has been assessed and been put into its correct TNMG category, can the appropriate treatment be decided. The *T category* represents the local state of the tumour and is assessed by clinical examination, urography, cystoscopy, bimanual examination under anaesthesia and by biopsy or transurethral resection of the tumour. The *N category* represents the state of the regional and juxtaregional lymph glands and is assessed by clinical examination and radiography including lymphography and urography. The *M category* represents the presence or absence of metastases and is assessed by clinical examination, radiography and isotope studies. The *G category* represents histological grading (UICC, 1978).

The T categories (Fig. 27.20)

Tis A preinvasive carcinoma, carcinoma in situ or flat tumour.

Ta A papillary noninvasive carcinoma (confined to mucosa).

T1 A T1 tumour is often impalpable on bimanual examination but if it is palpable it is a freely mobile mass that can no longer be felt after complete transurethral resection. Microscopically the tumour does not invade beyond the lamina propria.

T2 On bimanual examination there is induration of the bladder wall which is mobile. There is no residual induration after complete transurethral resection of the lesion and/or there is microscopic invasion of superficial muscle.

T3 On bimanual examination a nodular mobile mass is palpable in the bladder wall and persists after transurethral resection of the exophytic portion of the lesion and/or there is microscopic invasion of deep muscle (T3a) or of extension through the bladder wall (T3b).

As attempts to resect too much of a T3 tumour can cause serious complications it is mainly on the results of bimanual examination that the decision is made whether the lesion is T3a or T3b.

T4 A T4 tumour is fixed or extends to neighbouring structures.

T4a The tumour infiltrates the prostate, uterus or vagina.

T4b The tumour is fixed to the pelvic wall or abdominal wall or both.

The suffix (m) may be added to the appropriate T category to indicate multiple tumours, e.g. T2(m)

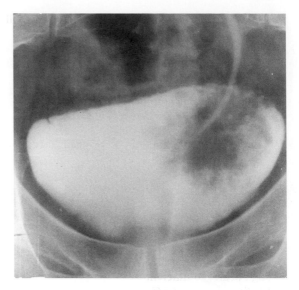

Fig. 27.19 Cystogram shows filling defect caused by a tumour in left side of the bladder

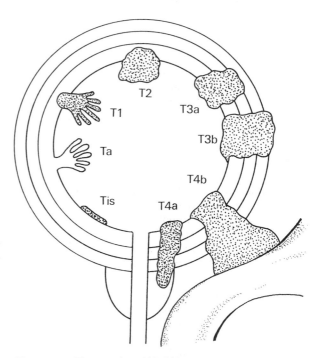

Fig. 27.20 T categories of bladder tumour

N category

N0 No evidence of regional lymph node involvement

N1 Evidence of involvement of a single homolateral regional lymph node

N2 Evidence of involvement of contralateral or bilateral or multiple regional lymph nodes

N3 Evidence of involvement of fixed regional lymph

nodes or there is a fixed mass on the pelvic wall with a free space between this and the tumour

N4 Evidence of involvement of juxtaregional nodes

NX The minimum requirements to assess the regional and/or juxtaregional lymph nodes cannot be met.

As pedal lymphangiography does not show the internal iliac nodes which are the regional glands of the bladder the N category is usually expressed as NX, meaning that the condition of the lymph nodes is unknown.

M category

M0 No evidence of distant metastases

M1 Evidence of distant metastases

G — histopathological grading

G0 Papilloma i.e. no evidence of anaplasia

G1 High degree of differentiation

G2 Medium degree of differentiation

G3 Low degree of differentiation or undifferentiated

GX Grade cannot be assessed.

Endoscopy

A careful endoscopy is carried out and must include urethroscopy because secondary tumours are frequently present in the urethra, particularly in the prostatic part. Assessment of the tumour includes its size, site appearance and number; the bladder is emptied, noting its capacity, the cystoscope is withdrawn and a bimanual examination carried out to determine the T category (which may be changed following the histologist's report).

After the bimanual examination, the endoscope is re-introduced and biopsies obtained using a resectoscope for proliferative tumours and pinch biopsy forceps (Fig. 27.21) for flat tumours. Three or four random mucosal pinch biopsies must be taken from other parts of the bladder because dysplastic mucosa or areas of carcinoma in situ may look normal when viewed through a cystoscope. Tumours of the bladder can be much more extensive than at first appears. Trans-urethral resection of the tumour provides a good biopsy which helps to assess the T category of the tumour and is a means of treating Ta, T1 and some T2 tumours, which can often be completely resected. (The specimen obtained should be submitted to pathology in two con-

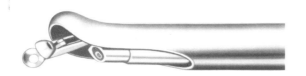

Fig. 27.21   Pinch biopsy forceps (Courtesy of Storz Ltd)

tainers; the bulk of the tumour in one, the base in the other, so that the depth of the tumour invasion can be determined). When resecting bladder tumours it is often necessary to resect well into the bladder wall (see Fig. 27.23b) and there is a risk of extravasation of large amounts of fluid. For this reason a continuous flow resectoscope should always be used.

Tis (carcinoma in situ)

The description suggests a very early stage of malignant disease and indeed, the changes are initially confined to mucosa and do not even extend into the lamina propria. However, in situ tumours of the bladder are frequently anaplastic (G3), much more widespread in the bladder than first appears, and often also involve the transitional epithelium of the urethra, ureters and pelvicaliceal systems. The bladder capacity is often reduced. In situ areas are flat and red, sometimes messy and often look infective rather than neoplastic. Furthermore, biopsies taken from mucosa that looks normal often reveal in situ or dysplastic changes and pinch biopsies must be taken from not only the suspicious areas, but also from selected normal areas in the bladder and prostatic urethra. To confuse in situ tumours with infection is particularly easy, because patients often complain, not of haematuria, but of frequency and dysuria, and it is, perhaps, not surprising that many are treated with antibiotics.

It is tempting to treat this stage of disease by resection or by electrocoagulation using an electrode through a cystoscope or a ball or roller loop through a resectoscope. But the change from dysplasia to in situ carcinoma and then to infiltrative carcinoma can be rapid, and patients treated in these ways must be carefully followed up by cytology, endoscopy and biopsy and treated more radically if the disease progresses or fails to respond. If the prostatic ducts are not involved, intravesical BCG may be considered; radiotherapy has little to offer, and many patients with in situ carcinoma of the bladder require cystectomy. When cystectomy is carried out, the cut ends of the ureters should be examined for in situ change by frozen section before the diversion procedure starts. If in situ changes are so extensive that healthy ureter is not available for the diversion, parenteral chemotherapy with Cyclophosphamide or Methotrexate may be considered postoperatively.

Ta tumours

These tumours are usually 3 cm or less in diameter, pedunculated and papillary. They can be resected easily and completely with one or two sweeps of the cutting loop of a resectoscope (Fig. 27.22) and the base can be coagulated with the cutting or ball loop. Larger ones can be excised by resecting the proliferative part of the tumour first and then the base which should be

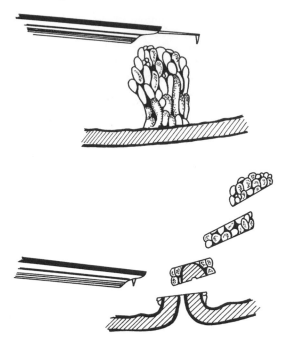

Fig. 27.22   Transurethral resection of Ta or T1 bladder tumour

kept separate from the proliferative part of the tumour when the specimen is sent to the pathologist.

T1 tumours

These tumours can also be completely resected and are often only recognized to be T1 rather than Ta ones when the pathologist reports that they involve the lamina propria.

Multiple tumours (Tam, T1m)

Ta or T1 tumours can be resected if they are solitary or few in number. If there are too many to resect and they do not involve the urethra, they can be treated by bladder instillations. Of the various substances available for this purpose Ethoglucid (Triethyleneglycol Diglycidyl, Epodyl) is as useful as any. 100 ml of a 1% solution is instilled into the bladder through a catheter which is then removed; the patient empties the bladder 1 hour later. This process is repeated weekly for 12 weeks then monthly for an indefinite period (Soloway, 1982). More radical treatment by X-ray therapy or cystectomy needs to be considered if multiple tumours do not respond, if the tumours are large or the prostatic urethra is involved.

Large T0 or T1 tumours

To resect large T0 or T1 tumours is possible but requires much time and patience and is often accompanied by severe haemorrhage which can be difficult to control. Bleeding vessels are best coagulated before

more cuts are made into the tumour and resecting part of the prostate or the bladder neck often facilitates the procedure, by rendering the base more accessible. The size of the tumour can often be reduced before resection by suction using a Wardill syringe through a resectoscope sheath or by the Helmstein distention method. Open diathermy is a poor alternative to resection as it seems to spread the tumour throughout the bladder or worse, into the suprapubic wound. Many large tumours considered to be T0 or T1 before resection prove to be T2 or worse when examined by the pathologist.

T2 tumours

T2 tumours involve the superficial muscle and are usually palpable on bimanual examination although some are considered T1 until the resected base of the tumour is examined under a microscope. They can be resected if the tumour is well or moderately differentiated (G1 or G2) (Fig. 27.23), but if the tumour is anaplastic (G3) it is wise to treat them like T3 tumours.

T3 tumours

T3 tumours have infiltrated the deep muscle of the bladder (T3a) or right through the bladder wall into the perivesical tissues (T3b), but remain mobile and are easily palpable. All of the tumour cannot be resected and attempts to do so will only perforate the bladder (Fig. 27.24). Although such perforations are usually extraperitoneal and heal if the bladder is kept empty for some time, they delay the radical treatment necessary to cure the tumour and it is necessary to resect only sufficient of the tumour for biopsy purposes. The treatment of T3 tumours, which causes much discussion and controversy, can be by X-ray therapy or by cystectomy or by cystectomy and X-ray therapy. Which treatment is offered depends upon the facilities available and the views of the surgeon and radiotherapist; although many believe that cystectomy preceded by a modified course of X-ray therapy gives better results than X-ray therapy or cystectomy alone, especially in patients under 65 years. The author treats patients with T3 tumours by a full course of X-ray therapy and carries out cystectomy later, if the tumour fails to respond. This decision is made only after some 3 to 6 months have elapsed since X-ray treatment has been completed.

T4 tumours

T4a tumours involve the prostate but are amenable to the same sort of treatment given to patients with T3 tumours because the prostate gland can be included in the X-ray field and is invariably removed at cystectomy. In women T4b tumours involving the vagina or uterus (which can be removed along with the bladder) can be

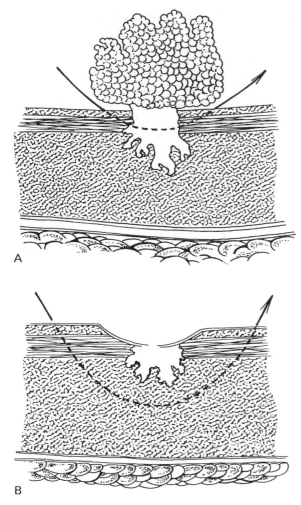

Fig. 27.23 Resection of T2 tumour

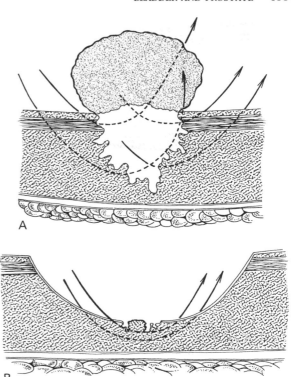

Fig. 27.24 Resection of T3 tumour. Although complete resection of T3a tumours is theoretically possible it is very unwise to attempt it

radically treated by surgery, but most T4b tumours are incurable because they are too large or too fixed and suitable only for palliative treatment.

Tumours in bladder diverticula

Tumours in bladder diverticula present special problems. Firstly, the extent or even the presence of the tumour may not be appreciated by endoscopy or on the pre- and postmicturition cystograms. These must be interpreted carefully because blood clot can produce filling defects indistinguishable from those of tumour. Secondly, since acquired diverticula have little, if any, muscle in their walls, a tumour becomes T3b as soon as it spreads through the lamina propria.

In diverticula, Ta, T1 or T3b tumours cannot be resected endoscopically and are best treated by excising the diverticulum together with a margin of bladder at its neck (p. 624); more serious tumours are treated by X-ray therapy or cystectomy.

PARTIAL CYSTECTOMY

This was once a popular operation for the treatment of bladder tumours that could be excised together with a 2.5 cm margin of healthy bladder, even if this included one ureteric orifice or part of the bladder neck. It is now only used to treat some tumours in the vault of the bladder which may be primary or secondary to rectal or colonic tumours, when the partial cystectomy is part (often a small part) of an operation which includes resection of rectum or colon.

Technique

For primary vault tumours, a transverse suprapubic incision is made and the peritoneum opened. The peritoneum is incised transversely over the back of the bladder so that the peritoneum on the vault will be excised with the tumour. The bladder is mobilized from peritoneum posteriorly by blunt dissection, except in the midline where it has to be cut away from peritoneum. Next the bladder is mobilized on each side by dividing the superior vesical pedicles and the bladder is opened anteriorly well away from the tumour. The tumour, with a 2.5 cm margin of healthy bladder, is excised together with the overlying peritoneum

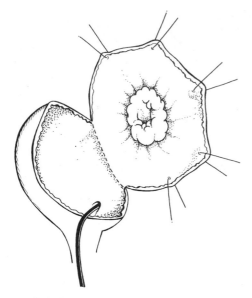

Fig. 27.25 Partial cystectomy. The tumour is excised together with a wide margin all round it of healthy bladder, without disturbing ureters or bladder neck

(Fig. 27.25). The bladder is closed in two layers with plain catgut and the wound closed in layers with drainage. The bladder should be kept empty for at least 7 or 8 days with a Foley catheter.

For the resection of bladder adherent to or infiltrated by rectal or colonic tumours, the technique varies with each case. In all it is important to find and secure both ureters at an early stage in the dissection; one or even both, may have to be reimplanted into the bladder once the procedure is completed. The bladder is sutured in two layers and kept empty with a Foley catheter.

TOTAL CYSTECTOMY (see Paulson, 1983)

The major indication for total cystectomy is malignant disease of the bladder which has not responded to or is unsuitable for less radical treatment. Thus the operation for malignant disease will be described although cystectomy may also be required for patients (fortunately now few) with severe haemorrhage from radiation cystitis or for patients with a neurogenic bladder who have previously had a urinary diversion and develop a *pyocystis* (a bladder filled with pus).

Preparation
The type of urinary diversion to be done will have been decided when the operation was discussed with the patient and this determines the preoperative preparation. Despite the disadvantages of an external fistula the author prefers an ileal loop diversion and will only do a ureterosigmoidostomy if the patient refuses to have an external opening.

Operation
A long lower left paramedian incision rather than a transverse one is recommended because it provides adequate exposure and does not interfere with the siting of the ileostomy opening in the right iliac fossa, nor with the wearing of the appliance. On opening the peritoneum, the bladder is examined to ensure that it can be removed, and the iliac, obturator and abdominal lymph glands and the liver are assessed for metastatic spread. In men an elliptical incision is made in the peritoneum behind the bladder so that the peritoneum on its vault can be removed with the bladder and the posterior aspect of the bladder is freed from peritoneum by a combination of blunt and sharp dissection. In women the uterus, cervix uteri and upper part of the vagina are removed together with the bladder and, in them, the posterior layer of the broad ligament is incised behind the uterus. Next the lateral aspects of the bladder are mobilized close to the side walls of the pelvis, dividing first the superior vesical pedicles and next the inferior vesical pedicles. In women, the round and the falciform ligaments are also divided. It should now be possible to demonstrate and secure the ureters with slings of tape or tube. These are divided about 2.5 cm above the bladder and the distal ends ligated. To prevent contamination of the wound with urine some surgeons temporarily put the proximal ends of the ureters into plastic bags. A long 6 or 8F polythene or silastic tube (a wider one if the ureter is very dilated) may be inserted some 10 cm into each ureter and secured to the cut end of the ureter with a suture, inserted in such a way that it does not interfere later with the ileo-ureteric anastomosis (p. 616). These tubes will eventually be brought through the ileal loop and out of the stoma (or put into the bowel if a ureterocolic anastomosis is done) and left for some days, but meantime they are drained into a plastic bag.

The steps of the operation can be modified by exposing and ligating the internal iliac arteries at an early stage of the operation as follows: once the peritoneum has been incised transversely behind the bladder in men (behind the uterus in women) the peritoneum (that is to remain) is incised upwards on each side along the line of the ureter as far as the brim of the pelvis and the ureters are secured with slings at or below the brim of the pelvis. Then the internal iliac arteries are mobilized and their anterior divisions are ligated and divided. Mobilization is continued down the lateral walls of the pelvis removing as much fascia and as many lymph glands as possible, dividing and ligating the deep vesical vessels and finally dividing the ureters.

If doing the operation for carcinoma in situ, sections from the proximal cut ends of the ureters are sent for frozen biopsy examination. If these sections show carcinoma in situ or severe dysplasia, the ureter is sectioned at a higher level and further sections are sent, continuing until normal ureter is obtained. Of course it may not be possible to do this, yet leave enough ureter for the diversion procedure. In men, once the lateral aspects of the bladder are fully mobilized and the posterior aspect partly mobilized, the anterior prostatic capsule is cleared of fat and veins and the puboprostatic ligaments are divided between right angled forceps, thus mobilizing the prostate gland which can now be pulled upwards to expose the membranous urethra. If the whole urethra is not being removed the membranous urethra is divided below the prostate. By dissecting from above and below, the prostate and seminal vesicles can be peeled safely off the anterior wall of the rectum and the specimen removed. If this is difficult, it is prudent to leave some of the seminal vesicles rather than remove some of the anterior rectal wall and produce a rectal fistula. In women the posterior part of the dissection is completed by incising the lateral and posterior vaginal fornices around the cervix. The specimen is now held only by the urethra, the anterior vaginal wall and the connective tissue and veins around the bladder neck. Once these are divided the specimen can be removed and one or two large packs are put into the pelvic cavity and left there while the diversion procedure (p. 613) is carried out. The packs are then removed, haemostasis secured and the wound closed in layers with drainage.

Urethrectomy

Some surgeons routinely excise the whole length of the urethra when removing the bladder for malignant disease. Others think it preferable only to do so if there is evidence of tumour within the urethra at the time of cystectomy. If tumour develops in the urethra later, a urethrectomy can be done then.

Operation

In women the entire urethra with a strip of vagina can be removed through two parallel vertical incisions 1 cm apart in the anterior wall of the vagina. In men the whole of the spongy part of the urethra can be mobilized through a transverse perineal incision. The bulbous part is mobilised and secured with a tape or tube. Applying traction to the tape or tube, the entire penile urethra can be mobilised by sharp dissection as the penis invaginates, without separately incising the penile skin. Once the urethra is freed it can be pushed upwards into the pelvis and removed with the specimen if urethrectomy is being done at the same time as cystectomy, otherwise it is just removed.

OPERATIONS TO EXPAND OR REDUCE THE CAPACITY OF THE BLADDER

Expansion operations

The problem of the contracted bladder is encountered much less frequently now than it was some years ago, but there are still patients whose bladder has been contracted by Hunner's ulcer (interstitial cystitis), radiotherapy, tuberculosis or bilharziasis and whose bladder capacity is so reduced that their lives are miserable. If their symptoms cannot be relieved by medical treatment, bladder instillation or hydrodistension, urinary diversion or some operation to increase bladder capacity has to be considered. The capacity of the bladder can be increased using an isolated ileal loop (made in the same way as for diversion). The loop is opened along its anti-mesenteric border and sutured to the margin of the bladder after the vault of the bladder has been excised. In tuberculosis and bilharziasis the ureteric orifices and lower ureters are often stenosed and are best reimplanted into the isolated ileal loop before it is sutured to the cut margins of the bladder.

The expansion operation should not be considered until the patient has been given an extensive trial with conservative measures and the advantages of a diversion operation have been discussed, since the operations used to expand the bladder are by no means always successful.

Reduction procedures (see Gow, 1980)

Patients with an atonic bladder must be assessed very carefully to decide if the cause is obstructive or neurological. With prolonged obstruction to the outflow of urine from the bladder, chronic retention occurs and the bladder loses contractility because its muscle fibres are overstretched. Its contractility recovers if it is kept empty for some time after the cause of the obstruction is treated. Parasympathomimetic drugs like Dystigmine bromide or myotonine chloride may accelerate this recovery.

With neurological causes of bladder atony, attempts to restore contractility by prolonged bladder drainage or drugs are often unsuccessful and permanent, intermittent or continuous drainage of the bladder by a urethral or suprapubic catheter is necessary; alternatively diversion or a bladder reduction operation is considered. Bladder reduction operations not only reduce bladder capacity but also improve contractility and the best of them is the one described by Vanwelkenhuyzen in which the bladder is double breasted (Fig. 27.26). The bladder is exposed through a generous transverse incision and mobilized extraperitoneally as far down as the bladder neck anteriorly and laterally and the interureteric bar posteriorly. A transverse incision is made through the front half of the bladder (a hemitransection)

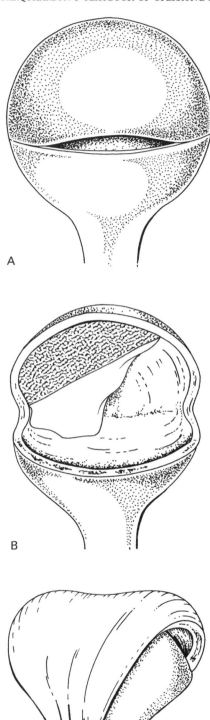

A

B

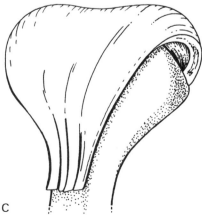

C

Fig. 27.26 Vanwelkenhuyzen's operation

about 6 cm above the bladder neck. The upper part of the bladder is stripped of its mucosa by sharp dissection. The lower cut surface of the bladder is sutured to the posterior wall of the bladder some 5 cm above the interureteric bar and some 5 cm below the upper cut margin in two layers, mucosa to mucosa, muscle to muscle. The posterior wall of the bladder already deprived of mucosa is now folded over the lower anterior wall and sutured to the bladder neck. The bladder is drained with a urethral catheter and the wound drained.

VESICAL FISTULAE

Colovesical fistula

This may occur in advanced diverticulitis of the pelvic colon — less frequently in carcinoma. A classical sign of the condition is the passage of faecal-smelling urine, accompanied by pneumaturia. The fistulous opening may show on cystoscopy, with gas or intestinal material occasionally visible.

Depending upon the extent of the diverticulitis, and the amount of healthy bowel below the lesion, it may be possible to resect the affected segment of colon and to repair the bladder. In poor risk patients, with gross infection, it is better to perform a defunctioning transverse colostomy in the first instance, in order to divert the faecal contents proximal to the fistula, and in the hope that reparative surgery can be undertaken later. If the primary condition is a carcinoma, it is likely to be irremovable and in such cases the only available treatment may be a palliative colostomy.

Vesico-vaginal fistula

This may result from pressure necrosis affecting the contiguous walls of the bladder and vagina during prolonged labour, from injury to the bladder during a difficult hysterectomy, from advancing carcinoma of the cervix or from post-irradiation necrosis.

Sometimes a recent fistula of small size will heal if the bladder is kept empty by an indwelling urethral catheter. As a rule operative treatment is necessary, but this should be delayed until infection has been overcome by vaginal lavage and by antibiotics.

The operation consists in excision of the fistulous opening with surrounding scar tissue, and in separation of the vagina and bladder sufficiently to permit separate closure of each without tension.

Smaller fistulae are approached usually through the vagina, but when there is much scarring in the vagina or when the cervix has been removed a transvesical approach is more satisfactory. Often a combination of the two methods is employed. After operation the bladder should be drained by an indwelling urethral catheter in order to ensure that it does not become distended.

In cases where a fistula has recurred after local methods of repair, a more determined attempt at cure may be made through an abdominal approach. After the viscera have been separated from above, a pedicled flap of omentum may be packed into the space between them (Turner-Warwick, 1973).

Irreparable fistulae

In a proportion of cases vesicovaginal fistula results from radiation necrosis sustained during treatment of carcinoma of the cervix. This type of fistula is not amenable to any form of local repair. Such cases together with those in which operative repair has proved unsuccessful, should be treated by transplantation of the ureters to an ileal loop.

OPERATIONS ON THE PROSTATE GLAND

Anatomy

The prostate consists of glandular tissue in a fibromuscular stroma and surrounds the beginning of the male urethra (see Fig. 27.40). It lies below the bladder, behind the pubis and in front of the rectum, through which some parts of it can be readily palpated. Its *base*, directed upwards, embraces the bladder neck; its *apex*, directed downwards, rests on the deep aspect of the external sphincter; its *posterior surface* is separated from the rectum by the two layers of the rectovesical fascia (Denonvillier) and divided by the ejaculatory ducts into an upper *middle lobe* and a lower *posterior lobe* which lies in the shallow median furrow separating the posterior aspects of the right and left lateral lobes (Fig. 27.27). The lateral lobes comprise most of the 6 or 7 g of the normal prostate and in front they are joined together by the anterior lobe which contains few, if any, glands. Only the posterior parts of the lateral lobes and the posterior lobe, in the median furrow between them, can be palpated through the rectum. The prostate contains two kinds of glands, an inner zone which surrounds the urethra and an outer zone which surrounds the inner zone, and which is separated from the loose pelvic fascia, containing the prostatic plexus of veins, by the thick fibrous capsule (Fig. 27.28). *Blood supply* to the prostate is from the internal iliac artery and *venous drainage* into the plexus around the front of the gland and thence into the internal iliac veins. *Lymph drains* first to nodes alongside the internal iliac or obturator vessels.

Benign simple prostatic hypertrophy

This disease is most frequently seen in men in the 7th, 8th or 9th decades of life, but also occurs in the 6th and even 5th decades. It is obviously related to, and probably caused by, changes that occur in hormone activity with age, but the precise cause has not yet been identified. Although medical treatment may alleviate symptoms by curing superadded infection, oedema or congestion, it does not prevent the disease nor alter the basic pathological changes; however, many safe and effective surgical methods of dealing with the disease are available for those patients who require treatment, and not all patients with the disease do require treatment. Benign hypertrophy begins in inner zone glands and consists of an increase in the number of glands (*adenosis*) some of which form small cysts because their ducts are blocked and their secretions retained, an increase in the number of cells forming the glands (*epitheliosis*) and an increase in the amount of fibrous tissue. If adenosis is the predominant change, the lobe or lobes affected enlarge and acquire the elastic consistence associated with benign hypertrophy. If *fibrosis* predominates, the prostate may be no bigger than normal,

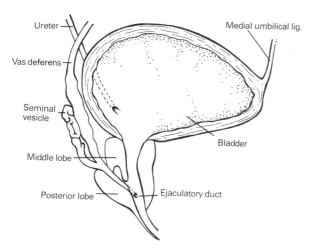

Fig. 27.27 A sagittal section of the bladder, urethra and prostate. It shows the relationships of the middle and posterior prostatic lobes to the ejaculatory duct and to each other

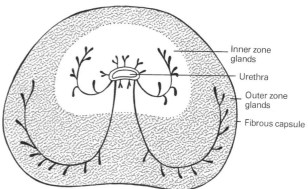

Fig. 27.28 Transverse section of the prostate

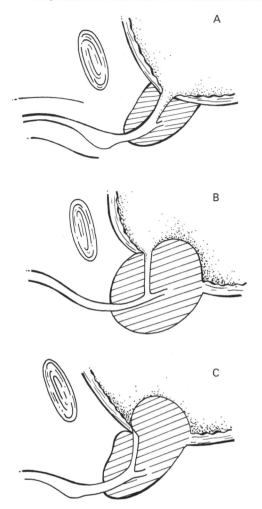

Fig. 27.29 Sagittal sections of (A) the normal prostate; (B) the hypertrophied prostate in which both lateral and middle lobes are involved; and (C) the hypertrophied prostate in which only the middle lobe is involved

yet can obstruct the outflow of urine from the bladder as much as the largest gland. The changes of benign hypertrophy may involve one or more lobes of the prostate (Fig. 27.29). Involvement of the lateral lobes can be appreciated by rectal examination (unless fibrosis predominates) whereas involvement of the middle lobe cannot, no matter how extensive the change becomes. When the middle lobe enlarges it bulges forwards into the bladder, not backwards into the rectum, yet can severely obstruct the outflow of urine by impacting in the bladder neck like a ball valve when the bladder contracts. Benign prostatic hypertrophy obstructs the outflow of urine from the bladder by narrowing, distorting and elongating the urethra or narrowing the bladder neck. The bladder responds to obstruction (Figs 27.30–27.33) by hypertrophy called *trabeculation*, and saccules and sometimes *diverticula* develop between

the bundles of hypertrophied muscle fibres (Fig. 27.32). In the early stages the increased contractility of the bladder compensates for the increased resistance in the urethra and the bladder is still able to empty. Later, however, the bladder fails to empty completely so that residual urine remains in it after micturition and gradually and progressively increases in quantity. Later still the flow of urine from the kidney to the bladder through the ureters is hindered by a combination of factors, which include obstruction and vesicoureteric reflux, and hydroureter, hydronephrosis and chronic renal failure ensue.

Treatment

Treatment is not required because the gland is large or fibrous, but because it is obstructing the outflow of urine from the bladder. In the early stages of obstruction the patient may have no complaints, but later he finds that micturition is slow to start, and difficult to stop so that terminal dribbling occurs; that the urinary stream is poor in force and calibre and the need to micturate is frequent, especially at night and often urgent. The symptoms usually become gradually worse and in time the patient develops chronic or acute retention. In *chronic retention* the residual urine has slowly, progressively and insidiously increased over some time; the patient presents with increased frequency, overflow incontinence and sometimes enuresis, and is often quite unaware that his bladder is very distended and still contains a litre or more of urine after micturition. Most patients with chronic urinary retention have dilated upper urinary tracts and some degree of chronic renal failure. *Acute retention* may be the culmination of increasing difficulties with micturition or superimposed on chronic retention, but often occurs in patients who have had little, if any, previous trouble. The sudden increase in prostatic size that causes acute retention in such patients may be due to infection or to oedema and congestion such as occurs in cardiac failure and in some patients who suppress the need to micturate rather than interrupt a meal or journey. As obstruction interferes with the free flow of urine, it inhibits the ability of the urinary tract to decontaminate itself of organisms and thus some patients have, and may indeed present with, recurrent or chronic bladder infections or stones.

In some patients the history and physical examination provide overwhelming evidence of obstruction, and it is apparent without any further investigations that treatment is needed; in others, it is less obvious and obstruction must be confirmed before proceeding with treatment. The author is not convinced that prostatectomy is a good prophylactic operation, even though many patients say 'surely it is better to have the operation now while I'm fairly young and fit, rather

Figs 27.30–27.33 *Effects of obstruction upon the bladder (diagram of cystoscopic appearance and cross section)*

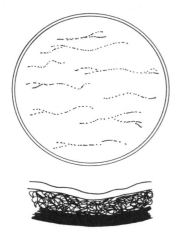

Fig. 27.30   Normal bladder

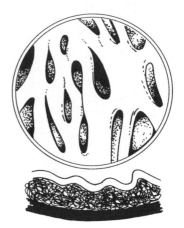

Fig. 27.31   Early trabeculation

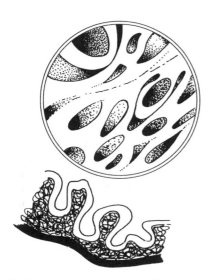

Fig. 27.32   Severe trabeculation with saccules

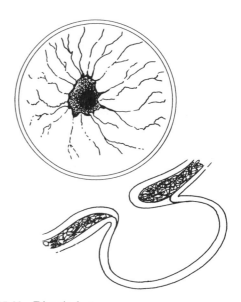

Fig. 27.33   Diverticulum

than in 10 years time, when I'll not be so young and may not be so fit'. What objective evidence of obstruction should be sought?

Rectal examination

The normal prostate is felt as a low lying elevation in the anterior wall of the rectum just within the anal orifice. It is smooth in outline, elastic in consistence and its lateral edges and upper limit are clearly defined. The shallow furrow, easily felt in the midline between the two lateral lobes, is the posterior lobe. Neither anterior nor middle lobes can be felt, even if they are abnormal. The rectal mucosa over the gland is mobile. In benign enlargement the prostate is enlarged, smooth

and bulges backwards into the rectum on either side of the median furrow if the lateral lobes are involved, but feels normal if the middle lobe alone is involved. A fibrous prostate is not normally enlarged and, though it may be firmer than the healthy gland, often feels surprisingly normal in consistence and morphology. A malignant prostate becomes hard, nodular, irregular, fixed and infiltrates the surrounding structures, obliterating the median furrow, but in its early stages may feel normal (p. 651). In benign enlargement there is no correlation between the size of the gland assessed rectally, and the degree of obstruction, since a small prostate may cause severe obstruction, and a large one little, if any.

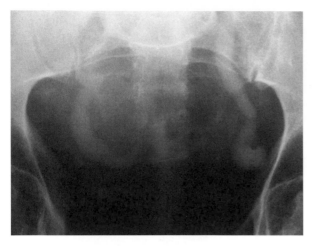

Fig. 27.34 Intravenous urogram. The patient has a distended bladder but it is not clearly seen because the dye entering it has been diluted by the large amount of urine within. Both ureters are dilated and their lower ends show the characteristic 'hooking' associated with a large prostate and distended bladder

Intravenous urography (Fig. 27.34)
This provides a good assessment of renal function, and will reveal dilatation of the ureters and pelvicaliceal system (if such exist), trabeculation, sacculation, diverticula of the bladder and the amount of residual urine. It may also reveal problems unrelated to the prostate such as a space occupying lesion in the kidney, and thus suggest the need for further investigations.

Residual urine
Inability to empty the bladder completely is an important sign of bladder outflow obstruction, and the measurement of residual urine (i.e. the volume of urine that remains in the bladder after micturition) can be useful if carried out after the patient has passed urine because he needed to; it is useless if done when the patient tries to pass urine, because he is told to do so. The intravenous post micturition cystogram is not a reliable means of assessing residual urine because the patient is dehydrated, has usually emptied the bladder before the examination, and has difficulty attempting to pass completely the small volume of urine the bladder usually contains when a cystogram is being done.

Cystourethroscopy
This may reveal evidence of obstruction, trabeculation, sacculation, diverticula or stones, and provides a satisfactory way of determining the size of the prostate including the middle lobe, and its effect upon the urethra. However, the procedure may make the prostate oedematous and aggravate urinary symptoms, or even cause acute urinary retention in patients with a large prostate.

Urodynamics
The measurement of flow by uroflowmeter is a useful test provided the rate is measured when the patient's bladder is filled to the extent that he wants to pass urine. In outflow obstruction the flow rate is reduced. Diseases other than obstruction may cause a low flow rate, but only in obstruction is it associated with a high detrusor pressure.

In summary, then, patients with prostatic hypertrophy only require treatment if they have bladder outflow obstruction. That there exists such obstruction may be obvious from the patient's history and the findings on physical examination; if not, further evidence of obstruction should be sought in the intravenous urogram or by measuring residual urine, flow rates or bladder pressures or by cysto-urethroscopy. If there is no evidence of obstruction, or the evidence is slight, some other cause of the patient's symptoms should be suspected.

Choice of operation
It is not easy to describe operations on the prostate gland in a manner which will find general acceptance, because widely divergent views are held on the choice of operation and on pre- and postoperative treatment.

Three methods of prostatectomy — transurethral, suprapubic and retropubic, and will be considered, and the detailed technique of each described. With all three methods of prostatectomy the same end result is produced, but the approach is different. In all operations the hypertrophied part of the prostate together with the prostatic urethra is removed leaving a cavity which is lined by the compressed outer group glands and the fibrous capsule (Fig. 27.35). The cavity contracts and its raw surface is gradually covered by epithelium growing downwards from the bladder and upwards from the urethra. In transurethral prostatectomy the plane between the hypertrophied part of the gland, which is being removed, and the capsule, which must be left, can be clearly seen. In open prostatectomy, the plane between the hypertrophied part of the gland and the compressed outer glands is easily felt and can be extended with a finger (like separating an orange from its skin) until the hypertrophied part is all freed or enucleated and can be removed. In the suprapubic prostatectomy, popularized by Freyer in 1901, the prostate is approached through the bladder and it is the simplest and safest method. In the retropubic prostatectomy which attained considerable popularity with the work of Millin, a suprapubic incision is made, but the bladder is not opened. Instead the prostate is approached behind the pubis and removed through the anterior aspect of the prostatic capsule. In the transurethral operation a resectoscope is used to remove the prostate in a series of small pieces or chips through the urethra,

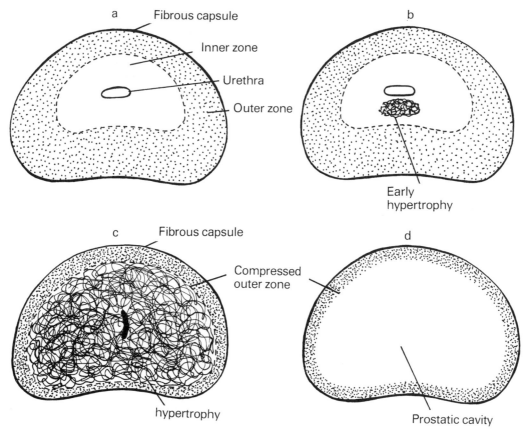

Fig. 27.35   Transverse sections of the prostate. (a) The normal prostate. (b) Early benign prostatic hypertrophy, the change beginning in the inner zone glands. (c) Marked benign prostatic hypertrophy. The prostatic urethra is squashed and displaced. The hypertrophied gland has compressed the outer zone glands into a false capsule. (d) After prostatectomy the cavity is lined by the compressed outer zone glands and the true fibrous capsule of the prostate

thus avoiding some of the hazards of an open operation, though bleeding, infection and strictures can still occur.

Ligation or division of the vas deferens
Epididymitis caused by the direct spread of infection from the prostatic bed down the vas used to be a common postoperative complication of any form of prostatectomy. Many urologists considered bilateral vasectomy a part of the operation of prostatectomy. It inflicts no additional disability, since after prostatectomy the ejaculate, if any, refluxes into the bladder. This operation is described on page 681 but is now rarely, if ever, done as part of prostatectomy.

TREATMENT OF PROSTATIC RETENTION OF URINE

About 20% of patients needing prostatectomy have acute or chronic retention of urine. The need to carry out a preliminary suprapubic cystostomy has long since been abandoned. The treatment of choice now, for patients in good general health without serious infection or renal insufficiency, is urethral catheterization followed a day or two later by prostatectomy if they have acute retention. If they have chronic retention they are catheterized before operation only if they have a serious degree of chronic renal failure.

TRANSURETHRAL PROSTATECTOMY

Although for the large benign prostates a retropubic or transvesical prostatectomy is a satisfactory alternative to a transurethral resection, the latter is preferable for the smaller benign prostates, for the fibrous or malignant prostates and for bladder neck contractures. Any surgeon who practices urological surgery must learn to use a resectoscope for these procedures and for the treatment and assessment of bladder tumours (p. 629). The largest prostates he can remove by open operation and, the more experienced he is with the resectoscope, the larger the prostates he will resect. Any surgeon, reasonably experienced in endoscopy, can learn to use a resectoscope from the many books, pictures, videos, and films about it, although of course instruction from an experienced resectionist is invaluable.

Position

The patient is placed in the appropriate position for endoscopy. A 'steridrape' or similar drape is applied. This is a plastic sheet one edge of which is adherent and sticks to the abdominal wall. The penis is brought through a hole in the centre of the sheet; below this hole is a finger cot which is lubricated and inserted into the rectum. The drape enables the surgeon to use the rectum to examine the prostate and facilitate resection without becoming unsterile. First the urethra, prostate and bladder are examined by cysto-urethroscopy, looking for strictures, diverticula, stones or tumours, which may have been unsuspected from the clinical examina-

tion. Next prostatic size is assessed and a decision made whether to proceed with a transurethral or an open procedure.

Assessment

The assessment of prostatic size is made partly by endoscopy, and partly by bimanual examination, which is best done while the cystoscope is in the bladder. Endoscopically the size of the middle lobe is estimated by the extent to which it bulges into the bladder and the size of the lateral lobes by the amount they encroach into the urethra, the length of contact between them and the length of the prostatic urethra from the bladder neck to the verumontanum. This length is about 2.5 cm (1 field of the cystoscope using a 70° telescope) for the normal prostate; it increases to about 5.0 cm (2 fields) with the 25 gm prostate and to about 7.5 cm (3 fields) with the 50 gm prostate. This endoscopy should be done in a theatre, where transurethral or open prostatectomy can be done so that operation need

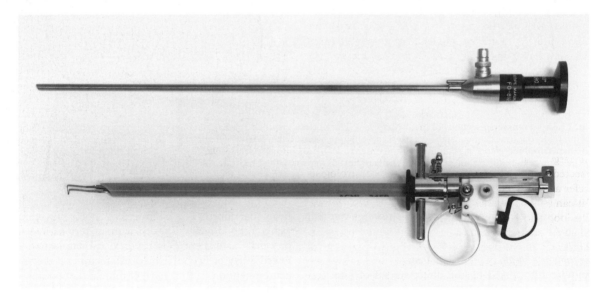

A

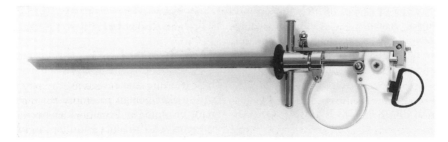

B

Fig. 27.36 Resectoscope. (A) Telescope and resectoscope sheath with loop extruded. (B) Sheath with loop retracted

not be deferred until another day. Two units of blood should be available, but are rarely used.

Resectoscope

A resectoscope sheath with its obturator is passed into the bladder choosing a 26F or 24F sheath depending on the ease with which it will pass. The sheath may be all fibreglass or metal with a fibreglass beak and the obturator is either straight or has a flexible tip (Timberlake obturator), which can be bent to facilitate introduction of the sheath into the bladder. If it proves difficult to pass even a 24F resectoscope sheath the urethra must first be enlarged by dilating with bougies, or better, by carrying out an internal urethrotomy with an Otis urethrotome. Once the sheath has passed into the bladder, the obturator is removed and replaced by the working element of the resectoscope, which has a channel for the fore-oblique or direct view telescope, (a 0° or 12° or 30°, depending upon the make of the instrument) and one for the loop electrode. Different working elements have different mechanisms for moving the loop backwards and forwards but most are now one handed, i.e. the instrument is held with the fingers and the loop is manipulated with the thumb of the same hand and most have a spring which assists either the cutting action or the return of the loop after cutting (cutting is done as the loop is drawn towards the operator) (Fig. 27.36). Cutting loops vary in size and are colour coded. One uses a 24F loop with the 24F sheath, because a loop will obviously not move freely in a sheath which is smaller. The larger the loop, the larger the chips or piece of prostate that can be resected in one cut, and for this reason most urologists prefer a 26 or 27F sheath to a 24 or 25F one, but only if it can be passed easily without damaging the urethra. The loop consists of the cutting wire, supported on an insulated stem by an insulated fork, which often incorporates a stabilizing device. The proximal end of the loop fits into the insulated block of the working element, which is attached to the diathermy machine by the diathermy cable. Loops, other than the cutting ones, are available; some have balls or rollers for coagulating, and others have knives for incising the bladder neck or ureteric orifice. The tap on the resectoscope sheath is connected to the source of the irrigating fluid, which is usually in plastic containers. If two bags are connected to the resectoscope via a Y connection (Fig. 27.37) there need be no delay in changing over when one bag is empty. Sterile saline cannot be used for transurethral resection because it forms an electroconductive solution which interferes with the electrocutting coagulation current. During resection large volumes (10 or more litres) of irrigating fluid are used and considerable amounts may be absorbed into the veins opened during resection. Since water reduces

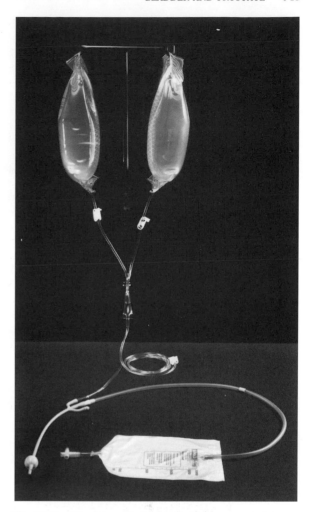

Fig. 27.37 Two bags of irrigating fluid are connected to a single tube by a Y connection. The single tube can then be attached to either resectoscope or, as in the illustration, to a catheter. The irrigation is carried out from only one bag at a time but, as soon as that bag is empty, irrigation can be continued from the other without delay

osmotic pressure and causes haemolysis it should not be used. Of the various isotonic or near isotonic fluids available, 1.5% glycine is as good as any. The irrigating fluid is allowed to run into the bladder as cutting takes place and washes blood and the resected chips into the bladder.

Irrigation

The working element has to be removed from the sheath at regular intervals to empty the bladder. Cystoscopes with continuous irrigation are available (Fig. 27.38). They have a double sheath; the fluid flowing in through one by gravity is sucked out of the other by a suction pump, but many urologists still prefer the conventional nonirrigating resectoscopes. The author uses a diathermy

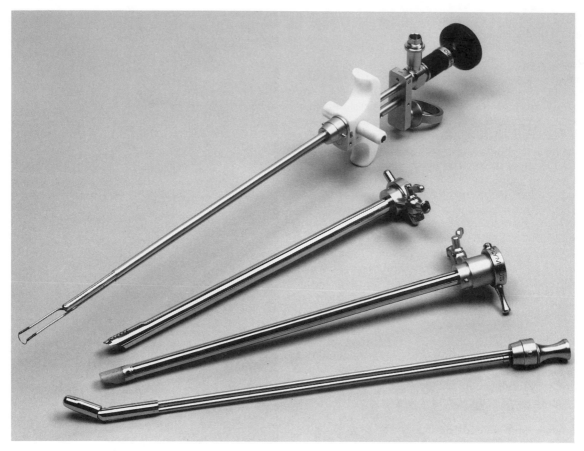

Fig. 27.38   Continuous irrigating resectoscope. The instruments shown are (from above downwards) the working element with loop and fore-oblique telescope, the inner sheath (24F), the outer sheath (26F), and the deflecting or Timberlake obturator (Courtesy of Key Med)

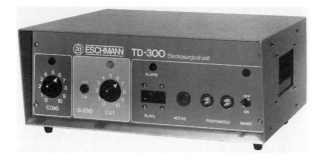

Fig. 27.39   Electrosurgical unit. This unit has two circuits, one for coagulating and one for cutting each activated by its own pedal. The machine also has a facility for blending (Courtesy of Eschmann Co.)

machine (Fig. 27.39) with separate cutting and coagulating circuits with a separate pedal for each, although cutting can be done with high coagulation current from older machines. The appropriate machine settings can only be worked out by practice. The blending of cutting and coagulating currents is probably best avoided.

Cutting

The loop moves about 2.5 cm and this is the maximum length of the chip if the sheath is not moved apart from tilting it while the cut is made. It is possible to cut larger chips by moving the resectoscope as well as the loop, but this can only be done with experience. It is far safer to keep the sheath steady while making the cut. The knack of cutting and the strength of diathermy needed can be estimated and practised by cutting soap and meat.

Before resection begins it is essential to recognise the two vital landmarks, the bladder neck above, the verumontanum below. No cuts must be made below the verumontanum (Fig. 27.40) which marks the level of the external sphincter, and no cuts must be made higher than the bladder neck. At the start of the procedure the muscle fibres of the bladder neck are exposed by resecting the middle lobe from 5 o'clock to 7 o'clock (Fig. 27.41). Next the lateral lobes are resected, exposing the bladder neck muscle fibres and the reticulate pattern of the inner aspect of the prostatic capsule. Of the many ways in which this can be done, it is best

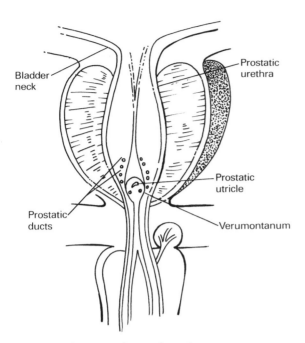

Fig. 27.40 Anatomy of prostatic urethra

to finish one lobe before starting on the other, and to commence cutting about 1 o'clock for the left lobe and 11 o'clock for the right (Fig. 27.42). Enough chips are cut in each position to expose the muscle of the bladder neck and capsule, and haemostasis is secured before rotating the instrument and making the next move; this is repeated until one is back at 5 o'clock or 7 o'clock depending which lobe is tackled first. Resection is continued until only apical tissue remains (Fig. 27.43) before proceeding to the other lateral lobe (Fig. 27.44). Finally the apical tissue is resected on both sides (being extremely careful not to go beyond the verumontanum and so damage the external sphincter) and the anterior lobe between 11 o'clock and 1 o'clock (where the wall is very thin and easily perforated). Although it is tempting to keep cutting if the bleeding does not hinder vision it is better, though slower, to secure haemostasis after each cut or after the cuts needed to form a trench deep enough to expose the muscle of the bladder neck and the prostatic capsule. Do not leave haemostasis to the end, when rebound bleeding can make recognition of the source and site of bleeding extremely difficult. Once the resection is complete, the chips which have not escaped when the working element was removed and the bladder emptied, are removed by washing the bladder out with an Ellik evacuator (Fig. 27.45). The working element is then reinserted and haemostasis secured, although of course many bleeding vessels will have already been dealt with during the resection; any remaining ones can often be coagulated more easily with a ball or roller electrode. Bleeding from veins

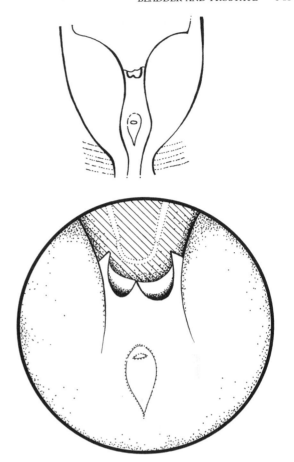

Fig. 27.41 Transurethral resection of prostate. The procedure starts by exposing the muscle fibres of the bladder neck by resecting the middle lobe from 5 to 7 o'clock

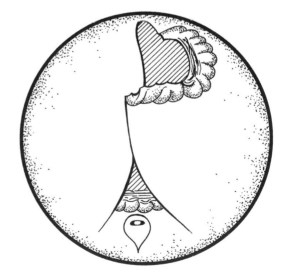

Fig. 27.42 Transurethral resection of prostate. A trench is dug into the left lateral lobe at 1 o'clock until the muscle fibres of the bladder neck and the criss-cross pattern of the prostatic capsule are exposed

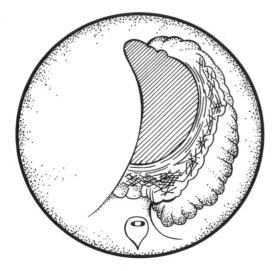

Fig. 27.43 Transurethral resection of prostate. The left lateral lobe has all been resected apart from apical tissue

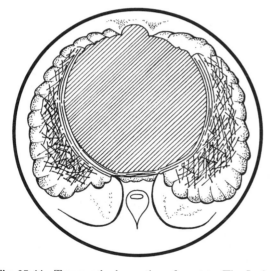

Fig. 27.44 Transurethral resection of prostate. The final stage consists of resection of the apical tissue seen on either side of the verumontanum. It is during this stage that great care must be taken to avoid damage to the external sphincter

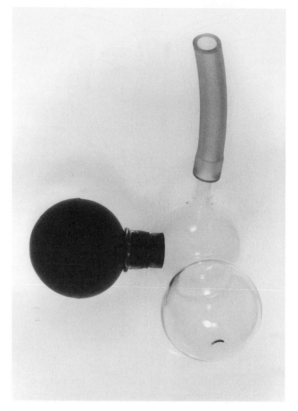

Fig. 27.45 Ellik evacuator (Courtesy of GU Manufacturing Co. Ltd)

opened when cuts are made close to, or even through, the prostatic capsule are more easily controlled by the Foley catheter than diathermy. Once all chips have been removed and bleeding reasonably controlled, a three-way 22 or 24F Foley catheter of haematuric type is introduced on a curved introducer to prevent the catheter passing behind the trigone of the bladder into the perivesical tissues. Its entry into the bladder can be readily confirmed if some fluid is left in the bladder when the resectoscope sheath is removed. The bladder is then continuously irrigated through the catheter with sterile water or saline. Haemostasis is often improved if the catheter, with 30 ml in the balloon, is pulled down so that the balloon compresses the bladder neck by traction (Fig. 27.46).

Precautions

1. Do not resect below the verumontanum nor above the muscle fibres of the bladder neck (exposed by resecting the middle lobe from 5 to 7 o'clock at the start of the operation).

2. Hold the resectoscope sheath still while resecting, so that only the loop moves and all cutting is done under vision.

3. Achieve haemostasis after each cut, or at least before rotating the sheath to dig another trench.

4. Do not cut unless you can see clearly; abandon the procedure, if you can not. One can always go back later and resect more, or do open procedure. You can not go back later and replace bits of the external sphincter or ureteric orifices.

Continuous irrigation is maintained through the three-way Foley catheter for 24 to 48 hours, depending how much bleeding occurs. The catheter is removed a day or two later. In patients with chronic retention,

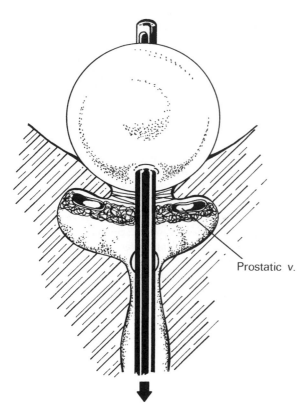

Fig. 27.46 Transurethral resection of prostate. A Foley catheter has been passed and its balloon inflated in the bladder. When traction is applied to the catheter, the prostatic cavity is squashed and open veins compressed

the bladder is usually hypotonic or even atonic and the catheter should be left in longer.

Complications of prostatic surgery

Clot retention

This is one of the most serious immediate complications of any prostatectomy and may occur if the catheter or other drainage tube becomes blocked by blood clot and is not expeditiously dealt with. It is unlikely to occur while the bladder is being irrigated through a three-way Foley catheter, provided that any blockage is detected and treated early. Small clots can be cleared by using a bladder syringe or just milking the catheter and these measures may be adequate to empty the bladder and restore drainage even if the bladder is distended by clot and fluid (irrigating fluid may continue to run in even if it is not running out).

If these measures are unsuccessful the patient should be taken to theatre and a large bore catheter or resectoscope sheath passed under general anaesthesia to allow evacuation of the clot by vigorous irrigation with a Wardill's all-glass or Ellik syringe. If even this fails, the bladder must be opened or reopened, although that is

rarely necessary. *Secondary haemorrhage* may occur on the 7th to the 10th day after any form of prostatectomy, but is perhaps more common after transurethral procedures; if the patient goes home before the 10th postoperative day, he should be warned that it might happen. In some patients secondary haemorrhage is enough to cause clot retention.

Stricture

Strictures, especially those at the external meatus, often result from forcing a catheter or resectoscope through the meatus. A smaller catheter or resectoscope sheath is tried, and if that will not pass easily, carry out a meatotomy or a urethrotomy with the Otis urethrotome first. The patient who has difficulty passing urine after prostatectomy, is not likely to be helped when told that it is no longer the prostate causing his trouble, but a stricture (and strictures may be more difficult to treat).

Incontinence

Some patients have stress or urge incontinence for some days after operation, but permanent incontinence is very uncommon unless the external sphincter has been damaged and this should not happen. Prostatectomy can cure the overflow incontinence of chronic retention once bladder contractility is restored, but is not advised for patients who have other sorts of incontinence unless it is certain that their problems are obstructive and not neurological.

Infection

Epididymitis is now an uncommon complication and few surgeons do a vasectomy to prevent it. Bladder infection may ascend to the kidneys causing pyelonephritis and even endotoxaemia and, with open prostatectomies, wound infection still occurs and should be treated appropriately. There is some evidence that prophylactic antibiotics given before or at the time of operation speed recovery.

Perforation of the prostatic capsule

It is easy to make a small perforation during prostatic resection and expose veins and sometimes fat. If a large perforation occurs the irrigating fluid leaks into the extravesical space, fluid fails to return through the resectoscope, the patient's abdomen swells and becomes cold (unless the irrigating fluid is warmed) and the anaesthetist appears concerned. The resection must be abandoned, a urethral catheter passed and the retropubic space drained through a transverse suprapubic incision, opening the peritoneum if intraperitoneal extravasation is suspected.

Transurethral resection (tur) syndrome

Large volumes of irrigating fluid may be absorbed into

the general circulation through open veins. If water has been used, severe haemolysis with acute renal failure can occur. Even isotonic fluids like Glycine may cause problems by expanding the blood volume which causes hypertension, and reduces electrolyte concentration, with resultant neuromuscular disturbances such as fits and temporary paralysis.

TRANSVESICAL PROSTATECTOMY

The patient is placed in the supine position on the operating table with a slight Trendelenburg tilt. Suitable illumination is arranged and the surgeon stands at the patient's left side. The external genitals and the abdominal wall are thoroughly washed. Towels are arranged so that the penis is accessible as well as the suprapubic area. The bladder is exposed through a transverse incision as described for the operation of suprapubic cystotomy (p. 622) and opened between stay sutures. A self retaining retractor is introduced. The bladder interior and the prostate gland are carefully inspected and the presence of calculi, diverticula or tumour determined. The self retaining retractor is then removed, and the margins of the bladder wall are held up by the sutures.

Technique of enucleation
The simplest method of finding the correct plane of cleavage between the hypertrophied part of the gland and false capsule is to introduce the index finger into the bladder neck and prostatic urethra and then to split the anterior commissure (the junction between the two lateral lobes) forwards until an obvious plane of cleavage is reached. The index finger is now swept round the prostate first on one side and then on the other, until the gland has been freed on both sides; enucleation continues on the anterior aspect, until the gland has been completely freed anteriorly and on each side. The urethra is now torn across from before backwards at the distal level of the plane of cleavage obtained, which is at the apex of the prostate. The tear occurs obliquely upwards and backwards above the verumontanum, so that the posterior lobe, the ejaculatory ducts, and much more importantly, the external sphincter, are undisturbed. The enucleation is completed by separating the posterior surface of the gland from the fibrous capsule which should also remain intact. Great care must be taken to keep the correct plane of cleavage within the false capsule, otherwise considerable venous bleeding may be encountered and the seminal vesicles, ejaculatory ducts or sphincter damaged. If the mucosa of the bladder neck remains adherent to the prostate and is liable to be stripped upwards from the trigone as the gland is removed, it should be divided close to the

gland with scissors or a diathermy knife. If enucleation is difficult posteriorly due to fibrosis it can be completed under vision. For this purpose the self-retaining retractor is reinserted, the partially separated lobes are pulled into the bladder with tissue forceps and held apart to display the floor of the prostatic urethra, which can be divided immediately above the verumontanum with diathermy or scissors, when enucleation can usually be completed without difficulty. If access is difficult, the operation can be facilitated if an assistant introduces an index finger into the rectum to steady and push forward the gland against the enucleating finger of the surgeon. This manoeuvre however, is seldom necessary.

Although it is usually possible to assess the size and determine the pathology of the prostate gland accurately before operation and to decide that enucleation at open operation rather than transurethral resection is the best treatment, sometimes no plane of cleavage is found at operation because the prostate is smaller and more fibrous than anticipated or even malignant. It is usually better to do something than abandon the procedure in favour of a resection at a later date. For the fibrous prostate careful enucleation can be attempted but it is safer to dilate the prostatic urethra and excise a wedge from the back of the bladder neck. For some malignant prostates enucleation is possible because the malignant process is confined to the interior of a benignly hypertrophied gland; for others enucleation is impossible because the malignancy has extended through the capsule and no more than a wedge resection should be attempted.

Haemostasis
As soon as enucleation has been completed, one or more packs are packed tightly into the prostatic bed for 5 minutes. A self retaining retractor is then reinserted and the bladder cavity is dried out with suction and swabs. The pack in the prostatic bed is cautiously withdrawn, the cavity inspected and tags of mucosa or remnants of prostatic tissue are carefully removed.

Bleeding vessels are secured with long artery forceps and sealed by diathermy coagulation or underrun with sutures. With care, patience and good illumination (preferably from a lighted retractor) major blood vessels can be secured and the haemorrhage reduced to an ooze. A Foley catheter is passed through the urethra into the bladder. Its balloon is inflated in the bladder or within the prostatic cavity, where it acts like the gauze pack which used to be left in the prostatic bed for some days after operation.

Removal of a posterior wedge from the bladder neck (trigonectomy)
A wedge of mucosa and muscle can be cut from the posterior aspect of the bladder neck with a diathermy

electrode or scissors if it overhangs the prostatic cavity. The apex of the wedge extends up between the ureteric orifices which must first be identified and carefully safeguarded. The wedge resection also facilitates inspection of the prostatic cavity and identification of bleeding points.

Suprapubic drainage of the bladder is now thought to be unnecessary and most urologists insert a three-way Foley catheter, close the bladder, and continuously irrigate it for a day or two after operation, but if you are doubtful about haemostasis and fearful of clot retention, even while irrigating the bladder through the three-way Foley, you can leave a suprapubic tube in the bladder for a few days. A drain is brought out from the pre-vesical space. Usually normal micturition is restored following catheter removal about the sixth day and the suprapubic wound has healed within 7 to 10 days of operation.

Second stage prostatectomy

This means prostatectomy after a previous suprapubic cystostomy and nowadays is a rare procedure. As the first step in the operation the suprapubic fistula and scar tissue are excised, safeguarding if possible the peritoneum; the bladder is separated from the abdominal wall to which it is usually adherent, and opened downwards from the cystostomy opening. The prostate is enucleated as described. If, as is frequently the case, the bladder is contracted and immobile, it may be difficult to introduce a self retaining retractor, and impossible, therefore, to arrest haemorrhage by securing individual vessels but the latter can usually be controlled by inflating the balloon of the three-way Foley catheter in the prostatic cavity and applying traction to it.

RETROPUBIC PROSTATECTOMY

This operation provides direct access to the prostatic cavity, facilitates haemostasis, is followed by a relatively short convalescence, restores micturition early and has a low incidence of complications, but is more difficult to do than the suprapubic operation.

Technique

Cystourethroscopy is essential at some stage before operation otherwise associated bladder conditions such as stone, neoplasm or diverticula can be missed. It can be done immediately before operation or some days previously. The bladder, which is emptied before operation, is exposed by the usual suprapubic approach (Fig. 27.47). A transverse approach is used and the lower rectus sheath flap split vertically to the pubis (Fig. 27.48). The prevesical fat and the peritoneum are gently stripped upwards. A Millin self retaining

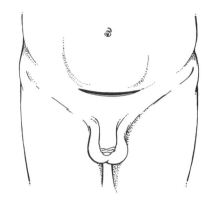

Fig. 27.47 Retropubic prostatectomy. The transverse suprapubic incision is made in a skin crease

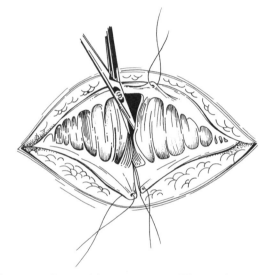

Fig. 27.48 Retropubic prostatectomy. The anterior rectus sheath has been divided in the line of the skin incision and separated from the underlying rectus and pyramidalis muscles. The lower flap has been split vertically to the pubic bone

retractor is inserted, the lateral blades spreading the recti, and the upper blade depressing the bladder neck which is protected by a folded gauze pack or two swabs. This opens up the retropubic space but the prostate is obscured by fat and veins. By gentle dissection the anterior surface of the prostatic capsule is completely cleared of fat and veins which are displaced laterally or divided, coagulated, ligated or clipped and divided. The later stages of the operation are very difficult unless the anterior prostatic capsule is properly exposed but considerable care is needed when dealing with the preprostatic veins which are often large and which can retract out of the field unless they are firmly secured before they are divided. Small gauze packs can be introduced into each lateral recess, but are not usually necessary. Using a long handled scalpel, a 2.5 cm incision is made through the anterior fibrous and false capsule of the prostate about 1 to 2 cm below its junction with the bladder, between two stay sutures one inserted at the lower part of the exposed prostatic capsule and the other at the bladder neck (Fig. 27.49). The incision is deepened through the capsule, which is often surprisingly thick, until the typical white colour of the 'adenoma' is seen (Fig. 27.50). The capsular flaps are undermined with curved scissors, freeing the anterior and lateral parts of the hypertrophied gland. The lower limits of the lateral lobes are defined by retracting the lower capsular flap and the urethra is divided at the apex of the prostate as close to the lateral lobes as possible with blunt ended scissors (Fig. 27.51). All packs

and the retractor are now removed. While the assistant holds and elevates the proximal stay suture with his left hand and uses the sucker or a swab on a forceps with his right hand, the surgeon holds and elevates the distal stay suture with his left hand and, using the index finger on his right hand, frees the adenomatous mass posteriorly, and finally removes it by dividing the mucosal cuff connecting it to the bladder, with scissors (Fig. 27.52).

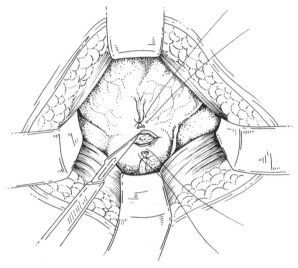

Fig. 27.49   Retropubic prostatectomy. After the anterior prostatic capsule has been completely cleared of fat and veins it is incised transversely between stay sutures

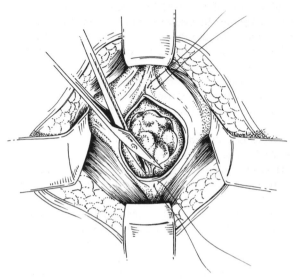

Fig. 27.51   Retropubic prostatectomy. The hypertrophied part of the prostate has been mobilized anteriorly and at both sides. It is pulled up by the fingers of the left hand (which have been omitted from the diagram) while the urethra at its apex is divided by scissors

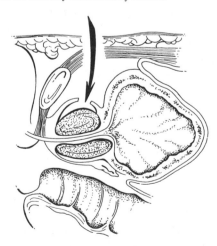

Fig. 27.50   Retropubic prostatectomy. Sagittal section of bladder and prostate. The incision in the anterior prostatic capsule goes through fibrous and false capsules to expose the adenoma which has a whiter colour than the surrounding tissues

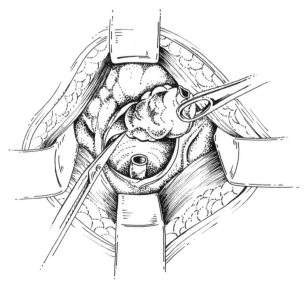

Fig. 27.52   Retropubic prostatectomy. The hypertrophied prostate has now been freed posteriorly and is being separated from the mucosa of the bladder neck by sharp dissection, thereafter it will be completely removed

A gauze pack is placed temporarily into the prostatic bed to control haemorrhage and the Millin retractor is reinserted. The pack is gently withdrawn and any remaining nodules of prostatic tissue or loose tags of capsule are removed. The bladder neck spreader is inserted into the bladder neck and held open by the assistant. The ureteric orifices are identified and protected while a generous wedge is excised from the back of the bladder neck (Fig. 27.53). Four or five interrupted sutures of No. 1 plain catgut are inserted into the cut edges of the wedge pinning down the bladder neck mucosa to the back of the prostatic capsule. A 22F three-way Haematuric Foley catheter is introduced into the urethra, and guided through the prostatic bed into the bladder. About 5 ml water is injected into the balloon at this stage (a further 15 ml is injected after the capsule is closed). After a final inspection to ensure that haemorrhage has been arrested, the capsular incision is closed with a continuous catgut suture (Fig. 27.54) placing the stitches close enough together to arrest haemorrhage especially at the lateral angles. Although this suture and the stay sutures used at an earlier stage can be inserted with a boomerang needle, the author prefers to use No 1 plain catgut on an ordinary needle with a Stratte needle holder. A drain is left in the retropubic space and the wound is repaired in layers. As soon as the operation has been completed, the bladder is washed out with water and some is left in the bladder until irrigation can be started. Irrigation is maintained as long as there is significant bleeding and the urethral catheter is removed on the third to fifth day after operation.

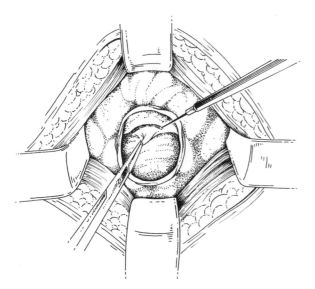

Fig. 27.53 Retropubic prostatectomy. The bladder neck has been grasped with tissue forceps and a V shape wedge with its apex superiorly is being excised; cutting diathermy is being used in this case although scissors may be used

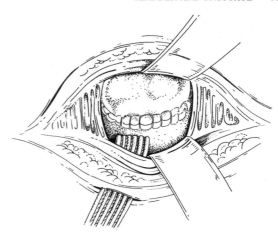

Fig. 27.54 Retropubic prostatectomy. The anterior prostatic capsule has been closed with a continuous catgut suture and a drain inserted into the retropubic space

CARCINOMA OF THE PROSTATE

At one time, nearly all patients with prostatic carcinoma were treated by hormone manipulation. Nowadays, the treatment depends on the category of the disease according to the TNMG system. The *T category* represents the local extent and is assessed by clinical examination, urography, endoscopy and biopsy (UICC, 1978).

Tis Preinvasive carcinoma (carcinoma in situ)

T0 No tumour palpable (includes the incidental finding of carcinoma in an operative or biopsy specimen)

T1 Tumour intracapsular surrounded by palpably normal gland

T2 Tumour confined to the gland. Smooth nodule deforming contour but lateral sulci and seminal vesicles not involved

T3 Tumour extending beyond the capsule with or without involvement of the lateral sulci or seminal vesicles or both

T4 Tumour fixed or infiltrating neighbouring structures (Fig. 27.55)

The *N category* represents the state of regional and juxtaregional lymph nodes and is assessed by clinical examination and radiography.

N0 No evidence of regional lymph node involvement

N1 Evidence of involvement of a single homolateral regional lymph node

N2 Evidence of involvement of contralateral or bilateral or multiple regional lymph nodes

N3 Evidence of involvement of fixed regional lymph nodes (there is a fixed mass on the pelvic wall with a free space between this and the tumour)

N4 Evidence of involvement of juxtaregional nodes

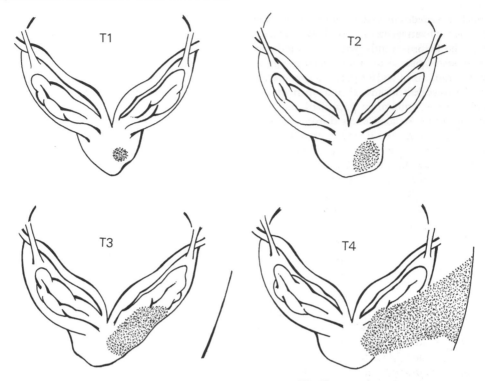

Fig. 27.55 Carcinoma of the prostate. The T categories

NX The minimum requirements to assess the regional and/or juxtaregional lymph nodes cannot be met

The *M category* represents the presence or absence of distant metastases and is assessed by bone scan, radiography and at least two estimations of the serum acid phosphatase.
M0 No evidence of distant metastases
M1 Evidence of distant metastases or raised serum acid phosphatase or both (Fig. 27.56)

The *G category* represents histopathological grading
G1 High degree of differentiation
G2 Medium degree of differentiation
G3 Low degree of differentiation or undifferentiated

As lymphangiography is of no value in demonstrating internal iliac glands most carcinomas of prostate are categorised NX.

Treatment
In all patients a biopsy is taken, either transperineally or transrectally with a Trucut needle or by transurethral resection. A transurethral resection is done in nearly all patients, not only to obtain a biopsy but also to create or enlarge the channel through the tumour and allow the patient to pass urine more easily.

The *management* of prostate cancer has become increasingly controversial because, although increasing

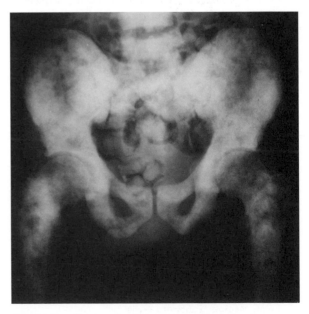

Fig. 27.56 Carcinoma of prostate. An X-ray showing widespread osteosclerotic prostatic metastases in femora, pelvis and lumbar spine

numbers of men are dying from the disease, the histological prevalence is nevertheless far in excess of the clinical disease. It is thus difficult to select those men who will truly benefit from treatment. For localized cancer, radical prostatectomy offers cure for some men but there is a risk of overtreatment especially in cases of well differentiated lesions in older men. For locally advanced or metastatic disease the most usual treatment is to deprive the tumour of androgens either by hormonal treatment or by orchidectomy. Hormonal treatment aims to limit the production of androgens or neutralise their effects, and some 80 to 90% of patients respond (for a time anyway) to this treatment. Stilboestrol 1 to 3 mg daily is effective but cannot be used in patients with cardiovascular or thromboembolic disease. The antiandrogen cyproterone acetate inhibits the binding of testosterone to its receptors. Although expensive, it does not have the side effects of oestrogens and may preserve some potency. In most cases, hormonal treatment is best accomplished with a Gonadotrophin Releasing Hormone (GnRH) analogue such as Goserilin; this inhibits pituitary stimulation of testosterone production by the Leydig cells (after an initial surge) and is equivalent to medical castration. Adrenal androgens are not inhibited, however, and there is some evidence that younger patients with small volume metastatic disease benefit by the addition of flutamide, a substance which inhibits the action of androgens at target cell. The alternative to monthly injections of Goserilin is subcapsular orchidectomy (p. 678).

What of patients whose tumour is not controlled by hormone manipulation after an initial response or who do not respond at all? To change the oestrogen helps little although Tetrasodium Fosfestrol and others can be tried. Non hormonal treatment of advanced prostatic cancer using a variety of chemotherapeutic agents, including cyclophosphamide, 5 fluorouracil, estramustine (a drug combining an oestrogen and an alkylating agent) and more recently Cisplatinum have been tried but results await evaluation before the treatment can be recommended.

PROSTATIC CALCULI

True prostatic calculi develop in stagnant or infected acini by the deposition of calcareous material on the corpora amylacea (small bodies of amorphous debris and desquamated epithelium which lie in the acini of the prostatic glands), and are usually found in men between the ages of 50 and 65. They are generally small and multiple, and found in infected glands or in the compressed outer zone or capsule of a hypertrophied gland.

Calculi themselves rarely cause symptoms, and are detected only on X-ray examination or during prostatectomy for benign hypertrophy. The clinical features of prostatic calculi are those of the associated simple hypertrophy or chronic infection although on rectal examination a gland containing calculi is hard and irregular and crepitus may be elicited.

Prostatic stones can be removed transurethrally, or at the time of prostatectomy. They are usually small enough to wash out without first crushing them.

REFERENCES

Gosling J A, Dixon J S, Humpherson J R 1982 Functional anatomy of the urinary tract. Churchill Livingstone, Edinburgh

Gow J G 1980 Bladder too small/too large. In: Chisholm G D (ed.) Urology. Heinemann, London, p 434

Husain I 1984 Tropical urology and renal disease. Churchill Livingstone, Edinburgh

Mitchell J 1981 Endoscopic operative urology. John Wright, Bristol

Paulson D F 1983 Radical cystectomy. In: Glenn J F (ed.) Urological Surgery, 3rd edn. Lippincott, Philadelphia, p 583

Soloway M S 1982 Intravesical chemotherapy for superficial bladder tumours. In: Spiers A S D (ed.) Chemotherapy and urological malignancy. Springer Verlag, Heidelberg, p 50

Turner-Warwick R 1973 Observations on the treatment of traumatic urethral injuries and the value of the fenestrated urethral catheter. British Journal of Urology 60: 775

UICC 1978 TNM Classification of Malignant Tumours, 3rd edn. International Union against Cancer, Geneva

FURTHER READING

Blandy J P 1978 Handbook of urological endoscopy. Pitman-Medical, Tunbridge Wells

Blandy J P 1984 Operative urology, 2nd edn. Blackwell, Oxford

Clark P 1985 Operations in urology. Churchill Livingstone, Edinburgh

Hohenfellner R, Wammack R (eds) 1992 Societie international d'urologie reports. Churchill Livingstone, Edinburgh

Mauermayer W 1983 Transurethral surgery. Springer Verlag, Berlin/Heidelberg

Paulson D F 1984 Genitourinary surgery. Churchill Livingstone, Edinburgh

Zingg E J, Wallace D M A 1985 Bladder cancer. Springer Verlag, Berlin/Heidelberg

28

Male urethra and genital organs

J. M. S. JOHNSTONE & T. B. HARGREAVE

OPERATIONS ON THE URETHRA

Anatomy of the urethra

The male urethra is about 20 cm long and is divided into prostatic, membranous and spongy parts (Fig. 28.1). *The prostatic part* is about 3 cm long and is the widest part of the urethra. It is surrounded by the prostate gland. The prostatic ducts (10 to 15 in number) open onto its posterior wall on either side of a longitudinal ridge called the urethral crest. At the lower end of this crest there is a rounded elevation called the verumontanum, on which lie the openings of the prostatic utricle and the ejaculatory ducts. The verumontanum marks the position of the external sphincter and it is a most important landmark when resecting the prostate.

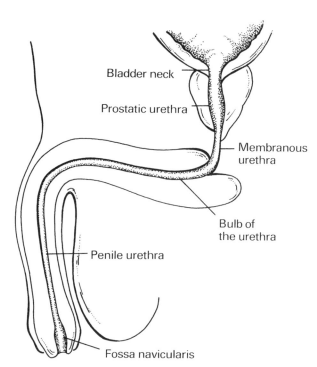

Fig. 28.1 A sagittal section of the male urethra

Bladder neck

Prostatic urethra

Membranous urethra

Bulb of the urethra

Penile urethra

Fossa navicularis

The membranous part, 1 cm in length, is surrounded by fibres of the external sphincter and passes through the perineal membrane to become continuous with the spongy part.

The spongy part is about 15 cm long and traverses the corpus spongiosum from the bulb (where it is wide) to the external meatus (which is the narrowest part of the whole male urethra). The ducts from the bulbo-urethral glands, which lie behind the membranous urethra, pierce the perineal membrane and open into the spongy urethra.

Injuries of the urethra: general considerations

The early signs of urethral injury are urethral bleeding, bruising and swelling in the perineum and an inability to pass water. Later the bladder distends and later still urine extravasates into the extraperitoneal tissues or the superficial perineal pouch depending upon the site of injury. The general principles of treatment are to prevent extravasation of urine by draining the bladder with a urethral or suprapubic catheter and to allow or encourage the urethra to heal with as little fibrosis and deformity as possible.

Injuries of the anterior urethra (see Newsam, 1980)

Injuries of the anterior urethra usually involve the bulbous part of the urethra in the perineum and are caused by blows or kicks or falling astride a hard object, such as a wooden plank. After such an injury blood leaks out of the external urinary meatus, and into the perineum. Spasm of the sphincter prevents the patient passing urine and urine only extravasates when the bladder distends and overflows. For that reason the patient can be left safely for some 24 hours after injury to see whether or not he can pass urine. If he is able to do so the injury probably consists of no more than a bruise and requires no active treatment. If he is unable to do so the injury is probably more serious and a complete or partial tear of the urethra is suspected. One cautious attempt is made to pass a *soft* 12 or 14F catheter through the urethra into the bladder with the strictest of aseptic techniques.

If successful, the catheter is left in situ; if not, a suprapubic cystostomy is required. On no account should attempts be made to pass a stiff plastic or metal catheter or a catheter on an introducer for fear of damaging the urethra further by converting a partial tear into a complete one. If there are obvious signs of extravasation in the superficial perineal pouch the extravasated urine must be drained. After 10 to 12 days the catheter is removed or the suprapubic tube clipped. If the patient passes urine satisfactorily no more need be done for 3 months when urethroscopy and urethrography will reveal any stricture. If the patient cannot pass urine satisfactorily these investigations are done earlier and the stricture, which is usually short, treated appropriately.

Injuries of the membranous urethra

Injuries of the membranous urethra are usually associated with a fractured pelvis and occur at the junction of prostatic and membranous parts. Tears are often complete because the urethra is damaged by the splintered rami. If the perineal membrane and the puboprostatic ligaments are also torn, the prostate and the neck of the bladder dislocate upwards and backwards and continuity of the urethra is completely lost (Fig. 28.2). About 10% of patients with injuries of the membranous urethra also have injuries of the bladder. The internal sphincter goes into spasm and urine extravasates into the extraperitoneal tissues only when the bladder becomes distended, unless of course the bladder is also injured. Many patients require blood transfusion and other resuscitative measures and have serious other injuries to abdomen, chest or pelvis that take precedence over the urethral injury. Fortunately, there is no urgency in treating the urethra. One attempt is made to pass a small soft catheter through the urethra; if it passes into the bladder and clear urine emerges, it is certain that little damage has occurred to either urethra or bladder. Nevertheless, it may be useful to leave the catheter in for a few days to measure the urinary output if the patient has serious other injuries. If the catheter appears to pass into the bladder but nothing more than blood or a little blood stained urine emerges, a cystogram is done to see if there is an extraperitoneal rupture of the bladder. If the catheter does not pass into the bladder a partial or complete tear of the urethra must be suspected. The bladder is drained by a suprapubic cystostomy if the patient is ill but more can be attempted if the patient is fit.

Operation

A transverse suprapubic incision is made although a midline or paramedian one is better if it is necessary to inspect the peritoneal cavity also. The prevesical and retropubic spaces are gently cleared of blood and urine,

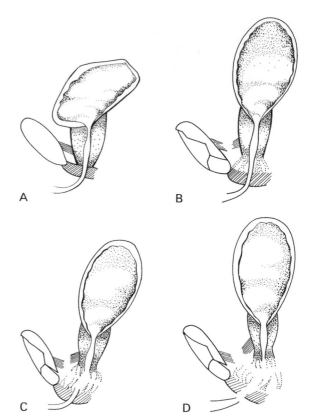

Fig. 28.2 Injuries of the urethra (A) The normal anatomy of the bladder, prostate, perineal membrane and puboprostatic ligaments. (B) The pelvis is fractured and the puboprostatic ligament ruptured but the urethra is only stretched and bruised. (C) The pelvis is fractured, the puboprostatic ligament disrupted and there is a complete tear through the membranous part of the urethra but the perineal ligament is intact. (D) The pelvis is fractured, both puboprostatic and perineal ligaments are disrupted and there is a complete tear which involves the membranous and bulbous part of the urethra with an upward and backward dislocation of the prostate and bladder

taking great care not to open or reopen any of the pelvic veins. If the bladder is empty the injury is probably vesical although the urethra may also be damaged. If the membranous urethra is injured it is necessary to realign the ruptured ends, which may be widely separated from each other, and maintain them in a satisfactory position until healing occurs. To suture the cut ends together or to suture the upper cut end to the perineal membrane is seldom possible and reliance must be placed on the splinting effect of an indwelling catheter. To achieve this the bladder is opened and a soft 12 or 14F catheter passed through the bladder neck and down the urethra until it emerges at the site of injury. A silastic Foley catheter is then passed up the urethra from the external meatus. When its tip emerges from the site of injury it is tied to the tip of the catheter passed from above. By withdrawing the upper one out of the urethra and out of the bladder the Foley catheter is negotiated into the bladder and its balloon inflated. By applying traction to the catheter the balloon pulls the prostate down to the perineal membrane opposing the cut ends of the urethra. The procedure can also be accomplished by using two bougies instead of two catheters. One is passed down the urethra from within the open bladder to the injury. The second is passed retrogradely to the injury through the external urinary meatus. By preserving contact between the tips of the two bougies the second one is manoeuvred into the bladder by withdrawing the first. A catheter is attached to the tip of the second bougie as it lies in the bladder and manoeuvred through the whole length of the urethra by withdrawing the bougie out of the external meatus. A Foley catheter can then be attached to the tip of this catheter and withdrawn back into the bladder. With both procedures it is wise to drain the bladder with a suprapubic tube.

Urethral strictures (see Turner-Warwick, 1983)

Congenital strictures are found at the external urethral meatus in boys, often secondary to hypospadias, but are uncommon elsewhere in the urethra. (Congenital lesions causing obstruction consist of either bladder neck contracture or posterior urethral valves.) Malig-

nant strictures are uncommon but can occur in patients who have a urethral tumour secondary to tumour of the bladder or prostate. They usually occur in the spongy part of the male urethra and are often palpable or even visible. Most urethral strictures are post inflammatory or post traumatic.

Post-inflammatory strictures

Non specific urethritis is caused by *Chlamydia trachomatis*, ureaplasma urealyticum, candida species, trichomonas or herpes and rarely causes strictures because the infection never extends more deeply into the urethral wall than the mucosa. Gonorrhoea on the other hand involves not only the mucosa of the urethra but also the submucosa and corpora spongiosa, and, unless effectively and rapidly treated, causes strictures in the bulbous part of the spongy urethra. Postgonococcal strictures are often multiple and complicated by sinuses, fistulae and false passages.

Post-traumatic strictures

Injuries in the perineum may cause strictures of the bulbous part of the spongy urethra which are usually short, straight and uncomplicated unless previously maltreated. Fractures of the bony pelvis can cause strictures of the membranous urethra which can be severe and complicated; endoscopic procedures and open

Figs 28.3 & 28.4 *False urethral passages*

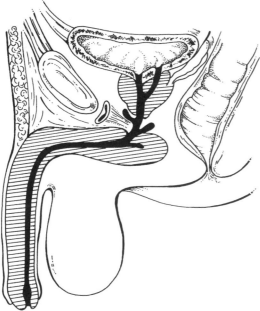

Fig. 28.3 Sites where false passages may occur. The lower three are sinuses, the upper one is a fistula forming an abnormal communication between bladder and prostatic urethra

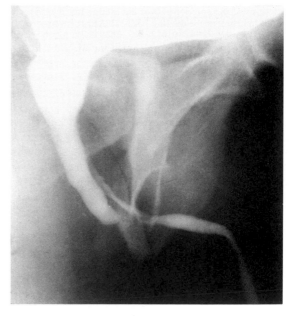

Fig. 28.4 Descending urethrogram showing false passage between prostatic urethra (which is dilated) and spongy urethra

operations on the rectum, colon, prostate and bladder may injure the urethra and cause or aggravate strictures. Even catheterization may cause a stricture of the external meatus.

Assessment

Strictures obstruct the outflow of urine from the bladder causing symptoms similar to those of prostatic diseases (p. 637); furthermore there may be local complications such as sinuses, abscesses, fistulae and false passages (Figs 28.3 & 28.4).

The diagnosis is sometimes made from the patient's history especially if the stricture is of traumatic origin, but confirmation of its extent and effects on the urinary tract requires investigation such as *urethroscopy,* ascending and descending *urethrography* and *intravenous urography.* The methods available for treating urethral strictures consist of:

1. urethral dilatation
2. external urethrostomy
3. internal urethrotomy — blind or optical

4. excision and suture
5. urethroplasty
6. urinary diversion.

Urethral dilatation by graduated bougies (Figs 28.5–28.7)

This used to be the standard treatment and there were few strictures to which it was not applied. Metal bougies can be more easily controlled than plastic ones and if used carefully and gently do no more damage. The procedure can usually be accomplished by anaesthetizing the urethra with 1 or 2% *Lignocaine gel.* If general anaesthesia is used, dilatation must be carried out even more carefully and gently. If records of previous urethral dilatations are available it is wise to choose a bougie three or four sizes smaller than the largest one passed on the previous occasion, remembering that false passages are more likely to be made by small bougies. The bougie is introduced by the following technique. Its tip is kept on the floor of the anterior urethra until the bulb is reached; then, the instrument is rotated, depressed and very gently pushed upwards towards the bladder with its tip in contact with the roof. If the first bougie arrests and cannot be passed, smaller ones are tried successively until the stricture is negotiated. Thereafter the scale of bougies is ascended until the patient complains of discomfort or dilatation is considered adequate. The last bougie, usually 26 or 28F, should be left in place for a few minutes if the maximum benefit is to be obtained from the dilatation. To overstretch the urethra causes bleeding and stimulates fibrosis. No stricture is cured by dilatation and it has to be repeated at intervals which vary from three

Figs 28.5–28.7 *Urethral bougies (*Courtesy of G U Manufacturing Co Ltd)

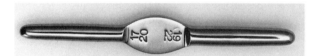

Fig. 28.5 Canny-Ryall bougie. This is used for dilating strictures of the anterior part of the urethra but is also a useful instrument for dilating perineal urethrostomies or nephrostomies

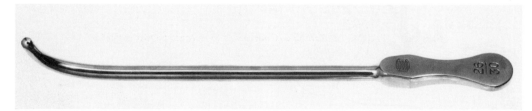

Fig. 28.6 Clutton bougie

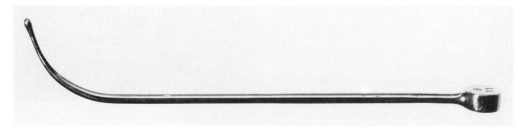

Fig. 28.7 Lister bougie

weeks to a year or more. Nevertheless, urethral dilatation remains a sensible means of treating strictures if the patient is old; the procedure easily accomplished, and unassociated with haemorrhage, infection, or other reaction; the intervals between treatments at least 6 months and the patient content. Strictures at the external meatus are usually caused by an endoscope or catheter and can often be cured by one or two dilations; if not, they should be treated by *meatotomy*.

Acute retention of urine due to stricture
A urethral stricture should be suspected as the cause of acute retention if the patient is young, has a normal prostate, or has had previous operations on the urethra or prostate; it is confirmed as the cause when a small catheter is arrested in the region of the bulb or membranous urethra. An attempt is made to negotiate the stricture with a metal bougie, and thereafter introduce a catheter. If this is not easily possible, the bladder is drained suprapubically, and the stricture treated in the appropriate way later.

Urethrostomy
External urethrostomy means entering the urethra through an incision in the skin. On the rare occasions when this is done, the patient is more likely to be suffering from urethral stone than stricture. However,

in an elaborate form, it is the first part of a two stage urethroplasty.

Internal urethrotomy
This can be done blindly or optically.

Blind urethrotomy
Of the several urethrotomes available, the Otis (Fig. 28.8) or one of its several modifications is the most popular. The Otis urethrotome is a 13F instrument which can be expanded from 13F to 43F by rotating the wheel at its proximal end. The instrument is passed beyond the stricture, which is usually possible only if the tip of the urethrotome has been modified to screw on to a filiform bougie which is passed first. Once beyond the stricture, the wheel of the urethrotome is rotated and the stricture dilated. Then the knife, hidden within the instrument, is withdrawn cutting the narrowed parts of the urethra lineally to a depth of 3 mm. (This instrument is also used before transurethral prostatic resections if the urethra does not easily accept the 26F resectoscope sheath and some surgeons use it routinely before all prostatic resections.)

Visual urethrotomy
Most firms now make an optical urethrotome (Fig. 28.9). It consists of a straight metal sheath with

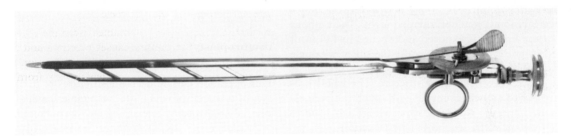

Fig. 28.8   The Otis urethrotome (Courtesy of G U Manufacturing Co Ltd)

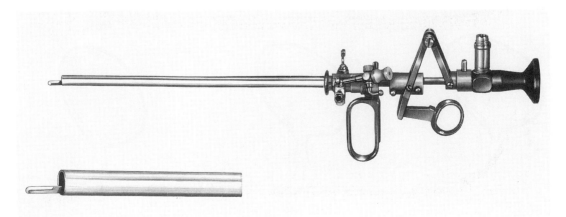

Fig. 28.9   Optical urethrotome (Courtesy of Stortz Ltd)

a side opening through which a ureteric catheter can be passed. An Iglesias resectoscope working element, modified to take and move a long knife instead of a loop electrode, is passed into the sheath, and vision obtained with a fore-oblique or direct view telescope. Under vision, the instrument is passed into the urethra, which is continuously, but slowly, irrigated through the side tap to separate the walls of the urethra. The stricture can be seen clearly. A ureteric catheter is passed through the side opening of the sheath, and on through the stricture into the bladder and acts as a guide for the knife which is then used to incise the stricture at 12 o'clock. Thereafter, a silastic Foley catheter is passed into the bladder and left for at least 2 weeks, although some surgeons leave it longer. Only the fibrous tissue of the stricture is cut but if the cut is made too deeply the corpora spongiosa is opened and much bleeding and bruising occurs. The optical urethrotome is proving of considerable value in the treatment of urethral strictures, and seems destined to replace urethral dilatation and many types of urethroplasty as the standard method of treatment (Chilton, 1983).

Excision of the stricture and reanastomosis

Short uncomplicated strictures of the bulbar part of the urethra often respond to dilatation or optical urethrotomy; if not, they can be excised and the cut urethral ends anastomosed (Fig. 28.10). The patient is placed in the semilithotomy position, and a vertical or ∩-shaped incision is made in the perineum. The bulbous part of the urethra is exposed and opened just in front of the stricture by cutting against the tip of a bougie passed from the external meatus. The urethra is opened again just behind the stricture. The whole procedure can often be accomplished through the perineal incision; if not, the bladder is exposed through a suprapubic incision and a second bougie passed through the bladder neck and down the urethra. The stricture and the fibrosed corpora spongiosum, which may extend

beyond the stricture, are excised. The anterior segment of urethra is mobilized and displaced backwards to permit a tension free end-to-end anastomosis with the proximal segment. The ends should be spatulated and sutured with 3/0 catgut. A small silastic Foley catheter is passed into the bladder and the wound is sutured.

Strictures of the membranous urethra are usually short in length, but difficult to treat because they are S shaped. They can often be managed by dilatation or by internal visual urethrotomy, which may be done more safely and effectively if the bladder is first opened and a cystoscope or bougie is passed down the urethra to the proximal level of the stricture.

Pull through operation (Badenoch)

This operation was described for strictures of the membranous urethra. The urethra is exposed by a perineal incision and divided transversely just below the stricture. The bladder is opened and the bladder neck and the prostatic and membranous parts of the urethra are dilated from above. A catheter is passed down the urethra from the bladder until its tip appears in the perineal wound. The tip of this catheter is sutured to the cut end of the distal urethra, which is pulled up to the bladder neck through the dilated prostatic and membranous urethra as the catheter is withdrawn into the bladder. By suturing the catheter to the suprapubic wound, the urethra is retained in its new position. The catheter is removed after 2 weeks.

Urethroplasty

One-stage skin patch operation

This operation can be used for strictures of the bulbar part of the urethra which are unsuitable for dilatation, internal urethrotomy or excision and are uncomplicated by fistulae or sinuses. The stricture and the healthy urethra and corpora spongiosum proximal and distal to it are exposed through a vertical or ∩ incision. The stric-

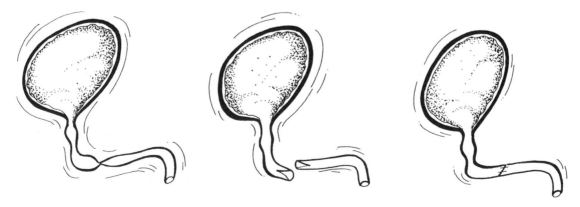

Fig. 28.10   Excision of urethral stricture and end-to-end anastomosis

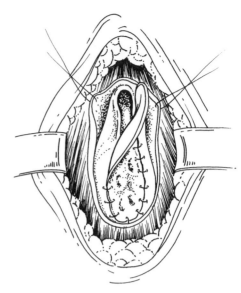

Fig. 28.12 Urethral stricture. Graft almost completed

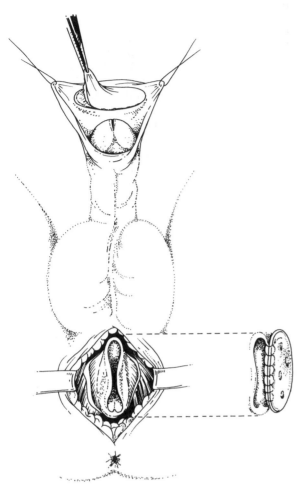

Fig. 28.11 Urethral stricture. A free full thickness graft taken from the prepuce is applied and sutured to the urethra, which has been laid open throughout the length of the stricture

ture is widely opened and the urethral defect is covered by a full thickness skin graft (Fig. 28.11) (the epidermis on the inside forming urethral lumen) secured all round with 4/0 absorbable sutures (Fig. 28.12). The skin patch can be a free one taken from the prepuce or penis or a pedicled one attached by the dartos muscle and taken from the side of a vertical skin incision or from the front of an ∩ one. A small silastic catheter is passed through the urethra into the bladder at the conclusion of the operation.

Two-stage urethroplasty

A number of two-stage operations have been described and perhaps the best of these is the scrotal flap procedure. This is indicated for strictures of the bulbar urethra complicated by fistulae, sinuses, or excessive scar tissue from infection or previous operations.

First stage (Figs 28.13–28.15). An ∩ incision is made in the perineum and extended vertically forwards be-

tween the two halves of the scrotum. The perineal flap of skin and fat is separated and allowed to fall backwards. The bulbospongiosum muscle is split in the midline and carefully separated from the spongy tissue and the underlying urethra. The urethra is incised vertically onto a bougie passed down from the external meatus. The incision into the urethra is continued forwards and backwards until the stricture is completely divided and healthy corpora spongiosum exposed. The front edge of the scrotal flap is then stitched to the proximal edge of the healthy urethra using 3 or 4/0 nylon sutures. The urethra is sutured to the skin edges and a catheter is passed through the exposed part of the urethra into the bladder.

Second stage (Figs 28.16 & 28.17). A bougie or catheter is passed through the urethra into the bladder. An incision is made around the exposed part of the urethra forming a skin tube which is loosely sutured over the bougie or catheter to reform the urethra. The skin edges are then undermined and closed over the skin tube.

Diversion

Urine is temporarily diverted from the urethra by perineal urethrostomy or suprapubic cystostomy for some of the repair operations just described; a permanent diversion by perineal urethrostomy, suprapubic cystostomy, ileal loop or ureterocolic anastomosis should rarely if ever be necessary.

Other urethral conditions

Urethral fistulae

Urethral fistulae may develop from peri-urethral ab-

Figs 28.13–28.17   *Two stage urethroplasty*

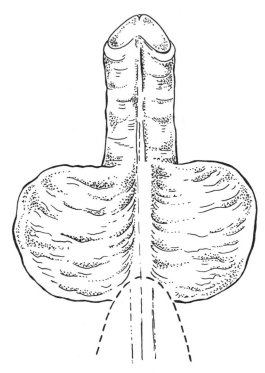

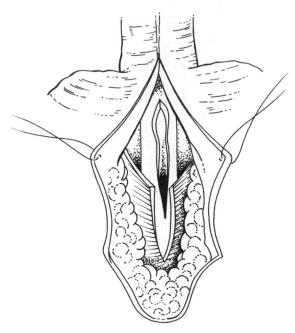

Fig. 28.14   The urethra is laid open until healthy urethra and healthy corpus spongiosum are demonstrated distally and proximally

First stage
Fig. 28.13   An ∩ incision is made in the perineum and extended forwards in the midline along the urethra

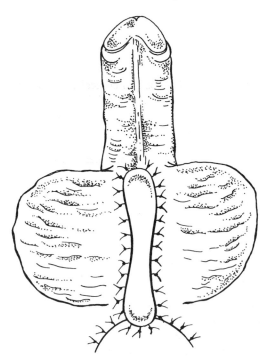

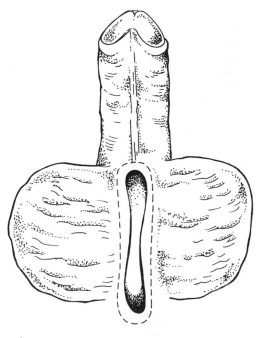

Fig. 28.15   The proximal end of the laid open urethra is sutured to the apex of the flap, the rest to the skin margin

Second stage
Fig. 28.16   An incision is made around the exposed open urethra

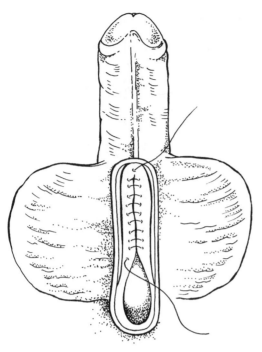

Fig. 28.17 The skin tube thus formed is loosely sutured over a bougie or a catheter to reform the urethra. The skin edges are then undermined and closed over the skin tube

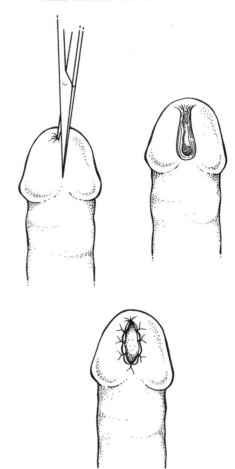

Fig. 28.18 Meatotomy

scesses, which can complicate urethral trauma or infection. They occur most commonly at the penoscrotal angle or in the perineum and are usually associated with strictures. If the stricture is treated and the urethral obstruction relieved the fistula often heals. If it does not, the fistulous tract can be excised together with surrounding scar tissue down to the urethral wall, and the defect closed in layers or covered with a full thickness skin graft.

Urethral stones
Stones that pass through the bladder neck into the urethra usually pass right through without difficulty. Occasionally they impact at the external meatus or behind a stricture more proximally in the urethra. Stones that impact immediately proximal to the external urinary meatus can usually be removed after a meatotomy (Fig. 28.18) has been carried out. Stones that impact in the urethra proximal to a stricture are more difficult to manage. It is probably best to push them back into the bladder with an endoscope or bougie and treat them appropriately (p. 626).

OPERATIONS ON THE PENIS

Anatomy

The penis has three parts, the glans, the body and the root. The *glans* is the enlarged conical extremity which bears the external urinary meatus. It has a basal oblique rim called the *corona* and it is covered to a variable extent by the *prepuce*. The prepuce has two layers: the outer layer is an extension of the hairless skin of the penis; the inner layer is thin and delicate and fuses at the corona with the epithelium covering the glans. The *frenulum* is a thin median fold of skin connecting the inner layer of the prepuce with the glans immediately below the external urinary meatus and it contains the main artery. The rest of the mobile part of the penis is called the *body*. The *root* of the penis is fixed and buried in the perineum. The penis consists of three longitudinal columns of cavernous erectile tissue, the two corpora cavernosa and the corpus spongiosum, bound together by fibrous tissue (Buck's Fascia) and covered with skin. The *corpora cavernosa* lie dorsally side by side in the body of the penis and diverge posteriorly to become the *crura* which are firmly adherent to the inferior rami of the pubis. The *corpus spongiosum* contains the urethra and lies anteriorly in a groove formed by the corpora cavernosa: inferiorly it expands to form the glans, posteriorly it expands to form the *bulb of the penis* which lies on the perineal membrane. The *suspensory ligament* holds the posterior part of the body of the penis against the front of the symphysis pubis.

Blood supply
The penis is supplied by three *arteries*, all derived from the internal pudendal artery; the artery of the bulb runs within the corpus spongiosum, the deep arteries run within the corpora cavernosa and the dorsal artery runs superficially. The *veins* correspond to the arteries except that the dorsal veins are superficial and deep not right and left. The superficial dorsal vein divides into right and left branches which drain by the external pudendal veins into the long saphenous vein; the deep dorsal vein joins the prostatic venous plexus. *Lymph vessels* follow superficial veins to the inguinal lymph nodes.

Circumcision

The common indications for circumcision are the presence of phimosis and recurrent balanitis; the former is a narrowing of the opening of the prepuce and the latter an infection in the subprepucial space. These two conditions are often related and are both associated with incomplete retraction of the prepuce. Phimosis makes hygiene difficult, may cause discomfort during coitus and predisposes to balanitis and carcinoma. Following an erection, which can be painful, paraphimosis may occur. Circumcision is still performed extensively for cultural reasons although the removal of a normal prepuce is of no medical benefit.

Phimosis in the child may impede micturition with spraying of urine and ballooning of the foreskin but repeated retraction of the prepuce probably aggravates the situation and parents should not be encouraged to do this. In the infant, adhesions between the prepuce and the glans may prevent retraction of the prepuce and give the appearance of a phimosis. However, the difference becomes apparent when the prepuce is pulled forward from the glans rather than retracted and an adequate opening can then be seen. Prepucial adhesions rarely persist after 3 years of age but are physiological in infancy. Balanitis is usually caused by infection of smegma or debris trapped under the prepuce. Infection is often recurrent but in some children adhesions retaining smegma can be broken down and, in the absence of phimosis, the condition will then resolve. Balanitis must be distinguished from ammoniacal dermatitis as both may present with inflammation of the prepuce. In the latter, however, the prepuce serves to protect the glans and a circumcision is therefore contraindicated.

In *children* the surgical management of phimosis and recurrent balanitis is by circumcision. Occasionally minor adhesions causing pain or recurrent infection may be successfully freed in outpatients after application of anaesthetic cream. In *adults,* circumcision is advisable for phimosis and is also required in the assessment and treatment of patients with carcinoma of the penis.

Circumcision in the child
The operation is performed under general anaesthesia with the child supine. The prepuce is first fully retracted to expose the coronal sulcus and retained smegma removed. To allow retraction it may be necessary to stretch the opening of the prepuce and to free adhesions by sweeping back the inner layer of the prepuce from the glans with a blunt probe. The prepuce is then returned to its normal position and the skin marked at the level of the corona, to serve as a guide to the line of dissection. Excessive suprapubic fat may carry abdominal skin onto the shaft of the penis and, before marking, this should be pushed firmly down onto the pubic symphysis so that the shaft is covered only by penile skin (Fig. 28.19). The tip of the prepuce is then grasped with two forceps and pulled forward with light traction. A narrow clamp is placed obliquely across the prepuce distal to the glans and parallel to the corona and the prepuce then divided immediately distal to the clamp (Fig. 28.20). As the clamp is released the outer layer will retract, leaving the inner layer partly covering the glans. The inner layer is then pulled forward with three clamps and trimmed so as to leave a cuff approximately 0.3 cm long which just covers the corona of the glans. This is most easily done by making a dorsal incision from the free margin of the inner layer to the level of the corona (Fig. 28.21); the point of dissection is then carried round both sides of the glans (Fig. 28.22) to the frenulum. Haemostasis is then secured with particular attention being paid to the dorsal vein. Only bipolar diathermy should be used. Finally the inner and outer layer of the prepuce are closed with fine interrupted absorbable sutures (Fig. 28.23); a ventrally placed mattress suture between skin and frenulum will control bleeding from frenular vessels.

A number of devices, of which the Hollister Plastibell is the best known, are available for circumcising the small infant and they make the operation simpler and quicker. The Plastibell is pushed into the space between glans and prepuce and the ligature, supplied with the kit, is applied around the lip of the bell. The prepuce is cut off with scissors and the plastic device extruded.

Circumcision in the adult
Although the operation can be done under local anaes-

Figs 28.19–28.23 *Circumcision in the child (see text)*

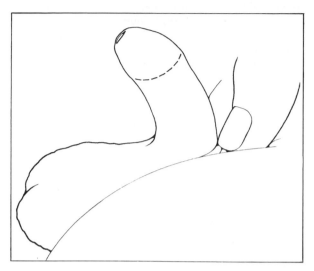

Fig. 28.19

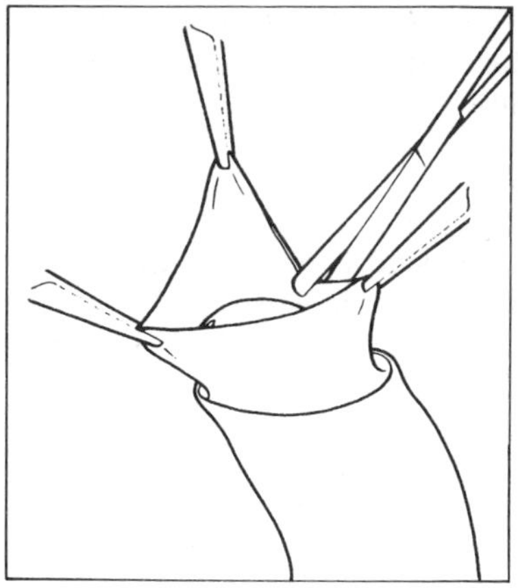

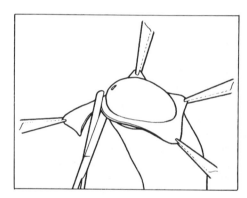

Fig. 28.21

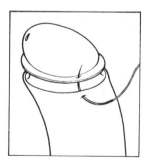

Fig. 28.22

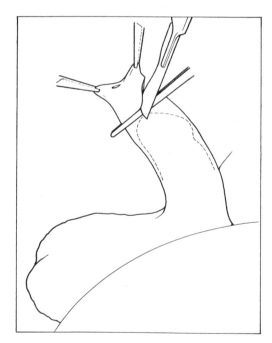

Fig. 28.20

Fig. 28.23

thesia by injecting 1% Lignocaine solution subcutaneously around the body of the penis and into the sensitive region near the frenulum, it is best done under general anaesthesia. Since the prepuce is seldom as long in the adult as in the child, and is much more vascular, the clamp method is unsuitable. Three small artery forceps are applied to the edge of the prepuce, one in the midline ventrally, two (side by side) in the midline dorsally. Adhesions between the prepuce and the underlying glans are separated and the prepuce in the mid dorsal line is slit between the two dorsally placed artery forceps as far as the corona, taking great care not to enter the urethra. After smegma has been removed the redundant part of the prepuce is cut off parallel to the corona. The underlying inner layer of the prepuce is trimmed in the same way leaving it about

0.5 cm longer than the skin. All bleeding vessels are ligated with 4/0 absorbable sutures and the cut edge of the skin is sutured to the cut edge of the inner layer of the prepuce with the same material (Fig. 28.24). Painful erections are rarely a problem during convalescence but can be prevented with chlorpromazine.

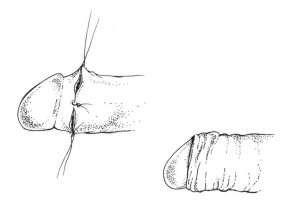

Fig. 28.24   End result of circumcision in the adult

Paraphimosis
Paraphimosis occurs when a tight prepuce has been forcibly retracted behind the corona and remains there as a constricting ring beyond which the inner layer of the prepuce swells rapidly to form an oedematous collar which prevents reduction. In most cases manipulative reduction should be attempted before operation is considered. An attempt is made to dispel some of the oedematous fluid by squeezing; then the glans is compressed and elongated with the thumb and first two fingers of the right hand and an attempt is made to draw the prepuce down over it with the fingers and thumb of the other hand. It is a mistake to try and push the glans upwards through the constricting ring. If manipulation fails, the constricting ring should be divided with a short longitudinal dorsal incision after which the prepuce can easily be drawn down. The incision is left unsutured. Circumcision should be carried out at a later date when all oedema and reaction has disappeared because a paraphimosis often recurs.

Tumours of the penis (see Lloyd-Davies, 1983)
Of the benign tumours the venereal wart (condyloma acuminatum), coronal papillae and the Buschke-Loewenstein tumour are the commonest. The common wart is viral in origin and found most frequently on the glans penis around the corona or at or just within the urethral meatus. Cases have been described however in which the warts have involved the whole of the urethra and even the bladder when it may be difficult to distinguish them from transitional cell tumours. Warts can be treated with 10% podophyllin or electro-

coagulation although those inside the meatus may have to be exposed by a meatotomy. Coronal papillae appear as tiny pale papillary processes along the edge of the corona and they can be disregarded. Buschke-Loewenstein tumours look like enormous common warts but tend to infiltrate deeper tissues. They are not considered to be malignant because they never metastasize and they can be treated by electrocoagulation or local excision.

The malignant tumours consist of in situ carcinoma called Paget's Disease, Bowen's Disease and the Erythroplasia of Queyrat and can only be distinguished from benign skin disorders by biopsy: epithelial carcinoma of which the vast majority are squamous; connective tissue tumours like sarcomas and lymphomas are rare as are secondary tumours which have metastasized from prostate or bladder. Squamous cell carcinoma usually begins near the corona and is easily overlooked in the early stages because it is usually hidden beneath the prepuce (which is often phimotic) or obscured by secondary infection. Many patients only seek advice when the tumour has spread down the body of the penis or to the inguinal glands. Penile carcinoma must be suspected when an elderly male patient presents with an offensive or blood stained discharge from the preputial orifice. In such cases a biopsy must be taken from the glans and the corona although it may be possible to do this only after a dorsal slit or a circumcision. The latter procedures also facilitate treatment of the local infection which is often severe.

Of the various ways of *staging* carcinoma of the penis clinically, the TNM system is probably the best although it is little used. It considers the local extent of the tumour (*T category*) separately from the state of the regional lymph nodes which are the inguinal ones (*N category*). With the other methods, the stage is decided after considering the local extent of the tumour and the state of the regional lymph nodes together. The treatment depends upon the local extent of the disease.

Carcinoma in situ
Carcinoma in situ can be treated by radiotherapy, by excision or by chemotherapy. Most surgeons would treat it first by radiotherapy because it can always be excised later if it fails to respond. If the lesion is excised the defect has usually to be covered with a skin graft. For chemotherapy 5-fluorouracil is applied locally but the treatments have to be continued for a long time and local reactions may be severe.

Carcinoma of the penis
If the growth is confined to the prepuce it may all be removed by circumcision. More often the tumour involves the glans as well as the prepuce and can be treated by X-ray therapy or partial amputation of the

penis. It is worth considering X-ray therapy because amputation can still be carried out at a later date if the tumour fails to respond. If the tumour has extended to the shaft of the penis, X-ray therapy can still be considered but is likely to be less successful than it is with the earlier tumours. Partial amputation may be possible if enough healthy tissue can be left between the edge of the tumour and the incision otherwise a total amputation should be carried out particularly if the tumour has recurred after a previous partial resection.

Amputation of the penis

Before partial or total amputation of the penis the patient will already have had a dorsal slit or circumcision and biopsy and some treatment to ameliorate the local infection.

Partial amputation (Figs 28.25–28.28)

A *flap* method (Fig. 28.25) is commonly employed. A fine catheter, a piece of soft rubber tubing or a non crushing intestinal clamp is applied around the base of

Figs 28.25–28.28   *The operation of partial amputation of the penis for carcinoma by the flap method*

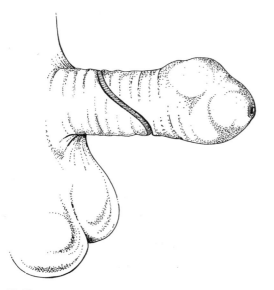

Fig. 28.25

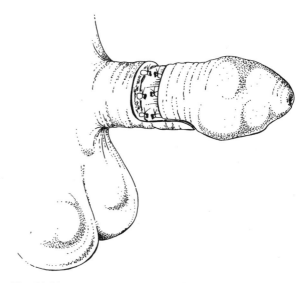

Fig. 28.26

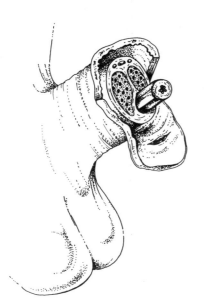

Fig. 28.27

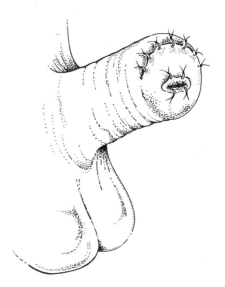

Fig. 28.28

the penis as a tourniquet. The combined lengths of the two flaps, the cut edges of which must be at least 2.5 cm clear of the growth, should be a little more than the diameter of the penis. The inferior flap should be longer than the superior one so that the suture line is at a higher level than the urethra which is brought out through a stab incision in the inferior flap. The flaps are fashioned by incising skin and subcutaneous tissue. down to Buck's fascia which covers the corpora cavernosa and the corpus spongiosum and reflecting them back to their bases. The corpora cavernosa are divided at this level but the corpus spongiosum and the urethra are divided some 1.5 to 2 cm more distally. The tourniquet is now removed and all bleeding vessels secured. The stump of the urethra is brought through a suitably placed stab wound in the inferior skin flap. The end of the emerging urethra is split into two halves by short lateral incisions and each half is sutured beyond the margin of the stab wound so that the urethra protrudes slightly beyond the skin. If haemostasis proves difficult the wound can be drained. A selfretaining catheter is introduced into the bladder and removed some 4 or 5 days later. The new external urinary meatus may have to be dilated periodically with bougies but, unless the stump of the penis is very short, the patient should experience no difficulty with micturition.

Total amputation of the penis
The patient is placed in the lithotomy-Trendelenberg position and the penis is enclosed in a polythene or rubber glove to allow cleaning of the whole area. A racquet incision is made encircling the base of the penis and is carried backwards in the midline of the scrotum and perineum to a point some 2–3 cm in front of the anus. Alternatively, an inverted U scrotal flap is used extending the incision forwards to encircle the base of the penis. By dissection exactly in the midline towards a bougie which has been placed in the urethra, the scrotum is split into two halves which are retracted laterally. The penis is then mobilized anteriorly by dividing the suspensory ligament and ligating the dorsal vessels. The penis is further separated from the pubic arch, and the deep vessels (especially the deep dorsal vein of the penis) ligated. The perineal part of the incision is deepened to expose the bulb of the penis (covered by the bulbospongiosus muscle) and the crura (each covered by the ischiocavernosus muscle). The bulb is separated from the anterior part of the perineal membrane, and the crura are detached from the margins of the pubic arch and divided, leaving a thin rim of tissue which is secured with sutures to control bleeding. The bougie is now removed; the urethra is dissected out of the muscular fibres surrounding the bulb and is divided about 5 cm below the perineal membrane.

The anterior part of the wound is repaired by suturing the skin flaps together in the midline; the posterior part is sutured around the stump of the urethra so that this now pursues a direct course from the bladder neck to the perineum and protrudes some 5 cm beyond the skin. The protruding part of the urethral stump is split into two halves by making short anterior and posterior incisions; these are then separated and loosely sutured to overlap the surrounding skin edges. A catheter is left in the bladder for some days. The perineal urethral meatus functions well and seldom becomes stenosed.

In the operation described, the scrotum and testes are retained. Many patients find that the perineal urethrostomy is difficult to manage so long as the scrotum remains, because it tends to get in the way of the urinary stream and becomes wet and excoriated. It may be preferable, therefore, to remove the scrotum and testes as part of the procedure.

Treatment of the inguinal lymph nodes in penile carcinoma
Few surgeons remove the inguinal lymph nodes at the time of amputation of the penis because lymph node enlargement is often due to secondary infection and subsides after the primary growth is removed. If the glands remain enlarged for some weeks after the operation — particularly if they feel hard — biopsy is advisable. If this confirms metastatic disease and if there is no reason to suppose from pedal lymphangiography or CAT scan that deeper glands are also involved, a block dissection of the inguinal glands can be carried out or they can be treated by X-ray therapy.

Anatomy of the inguinal lymph nodes
The *superficial nodes*, which are numerous and large, are often palpable even when healthy. They form two chains forming the letter T; a horizontal chain immediately below the inguinal ligament, and a vertical one along the upper 5–8 cm of the long saphenous vein. They receive lymph from the superficial tissues of the greater part of the abdominal wall and lower limb, from the external genitalia, the buttocks and the anal canal. The *deep nodes*, 4 or 5 in number, lie alongside the proximal end of the femoral vein, the uppermost one being within the femoral canal. They receive lymph from the superficial glands and from the deep tissues of the lower limb and drain to nodes around the external and common iliac vessels.

Biopsy of the inguinal lymph nodes
Biopsy from enlarged inguinal lymph nodes or from clinically normal nodes should be taken from the superficial nodes which lie superomedially and can be carried out through an incision or by percutaneous aspiration.

Inguinal gland dissection

An incision is made 2 cm above and parallel to the whole length of the inguinal ligament. The upper skin flap is reflected and the incision is deepened through the fat to expose the external oblique aponeurosis some 5 cm above the ligament. All fascial and glandular tissue is then stripped cleanly off the aponeurosis down to the level of the inguinal ligament, securing three small arteries, the superficial circumflex iliac, the superficial epigastric and the superficial external pudendal together with their accompanying veins. The lower margin of the wound is strongly retracted; the long saphenous vein is divided between ligatures at least 10 cm below the ligament, and its stump is turned upwards together with all surrounding fat and lymph glands. The partially separated tissue is now stripped off the inguinal ligament from lateral to medial side. As this dissection proceeds, the small arteries already secured and the long saphenous vein are divided again at their junctions with the femoral vessels, which are now left clearly exposed. All fatty and glandular tissue is cleared away from the medial side of the femoral vein and from the femoral canal.

There is usually profuse discharge of lymph after operation and free drainage of the wound should always be provided. Sepsis often occurs and lymphoedema of one or even both legs is common. Healing of the wound is facilitated if the skin incision is not a simple linear one above and parallel to the inguinal ligament, but a flap incision (Fig. 28.29), which leaves intact the superficial inguinal, the superficial external pudendal and the superficial circumflex iliac arteries.

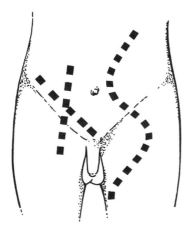

Fig. 28.29 The incisions used for inguinal lymph node dissection. On the patient's right side is shown the oblique incision just above the inguinal ligament and the vertical incision. On the left is shown the flap incision which heals better because the blood supply to the medial flap is preserved

Curvature of the penis

Curvature of the penis may be congenital or acquired. The congenital forms are often associated with epispadias or hypospadias (see p. 670). The most common acquired form is Peyronie's disease which is an inflammatory process with fibrotic changes in the elastic connective tissue of the corpora cavernosa of unknown aetiology. 10% of patients with Peyronie's disease also have Dupuytren's contracture and some 3% of patients with Dupuytren's contracture also have Peyronie's disease. The disease usually begins in middle life but is sometimes found in younger men. Most patients present complaining of angulated and painful erection but some complain of a lump in the penis. The lump consists of a plaque of fibrous tissue which replaces some of the elastic tissue of the corpora cavernosa. This plaque of fibrous tissue does not elongate as the penis expands with erection. The penis therefore becomes angulated and painful when erect. Although impotence is not a feature of Peyronie's disease, the penis beyond the plaque does not become as erect as the rest of the penis and some patients develop psychological impotence if they have had the disease a long time.

The patient must be reassured that the disease is not cancer and that there is every reason to believe that it will improve although it may take a long time in doing so. It is doubtful if the disease should be treated unless it is causing pain or interfering with intercourse. If treatment is required a number of drugs are available including Alpha Tocopherol Acetate (Vitamin E), Potassium Amino Benzoate (Potaba), Phenylbutazone and Corticosteroids which can be injected locally or given parenterally and they should probably be tried in that order. Operation should only be considered in patients who remain incapacitated a year or more after the condition was first diagnosed, because the disease has not resolved or has failed to respond to medical treatment.

Operations aimed at removing the fibrous plaque and replacing it with a skin graft are nearly always unsuccessful and frequently make the condition worse. The best operation is the Nesbit procedure in which a wedge of Buck's fascia is excised from the convex aspect of the curve without damaging the corpora cavernosa or corpus spongiosum and without touching the fibrous plaque, the effect being like that of an osteotomy (Pryor, 1979).

Operation

A Foley catheter is first passed into the bladder along the urethra. A circumferential incision is made through the penile skin 1 cm proximal to the corona and the prepuce is excised unless the patient has already been circumcised. The skin can now be drawn back easily, like a sleeve, to the base of the penis exposing Buck's fascia, which is the extension into the penis of the membranous layer of superficial fascia. Buck's fascia is incised longitudinally to expose the corpus spongiosum (which contains the urethra) and the thick fibrous tissue of the tunica albuginea which surrounds and binds together the corpora cavernosa. The corpus spongiosum is separated from the corpora cavernosa for some 5 cm by sharp dissection, avoiding damage to the erectile tissue and the urethra. The corpus spongiosum can now be secured with tapes or Paul's tubing and retracted. To determine precisely the site and size of the wedge, it is now necessary to produce an artificial erection by injecting or infusing into the corpora cavernosa about 100 ml or more of sterile saline after temporarily excluding the venous return from the penis by applying a light occlusion clamp across its base or by compressing the crura against the under surfaces of the pubic rami. The most convex aspect of the artificially erected penis is marked with a stitch in the tunica albuginea. Two parallel incisions, 0.5 cm to 1 cm apart depending on the degree of angulation, are made through the tunica albuginea for about half the circumference of the penis centred on the point of greatest convexity. The tunica is excised between the incisions and the cut edges are sutured together using polyglycolic acid, catgut or polydioxanone sutures in such a way that the knots lie deeply. Alternatively the intervening tunica can be buried and not excised. The skin is drawn back to the tip of the penis and sutured as after a circumcision. The urethral catheter is removed 24 hours later.

Hypospadias

Hypospadias is a congenital malformation in which incomplete fusion of the urethral folds results in an ectopic urethral meatus on the ventral aspect of the penis proximal to the normal opening. Depending on the position of the meatus, the condition may be described as *glandular, coronal, penile, penoscrotal, scrotal or perineal*. The meatus is often stenosed though it may be of normal size. The prepuce fails to fuse along the ventral aspect and has a characteristic hooded appearance. The penis may be bowed (*chordee*) in part by foreshortening ventral skin and in part by fibrosis and splaying of an incompletely formed corpus spongiosis distal to the ectopic meatus. The bowed appearance is exaggerated and, indeed, may only be apparent when the penis is erect. There is an increased incidence of undescended testes in boys with hypospadias although there is no significant increase in upper urinary tract abnormalities. Problems of intersex must be considered in boys with scrotal or perineal hypospadias and the scrotum must be carefully examined to confirm that normal testes are present.

A glandular or coronal hypospadias may cause no problem. However, when the malformation is more severe, urine may be sprayed downwards and backwards during micturition and bowing of the penis may prevent normal coitus. Depending on the severity of the lesion, three stages may be necessary to correct the malformation; meatotomy for meatal stenosis, straightening of the penis by release of chordee, and urethroplasty.

Meatotomy

This can easily be performed by introducing a blade of pointed scissors into the urethra and cutting back in the midline through the ventral wall of the urethra and the overlying skin. The cut margins of urethral mucosa and skin are then sewn together with fine absorbable sutures.

Reconstruction of the urethra

Many techniques of urethroplasty depend on the concept that a buried skin strip forms an epithelial tube by proliferation from the edges. Thus, a distal urethra can be created by fashioning a 1 cm strip that runs from the ectopic meatus to the end of the glans and by covering that strip with skin taken from elsewhere on the penis. In Van der Meulen's operation (1977) use is made of excessive skin from the dorsum of the prepuce whilst in the Denis Browne operation (1949) skin is mobilized from the shaft of the penis. More recently, techniques in which a tube is fashioned from a skin flap have become popular, such as the transverse preputial island flap (Duckett, 1980).

Van der Meulen's operation is particularly suitable when the meatus lies in the distal half of the penis. Chordee if present, however, must be corrected at a preliminary operation. A circumferential skin incision is made starting just proximal to the ectopic meatus, running distally on either side of the midline towards the corona so as to leave a strip of skin 1 cm wide and then extended along the free margin of the prepuce (Fig. 28.30). The skin strip from the ectopic meatus is then extended along the length of the glans by excising two triangular areas of skin from the ventral surface on either side of the midline (Fig. 28.31). The skin is undermined along the length of the shaft of the penis and rotated so that the skin from the dorsal aspect of the prepuce comes to cover the ventral surface of the glans (Fig. 28.32). An oblique incision on the dorsum of the penis allows the flap to be rotated more freely. Using fine absorbable sutures the skin flap is then sewn to the outer margin of the triangles (Fig. 28.33). The rotation creates a deficiency on the dorsum of the penis which is filled by folding back the inner layer of the prepuce. The skin margins around the remaining circumference of the penis can then be sewn together with ease.

Figs 28.30–28.33 *Van der Meulen's operation for hypospadias (see text)*

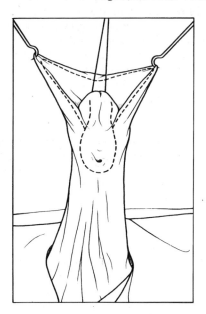

Fig. 28.30

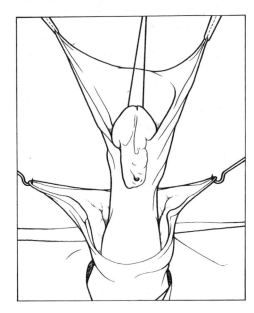

Fig. 28.31

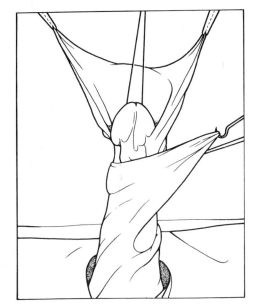

Fig. 28.32

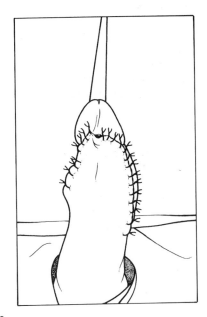

Fig. 28.33

In Duckett's transverse preputial island procedure an isolated flap with pedicle is created by separating the inner layer of the prepuce from the outer layer, taking advantage of an independent vasculature. The inner layer can then be fashioned into a tube and swung ventrally on its vascular pedicle. One end of the tube is anastomosed to the ectopic meatus and the other end is tunnelled through to the tip of the glans. The outer layer of the prepuce is then split longitudinally in the midline and the resulting flaps are brought round on either side so as to cover the skin deficit on the ventral surface.

THE TESTES, THE SPERMATIC CORD AND THE SCROTUM

Anatomy

The testis is oval in shape and measures about 4 cm by 2.0 cm by 2.5 cm. Dense fibrous tissue, the *tunica albuginea,* encloses the testis and projects posteriorly into it as the *mediastinum testes* which is pierced by the efferent ducts of the testes and by blood vessels and lymphatics (Fig. 28.34). The *epididymis,* crescentic in shape and attached to the posterior border of the testis, has a head, body and tail. The tail becomes the vas deferens which runs upwards behind the testis to join the spermatic cord. The *tunica vaginalis,* which is derived from peritoneum, surrounds the testis and epididymis and extends upwards for a short distance into the spermatic cord. It has a *parietal* layer that lines the scrotal cavity and a *visceral* layer that covers the testis and epididymis. The two layers become continuous posteriorly forming a broad ligament called the *mesorchium* that attaches the testis and epididymis to the posterior wall of the scrotum. The testis is covered by the external spermatic fascia, the cremasteric muscle and fascia and the internal spermatic fascia, all of which are derived from the abdominal wall.

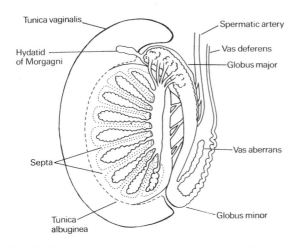

Fig. 28.34 A sagittal section of the testis and epididymis

Blood supply

The testis is supplied not only by the testicular artery, which arises from the aorta at the level of the first lumbar vertebra, but also by the cremasteric artery, the artery to the vas deferens, and the posterior scrotal arteries. Veins from the testis form the *pampiniform plexus* which drains into the testicular vein. The right testicular vein joins the inferior vena cava, the left one joins the left renal vein. *Lymphatic vessels* from the testis run upwards in the spermatic cord alongside the veins and

end in the para-aortic lymph nodes at the level of the first lumbar vertebra (Smith, 1983).

The spermatic cord and its coverings (which are those of the testis also) have been described on page 523.

The scrotum is composed of skin, muscle and fascia. It is divided by a median septum into two compartments. The superficial fascia is devoid of fat, and is largely replaced by a thin sheet of unstriped muscle, the *dartos.*

The wall of each scrotal chamber consists from without inwards of skin, dartos muscle, the three coverings of the testis and the parietal layer of the tunica vaginalis. These structures are traversed in aspiration of a hydrocele, or in exposure of the testes through the scrotum.

Lymphatic drainage of the scrotum takes place to the inguinal glands.

Imperfect descent of the testes

Imperfect descent of one or both testes in boys is relatively common, the incidence being approximately 0.3% of the male population. Several problems are associated with the condition of which the two most important are impaired spermatogenesis and an increased incidence of testicular tumour. Because of these problems, such children should undergo orchidopexy, an operation in which the testis is transferred from the abnormal site to the scrotum.

Embryology. The testis develops in the embryo from the genital ridge in the germinal epithelium and can be recognized in the upper lumbar region and in front of the mesonephros at 6 weeks. The testis then migrates caudally and comes to lie in the iliac fossa at 3 months. Little further movement takes place until the seventh or eighth months when the testis, preceded by the tunica vaginalis and following the line of the gubernaculum, passes through the inguinal canal to the scrotum. The factors responsible for descent are not understood but placental chorionic gonadatrophins and interstitial cell function influence the final stages.

Classification. The testis may be absent from the scrotum because of imperfect descent or because of retraction into the abdominal wall by cremaster muscle. The distinction is important since the retractile testis will come to lie in the scrotum in due course and should be regarded as a variant of normal. The imperfectly descended testis is abnormal and may be either incompletely descended or ectopic. The *incompletely descended testis* lies along the line of normal descent and may therefore be found in the abdomen, the inguinal canal, the superficial inguinal tissues or immediately above the neck of the scrotum. The *ectopic testis* is said to have deviated from the normal line of descent; it is usually found in the superficial inguinal pouch, above and lateral to the external inguinal ring, but may occasionally lie in the femoral or perineal tissue or at the base of the penis.

Associated problems. A number of problems are associated with imperfect descent of the testes. Spermatogenesis is impaired, there is an increased incidence of testicular tumour, the risk of both torsion and trauma are greater, inguinal herniae are more common and, finally, the appearance may be the cause of embarrassment.

Impaired spermatogenesis in a male with bilateral imperfect descent of the testes is likely to be the cause of infertility. Early changes indicating impaired development are present by 5 years of age and become increasingly evident with time. Failure of maturation may be related to the temperature differential between the abdomen and the scrotum or to primary tissue dysplasia. The value of orchidopexy with regard to spermatogenesis is difficult to assess; it is doubtful that established changes in the testis are reversed but it is quite probable that further deterioration is prevented.

The association of malignant change and imperfect descent of the testis is well established; the incidence of tumour developing in an abnormal testis is 30 times greater than normal and it is interesting to note that the abdominal testis is particularly at risk. Curiously, the incidence of malignant change in the normal testis of a man with unilateral descent is also greater than normal. The advantage of orchidopexy in averting malignancy is difficult to assess; it is doubtful that the operation carried out after puberty alters the prognosis but it is suggested that the procedure carried out in a younger child may be of value.

Clinical evaluation. The condition usually presents in childhood but surprisingly often remains unnoticed until the first school medical examination. Less often the patient presents for the first time in adult life. The clinical assessment of a child needs to be carried out with great care. Questions should be asked about torsion, trauma, orchitis and mumps. Both the weight and height should be recorded on percentile charts. The child should be warm and relaxed and placed supine on an examination couch with the legs slightly apart. It is important to note the development of the penis and scrotum as bilateral impalpable testes in association with microgenitalia raises the possibility of endocrine or chromosome abnormality. The scrotum should be examined next as, not infrequently, two normal testes are found.

An attempt is then made to locate the testis and to push it down into the scrotum so that a distinction can be made between imperfect descent and retraction. First the superficial inguinal and prepubic tissue is palpated. If no testis is found, as is particularly common in the obese child, an attempt is made to displace the gonad from the superficial inguinal pouch or the inguinal canal towards the neck of the scrotum where it can be felt more easily. This is achieved by sweeping fingers of one hand firmly across the inguinal region from the anterior superior iliac spine towards the pubic tubercle and placing the fingers of the other hand at the neck of the scrotum. If the testis can be pushed through the neck of the scrotum it should be lightly grasped and pulled down towards the normal position. The testis which remains impalpable may either lie in one of the less common ectopic positions or it may be intra-abdominal, hypoplastic or absent.

The typical ectopic testis lies above and lateral to the external inguinal ring; it can be felt with relative ease both with abdominal muscles relaxed and, when pushed towards the scrotum, will run down and lateral to the neck of the sac. The incompletely descended testis often lies in the inguinal canal; it may be difficult to feel initially but, with manipulation, may be pushed through the external ring towards the neck of the scrotum. The retractile testis lies in the superficial inguinal tissues and can be drawn down into the middle or lower thirds of the scrotum; the testis remains temporarily within the scrotum when pressure is released but is promptly withdrawn into the abdominal wall when the cremaster reflex is stimulated by touching the inner aspect of the thigh. When there is doubt it is helpful to ask the child to squat down as, in this position, the cremaster reflex is diminished and the testis may move spontaneously into the scrotum. In some children the testis lies in the superficial inguinal tissues, can be manipulated into the upper third of the scrotum but retracts when pressure is released. In this group it is difficult to distinguish between imperfect descent and a retractile testis; if the latter seems more probable the child can safely be reviewed at a later date.

Management

Investigation of a child with imperfect descent of testes is rarely necessary unless a chromosome or endocrine abnormality is suspected. Hormonal therapy using intramuscular testosterone to provoke testicular descent has some advocates but doubtful efficacy; side effects and the discomfort of the injections have discouraged more general acceptance. More recently luteinizing hormone releasing hormone, which stimulates pituitary gonadotrophins, has become available as a nasal spray and this may prove more acceptable. Orchidopexy should, under normal circumstances, be recommended for all children with incomplete descent of the testis. Orchidectomy should not be considered before puberty as interstitial cell function remains although spermatogenesis is impaired. It is important that orchidopexy should be performed before the child is 5 years old (Ashby, 1980).

The object of orchidopexy is that the testis should be

mobilized and placed in the scrotum without tension on the testicular vessels. Occasionally mobilization may be inadequate to allow the testis to be placed in the scrotum; the testis should then be fixed at a point in the normal line of descent and a second operation may be performed at a later date. If at operation no testicle is found, a search should be made of the inguinal canal for a structure resembling a vas deferens which may lead distally to a hypoplastic gonad that can be excised. In the absence of a vas deferens it can be assumed that the testis is intraabdominal or absent. It is then prudent to continue the search in the extraperitoneal tissues (Jones, 1979) through an incision 2 cm above the deep ring as described in the operation for varicocoele on p. 681.

Orchidopexy

A skin crease incision is made 1 cm above and parallel to the medial two thirds of the inguinal ligament. The subcutaneous tissue is explored with care as the testis may lie in the superficial inguinal pouch immediately deep to Scarpa's fascia. Once found, the tunica of the testis is cleared of adherent tissue and the gubernaculum at the lower pole divided. Artery forceps are then applied to the tunica and, with gentle traction, the

spermatic cord will be seen emerging from the external inguinal ring. The inguinal canal is then opened by dividing external oblique aponeurosis in the line of its fibres. Cremasteric fascia is cleared from the spermatic cord by blunt gauze dissection so that the cord lies free up to the internal ring (Fig. 28.35).

The covering of the cord is then divided longitudinally and the free margins held apart with forceps so as to expose the contents. A hernial sac will usually be found and, using the technique described on p. 525, an inguinal herniotomy is performed. In the proximal part of the cord the vas deferens and testicular vessels are dissected free from surrounding tissue. The vas and vessels are then held to one side and the remaining tissue divided transversely (Fig. 28.36).

At this stage the testis is suspended from the internal ring only by the vas and vessels and can usually be placed within the scrotum. However, if needed, greater length can be provided by retroperitoneal dissection of

Figs 28.35–28.37 *Mobilization of the testis and spermatic cord for orchidopexy*

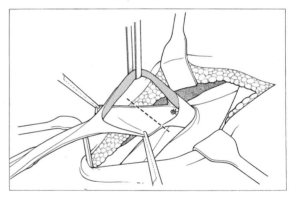

Fig. 28.36

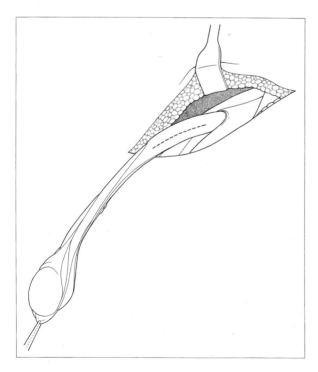

Fig. 28.35

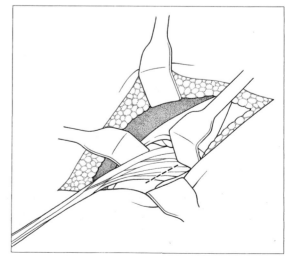

Fig. 28.37

Figs 28.38–28.42   *Dartos pouch method of fixation*

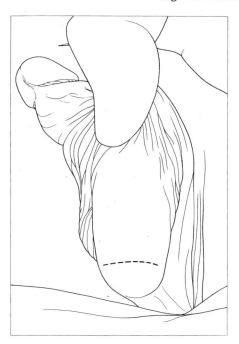

Fig. 28.38

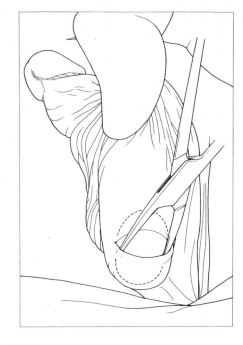

Fig. 28.39

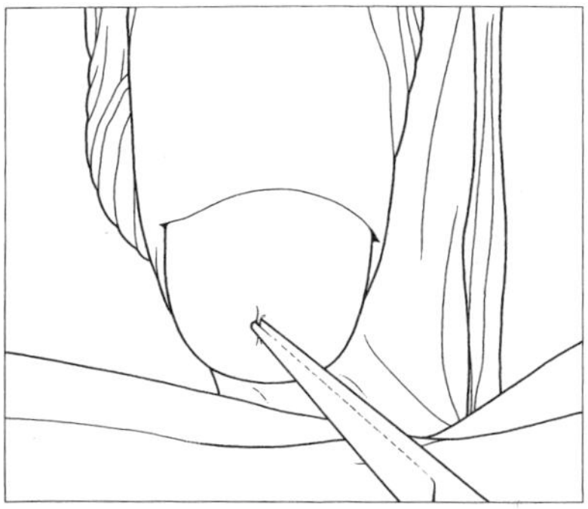

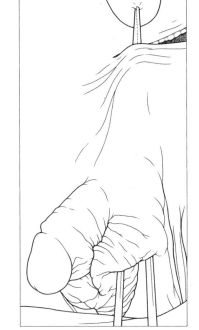

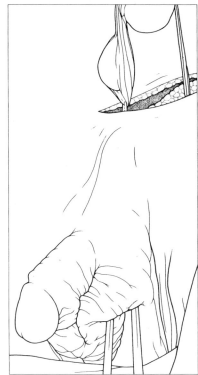

Fig. 28.40

Fig. 28.41

Fig. 28.42

the vessels and by releasing the fascia restricting the vas at the medial margin of the internal ring. The vessels are tethered by the overlying peritoneum and by fascial bands that run laterally in a retroperitoneal plane. The peritoneum is lifted free by blunt dissection using a finger or gauze pledget and the bands, which are clearly seen when the vessels are under traction, are divided (Fig. 28.37).

The testis should only be placed in the scrotum when it lies without tension on the vessels. To prevent accidental displacement, it is usual to fix the testis in place and a dartos pouch (Figs 28.38–28.42) provides a convenient method. First a finger is pushed through the inguinal wound to break down fascia occluding the neck of the scrotum and to stretch the corrugated skin. With the finger still in place, the skin over the lower part of the scrotum is incised and a pouch made between the skin and dartos fascia. An artery forceps is then pushed through the dartos fascia, through the scrotum and up to the inguinal wound where the testis is grasped. By withdrawing the forceps, the testis is pulled down through the dartos fascia into the pouch and is retained in position by the narrow opening in the fascia. The scrotal skin is then closed over the testis with absorbable interrupted sutures.

A final check is made of the testicular vessels and vas in the inguinal canal to exclude tension or torsion and the inguinal wound is closed in layers.

Torsion of the testis (or torsion of the spermatic cord)

The testis and epididymis are suspended in the scrotum by the spermatic cord which passes through the mesorchium. If the mesorchium is abnormally long or narrow (bell-clapper type of testis) torsion can occur within the tunica vaginalis and this is called *intravaginal* torsion (Fig. 28.43). *Extravaginal* torsion occurs when the cord twists above the mesorchium and the whole tunica (including the parietal layer) rotates within the scrotum but is rare. Torsion occurs most commonly in adolescents between the ages of 12 and 16 and in a distressingly large proportion of cases is misdiagnosed. It is often considered to be epididymitis, because the signs are similar to those of acute inflammation, but infarction and atrophy of the testis inevitably results if it is treated as such. The age of the patient distinguishes torsion from epididymitis because epididymitis is rare before the age of 20. The onset of torsion is sudden with pain, often referred to the iliac fossa, and swelling in the scrotum associated with nausea. The affected side becomes tender and red with oedematous and sometimes bruised skin. Because the cord is twisted and shortened, both epididymis and testis lie at a high level in the scrotum but it is usually impossible to distinguish by palpation one from the other. It

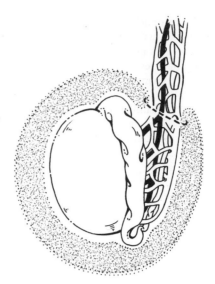

Fig. 28.43 Intravaginal torsion of the testis. Note the narrow mesorchium compared with Fig. 28.34

is a good rule that *a swollen and painful testis in a boy in his 'teens is a torsion until proved otherwise by operation.* Torsion is much less common in adults but may be suspected if an acute scrotal condition develops without obvious cause. Torsion of an undescended testis may be mistaken for a strangulated inguinal hernia but the true diagnosis should be reached by operation.

Immediate operation should be undertaken on *suspicion* alone, since the testis cannot survive more than 6 hours ischaemia. As the torsion is usually intravaginal, it is best approached through a scrotal incision and is untwisted. The direction of torsion is usually obvious at operation and generally anticlockwise on the left and clockwise on the right. If the testis seems viable it is returned to the scrotum and anchored to the scrotal wall with two or three sutures to prevent recurrence. If the testis is obviously nonviable, it should probably still be replaced in the scrotum, even though it will atrophy because sufficient interstitial cells may survive to produce some testosterone. The anomaly that predisposes to torsion is usually bilateral and, if torsion occurs in one testis, it is very likely to occur at a later date in the other which must also be fixed. Fixation of both testes should of course be advised if the torsion reduced spontaneously without operation.

Technique

To fix a testis in these circumstances, an incision 1 cm long is made through skin, scrotal coverings and into the tunica albuginea. A few 3/0 catgut sutures are then inserted through skin and tunica albuginea, and tied, so that the testis is secured to the skin of the scrotum.

Torsion of the appendix testis

The appendix testis, or Hydatid of Morgagni (Fig. 28.34) is a small pedunculated structure attached to the tunica albuginea on the anterior aspect of the testis and it is a remnant of the Müllerian or paramesonephric duct. The clinical features of torsion of the appendix testis are similar to, but less severe than, those of torsion of the testis. The pain is severe, but localized and the twisted appendix can usually be palpated, or even seen through the scrotal skin. The testis and epididymis can be recognized as normal, unless a hydrocele forms. The lesion is treated by excising the twisted appendix testis through a small scrotal incision.

Orchidectomy

There are a number of indications for the removal of a testis, but malignant disease is the principal one. Orchidopexy (p. 674) is the operation of choice for the ectopic or undescended testis before puberty, but orchidectomy is best after puberty unless the condition is bilateral, when orchidopexy should still be attempted. The repair of large indirect or direct inguinal herniae in elderly men is often facilitated if the testis is removed and the inguinal canal obliterated. Orchidectomy is the operation of choice in the rare granulomatous disease of the testis, and, in carcinoma of the prostate, orchidectomy is frequently advocated but usually done by the subcapsular method (p. 678).

Malignant disease (see Peckham, 1987)

Most patients with a testicular tumour present with a painless lump in the testis. Lumps in the testis should always be explored if doubt exists as to their nature.

Apart from malignant disease only syphilis, granulomatous lesions and mumps produce lumps in the testis and only the last of these can be confidently diagnosed without operation (and then only if the patient has or has recently had mumps in one or more salivary glands). It is important not to be misled by a history of trauma, of variations in the size of the lump and of its response to tablets. Before operation, the tumour markers, Human chorionic gonadotrophin (HCG), Alphafetoprotein (AFP), and Lactic dehydrogenase (LDH) must be estimated in the blood, since changes in their levels after orchidectomy can be a useful means of monitoring the progress of the disease. Chest X-ray, intravenous urography, CAT scans and lymphangio-

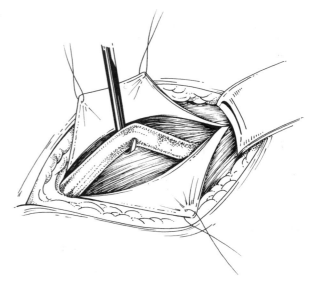

Fig. 28.45 The inguinal canal is opened and the spermatic cord is gently mobilized upwards to the deep inguinal ring

Figs 28.44–28.46 *Left orchidectomy*

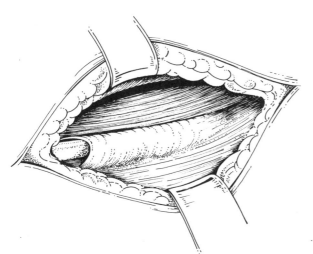

Fig. 28.44 The skin is incised parallel to the inguinal ligament and the external oblique aponeurosis exposed

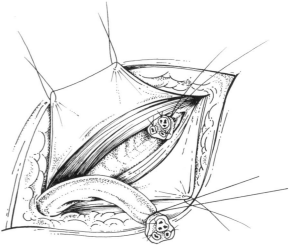

Fig. 28.46 The cord is ligated at the deep inguinal ring and divided

graphy can all be deferred until after operation unless it is proposed that the para-aortic lymph nodes should be removed at the time of orchidectomy. Orchidectomy for nonmalignant disease can be carried out through a scrotal or an inguinal incision, but for malignant disease a more radical procedure is done through an inguinal incision.

Orchidectomy for malignant disease (see Peckham, 1987)
Through an incision (Fig. 28.44) above the appropriate inguinal ligament, the inguinal canal is opened. (Fig. 28.45). The spermatic cord is freed from the internal spermatic fascia and mobilized to the deep inguinal ring where it is divided between ligatures (Fig. 28.46). The cord and testis are then mobilized and removed. If the tumour is large, removal is facilitated by extending the skin incision into the neck of the scrotum, but scrotal skin need only be excised with the tumour if it is adherent.

If the nature of the swelling is uncertain, the testis may be examined and a frozen section taken before proceeding to orchidectomy. Instead of dividing the spermatic cord between ligatures, the vessels are occluded with a Potts or Craaford arterial occlusion clamp. The cord and the testis can then be mobilized and delivered through the wound. Unless the diagnosis is obvious, a biopsy can be taken, making sure that no cells spill into the wound. If the lesion is malignant it is easy to ligate and divide the cord. The wound is sutured in layers and not usually drained. Some surgeons have reported dysplasia or carcinoma in situ of the normal (contralateral) testis in a significant proportion of patients with testicular tumour. However, it is not yet common practice to take a biopsy from the normal testis unless it feels abnormal.

Subcapsular orchidectomy
Removal of testicular substance from within the tunica vaginalis is frequently carried out in patients with M1 category carcinoma of the prostate instead of (and sometimes as well as) giving oestrogens and is now generally regarded to be as satisfactory a method of treating this disease as a formal orchidectomy.

It can be carried out through a scrotal incision. The tunica albuginea is exposed and incised anteriorly from top to bottom revealing the seminiferous tubules (Fig. 28.47). These are easily freed from the inside of the tunica with a swab or pledget except posteriorly, where the vessels enter. The vessels are clamped and the tubules severed from their attachments. The tunica is plicated with a catgut stitch (Fig. 28.48), and the wound is closed. The same procedure is carried out on the other testis through another scrotal incision.

Epididymectomy
This operation is rarely if ever done now but it may be indicated for a tuberculous infection of the epididymis when no other active focus can be discovered, and when it shows no response to the appropriate chemotherapy. The testis is exposed through an inguinal or a scrotal incision. The tunica vaginalis is opened and it is confirmed that the disease is confined to the epididymis. Separation of the epididymis from the body of the testis and from the tunica vaginalis is commenced at its lower pole taking care not to damage the testicular vessels entering the mesorchium. The vas deferens may be divided at the upper pole of the epididymis, but if it also is involved it should be divided as close to the deep inguinal ring as possible.

Hydrocele
A hydrocele is a collection of clear fluid within the

Figs 28.47 & 28.48 *Subcapsular orchidectomy*

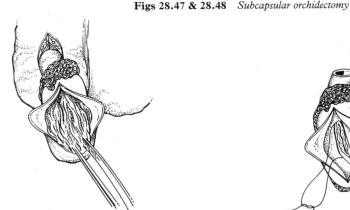

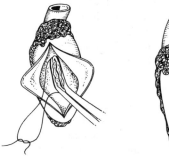
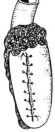

Fig. 28.47 The testis has been exposed through a scrotal incision and the tunica albuginea incised vertically (to expose the seminiferous tubules). The seminiferous tubules are separated from the inside of the tunica with a swab or pledget.

Fig. 28.48 The seminiferous tubules are removed and their blood vessels clamped and ligated. The tunica albuginea is then repaired with a catgut stitch.

tunica vaginalis. Hydroceles can be classified as congenital, encysted, infantile or vaginal (idiopathic). The vaginal or idiopathic hydrocele occurs in a normally formed tunica vaginalis and is by far the commonest. The other varieties occur when the tunica is abnormal and the processus vaginalis fails to close in whole or in part. In the congenital hydrocele the tunica communicates with the peritoneal cavity, and the fluid disappears into the abdomen when the scrotum is elevated (indeed the fluid in the hydrocele may be ascitic fluid). The emptied congenital hydrocele forms a smooth oval swelling associated with the spermatic cord, and is often mistaken for a hernia. An infantile hydrocele extends as far as the deep inguinal ring but does not communicate with the peritoneal cavity. In the child, excision of the processus vaginalis within the inguinal canal resolves *congenital hydrocele or hydrocele of the cord* (p. 525).

Vaginal hydrocele

The condition is called idiopathic because the pathogenesis is obscure, but it may be associated with disease of the testis or epididymis, or follow an operation for hernia or varicocele. Many patients with small hydroceles seek reassurance that the condition is not serious, rather than treatment; others require treatment. Cure of an adult hydrocele by operation is usually advised but aspiration (tapping) with or without injection treatment may be preferred. Aspiration is painless, can be carried out in an ambulant patient and rarely causes haematoma, but gives only temporary relief because the fluid inevitably reaccumulates.

Aspiration. The position of the testis, which usually lies posteriorly, is confirmed by palpation and transillumination. The scrotum is grasped so that the fluid is pressed towards the lower anterior part of sac, rendering it tense. A small wheal of local anaesthetic solution is raised in an area of the scrotal skin that is free of visible vessels, and well clear of the testis. A fine trocar and cannula (or needle cannula, Fig. 2.2) is thrust through it into the sac. After all fluid has been evacuated and the cannula withdrawn, the testis is carefully examined to ensure that it is healthy.

Injection treatment. The solution most commonly employed is made up to the following formula:

Quinine hydrochloride	4 g
Urethane	2 g
Water for injection	30 ml

10 ml of this solution is injected through the cannula into the cavity of the tunica vaginalis when all the hydrocele fluid has been evacuated. Gentle massage is employed to disperse the solution throughout the cavity of the tunica, and the scrotum is supported for some days with a suspensory bandage. The procedure may be repeated at a later date if necessary, using 5 ml of the solution. An alternative solution is 2 ml sodium tetradecyl (see p. 558) used for sclerotherapy.

Inguinal approach

The incision is placed over the superficial inguinal ring. A finger is passed downwards and swept around the hydrocele sac to separate it from the inside of the scrotum. The sac together with the testis and epididymis is pushed out of the scrotum into the wound. If the sac is very large, its fluid content can be aspirated before it is pushed out of the scrotum. After the coverings have been stripped aside an opening is made into the tunica vaginalis and the testis is carefully examined. If it is healthy the hydrocele alone requires treatment. If the hydrocele is small and the sac thin walled the Jaboulay procedure is the operation of choice. It consists simply of turning the sac inside out (*eversion*) so that it lies entirely behind the testis and inserting a few sutures to retain it in position. These sutures must not pull the margins of the sac too tightly around the cord otherwise the blood supply to the testis may be impaired. If the hydrocele is large or the sac thick walled, the sac is better *excised* by cutting it off closely around its attachment to the testis. The bleeding points on the small remaining fringe of sac must be secured by ligatures or a running stitch, otherwise a haematoma will form. After both these operations haemostasis is secured, and the testis is returned to the scrotum from which a drain is brought out through the wound. As a further precaution against haematoma formation, the scrotum should be well supported with a compression bandage.

Scrotal approach

A scrotal approach can be used instead of an inguinal one for either of these two operations and is preferable. For the operation described by Lord, a scrotal approach must be used. Lord's procedure is virtually bloodless, and considerably reduces the risk of a scrotal haematoma, which is, unfortunately, very common after the other operations. The hydrocele is grasped in the left hand and the anterior scrotal skin stretched. An incision, about 4 cm in length, is made through the skin and dartos muscle avoiding, as far as possible, the superficial vessels, which are easily seen through the stretched skin. The tunica vaginalis is opened by an incision of the same length, but neither mobilized nor separated from the inside of the scrotum and the hydrocele fluid is evacuated. The testis is then lifted out through the incision in the tunica vaginalis. Five or six 'gathering' stitches are now inserted into the evaginated tunica, radiating outwards from its attachment to the testis towards its cut edge (Fig. 28.49). When these are tied, the tunica is plicated and forms a collar around the junction of testis and epididymis. Finally, the testis is

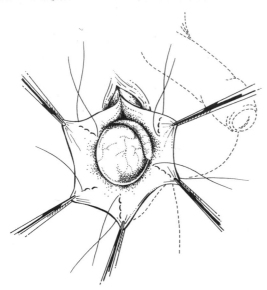

Fig. 28.49   Lord's procedure for hydrocele

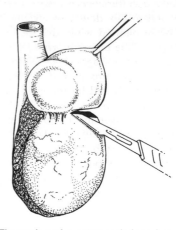

Fig. 28.50   The testis and spermatocele have been exposed through a scrotal incision and removal of the spermatocele begun

returned to the scrotum, and the dartos muscle and skin are closed as one layer by stitches or clips.

Haematocele

A haematocele (an effusion of blood into the tunica vaginalis) results from direct injury or follows an operation on the scrotum such as vasectomy. Operation is probably advisable in all but the mildest cases if the condition is recognized at an early stage before the clot has organized. A haematocele is best evacuated by a direct approach through the anterior wall of the scrotum, but it is often disappointing how little clot one is able to remove. The lower part of the scrotal wound should be drained.

Spermatocele

A spermatocele is a retention cyst arising from either the vasa efferentia of the testis or from the epididymis and when large it is frequently mistaken by the patient for a third testis. It is normally situated above and behind the testis, and contains white opalescent fluid and spermatozoa. Small spermatoceles are usually symptomless and do not require treatment. Larger ones, and those which cause symptoms, may be dealt with by injection (on the same lines described for hydrocele) or by operation. At operation the sac is excised through a scrotal incision (Figs 28.50–28.52).

Varicocele

This is the name given to varicosity of the pampiniform plexus. It is usually idiopathic and occurs almost exclusively on the left side, doubtlessly due to the anatomical differences in the venous drainage of the testis on the two sides (p. 672).

Some left sided varicoceles are secondary to an

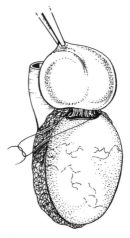

Fig. 28.51   The vessels supplying the spermatocele are ligated and excision continues

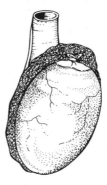

Fig. 28.52   The final result

obstructed renal vein in patients with carcinoma of the kidney. Secondary varicoceles are usually obvious even when the patient lies down, whereas idiopathic ones can only be recognized while the patient is standing. Some fullness of the pampiniform plexus is normal in healthy men and the diagnosis of a small varicocele is not easy. The symptoms of slight aching or dragging pain, are usually relieved by the wearing of a suspensory bandage, although operation may fail to relieve the symptoms in some patients. The operative treatment of varicocele does have a definite place in the treatment of some subfertile men (Nilsson, 1983). Otherwise operation should only be advised if gross varicosity is present, or if the patient is convinced that his symptoms are due to the varicocele and unlikely to be relieved by conservative treatment and reassurance.

The classical operation for varicocele is carried out through an inguinal approach, the inguinal canal being opened and the spermatic cord delivered. The coverings are incised and the vas deferens, the arteries and two or three veins, are carefully separated from the main mass of dilated vessels. The latter are freed for a short distance upwards and downwards, and excised between ligatures placed some 5 cm apart. Approximation of these ligatures shortens the cord so that the testis is suspended at a higher level. An alternative method is to dissect out the selected veins right down to the level of the testis, but it is doubtful whether this confers any additional advantage, because bleeding is more troublesome and a scrotal haematoma is more liable to complicate convalescence. Some surgeons open and evert the tunica vaginalis (Jaboulay) to prevent subsequent hydrocele formation.

Paloma described an operation carried out *above* the inguinal canal for the cure of varicocele. A transverse or oblique incision is made 3 cm above the level of the deep ring, the external oblique aponeurosis is incised in the line of the incision, and the lateral edge of the rectus sheath nicked to expose the underlying transversalis fascia. The internal oblique and transversus muscles and transversalis fascia are then split as in the classical gridiron incision. Extraperitoneal fat and peritoneum are swept forwards to expose the psoas major muscle on the posterior abdominal wall. The testicular veins, usually two in number, are found as they lie on the posterior abdominal wall, lateral to the external iliac artery. They are usually lifted forward with the peritoneum, but can generally be identified in the extraperitoneal fat, even in a fat person. (The ureter lies more medially and is not usually seen). The testicular veins are identified and divided between ligatures, preserving the testicular artery which at this level is usually well separated from the veins (Fig. 28.53). Care must be taken not to ligate the inferior epigastric vein instead of the testicular vein.

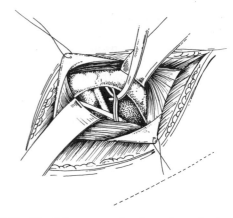

Fig. 28.53 The Paloma operation for varicocoele. A gridiron incision has been made and the peritoneum retracted medially exposing the testicular artery and the testicular veins which are being held up with an artery forceps

Ligation or division of the vas deferens (vasectomy)

Vasectomy is carried out to effect sterilization, and is rarely performed now to prevent infection spreading from the posterior urethra to the epididymis along the vas or its lymphatics after prostatectomy.

Technique

The operation is usually done under local anaesthesia; general anaesthesia is preferable if the patient has had a previous scrotal or inguinal operation or when the vas cannot be easily distinguished by touch from the other cord structures. The vas is identified, then grasped and steadied under the skin with the thumb and index finger of one hand. A small bleb is raised in the skin over the vas by injecting 1 or 2 ml 1% Lignocaine; the needle is then passed through the bleb and a further 2 or 3 ml of local anaesthetic injected into the cord. A 1 cm transverse incision is made through the bleb overlying the cord, and the cord enclosed in its fibrous sheath is picked up with an Allis or Poirier tissue forceps and released from its grip by thumb and index finger. (If holding the vas for this time proves difficult, the needle used for injecting the local anaesthetic can be passed underneath the vas and out through the skin beyond, while injecting the local anaesthetic.) The fibrous sheath of the cord is incised and the vas itself grasped with small artery forceps and lifted out. A window is made in the 'mesentery' of the vas and the proximal end is ligated and divided (the author uses 2/0 absorbable material). The distal end is ligated about 1½ cm away and the intervening section excised. If the distal ligature is now tied around the point of an artery forceps applied to the dartos muscle, the proximal end is buried underneath the dartos and the distal end kept between it and the skin. The same procedure is then done on the other side. It is important to separate the cut and ligated ends of the vas by a gap and a tissue plane in the way described because regeneration, either directly or through a granuloma, can occur. After haemostasis has been secured, the skin is loosely sutured with a catgut stitch. The operation can be done through one anterior median incision or two lateral incisions, one for each vas. It is important to tell patients requesting vasectomy that they must regard themselves fertile, and take other contraceptive precautions until two negative seminal analyses have been obtained (the first at least 3 months after the operation and the second at least 3 weeks after the first); that occasionally the fluids do not become negative, and the operation has to be redone, and that 1 or 2% of patients get more bruising than others and may be uncomfortable for some time.

Reversal of vasectomy

A reversal of vasectomy is occasionally requested. The presence of antisperm antibodies in serum or seminal plasma are not a contraindication to operation but make its success less likely. The operation is usually done under general anaesthetic, but is possible under local. The vas is easily palpable after vasectomy because the cut ends are buried in a granuloma (which varies in size) and closer together than might be expected. An incision is made over the vas and the granuloma picked up with Allis forceps and excised to expose normal vas above and below. An end-to-end or side-to-side anastomosis is made using interrupted 6/0 nylon or prolene sutures. As the lumen of the vas is small, anastomosis is facilitated if a splint, such as a

piece of No. 1 nylon, is used and left in for some days after operation. The author passes one end of the splint some 5 cm into the distal end of the vas and passes the other end on a needle, into the proximal lumen, bringing it out through the side wall of the vas and the skin, to which it is secured with a button or bead. The skin incision is closed with catgut and the splint removed after 7 days.

Vaso-epididymostomy

In patients with azoospermia, the cause is either testicular dysfunction or a congenital obstruction situated usually at the tail of the epididymis as it becomes continuous with the beginning of the vas. If the history, the physical examination and the results of hormone assays and testicular biopsy suggest that the cause of

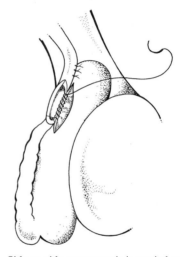

Fig. 28.55 Side-to-side anastomosis is carried out using 6/0 prolene sutures

Figs 28.54–28.56 *Vaso-epididymostomy*

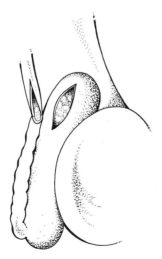

Fig. 28.54 The vas has been mobilized, incised and offered to a deep incision in the head of the epididymis

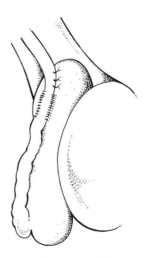

Fig. 28.56 The operation is completed

azoospermia is obstruction, it is worth exploring the scrotum and carrying out the operation of vaso-epididymostomy. The patient should be told that the chances of success are not high. The operation is carried out through two scrotal incisions, one for each side. The vas is exposed and mobilized so that it can be brought alongside the head of the epididymis without tension. A deep incision is made into the head of the epididymis until creamy fluid, which usually contains spermatozoa, appears. An incision of similar length is made in the side wall of the vas and a side-to-side anastomosis carried out between the head of the epididymis (Fig. 28.54) and the vas using 5 or 6/0 prolene sutures (Figs 28.55 & 28.56).

Operations on the scrotum

Avulsion of the scrotal skin, a not uncommon accident, requires careful treatment, especially if the testes are exposed. All available fragments of scrotal skin should be utilized to cover the testis and split skin grafts can be applied where deficiencies remain. *Carcinoma of the scrotum* is treated by radical excision of the local lesion and block dissection of the inguinal glands if they are involved. *Elephantiasis of the scrotum* is caused by fila-riasis and surgery is the only treatment of avail. The greater part of the oedematous scrotum is excised, preserving the penis, the urethra and the testes. Flaps of scrotal skin are preserved to form a pocket for the testes, and a covering for the penis. Deficiencies are covered with split skin grafts.

Fournier's gangrene (idiopathic gangrene of the scrotum)

This is an acute fulminating cellulitis of the scrotum which develops suddenly and often without any apparent cause. Infection is usually mixed, with haemolytic streptococci and *Clostridium welchii* predominating. Gangrene probably due to thrombosis of cutaneous vessels of the scrotal skin occurs early and, if uncontrolled, the infection spreads upwards into the abdominal wall. Early cases can be aborted by intensive chemotherapy but if gangrene develops, no time should be lost before excising the necrotic tissue. One or both testes may be exposed by the excision of scrotal tissues, but seldom suffer damage. As soon as the wound is clean and the patient's condition is satisfactory, the scrotum is repaired by secondary suture and skin grafting.

REFERENCES

Ashby E C 1980 Maldescended testis. In: Taylor S(ed) Recent advances in surgery, No. 10. Churchill Livingstone, Edinburgh, ch 15

Browne D 1949 An operation for hypospadias. Proceedings of the Royal Society of Medicine 42: 466

Chilton C P, Shah P J R, Fowler C G, Tiptaft R C, Blandy J P 1983 The impact of optical urethrotomy on the management of urethral strictures. British Journal of Urology 55: 705

Duckett J W 1980 Hypospadias. Clinics in Plastic Surgery 7: 149–160

Jones P F, Bagley F H 1979 An abdominal extraperitoneal approach for the difficult orchidopexy. British Journal of Surgery 66: 14–18

Lloyd-Davies R W, Gow J G, Davies D R 1983 A colour atlas of urology. Wolfe, London, ch 11

Newsam J E, Buist T A S 1980 Trauma. In: Chisholm G D (ed) Urology. Heinemann, London p 389

Nilsson S 1983 Varicocele. In: Hargreave T B (ed) Male infertility. Springer Verlag, Heidelberg, p 199

Peckham M J, Hendry W F 1987 Testicular cancer. In: Hendry W F (ed) Recent advances in urology — 4. Churchill Livingstone, Edinburgh, p 279

Pryor J P, Fitzpatrick J M 1979 New approach to correction of penile deformity in Peyronie's disease. Journal of Urology 122: 622

Smith J W, Murphy T R, Blair J S G, Lowe K G 1983 Regional anatomy illustrated. Churchill Livingstone, Edinburgh

Turner-Warwick R 1983 Urethral stricture surgery. In: Glenn J F (ed) Urological surgery, 3rd edn. Lippincott, Philadelphia, p 689

Van der Meulen J C M 1971 Hypospadias and cryptospadias. British Journal of Plastic Surgery 24: 101

FURTHER READING

Blandy J P 1984 Operative urology, 2nd edn. Blackwell, Oxford

Clark P 1985 Operations in urology. Churchill Livingstone, Edinburgh

Mitchell J P 1984 Urinary tract trauma. Wright, Bristol

Paulson D F 1984 Genitourinary surgery. Churchill Livingstone, Edinburgh

Whitaker R H, Woodward J R (eds) 1984 Paediatric urology. Butterworth, London

29

Gynaecological encounters in general surgery

J. R. B. LIVINGSTONE

Not infrequently the general surgeon, when performing a laparotomy, encounters an unexpected gynaecological condition, the correct management of which may cause him some doubt and anxiety. In a large hospital, he can usually call upon the assistance of a gynaecological colleague and should do so if at all possible. Unfortunately, there have been many occasions when an essentially normal ovary has been removed by an inexperienced surgeon, who has mistaken follicular or luteal cysts for disease. Furthermore, in cases of suspected or unsuspected ovarian malignancy, surgery has very often been incorrect or incomplete in inexperienced hands. However, in a small hospital without access to gynaecological opinion, the general surgeon himself has to accept responsibility for deciding what, if any, operative procedure is indicated and of mastering the techniques required. It is for his guidance that this chapter is written.

Anatomy

The uterus is a thick-walled muscular organ, situated between the bladder and the rectum; in its normal position of anteversion it lies obliquely overhanging the bladder. It is piriform in shape and flattened anteroposteriorly. It is about 7.5 cm long, 5 cm broad, and 2.5 cm thick. Its upper part or *body* projects upwards into the pelvic cavity and has a complete peritoneal covering. Anteriorly, the peritoneum is reflected on to the upper surface of the bladder, with the shallow *uterovesical pouch* between; posteriorly, it sweeps downwards to form the *rectouterine pouch* (of Douglas); laterally on each side, it forms the broad ligament. The rounded upper end of the uterus is called the *fundus;* this is demarcated from the body by the entrance of the uterine tube at each side. The lower part of the uterus or *cervix* lies mainly below the peritoneum, and is invaginated into the vaginal vault, so that it is divided

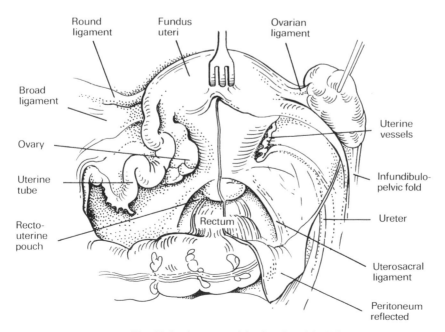

Fig. 29.1 Anatomy of the female pelvis (After Anson)

into supra- and intravaginal parts. The body and cervix are separated by a circular constriction called the *isthmus*. The supravaginal part of the cervix is related anteriorly to the bladder, to which it is connected by some loose fibrous strands, the *uterovesical fascia*. Laterally, it is related to the *transverse cervical ligament*, which runs to the side wall of the pelvis; posteriorly, it is joined to the sacral fascia by the *uterosacral ligaments*, which pass backwards on each side of the rectum, raising folds in the peritoneum of the pelvic floor.

The broad ligament is a double fold of peritoneum stretching from the lateral border of the uterus to the side wall of the pelvis. The ovary is attached to the lateral part of its posterior surface. Its upper free border contains the uterine tube in its medial four-fifths; its lateral one-fifth, containing the ovarian vessels, constitutes the *infundibulopelvic ligament*. The uterine vessels lie between the layers of the ligament, first at its base, and then close to its attachment to the uterus. Other contents of the broad ligament, beside lymph vessels and glands, are the *round ligament* of the uterus, which raises a ridge on its anterior surface as it passes towards the inguinal canal, and the *ovarian ligament*, which joins the ovary to the uterus, and raises a small ridge on its posterior surface. Some vestigial tubules, remnants of the Wolffian body, may also be present within the ligament. The part of the broad ligament between the uterine tube and the ovary is termed the *mesosalpinx*.

The vagina (intrapelvic part)
The space between the intravaginal part of the cervix and the vaginal wall is divided into *fornices* — anterior, posterior, right and left lateral. The posterior fornix is in direct contact with the peritoneum of the pelvic floor. The ureter passes forwards immediately above the lateral fornix.

The ovary
Each ovary is about the size and shape of a very large almond, measuring 3–5 cm in its long axis. It is greyish-white in colour but its size, shape and surface can vary considerably depending on whether the patient is pre- or postmenopausal, and on the time of the menstrual cycle. In prepubertal girls the surface is smooth but following puberty the surface becomes wrinkled and scarred, and it may contain several or single cysts. (Failure to recognise that these changes may be physiological has led to countless ovaries being sacrificed needlessly.) It lies against the posterior surface of the broad ligament, part of which is drawn outwards to form the *mesovarium* containing the ovarian vessels. It is connected to the side wall of the pelvis by the infundibulopelvic ligament, and to the uterus by the ovarian ligament. The open end of the uterine tube overlaps its medial surface.

The uterine tube
Each tube is about 10 cm long, and 6–7 mm in diameter. It lies along the upper free border of the broad ligament in its medial four-fifths. Medially, it traverses the lateral wall of the uterus between body and fundus, to open into the upper angle of the uterine cavity. Laterally, it emerges through the posterior layer of the broad ligament, and opens into the peritoneal cavity, where it overlaps and is attached to the medial surface of the ovary. Its medial part is narrow and is called the *isthmus;* its lateral part is wider and is called the *ampulla*. Its open lateral end or *infundibulum* is divided into several finger-like processes termed *fimbriae*, the largest of which is attached to the ovary.

Vessels
The uterine artery arises from the anterior division of the internal iliac; it runs forwards to the base of the broad ligament, and then medially within it above the lateral fornix of the vagina, where it crosses the ureter 1–2 cm lateral to the supravaginal part of the cervix; finally, it runs upwards along the lateral margin of the uterus, to which it gives numerous branches, including one to the uterine tube. *The ovarian artery* arises from the aorta, a little below the renal, and runs down the posterior abdominal wall; it then passes forwards and medially to reach the ovary via the infundibulopelvic ligament. There is an anastomosis between the uterine and ovarian arteries in the mesosalpinx at the lower border of the tube, and this anastomosis is important because it allows an alternative blood supply to the uterus when internal iliac artery ligation is required to control uterine haemorrhage.

Veins correspond to the arteries, but the right ovarian vein enters the inferior vena cava, and the left, the left renal vein.

CONDITIONS AFFECTING THE UTERINE TUBE

Ruptured ectopic pregnancy
The rupture occurs commonly between the 6th and the 10th week, although it may occur earlier or later. There is usually a history of at least one missed period, but this is not necessarily the case, and in 30% of patients a clear history of amenorrhoea is absent. Classically, the patient shows signs of internal haemorrhage with shock, but much more commonly the development of symptoms and signs is more insidious, due to the fact that most ectopic pregnancies end in tubal abortion with less bleeding than that associated with tubal rupture. Thus these signs may be absent, and not infrequently the case is diagnosed as one of acute appendicitis or of some other general surgical emergency.

However, if the possibility of ectopic pregnancy is seriously entertained (and this diagnosis can frequently be confused with salpingitis which should be treated conservatively) then it can be confirmed or excluded by laparoscopy — a relatively simple procedure which may save the patient from laparotomy.

Laparoscopy

This is usually carried out under general but may be performed under local anaesthesia. Apart from its extensive use in gynaecology, for the diagnosis and treatment of ectopic pregnancy and also for the investigation of infertility, the operation of laparoscopy is proving increasingly popular in general surgery. As a method of minimally invasive surgery, laparoscopic cholecystectomy is routine in many centres and other uses for the laparoscope are being devised. The basic technique for inserting the instrument has changed little from the method devised by the gynaecologist.

The patient is catheterized and is then placed in the Trendelenburg position and a site is selected at the lower margin of the umbilicus if this can be sterilized adequately. At this point a Veres needle (Fig. 29.2), with the cannula retracted, is thrust obliquely through the skin, superficial fascia and rectus sheath. Once the rectus sheath has been penetrated, the spring on the cannula is released and it is then thrust boldly through the parietal peritoneum towards the midpoint of the pelvic brim and into the peritoneal cavity. In very obese women, the Veres needle should be thrust more perpendicularly through the abdominal wall, otherwise there is a likelihood that the extraperitoneal space will be insufflated instead of the peritoneal cavity. In slim women, the Veres needle should be inserted at an angle as shown in Figure 29.3, since there is a serious risk, if it is inserted too vertically, of damaging the aorta. A gas source is then connected to the cannula and either carbon dioxide or nitrous oxide is passed into the peritoneal cavity at a pressure of no more than 60 cm water and a rate of approximately 1 litre per minute. About 3 litres of gas are usually required to distend the abdomen and to lift the anterior abdominal wall from the intestinal contents. The abdominal distension should be even, but if it is asymmetric then insufflation of the extraperitoneal space or even of bowel must be suspected. The Veres needle is then withdrawn, and a

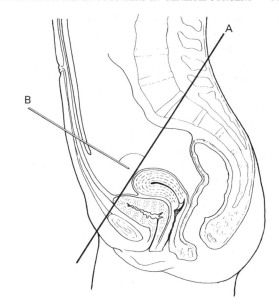

Fig. 29.3 Median section of Female abdomen showing (A)the angle of inclination of the pelvic brim and (B)the preferred angle of insertion of the Veres needle and of the trocar and canula

small transverse incision 1.5 cm long is made along the lower margin of the umbilicus and carried obliquely down to the rectus sheath where a similar small transverse incision is made. This allows the subsequent easy and less traumatic passage of the trocar and cannula (Fig. 29.4). Some surgeons prefer to make the skin incision before introducing the Veres needle but others find that the 'feel' which is experienced on passing the needle through the skin and layers of the abdominal wall allows better appreciation of entry into the peritoneal cavity. The trocar is then withdrawn and the laparoscope, connected to a fibre-optic light source, is passed through the cannula. This allows very accurate inspection of the pelvic cavity but if vision is obscured by omentum or adhesions, the uterus, tubes and ovaries may be manipulated by passing a pair of Palmer's biopsy forceps through a trocar and cannula inserted through a separate 1 cm incision made in the lower abdomen. Preferably this should be made near the midline so as to avoid the inferior epigastric artery.

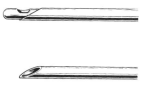

Fig. 29.2 Veres needle showing the tip in detail

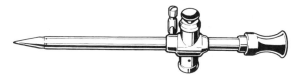

Fig. 29.4 Trocar and cannula with inlet for gas insufflation

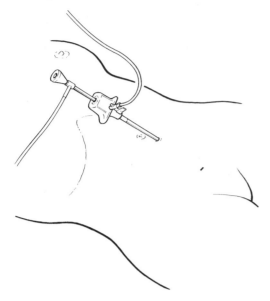

Fig. 29.5 Double puncture laparoscopy — pelvic operation showing site of incision for auxiliary instruments

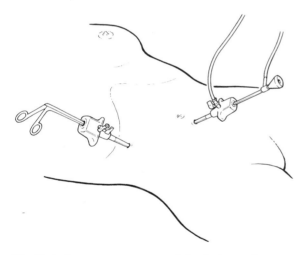

Fig. 29.6 Laparoscopy — upper abdominal procedure showing separate operative instrument in position

Complications of laparoscopy

(a) *Immediate:* because the insertion of the Veres needle and the trocar and cannula has to be done blindly, it is not surprising that damage to underlying viscera, blood vessels and even the ureters has been described. Perforation of the viscera can be recognised by a faecal smell following introduction of the Veres needle (or trocar and cannula) or occasionally by the presence of intestinal contents on the tip of the needle or trocar. Uneven distension of the abdomen on peritoneal insufflation may also alert the surgeon to damaged viscera. Injury to a major vessel can be recognised by backflow of

blood through the cannula and, if this occurs, the instrument should be left in situ and the trocar immediately replaced to control haemorrhage before emergency laparotomy is undertaken.

(b) *Late:* peritonitis following damage to viscera and, rarely, herniation through the laparoscopic incision may occur.

Laparotomy (see p. 364)

Sometimes the diagnosis of ectopic pregnancy can be made clinically with such certainty that laparoscopy can be omitted and at operation, if profuse bleeding has occurred into the peritoneal cavity, this will be apparent from the blueish tinge of the peritoneum as soon as the muscles have been separated. After the peritoneal cavity has been entered, it may be difficult, because of the amount of blood in the pelvis, to identify the affected tube, unless much time is wasted in scooping out blood clot. It is better to insert the hand, to seize the fundus of the uterus, and to draw it up to and out of the wound. The affected tube is now readily identified. The broad ligament is compressed with the fingers in order to arrest haemorrhage; forceps are then applied, first to the uterine end of the affected tube, along which passes its main arterial supply derived from the uterine artery, and then to that part of the broad ligament connecting the tube to the ovary, i.e. the mesosalpinx (Fig. 29.7). The tube is now removed, the pedicles are tied off, and the stumps invaginated. If the ovary is healthy, it is not necessary to remove it, but consideration should be given to doing so if there has been a history of subfertility. By removing the ovary on the affected side the patient is left with a normal tube and ovary on the other side so that ovulation subsequently will always take place from the ovary adjacent to the remaining tube. This must only be considered

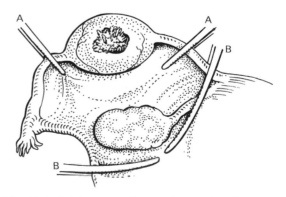

Fig. 29.7 Salpingectomy for ectopic gestation. Clamps are placed on the mesosalpinx and on the uterine end of the tube (AA). The infundibulopelvic ligament, carrying the ovarian vessels, is preserved. If the decision is made to remove the ovary along with the tube, then the tissue between clamps BB would be excised

when the remaining tube and ovary appear perfectly normal. If the ovary is unhealthy on the affected side, e.g. involved in endometriosis, then again it should be removed together with the tube.

Preservation of the tube is not normally recommended, because there is a considerable risk of a further ectopic pregnancy in the already abnormal tube. If, however, the opposite tube is hopelessly diseased, or has been removed, and if the patient is very anxious for a further pregnancy, an attempt may be made to conserve the tube. In such cases, the gestation is evacuated either through a longitudinal incision in the wall of the tube (which is thereafter repaired by 4/0 Dexon interrupted sutures, taking care to exclude the mucosa), or by milking it through the ampulla and inducing a tubal abortion. Continued bleeding thereafter, however, can be a problem.

Provided that the patient's condition allows, an effort should be made to remove all blood within the peritoneal cavity. Before the abdomen is closed, therefore, the patient should be tilted into the feet-down position so that any blood in the upper abdomen will gravitate into the pelvis from which it can be removed by swabbing or by suction. In some parts of the world where facilities for blood transfusion are scarce this blood can be returned to the patient by means of the autotransfusion pump.

Occasionally, the rupture of an ectopic pregnancy takes place within the broad ligament, leading to the development of a haematoma between its layers. In such cases, the tube should first be removed; thereafter, the haematoma may be evacuated by incising either the anterior or the posterior layer of the broad ligament. Sometimes placental tissue will be found to be adherent and serious bleeding can be provoked by injudicious attempts at removal. In these cases the remaining placental tissue should be left undisturbed.

Salpingitis

When this is found at laparotomy, conservation is usually called for, especially since the infection is likely to be bilateral. Unless peritonitis has developed, it is usually sufficient to take a swab from the abdominal osteum of the tube and from any pelvic exudate for bacteriological examination (Cameron, 1976). The wound is closed without drainage and antibiotic therapy is instituted. If, however, a spreading peritonitis is present, and if only one tube is involved, its removal may be considered. The ovary, if healthy, should be preserved.

CONDITIONS AFFECTING THE OVARY

Simple ovarian cysts

A normal healthy ovary, during the childbearing period, contains Graafian follicles and corpora lutea. Both of these may become cystic and may project from the surface of the ovary. Such cysts may be single or multiple, very small or as large as the ovary itself. They are common in women who have no symptoms referable to them, and are in no way pathological. Corpus luteum cysts are often associated with menstrual disturbances, and contain blood. If they rupture, a quantity of blood may be present in the peritoneal cavity, and the symptoms may be taken for those of acute appendicitis. No treatment of such cysts is required, unless bleeding is still taking place from a ruptured cyst, when it may be arrested by one or two sutures placed in the ovarian substance.

When a cyst is of significant size, i.e. more than 5 cm in diameter, it is in the patient's interests that it should be removed. If the ovary itself is healthy, and if the patient is under 45, as much of it as possible should be preserved. In the operation of *ovarian cystectomy,* an incision is made through the ovarian cortex around the base of the cyst, which is then shelled out by sharp dissection, after which the wound in the ovary is sutured either by interrupted or continuous 2/0 catgut taking care to abolish the dead space (Fig. 29.8.) In the case of larger cysts, where it is thought that little functioning ovarian tissue remains, *oophorectomy* should normally be performed — that is, provided that the other ovary is healthy. Clamps are applied as shown in Figure 29.9. In still larger cysts, the uterine tube is often stretched out over the surface of the cyst so that it is best removed. The incision should be enlarged, or a fresh incision made, so that the cyst can be brought out of the wound and removed intact by division of its pedicle. The lateral part of the pedicle is formed by the infundibulopelvic ligament containing the ovarian vessels, which in the case of a large cyst are likely to be much dilated; the medial or uterine part contains the

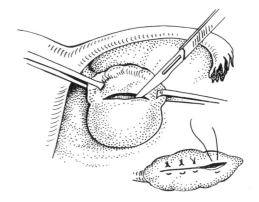

Fig. 29.8 Ovarian cystectomy, the cyst being shelled out through an incision in the ovarian cortex around its base. The ovary is then repaired by suture

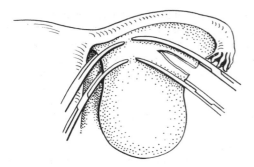

Fig. 29.9 Oophorectomy for a cystic ovary containing little functioning tissue. The infundibulopelvic fold and the ovarian ligament are divided between clamps

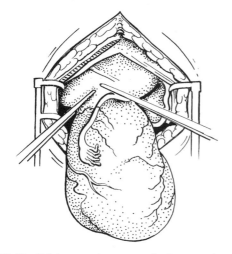

Fig. 29.10 Salpingo-oophorectomy for large ovarian cyst. On the lateral side of the pedicle, the infundibulopelvic fold, containing the dilated ovarian vessels, is divided between clamps, two being placed on the proximal side. On the uterine side a clamp has been placed across the ovarian ligament and the uterine tube, which is usually stretched out over the surface of the cyst

uterine tube and the ovarian ligament (Fig. 29.10). These structures are divided between clamps. For the lateral part of the pedicle (containing the vessels) it is advised that two clamps should be placed proximal to the level of division, and that a transfixing ligature should be employed. This is advised because, if the clamp or ligature slips, the cut ovarian artery may retract behind the peritoneum, causing very troublesome haemorrhage.

Torsion of an ovarian cyst may well be misdiagnosed as a case of acute appendicitis, especially in stout women. The incision should be enlarged sufficiently, or a fresh incision made, so that the cyst can be untwisted under vision and removed intact. Rarely in prepubertal girls and teenagers, torsion of a normal tube and ovary may occur. In such cases the affected tube and ovary

may be untwisted and infarcted blood can be removed from the ovary by incising the cortex which is then repaired. If, thereafter, the tube and ovary recover viability, they may safely be left in situ and function may be preserved.

Endometrial cysts of the ovary are essentially benign but come into a special category. The cyst rarely exceeds 10 cm in diameter, its capsule is thick, firm and white in colour frequently mottled with brown, and adhesions bind it to adjacent structures. Often the cyst bursts while adhesions are being separated and the escape of chocolate-coloured or tarry fluid establishes the diagnosis. Additional confirmation may be obtained from the presence of vascular adhesions on the surface of the ovary or of endometrial deposits in other parts of the pelvis (p. 693).

Tumours of the ovary

Serous cystadenoma is the commonest tumour or pathological cyst of the ovary. It is usually unilateral and unilocular and is thin walled and pearly white in colour. Pseudomucinous cystadenoma is the next commonest; as a rule it is mainly cystic, containing pseudomucinous material. It is pearly white in colour, bossed or loculated, and may reach very large dimensions. Sometimes there is little functioning ovarian tissue on the affected side and oophorectomy should then be performed together with salpingectomy if the tube has been unduly stretched over the surface of the cyst. Every effort should be made, however, to determine whether the cyst is simple or malignant, and for this reason it should be cut open immediately after removal.

Pseudomyxoma peritonei may result from intraperitoneal rupture of a pseudomucinous cyst of the ovary, and the whole of the peritoneal cavity may then be filled with pseudomucinous material. The treatment advised is bilateral oophorectomy, and (if the operator has the necessary experience) total hysterectomy.

Ovarian carcinoma

The classical picture of malignant disease is that the ovarian swellings are bilateral — one being much larger than the other. They are mainly solid, but may contain cystic spaces; their internal structure is necrotic in appearance and consistency. When malignancy is suspected a careful exploration of the pelvis and abdominal cavity should be made and the observations noted so that a base-line may be established on which to plan, monitor and evaluate appropriate adjuvant therapy. If the disease appears to be unilateral in Stage I A(i) and the patient desires to maintain reproductive function then a salpingo-oophorectomy can be carried out on the affected side and no further treatment is required if a biopsy from the contralateral ovary taken at the same time is normal. If reproductive function is no longer desired or if the ovarian cancer is more advanced a bilateral salpingo-oophorectomy and total hysterectomy should be performed if at all possible. Omentectomy and removal of any bulk disease should also be carried out and any spread to the undersurface of the diaphragm, pelvic or para-aortic lymph nodes or elsewhere in the peritoneal cavity together with an estimate of the maximum volume of any remaining bulk disease should be carefully noted. There is no doubt that the effect of chemotherapy is considerably enhanced if residual disease can be kept to a minimum. In many cases, however, the ovarian tumours may be so densely adherent to surrounding structures that their removal is fraught with such hazards that they are inoperable. In such cases a biopsy should be taken and, depending on the type of tumour, treatment with radiotherapy or chemotherapy can be instituted and a significant number may then become operable.

HYSTERECTOMY

The general surgeon will seldom be called upon to perform a hysterectomy, but the unexpected necessity or indication may occasionally arise. In an operation for excision of the rectum (especially with conservation of the sphincter) an unusually bulky uterus, or one that is the seat of fibroids, may so obstruct the operative field that its removal is imperative. A carcinoma of some neighbouring organ, such as the rectum, the pelvic colon or the bladder, may involve the uterus, so that this may require to be removed as part of any operation which aims at radical cure. Endometriosis also is an occasional indication for hysterectomy — but not in the hands of the inexperienced.

Total hysterectomy

This has now almost entirely replaced the older subtotal operation. As a rule there is nothing to be gained by leaving the cervix, and indeed some risk is incurred, for it may be the seat of existing or subsequent disease, e.g. carcinoma. The total operation involves a deeper dissection into the pelvis and entails a greater risk of damage to the ureter but, unless the dissection is rendered unusually difficult by the presence of dense adhesions, the risk is not a serious one, provided that reasonable care is taken.

Technique

The incision is enlarged if necessary or a fresh incision made. The patient is placed in the Trendelenburg position (p. 337), small bowel is packed off into the upper abdomen, and self-retaining retractors are inserted. If the ovaries are healthy, and if the patient is under 45, it is best to leave them; otherwise, they are

removed. The fundus of the uterus is grasped with a vulsellum forceps, and is drawn upwards and to the left, so that the right appendages come into view. When the ovaries are to be preserved, the upper part of the broad ligament, containing the uterine tube, the round ligament, the ovarian ligament and anastomoses between ovarian and uterine arteries, is divided between clamps close to the uterus, the round ligament being clamped separately from the uterine tube and ovarian ligament. The clamps are at once tied-off, since they would get in the way of the rest of the operation. The peritoneal incision in the anterior leaf of the broad ligament is carried downwards close to the uterus towards the base of the ligament, and is then continued towards the left across the utero-vesical pouch at the level of the isthmus, where the peritoneum is loose. The anterior peritoneal flap is raised to expose the bladder, which is joined to the cervix by fascial strands (uterovesical fascia). This fascia is divided (Fig. 29.11) in order to open up the plane of cleavage between bladder and cervix. The bladder is now pushed downwards off the cervix and upper part of the vagina. This carries the ureter downwards with the bladder to below the level of the

Figs 29.11–29.14   *Hysterectomy (after Shaw)*

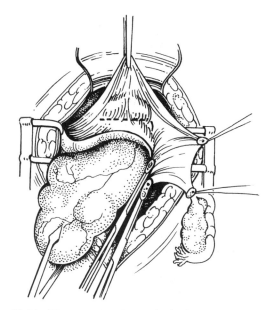

Fig. 29.11   The uterus has been seized with a vulsellum and drawn upwards to expose the appendages on the right side. The uterine tube and the ovarian ligament have been divided between one pair of clamps, and the round ligament between another; the laterally placed clamps have been tied-off. The incision in the broad ligament has been extended across the peritoneum of the uterovesical pouch at the level of the isthmus. The uterovesical fascia (shown by broken line) must next be divided

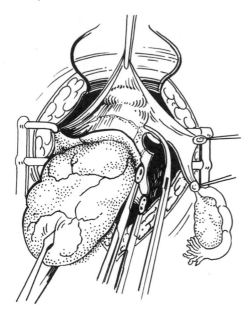

Fig. 29.12   The uterovesical fascia has been divided, to open up the plane of cleavage between the bladder and cervix. The bladder has been mobilized and displaced downwards, first from the cervix and then from the vagina. This carries the ureter downwards, clear of the uterine artery, which is then clamped as shown — *close to the uterine wall.* Before the clamp is applied, it is usually advised that the ureter should be identified as it passes forwards and medially to the bladder at a lower level

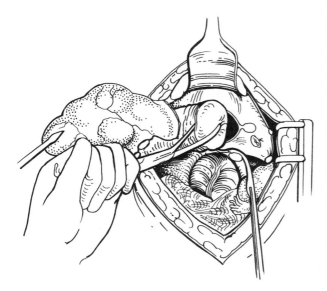

Fig. 29.13   A similar dissection has been carried out on the left side, and the uterine artery secured. The vagina is now opened posterolaterally on the right side, after cutting through the transverse cervical and uterosacral ligaments (to which a clamp is shown attached), and the incision is carried round to the front of the vaginal vault close to the cervix. A vulsellum forceps has been applied to the cervix for traction so that division of the vagina can be completed on the opposite side. The uterus may then be lifted out

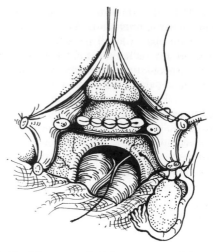

Fig. 29.14   After removal of the uterus, careful attention is paid to haemostasis, vessels in the vaginal wall and in the parametrial tissues around the uterosacral ligaments being secured. The vagina is now closed by suture, and the peritoneum of the pelvic floor is reconstituted, the several ligatured stumps being invaginated beneath the flaps. If complete haemostasis has not been secured, it is better *not* to suture the vagina, but to bring out a gauze pack through it from below the sutured peritoneum

uterine artery, and should safeguard it when this vessel is clamped. The stripping, however, must be done gently, especially on the lateral side of the cervix, where the parametrial venous plexuses may be torn; injudicious clamping of these veins may result in damage to the ureter. It is advisable, therefore, that, before the stripping is carried too far, the ureter should be identified, as it runs forwards and medially above the lateral fornix of the vagina to enter the bladder. As soon as this has been done, the uterine artery should be clamped close to the uterus (Fig. 29.12).

A similar dissection is now carried out on the left side of the uterus, the uterine artery being clamped and divided after the ureter has been safeguarded. At this stage after dividing the pedicle right to the points of the forceps, the clamps containing the uterine vessels may be pushed downwards and laterally on each side for a distance of about 1 cm. This manoeuvre exposes the transverse cervical ligament and uterosacral ligament which may be clamped (either together or separately depending on the size) by curved Kocher's forceps which are applied so that the ends of the forceps reach the lateral fornix of the vagina on each side. A long handled knife is then used to divide these pedicles and this incision is carried across the vault of the vagina, thus removing the uterus together with the cervix. Care must be taken at this stage to avoid injuring the rectum which may be adherent to the back of the posterior fornix. The vault of the vagina is then closed with a continuous No. 1 Dexon suture to reduce the risk of postoperative vault granulations developing and thereafter the parametrial and uterine pedicles are ligated. Careful haemostasis is secured and the pelvic peritoneum is reconstituted with a continuous stitch taking care not to damage or kink the ureter.

Sub-total hysterectomy

In this operation, the dissection is not carried so deeply into the pelvis, and the bladder is not separated from the vaginal vault. The uterine artery is secured as in total hysterectomy, the ureter being safeguarded. The cervix is then divided just below the isthmus; its remaining part is closed by two or three interrupted sutures, and the stump is buried below the peritoneal flaps.

OTHER GYNAECOLOGICAL CONDITIONS

Endometriosis is a term used to denote the presence of ectopic endometrial tissue in various organs within the pelvis. The ovaries, the uterine tubes, the uterosacral ligaments and the peritoneum of the recto-uterine pouch are areas commonly affected. The condition occurs also on the posterior surface of the uterus and within its muscular wall. The endometrial tissue presents in the early stages of the condition in the form of dark brown or purplish nodules, which are charac-

teristically the size of lead shot. Around each nodule the peritoneum may be drawn into a series of puckers. In more advanced cases, there may be an inextricable mass of adhesions, completely obliterating the recto-uterine pouch and binding together all the pelvic structures; bowel and omentum may also be involved. The ovaries are white and opaque, and may show puckered scars on their surface; alternatively they may be cystic, containing altered blood — the so-called 'chocolate' or 'tarry' cysts.

Fortunately, endometriosis can often be cured by abolishing ovarian function. It is essentially a benign non-neoplastic condition, but malignant degeneration has occasionally been reported. In women near the menopause, bilateral oophorectomy can be performed. Hysterectomy may be carried out at the same time, provided that the operator is experienced in gynaecological surgery, but, if dense adhesions are present, the uterus is best left alone, since there is a serious risk of damaging adherent bowel. In young women, bilateral oophorectomy is obviously undesirable but, if one ovary is extensively diseased, it may be removed and the other left. At the same time, obvious and readily removed areas of disease may be excised and their beds cauterised.

The general surgeon, who unexpectedly discovers the condition of endometriosis at laparotomy, should suffer no reproaches if he simply closes the abdomen for the condition can often be improved if not cured by hormone therapy. A further operation can then be undertaken if necessary.

Parovarian (broad ligament) cysts

These cysts, which are probably derived from vestigial remnants of the Wolffian body, lie within the broad ligament, usually between the uterine tube and the ovary. They contain clear watery fluid and are usually unilocular. They never attain any great size and are of

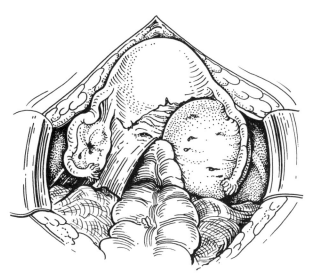

Fig. 29.15 Typical appearances of endometriosis. Dense adhesions, obliterating the recto-uterine pouch and binding the uterus to the rectosigmoid, have been separated, leaving extensive raw areas on these structures. The left ovary shows a puckered scar, the right ovary an endometrial cyst. Scattered nodules are present elsewhere over a wide area in the pelvis

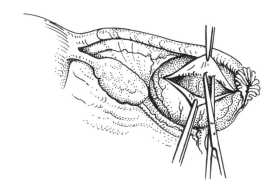

Fig. 29.16 Removal of a broad ligament cyst after incision of the peritoneum of the ligament

little clinical significance. Owing to their situation within the broad ligament, they cannot be delivered at the wound.

If such a cyst is found at laparotomy, and appears to be reasonably accessible, it may be removed. The broad ligament is incised over the cyst, which is then shelled out by dissection close to its wall, with due regard to the proximity of the ureter and the ovarian vessels (Fig. 29.16). Haemorrhage is arrested, and the broad ligament is repaired by suture.

REFERENCE

Cameron M D 1976 Gynaecological problems and the general surgeon. In: Hadfield J, Hobsley M (eds) Current surgical practice, vol. 1. Arnold, London, ch 15

Index